Review of
Preventive and Social Medicine
(Including Biostatistics)

Review of
Preventive and Social Medicine
(Including Biostatistics)

(Thoroughly revised and updated edition including latest exam-pattern questions)

15th Edition

Vivek Jain
MBBS (Maulana Azad Medical College), Delhi, India
MD Community Medicine (PSM) (Lady Hardinge Medical College), Delhi, India

Formerly
Consultant UN Office on Drugs & Crime–South Asia
Senior Resident UCMS & GTBH, VMMC & SJH, Delhi
Faculty GFIMSR, Faridabad, Haryana, India

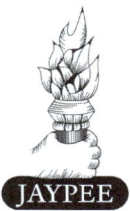

JAYPEE BROTHERS MEDICAL PUBLISHERS
The Health Sciences Publisher
New Delhi | London

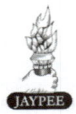

Jaypee Brothers Medical Publishers (P) Ltd

Headquarters
Jaypee Brothers Medical Publishers (P) Ltd
EMCA House, 23/23-B
Ansari Road, Daryaganj
New Delhi 110 002, India
Landline: +91-11-23272143, +91-11-23272703
+91-11-23282021, +91-11-23245672
Email: jaypee@jaypeebrothers.com

Corporate Office
Jaypee Brothers Medical Publishers (P) Ltd
4838/24, Ansari Road, Daryaganj
New Delhi 110 002, India
Phone: +91-11-43574357
Fax: +91-11-43574314
Email: jaypee@jaypeebrothers.com

Overseas Office
JP Medical Ltd
83 Victoria Street, London
SW1H 0HW (UK)
Phone: +44 20 3170 8910
Fax: +44 (0)20 3008 6180
Email: info@jpmedpub.com

Website: www.jaypeebrothers.com

Website: www.jaypeedigital.com

© 2023, Jaypee Brothers Medical Publishers

The views and opinions expressed in this book are solely those of the original contributor(s)/author(s) and do not necessarily represent those of editor(s) or publisher of the book.

All rights reserved. No part of this publication may be reproduced, stored or transmitted in any form or by any means, electronic, mechanical, photocopying, recording or otherwise, without the prior permission in writing of the publishers.

All brand names and product names used in this book are trade names, service marks, trademarks or registered trademarks of their respective owners. The publisher is not associated with any product or vendor mentioned in this book.

Medical knowledge and practice change constantly. This book is designed to provide accurate, authoritative information about the subject matter in question. However, readers are advised to check the most current information available on procedures included and check information from the manufacturer of each product to be administered, to verify the recommended dose, formula, method and duration of administration, adverse effects and contraindications. It is the responsibility of the practitioner to take all appropriate safety precautions. Neither the publisher nor the author(s)/editor(s) assume any liability for any injury and/or damage to persons or property arising from or related to use of material in this book.

This book is sold on the understanding that the publisher is not engaged in providing professional medical services. If such advice or services are required, the services of a competent medical professional should be sought.

Every effort has been made where necessary to contact holders of copyright to obtain permission to reproduce copyright material. If any have been inadvertently overlooked, the publisher will be pleased to make the necessary arrangements at the first opportunity.

Review of Preventive and Social Medicine (Including Biostatistics)

Third Edition: 2011
Fourth Edition: 2012
Fifth Edition: 2013
Sixth Edition: 2014
Seventh Edition: 2015
Eighth Edition: 2016
Ninth Edition: 2017
Tenth Edition: 2018
Eleventh Edition: 2019
Twelfth Edition: 2020
Thirteenth Edition: 2021
Fourteenth Edition: 2022

Fifteenth Edition: 2023, Reprint: 2024

ISBN: 978-93-5696-300-9

Printed at Rajkamal Electric Press, Kundli, Haryana.

Preface

Dear Students,

Let me first thank you for your overwhelming support to the previous editions of the book, making it the **Best-seller book on the subject in India since last 14 golden years**. It again reiterates my belief that good content by a subject-specialty author is always appreciated by students. It now gives me immense pleasure to share with you the NEW (Fifteenth) edition of the book.

Key features of Fourteenth edition retained in Fifteenth edition
- **Theory given at start of each chapter** (Theory divided chapter-, topic-, sub-topic wise – Small/one-liner points in each topic/ Important previous MCQs marked as^Q)
- **Key REVISION Point Boxes given on side of each topic** for **MUST-KNOW MCQ** facts
- **New/Recent Examination-based pattern has been adopted chapter-wise** [Focus on Wider coverage, Concept development, One-liner approach, Value-based MCQs, Applied aspect MCQs, Image-based MCQs, Updated previous year questions (PYQs)]

In the Fifteenth edition of the book following NEW ADDITIONS have been done to make a student stay ahead in this competitive era with changing pattern of examinations.
- NEW chapter-wise image-based MCQs with explanatory answers
- NEWLY added 130+ Images, flowcharts and diagrams
- Recent most solved MCQ papers
  - AIIMS 2019–2020, INICET 2020–2023
  - ALL "NEET Pattern Questions" of PGMEE 2012–2023
- Recent/New topics and Changing concepts in PSM
  - NEW Topics in Public Health: Monkeypox, Coronavirus & COVID-19 disease, Mucormycosis, Emerging & Re-emerging pathogens, Air Quality Index (AQI), Global Hunger Index (GHI), Tribal Health in India, Health Index of India, BMW categorization, Nutrition Rehabilitation Centres (NRCs), Contraception and Adolescence, Health Care and System, Adjuvants in Vaccines
  - NEW Initiatives (Indian): IPHS Guidelines 2022, Nikshay Mitra Initiative 2022, SUMAN 2019, SAANS 2019, AAROGYA SETU 2020, PMSMA, PMMVY 2017, DAKSHTA 2015, Ayushman Bharat 2018, Anemia Mukt Bharat 2018, Swachh Bharat Mission, National Nutrition Mission (NNM) 2017–18, Td Vaccination Guidelines 2018–19
  - NEW Initiatives (Global): Global Alliance for Ending Aids in Children by 2030, Global Programme to Eliminate Lymphatic Filariasis (GPELF), Global Health Sector Strategy on Viral Hepatitis 2016–2021, EYE Strategy, Global Eye Health Action Plan 2014–19, Integrated Global Action Plan for Prevention and Control of Pneumonia & Diarrhoea (GAPPD), Global Technical Strategy for Malaria (2016–2030)
  - NEW Topics in Disease Control: New Anti-Cervical Cancer Vaccines, New Anti-Rabies Vaccines, COVID-19 Vaccines, Measles treatment, Diphtheria treatment, Chicken pox vaccines, TB Facts Epidemiology, TB and Co-morbidities, IPV vs fIPV, Treatment of Severe/Complicated Malaria, Active Surveillance in Kala-azar, Lifestyle Modifications to Manage Hypertension, Vision Impairment, Oral diseases, WHO Hand Hygiene Guidelines
  - NEW National Lists of Essential Medicines (NLEM) 2022
  - NEW National Programme on AMR Containment
  - NEW ARV PEP Guidelines for HIV NACP 2021–22
  - NEW NTEP Guidelines 2020–21: Diagnosis algorithms, Treatment
  - NEW Rabies Notification Guidelines 2021–22
  - NEW NPCBVI Guidelines 2021–22
  - NEW NDHM 2020–21
  - NEW Covid BMW Management Guidelines 2021–22
  - NEW MTP Act Guidelines 2021–22
  - NEW Nutrition Guidelines 2021–22
  - NEW NMC Guidelines 2020–21
  - NEW WHO IHR Guidelines 2021–22
  - NEW NTEP Guidelines 2020–21
  - NEW NPEP Guidelines 2018–19: AFP Surveillance Indicators
  - NEW RCH Programme Guidelines 2018–19: New Initiatives in Family Planning, National Family Planning Indemnity Scheme, Post-natal visits guidelines
  - NEW NACP Guidelines 2018–19: CD4 treatment criteria
  - NEW NVBDCP Guidelines 2018–19: Kala-azar treatment, Malaria treatment
  - NEW H1N1 Categorization Guidelines in India 2018–19

- NEW National Immunization Schedule (NIS) 2020–21
- NEW BMW Treatment Standards in India 2018–19
- NEW Incentive Packages under National Health Programmes 2018–19
- NEW Emergency Response Support System (ERSS) 2019–20
- NEW Specific Targets for SDG Target 3.3 on Infectious Diseases
- NEW Developed Vaccines: Dengue, Leprosy, Malaria, Rabies, MR
- NEW WHO Rabies Vaccination Guidelines 2018
- NEW WHO Uniform MDT Guidelines 2018–19
- NEW WHO-UNICEF BFHI Guidelines 2018–19
- NEW WHO ICD-11 Classification 2018
- NEW International Death Certificate (IDC) Format 2018–19
- NEW Goalposts to construct HDI Index 2018–19
- NEW Poverty Criteria: Multidimensional Poverty Index (MDPI)
- NEW AHA Revised Jones Criteria for Diagnosis of Rheumatic Fever 2015
- NEW Policies and Legislations: Open Vial Policy 2015, The Rights of Persons with Disabilities Bill 2016–17, National Health Policy 2017
- **UPDATED Concepts:** Evidence Based Medicine, Meta-analysis, Systematic reviews
- **Other New Inclusions/Upcoming Topics:** Triangle of Epidemiology & Advanced Model of Epidemiological Triangle, Ottawa Charter - Health Promotion, VDPV vs VAPP, QALY, YPLL, New Sterilization Guidelines, New Semen analysis (WHO) guidelines, Newer Visual Impairment guidelines, National Abortion Guidelines, DASH diet, Latent TB, Danger Signals of Cancer, Haddon matrix, H1N1 Categorization, Oseltamivir Dosages, New Establishments (NITI Aayog, NIRT, NIE, NIDM, NDRF), Twelfth Five Year Plan 2012–17, Changes in National Health Programs (NRHM, MDMP, JSSK, HNBC, ICDS), Changes in Epidemiology of various diseases, New Protein Quality Assessment Guidelines 2015, New/Emerging Diseases (H5N6, H7N9, Ebola, MERS-CoV), Recent Schemes (NIKSHAY, Swajaldhara, Link worker, Ujjwala, ICPS), Recent Health programs (NHM, RBSK, NSSK, RKSK, PMJDY, PMSSY, NUHM), Recent strategies (RMNCH+A, STOP/End-TB, NLEP 2012–17), Recent Initiatives (TB Mission 2020, ALL-IN Initiative, HIV-PEP), Recent Guidelines (RTI/STI Treatment Guidelines, Rabies Prophylaxis), New BPL Criteria (WHO), Health Economics India Data, Trachoma-free India, Intensified Mission Indradhanush, M-Diabetes, DOTS-99, AMRIT, LaQshya, Pradhan Mantri Surakshit Matritva Abhiyan (PMSMA), Mission Parivar Vikas, National Nutrition Mission (NNM), ESI Guidelines & Criteria 2017–18, List of Emerging Diseases (WHO) & Zika Virus disease, Blood Pressure Classification 2018
- NHP 2017, SDGs 2015–2030
- Rural Health Statistics India 2020–21
- Covid Situation Update, Newer Covid Vaccines Updates 2023–24
- An Updated compilation of Public Health Statistics of India 2023–24 (Including NFHS-5, 2019–21)

'Understanding PSM is difficult, owing to the vastness of the subject, but enjoyable, if you come across a good teacher and a useful book!'

A student

While preparing for PG entrance examination, I myself realised that most of the PSM MCQs, related text and even the referenced answers given in books were invariably unable to satisfy me as a student. Most of the times, there were questions from '*topics not given in standard textbooks*' (e.g., nested case control study, case series report, statistical errors, probability, odds and likelihood ratios, health legislations, water washed diseases, Golden rice, COPRA, Punnett square, Dixon's Q-test, Evidence based Medicine, etc. – all together just the tip of an iceberg of such MCQs). Every year there were '*new unheard questions from unexplored fields*', overlapping choices of MCQs from other fields of medicine accompanied with futile search for '*recent most data of Public Health Statistics*', etc. This all made me realize that PSM is a vast and varied subject to conceptualise and memorize. Elaborate books also confused me regarding the relative importance of each topic in the subject. I also realised that students face maximum difficulty in understanding the concepts of '*Biostatistics*' and in obtaining precise, concise and useful data from '*National Health Programmes of India*'.

Also, PG entrance examinations have a sizeable chunk of direct MCQs from PSM subject (Just 1 subject out of 19 total subjects), ranging from 10 to 14% of total (20–25% in CMS-UPSC). Moreover, PSM helps in solving several allied questions (partly or totally) of Pediatrics, Obstetrics, Pharmacology, Medicine, Microbiology, Ophthalmology, etc.

So, there is no denying the fact that '*PSM is of paramount importance*' to successfully tackle any PG Entrance Examination. Thus, I have written this book keeping a student's, a teacher's and an examiner's perspective in mind.

Each chapter divided into topics and sub-topics, **Theory and MCQs arranged section-wise** for more comprehensive understanding of topics. In Theory, **Important previous years MCQs highlighted** (as^Q) and MUST-KNOW facts given separately. Book includes PG Entrance Examination MCQs of **AIIMS (1991–2019)** and **AIPGME/DNB/NEET-PG (1991–2012 + "NEET Pattern MCQs 2012–2022")** with referenced, authenticated, full explanatory answers. Solved explanatory MCQs from **PGI, JIPMER PG Entrance Examinations (2000–2019), INICET (2020–22)** added to help students grasp subject better. Over 3,000 solved MCQs from

UPSC CMS & Several **State Medical PG Entrance Examinations** (Rajasthan, MP, Andhra Pradesh, Tamil Nadu, Maharashtra, Bihar, DNB, JIPMER, Kolkata, and Karnataka PGMEE) added for wider coverage. Recent most changes in National Health Programs with updates in Communicable and Non-communicable diseases provided for competitive edge. Many answers are followed by a section on '**Also Remember**'- A compilation of various important noteworthy points based on previous questions from several fields. **PYQs (Chapter-wise)** have been included for a quick revision just before the examination. Several **Annexures** (Incubation period and Modes of transmission of diseases, Important days of Public Health, Instruments of importance in public health, Important health legislations and programs in India, Vectors, NHP 2017 & NPP 2000, BMW Guidelines 2018, Updated Public Health related statistics of India) have been included towards the start of the book to given the student an edge over others.

Please remember there is no substitute to Theory books, but hopefully you will find all relevant theory in this user-friendly book.

Despite every possible effort been undertaken to ensure no technical or typographical errors in the book, such are bound to be present in any book. If you come across another such error or if you have any comment, suggestions, queries or views, you are most welcome to e-mail to me for a prompt response. All contributions will be duly acknowledged. Do share your experiences while reading this book and the subject.

Hope you have a successful career ahead.

Wish you Success, *not just in PSM but in Life!*

Dr Vivek Jain
MBBS MD (Community Medicine)
Email: docvivekjain2@gmail.com
docvivekjain3@gmail.com
India 2023–24

Author E-support Get regular updates on PSM

- **Instagram** Follow "**vivekjainpsm**"
- **Facebook** Type <**Dr Vivek Jain** > in Search box: Like, Follow the posts
- **Telegram** Type "**Dr Vivek Jain Sir PSM**" in Search Box and Join. To receive an invite, send a message on
  Telegram/WhatsApp to **+91-9871960266**
- **YouTube** Subscribe "**Dr Vivek Jain**"
- **Website** Visit the webpage **www.vivekjainpsm.com**
- **Twitter** Follow '**Vivek Jain @docvivekjain**'

Acknowledgements

I am sincerely thankful to Late Mr RD Jain, my maternal grandfather and my wife Dr Rashmi Naudiyal for being a constant source of inspiration for completion of this book. Without support of Dr Rashmi and Baby Mischka, this book would not have seen light of the day. Without the blessing of my Parents, Family, Parents-in-laws and God this endeavour would not have been successful.

Firstly I thank PadmaShree Dr Jagdish Prasad, DGHS for organising a grand launch of first edition of the book at New Delhi.

I am grateful to Dr Saudan Singh, Director—NOTTO & Director—Professor, Department of Community Medicine, Vardhman Mahavir Medical College (VMMC), New Delhi, Former DG (Medical Education), Government of Uttar Pradesh, for being a source of support, guidance and motivation for myself.

I am thankful to Dr SK Pradhan, former Director—Professor, Department of Community Medicine, VMMC, New Delhi for providing me with academic opportunities to help me understand the finer nuances of the subject throughout my PGship and SRship.

I also appreciate the support and encouragement by Dr DK Raut, former Director—Professor, VMMC SJH, Dr AT Kannan, former Director—Professor and Head, Department of Community Medicine, UCMS, Dr GK Ingle, former Director—Professor and Head, Department of Community Medicine, MAMC, Dr Vibha, former Professor and Head, Department of Community Medicine, LHMC, Dr SK Rasania, Director—Professor & Head, LHMC and respected Faculty of Department of Community Medicine of these colleges respectively.

Dr Rajesh Kumar—Professor MAMC, always inspiring me to excel academically, has been a guiding light for me!

I am sincerely thankful to Dr P Sai Kumar, MPH (UK), for motivating me to write this book, and for his unparallel support as my mentor. I am ever thankful to Dr Surabhi, Dr Shagun, Dr Isha and Dr Nidhi, former undergraduates and other students of LHMC and VMMC, for helping me develop my teaching capabilities.

Words of thanks to Mr Rajesh Sharma (PG-DIAMS), Dr Sumer Sethi (DAMS) and Dr Bhatia (DBMCI) for helping me gain entry into the competitive world of academics.

I am highly grateful to Shri Jitendar P Vij (Group Chairman) M/s Jaypee Brothers Medical Publishers (P) Ltd, New Delhi, India for his wholehearted support in publication of this book. I thank Ms Chetna Malhotra (Senior Director—Professional Publishing, Marketing, and Business Development), Ms Pooja Bhandari (Director—Production), Ms Ruby Sharma (Business Manager), Ms Kamlesh Visht, Mr Jyotindra Mohan Jha, Ms Rekha Kumari and their Team at Jaypee Brothers Medical Publishers (P) Ltd, New Delhi, India for commendable work and inputs for the current edition.

A special personal word of thanks for Dr Prashaant Bhatnagar, Assistant Professor (Community Medicine), LLRM Medical College, Meerut, UP for being a source of constructive criticism and continuous support!

Acknowledgement is also due to Mr Anurag (Book Store, LHMC), Mr Varish (Book store MAMC) and Mr Nikhil (Book store Jain Stationery, Gautam Nagar, Delhi) for their constructive suggestions.

I also take this opportunity to thank the following students/doctors for sharing their invaluable constructive criticisms for the improvement of the book:

- Dr Aanchal Jain, GMC, Nagpur
- Dr Aarav Kumar
- Dr Abhilasha Prasad
- Dr Abhishek Prasad Dash, Bhubaneswar, Odisha
- Dr Aditya Jadhav
- Dr Afeefa Hanif, MES Medical College, Kerala
- Dr Ajeet Singh, Patna Medical College
- Dr Akanksha Jain, MVPs Dr Vasantrao Pawar Medical College
- Dr Amit Kumar Gupta, DNB Family Medicine, Maharaja Agrasen Hospital, Delhi
- Dr Amit Kumar Yadav, PTJNM Medical College, Raipur
- Dr Amit Polara, Civil Hospital, Surat
- Dr Ananta Narayan Panda
- Dr Animesh Agrawal
- Dr Ankit Madan
- Dr Ankit Thukral, SGRRIHMS, Dehradun
- Dr Anubhav Srivastava, SNMC, Agra
- Dr Ankita, JJMMC, Bengaluru
- Dr Ankush Koul, Darbhanga Medical College, Bihar
- Dr Anoop Shanbhag
- Dr Anuj Malhotra
- Dr Anupriya Thadani, Era's Medical College and Hospital, Lucknow

- Dr Anurag Gour
- Dr Apurv Gupta, Delhi
- Dr Archita Makharia, AFMC
- Dr Arpan Ray, Birbhum, West Bengal
- Dr Arvinder, DMC, Ludhiana
- Dr Ashutosh Sahu
- Dr Ashwini Gupta, Darbhanga Medical College and Hospital
- Dr Avi Singh
- Dr Avinash Ashok
- Dr Bharat Vantekunta, Kakatiya Medical College, Warangal
- Dr Bindhiya Mak, Wuhan University School of Medicine, China
- Dr Deepa Grover, GMC, Miraj, Maharashtra
- Dr Duvvuru Sai Tharun, Kurnool Medical College
- Dr Eftekhar Mohd.
- Dr Farjana Habiba Ahmed, Silchar Medical College and Hospital
- Dr Gagan Prakash, BMCRI, Bengaluru
- Dr Gopal Singh Bhati, SMS, Jaipur
- Dr Gurpreet Singh Gill, VMGMC, Solapur
- Dr Himanshu Agrawal, GSVM, Kanpur
- Dr Indraneel Sharma, Guwahati
- Dr Jeyakumar Meyyappan
- Dr Jujhar Singh Mann, Rajshahi University, Bangladesh
- Dr Kanika Kachhwaha, SSG, Vadodara
- Dr Kathan Acharya, BJMC, Ahmedabad
- Dr Khatri Mehul, PDU Medical College, Rajkot
- Dr Kumar Rohit, SKMCH, Muzaffarpur
- Dr Kunal Tatte
- Dr Lucky Singh, Kanpur
- Dr Mahanthesh Gidaveer
- Dr Mahendra, SIMS, Karnataka
- Dr Mahender Kumar
- Dr Malvika Nagpal, Delhi
- Dr Manish Choudhary, Kasturba Medical College, Manipal
- Dr Manish Sahu, JNMC, Raipur
- Dr Manosij Maity
- Dr Manpreet Singh
- Dr Mareddy Mahesh, Dali University
- Dr (Md) Matin Khan, MGM Medical College, Jamshedpur
- Dr Narendra HR
- Dr Navin Chaudhary, Bhuj
- Dr Neel Choksi, BJ Medical College, Ahmedabad
- Dr Nilesh Sonawane, Civil Hospital, Sangli
- Dr Nissy Motupalli
- Dr Om Shrivastava, CIMS, Bilaspur
- Dr Opalina Roy, Burdwan Medical College
- Dr Partha Jana
- Dr Piyush Gadegone
- Dr Piyush Singh, Bengaluru
- Dr Poonam Choudhary GMC, Surat
- Dr Prashant Shukla, RIMS, Imphal
- Dr Pratik Khare NSCB Medical College, Jabalpur
- Dr Praveen K, Calicut Medical College
- Dr Preeti Chopra
- Dr Prerna Upadhyay
- Dr PV Rajesh, Chongqing Medical University, China
- Dr Puneet Aggarwal, Nepalgunj Medical College
- Dr Rachit Kapoor, Regional Advisor The Lancet Student
- Dr Rachit Singhania, West Bengal University of Health Sciences
- Dr Raghvendra Singh, MIMSR College and Research Centre
- Dr Rakesh Kumar Jha, Darbhanga Medical College & Hospital, Bihar

Acknowledgements

- Dr Rashmi Lohia
- Dr Ravi Kumar Gupta, R.U.H.S and RNT Medical College, Udaipur
- Dr Rinku Sharma, NCDC, Delhi
- Dr Ronak Jain, TNMGR University, Chennai
- Dr Ronak Patel, University of Northern Philippines
- Dr Rupesh Sharma, Southern Medical University, China
- Dr Ruchir Rustogi, SR, MAMC
- Dr Sachin Harit, Delhi
- Dr Sagar Gandhi, NKP Institute of Medical Sciences
- Dr Sagar Mahapatra, Berhampur, Odisha
- Dr Saikat Mitra, Kolkata
- Dr Sakil Ahmed
- Dr Saksham Pandey, Delhi
- Dr Samcy Arora
- Dr Sandeep Ghanghas, Panipat
- Dr Sanjiv Sharma, RIMS, Imphal
- Dr Sanket Agrawal
- Dr Saraswata Mitra, Grodno State Medical University, Belarus
- Dr Sarweshwar Sripada
- Dr Saurabh Daseda, GMC, Surat
- Dr Shameema Farook, Madras Medical College
- Dr Sharaff Dileep, Dalian University, China
- Dr Sharath Kumar Reddy, Gandhi Medical College
- Dr Shashank Saurabh
- Dr Sherinsha Sharafudeen
- Dr Shraddha Shejekar, BIMS, Belgaum
- Dr Shyamsundar Punia, Lugansk-State-Medical-University
- Dr Siddharth Jain, BJMC, Ahmedabad
- Dr Silky Priya
- Dr Siva Vicky
- Dr Surabhi Jain, Pune
- Dr Surendra Chaudhary, China Medical University
- Dr Swati Verma Attam, Consultant Gynecologist & Obstetrician, Noida
- Dr Taanya Joseph
- Dr Tapaprakash Behera, VSS Medical College, Burla
- Dr Teju High, JLMNC, Bhagalpur
- Dr Uma Shankar KIMS, Bengaluru
- Dr Vikas Gupta, Pilibhit
- Dr Vishnu M Satheesan, Thiruvananthapuram, Kerala
- Dr Vismay Deshani, Smolensk State Medical Academy, Russia
- Dr Vitrag N Shah, New Civil Hospital, Surat
- Dr Yash Gore Lokmanya Tilak Municipal General Hospital
- Dr Yash Tripathi, GSVM Medical College, Kanpur, UP

Last but definitely not the least, no words can describe the role of **ALL MEDICAL STUDENTS**, with whom I ever have had interacted, in helping me give this book, its final shape!

From the Publisher's Desk
We request all the readers to provide us their valuable suggestions/errors (if any) at:
jaypeemcqproduction@gmail.com
so as to help us in further improvement of this book in the subsequent edition(s).

Contents

Section 1: Previous Year Questions (PYQs)

A.	Image-based Questions (2019–2023)	3
B.	NEET FMGE Pattern PYQs (2005–2023)	17

Section 2: Annexures

Annexure 1:	Incubation Period of Diseases	37
Annexure 2:	Important Days of Public Health Importance	39
Annexure 3:	Instruments of Importance in Public Health	40
Annexure 4:	Mode(s) of Transmission of Diseases	41
Annexure 5:	Some Important Health Legislations Passed in India	42
Annexure 6:	Some Important Health Programmes of India	43
Annexure 7:	Vectors and Diseases Transmitted	44
Annexure 8:	New Tuberculosis Management (NTEP/RNTCP) Guidelines (2020 Onwards)	45
Annexure 9:	National Population Policy (NPP) 2000	51
Annexure 10:	National Health Policy 2017 (NHP 2017)	52
Annexure 11:	Sustainable Development Goals (SDGs)	53
Annexure 12:	New Malaria Treatment Guidelines in India (2013 Onwards)	55
Annexure 13:	New Biomedical Waste Management Guidelines 2016	57
Annexure 14:	Current Public Health-related Statistics of India	58
Annexure 15:	Honors in Health and Medicine	62
Annexure 16:	Incentives under National Health Programs	63
Annexure 17:	High Level Expert Group (HLEG) Report on Universal Health Coverage (UHC)	64
Annexure 18:	Health Index of India, Hii (Niti Aayog)	66
Annexure 19:	Ayushman Bharat Program 2018	67
Annexure 20:	Swachh Bharat Mission (SBM) 2014	68
Annexure 21:	Anemia Mukt Bharat	69
Annexure 22:	NEW WHO Rabies Vaccination Guidelines	71
Annexure 23:	NEW WHO Guidelines for Treatment of Leprosy: Uniform MDT	73
Annexure 24:	Tribal Health in India	74

Section 3: Topic-wise Theory, MCQs and Explanations

Chapter 1 History of Medicine 77
Theory and NEET-PG Pattern PYQs 77
Multiple Choice Questions 82
Explanations 85

Chapter 2 Concepts of Health and Disease 87
Theory and NEET-PG Pattern PYQs 87
Multiple Choice Questions 99
Explanations 106

Chapter 3 Epidemiology and Vaccines 115
Theory and NEET-PG Pattern PYQs 115
Multiple Choice Questions 158
Explanations 185

Chapter 4 Screening of Disease 224
Theory and NEET-PG Pattern PYQs 224
Multiple Choice Questions 230
Explanations 237

| Chapter 5 | Communicable and Non-communicable Diseases | 247 |

Theory and NEET-PG Pattern PYQs 247
Multiple Choice Questions 329
Explanations 364

| Chapter 6 | National Health Programmes, Policies and Legislations in India | 407 |

Theory and NEET-PG Pattern PYQs 407
Multiple Choice Questions 455
Explanations 470

| Chapter 7 | Demography, Family Planning and Contraception | 493 |

Theory and NEET-PG Pattern PYQs 493
Multiple Choice Questions 520
Explanations 530

| Chapter 8 | Preventive Obstetrics, Pediatrics and Geriatrics | 545 |

Theory and NEET-PG Pattern PYQs 545
Multiple Choice Questions 563
Explanations 571

| Chapter 9 | Nutrition and Health | 584 |

Theory and NEET-PG Pattern PYQs 584
Multiple Choice Questions 605
Explanations 617

| Chapter 10 | Social Sciences and Health | 633 |

Theory and NEET-PG Pattern PYQs 633
Multiple Choice Questions 641
Explanations 645

| Chapter 11 | Environment and Health | 651 |

Theory and NEET-PG Pattern PYQs 651
Multiple Choice Questions 671
Explanations 683

| Chapter 12 | Biomedical Waste Management, Disaster Management, Occupational Health, Genetics and Health, Mental Health | 699 |

Theory and NEET-PG Pattern PYQs 699
Multiple Choice Questions 716
Explanations 726

| Chapter 13 | Health Education and Communication | 739 |

Theory and NEET-PG Pattern PYQs 739
Multiple Choice Questions 745
Explanations 747

| Chapter 14 | Health Care in India, Health Planning and Management | 750 |

Theory and NEET-PG Pattern PYQs 750
Multiple Choice Questions 760
Explanations 767

| Chapter 15 | International Health | 776 |

Theory and NEET-PG Pattern PYQs 776
Multiple Choice Questions 780
Explanations 782

| Chapter 16 | Biostatistics | 787 |

Theory and NEET-PG Pattern PYQs 787
Multiple Choice Questions 805
Explanations 821

Section 4: PYQs (2012–2018): Image-based Questions

Image-based Questions 855

Key Topics in PSM for PGMEE

Chapters	NEET-PG, FMGE, UPSC patterns	INI-CET patterns
1. History of Medicine	• Theories of disease causation • Names of Scientists • Names of epidemiologists	—
2. Concepts of Health and Disease	• PQLI/HDI • Levels of prevention • ICD-10, 11 • Types of epidemics	HPI/Multidimensional poverty
3. Epidemiology	• Cohort-RR, Adv/Disdv • Case control-OR, Adv/Disdv • RCT • Clinical trials	• Retrospective/Mixed cohort • Nested case control • RCT • Meta-analysis • Evidence-based medicine
3. Vaccines and Cold Chain	• Types of vaccines • National schedule • Contraindications • Cold chain • COVID-19 vaccines	• AEFIs • COVID-19 Vaccines • Newer Vaccines
4. Screening of Disease	• Sensitivity/Specificity • Names of Screening tests • Names of diagnostic tests	• Validity/Reliability • Likelihood ratio • ROC curve • Bayes' theorem
5. Communicable Diseases	• Measles, Rubella, Influenza, TB • Typhoid, Cholera, ORS • Hepatitis A/E • HIV • Malaria/Dengue • Rickettsial Diseases • COVID-19 disease	• TB, H1N1 • Cholera epidemic • Hepatitis B • STDs/HIV • Malaria, Dengue • COVID-19, Monkeypox disease • Mucormycosis
5. Non-communicable Diseases	• Blindness • Obesity • Cancers	Blindness
6. National Health Programmes, Policies and Legislations in India	• NTEP, RNTCP, NVBDCP, NLEP, NACP • MTP	• NHM, NRHM, NTEP, RNTCP, NVBDCP, NLEP, NACP, NPCDCS, • RBSY, NREGA, MTP, PNDT
7. Demography	• Definitions & values • Formulae • Census • Fertility Indicators	• Data collection systems • Definitions
7. Family Planning and Contraception	• Methods in RCH Programme • Pearl index • Composition, Adv/Disadv	Newer methods
8. Preventive Obstetrics, Paediatrics and Geriatrics	• Values • RCH Programme components • Pneumonia control • School health, IQ level • ICDS	• RCH Programme components • JSSK • School health
9. Nutrition and Health	• RDA of nutrients NEW Guidelines • References man/woman • Vitamin deficiencies • Midday meal program	• Uncommon Nutrient Deficiencies • New Nutrition Guidelines 2020–21
10. Social Sciences and Health	• Definitions • SES scale—Kuppuswami	Theories of diseases (Sociology)
10. Health Economics	Definitions—GDP, NNP, GNI	Values—GDP Growth, Health expenditure

Chapters	NEET-PG, FMGE, UPSC patterns	INI-CET patterns
11. Environment and Health	• Values • Water—Chlorination, Quality • Air—Quality • Entomology—Vectors	• Water—Chlorination, Quality • Air—Quality • Waste disposal • Entomology—Vectors, Control
12. Biomedical Waste Management	Wastes segregation, disposal	Newer methods, Covid BMW
12. Disaster Management	Triage, Post Disaster Phase	Worst disasters in history, START triage
12. Occupational Health	• Pneumoconioses • Lead poisoning • ESI/Factory Act	• ESI Act • Occupational cancers
12. Genetics	• ABO system • Hardy Weinberg law	—
12. Mental Health	• Epidemiology in India • Suicide	Mental health care Act
13. Health Education and Communication	• Didactic/Socratic methods • Definitions of methods	Health propaganda
14. Health Care System	• Health centres • Health workers • Primary health care – Definition	Primary health care—Definition, Elements, Principles
14. Health Planning and Management	• H. committees • H. management techniques	Universal health coverage
15. International Health	• International health regulations • WHO, UNICEF	• Bioterrorism agents • International surveillance
16. Biostatistics	• Central tendency • Dispersion • Normal distribution • Statistical graphs • Variables • Chi-square test/Paired t-test	• Central tendency • Dispersion • Normal/skewed distribution • Statistical graphs • Scales • Sampling—Methods/Size • Correlation/Regression • Statistical tests • Statistical errors • Confidence level/intervals
Images	1–2	1–5

(Indicative list prepared by Dr Vivek Jain based on his 20 + years teaching experience)

Best wishes for Exam!
Dr Vivek Jain

SECTION 1

Previous Year Questions (PYQs)

SECTION OUTLINE

- A. Image-based Questions (2019–2023)
- B. NEET FMGE Pattern PYQs (2005–2023)

A. Image-based Questions (2019–2023)

1. Identify the causative agent of the Rickettsial disease transmitted by vector shown in the image:
   [INICET May 2023, AIIMS November 2019]

   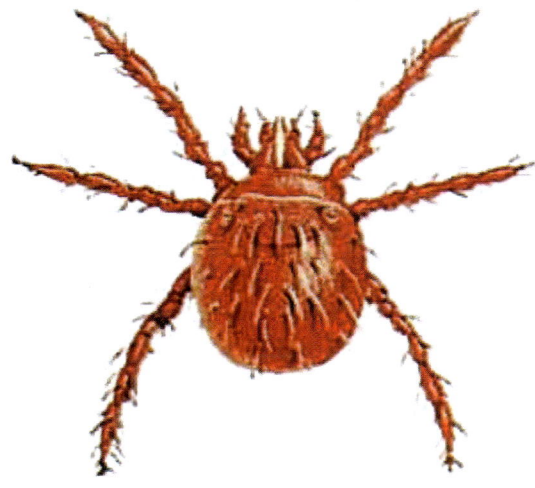

   (a) R. prowazekii
   (b) R. typhi
   (c) Coxiella burnetii
   (d) Orientia tsutsugamushi

2. Water from a broken septic tank is collected in a container and breeding mosquitoes are seen. The image of the larva is given below. Identify the species of the mosquito.
   [INICET November 2022]

   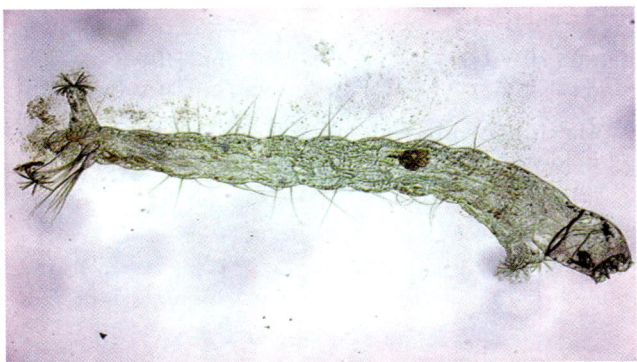

   (a) Anopheles
   (b) Aedes
   (c) Mansonia
   (d) Culex

3. Which of the following models of disease causation is depicted in the image below? *[INICET November 2022]*

   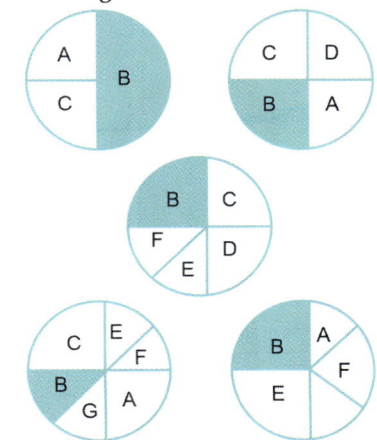

   (a) Sufficient component cause model
   (b) Epidemiological triad
   (c) PERT model
   (d) Web of causation model

4. The drug shown in the image below is administered for:
   [INICET November 2022]

   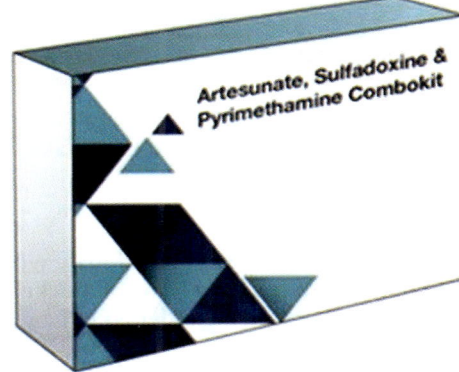

   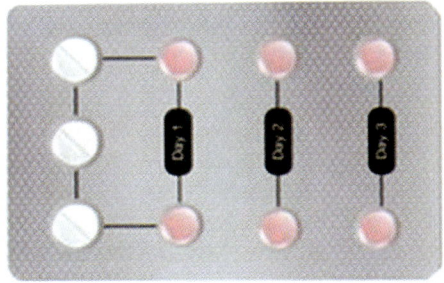

(a) Malaria
(b) Dengue
(c) Sexually transmitted infections
(d) AIDS

5. Which of the following is correct about the given image?
   [INICET November 2022]

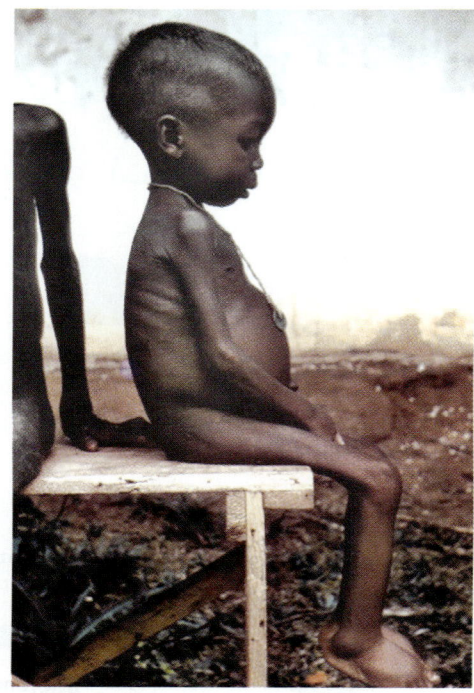

(a) Kwashiorkor due to less energy intake
(b) Kwashiorkor due to less protein intake
(c) Marasmus due to less energy intake
(d) Marasmus due to less protein intake

6. Mr Mayitree Sarkar is 38-year-old male with single stellate hypopigmented skin lesion and thickening of nerve. Which dose is to be given under NLEP?
   [INICET May 2022]

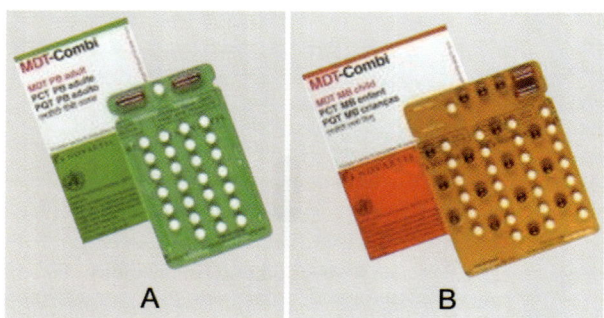

(a) A blister pack × 6 months
(b) A blister pack × 12 months
(c) B blister pack × 6 months
(d) B blister pack × 12 months

7. Identify the vitamin deficiency as shown in the image below:
   [NEET PG Pattern 2022]

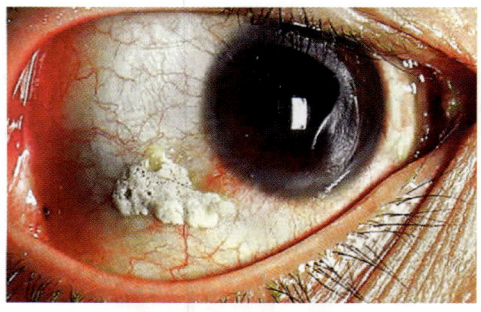

(a) Vitamin A
(b) Vitamin C
(c) Vitamin B_3
(d) Vitamin D

8. A female presented with anogenital wart. With gene study, they came to know she is having high risk of cancer cervix. Which is most likely responsible for high risk of cervical cancer?
   [NEET PG Pattern 2022]

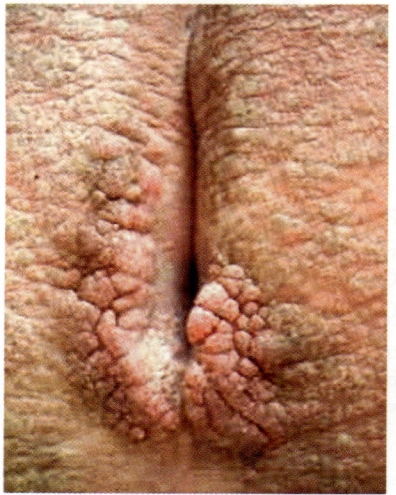

(a) HPV 1
(b) HPV 5
(c) HPV 11
(d) HPV 18

9. Match the correct option according to the image given below:
   [INICET November 2021]

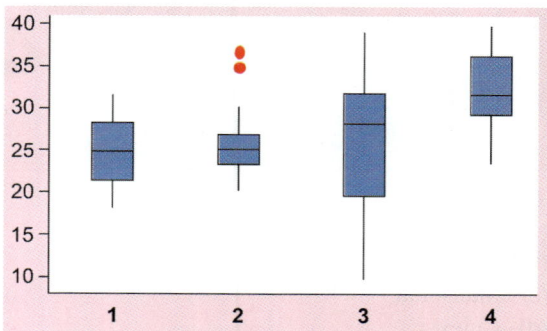

(a) Normal, positive skew, negative skew, outliers
(b) Positive skew, normal, negative skew, outliers
(c) Normal, outliers, negative skew, positive skew
(d) Normal, outliers, positive skew, negative skew

10. See the image given and identify: *[FMGE Pattern June 2022]*

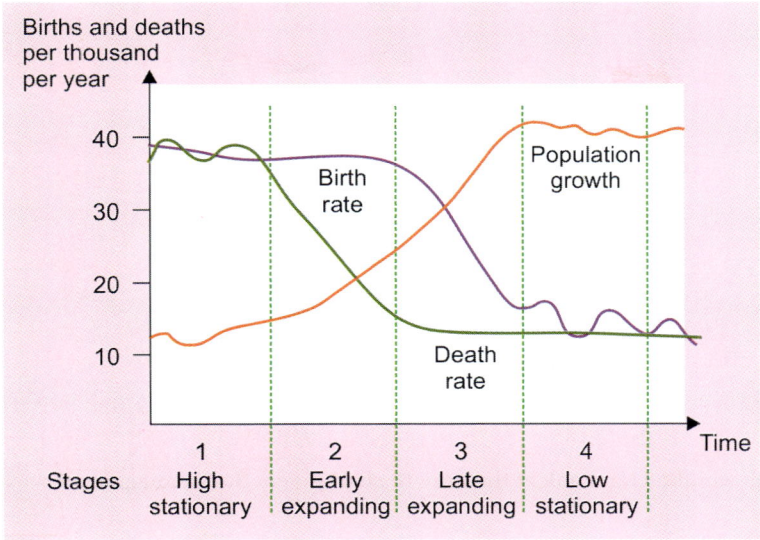

(a) Population cycle
(b) Demographic processes
(c) Registration of births
(d) Demographic transition

11. Correct statement about the double histogram of population pyramid shown is: *[FMGE Pattern June 2022]*

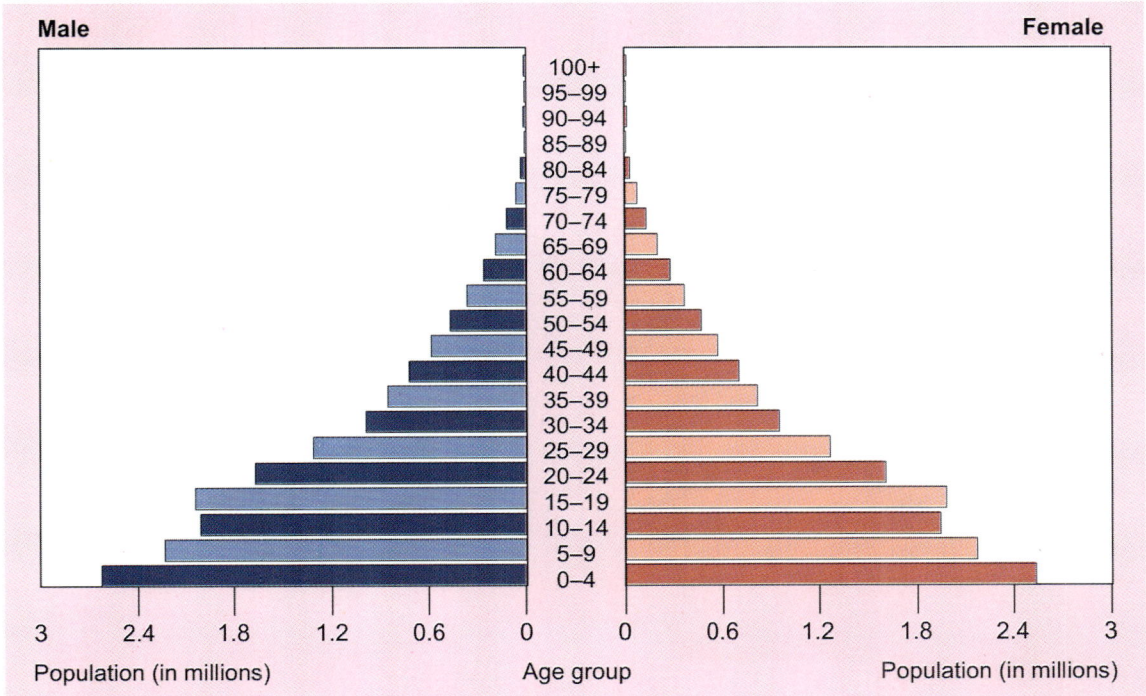

(a) Increased height means low life expectancy
(b) Middle part Males > Females
(c) Broad base represents high fertility and high dependency
(d) Broad base means more working population

12. What is the percentage of 1SD in the given graph? *[FMGE December 2021]*

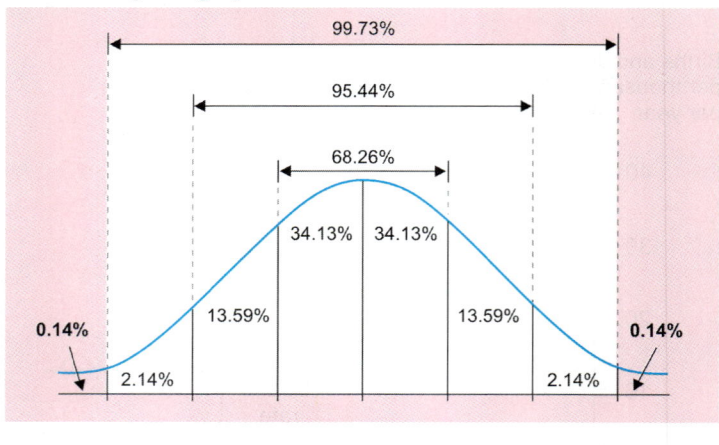

(a) 68.3%   (b) 75.4%   (c) 98.5%   (d) 99.7%

13. A 16-month-old child has weight 8 kg. Look at the growth chart given. Best management will be:
[NEET PG Pattern September 2021]

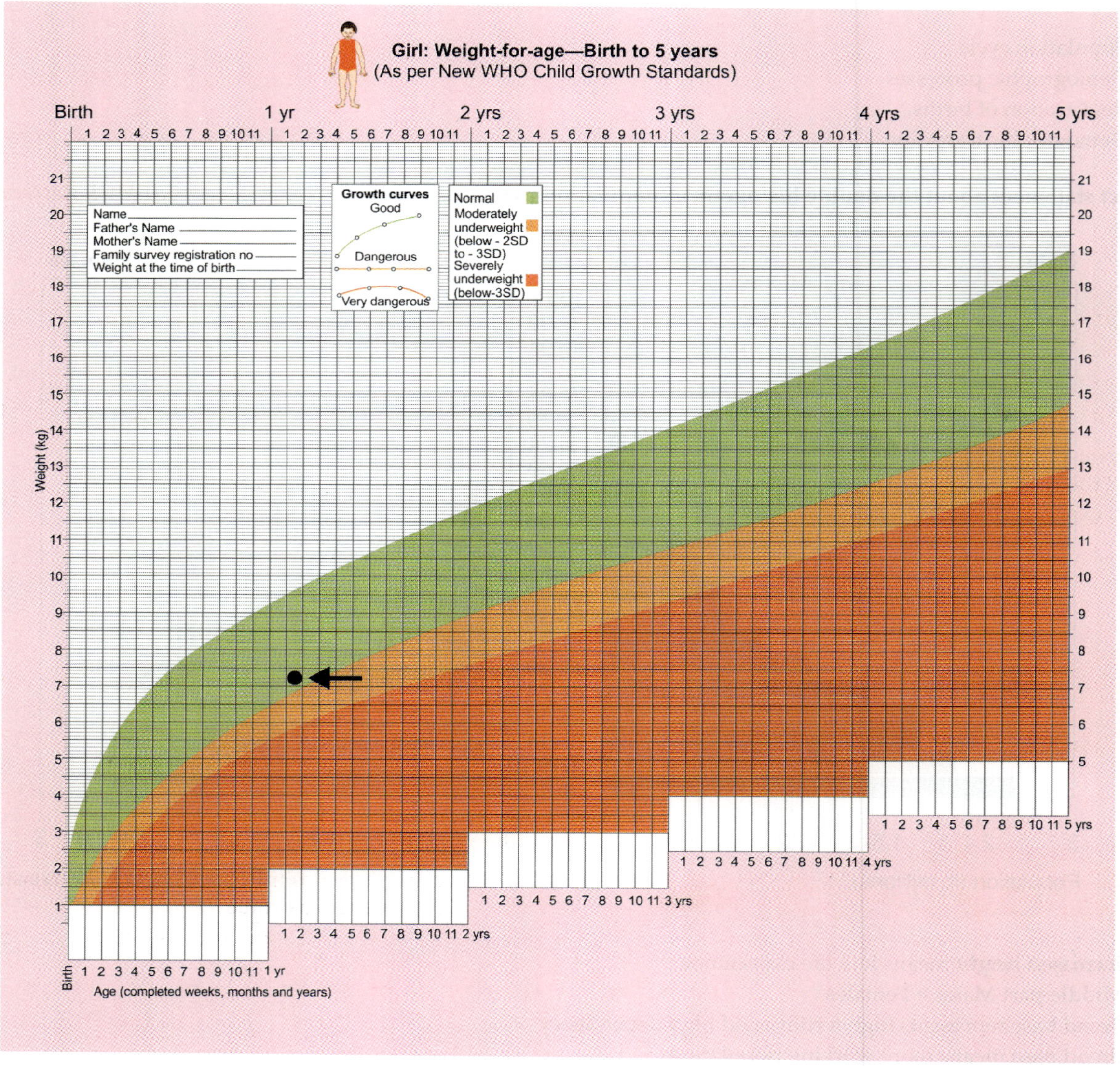

(a) Child is healthy, no advice required further
(b) Child moderately undernourished (MAM), mother given advice
(c) Child severely malnourished (SAM), mother given advice
(d) Child severely malnourished (SAM), referral to nutritional rehabilitation center (NRC)

14. A study conducted in 30,000 women where Researcher wanted to find out if there is any relationship between CRP levels and risk of MI/Stroke. The study subjects were divided into five groups of 6000 subjects each. RR of MI/Stroke was plotted against CRP levels. See the image given below and interpret your findings:
   [NEET PG Pattern September 2021]

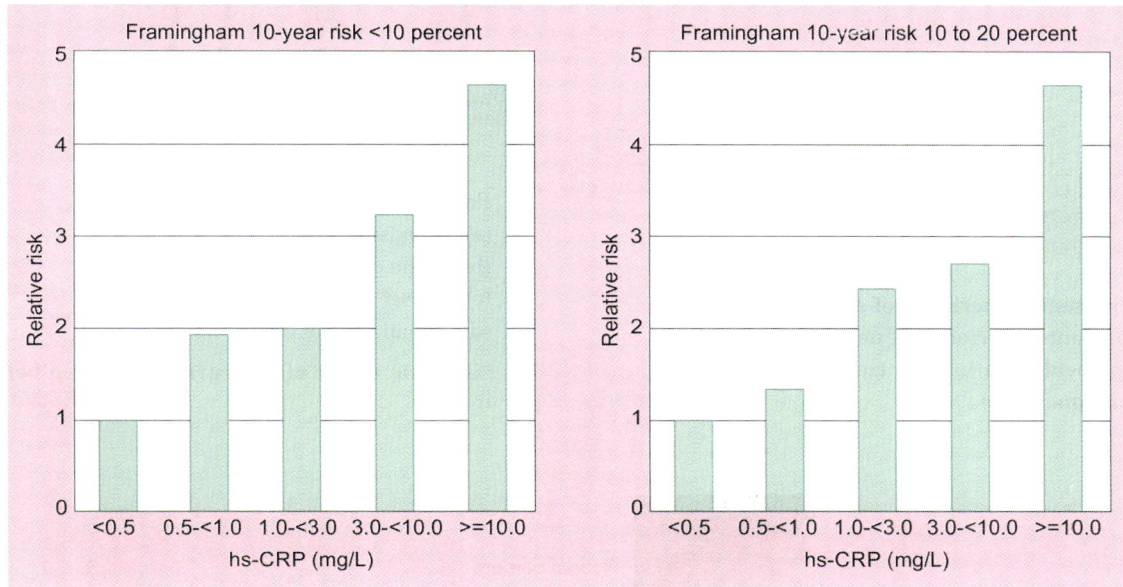

(a) CRP has no relation to MI/Stroke risk
(b) Increase in CRP decreases MI/Stroke risk
(c) Increase in CRP levels increases MI/Stroke risk
(d) Decrease in CRP levels increases MI/Stroke risk

15. A 34-year-old patient presented to OPD with lesion around the neck (See image). Which other manifestations do you expect? *[NEET PG Pattern September 2021]*

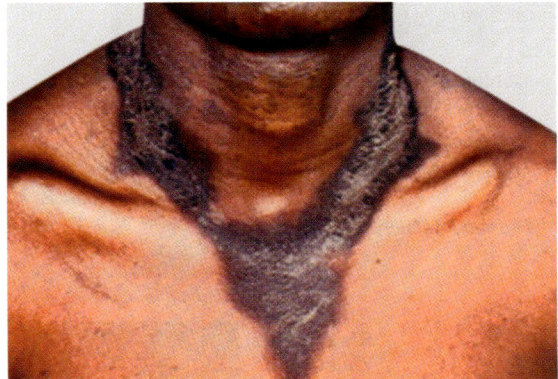

(a) Diarrhoea, dementia
(b) Diarrhoea, memory impairment
(c) Diarrhoea, arthritis
(d) Diarrhoea, disability

16. A study was conducted to see the effect of pulse oximeter readings in neonates with and without micropore. A plot between the two values was made as shown in the figure below. What conclusion can be drawn from the plot?
   [INICET July 2021]

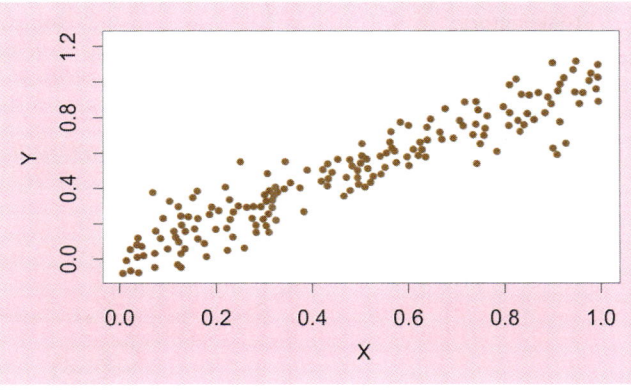

(a) There is a positive correlation with constant 3% increase in Y-axis value
(b) There is a constant negative correlation between two variables
(c) There is a constant positive correlation between two variables
(d) There is no correlation

17. Regarding the equivalence margin graph consider the following statements:

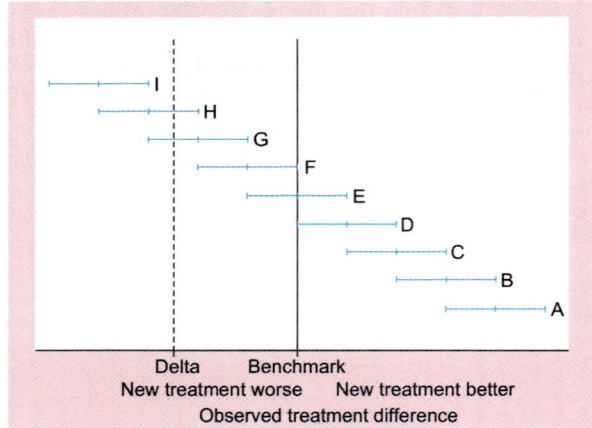

1: 'A' represents superiority of new treatment
2: 'I' represents inferiority of new treatment
3: 'E' represents non-inferior treatment
4: 'C' is inconclusive

Which of the statements are correct? [INICET July 2021]
(a) 1, 2 only
(b) 1, 2, 3 only
(c) 1, 2, 3, 4
(d) 4 only

18. See the image of natural history of disease: [INICET July 2021]

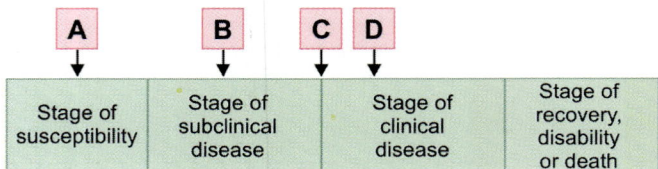

Point 'C' indicates
(a) Exposure time
(b) Time of pathological changes
(c) Onset of symptoms
(d) Usual time of diagnosis

19. Life cycle Image of an organism is given below. Identify it. [INICET November 2020]

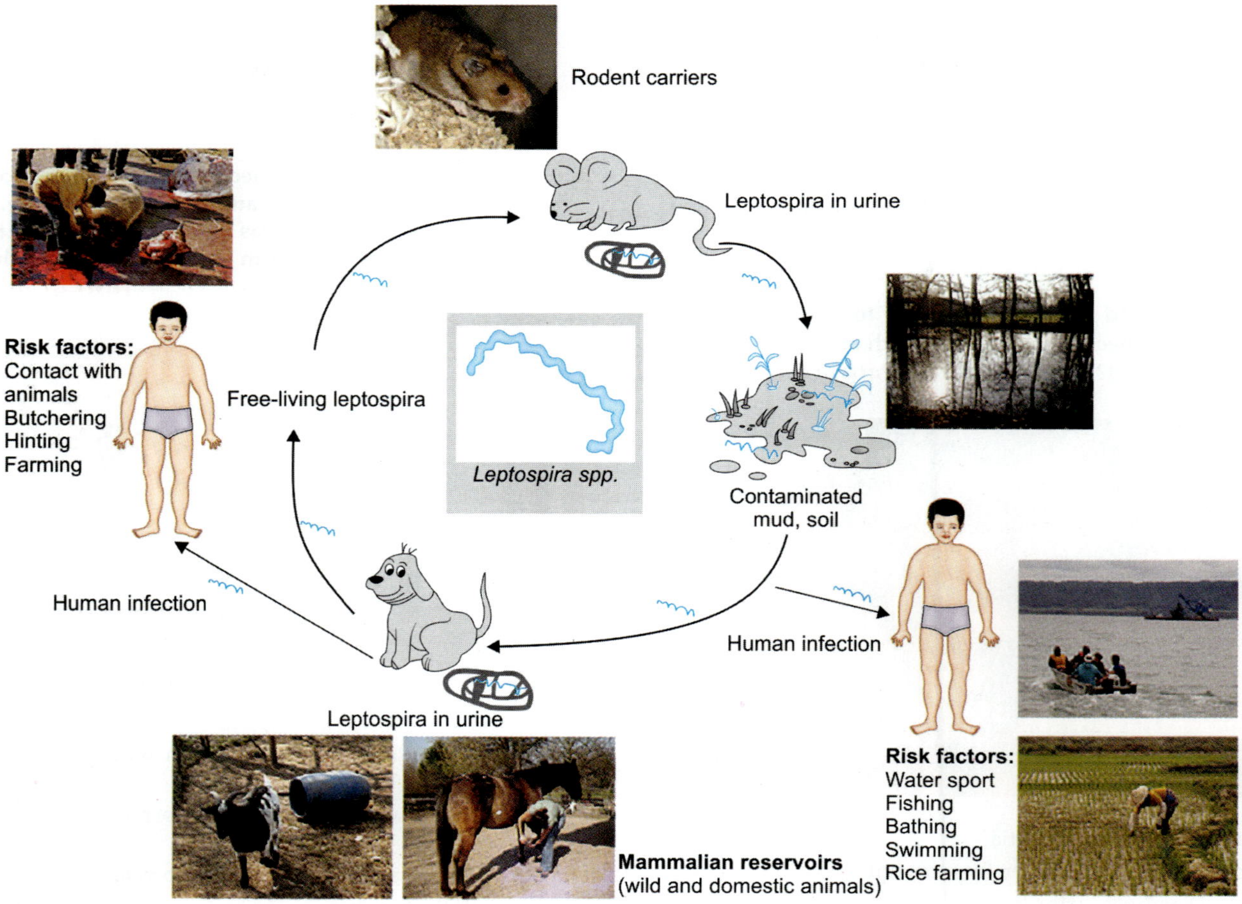

(a) Hantavirus
(b) Leptospirosis
(c) Yersinia pestis
(d) Rickettsia

20. Transplacental transmission with microcephaly. Identify the organism: *[INICET November 2020]*

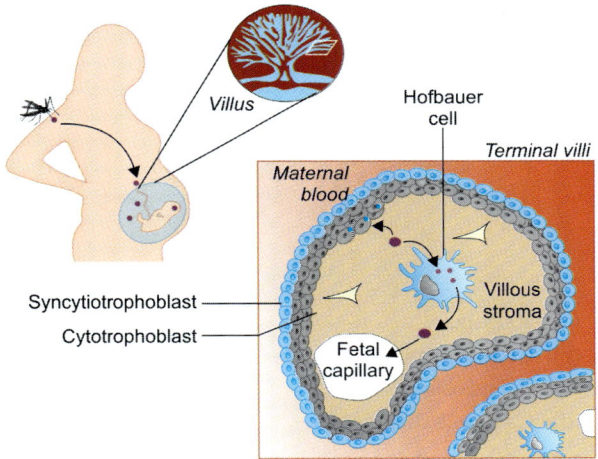

(a) Rubella virus (b) Zika virus
(c) CMV (d) Parvo virus

21. Identify the worm infestation: *[INICET November 2020]*

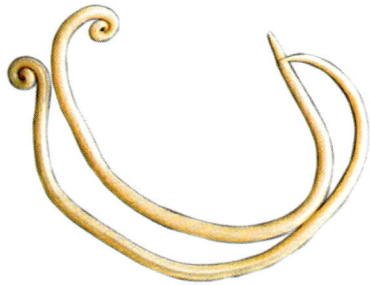

(a) Roundworm
(b) Ancylostoma duodenale
(c) Necator americanus
(d) Enterobius vermicularis

22. Study the life cycle image given below and identify the vector with transovarial transmission: *[AIIMS June 2020]*

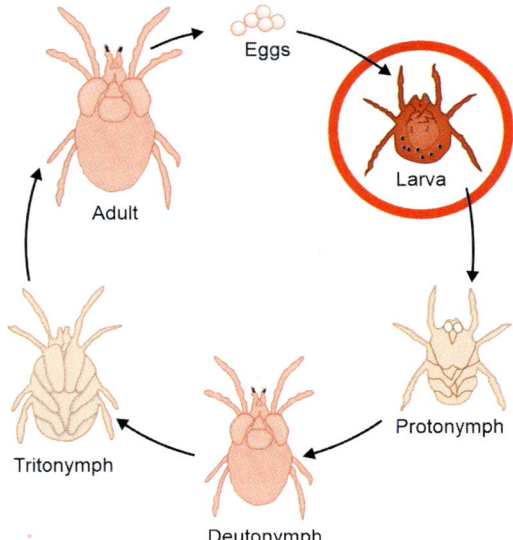

(a) Hard tick
(b) Soft tick
(c) Louse
(d) Trombiculid mite

23. Study the natural history of disease shown below. Identify the disease: *[AIIMS June 2020]*

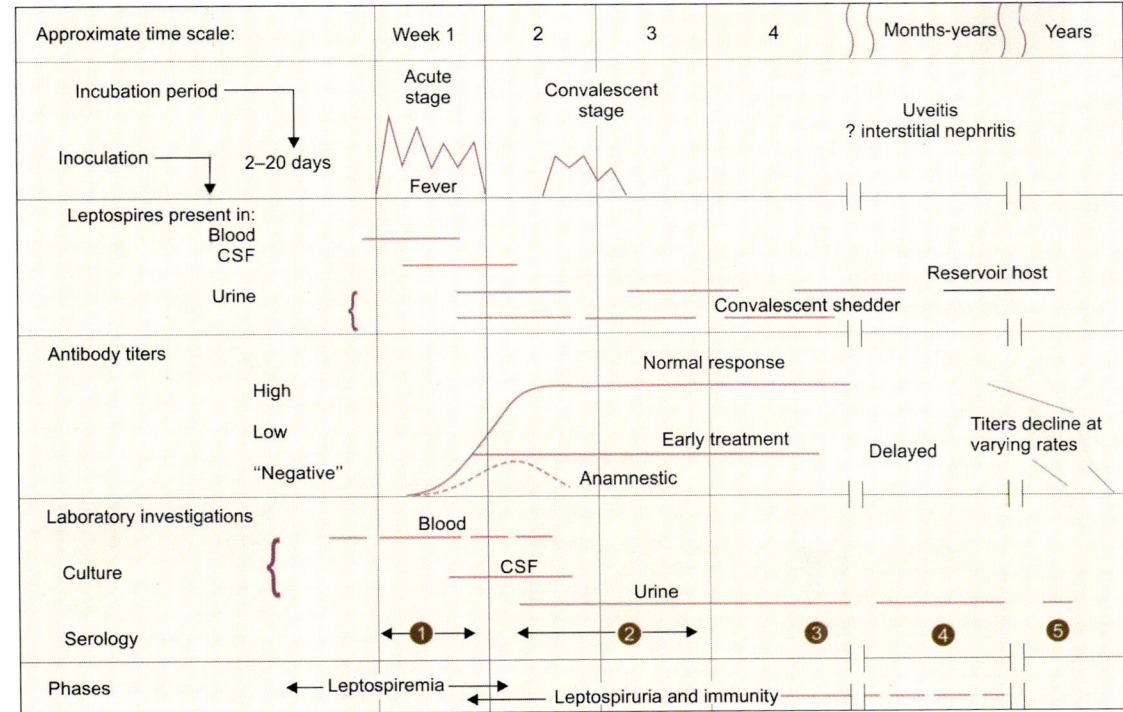

(a) Typhoid
(b) TB
(c) Cerebral malaria
(d) Leptospirosis

24. Identify the contraceptive method shown in the photograph below: [NEET PG Pattern January 2020]

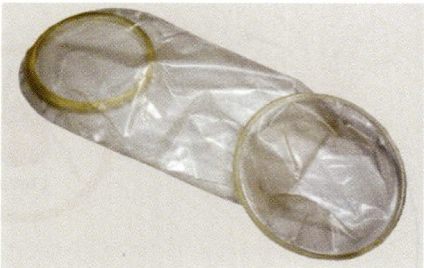

(a) Male condom
(b) Diaphragm
(c) Vaginal sponge
(d) Female condom

25. Patient presented with features of diarrhea, dementia, dermatitis and clinical features as suggested in image. What is the diagnosis? [NEET PG Pattern January 2020]

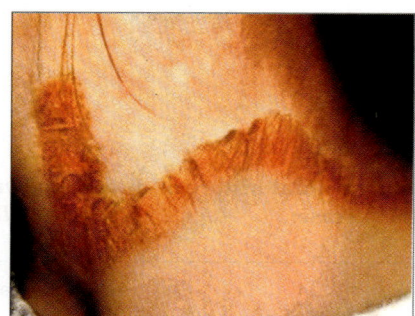

(a) Vitamin B_1
(b) Vitamin B_{12}
(c) Niacin
(d) Pyridoxine

26. Graph as shown in the photograph below belongs to a patient with resolved hepatitis B infection. Curve (Green upper most curve) represents: [AIIMS November 2019]

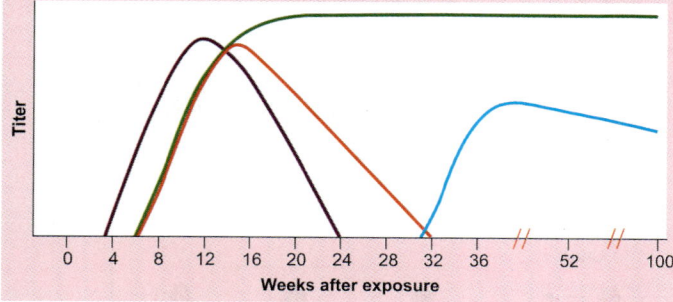

(a) HBsAg
(b) HBeAg
(c) Anti-HBsAg
(d) Anti-HBcAg

27. Which of the following diseases is NOT transmitted by vector shown in photograph? [AIIMS May 2019]

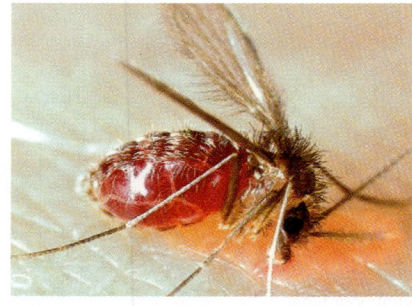

(a) Kala azar
(b) Chandipura encephalitis
(c) Babesiosis
(d) Carrion's disease

28. A study was done to assess the risk factors for breast cancer in 100 females from Urban cities for which image is shown below. How many actual risk factors may be ascertained correctly from the statistical analysis of the research? [AIIMS May 2019]

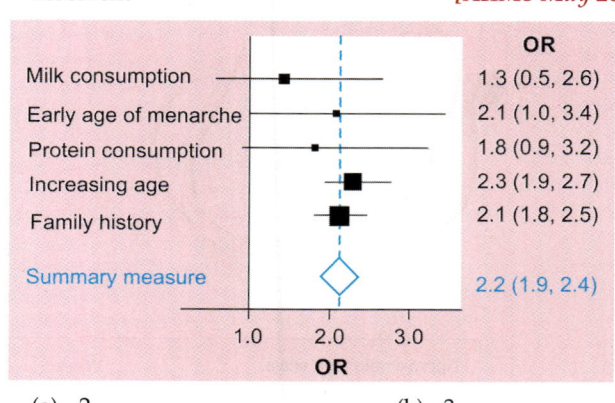

(a) 2
(b) 3
(c) 4
(d) 5

29. Look at the image below and find the correct corresponding option: [AIIMS May 2019]

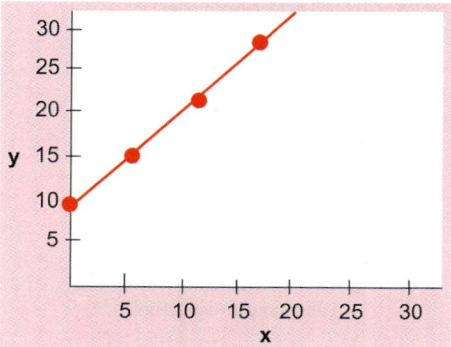

(a) y = x + 10
(b) x = 11 + 2y
(c) x = 10 + y
(d) y = 11 + 2x

30. Bone mineral density (SOS) along with gestational age and birth weight is plotted from 2 different researchers. Which of the following is true for the relation between BMD & GA, and BMD & BW? *[AIIMS May 2019]*

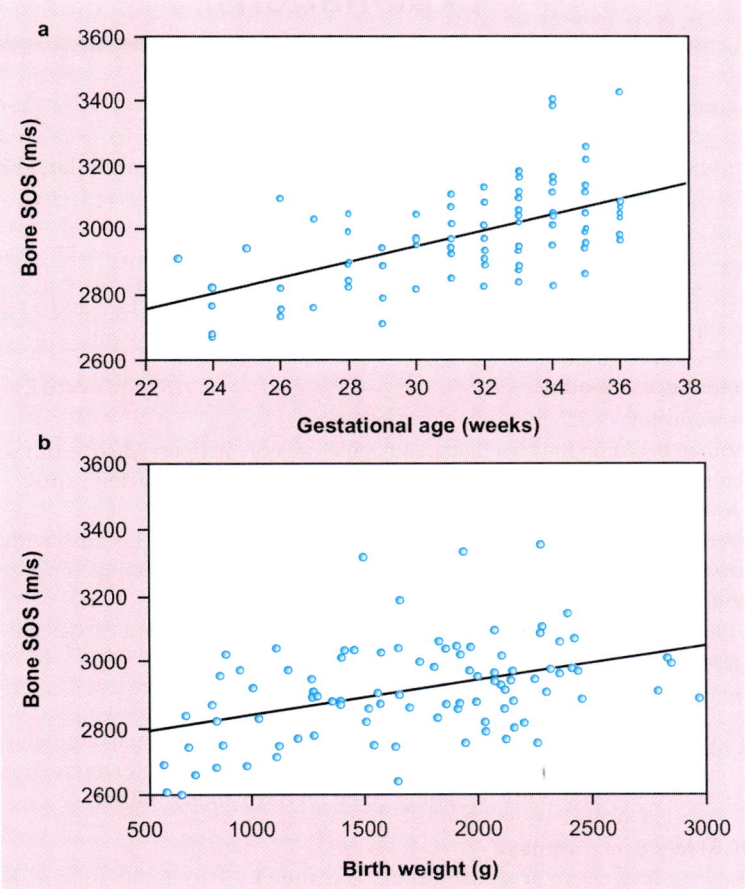

(a) Strength of relation is same in a and b
(b) Strength of relation is more in a than b
(c) Strength of relation is more in b than a
(d) Variation is more with a than with b

Explanations

1. **Ans. (d) Orientia tsutsugamushi**   *[Ref. Park 27/e p347]*
   - Vector shown in the image is Trombiculid mite, so the disease is scrub typhus
   - Orientia tsutsugamushi, the causative agent of scrub typhus, is an obligate, intracellular, gram-negative bacterium

2. **Ans. (d) Culex**   *[Ref. Park 27/e p896]*
   - The species of mosquito that breeds in dirty water is Culex
   - It can be identified by the presence of unspotted wings and hunched back
   - The larva has a head that is suspended downwards at an angle to the water surface and a siphon tube is present
   - It breeds in dirty water collections like stagnant drains, septic tanks, and burrow pits

3. **Ans. (a) Sufficient component cause model**   *[Ref. Modern Epidemiology by Rothman 3/e p9]*
   Sufficient component cause model
   - It was developed by Rothman based on the idea that an outcome can only happen when a sufficient cause is present
   - The complete pie, which might be considered a causal pathway, is called a sufficient cause
   - The individual factors are called component causes
   - A component that appears in every pie or pathway is called a necessary cause, because without it, disease does not occur
   - A disease may have more than one sufficient cause, with each sufficient cause being composed of several component causes that may or may not overlap

   In the given model, each pie chart represents a sufficient cause made of component causes. Since B is present in all the charts, it can be considered a necessary cause

4. **Ans. (a) Malaria**   *[Ref. Park 27/e p307]*
   - Artemisinin-based combination therapy (ACT) is used in the treatment of Falciparum malaria
   - ACT consists of Artesunate given for 3 days and Sulphadoxine-pyrimethamine given for 1 day
   - Primaquine with dose of 0.75 mg/kg of body weight is given on day 2 along with it.

5. **Ans. (b) Kwashiorkor due to less protein intake**   *[Ref. Park 27/e p755]*
   - The following given image is suggestive of kwashiorkor, as it shows a bulging abdomen and pedal edema along with thin limbs and prominent ribs
   - Kwashiorkor occurs as a result of less protein intake, whereas marasmus occurs due to less calorie intake.

Kwashiorkor	Marasmus
Occurs due to protein deficiency	Due to deficiency of calories and proteins
Edema is present	Edema is absent
Poor appetite	Voracious appetite
Apathy and lethargy seen	Active child
Hepatomegaly seen	Hepatomegaly is usually not seen

6. **Ans. (a) A blister pack × 6 months**   *[Ref: Park 27/e p371]*
   Single skin lesion with thickening of nerve in 38 years old male indicate Paucibacillary Leprosy (PBL case) who will get 2 drug multidrug therapy (Dapsone, Rifampicin) for 6 months
   Blister packs colour coding under NLEP

MDT blister pack	Colour
PBL adult	Green color
MBL adult	Red color
PBL child	Blue color
MBL child	Yellow colour

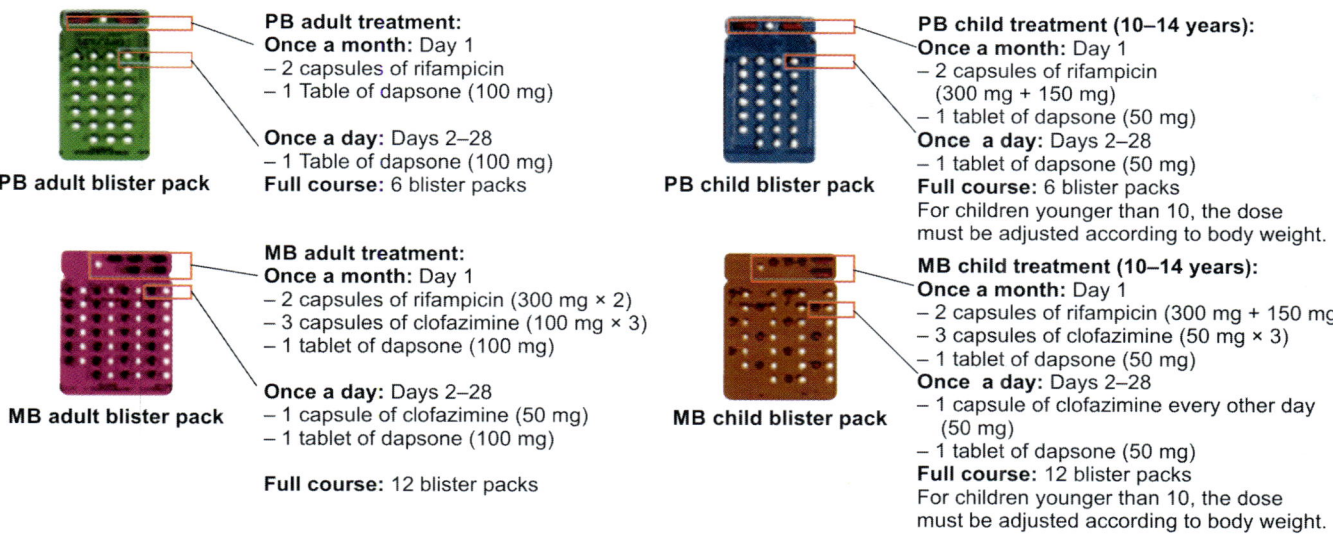

7. **Ans. (a) Vitamin A** [Ref: Park 27/e p731]
   - Bitot's Spots' are triangular, pearly-white or yellowish, foamy spots on bulbar conjunctiva, on either side of cornea (X1B category in WHO Classification)
   - In young children they indicate Vitamin-A deficiency, whereas in adults they are often inactive sequelae of earlier disease

8. **Ans. (d) HPV 18** [Ref: Human Papillomavirus and Cervical Cancer by Burd, Clin Microbiol Rev. 2003 Jan; 16(1): 1–17]

Disease	MC HPV associations
Recurrent respiratory papillomatosis	6,11
Condyloma acuminata (genital warts)	6,11
Cervical intraepithelial neoplasia (low risk)	6,11
Cervical intraepithelial neoplasia (high risk)	16,18
Cervical carcinoma	16,18

   (Table © Vivek Jain 2022-23)

9. **Ans. (c) Normal, outliers, negative skew, positive skew** [Ref: Business Statistics by Black, 7/e p85]
   Box and whisker plot
   - Description: A convenient way of graphically depicting groups of numerical data through their quartiles
   - Edges of box: 1st and 3rd Quartile
   - Line in Box: 2nd Quartile (Median)
   - Whiskers end: Minimum & maximum values
   - Outlier: A data point that is located outside the whiskers of the box plot

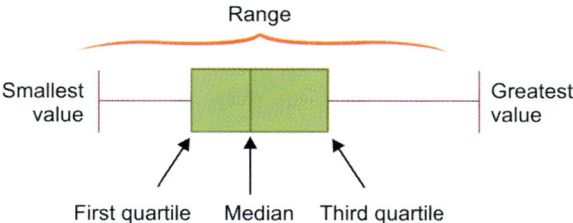

10. **Ans. (d) Demographic transition** [Ref: Park 27/e p554]
    Demographic transition: is a model used to explain the process of transition from high BR and high DR (Stage 1 demographic cycle – High stationary) to low BR and low DR (Stage 4 Demographic cycle – Low stationary) as part of the economic development of a country from a pre-industrial to an industrialized economy

11. **Ans. (c) Broad base represents high fertility and high dependency** [Ref: Park 27/e p557]
    Population pyramid
    - Age-sex pyramid (age structure diagram) is a graphical illustration that shows the distribution of various age groups in a population which normally forms the shape of a pyramid (Double histogram)
    - Expansive pyramid (Upright triangle, developing countries): A population pyramid showing a broad base, indicating a high proportion of children (high fertility, high dependency), a rapid rate of population growth, and a low proportion of older people

12. **Ans. (a) 68.3%** [Ref: Park 27/e p977]
    Normal (Gaussian/Standard) distribution
    - Mean ± 1SD ($\mu \pm 1\sigma$) covers 68.3% values
    - Mean ± 2SD ($\mu \pm 2\sigma$) covers 95.4% values
    - Mean ± 3SD ($\mu \pm 3\sigma$) covers 99.7% values

13. **Ans. (b) Child moderately undernourished (MAM), mother given advice**
    [Guidelines for Management of SAM Children at NRC Guidelines NHM 2012, p22]
    - No Severe Acute Malnutrition (SAM) is MUAC > 115; or WFH > –3SD; and no bilateral pedal oedema: Nutrition counselling to mother/caregiver
    - Severe Acute Malnutrition (SAM) is WFH < –3SD/ and/or severe visible wasting and/or bilateral pedal oedema and/or MUAC < 115 mm
        - No medical complications: Refer to VHND or subcenter to be further assessment and counseling by ANM
        - Any one medical complication: Immediate referral to NRC
    - Medical complications include poor appetite, visible severe wasting, edema of both feet, severe palmar pallor, any sick young infant (<2 months old), lethargy, drowsiness, unconsciousness, continually irritable and restless, any respiratory distress, signs suggesting severe dehydration in a child with diarrhoea
    In the given question, Growth chart wise child falls into category of mild-moderate malnutrition (between –2SD and –3SD, yellow zone)

14. **Ans. (c) Increase in CRP levels increases MI/Stroke risk** *[Ref. C-reactive Protein and Cardiovascular Disease by Ridker 1/e]*
    - High-sensitivity C-reactive protein (hsCRP) is a marker of inflammation that predicts incident myocardial infarction, stroke, peripheral arterial disease, and sudden cardiac death among healthy persons without a history of cardiovascular disease, as well as recurrent events and death in patients with acute or stable coronary syndromes
    - hs-CRP is a stronger predictor of heart attack and stroke than LDL cholesterol
    - **Interpretation of the graphs given** - As the hs-CRP level increase, the risk of MI/Stroke development also increase

    [**Kindly Note:** Some students suggested that Question asked interpretation of RR = 1. Please remember RR = 1 implies No Association]

15. **Ans. (a) Diarrhoea, Dementia** [Ref: Park 26/e p709]
    - Pellagra is characterized by 4 D's: Diarrhoea, dementia, death, dermatitis
    - Skin rash in pellagra may appear as pigmented and scaly in areas exposed to sunlight. esp. neck when it is known as 'Casal's Necklace' (See image)

16. **Ans. (c) There is a constant positive correlation between two variables** [Ref: Park 27/e p975]
    - Scatter of DOTS show a positive slope, so its positive correlation
    - Correlation coefficient will lie between 0 and +1

17. **Ans. (b) 1, 2, 3 only**
    [Ref: Leung JT, Barnes SL, Lo ST, et al. Non-inferiority trials in cardiology: what clinicians need to know. Heart 2020;106:99-104]

    Three types of trials are superiority trials (New drug is better than older drug), Non-inferiority trials (New drug is as good as older drug) and equivalence trials (New drug is same as older drug)
    - Maximum success has been reported with non-inferiority (NI) trials
    - Equivalence margin graph is a Forest graph type of plot used in NI trials
    - Right side is new treatment/drug better and left side represents new treatment/drug as worse
        - Benchmark solid vertical line is RR = 1 (No difference)
        - Dashed vertical line is Delta (NI margin) indicates smallest evidence of inferiority of New treatment/drug (Its not acceptable)

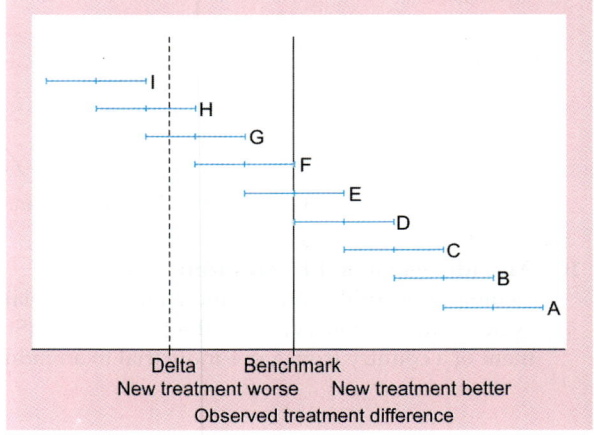

- If results lie on right side (Lines A, B, C, D): New treatment/drug is superior to older
- If results cross Benchmark line and lie towards Delta also (Line E, F): NI of New treatment/drug
- If Results do not cross Benchmark (RR = 1) as well as do not lie beyond Delta (Line G, H): Inconclusive results
- If results lie beyond Delta margin (Line I): New treatment/drug is inferior to older

18. **Ans. (c) Onset of symptoms** *[Ref. Principles of Epidemiology in Public Health Practice. CDC. 3/e Lesson 1]*
    Natural history of disease
    - A - Exposure time
    - B - Time of pathological changes
    - C - Onset of symptoms
    - D - Usual time of diagnosis

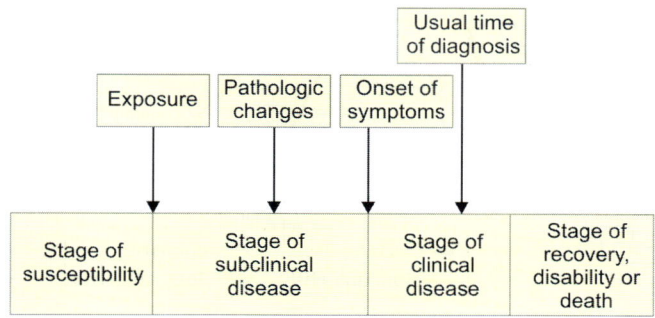

19. **Ans. (b) Leptospirosis** *[Ref. Park 27/e p338]*
    - Leptospirosis results from a mild febrile illness to severe fatal disease with liver/kidney involvement
    - Route of transmission is direct skin contact with infected rat's urine
    - Occupational exposure at risk: Agricultural and lives tock farmers (rice fields, sugarcane fields, underground sewers, abattoir workers, meat/animal handlers, veterinarians)

20. **Ans. (b) Zika virus** *[Ref. Park 27/e p321]*
    - Clinical picture of Zika viral infection: Fever, fatigue, myalgia, headache, rashes, conjunctivitis, retro-orbital pain
    - In some cases, stillbirth, microcephaly, intracranial calcifications, and Guillain-Barré syndrome are also manifested
    - In Zika viral infection there is downregulation of neurogenesis and upregulation of apoptosis which leads to impaired brain growth culminating in microcephaly

21. **Ans. (a) Roundworm** *[Ref. Park 27/e p285]*
    Ascariasis/Roundworms
    - Soil transmitted helminths (man is the only reservoir) with faecal-oral route of transmission
    - males are 12–30 cms long, females 20–35 cms
    - Female lays 240,000 eggs per day
    - Life span is 6–12 months

22. **Ans. (d) Trombiculid mite** *[Ref. Park 27/e p347]*
    Trombiculid Mite (Leptotrombidium deliense)
    - Disease transmitted: Scrub typhus (Cause: R. tsutsugamushi)
    - Synonyms: Berry bugs, Chiggers
    - Larvae have 3 pairs of legs, adults have 4 pairs
    - Larval stage act as Reservoir as well as Vector

23. **Ans. (d) Leptospirosis** *[Ref. Park 27/e p338]*
    - Acute interstitial nephritis (AIN) is a renal lesion that typically causes a decline in kidney function and is characterized by an inflammatory infiltrate in the kidney interstitium
    - AIN, most often induced by drug therapy, is also caused by autoimmune disorders or other systemic disease (SLE, Sjögren's syndrome, sarcoidosis), a variety of infections remote to the kidney (Legionella, Leptospirosis, and streptococcal organisms), and Tubulointerstitial nephritis with uveitis (TINU) syndrome
    - IP Leptospirosis is 4–20 days (Median IP 10 days)

24. **Ans. (d) Female condom** *[Ref. Park 25/e p546]*
    Female condom is a Polyurethane pouch which lines the vagina, internal ring covering cervix and outer ring remain outside vagina

25. **Ans. (c) Niacin** *[Ref. Park 25/e p676]*
    - Pellagra is characterized by 4 D's: Diarrhoea, dementia, death, dermatitis
    - Skin rash in pellagra may appear as pigmented and scaly in areas exposed to sunlight. esp. neck when it is known as 'Casal's Necklace'

26. **Ans. (d) Anti-HBcAg** [Ref. Park 25/e p]

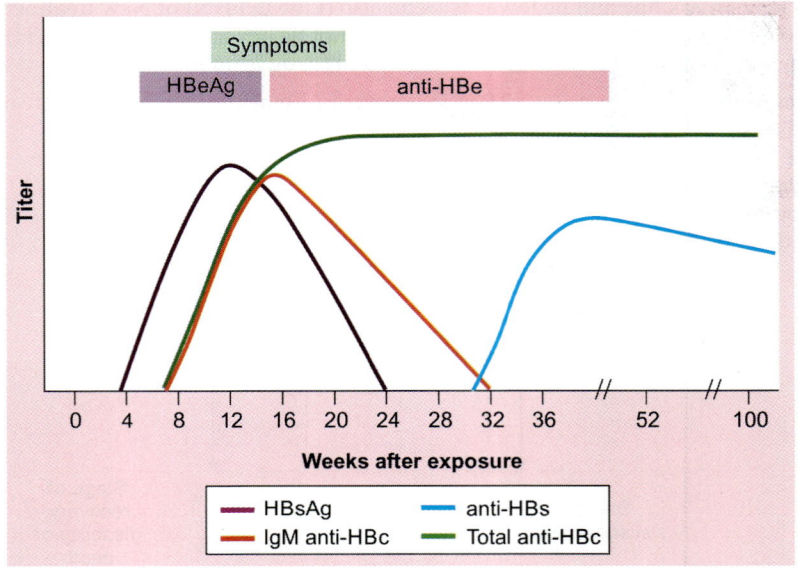

27. **Ans. (c) Babesiosis** [Ref. Park 25/e p835]
    Sandfly vector (Photograph) can transmit Kala azar, Oriental sore, Sandfly fever. Oraya fever, Chandipura virus, Carrion's disease, Changuinola virus, Summer meningitis, Vesicular stomatitis, Naples virus, Toscana virus, Sicilian virus, Cyprus virus, Turkey virus, Puntotora virus, Vesiculo virus

28. **Ans. (a) 2** [Ref. Confidence Intervals by Smithson Issue 140 p10]
    Forest Plot (Blobbogram)
    - A graphical display of estimated results from a number of scientific studies addressing the same question, along with the overall results
    - **In the given question,** 5 risk factors of breast cancer are chosen for evaluation – Milk consumption, early age of menarche, protein consumption, increasing age, family history
    - Each factor has OR given with confidence intervals
    - All 5 factors have OR >1 (Each factor has association present with breast cancer)
    - If confidence interval include 1 in its range (as seen in milk consumption, early age of menarche, protein consumption) it indicates insufficient evidence to conclude that the groups are statistically significantly different (or in this case association)
    - **Hence,** only 2 factors: Increasing age, family history have significant association with breast cancer

29. **Ans. (a) y = x + 10** [Ref. Park 25/e p916]
    Simple Linear Regression
    - y = a + bx
    - Looking at the diagram given in question
    - If x is 0, then y is 10
    - **So,** if x is taken as 5, 10, 15 then y will be 15, 20, 25 respectively
    - **Therefore** for every increase of 5 VALUES in x, leads to increase Y linearly by 5 values
    - **So,** answer is y = x + 10

30. **Ans. (b) Strength of relation is more in a than b** [Ref. Park 25/e p909-910]
    - In graph a, bone mineral density (SOS) is plotted against gestational age (weeks) on a scatter diagram and line is having positive slope, hence it depicts positive correlation
    - In graph a, bone mineral density (SOS) is plotted against birth weight (grams) on a scatter diagram and this line is also having positive slope, hence it depicts positive correlation too
    - In graph a, slope is higher so its coefficient of correlation is higher as compared to graph b (r value in graph a > r value in graph b)
    - Interpretation: BMD (SOS) has a higher degree of correlation with gestational age (weeks) as compared to birth weight (grams)

B. NEET FMGE Pattern PYQs (2005–2023)

PYQs: NEET FMGE Pattern January 2023

Washing hands in COVID-19 is which level of prevention	Primary
Since many people are dying with cancer in association with tobacco use, Government of India made an act to prevent the use of tobacco in community, level of prevention is	Primary
Ground glass appearance on chest X-ray is seen in	Asbestosis
Minimum per capita space should be available for children in school	>10 sq. feet
A child presented with white patches on the anterior incisors later it turned into brown color, component responsible is	Fluorine
Which is not a micronutrient?	Selenium, copper
A study was conducted to compare MMR vaccine history in children with autism and children without autism. What kind of study is being done here?	Case control study
Shelf life of CuT 380 A is	10 years
S in SAFE strategy of trachoma stands for	Surgery
Eligible couple register is maintained at which level	Sub-centre level
A person living with his wife who is pregnant and also has a less than 3 years old child. His brother and his wife came for winter vacation for 1 month and staying together. Now you went to survey their family, this is a type of	Nuclear family
A child presenting with dryness of the eyes which vitamin deficiency is associated with it	Vitamin A
A 9-month-old child is presents to you after MMR vaccination. What is the dose of vitamin A you will provide him?	1 Lac IU
Which of the following help in collagen synthesis?	Ascorbic acid and copper
As a doctor you are advised to explain a community that vaccination will not cause impotency; as a doctor you are overcoming which type of barrier?	Cultural barrier
A 2nd trimester pregnant female, having a 2-year-old child, presents for vaccination. She was vaccinated completely in her previous pregnancy. What is the recommended regime?	Td booster dose
After vasectomy, till how many months you will advise use of barrier methods?	12–16 weeks
Denominator in infant mortality rate	1000 Live births
Infectivity is also termed as	Secondary attack rate
A patient came with Class 3 bite by a stray dog to OPD. Also, recently she took post-exposure vaccination for monkey-bite 6 months ago. What is the management you will provide?	Wound care + IM vaccine 0, 3 days
A maize eater is presenting with symptoms of diarrhea, dermatitis and dementia, which deficiency may lead to this?	Niacin
Not a components of RCH program	Women education and empowerment
In which demographic cycle stage, is the birth rate highest	Stage 1
True for single exposure point source epidemic	Explosive in nature
A pregnant woman of 8 weeks, working in an industry consults the doctor. According to the ESI act, how long the maternity leave will be provided?	26 weeks
You are planning to do a study in Urban Delhi on diets in different religions. On 3000 families you are conducting this study, which type of sampling you will use for this diet study?	Stratified random sampling
Sickness absenteeism of workers in the industry is used to evaluate	State of health of workers
School health does not include the following component	A doctor on school premises
In a village you are asked to educate the people regarding washing wound after dog bite, which method you will prefer use to teach the community?	Demonstration
Health propaganda refers to	Trying to make them conscious for themselves
Oxidation pond uses which method	Aerobic during day time and anaerobic during night time

PYQs: NEET FMGE Pattern June 2022

According to WHO, maternal mortality is defined as	Death antenatal to within 6 weeks of delivery
There are 30 people at a small camping site. How will they manage their garbage?	Burial
Nutrient deficient in breast milk is	Vitamin D
Counselling and screening is done for tuberculosis in a HIV positive patient at ICTC Centre (NACP programme). This is which level of prevention?	Secondary
More than one Doctor's opinion is required for doing MTP (As per latest regulations 2021)	20–24 weeks
Which of the following is not a health worker at village level?	ANM
Role of social factors in disease causation is studied under	Social pathology
Patients from different age groups from a village in West Bengal came to clinic with illness. On examination, it is noted that all of them were having edema. On history it was found that they were consuming mustard seed bought from the same local shop. Which is the best probable diagnosis?	Epidemic dropsy
If Arhar dal is found to be contaminated with Khesari dal, which of the following will be done?	Ban the crop; give vitamin C prophylaxis; remove toxin
In a European country there is low births and high deaths reported. Which stage of demographic cycle will be present?	Declining stage
Blood bag should be deposited in which category bag	Yellow
A patient presented with neurological deficit and history of chronic alcohol intake. It is due to deficiency of	Thiamine
Measles vaccine given at 7 months age to a boy. When will be the next dose?	9 months age
Relative risk (RR) is calculated in which study	Cohort study
Substance chemical used in 'Today' contraceptive	Nonoxynol 9
Which vaccine is given at birth?	BCG, OPV birth dose, Hep B birth dose
Patient presented with blue lines on gums, abdominal pain, constipation. How will you manage the patient?	EDTA + Dimercaprol
Vitamin deficiency in pellagra	Niacin
Women who recently delivered baby comes to clinic for contraception plan for the next 3 years. Best contraceptive in this case	Copper T
In villages, first contact of people to medical health care is	Subcentre
At subcenter birth care is done by all of following except	TBA
Which of the following vaccine is recommended at birth	BCG
TB sputum assessment comes under which type of mode of prevention	Secondary
Trend of diarrhoeal diseases can be plotted on	Line chart
A child presents with normal height but weight was lesser than expected for that height. He will be classified as a case of	Wasting
Before blood transfusion all of the following are tested except	HAV
NOT true for PHC	First referral centre
NOT present at CHC	Intensive neonatal care
How to compare life expectancy of two different countries?	DALY
On World Health Day, 4–8 persons are sitting in front of an audience and they are discussing a health topic. CEO Director of hospital welcomes everyone, opens meeting and introduces speakers. He then introduces topic briefly and invites speakers to present their point of view. This is a type of	Panel discussion
A patient presents with typically dry-appearing triangular patches of conjunctiva with a layer of foam on the surface, usually located temporal to the cornea. This is	Conjunctival xerosis
A person working in an industry lost his hand. He is unable to do his daily activities including writing and machine working. Which is an impairment in this guy?	Loss of anatomical structure
Best radically new approach for health education is	Primary healthcare approach
A couple goes to hospital and told Doctor that they are prone to have anencephaly in their baby. Then they asked Doctor how to prevent it. Most likely response by Doctor	Give folic acid antenatally

PYQs: NEET FMGE Pattern June 2022 (Continued)

A baby has come to PHC OPD for routine checkup. His growth chart shows Weight of the baby between 85 and 95th percentile. He is	Over-weight
A 2-year-old child is brought to PHC OPD with fever and cough since last 2 days. On examination, chest indrawing is present. RR is 38 per minute. Management will be	Pneumonia – Clinical treatment at PHC
A group organized a mass gathering on handwashing awareness. Logical sequence will be	Awareness – Interest – Evaluation – Adoption
If wide range of values are present in a community then best measure of central tendency will be	Median
If old people die then dependency ratio will	Decrease
A 32-year-old male presented to OPD with progressive black discoloration of nose. He was subsequently diagnosed as a case of mucormycosis. Treatment will include	Amphotericin B
Under biomedical waste management guidelines, following could be used for blood spillage	Sodium hypochlorite

PYQs: NEET FMGE Pattern December 2021

Most common cause of blindness among children in India	Vitamin A deficiency
Best method of teaching villagers about ORS is	Demonstration
How would you demonstrate balance diet to uneducated patient's relatives and family pictorially?	Pie chart
Highest content of sodium is found in	Loaf of bread
Minimum antenatal visits according to WHO	8
In a population of 10,000 the sex ratio is more than 1000. What is the correct option from below?	Males less than 5000
In 14th century, during outbreak of Plague, quarantine of ship sailors was done for	40 days
Which of the following food has the lowest glycemic index?	Sweet corn
Which coloured bag is used to dispose cotton swab contaminated with blood?	Yellow
A patient is resistant to isoniazid, rifampicin, ofloxacin and kanamycin. What type of resistance is being shown by the patient?	Extensively drug resistant
Colour coded STD kit used for female with vaginal discharge and lower abdominal pain	Kit 6 - Yellow
No. of maternal deaths due to pregnancy related process expressed per 1,00,000 live births is known as	Maternal mortality ratio
A women 25–45 years, 8th pass, married/divorced, belongs to the same village community, with well communication skill/leadership quality. Selected by village personnel. She is eligible to work as	Accredited Social Health Activist
As a Medical Officer of a PHC, you want to talk and discuss some health related issue with Antenatal mothers. How many members will you include in focal group discussion?	6–12
Which is the home-based pregnancy test kit provided by GOI?	NISCHAY
For the population of 10000, Trench method sanitary landfill pit of depth 2 m is to be constructed. How much land area is required per year?	1 acre
A child more than 12 months old less than 8 kg weight, Malnourished with Vitamin A deficiency, oral dose required is	1 lakh IU
In a study, a doctor wants to check incidence of some disease in workers band managers after sound exposure for 1 year between exposed and non-exposed group. Which study design is used?	Cohort study
To prevent neural tube defects in a woman with history of NTD, dose of folic acid to be given to woman is	4 mg
Case history of child with swelling on face and also with swelling in scrotum. He cannot chew properly/open mouth	Mumps
Causative organism of Donovanosis (Granuloma inguinale) is	Klebsiella granulomatis

PYQs: NEET FMGE Pattern December 2021 (Continued)

Secondary/Re-infection of this virus cause severe disease due to antibody response	Dengue virus
Absolute contraindication of IUD	Unexplained uterine bleeding; Previous ectopic pregnancy history; History of PID
Under MTP Act 2021 New update, MTP is permitted up to	24 weeks
Vitamin K at birth is given to prevent	Hemorrhagic disease of newborn
All are present in Colostrum	Low sugar and fat; Thick n yellow color (Deep lemon colour); High IgA; High amino-acids and minerals
A maize eater case presents with dermatitis, diarrhoea. Mental issues present. Diagnosis is	Pellagra
All are true about Vasectomy	Recanalization possible; Use contraceptive for 3 months; Permanent method of contraception
Poor man with gum bleeding is seen in deficiency of	Vitamin C
A farmer's wife ate Bajra in meal and developed allergy. The farmer brought the Bajra gains to a doctor who noticed black grains mixed in that. How will you separate the adulterant from the food?	20% salt solution
A person from Delhi went to Assam for a trip and is now suffering from malaria for 4 days. He has now developed vomiting, altered sensorium and hallucinations. Blood smear tests show plasmodium falciparum. What drug should be given?	IV artesunate
A married couple has 1 child birth recently. They belong to which phase of family cycle?	Extension
A doctor is doing a clinical trial which there is error in clinical overreporting of disease in one group. The Selection bias removal can be done by	Randomisation
In rural areas, patient don't have insurance. But under ESI, Registered medical practitioner can give which of the following service to beneficiary?	Indirect pattern medical benefit
A couple brought their son to doctor. They were worried because their son likes to eat foods from multinational companies. What we will call this shift from consumption of traditional natural foods to western fast foods?	Acculturation
Registration of births to married couples on State and National level is done by	Civil registration system
Burden of disease in a society is best indicated by	DALY

PYQs: NEET FMGE Pattern June 2021

Recent transmission of malaria can be calculated from	Infant parasite rate (IPR)
Which is NOT a principle of Primary health care?	Family mobilisation
Which is the largest fund for Population and Reproduction related programs?	UNFPA
Which agency promote health awareness in India?	CHEB Central Health Education Bureau
Sustainable development goals (SDGs) are under which health organization?	UNDP
Which organization funds for National TB Program of India?	SIDA, WHO, World Bank
Identify the following diagram as given in the Image below (Image-based)	Component bar diagram
Disease transmitted by Vector shown in the Image is (Image of Culex)	Japanese encephalitis
An ANM receives two open vaccine vials – One MR vaccine vial and another Pentavalent vaccine vial. Which can be used for the immunization round?	Discard MR and use Pentavalent
A person with history of 30 years working in cardboard manufacturing industry, develops breathlessness and cough. X-rays show mottling in lungs. Disease most likely is	Bagassosis
Which biomedical waste color bag is disposed by incineration?	Yellow bag
Ortho-toluidine test is used for measuring which of the following compounds?	Free chlorine, combined chlorine
Man working in a place where they store ground-nuts has some poisoning. Most likely it is	Aflatoxicosis

PYQs: NEET FMGE Pattern June 2021 (Continued)

Low stationary growth is in which stage	Stage 4
Health check-up in village school is the responsibility of	PHC
Under Ayushman Bharat Scheme, how much money can a family get per year as insurance?	₹5 Lacs
A person with vision <3/60 in right eye and perception of light present in left eye presents to PHC OPD. He belongs to which category?	Social blindness
For screening of cervical cancer which is most cost effective method?	VIA - Visual inspection with 5% acetic acid
First Referral units in India	CHC, sub-district hospitals
Man returning from China on Jan 2020 was taken swab test. Look at the image given. What is the screening done on him? (Image-based)	Real time RT-PCR
A 2-year-old child - bottle fed, irritable and extreme thirsty since 2 days brought to PHC. 14 episodes of diarrhoea in last week. Child was eager to drink. what should be done	ORS
Refer to the image given below. Bull neck is seen in (Image-based)	Diphtheria
A person who had been working in dye industry, now presents to OPD with symptoms of bladder problems. Most probable diagnosis is	Transitional cell carcinoma
Health Worker female is going out in public once every 15 days for malarial surveillance. This is which type of surveillance?	Active surveillance
MC cancer of Head and Neck region in India is	Oral cavity
A pregnant female scratched by a street dog, Treatment given	Rabies vaccine plus local treatment
Most popular fertility indicator among the following is	TFR
The average number of children that is born to a women over her reproductive life span refers to	Total fertility rate
Vitamin which increases Iron absorption is	Vitamin C
A boy returned from Assam. After few days he developed fever, malaise, confusion and arthralgia. Plasmodium falciparum diagnosis was being made. Treatment regimen will include	Artemether
An intern has to study relationship between Ordering food online and Development of obesity using a Case control study. Best study groups to be selected include	Obese and non-obese persons
Open vial policy is not applicable for	Pentavalent vaccine
Demographic bonus is	Increase in productive-age population
Vaccine with faster sero-conversion time as compared to Incubation period	Measles vaccine
Total fertility rates of four cities are a – 2.1, b – 2.6, c – 2.7, d – 2.8. Which of the cities has achieved desirable TFR?	a
Orchitis is a complication of	Mumps
Identify the organism as shown in the photograph (Image-based)	HIV
In a hospital, the management wants to know that how much time each doctor is spending with patient on an average. They want to increase/decrease number of doctors, as per requirement, to improve the quality of care. The Management technique they should use is	Work sampling
For immunization survey in a community. What is first step to be done?	Census data of community
Study the graphs given below for different occupational groups. Analyse and mark-who has the highest chance of developing fever? (Image-based)	White collar jobs

PYQs: NEET FMGE Pattern December 2020

Identify logo (Image-based)	Suraksha clinic
Rabies-free state in India is	Andaman & Nicobar Islands
Training is given to an ANM worker. Now you have to check her ability to do immunization. You are the medical officer. She is having cotton, lunch box and syringe-needle after immunization of a child. Which of the following is true?	Cotton swab in Yellow bag

PYQs: NEET FMGE Pattern December 2020 (Continued)

NITI Aayog has replaced	National Planning Commission (NPC)
A screening test is used for a disease in a population. B-C represents (A = Disease onset, B = First possible detection, C = Critical point, D = Usual time of diagnosis, E = Final outcome)	Screening time
ASHA worker in rural areas is designated for how much population?	1000
Calculate Neonatal mortality rate from the data given. Total live births were 4000. Total deaths among day 0–7 babies: 40, day 7–28: 40, more than one month age: 40 and in-utero (perinatal): 40	20
A research study is being conducted on patients in rehabilitation where impact of addiction among young adults was assessed on their subsequent divorce. Among two groups of study subjects, divorced and non-divorced, history of alcohol/drug use was assessed. What kind of study was done?	Case control study
Sample registration system does not include	NONE
Mortality is taken into consideration in	Net Reproduction Rate (NRR)
White bag is used for disposal of	Sharp waste
STD Kit colour for female with vaginal discharge	Kit 2 GREEN
STD Kit colour for male urethral discharge is	Kit 1 GREY
A new drug is introduced in the market after which phase of clinical trials?	Phase 3
A health worker nurse got an accidental prick with HIV+ needle. Parameter used to test for confirmatory diagnosis is	Western blot assay
Students of the same boarding school have been eating from the same canteen. One student develop abdominal pain, jaundice and fever. Soon other students presented with similar symptoms. Hostel medical officer will investigate for which of the following parameters to establish diagnosis?	IgM for Hepatitis A
A patient presented with rash and diarrhoea since 2 months. Identify the deficiency as shown in the Image below (Image-based)	Niacin deficiency
Minimum thickness of Lead apron required is	0.5 mm
A woman who is lactating came to OPD 6 weeks after delivery, for check-up and to get advice for the contraception. Which of the following is not advised?	Combined OCP
22 years old low socioeconomic female worker present within 8 hours of sexual assault on 13th day of cycle and asked for emergency contraception. What will be your advice?	LNG 1.5 milligram
Contraindications of the device shown in image below include (Image of IUD given)	PID
A child has an IQ level of 55. He is having	Mild Mental retardation
Vector of Zika virus disease is	Aedes aegypti
Urban Heart is	Urban Health Equity Assessment and Response Tool
Relative risk for two vaccines A and B is 0.5 and 2.0 respectively, used to prevent COVID-19 among Health workers. Identify the graph(s) which represent correctly (Image-based)	A and B
Which agency collects data and publishes large scale surveys continuously regarding morbidity, family planning, vital events?	National Sample Survey
Prevalence is associated with	PPV
Best high-level disinfectant is	Glutaraldehyde
Newborn birth rate is 25 per 1000 population in a village with total population of 5000. The total number of pregnancies per year is	138
Under ESI, after certification by Medical Officer, beneficiaries get 70% wages for 3 months under	Sickness benefit
There is a group of 200 hypertensive patients. First group of 100 patients follow Medical advice whereas Second group of 100 patients follow Lifestyle advice. There is test for both the groups after 3 months. Which of the following is best test for significance to compare Blood pressure levels in both the groups?	Unpaired Students t-test
Which of the following are included in NPCDCS?	CVD, cancer, diabetes, stroke
A Doctor is teaching an Intern about Knee reflex demonstration. What type of learning is this?	Psychomotor learning
Under ICDS, Intersectoral coordination is found with	NRHM

PYQs: NEET FMGE Pattern August 2020

Minimum number of antenatal visits required are	04
A man came for checkup after his father had a cerebrovascular accident due to hypertension. What type of prevention?	Secondary
Mid-year population is taken on	01 July
Histogram is (Image-based)	Quantitative continuous data
BIS is (Image-based)	Bureau of Indian Standards
In a School scenario, School health guidelines include	Minus type desks
Researcher was conducting study in relation of depression associated with history of social media usage. One group had social media users with depression and another group had social media users without depression. Which type of study design is used?	Case control study
Delphi technique used for collective opinion of	Group
A Researcher did study on staff, nurses and JRs doing yoga (Divided into male and female). Yoga shows 25% decreased risk of infections. Which is the best test to test the significance of the result?	Chi-square test
A Researcher undertakes follow-up study for a certain time period duration, and tells that the people increasingly develop the disease with time, then it expressed as	Cumulative incidence
Not included in Principles of Primary Health Care	Appropriate facility
In graphs, Secular trend of a Disease is best represented by	Line diagram
Following is Indicative of Severity/lethality of disease	Case fatality rate
In a hospital, systematic observation and recording of doctors spending time with patients care and time without patients care is calculated for future management purposes. The type of management technique used is	Work sampling
WHO definition of blindness is	<3/60 in better eye
A child reported to a PHC with runny nose and fever since last 3 days. Rash started on face and then covered the trunk part of body. What's the most likely diagnosis?	Measles
Which of the following is NOT constrained by Time or Existing resources?	Goal
Newborn Health Mission component do not include	Target of infant mortality to double digit by 2030
Identify the image (Image-based)	CuT 380 A
If you are posted as a Medical officer in an area under NVBDCP, and you will be advised to spray Malathion for malaria prophylaxis. What could be the probable decision you will take regarding frequency of Malathion spray?	Once every 3 months
A country is suspecting a severe disease. What is the probable time within which one should report it to WHO?	24 hours
Least Iron content is present in	Milk
A nurse spilled blood on floor. Used to disinfect it	1% Sodium hypochlorite
In a train accident, there were 74 dead, 64 were severely injured, 20 moderately injured and 32 mildly injured. Colour coding in Triage Highest to Lowest category is	Red – Yellow – Green – Black
A healthy person got in contact with an infected case, and they have to separate him not more than the incubation period of disease. This is	Absolute quarantine
A male underwent Vasectomy and after 3 months his wife got pregnant. What advice should have been given to him post-vasectomy?	Usage of Barrier methods for 3 months after the procedure
First investigation for TB Diagnosis	Sputum smear examination
First investigation for TB Diagnosis among HIV positives	CBNAAT
In ORS, Sodium is given along with Glucose for	Co-transport
A factory workers had a history of frequent exposure to groundnuts. Subsequently he develops Hepatocellular carcinoma. Most likely exposure association is	Aflatoxin
A Medical officer examines workers in mines and diagnosed Silicosis. What should be his comments?	TB screening should be done at regular intervals
A person returning from malaria endemic country should continue chemoprophylaxis for how long?	4 weeks

PYQs: NEET FMGE Pattern August 2020 *(Continued)*

An infant is given Buffalo milk. It is superior because	High calories and high protein
Long-term changes/sequelae of a disease are seen in	Secular trend of disease
A 5-year-old child came into OPD with fever, rashes on the body. There were rashes on the axilla and flexor surface with various macules, papules and vesicles. Rashes and blisters are in different stages and non-uniform. Most probable diagnosis is	Chicken pox

PYQs: NEET FMGE Pattern 2005–2020

Concepts of Health and Disease	
Human living standards can be compared in different countries by	HDI
In construction of Educational Index in HDI which is not true?	Gross enrollment of secondary education is considered and not primary education
Indicator used to measure disability rates in a community	DALY
Health indicators are used for	Health status of community
In Advanced Epidemiological triad, agent is replaced by	Causative factors
Decrease in the incidence of a disease to a level where it ceases to be a public health problem is	Control
Sentinel surveillance is used for	Supplementary to routine notification
An example of Disability limitation in poliomyelitis	Resting affected limbs in neutral position
Primordial prevention for NCDs (non-communicable diseases)	Preservation of traditional diet in low NCD area
Childhood obesity prevention to a type of	Primordial prevention
Which one of the following is primary prevention?	Vaccination
Not allowing the emergence or development of the risk factor itself is which level of prevention?	Primordial
All of the statements about quarantine are true except	It is synonymous with Isolation
There has been a gradual increase in number of cases of Non communicable diseases as compared to previous years. This trend is called as	Secular trend
Carriers are not found in	Whooping cough
Epidemiology and Vaccines	
False about 'Evidence-based medicine'	Evidence is generated from weak and poor studies
Studying distribution of disease or health related characteristics in human population and identifying the characteristics with which disease seem to associated is	Descriptive epidemiology
All are true for standardized mortality ratio (SMR) except	Is a form of direct standardization
All the statements are true about standardization except	The national population is always taken as the standard population
Age specific death rates can be used for all of the following except	Comparison between different sexes in relation to injuries/accidents
If the prevalence is very low as compared to the incidence for a disease, it implies	Disease is very fatal and/or easily curable
True about incidence is	Not affected by duration
Attack rate is	Incidence of the disease
Secular trends are	Progressive changes occurring over a long period of time
All of the following help reduce bias except	Ethical considerations
Matching is done for removal of	Known confounding
False about odds ratio is	It is always >1
Analytical study with population as Unit of Study is	Ecological study

PYQs: NEET FMGE Pattern 2005–2020 (Continued)

Relative risk of a disease measures the	Strength of association between suspected cause and effect
Confounding bias is reduced by all except	Blinding
Cross-sectional study is	Vertical study
Definition of population attributable risk	Estimated amount of disease that can be reduced if risk factor is modified/eliminated
Not true about cohort study is	Less time consuming
Case control studies help in calculation of	Odds ratio
Not true in a randomized control trial (RCT)	The dropouts from the trial should be excluded from the analysis
HIV cases are reported from all over the world. This is called as	Pandemic
Subclinical infection is not seen in	Rabies
Presence of infectious arthropod agent on clothes or dressing is	Contamination
Which is indirect mode of transmission?	Vector-borne
Carrier has no role in transmission of which of the following disease	Measles
Strain used for BCG vaccine	'Danish' 1331
The following statements are true about DPT vaccine except	Presence of acellular pertussis component increases its immunogenicity
Active and passive immunity should be given together in all except	Measles
Live vaccine includes	BCG, Yellow fever, Mumps
How many fully frozen ice packs should a vaccine carrier contain?	Four
True about polio vaccination is all except	Follow up of AFP every 30 daps
Live attenuated vaccine can be given to	Children under 8 years
Storage at a cool place means a temperature of	8–15°C
Storage time for reconstituted JE vaccine is	4 hours
Storage temperature for vaccine is	+2°C to 8°C
Toxoid vaccines	Micro-organism produces exotoxins
Human immunoglobulin is given in all except	Measles
Sputum is sterilized by all except	Chlorhexidine
Disinfectant is one which	Kills bacteria only
Iron and folic acid supplementation forms	Specific protection
Hospital based study among following is	Case control study, cross over study
Screening of Disease	
All comprise inherent properties of a screening test except	Yield
Diagnostic power of the test is reflected by	Predictive value
Which one of the following relationships shown between different parameters of a performance of a test is correct?	Sensitivity is inversely proportional to specificity
If prevalence is increased, which of the following will be seen?	Increase positive predictive value
True negatives in a screening test is	d/b+d
Usefulness is	True positive/True positive + false negative
Not a part of National Screening programme	Dental caries
Epidemiological survey of 'at risk' is called	Screening
Communicable Diseases and Non-communicable Diseases	
False about chickenpox is	Crusts contain live virus
Most serious complication of measles is	Meningoencephalitis
The incubation period of measles is	10 days

PYQs: NEET FMGE Pattern 2005–2020 (Continued)

Rubella features include all except	Incubation period <10 days
Incubation period of Swine flu	1–3 days
Positive Schick test indicates	Susceptibility to diphtheria
The usual incubation period for pertussis is	7–14 days
The following statements about Meningococcal meningitis is false	Source of infection is mainly clinical cases
MC serotype of Meningococcus causing epidemics worldwide is	A
Which of the following is true about Tuberculin test?	It may be negative in dissociated tuberculosis
Which of the following is True about annual risk of TB?	It is assessed by Tuberculin conversion in previously non-vaccinated children
Sputum positive TB is	1 out of 2 sputum sample positive
In Tuberculosis combination of antimicrobials is used for	To delay the development of resistance
Incubation period of vaccine associated paralytic poliomyelitis is	4–30 days
Marker for infectivity of in Hepatitis B is	HBeAg
Most important in diagnosing Acute Hepatitis B is	IgM Anti-HBc
The best approach to prevent cholera epidemic in a community is	Safe water and sanitation
Antibiotic of choice for treating cholera in an adult is a single dose of	Doxycycline
Reservoir of enteric fever is	Man
In oral rehydration solution, least amount is of	Potassium chloride
Dengue shock syndrome is not characterized by	Decreased hemoglobin
Which of the following statement(s) is/are true about Dengue?	Increased haematocrit, decreased platelet, positive tourniquet test, vector aedes aegypti usually bite during day time, pleural effusion present
Classical Dengue fever is transmitted by	Aedes aegypti
Urban malaria is transmitted due to	Anopheles stephensi
Malaria recrudescence is	Reappearance of sexual stage parasitemia after treatment
Incubation period of Plasmodium vivax is	10–14 days
Class II exposure in animal bites includes the following	Scratches without oozing of blood
Virus is used to produce Rabies vaccine is	Fixed virus
Not true about Rabies virus is	It is a DNA virus
Yellow fever certificate of vaccination is valid for	Lifelong
JE virus life cycle in nature run between	Pigs-Mosquito
Kyasanur forest disease in transmitted by	Hard tick
Plague is transmitted by	Rat flea
R. rickettsii causes	Rocky mountain spotted fever
True about Trench fever are all except	Also called 7-day fever
False about Leishmaniasis is	Aldehyde test of Napier is a good test for diagnosis
False about Kala-azar is	Man has flagellar stage of organism
Single drug treatment recommended for Trachoma control in India is	Azithromycin
Drug of choice for Tetanus is	Metronidazole (NOW)
Which of the following statements about lepromin test is not true?	It is a diagnostic test
Elimination of leprosy is defined as prevalence.	<1 per 10000
In Multibacillary leprosy, the follow-up examination after adequate Rx should be done yearly for	5 years
Most common mode of HIV transmission in India is	Sexual transmission

PYQs: NEET FMGE Pattern 2005–2020 (Continued)

Criteria included in AIDS Surveillance definition include	Extrapulmonary, Cryptococcosis, Candidiasis, Kaposi sarcoma
Most effective to prevent HIV vertical transmission	HAART
In a HIV infected child which vaccine should not be given	OPV
Not a STD agent	Chlamydia psittaci
All of the following are Zoonoses except	HIV
Following arboviral disease has not been reported in India	Yellow fever
WHO vaccination strategy of Catch-up, keep-up and follow-up is for	Measles
Arboviral disease are	Yellow fever, Japanese encephalitis
False about Japanese Encephalitis is	Overhead tanks severe as breeding sites
Arboviral infection(s) include	CGF, West Nile fever, JE, Sandfly fever
Zoonotic disease(s) transmitted by arthropods is/are	Plague, Rabies, Leishmaniasis
Chemoprophylaxis is not required in	Typhoid
Transplacental transmission is not seen in	Hepatitis A
Staphylococcus food poisoning causes all except	Fever is common
All are Zoonotic disease except	Scabies
Cyclops is an intermediate host for	Guineaworm disease
Yaws is a disease caused by	Treponema pertenue
False about SARS is	Effective vaccine with 82% efficacy
Clinical Goal of "Cholesterol/ HDL ratio" for CHD prevention is	<3.5
Modifiable risk factor for hypertension is	Obesity
Rheumatic heart disease can be prevented by	Screening of school going children
HPV vaccination false is	2 primary doses req for immunization, recommended for age group 20–40 years
Early warning signs of Cancer that public should be aware does not include	Unexplained weight gain
For Asian populations, the Normal BMI (body mass index) range is	18.5–22.99
Overweight BMI	25–29.99
Site not used for measurement of skin fold thickness	Gluteal area
Most common cause of blindness in India is	Cataract
Blindness rate in India due to refractive errors	19.7%
Accidents happening during weekends is	Cyclic trends
Smoking is preventive for	Ulcerative colitis
Smoking is not associated with the following respiratory lesion	Sarcoidosis
National Health Programmes, Policies and Legislations in India	
Sputum examination under DTP is done when the patient present with	Hemoptysis
Drugs not included in continuation phase of category II under RNTCP	Pyrazinamide
Disadvantage of INH prophylaxis are all of the following except	Cannot prevent disease in infected person
Acute flaccid paralysis is reported in a child aged	0–15 years
IMNCI differs from IMCI in all except	Sick neonates are preferred over sick older children, treatment is aimed at more than one disease (condition) at a time
Screening tests used in antenatal mothers in RCH-II is	Hemoglobin level
RCH-II includes	Low osmolar ORS, adolescent health, exclusive breastfeeding
Most cost-effective method for cataract surgery in India is	NGO organized Screening camps followed by Surgery at base hospital

PYQs: NEET FMGE Pattern 2005–2020 (Continued)

Which of the following Health organization is not a part of Vision 2020?	UNICEF
Mobile eye care services are not done at which levels	Tertiary care
Which of the following RTI/STI Colour coded kits wrongly matched?	Kit 4 – Red
Helping for AIDS can be reached by dialing	1097
Insecticide treated bed nets (ITBN) are treated with	Deltamethrin and Cyfluthrin
Burden of malaria is best estimated by	API
Larvicide used under Urban Malaria Scheme is	Abate
Not included in National Rural Health Mission (NRHM)	Formation of family health and social welfare societies
ASHA is located at	Village level
ASHA worker duty includes which of the following	Escort all pregnant mothers to hospitals/health facility for delivery
Survey education and treatment center (SET centers) cover a population of	20–25000
Target for cure rate for multi-bacillary leprosy under program implementation plan for 12th five-year plan period	>95%
STEPS done for	Surveillance of risk factors of non-communicable diseases
Laboratory report of diseases sent as 'L-form' in IDSP is	Confirmed diagnosis
Treatment of Lepromatous leprosy is	Rifampicin + Dapsone + Clofazamine
Which of the following programmes were started before 1960?	Malaria, Filaria, Leprosy
National Health Policy is based on	Primary health care
Transplantation of Human Organs Act was passed by Government of India in	1994
Act passed before 1980	ESI, Factory, MTP, Children's Act
Act(s) passed after independence in India is/are	MTP act, ESI act, Factory act
RTI act was passed in	2005
National Health Programmes, Policies and Legislations in India	
Early Expanding stage is denoted by	Unchanged birth rate, decreased death rate
If birth rate 42 and death rate 31, then annual growth rate	1.1%
In calculating Dependency Ratio, the numerator is expressed as	Population under 15 years and 65 above
True about 'Total fertility rate' is	Completed family size
Denominator is General fertility rate is	Reproductive women 15–45 years mid-year population
Census population count is in reference to	1st March
True regarding Census of India is/are	Done by Ministry of Home Affairs, Census Commissioner is the Supreme head
All are true regarding sample registration system (SRS) except	Survey should be done every year
Scope of Modern Concept of family planning services does not include	Screening for HIV infection
Unmet is need of contraceptive for	Family planning in those who are not using any contraception
Barrier methods are all except	Lippes loop
False about Intrauterine devices (IUD)	Multiload Cu-375 is 3rd generation IUD
True about IUCD	Progestasert is 3rd generation IUCD
False about Centchroman	Useful for females with PCOD
Non-contraceptive benefits of combined oral pills is/are reduction of	Iron deficiency anaemia, ovarian cancer, PID, ovarian cysts
All are non-contraceptive advantages of oral contraceptive pills except	Hepatic adenoma

PYQs: NEET FMGE Pattern 2005–2020 (Continued)

Yuzpee and Lancee regimen must be administered within maximum	72 hours
Most cost-effective family planning method is	Vasectomy
Which of the fertility rates have mid-year population as denominator?	Crude birth rate, general fertility rate, general marital fertility rate, age-specific fertility rate, age-specific marital fertility rate
Preventive Obstetrics, Pediatrics and Geriatrics	
Average weight gain during pregnancy in poor Indian women is about	6.5 kg
For a given population, minimum no. of newborns to be examined for calculating percentage of LBW babies is	500 babies
After birth, care of eye of newborn is by	$AgNO_3$ eye drop
Maternal mortality ratio is calculated by	Maternal deaths/100000 live births
Commonest cause of neonatal mortality in India is	Low birth weight and Prematurity
Numerator in Infant mortality rate is	Less than 1 year
As compared to Cow's milk, human milk has	More iron
Deficit in weight for height in a 3-year-old child indicates	Acute malnutrition
Type of Growth Charts used by Anganwadi workers (ICDS) for growth monitoring	MRGS
Best indicator of long term nutritional status	Height for age
Lower limit of the normal range in a growth chart curve is	80% median weight
Guidelines according to baby friendly hospital initiative does not include	Mother to initiate breastfeeding within 4 hours of normal delivery
In ICDS, not included is	Prevention of iodine deficiency disorder
Known as 'The Medical Discovery of 20th century'?	ORS
Ujjwala scheme is for prevention of	Child trafficking
Gerontology is study of	Old age
Nutrition and Health	
False about Reference Indian Male	Age 18–35 years
Qualitative assessment of proteins can be done by	Net protein utilization (NPU)
Pulses are deficient in	Methionine and Cysteine
Reference protein is	Egg
Cereals and proteins are considered complementary since	Cereals are deficient in methionine and pulses are deficient in lysine
Glycemic index denotes	Food's ability to raise blood sugar
Physiologically most active form of Vitamin D is	Calcitriol
Following is supposed to prevent congenital neural tube defect	Folic acid
Decreased level of serum Vitamin B_6 is seen in	INH therapy
Iron is maximum in	Dried pumpkin seeds > Pistachio
'Twin fortified salt' contains	Iodine plus Iron
Energy yielded by one ml of alcohol in the body is	7 calories
Daily elemental calcium requirement for an elderly woman is	1200 mg
Zinc deficiency is characterized by	Sexual infantilism, poor growth, poor wound healing
What is not found in an Egg?	Vitamin C
Milk borne disease are	Brucellosis, TB, Q-fever, Leptospirosis
Phosphatase test in milk is done to know	Quality of Pasteurization
Soyabean contains protein to the tune of	43%
Parboiling refers to	Partial cooking in steam
Maximum calories per 100 gm are in	Jaggery

PYQs: NEET FMGE Pattern 2005–2020 (Continued)

Endemic ascites is caused by	Jhunjhunia seeds
Food standards in India have to achieve a minimum level of quality	PFA standards
Shakir's tape is a useful method employed in the field to measure	Mid arm circumference
Regular drinking to help prevent urinary tract infection (UTI)	Cranberry juice
Vegans are those who?	Neither eat dairy products nor eggs
Prudent diet is	Diet for dietary goal achievement
Social Science and Health	
Sociology is	Study of human relationship and behaviour
The behavioral science used extensively in PSM is	Anthropology
Maslow hierarchy is	Physiological, safety, belonging, esteem, self-actualization
Reading and writing skills of a moderate mentally retarded child	Should be basic skills
Socio-economic/housing scale developed for rural setup is	Udai Pareek Scale
Income generated within a country is known as	Gross domestic product (GDP)
Most powerful example of social cohesion is	Family
Environment and Health	
Temporary hardness of water is primarily due to the presence of	Calcium and magnesium bicarbonates
Bleaching powder required to disinfect 455 litres of water if 4, 5, 6 cup shows distinct colouration in Horrock's apparatus?	8 grams
Softening is recommended when hardness of water is more than	150 mg/litre
Minimum residual chloride level post-epidemic	0.5 mg/L
Bacteriological quality of drinking water is small community is acceptable up to	No coliform bacteria in water
Drawback of ozone as water disinfectant is	No residual action
'Cooling Power' of air is measured by	Kata thermometer
Air velocity is measured by	Anemometer
Number of air changes in a drawing room per hour should be at least	2–3
The decibels above which auditory fatigue occurs is	85 dB
A good trap should have effective seal of	2.5 cm
Heart of activated sludge process is	Aeration tank
Trickling filter is used in	Secondary treatment of sewage
Acceptable safe dose of radiation during pregnancy is	0.5 rads
Lice are not the vectors of	Q fever
Dengue fever is transmitted by	Tiger mosquito
Sandfly does not transmit	Trench fever
Organophosphate insecticide is all except	Dieldrin, Propoxur, Lindane
Vectors do not transmit infection by	Ingestion
Sanitary toilets can decrease incidence of all except	Malaria
Which of the following viral infections is transmitted by tick?	Kyasanur forest disease (KFD)
DDT is a	Organochlorine compound
Which of the following diseases is transmitted by soft tick?	Q fever
Disease(s) spread by ticks include	RMSF, Crimean Congo Fever
Range of flight of Aedes mosquito is?	Less than 100 m
Average no. of mites found on a person's Scabies is	10–15
Most efficient anti-larval measure to prevent urban malaria is	Cover overhead tanks properly

PYQs: NEET FMGE Pattern 2005–2020 (Continued)

BMW, Disaster Management, Occupational Health, Genetics and Health, Mental Health	
Which of the following biomedical wastes can be Incinerated?	Human anatomical waste
Incineration not done for	Radioactive waste, PVC, Heavy metals
Incineration is done for BMW categories	1, 2, 3, 6
Urine bags and catheters biomedical waste will be disposed in	Red bag
"3-D" means in hospital waste management is	Disinfection, Disposal, Drainage
In draughts, commonly noticed vitamin deficiency is	Vitamin A
Natural disaster causing maximum deaths	Hydrological
In disaster management all are true except	Response in pre-disaster phase
Indian constitution has declared that children less than _____ years should not be employed in factories or mines	14
Periodic examination of factory workers is a type of	Secondary prevention
Nearly 3/4th of occupational cancers is	Skin cancer
Financial contribution for ESI comes from	Employers', State and Central government
The benefits of ESI act include the following except	Nutritional allowance
Silicosis occurs with	Silica fibres
Dust particle, in an industry is a	Chemical hazard
Minimum duration to developing coal miner pneumoconiosis	>12 years
Which of the following is true about ESI act (1948)?	State government share 1/8, ESIC 7/8
Haemophilia, genetic disorder of coagulation seen in males, is transmitted as	X-linked recessive
Population genetics is related with	Hardy Weinberg law
Not a components of District Mental Health Program	Screening
Health Education and Communication	
Which one is an example of ONE-WAY communication?	Didactic method
GATHER Approach is useful for	Contraceptive counselling
Following are the Group health education approach except	Documentary
Principles of Health Education include all except	Punishment
Most persuasive and effective media system for communication is	Interpersonal communication
Counselor must have all except	Sensitivity
Health Care in India, Health Planning and Management	
Principal Unit of Administration in India is	District
Function of Health worker females	Perform 50% of delivers, Trains dais, Collectors of urine sample
Highest level of integration in health service is	District hospital
Optimum unit of preventive, curative and promotive services in health care is known as	Comprehensiveness
As per IPHS norms, the proposed number of female health worker at Sub-center	2
Which of the following conditions must be fulfilled for a PHC to become a First referral unit?	Emergency obstetric care
An example of Secondary health care level would be	Community health center (CHC)
Under NHP 2002, all of the following are correctly matched except	Achieve zero level growth of HIV/AIDS-2010
Integration of health services was first proposed by	Jungalwalla committee
Not used in health care planning	Increasing demands for resources
Time taken for any project is estimated by	Network analysis
True about "Zero base budgeting" is	Relies on data of previous budget

PYQs: NEET FMGE Pattern 2005–2020 (Continued)

Graphic plan of all the events and activities to be completed in order to reach an end objective is called	Network analysis
Cost-benefit is best analyzed by	Network analysis
Antenatal support is not delivered by	Traditional birth attendant
International Health	
WHO formation day is	7 April
UNDP works as	Main source of funds for technical assistance
Quarantine was originally introduced as a protection against	Plague
Who among the following has/have received Nobel prize?	Taum and Lederberg, Ronald Ross, Kary Mullis
Quarantine is required for	Yellow fever, Cholera, Plague
Biostatistics	
Mean and standard deviation can be worked out only if data is on	Interval/Ratio scale
The response which is graded by an observer on an agree or disagree continuum is based on	Likert scale
Nominal data example is	Types of hospitals
An old man with hypertension and BP 210/110 mm Hg is classified into severe hypertension. Scale used is	Ordinal
Histogram is used as method of group presentation for	Quantitative continuous data
Median is important for all except	Blood pressure
Values are arranged in ascending and descending order to calculate	Median
A measure of location that divides the distribution in the ratio of 3:1 is	Third quartile
If each value of a given group of observation is multiplied by 10, the standard deviation of the resulting observation is	Original standard deviation ×10
Measuring variation between two different units is done through	Coefficient of variation
Z score criteria applicable to	Normal distribution
A normal distribution curve depends on	Mean and standard deviation
If the systolic blood pressure in a population has a mean of 130 mm Hg and a median of 140 mm Hg, the distribution is said to be	Negatively skewed
In normal curve	Mean = Median
Q-test is used for detecting	Outliers
Simple random sampling is ideal for	Homogenous population
Simple random sampling	Equal chance to each for collection of certain number for a sample
In a study, variation in cholesterol was seen before and after giving a drug. The test which would give the significance is	Paired t-test
While applying Chi-square test to a contingency table of 4 rows and 4 columns, the degrees of freedom would be	9
For testing the statistical significance of the difference in heights of school children	One way analysis of variance (one way ANOVA)
Tests of significance include all except	SD
Chi-square test is used to measure the degree of	Significance of difference between two proportions
ANOVA is used	To compare means in 3 or more groups
Which of the following is not true about 'Correlation'?	Correlation can measure risk
A coefficient of correlation value of "r = +0.8" indicates	Strong direct relationship between two variables

PYQs: NEET FMGE Pattern 2005–2020 *(Continued)*

Type I sampling error is classified as	Alpha error
Statistical power of a trial is equal to	$1-\beta$
When we say that "the difference is significant", it means that	It is unlikely by chance and when $p < 0.05$
Person or spearman coefficient is used for evaluation of	Correlation
Intraocular pressure (IOP) was measured in 400 people. Mean was found to be 25 mm Hg and Standard deviation was recorded 10 mm Hg. 95% confidence interval would be?	24–26

Notes

Notes

Notes

SECTION 2

Annexures

SECTION OUTLINE

- Incubation Period of Diseases
- Important Days of Public Health Importance
- Instruments of Importance in Public Health
- Mode(s) of Transmission of Diseases
- Some Important Health Legislations Passed in India
- Some Important Health Programmes of India
- Vectors and Diseases Transmitted
- New Tuberculosis Management (NTEP/RNTCP) Guidelines (2020 Onwards)
- National Population Policy (NPP) 2000
- National Health Policy 2017 (NHP 2017)
- Sustainable Development Goals (SDGs)
- New Malaria Treatment Guidelines in India (2013 Onwards)
- New Biomedical Waste Management Guidelines 2016
- Current Public Health-related Statistics of India
- Honors in Health and Medicine
- Incentives under National Health Programs
- High Level Expert Group (HLEG) Report on Universal Health Coverage (UHC)
- Health Index of India, HII (NITI Aayog)
- Ayushman Bharat Program 2018
- Swachh Bharat Mission (SBM) 2014
- Anemia Mukt Bharat
- NEW WHO Rabies Vaccination Guidelines
- NEW WHO Guidelines for Treatment of Leprosy: Uniform MDT
- Tribal Health in India

ANNEXURE 1

Incubation Period of Diseases

Disease	Causative organism	IP
Small pox	Variola virus	7–14 days
Chicken pox	Human (alpha) herpes virus 3	14–16 days
Measles (Rubella)	RNA paramyxovirus	10–14 days
Rubella (German Measles)	RNA Togavirus	14–21 days
Mumps	RNA Myxovirus	14–21 days
Influenza	Orthomyxovirus	18–72 hours
Diphtheria	Corynebacterium diphtheriae	2–6 days
Pertussis (Whooping cough)	Bordetella pertussis	7–14 days
Meningococcal meningitis	Neisseria meningitis	3–4 days
SARS	Corona virus	3–5 days
Tuberculosis	Mycobacterium tuberculosis	Weeks–years
Poliomyelitis	Poliovirus	7–14 days
Hepatitis A	Enterovirus 72 (Picornavirus)	15–45 days
Hepatitis B	Hepadnavirus	45–180 days
Hepatitis C	Hepacivirus	30–120 days
Hepatitis D	Deltavirus	30–90 days
Hepatitis E	Calicivirus	21–45 days
Cholera	Vibrio cholerae	1–2 days
Typhoid fever	Salmonella typhi	10–14 days
Staphylococcal food poisoning	Staphylococcus aureus	1–6 hours
Ascariasis	Ascaris lumbricoides	2 months
Ancylostomiasis (Hookworm)	A. duodenale	5 weeks–9 months
Guinea worm (Dracunculiasis)	Dracunculus medinensis	1 year
Dengue	Arbovirus	3–10 days
Malaria	Plasmodium vivax	8–17 days
Malaria	Plasmodium falciparum	9–14 days
Malaria	Plasmodium malariae	18–40 days
Malaria	Plasmodium ovale	16–18 days
Lymphatic filariasis	Wuchereria bancrofti	8–16 months
Rabies	Lyssavirus type 1 (Rhabdovirus)	3–8 weeks
Yellow fever	Flavivirus fibricus	2–6 days
Japanese encephalitis	Group B arbovirus (Flavivirus)	5–15 days
KFD	Arbovirus (Flavivirus)	3–8 days
Chikungunya fever	Chikungunya virus (Arbovirus A)	4–7 days
Leptospirosis	Leptospira interrogans	4–20 days
Bubonic plague	Yersinia pestis	2–7 days

Contd...

Contd...

Disease	Causative organism	IP
Pneumonic plague	Yersinia pestis	1–3 days
Septicemic plague	Yersinia pestis	2–7 days
Scrub typhus	Rickettsia tsutsugamushi	10–12 days
Q fever	Coxiella burnetii	2–3 weeks
Taeniasis (Tapeworms)	T. solium, T. saginata	8–14 weeks
Leishmaniasis (Kala azar)	L. donovani	1–4 months
Trachoma	Chlamydia trachomatis	5–12 days
Tetanus	Clostridium tetani	6–10 days
Yaws	Treponema pertenue	3–5 weeks
HIV/ AIDS	HIV/HTLV–III/LAV	Months–10 years
Swine flu	H_1N_1 Type A Influenza	1–4 days
Crimean Congo Fever	Nairovirus	1–3 days
NIPAH Virus	Hendra/Henapi virus	14–16 days
Ebola Virus	Ebola virus	2–21 days
Anthrax	Bacillus anthracis	1–7 days
Brucellosis	Bacillus melitensis	5–60 days
Zika Virus Disease	Zika virus	3–14 days
H_7N_9 Avian Influenza	H_7N_9 Type A Influenza	1–10 days
H_5N_1 Avian Influenza	H_5N_1 Type A Influenza	2–5 days
COVID-19 disease	SARS Coronavirus -2	2–14 days (5.1 Days)
Monkey pox	Monkey pox virus	3–17 days
Mucormycosis	Mucormycetes	7–14 weeks

ANNEXURE 2: Important Days of Public Health Importance

30th January	Anti-Leprosy Day^Q
4th February	World Cancer Day
2nd Wednesday of March	No Smoking Day
8th March	International Women's Day
15th March	World Disabled Day
24th March	Anti-TB Day^Q
7th April	World Health Day^Q
25th April	World Malaria Day^Q
8th May	World Red Cross Day
31st May	No Tobacco Day^Q
5th June	World Environment Day^Q
14th June	World Blood Donor Day
26th June	International Day Against Drug Abuse and Illicit Trafficking
1st July	Doctors Day
11th July	World Population Day
28th July	World Hepatitis Day
8th September	World Literacy Day
28th September	World Rabies Day
29th September	World Heart Day^Q
1st October	International Day for Older Persons
1st October	National Voluntary Blood Donation Day
2nd Wednesday of October (Now 13 October)	World Disaster Reduction Day
9th October	World Sight Day
10th October	World Mental Health Day
16th October	World Anesthesia Day^Q
24th October	UN Day
10th November	Universal Immunization Day
14th November	World Diabetes Day^Q
17th November	National Epilepsy Day^Q
25th November	International Day for Elimination of Violence against Women
1st December	World AIDS Day^Q
3rd December	International Day of Disabled Persons
10th December	Human Rights Day
Last Week of April	World Immunization Week
1–7th May	Anti-Malaria Week^Q
1–30th June	Anti-Malaria Month^Q
1–8th August	World Breast Feeding Week^Q
25th August–8th September	Eye Donation Fortnight^Q
15–21st November	Newborn Care Week

ANNEXURE 3: Instruments of Importance in Public Health

Instrument	Use
Ice Lined Refrigerator (ILR)	Cold chain temperature maintenance
Dial Thermometer^Q	Cold chain temperature monitoring
Horrock's Apparatus^Q	Chlorine demand estimation in water
Chlorinator, Chloronome	Mixing/regulating the dose of chlorine in water
Chloroscope^Q	Measuring level of residual chlorine in drinking water
Winchester Quart bottle^Q	Assess physical and chemical quality of drinking water
Kata Thermometer^Q	Assess cooling power of air and air velocity (Latter Currently)
Anemometer	Assess air/wind velocity
Hygrometer and Sling Psychrometer^Q	Assess air humidity (moisture content of air)
Assman Psychrometer	Assess air humidity (moisture content of air)
Mercurial Barometer	Atmospheric pressure
Anaeroid Barometer	Atmospheric pressure
Wind Vane	Assess air/wind direction
Salter's scale^Q	Field Instrument for Low Birth Weight (LBW)
Infantometer^Q	Length of infants
Stadiometer	Height of adults
Shakir's Tape^Q	Mid-Arm Circumference (MAC)
Sound Level Meter	Measures intensity of sound
Band Frequency Analyzer	Characteristic of sound (pitch)
Audiometer	Hearing ability assessment

ANNEXURE 4

Mode(s) of Transmission of Diseases

Disease	Mode(s) of transmission	Remarks
Chicken Pox	Droplet infection, droplet nuclei	Face to face transmission
Measles	Droplet infection, droplet nuclei, through conjunctiva	4 days before rash to 5 days later
Rubella	Droplet infection, droplet nuclei, vertical	1 week before rash to 1 week later
Mumps	Droplet infection, direct contact	
Influenza	Droplet infection, droplet nuclei	
Diphtheria	Droplet infection, direct contact, fomite borne	95% transmission from carriers
Whooping Cough	Droplet infection, direct contact, fomite	
Meningococcal	Droplet infection	Carriers most important source of infection
TB	Droplet infection, droplet nuclei	Not Fomite borne
COVID-19	Droplet infection, contact	
Poliomyelitis[Q]	Faeco-oral, droplet infection	
Hepatitis A[Q]	Faeco-oral, parenteral, sexual	
Hepatitis B	Perinatal, parenteral, sexual, horizontal	
Hepatitis C	Perinatal, parenteral, sexual	
Hepatitis D	Perinatal, parenteral, sexual	Super-infection/co-infection to HBV
Hepatitis E[Q]	Feco-oral	
Cholera	Feco-oral, contaminated foods/drinks, direct contact	
Typhoid	Feco-oral, urine-oral	
Amoebiasis	Feco-oral	
Ascariasis[Q]	Feco-oral	
Ancylostomiasis[Q]	Direct penetration(skin), oral	Transmission may be perennial
Dracunculiasis[Q]	Consumption of water containing cyclops	Water based disease
Dengue[Q]	Aedes bite	Water breeding disease
Leptospirosis[Q]	Urine, feces, tissues of rats	Direct skin contact
Nipah virus[Q]	Consumption of bats-eaten fruits	Person-to-person in India
Ebola virus[Q]	Body fluids (blood, semen, urine, feces, vomit, tears, sweat, saliva)	–
Brucellosis[Q]	Direct contact, food borne, air borne	Aborted foetus, placenta can transmit
Zika Virus[Q]	Aedes bite, vertical, sexual	Microcephaly in fetus

ANNEXURE 5: Some Important Health Legislations Passed in India

- The Quarantine Act, 1870^Q
- The Vaccination Act, 1880
- The Epidemic Disease Act, 1897
- The Child Marriage Restraint (SARDA) Act, 1929^Q
- The Employees State Insurance (ESI) Act, 1948^Q
- The Factories Act, 1948^Q
- The Prevention of Food Adulteration (PFA) Act, 1954
- The Hindu Marriage Act, 1955
- The Immoral Traffic (Prevention) Act, 1956
- The Indian Medical Council (Prof. Conduct and Ethics) Act, 1956^Q
- The Dowry Prohibition Act, 1961
- The Maternity Benefit Act, 1961^Q
- The Insecticides Act, 1968
- The Registration of Births and Deaths Act, 1969^Q
- The Medical Termination of Pregnancy (MTP) Act, 1971^Q
- The Narcotic Drugs and Psychotropic Substances Act, 1985
- The Consumer Protection Act (COPRA), 1986^Q
- The Environmental Protection Act (EPA), 1986
- The Mental Health Act, 1987^Q (Repealed now)
- The Infant Milk Substitutes, Feeding Bottles and Infant Food (Regulation of production, supply and distribution) Act, 1992
- The Protection of Human Rights Act, 1993
- The Pre-conception and Pre-natal Diagnostic Techniques (Prohibition of Sex Selection) [PNDT] Act, 1994^Q
- The Transplantation of Human Organs Act, 1994^Q
- The Persons with Disabilities (Equal opportunities, Protection of Rights, Full Participation) Act, 1995
- The Biomedical Waste (Management and Handling) Rules, 1998^Q
- The Tobacco Control Act, 2003
- The Information Technology Act, 2000^Q
- The Disaster Management Act, 2005
- The National Rural Employment Guarantee Act (NREGA), 2005^Q
- The Protection of Women from Domestic Violence Act, 2005
- The Right to Information (RTI) Act, 2005^Q
- Prohibition of Child Marriage Act, 2006
- The Food Standards and Safety Act, 2006^Q
- The Protection of Children from Sexual Offences (POCSO) Act, 2012^Q
- The Sexual Harassment of Women at Work Place (Prevention, Prohibition and Redressal) Act, 2013
- The Juvenile Justice (Care and Protection of Children) Act, 2015
- The Rights of Persons with Disabilities Bill 2016
- The Mental Health Care Act, 2017^Q
- The HIV/AIDS (Prevention & Control) Act, 2017^Q
- The Mental Health Care (Rights of Persons with Mental Illness) Rules, 2018

Annexure 6: Some Important Health Programmes of India

- National Family Planning Programme: 1951
- National Malaria Control Programme (NMCP): 1953
- Lymphatic Filariasis Control Programme: 1955
- National Leprosy Control Programme: 1955
- National Malaria Eradication Programme (NMEP): 1958
- National Tuberculosis Programme (NTP): 1962
- National Goitre Control Programme (NGCP): 1962
- National Trachoma Control Programme: 1963
- Urban Malaria Scheme (UMS): 1971
- Integrated Child Development Services (ICDS) Scheme: 1975
- National Cancer Control Programme: 1975–76
- National Programme for Control of Blindness (NPCB): 1976
- Kala Azar Control Programme: 1977
- Modified Plan of Operation (MPO): 1977
- National Mental Health Programme: 1982
- National Leprosy Eradication Programme (NLEP): 1983
- National Guineaworm Eradication Programme: 1983–84
- National AIDS Control Programme (NACP): 1987
- Baby Friendly Hospital Initiative (BFHI): 1991
- Revised National Tuberculosis Control Programme (RNTCP): 1992
- Child Survival and Safe Motherhood (CSSM) Programme: 1992
- National AIDS Control Programme I (NACP I): 1992–97
- National Iodine Deficiency Disorders Control Programme (NIDDCP): 1992
- Yaws Eradication Programme: 1996–97
- Revised Lymphatic Filariasis Control Programme: 1996–97
- Enhanced Malaria Control Project (EMCP): 1997
- Reproductive and Child Health Programme I: 1997
- National Anti Malaria Programme (NAMP): 1999
- National Oral Health Project: 1999
- National Vector Borne Disease Control Programme (NVBDCP): 2003–04
- Integrated Disease Surveillance Project (IDSP): 2004–09
- Reproductive and Child Health Programme II: 2004–09
- National Rural Health Mission (NRHM): 2005–12
- Pradhan Mantri Swasthya Suraksha Yojana (PMSSY), 2006
- National Tobacco Control Programme (NTCP): 2007–08
- National Program for Prevention and Control of Cancer, Diabetes, Cardiovascular Diseases and Stroke (NPCDCS): 2008
- National Program for Health Care of the Elderly (NPHCE): 2011
- National Health Mission (NHM): 2013
- National AIDS Control Program IV (NACP IV): 2012–17
- Pradhan Mantri Jan Dhan Yojana (PMJDY), 2014
- National Programme for Prevention & Control of Viral Hepatitis, 2014
- Beti Bachao Beti Padhao Andolan, 2014
- Pradhan Mantri Suraksha Bima Yojana: 2015
- Pradhan Mantri Jeevan Jyoti Bima Yojana: 2015
- Pradhan Mantri National Dialysis Programme: 2016
- National Nutrition Mission, 2018
- Ayushman Bharat & National Health Protection Mission, 2018
- Emergency Response Support System, 2019
- The NMC Act, 2019

ANNEXURE 7

Vectors and Diseases Transmitted

Vector	Disease(s) transmitted
Housefly (Musca domestica)	Diarrhoeal and dysentrical diseases, Poliomyelitis, Yaws, Anthrax, Trachoma
Sandfly (Phlebotomus argentipes)	Kala azar (Visceral Leishmaniasis), Oriental sore (Cutaneous Leishmaniasis), Sandfly fever, Oroya fever
Tse-Tse fly (Glossina palpalis)	Sleeping sickness of Africa (African Trypanosomiasis)
Reduviid bug (Triatominae)	Chagas Disease (Sleeping sickness of America- American Trypanosomiasis)
Black fly (Simulium)	Onchocerciasis (River Blindness)
Soft tick	Relapsing fever, Q fever, KFD (outside India)
Hard tick	Tularemia, Babesiosis, KFD (India), Tick paralysis, Tick encephalitis, Tick hemorrhagic fever, Indian Tick Typhus, RMSF
Louse	Epidemic typhus, Trench fever, Relapsing fever
Mite	Scrub typhus, Rickettsial pox
Flea	Plague, Murine typhus
Anopheles mosquito	Malaria, Filaria (outside India)
Culex mosquito	Bancroftian Filariasis, Japanese Encephalitis, West Nile fever, Viral arthritis
Aedes mosquito	Yellow fever, Dengue, DHF, Chikungunya, Rift Valley fever, Filariasis (Outside India), Zika
Mansonoides mosquito	Malayan (Brugian) filariasis, Chikungunya

ANNEXURE 8: New Tuberculosis Management (NTEP/RNTCP) Guidelines (2020 Onwards)

Revised Technical and Operational Guidelines[Q]

- Revision in diagnostic algorithm with use of CXR in screening and early use of CBNAAT
- Systematic Active TB case finding strategy
- Transition from Intermittent (Thrice weekly) to daily regimen
- Treatment of all forms of drug resistant TB (DR-TB)
- Use of new drug Bedaquiline along with DST guided treatment
- Use of ICT enabled adherence support for patient centric care
- Single window delivery approach for HIV-TB coinfection care
- Improved TB surveillance strategy
- Effective strategies to reach TB patients.

Diagnosis of TB under RNTCP[Q]

- Microscopy[Q]:
  - ZN staining-based Conventional Microscopy (First main test performed)
  - Light Emitting Diode-based Fluorescence Microscopy (LED FM)
- Culture (Diagnosis)[Q]:
  - Solid Lowenstein Jensen (LJ) Medium
  - Automated Liquid Culture Systems (BACTEC MGIT 960, Bactialert, VersaTrek)
- Culture (Drug Sensitivity Testing):
  - Modified PST for MGIT 960 system (for both 1st and 2nd line drugs)
  - Proportional Sensitivity Testing (1%) Economic variant using LJ Medium (as back-up)
- Rapid Molecular Diagnostic Testing:
  - Line Probe Assay (MTB complex and INH/RIF resistance)
  - Cartridge based nucleic acid amplification test (CBNAAT–Xpert/MTB/Rif testing using GeneXpert system)
- Other Diagnostic Tests:
  - Chest X-ray (Mainly for screening. If used for diagnosis its known as Clinically diagnosed TB)
  - Standardized Tuberculin Skin Test (Complimentary test in children)
  - Interferon Gamma Release Assay (IGRA–Not recommended for adults in India)
  - Serological tests (Banned in India).

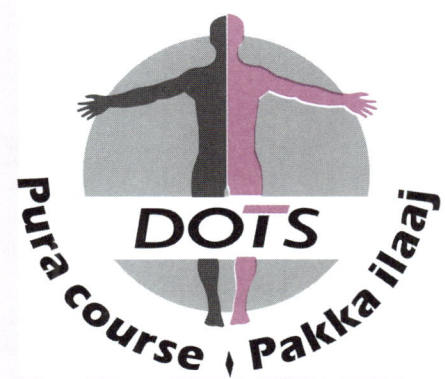

DOTS RNTCP

Two Sputum Smears Collection

- Two-day collection (Day 1: Spot sample and Day 2: Morning sample): 2 mL mucopurulent each
- One day collection (Day 1: Both Spot samples): 2 mL mucopurulent each.

Diagnostic Algorithm for Pulmonary TB^Q

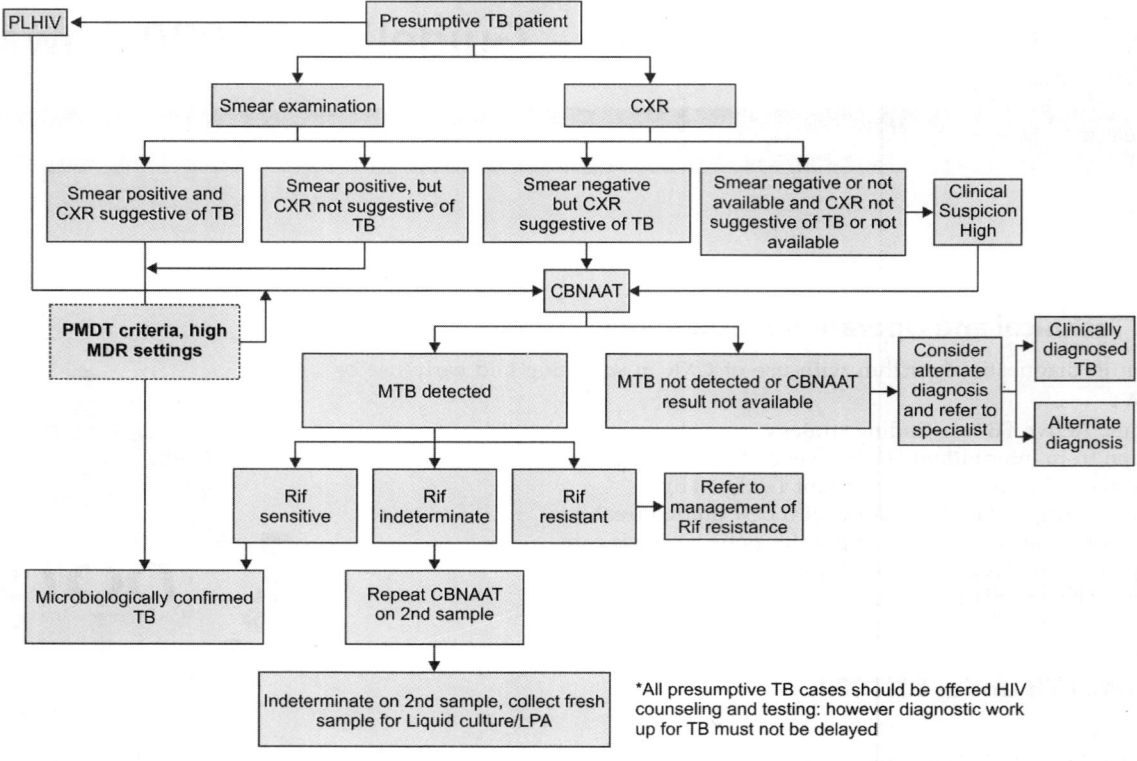

Diagnostic Algorithm for Extra-pulmonary TB (EPTB)

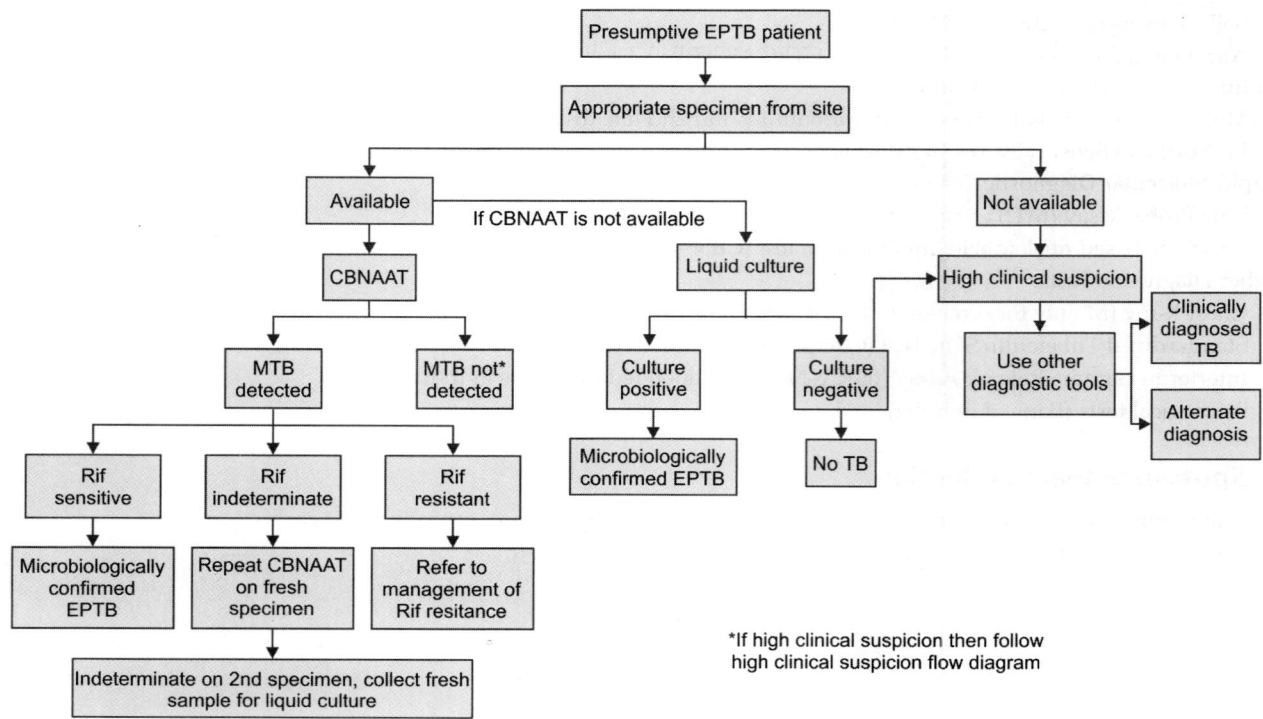

Diagnostic Algorithm for Paediatric Pulmonary TB

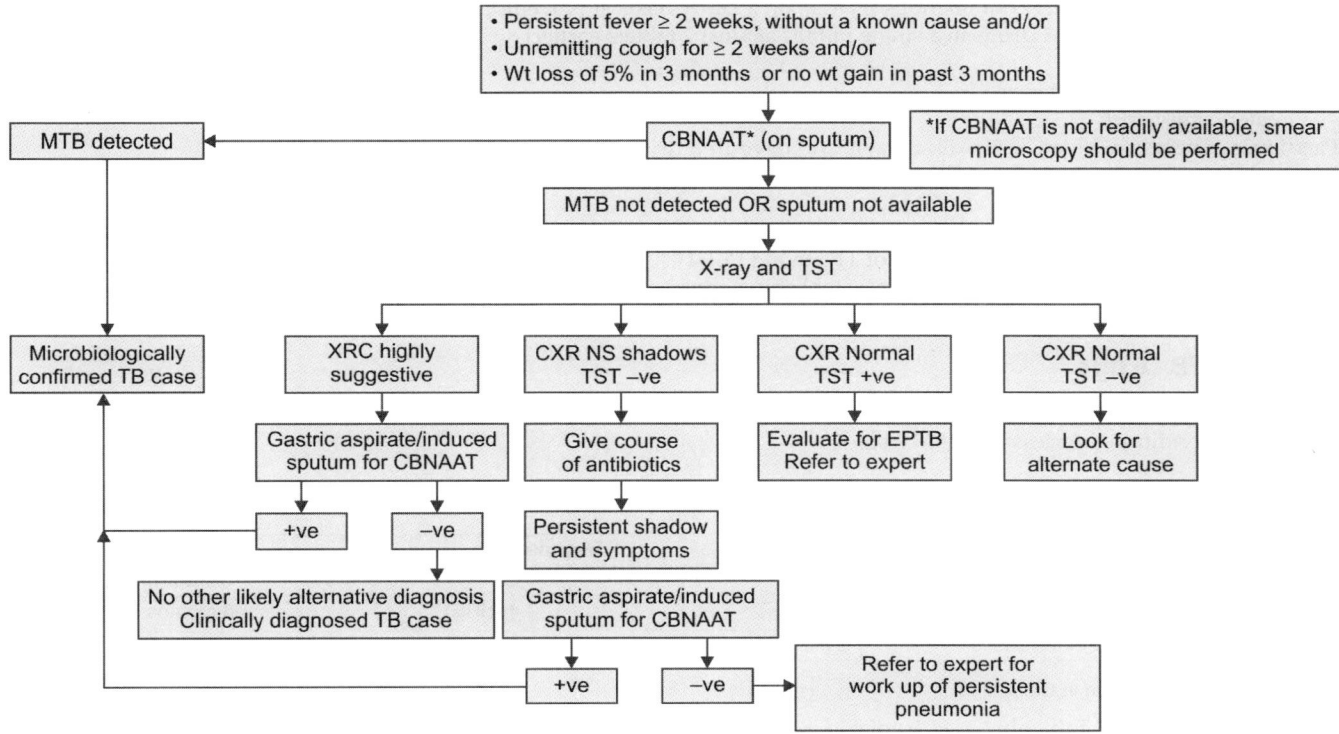

Diagnosis of Drug Resistant TB (DR-TB)
- Phenotypic drug susceptibility testing:
  - Solid culture media
  - Liquid culture media
- Genotypic testing of resistance:
  - Line probe assay (LPA): Detect resistance to both Rifampicin and Isoniazid
  - CBNAAT (Xpert/MTB/Rif test): Detect resistance to Rifampicin only.

Intensified TB Case Finding
- Provider initiated activity
- Aim: Early detection of TB cases (by Active case finding) and prompt treatment
- Targeted population:
  - Those seeking health care with/without signs/or symptoms of TB
  - Focus on high risk populations
- Screening strategies:
  - Community screening: Those with recent contact (Mobile/fixed facility based screening); Door-to-door screening
  - Institutional screening: Active screening of vulnerable individuals attending hospitals (Health care facilities); Active screening of vulnerable individuals (Shelters/Old age homes/Refugee camps/Correctional facilities/Workplaces)

Active Case Finding in TB in India[Q]
- Door-to-door screening of TB in India: 15-day campaign across the country for early detection, diagnosis and treatment of tuberculosis to eliminate the disease (December 2017)
- Active surveillance: Health department workers, ASHAs, TB supervisors will make door-to-door visits to find TB patients and give them free medical treatment till they are cured.

New Strategies in Treatment of TB (RNTCP)[Q]
- Daily regimen for treatment of TB (to gradually replace Thrice weekly Intermittent regimen)
- Use of Bedaquiline for treatment of drug resistant TB with drug susceptibility testing (DST) guided treatment
- Information communication technology (ICT)-based adherence support
- Post-treatment follow-up.

Treatment Protocol: NEW Guidelines[Q]

- Patients are given fixed drug combinations (FDCs), on a **Daily basis** (1 November 2017 onwards PAN-India)[Q]
  - Reduced pill burden: 3–4 drugs in a single pill (as against 7 tablets earlier)
  - Lesser relapses
  - Reduction in drug-resistance
  - Greater compliance
- Paediatric patients are given easily-dissolvable and flavoured drugs (instead of bitter tablets earlier)
- Weight bands: Patients get appropriate dosages as per body weight
- TB-HIV Coinfection:
  - 'Intensified TB case finding and appropriate treatment' through single window delivery of services from all ART centres
  - INH preventive therapy for prevention of TB among PLHIV
  - Implementation of Pharmacovigilance by establishing adverse drug reaction monitoring centres at ART centres
- Patients not registered under DOTS are provided Intermittent (alternate day OR **Thrice weekly**) regimen.

Newer Anti-TB Drugs

- Bedaquiline Conditional Access Program trials[Q]
- Delamanid Conditional Access Program trials

Daily Treatment Regimens[Q] (OLD Guideline)

Category	Type of patient	Regimens		Duration
		IP	CP	
Cat I	New cases	2 (HRZE)	4 (HRE)	6 months
Cat II	Previously treated cases	2 (HRZES) + 1 (HRZE)	5 (HRE)	8 months

(Category III has been merged in Category I)

- *Letters*: R-Rifampicin, E-Ethambutol, H-Isoniazid, S-Streptomycin, Z-Pyrizanamide
- *Numbers*: The numbers before letters refer to months of treatment (2 imply two months of treatment).
- *Seriously ill extrapulmonary TB*: Meningitis, disseminated TB, tuberculous pericarditis, peritonitis, bilateral or extensive pleurisy, spinal disease with neurological complaints, SS –ve TB with extensive parenchymal involvement, and intestinal and genitourinary TB.

NEW RNTCP Guidelines (December 2018) Onwards

- All Previously treated TB patients (Category II) shall now be treated with Standard First Line Anti TB Regimen "2HRZE/4HRE" as prescribed for New TB patients (Category I)
- Such patients will continue to be designated as "Previously treated TB patients"
- Follow-up schedule to be same as New TB patients
- DST to be at least conducted for Rifampicin for all Previously treated patients
- Do not wait for DST results for initiation of treatment
- Honorarium of Previously treated TB patients to be now same as New TB patients (₹ 1000/- instead of ₹ 1500/-)

NEW Regimens for Treatment of Drug Resistant TB (RNTCP 2017–18)

Regimens	Intensive phase	Continuation phase
H Mono/Poly DR-TB Regimen	3-6 (LKREZ)	6 (LREZ)
Shorter MDR-TB Regimen	4-6 (MhKEtCzZHE)	5 (MhCzZE)
MDR/RR-TB Regimen	6-9 (LKEtCsZE)	18 (LEtCsE)
MDR TB + FQ/SLI Resistance (With new drugs)		
MDR TB + FQ Resistance (With new drugs)	6-9 (KEtCsZLzCz) + 6 (Bq)	18 (LEtCsLz)
MDR TB + SLI Resistance (With new drugs)	6-9 (LCmEtCsZLzCz) + 6 (Bq)	18 (LEtCsLz)
MDR TB + FQ/SLI Resistance (Without new drugs)		
MDR TB + FQ Resistance (Without new drugs)	6-9 (MhKEtCsZLzCz)	18 (MhEtCsLzCz)
MDR TB + SLI Resistance (Without new drugs)	6-9 (LCmEtCsZLzCz)	18 (LEtCsLz)
XDR TB Regimen (With new drugs)	6-12 (CmEtCsLzLzCzE) + 6 (Bq)	18 (EtCsLzCzE)
XDR TB Regimen (Without new drugs)	6-12 (MhCmEtCsLzCzE)	18 (MhEtCsLzCzE)
Mixed pattern DR-TB (With new drugs)*	6-12 (CmEtCsZLzCzE) + 6 (Bq)	18 (EtCsLzCzE)

Contd...

Contd...

Regimens	Intensive phase	Continuation phase
Mixed pattern DR-TB (Without new drugs)		
H Mono/Poly + FQ/SLI/Lz Resistance (Without new drugs)	3-6 (REZCmEtLz)	6 (REZEtLz)
MDR/RR-TB + FQ/SLI + Lz/Other Resistance (Without new drugs)*	6-12 (MCmEtCsLzCzE)	18 (MEtCsLzCzE)

(© Table Dr Vivek Jain 2019-20)
(*1. Add Cm in IP if K-resistant; 2. MDR/RR + FQ resistance, XDR-TB, Mixed pattern resistance Mh to be added upfront, if new drug is not considered; 3. If found resistant, Replace Lz with suitable drug. Reclassify patient as Mixed pattern DR-TB)
(Drugs: Hh: High dose Isoniazid; E: Ethambutol; Z: Pyrazinamide; K: Kanamycin; Cm: Capreomycin; A: Amikacin; L: Levofloxacin; M: Moxifloxacin; Mh: High dose Moxifloxacin; Et: Ethionamide; Cs: Cycloserine; Cz: Clofazimine; Lz: Linezolid; Bq: Bedaquiline)

Weight Bands under RNTCP (with Drug Dosage)[Q]

- Adults cases under RNTCP: FOUR weight bands[Q]

Weight band (kg)	No of tablets (FDCs)		Inj. Streptomycin (gm)
	IP HRZE (75/150/400/275 mg)	CP HRE (75/150/275 mg)	
25–39 kg	2	2	0.5
40–54 kg	3	3	0.75
55–69 kg	4	4	1
≥70 kg	5	5	1

(IP: Intensive phase; CP: Continuation phase)

- Pediatrics cases under RNTCP: SIX weight bands[Q]

Weight band (kg)	No of tablets (Dispersible FDCs)			Inj. Streptomycin (mg)
	IP HRZ (50/75/150 mg)	IP E (100 mg)	CP HRE (50/75/100 mg)	
4–7 kg	1	1	1	100
8–11 kg	2	2	2	150
12–15 kg	3	3	3	200
16–24 kg	4	4	4	300
25–29 kg	3 + 1A*	3	3 + 1A*	400
30–39 kg	2 + 2A*	2	2 + 1A*	500

(IP: Intensive phase; CP: Continuation phase; A: Adult FDC–HRZE 75/150/400/275, HRE 75/150/275)

DOTS-99: ICT-based Adherence Support[Q]

- Low-cost approach for monitoring and improving TB medication adherence
- Each anti-TB blister pack is wrapped in a custom envelope, which includes hidden phone numbers that are visible only when doses are dispensed.
- After taking daily medication, patients make a free call to the hidden phone number, yielding high confidence that the dose was "in-hand" and has been taken.

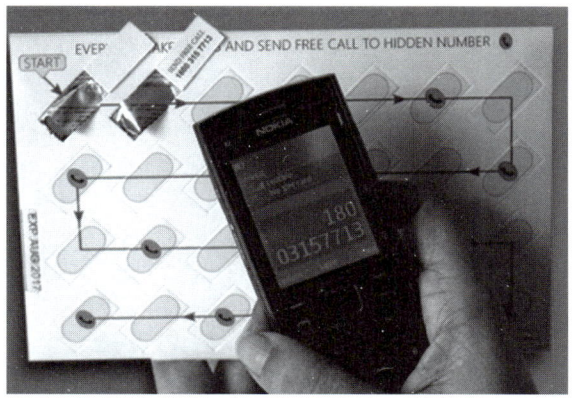

NIKSHAY: ICT-based Surveillance Support[Q]
- ICT enabled state-of-art surveillance system (Online monitoring software) to get notification of TB cases at diagnosis from both public and private sector including drug resistant TB patients
- Continuous monitoring and treatment adherence for all TB patients registered
- Enable tracking of all notified TB patients across TB care cycle, geographies, transfers and referrals.

New Definitions under RNTCP[Q]
- New case: Never had treatment for TB OR took anti-TB drugs for <1 month
- Previously treated patients: Received 1 month or more of anti-TB drugs in the past
- Recurrent TB case: Patient previously declared as successfully treated (cured/treatment completed) and is subsequently found to be microbiologically confirmed TB case
- Treatment after failure: Patients who have previously been treated for TB and whose treatment failed at the end of their most recent course of treatment
- Treatment after loss to follow-up: Patient previously treated for TB for 1 month or more and was declared lost to follow-up in their most recent course of treatment and subsequently found microbiologically confirmed TB case
- Other previously treated patients: Patients who have previously been treated for TB but whose outcome after their most recent course of treatment is unknown or undocumented
- Transferred in: Patient who is received for treatment in a Tuberculosis Unit, after registered for treatment in another TB unit is considered as a case of transferred in.

Other Must Know Facts of RNTCP[Q]
- Engagement of NGOs/Private Practitioners through Partnership Options
- National Strategic Plan (NSP) 2017–25 for elimination of TB: To rapidly decline TB incidence and mortality in India by 2025, five years ahead of the global End TB targets and Sustainable Development Goals to attain the vision of a TB-free India
- MDR/XDR treatment is started at the DOTS-plus sites where the patient is admitted for treatment for 2/3 weeks; After adjusting the medication the patient is sent back to continue his/her treatment at his respective chest clinic/DOTS provider
- Non-DOTS is available at all DOTS clinics in India, but preference is given to DOTS
- For pulmonary TB, CBNAAT is performed if Smear is negative but X-ray is suggestive of TB/If clinical suspicion is high/PLHIV/Paediatric group
- Extension of Intensive phase is NOT done under RNTCP now: Send the sample for CBNAAT/LPA for diagnosis of INH/RIF resistance[Q]
- Identified Tuberculosis patients across the country will get ₹ 500/- every month from the Centre as social support (December 2017)
- Incentives for DOTS-providers:[Q]
    - Providing treatment to Cat-I patients: ₹ 1000/-
    - Providing treatment to Cat-II patients: ₹ 1000/- (New proposed)
    - Providing treatment to Cat-IV/V patients: ₹ 5000/-

ANNEXURE 9

National Population Policy (NPP) 2000

Objectives of National Population Policy 2000	– *Immediate objectives:* To meet unmet need of contraception; to strengthen health infrastructure; to strengthen health personnel and to promote integrated service delivery for basic RCH care
	– *Mid-term objective:* 'To bring the total fertility rate (TFR) to Replacement Level; i.e. TFR to 2.1'
	– *Long-term objective:* To stabilize population by 2045
National Socio-demographic Goals of NPP 2000 (achieve by 2010)	– Address the unmet needs for basic reproductive and child health services, supplies and infrastructure
	– Make school education up to age 14 free and compulsory, and reduce drop outs at primary and secondary school levels to below 20 percent for both boys and girls
	– Reduce infant mortality rate to below 30 per 1000 live births
	– Reduce maternal mortality ratio to below 100 per 100,000 live births
	– Achieve universal (100%) immunization of children against all vaccine preventable diseases
	– Promote delayed marriage for girls, not earlier than age 18 and preferably after 20 years of age
	– Achieve 80 percent institutional deliveries and 100 percent deliveries by trained persons
	– Achieve universal access to information/counseling, and services for fertility regulation and contraception with a wide basket of choices
	– Achieve 100 percent registration of births, deaths, marriage and pregnancy
	– Contain the spread of Acquired Immunodeficiency Syndrome (AIDS), and promote greater integration between the management of reproductive tract infections (RTI) and sexually transmitted infections (STI) and the National AIDS Control Organisation
	– Prevent and control communicable diseases
	– Integrate Indian Systems of Medicine (ISM) in the provision of reproductive and child health services, and in reaching out to households
	– Promote vigorously the small family norm to achieve replacement levels of TFR
	– Bring about convergence in implementation of related social sector programs so that family welfare becomes a people centred programme

ANNEXURE 10: National Health Policy 2017 (NHP 2017)

Targets by 2017
- Eliminate Kala-Azar
- Eliminate Lymphatic Filariasis

Targets by 2018
- Eliminate Leprosy

Targets by 2019
- IMR 28

Targets by 2020
- MMR 100
- Achieve 90:90:90 for HIV/AIDS
- Reduction in prevalence of tobacco use by 15% (and 30% by 2025)
- Access to safe water and sanitation to all (Swachh Bharat Mission)
- Reduction of occupational injury by 50% in agricultural workers
- Increase State sector health spending to > 8% of their budget by 2020

Targets by 2022
- Establish DALY as a measure of burden/trend of disease

Targets by 2025
- Increase Life Expectancy at birth to 70
- TFR 2.1
- U5MR 23
- NNMR 16
- SBR "Single digit"
- TB cure rate >85%, TB Elimination
- Prevalence of blindness 0.25 per 1000 (Reduce burden by 1/3rd)
- Reduce premature mortality from CVDs, cancer, diabetes or chronic respiratory diseases by 25%
- Increase utilization of public health facilities by 50%
- Antenatal care coverage >90%, Skilled attendance at birth >90%
- 90% of the newborn are fully immunized by one year of age
- 90% Met need of family planning
- 80% of HTN and DM maintain "Controlled disease status"
- 40% reduction in prevalence of stunting of under-five children
- Health expenditure by Government from 1.15% to 2.5% of GDP

ANNEXURE 11

Sustainable Development Goals (SDGs)

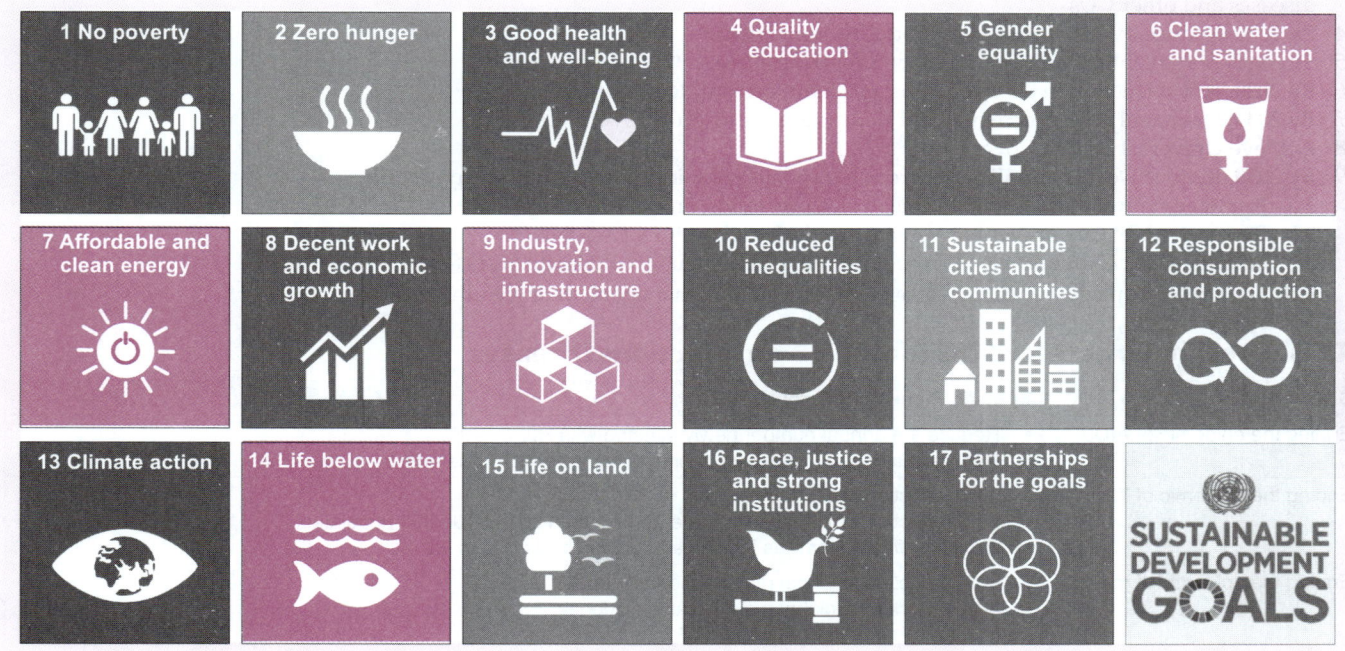

SDGs

Sustainable Development Goals (SDGs)

- 'Transforming our world: 2030 Agenda for Sustainable Development'^Q - An intergovernmental set of 17 aspiration Goals with 169 targets
- Post 2015 Development Agenda (successor to MDGs^Q)
- Directly Health related goals^Q: One (Goal 3)
- Directly Health disparities addressing goals: Six (Goals 1-6)
    1. End Poverty in all its forms everywhere
    2. End Hunger, achieve food security and improved nutrition and promote sustainable agriculture
    3. Ensure Healthy lives and promote well-being for all at all ages
    4. Ensure inclusive and equitable quality Education and promote lifelong learning opportunities for all
    5. Achieve Gender equality and empower all women and girls
    6. Ensure availability and sustainable management of Water and Sanitation for all
    7. Ensure access to affordable, reliable, sustainable and modern Energy for all
    8. Sustained, inclusive & and sustainable Economic growth, full and productive employment and decent work for all
    9. Build resilient infrastructure, promote inclusive and sustainable Industrialization and foster innovation
    10. Reduce Inequality within and among countries
    11. Make cities and Human Settlements inclusive, safe, resilient and sustainable
    12. Ensure sustainable Consumption and Production patterns
    13. Take urgent action to combat Climate change and its impacts
    14. Conserve and sustainably use the Oceans, Seas and Marine resources for sustainable development
    15. Protect, restore and promote sustainable use of Terrestrial ecosystems, sustainably manage forests, combat desertification, and halt and reverse land degradation and halt biodiversity loss

16. Promote peaceful and inclusive Societies for sustainable development, provide access to justice for all and build effective, accountable and inclusive institutions at all levels
17. Strengthen the means of implementation and revitalize the Global partnership for sustainable development

GOAL 3: Ensure Healthy Lives and Promote Well-being for All at All Ages

TARGETS^Q

3.1 By 2030, Global MMR <70 per 100,000 live births^Q
3.2 By 2030, End Preventable deaths of Newborns and Under-five children
   – NNMR 12 per 1,000 live births^Q
   – U5MR 25 per 1,000 live births^Q
3.3 By 2030, End Epidemics of AIDS, Tuberculosis, Malaria and Neglected tropical diseases and Combat Hepatitis, Water-borne diseases and other CDs
3.4 By 2030, Reduce by 33% Premature mortality from NCDs^Q
3.5 Strengthen Prevention and Treatment of Substance abuse
3.6 By 2020, 50% reduction in Global deaths and injuries from Road traffic accidents^Q
3.7 By 2030, Universal access to Sexual and Reproductive health-care services
3.8 Achieve Universal Health Coverage
3.9 By 2030, Reduce Deaths and illnesses from hazardous chemicals, air/water/soil pollution
   3.a Implementation of the WHO Framework Convention on Tobacco Control
   3.b Research and Development of Vaccines and Medicines for CDs & NCDs
   3.c Financing, recruitment, development, training and retention of Health workforce
   3.d Strengthen capacity for early warning, risk reduction, management of Health risks

SDGs–Specific Targets for SDG Target 3.3 on Infectious Diseases

SDG target	Specific Plan–Main Targets 2030
Ending the epidemic of AIDS	• Reduce the annual number newly infected with HIV by 90% • Reduce the annual number of people dying from AIDS-related causes by 80%
Ending the epidemic of TB	• 90% reduction in TB deaths • 80% reduction in TB incidence rate (to less than 20 per 100,000 population) • Zero TB-affected families facing catastrophic costs due to TB
Ending the epidemic of malaria	• 90% reduction in global malaria mortality rate • 90% reduction in global malaria case incidence • Malaria eliminated from at least 35 countries • Re-establishment of malaria prevented in all countries identified as malaria-free
Ending the epidemic of NTDs	• 90% reduction in the number of people requiring interventions against NTDs
Combat hepatitis	• 95% decline in new cases of chronic HBV infection between 2010-2030 • 80% reduction in new cases of chronic HCV infection between 2010-2030 • 65% reduction in HBV- and HCV-related deaths
Combat waterborne diseases	• No one practices open defecation (by 2025) • Everyone uses a basic drinking-water supply, hand-washing facilities at home • Everyone uses adequate sanitation when at home (by 2040) • All drinking-water supply, sanitation and hygiene services are delivered in progressively affordable, accountable and financially and environmentally sustainable manner

ANNEXURE 12: New Malaria Treatment Guidelines in India (2013 Onwards)

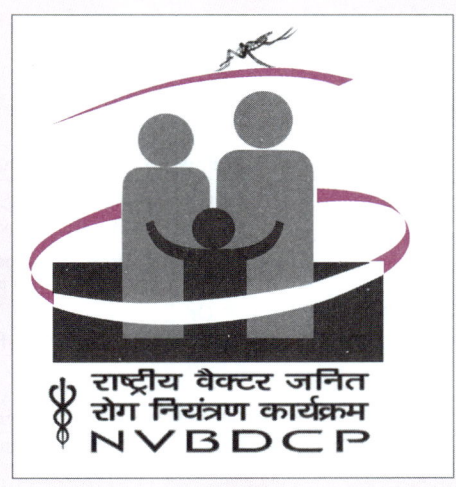

NVBDCP

I. VIVAX MALARIA
- Chloroquine × 3 days (10 mg per kg Day 1; 10 mg per kg Day 2; 5 mg per kg Day 3) +
- Primaquine × 14 days (0.25 mg per kg)

II. FALCIPARUM MALARIA
- *In Other States (Other than North-Eastern states)*:
  - Artemisinin-Based Combination therapy (ACT-SP)
    - Artesunate × 3 days (4 mg per kg) +
    - Sulfadoxine × Day 1 (25 mg per kg) +
    - Pyrimethamine × Day 1 (1.25 mg per kg)
  - Primaquine × Day 2 (0.75 mg per kg)
- *In North-Eastern states*:
  - Artemether based Combination therapy (ACT-AL)
    - Artemether × 3 days (80 mg BD) +
    - Lumefantrine × 3 days (480 mg BD)
  - Primaquine × Day 2 (0.75 mg per kg)

PLEASE NOTE:
- *Colour coding of age-wise blister packs for P. falciparum treatment*:

Age	Colour code for blister pack
0–1 year	Pink
1–4 years	Yellow
5–8 years	Green
9–14 years	Red
15+ years	White

- *Treatment of Uncomplicated P. falciparum in Pregnancy*:
  - 1st trimester: Quinine × 7 days (10 mg per kg TDS)
  - 2nd/3rd trimester: ACT-AL in NE states/ACT-SP in Other states

III. MIXED INFECTIONS (P. VIVAX + P. FALCIPARUM)
- *In Other States (Other than North-Eastern states):*
  - ACT-SP × 3 days
  - Primaquine × 14 days (0.75 mg per kg)
- *In North-Eastern states:*
  - ACT-AL × 3 days
  - Primaquine × 14 days (0.75 mg per kg)

IV. PLASMODIUM MALARIAE
- Treat as P. falciparum

V. PLASMODIUM OVALE
- Treat as P. vivax

VI. MIXED INFECTIONS
- Treat as P. falciparum
- Primaquine × 14 days

VII. SEVERE & COMPLICATED MALARIA

Treatment of Severe and Complicated Malaria

Initial parenteral treatment (Any 1 of 4 options)	Follow-up treatment (shift to Oral t/t)
- Quinine 20 mg/kg Loading dose + - Quinine 10 mg/kg Maintenance dose	- Quinine 10 mg/kg TDS + - Doxycycline/ Clindamycin* × 7 days total
- Artesunate - Artemether - Arteether	**Full oral course area-specific ACT** - ACT-SP (× 3 days) + PQ (Day 2) [NE India] Or - ACT-LM (× 3 days) + PQ (Day 2) [Other India]

VIII. CHEMOPROPHYLAXIS
- Short-term (≤ 6 weeks): Doxycycline OD (Start 1 day before travel; Continue for 4 weeks after return)
- Long-term (> 6 weeks): Mefloquine weekly (Start 2 weeks before travel; Continue for 4 weeks after entering endemic area)

ANNEXURE 13

New Biomedical Waste Management Guidelines 2016[Q]

- Ministry: Ministry of Environment and Forests
- Legislation: Sections 6, 8 and 25 of Environment (Protection) Act, 1986
- These rules shall not apply to Radioactive wastes, Hazardous chemicals, Municipal solid wastes, Lead acid batteries, Hazardous wastes, e-Waste, Hazardous micro-organisms, Genetically engineered microorganisms

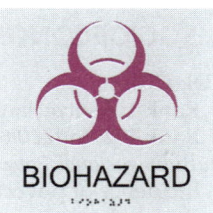

BMW

Category	Types of Waste [Older Cat no.]	Bag/Container	Treatment and Disposal options
YELLOW	(a) Human Anatomical Waste [1] (b) Animal Anatomical Waste [2]	Yellow non-chlorinated plastic bags	Incineration/Plasma Pyrolysis/Deep burial
	(c) Soiled Waste [6]		Incineration/Plasma Pyrolysis/Deep burial OR Autoclaving/Microwaving/Hydroclaving THEN Shredding/ Mutilation
	(d) Expired/Discarded Medicines [5] (e) Chemical Waste [10]	Yellow non-chlorinated plastic bags or containers	Incineration/Encapsulation/Plasma Pyrolysis
	(f) Chemical Liquid Waste [8]	Separate collection system leading to effluent treatment system	Pretreatment THEN Drain
	(g) Discarded linen, mattresses, beddings contaminated with blood or body fluid	Non-chlorinated yellow plastic bags or suitable packing material	Non- chlorinated chemical disinfection THEN Incineration/Plasma Pyrolysis/Energy recovery OR Shredding/Mutilation
	(h) Microbiology, Biotechnology, Clinical laboratory waste [3]	Autoclave safe plastic bags or containers	Pre-treat with Non-chlorinated chemicals THEN Incineration
RED	Contaminated Waste (Recyclable) [7]	Red non-chlorinated plastic bags or containers	Autoclaving/Microwaving/Hydroclaving THEN Shredding/Mutilation THEN Energy Recovery/Plastics to diesel or fuel oil/Road making
White (Translucent)	Waste sharps including Metals [4]	Puncture proof, Leak proof, tamper proof containers	Autoclaving/Dry Heat THEN Shredding/Mutilation/Encapsulation THEN Iron foundries/Sanitary Landfill/Waste sharp pit
Blue	(a) Glassware [4] (b) Metallic Body Implants	Cardboard boxes with blue colored marking	Sodium Hypochlorite/Autoclaving/Microwaving/Hydroclaving THEN Recycling

(Dear Students, although Older Category Numbers 1-10 are NOT USED in Newer classification, I have given them in [ ] so as to help you memorize better)

ANNEXURE 14

Current Public Health-related Statistics of India*

I. SOCIOECONOMIC INDICATORS

- HDI: (2015)
  - Rank 1: Switzerland 0.962–High Development
  - Rank 132: India 0.633–Medium Development
- *Multidimensional Poverty Index (MPI)*: 0.069 (2022)
  - Incidence of poverty: 16.4%
  - Population living below poverty line (BPL): 22% (Tendulkar Committee), 29.5%. (Rangarajan Committee)
  - Nigeria has highest no. of poor in the world
- *GDP per capita*: $ 2256
- *Income per capita*: ₹ 1,48,524/- per annum
- *Population with improved source of drinking water*: 94% (CIA 2017)
  - Urban: 97.1%
  - Rural: 92.6%
- *Population with improved sanitation facilities*: 39.6% (CIA 2017)
  - Urban: 62.6%
  - Rural: 28.5%

II. DEMOGRAPHY & FERTILITY INDICATORS

- *Crude birth rate (CBR)*: 19.5 per 1000 mid year population
- *Crude death rate (CDR)*: 6.0 per 1000 mid year population
- *School participation (primary level)*:
  - Male: 85%
  - Female: 81%
- *Median age at first marriage*:
  - Females: 17.2 years
  - Males: 23.4 years
- *TFR*: 2.0
  - Rural: 2.1
  - Urban: 1.6
- *Median interval between births in India*: 31 months
- *Contraceptive Prevalence Rate*: 67% (NFHS-5, 2019–2021)
  - Sterilization: 36% (Most common)
  - IUDs: 1.5%
  - Unmet need for Contraception: 13%
- *Primary Immunization Coverage*: 77%

III. MCH INDICATORS

- *IMR*: (SRS 2022)
  - India: 28 per 1000 Live Births
- *MMR*: (2022)
  - India: 97/Lac LB (SRS 2016)
- *U5MR*: (2022)
  - India: 32/1000 LB
  - UK/USA/Japan/Singapore: <10
  - World: 38

- *NNMR*: (2022)
  - India: 20/1000 LB
  - UK/USA/Singapore: <5
  - World: 17.1
- *PNMR*: (2022)
  - India: 18/1000 LB
- *Still birth rate (SBR)*: (2022)
  - India: 3/1000 Total births
- *≥4 visits in antenatal period*: 51%
- *TT coverage in pregnancy (2 doses)*: 89%
- *Institutional deliveries*: 79%
- *Delivery assisted by a health professional*: 81%
- *Exclusive breast feeding < 6 months age*: 55% (WHO recommendation: 6 months)
- *Average duration of breast feeding*: 25 months (WHO recommendation: 24 months minimum)
- *Infants with LBW (<2500 gms BW)*: 18%
- *Children's Nutritional Status*:
  - Underweight: 36%
  - Stunting: 38%
  - Wasting: 21%
- *Anemia*:
  - Women: 53%
  - Men (15–49 y): 23%
  - Children 6–59 months: 59%
- *AIDS comprehensive awareness*:
  - Men: 33%
  - Women: 21%
- *Domestic Violence (spousal) ever experienced by women*: 29%

IV. DISEASES

- *Human Avian Influenza H5N1*:
  - Global: 873 cases & 458 deaths in 16 countries (WHO 2023)
  - Zero confirmed cases in India
- *Human Avian Influenza H7N9*:
  - Global: 1567 cases & 615 deaths China, Malaysia (1), Cananda (2) (2019)
  - Zero confirmed cases in India
- *SARS*:
  - Global: 8422 cases with 916 deaths in 30 countries (WHO 2003)
  - 3 suspect cases in India
- *Middle-East Respiratory Syndrome–CoronaVirus (MERS-CoV)*
  - 2311 total cases with 811 related deaths (WHO 2019)
  - Zero confirmed cases in India
- *Malaria (2022)*:
  - 0.16 m cases (62% *P. falciparum* most common) with 90 deaths
  - API: 0.12
- *Leprosy (NLEP, 2022)*:
  - Prevalence rate: 0.41/10000 (Elimination achieved on Dec 2005)
  - ANCDR: 4.5/100,000
- *Tuberculosis (NTEP 2020–21)*:
  - Incidence TB cases: 2.7 million (27% of Global)
  - Mortality of TB: 4,40,000 (31% of Global)
  - Incidence HIV-TB: 92,000 (9% of Global)
  - Mortality of HIV-TB: 9,700 (4% of Global)
  - MDR-TB: 130,000 (24% of Global)
  - Children with TB: 342,000 (31% of Global)
- *HIV/ AIDS (NACO; 2021)*:
  - General adult population HIV+ prevalence: 0.21% (Mizoram 2.70% Highest)
  - No. of HIV+: 2.4 m (People on ART: 1.18 m)

- Maximum HIV cases: Maharashtra (16%)
- Highest prevalence: Mizoram (2.70%)
- *Poliomyelitis 2023*: [India declared 'POLIO-FREE' on 27 March 2014 by WHO]
  - No. of Polio cases: ZERO
  - No. of Vaccine derived Polio virus (VDPV) cases: Zero
  - No. of AFP cases: 9150
  - Non-polio AFP rate: 5.79

V. CENSUS OF INDIA 2011

- *Total population*: 1210 million population as on 00.00 hrs 1st March 2011
- *Sex ratio*: 943 females per 1000 males
  - *Child-sex ratio*: 919 girls per 1000 boys (0-6 yrs age)
- *Dependency ratio*: 54 per 100 (0.54)
- *Density of population*: 382 persons per square km
- *Literacy Level (aged 7 yrs and older)*: 74%
  - Males: 82%
  - Females: 65%
- *Growth rate*:
  - Decadal Growth Rate: 17.64%
  - Annual Growth Rate: 1.64%

VI. AGE DISTRIBUTION INDIA (2017–18)

- <10 years   :   17.4%
- 10–14 years   :   9.6%
- 15–49 years   :   56.6%
- 50–59 years   :   7.9%
- ≥60 years   :   8.5%

VII. FEW KEY FINDINGS OF NFHS-5, INDIA (2019–21)

- NFHS-5 2019-21, India: Key Parameters

Parameter	Value(s)
Population below age 15 years (%)	26.5%
Sex ratio of the total population (females per 1,000 males)	1,020
Sex ratio at birth (females per 1,000 males)	929
Births registered with the civil authority	89%
Deaths registered with the civil authority	71%
Households with an improved drinking-water source	96%
Households that use an improved sanitation facility	70%
Households using clean fuel for cooking	59%
Literacy levels (male, female)	84% (M), 71% (F)
Ever used Internet (male, female)	57% (M), 33% (F)
Total fertility rate (children per woman)	2.0
Infant mortality rate (IMR)	35
Neonatal mortality rate (NNMR)	25
Under-five mortality rate (U5MR)	42
Any method use for Family planning	66.7%
Total unmet need for Family planning	9.4%

VIII. UPDATED IMPORTANT PUBLIC HEALTH DATA OF INDIA 2022–23

- Infant Mortality Rate (IMR) India: 28 per 1000 Live births (SRS, May 2022)
- Maternal Mortality Rate (MMR): 97 per 100,000 Live births (SRS, March 2022)
- Under Five Mortality Rate (U5MR): 32 per 1000 Live births (SRS, September 2022)
- Neonatal Mortality Rate (NNMR): 20 per 1000 Live births (SRS, September 2022)
- Perinatal Mortality Rate (PNMR): 18 per 1000 Live births (SRS, September 2022)
- Still Birth Rate (SBR): 3 per Total births (SRS, September 2022)
- Crude Birth Rate (CBR): 19.5 per 1000 Mid-year population (SRS, May 2022)
- Crude Death Rate (CDR): 6.0 per 1000 Mid-year population (SRS, May 2022)
- Natural Growth Rate: 13.5% (SRS, May 2022)
- Human Development Index (HDI): 0.633 (Rank 132 Medium Development, 2021–22)
- Multidimensional Poverty Index (MDPI): 0.069 (16.4% Poor)
- GDP Per Capita: 2,257 US Dollars (2021)
- Total Fertility Rate (TFR): 2.0 (NFHS-5, 2019–21)

(*Compiled from Multiple sources by © Dr Vivek Jain 2023-24)

ANNEXURE 15: Honors in Health and Medicine

Honor(s)	Scientist
Father of Antisepsis/Modern surgery*	Joseph Lister
Father of Bacteriology*	Robert Koch
Father of Biochemistry	Carl Alexander Neuberg
Father of Biology/Zoology	Aristotle
Father of Computed Tomography (CT)	Godfrey Hounsfield
Father of Endocrinology	Thomas Addison
Father of Epidemiology/Modern Epidemiology, Greatest doctor	John Snow
Father of Evidence based Medicine	DL Sackett
Father of Genetics	Gregor Mendel
Father of Gynecology	J Marion Sims
Father of Histology	Marie-Francois Xavier Bichat
Father of Homeopathy	Samuel Hahnemann
Father of Indian Medicine	Charaka
Father of Indian Pharmacology	Ram Nath Chopra
Father of Indian Surgery/Plastic & Cosmetic surgery	Sushruta
Father of Interventional Radiology	Charles T Dotter
Father of Medical Ultrasound	John J Wild
Father of Medicine/Modern medicine, First True Epidemiologist	Hippocrates
Father of Microbiology	Louis Pasteur
Father of Modern medicine	William Osler
Father of Modern/Microscopic/Cellular pathology	Rudolf Virchow
Father of Modern anatomy	Andreas Vesalius
Father of Modern laparoscopy	Camran Nezhat
Father of Modern microbiology	Louis Pasteur
Father of Modern pharmacology	Oswald Schmiedeberg
Father of Modern toxicology	Mathieu Orfila
Father of Nutrition	Antoine Lavoisier
Father of Obstetric ultrasound	Ian Donald
Father of Pediatrics	Abraham Jacobi
Father of Physiology	Claude Bernard
Father of Psychoanalysis	Sigmund Freud
Father of Public health	Cholera
Father of Radiology/Diagnostic radiology/X-rays	WC Roentgen
Father of Sociology*	Karl Marx
Father of Surgery/Modern surgery	Ambroise Pare
Father of Veterinary medicine	Renatus Vegetius
Hindu God of Medicine	Dhanvantari

(*Multiple scientists have been given these honors)

ANNEXURE 16

Incentives under National Health Programs

KINDLY NOTE: Incentives are NOT uniform and state-wise variations exist in majority of Incentives covered under National Health Programs in India. They are updated time-to-time.

JSSK Package (National Health Mission)

Category	Rural area			Urban area		
	Mother's package	ASHA's package	Total package	Mother's package	ASHA's package	Total package
LPS	1400	600	2000	1000	400	1400
HPS	700	600	1300	600	400	1000

(LPS: Low performing states; HPS: High performing states)

Sterilization Incentive Package (RCH Program)

- 3-year Bachelor of Rural Health Care (BRHC) degree program (cadre of rural health care practitioners for recruitment and placement at SHCs)
- National Health and Medical Facilities Accreditation Unit (NHMFAU): Regulatory and accreditation body on management and institutional reforms
- Setting District Health Knowledge Institute: DHKI for districts with population >500,000

States	Operation	Acceptor	ASHA/H. worker	Others	Total
11 high focus states	Vasectomy	2000	300	400	2700
	Tubectomy	1400	200	400	2000
Other high focus states	Vasectomy	1100	200	200	1500
	Tubectomy	600	150	250	1000
Non high focus states	Vasectomy	1100	200	200	1500
	Tubectomy (BPL/SC/ST)	600	150	250	1000
	Tubectomy	250	150	250	650
Mission Parivar Vikas Districts	Vasectomy	3000	400	600	4000
	Tubectomy	2000	300	500	2800
	Tubectomy (PPS)	3000	400	600	4000
	Vasectomy (COT)	3000	400	1600	5000
	Tubectomy (COT)	2000	300	2200	4500

(11 High focus states: UP, BH, MP, RJ, CG, JH, OD, UK, AS, HR, GJ; Other high focus states: NE states, J&K, HP)

Incentives for DOTS-providers (RNTCP)

- Providing treatment to Cat-I patients: ₹ 1000/-
- Providing treatment to Cat-II patients: ₹ 1000/-
- Providing treatment to Cat-IV/V patients: ₹ 5000/-

ANNEXURE 17

High Level Expert Group (HLEG) Report on Universal Health Coverage (UHC)

DEFINITION OF UHC

- Ensuring equitable access for all Indian citizens to affordable, accountable, appropriate health services of assured quality as well as public health services addressing the wider determinants of health, with the government being the guarantor and enabler

FIVE LEVELS OF HEALTH CARE

- Level 1: Villages, Community level in Urban areas
- Level 2: Sub Health Centers (SHCs)
- Level 3: Primary Health Centers (PHCs)
- Level 4: Community Health Centres (CHCs)
- Level 5: District Hospitals, Medical Colleges, Other tertiary care institutions

URBAN HEALTH CARE SYSTEM

Urban Family Welfare Centres (UFWC)	Urban Health Posts (UHP)
Type I: 1 per 10000–25000 population Type II: 1 per 25000–50000 population Type III: 1 per >50000 population **Staffing Pattern:** Type I/II: 2 paramedical staff Type III: 6 staff including Medical officer	Type A: 1 per <5000 Type B: 1 per 5000–10000 Type C: 1 per 10000–20000 Type D: 1 per 25000–50000 **Hospital attachment:** Type A, B, C: Referral and supervisory services Type D: Sterilization, MTP, Referral

OTHER RECOMMENDATIONS

- 3-year Bachelor of Rural Health Care (BRHC) degree program (cadre of rural health care practitioners for recruitment and placement at SHCs)
- National Health and Medical Facilities Accreditation Unit (NHMFAU): Regulatory and accreditation body on management and institutional reforms
- Setting District Health Knowledge Institute: DHKI for districts with population > 500,000

KEY TARGETS OF HLEG ON UHC

Parameter/Norm	Target	Current situation
Beds per 1000 population	2 beds per 1000 population by 2022	0.9 per 1000 population
ASHA* per 1000 population	2 per 1000 per population	1 per 1000 population
Nurse/Midwives per 1 doctor	3 per 1 doctor by 2025	1.5 per 1 doctor
Doctor per 1000 population	1 per 1000 by 2027	0.5 per 1000 population
Health personnel per 10000 population	23 per 10,000 population	12.9 per 10,000 population
Staff at Sub Health Centre	2 ANM, 1 MHW + 1 BRHC	2 ANM, 1 MHW
Staff at PHC	Existing staff + 1 AYUSH doctor, 1 Dentist, 1 More allopathic doctor, 1 MHW	15 Total staff (including 1 allopathic doctor)

Contd...

Contd...

Parameter/Norm	Target	Current situation
Staff at CHC	Existing staff + Total 19 nurses, 1 Head nurse, 1 Physiotherapist, 1 MHW	30–31 Total staff
Government spending on Health care	2.5% of GDP by 2017 3% of GDP by 2022	1.2% of GDP
Public health expenditure on health care	7.0% of GDP by 2017 8.6% by 2022	4.1% of GDP

(*ASHA = Community Health Worker; #Doctors + Nurses + Midwives; BHRC Bachelor of Rural Health care; MHW Male Health Worker)

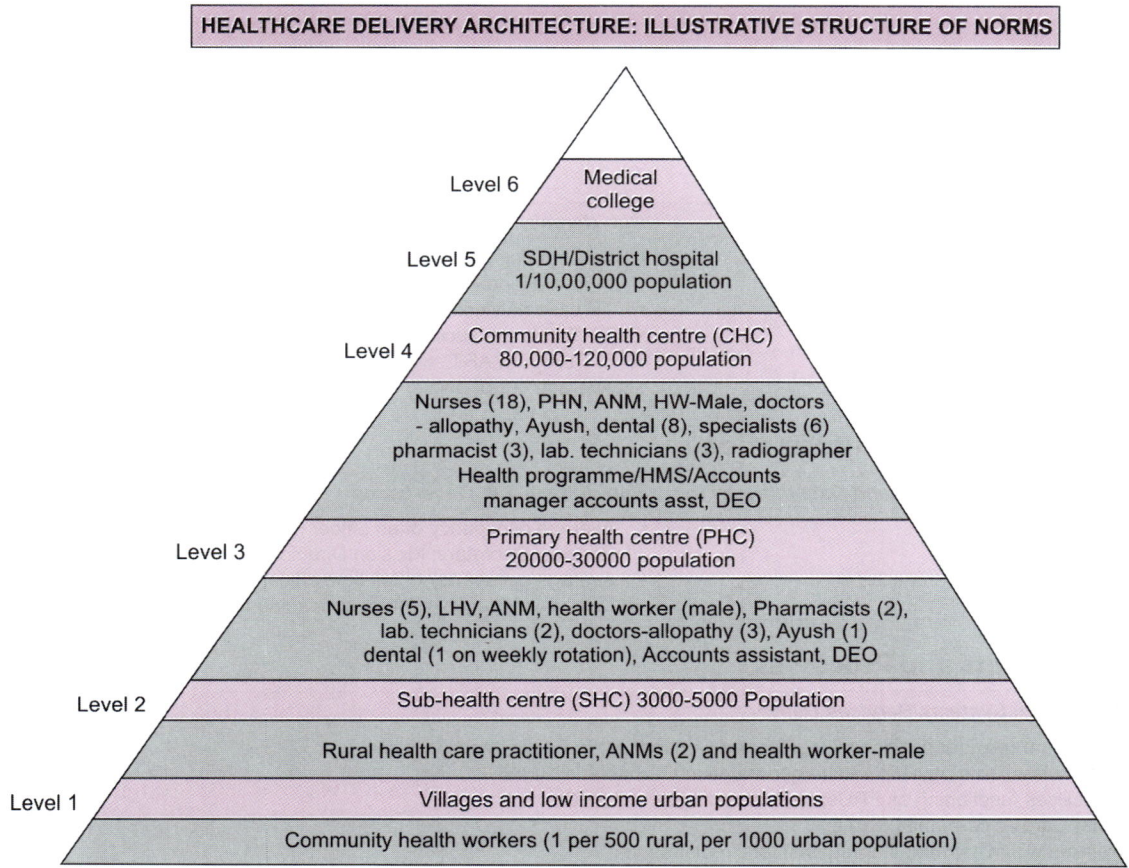

ANNEXURE 18: Health Index of India, HII (NITI Aayog)

DESCRIPTION

- Weighted composite index, based on indicators in 3 domains, namely Health outcomes (70%), Governance and Information (12%), and Key Inputs and Processes (18%)

Domain 1: Health Outcomes

Sub-domain 1.1: Key Outcomes	Sub-domain 1.2: Intermediate Outcomes
• NNMR • U5MR • TFR • % LBW • Sex Ratio at birth	• Full immunization coverage • % Institutional deliveries • TB case notification rate • TB Treatment success rate • % PLHIV on ART • Average out-of-pocket expenditure/ delivery in PHF

Domain 2: Governance and Information

Sub-domain 2.1: Health Monitoring and Data Integrity	Sub-domain 2.2: Governance

• Data Integrity measures
   – Institutional deliveries
   – ANC registered within 1st trimester
	• Average occupancy of an officer (months in last 3 years) at state level: Principal Secretary, Mission Director (NHM), Director (Health Services)
	• Average occupancy of full-time officer (months in last 3 years) in all districts: District CMO/equivalent (post heading District health services)

Domain 3: Key Inputs and Processes

Sub-domain 3.1: Health Systems/Services Delivery
• % Vacant healthcare provider positions (Regular and Contractual) in Public health facilities • % Total staff for whom an e-pay-slip can be generated in IT-enabled HRMIS • % Specified facilities functioning as FRUs; % Functioning 24 × 7 PHCs • % Districts with Cardiac care units (CCUs) • % ANC registered within 1st trimester (against total registrations) • Level of Registration of births • Completeness of P, L forms reporting under IDSP • % CHCs with grading above 3 points • % PHFs with Accreditation certificates by a Standard quality assurance program# • Av. no. days for Central NHM fund from State to Implementation agency (last year basis)

(NNMR: Neonatal mortality rate; U5MR: Under-five mortality rate; TFR: Total fertility rate; LBW: Low birth weight; PLHIV: People living with HIV; ART: Anti-retroviral therapy; PHF: Public health facility; ANC: Ante-natal clinic; NHM: National health mission; CMO: Chief Medical Officer; HRMIS: Human resource management information system; FRU: First referral unit; IDSP: Integrated disease surveillance program; CHC: Community Health Centre) (#NQAS, NABH, ISO, AHPI)

ANNEXURE 19: Ayushman Bharat Program 2018

HEALTH AND WELLNESS CENTRES (HWC)

- 1.5 Lac HWC centres
- Comprehensive health care (including MCH, NCDs)
- Free essential drugs and diagnostic services

NATIONAL HEALTH PROTECTION SCHEME (AB-NHPS)

- *Syn.* Pradhan Mantri Jan Aarogya Yojana (PMJAY)
- Main Aim: To provide a service to create a healthy, capable and content new India
- Goals:
  - Create a network of health, wellness infrastructure delivering comprehensive primary healthcare services
  - Provide insurance cover to >40% population deprived of secondary & tertiary care services
- Target (10.74 Crore families, **Total 50 crore people**)
  - Poor, deprived rural families
  - Identified occupational urban workers' families
- Apex Level: Chaired by Union Health & Family Welfare Minister
- Defined Benefit Cover:
  - **Rupees 5 lakh per family per year**
  - Secondary and Tertiary care hospitalization
  - To subsume the existing RSBY
  - No cap on the family size and age
  - Cashless and paperless scheme
  - Public hospitals and empanelled private hospitals
  - Include 1,354 packages (Including Bypass, stenting, knee replacements)
  - 15-20% cheaper rates than CGHS
- **Beneficiaries Criteria:**
  - Rural areas: Based on the deprivation categories (D1, D2, D3, D4, D5, D7) under the SECC database
  - Urban areas: 11 occupational criteria
  - RSBY beneficiaries in states where it is active
- Hospitalization Process:
  - No charges/premium for hospitalisation expenses
  - Include Pre- and Post-hospitalisation expenses
  - 'Ayushman Mitra' in each hospital to assist patients
- Hospital Eligibility:
  - All public hospitals
  - Empaneled private health care facilities
  - **Empanelment criteria: Hospital with >10 beds**

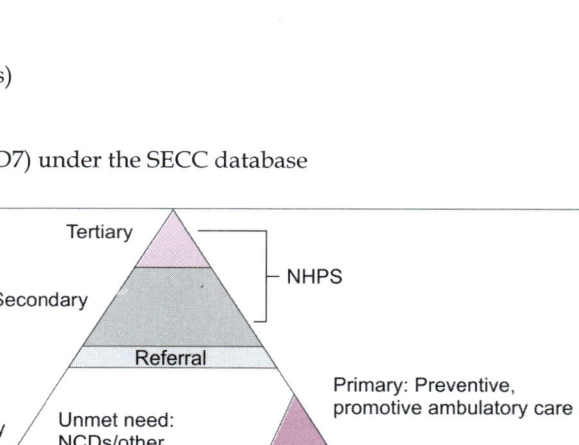

Ayushman Bharat—Continuum of Care NHPS/CPHC

Annexure 20: Swachh Bharat Mission (SBM) 2014

Syn. **Swachh Bharat Abhiyan**
- *Description*: National campaign to clean roads, streets and infrastructure of the country
- *Aim*: To eradicate/end open-defecation in India by 2019 by construction of 12 million toilets

Swachh Bharat Mission–Gramin (SBM-G)
- Key objectives:
  - Improve Quality of life by promotion of cleanliness, hygiene and elimination of open defecation
  - Accelerate sanitation coverage to achieve Swachh Bharat by 2 October 2019
  - Motivate communities and PRIs to adopt sustainable sanitation practices and facilities
  - Cost effective and appropriate technologies for ecologically safe, sustainable sanitation
  - Development of community managed sanitation systems (Solid and liquid waste management)
- Components:
  - Construction of toilets in Government schools (**Ministry of Human Resource and Development**)
  - Rural school sanitation- Separate Boys/Girls toilets (**Department of School Education**)
  - Construction of toilets in Anganwadi centers (**Ministry of Women and Child Development**)

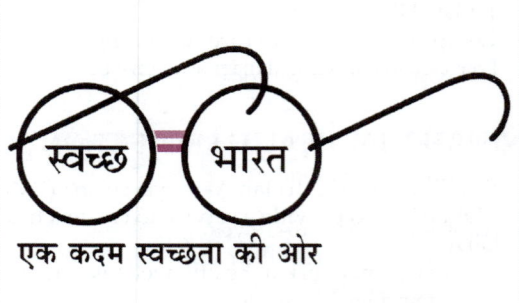

Swachh Bharat Mission–Urban (SBM-U)
- Key objectives:
  - Elimination of Open defecation
  - Eradication of manual scavenging
  - Modern and scientific municipal solid waste management
  - Behavior change regarding healthy sanitation practices
  - Awareness generation of sanitation and its linkage with public health
  - Capacity augmentation
  - Private sector participation
- Components:
  - Household toilets (and conversion of insanitary latrines to pour-flush latrines)
  - Community toilets
  - Public toilets
  - Solid waste management
  - IEC and public awareness
  - Capacity building
- Implementation by: Ministry of Urban Development

Annexure 21: Anemia Mukt Bharat

SYN. INTENSIFIED IRON-PLUS INITIATIVE

Main Aim
- To reduce prevalence of anemia by 3% points per year among children, adolescents and women in the reproductive age group (15–49 years), between the year 2018–2022

Anemia Mukt Bharat Beneficiaries
- Children (6–59 months)
- Children (5–9 years)
- Adolescent boys (10–19 years)
- Adolescent girls (10–19 years)
- Women of reproductive age (20–24 years)
- Pregnant women
- Lactating women

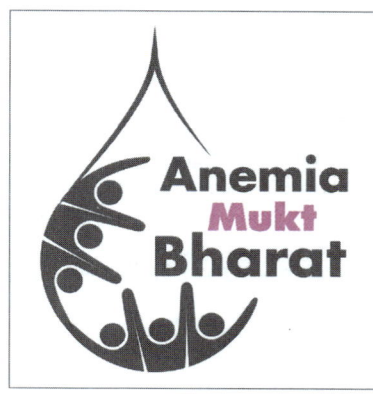

Anemia Mukt Bharat Anemia Reduction Targets for 2022

Age group	Anemia prevalence (%)	
	Baseline (NFHS 4)	National Target 2022*
Children (6–59 months)	58	40
Adolescent girls (15–19 years)	54	36
Adolescent boys (15–19 years)	29	11
Women of reproductive age	53	35
Pregnant women	50	32
Lactating women	58	40

(* at 3 percentage points per annum from baseline)

Anemia Mukt Bharat 6X6X6 Strategy

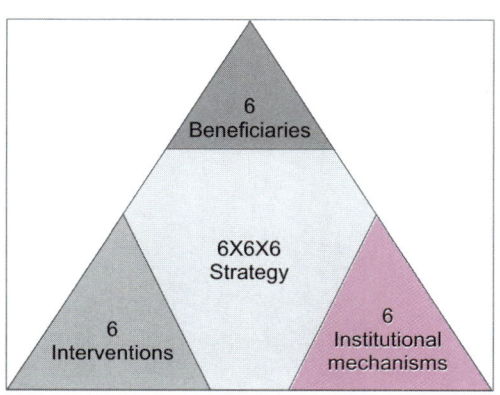

Interventions
- Prophylactic Iron Folic Acid supplementation
- Deworming
- Intensified year-round BCC Campaign including ensuring delayed cord clamping
- Testing of anemia using digital methods and point of care treatment
- Mandatory provision of Iron Folic Acid fortified foods in public health programmes
- Addressing non-nutritional causes of anemia in endemic pockets, with special focus on malaria, haemoglobinopathies and fluorosis

Prophylactic Dose and Regime for Iron Folic Acid Supplementation

Age Group	Iron (mg)	Folic acid (mcg)	Frequency	Remark
6–59 months Children	20 mg elemental	100 mcg	Biweekly	Bottle (50 mL^)
5–9 years Children	45 mg elemental	400 mcg	Weekly	Pink color tablet
10–19 years Adolescents*	60 mg elemental	500 mcg	Weekly	Blue color tablet
20–49 years Women (NPNL#)	60 mg elemental	500 mcg	Weekly	Red color tablet
Pregnant, Lactating mothers$	60 mg elemental	500 mcg	Daily	Red color tablet

(© Table Dr Vivek Jain 2019-20)
(^20 mg + 500 mcg = 1 mL; * Boys & Girls; # NPNL: non-pregnant, non-lactating; $ of 0–6 months child) (1 Iron and Folic Acid tablet starting from 4th month POG continued throughout pregnancy, minimum 180 days during pregnancy and to be continued for 180 days, post-partum)

Deworming with Albendazole 400 mg Tablet

Age Group	Tablet	Frequency
12–59 months Children*	½–1 tablet^	Biannual mass deworming$
5–9 years Children*	1 tablet	Biannual mass deworming$
10–19 years Adolescents*	1 tablet	Biannual mass deworming$
20–49 years Women (NPNL)	1 tablet	Biannual mass deworming$
Pregnant, Lactating mothers#	1 tablet	Once in 2nd trimester

(© Table Dr Vivek Jain 2019-20)
(*Anganwadis/Schools; # ANC clinics/VHND; $ National Deworming Day program; ^ ½ tablet 12–24 months & 1 tablet 24-59 months)

ANNEXURE 22: NEW WHO Rabies Vaccination Guidelines

ADMINISTRATION OF RABIES VACCINES

- ID injection sites (0.1 mL dose): Deltoid region/ Anterolateral thigh/Suprascapular regions
- IM administration sites (Entire vial): Deltoid area (for age ≥2 years), Anterolateral area of the thigh (Children aged <2 years)

1. Post-Exposure Prophylaxis (PEP)

Immediate Steps

- All bite wounds, scratches and RABV-exposure sites thorough washing and flushing of the wound for approximately 15 minutes, with soap or detergent and copious amounts of water, is required; Where available, an iodine-containing, or similarly viricidal, topical preparation should be applied to the wound
- A series of rabies vaccine injections should be administered promptly after an exposure
- RIG should be administered for severe category III exposures
- Wounds that require suturing should be sutured loosely and only after RIG infiltration into the wound

WHO Rabies Exposure Categories

- *Category I*: Touching or feeding animals, animal licks on intact skin (no exposure)
- *Category II*: Nibbling of uncovered skin, minor scratches or abrasions without bleeding (exposure)
- *Category III*: Single or multiple transdermal bites or scratches, contamination of mucous membrane or broken skin with saliva from animal licks, exposures due to direct contact with bats (severe exposure)

PEP Recommendations by Category of Exposure

Exposure	No previous immunization	If previously immunized
Category I	- Wash exposed skin surfaces - No PEP required	- Wash exposed skin surfaces - No PEP required
Category II	- Wound washing, Immediate vaccination - 2-sites ID (Days 0,3,7)^ Or - 1-site IM (Days 0,3,7,14-28)^^^ Or - 2-sites IM (Days 0,1) + 1-site IM (Days 7,21)^^^^ - RIG is not indicated	- Wound washing, Immediate vaccination* - 1-site ID (Days 0,3) Or - 4-sites ID (Day 0) Or - 1-site IM (Days 0,3) - RIG is not indicated
Category III	- Wound washing, Immediate vaccination - 2-sites ID (Days 0,3,7)^ Or - 1-site IM (Days 0,3,7,14-28)^^^ Or - 2-sites IM (Days 0,1) + 1-site IM (Days 7,21)^^^^ - RIG is Indicated	- Wound washing, Immediate vaccination* - 1-site ID (Days 0,3) Or - 4-sites ID (Day 0) Or - 1-site IM (Days 0,3) - RIG is not indicated

© Table Dr Vivek Jain 2019-20) (* except if complete PEP already received within <3 months previously)

- ^**Institut Pasteur du Cambodge (IPC) regimen:** 1-week, 2-site ID regimen, 2-2-2-0-0, Duration 7 days for entire PEP course
- ^^^**4-dose Essen regimen:** 2-week IM PEP regimen, 1-1-1-1-0, Duration 14-28 days for entire PEP course
- ^^^^**Zagreb regimen:** 3-week IM PEP regimen, 2-0-1-0-1, Duration 21 days for entire PEP course

Rabies Immunoglobulin (RIG) Administration

- Given only once, as soon as possible and not beyond Day 7 after the first dose of vaccine
- eRIG is less costly than hRIG, both have shown similar clinical outcomes
- eRIG products are now highly purified, skin testing before administration is unnecessary
- Maximum dose: 20 IU (hRIG) and 40 IU (eRIG) per kg body weight

- Infiltrate as much as possible into the wound; the remainder of the calculated dose of RIG does not need to be injected IM at a distance from the wound but can be fractionated in smaller, individual syringes to be used for other patients, aseptic retention given
- If RIG is not available, thorough, prompt wound washing, together with immediate administration of the first vaccine dose, followed by a complete course of rabies vaccine
- Vaccines should never be withheld, regardless of the availability of RIG
- If a limited amount of RIG is available, RIG allocation should be prioritized for exposed patients based on the following criteria: Multiple bites, deep wounds, bites to highly innervated parts of the body (such as head, neck and hands), severe immunodeficiency, the biting animal is a confirmed or probable rabies case, and bites, scratches or exposures of mucous membranes caused by a bat.

2. Pre-Exposure Prophylaxis (PrEP)

- Recommended for
  - Individuals at higher risk due to occupation
  - Sub-populations living in remote, rabies endemic areas, where access to PEP is difficult, the dog bite incidence is >5% per year or vampire bat rabies is known to be present
- For previously unimmunized: 2 sites ID Or 1-site IM vaccine (Days 0,7)
  - A routine PrEP booster or serology for neutralizing antibody titres is recommended only if a continued, high risk of rabies exposure remains.
  - Individuals with documented immunodeficiency should be evaluated on a case-by-case basis and best receive an ID Or IM PrEP schedule as above, plus a third vaccine (Days 21-28)
  - Additionally, in the event of an exposure, a complete PEP course, including RIG

ANNEXURE 23

NEW WHO Guidelines for Treatment of Leprosy: Uniform MDT

- **3-drug regimen of Rifampicin, Dapsone, Clofazimine for all leprosy patients**
  - Duration of treatment: 6 months (PB Leprosy); 12 months (MB Leprosy)
  - Advantage: Simplification of treatment (i.e. the same blister pack could be used for treating both types of leprosy) and reduced impact of misclassification of MB leprosy as PB leprosy
- *For Rifampicin-resistant leprosy*: At least two 2nd line drugs (Clarithromycin, Minocycline or a Quinolone) plus Clofazimine daily for 6 months, followed by Clofazimine plus one of these drugs for an additional 18 months
- *When Ofloxacin resistance is also present*: Fluoroquinolone should not be used as part of second-line treatment; the regimen of choice in such cases shall consist of 6 months of Clarithromycin, Minocycline and Clofazimine followed by Clarithromycin or Minocycline plus Clofazimine for an additional 18 months

Age	Drugs	Dose	PB duration	MB duration
Adult	Rifampicin	600 mg OAM	12 months	6 months
	Clofazimine	300 mg OAM and 50 mg OD		
	Dapsone	100 mg OD		
Children (10–14 years)	Rifampicin	450 mg OAM	12 months	6 months
	Clofazimine	150 mg OAM and 50 mg OD		
	Dapsone	50 mg OD		
Children<10 y or <40 kg	Rifampicin	10 mg/kg OAM	12 months	6 months
	Clofazimine	6 mg/kg OAM and 1 mg/kg OD		
	Dapsone	2 mg/kg OD		

(OAM: Once a month)

Recommended regimens for Drug-resistant Leprosy

Resistance type	Treatment First 6 months (daily)	Treatment Next 18 months (daily)
Rifampicin resistance	Ofloxacin 400 mg* + Minocycline 100 mg + Clofazimine 50 mg	Ofloxacin 400 mg* Or Minocycline 100 mg + Clofazimine 50 mg
	Ofloxacin 400 mg* + Clarithromycin 500 mg + Clofazimine 50 mg	Ofloxacin 400 mg* + Clofazimine 50 mg
Rifampicin and Ofloxacin resistance	Clarithromycin 500 mg + Minocycline 100 mg + Clofazimine 50 mg	Clarithromycin 500 mg Or Minocycline 100 mg + Clofazimine 50 mg

(*Ofloxacin 400 mg can be replaced by Levofloxacin 500 mg OR Moxifloxacin 400 mg)

ANNEXURE 24

Tribal Health in India

Scheduled Tribes [Article 366 (25)]
- Includes tribes or communities as deemed under Article 342
- List is State, Union Territory specific

Demographic and Health Profile

Parameter	Tribal Population	Country Population
Total population	104 million (705 tribes)	1340 million
% Total population of country	8.6%	100%
Rural: Urban distribution	90:10	69:31
High population states	MP > Maharashtra > Odisha	UP > Maharashtra > Bihar
Sex ratio (females /1000 males)	990	943
Child sex ratio (0-6 years age)	957	919
Literacy rate (%)	59% (M: 69%, F: 35%)	74% (M: 82%, F: 65%)
Life expectancy	63.9 years	68.6 years
Institutional deliveries	68%	79%
Deliveries by skilled personnel	71.5%	81%
Post natal care (<48 hours)	37%	N/A
IMR (per 1000 LB)	44.4	34
U5MR (per 1000 LB)	57.1	39.4
NNMR (per 1000 LB)	31.3	24

Burden of Disease in Tribal Population

Disease	Burden in Tribal Population	Burden in Country Population
Tuberculosis prevalence*	703/100,000 population	256 per 100,000 population
Leprosy	18.9% of total cases	1.35 Lac total new cases
Malaria	30% of Total cases 60% of Falciparum cases 50% of Total mortality	1.1 million total cases
Hypertension	25% tribal adults	–
Genetic disorders	1–40% prevalence SCA# 1–15% prevalence of G6PD	–
Tobacco use	72%	56%
Alcohol use	50%	–
Animal attacks	Snakes, dogs, scorpion bites	–
Violence in conflict areas	–	–

(*Mobile TB Diagnostic Van with X-ray/Sputum smear facility in 5 states; #SCA Sickle cell anemia)

Healthcare Infrastructure for Tribal Population
- 27–40% shortfall in Health care institutions
- 27% shortfall in Subcentres (11 states) (8% shortfall in UT Dadra and Nagar Haveli)
- 40% shortfall in PHCs (7 states)
- 31% shortfall in CHCs (10 states) (1 CHC shortfall in UT Dadra and Nagar Haveli)

SECTION 3

Topic-wise Theory, MCQs and Explanations

SECTION OUTLINE

- History of Medicine
- Concepts of Health and Disease
- Epidemiology and Vaccines
- Screening of Disease
- Communicable and Non-communicable Diseases
- National Health Programmes, Policies and Legislations in India
- Demography, Family Planning and Contraception
- Preventive Obstetrics, Pediatrics and Geriatrics
- Nutrition and Health
- Social Sciences and Health
- Environment and Health
- Biomedical Waste Management, Disaster Management, Occupational Health, Genetics and Health, Mental Health
- Health Education and Communication
- Health Care in India, Health Planning and Management
- International Health
- Biostatistics

CHAPTER 1

History of Medicine

PRIMITIVE MEDICINE

Homeopathy System of Medicine

- *Principles of Homeopathy system of medicine*:
  - *First principle – 'similia similibus curenter'*[Q]: Homeopathy is system of pharmaco-dynamics based on treatment of disease by use of small amounts of a drug that, in healthy persons, produces symptoms similar to those of the disease being treated (known as 'Human drug pathogenicity study')
  - *Second principle*: Single medicine at the time of treatment
  - *Third principle*: Minimum dose to be used
- *Founding Father of Homeopathy*: Samuel Hahnemann[Q] (Germany[Q])

Ayurveda System of Medicine

- Ayurveda means the *'science of life'*
- *Tridosha theory of disease*[Q]: Disease occurs when there is disequilibrium in three doshas (humors), namely, Vata (wind), Pitta (gall) and Kapha (mucus)

Siddha System of Medicine

- Siddha means *'achievement'*
- Is practiced in Tamil speaking parts in India and abroad
- Based on notion that medical treatment has to take into account the patient's environment, age, sex, race, physiological constitution, etc.

Unani System of Medicine

- Originated from Greece[Q]
- *'Based on the humoral theory'*[Q]: Blood, phlegm, yellow bile and black bile
- Patient's character: Sanguine, phlegmatic, choleric and malancholic

Profounders of Theories in Public Health

- *Germ theory of disease*[Q]: Louis Pasteur
- *Multi-factorial causation of disease*: Pattenkofer[Q]
- *Spontaneous generation theory*: Aristotle[Q]

Discoveries, Inventions and Developments

- *First vaccine developed*[Q]: Small pox (Edward Jenner)
- *Term 'Vaccination'*[Q]: Edward Jenner
- *Term 'Vaccine'*[Q]: Louis Pasteur
- *Vaccines – Anthrax, Rabies*: Louis Pasteur
- *First Polio Vaccine*: Jonas Salk
- *Penicillin (First antibiotic)*: Alexander Fleming[Q]
- *Growth Chart*: David Morley[Q]

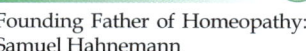

Founding Father of Homeopathy: Samuel Hahnemann

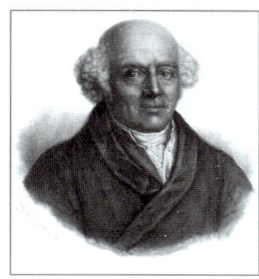

Samuel Hahnemann

Key points

Germ theory of disease: Louis Pasteur

Key points

First vaccine developed: Small pox

Key points

Life cycle of Plasmodium: Ronald Ross

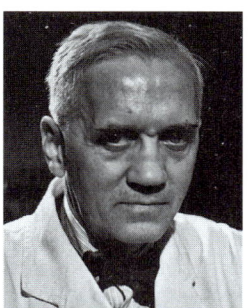

Sir Alexander Fleming

- *Homeopathy*: Samuel Hahnemann
- *Blood group types*: Karl Landsteiner
- *Citrus fruits in prevention of Scurvy*: James Lind
- *Transmission of Yellow fever*: Walter Reed
- *Life cycle of Plasmodium*: Ronald Ross[Q]

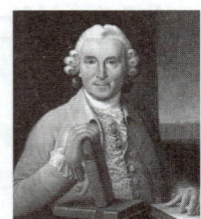
James Lind

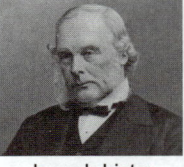
Joseph Lister

Authors of Important Books in Public Health
- *The Canon of Medicine*: Avicenna[Q]
- *The Book on Healing*: Avicenna
- *Antiseptic Principle of the Practice of Surgery*: Joseph Lister[Q]
- *Air, Water and Places*: Hippocrates[Q]
- *Ayurvedic Text Nidana*: Madhav
- *Charaka Samhita*: Charaka
- *Susruta Samhita*: Susruta

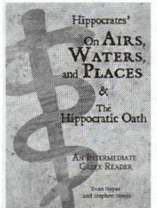
Air, Water and Places

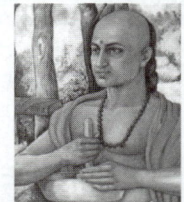
Charaka

> **Key points**
> The Canon of Medicine: Avicenna

Important Contributors in Public Health: Hippocrates
- Also known as: Father of Medicine, First True Epidemiologist[Q]
- Wrote book: Air, Water and Places[Q]
- First physician to reject superstitions, legends and beliefs that credited supernatural or divine forces with causing illness
- Hippocratic school held that all illness was the result of an imbalance in the body of the four humors, blood, black bile, yellow bile and phlegm
- First to describe clubbing

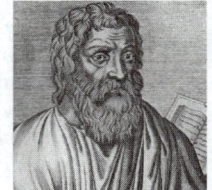
Hippocrates

> **Key points**
> Air, Water and Places: Hippocrates

Sushruta
- Wrote 'Sushruta Samhita'
- Is also known as 'Father of Plastic Surgery and Cosmetic Surgery'
- Is regarded as 'Father of Indian Surgery'[Q]

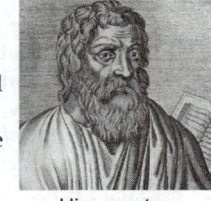
Sushruta

> **Key points**
> Hippocrates
> Also known as: Father of Medicine, First True Epidemiologist

SCIENTIFIC MEDICINE

John Snow
- *John Snow*, an English epidemiologist, studied Cholera[Q] (1848-54) and established the role of drinking water in its spread (Causative agent was identified much later)
- John Snow is also known as,
  - Father of Epidemiology/Modern Epidemiology[Q]
  - Greatest doctor
- John Snow studied and calculated dosages for use of ether and chloroform as surgical anesthesia

> **Key points**
> Sushruta
> Is regarded as 'Father of Indian Surgery'

History of Cholera
- *John Snow* (1813-1858): Found the link between cholera and contaminated drinking water (1854 using *Spot maps*[Q])
- *William Budd* concluded that spread of typhoid was by drinking water
- *Robert Koch* microscopically identified *V. cholerae* as bacillus causing the disease (1885)
- *Father of Public Health*: Cholera (Father of PH is a disease, *not a person*)

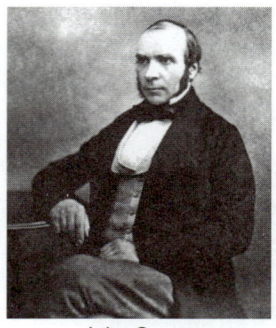
John Snow

Some Important Honours
- *Father of (Modern) Medicine*: Hippocrates[Q]
- *Father of Indian Medicine*: Charaka[Q]
- *Hindu God of Medicine*: Dhanvantari
- *Father of (Modern) Surgery*: Ambroise Pare
- *Father of Indian Surgery*: Sushruta[Q]
- *Father of Epidemiology/Modern Epidemiology*: John Snow[Q]
- *Father of Bacteriology*: Louis Pasteur[Q]
- *Father of Biology*: Aristotle
- *Father of Genetics*: Gregor Mendel[Q]
- *Father of (Modern) Anatomy*: Vesalius[Q]

> **Key points**
> John Snow
> Father of Epidemiology/Modern Epidemiology

> **Key points**
> Father of Public Health: Cholera

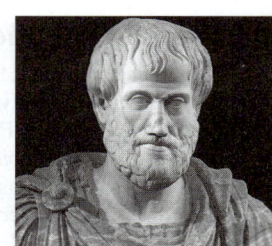
Aristotle

- *Father of Physiology*: Claude Bernard
- *Father of Psychoanalysis*: Sigmund Freud^Q
- *Father of Homeopathy*: Samuel Hahnemann^Q

Edward Jenner

- Discovered Small Pox vaccine in 1796
- Small pox vaccine was the *'First Vaccine'* to be discovered^Q
- Small Pox is the *'First and Only'* disease to be eradicated [Poliovirus 2 eradicated on 20 Sep 2015]
- Term *'Vaccination'* was coined by Edward Jenner

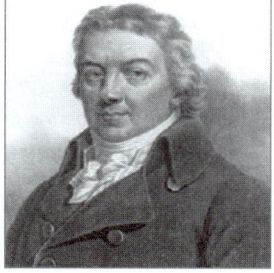

Edward Jenner

Louis Pasteur

- Gave the *'Germ theory of disease'*
- Coined term *'Vaccine'*
- Developed *'Vaccines for Rabies and Chicken Cholera'*
- Techniques of *'Sterilization'* and *'Pasteurization'*

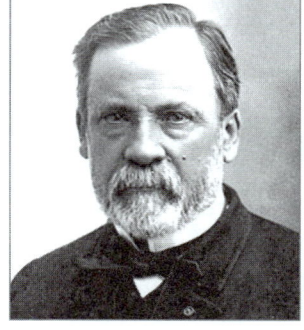

Louis Pasteur

MODERN MEDICINE

AYUSH^Q

- ISM&H (Indigenous Systems of Medicine and Homeopathy) have been now re-designated as *'AYUSH system'* of medicine
  - **A**yurveda
  - **Y**oga and Naturopathy
  - **U**nani
  - **S**iddha
  - **H**omeopathy
  - Sowa-Rigpa (Tibetan system of medicine): Recently added
- Mainstreaming of AYUSH is a key component of National Rural Health Mission (NRHM) 2005-12

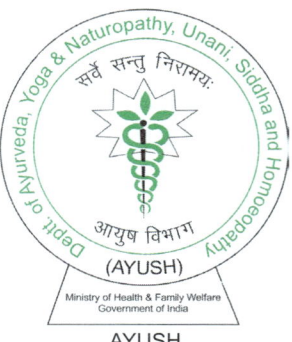

AYUSH

REVOLUTION IN MEDICINE

Types of Medicine

- *State Medicine*: Provision of free medical services to the people at government expense
- *Socialized Medicine*^Q: Provision of medical service and professional education by the State (as in state medicine), but the programme is operated and regulated by professional groups rather than by government
  - Prevents competition between practitioners and clients
  - Provision of medical services supported by state government
  - Ensures social equity that is universally operated by professional health services
- *Social medicine*: Study of the social, economical, environmental, cultural, psychological and genetic factors, which have a bearing on health

> **Key points**
> Socialized Medicine programme is operated and regulated by professional groups rather than by government

First Country Honours

- *First country to socialize medicine completely*^Q: Russia
- *First country to introduce compulsory sickness insurance*^Q: Germany
- *First country to start family planning programme*: India
- *First country to start blindness control programme*: India
- *First country to establish finger printing bureau*^Q: India (Calcutta, 1897)

> **Key points**
> First country to establish finger printing bureau: India

MISCELLANEOUS

Isolation & Quarantine

- *Isolation*' is the separation for the period of communicability, of infected persons from others in such places/conditions as to prevent/limit transmission to those susceptible
  - It applies to persons who are known to be ill with a contagious disease

- *'Quarantine'* (meaning *"40 Days"*) is the restriction of activities of apparently healthy persons who have been exposed to a case of communicable disease during its period of communicability
  - *It applies to those who have been exposed to a contagious disease but who may or may not become ill*
  - *Quarantine was first applied for plague*^{Q}
  - *Quarantine period for Yellow fever*^{Q}: 6 days (maximum IP)
  - *Quarantine currently has been 'replaced with active surveillance'*

	Isolation	Quarantine
Separation of	Cases	Healthy contacts of cases^Q
Done for	Cases themselves	Other persons around
Level of Prevention^Q	Secondary (Treatment)	Primary (Specific Protection)
Duration	Till recovery (period of communicability)	Till maximum incubation period^Q

> **Key points**
> Quarantine period for Yellow fever^Q: 6 days (maximum IP)

> **Key points**
> Quarantine period for Yellow fever^Q: 6 days (maximum IP)

> **Key points**
> WHO declared global eradication of smallpox^Q: 8th May 1980

> **Key points**
> 8th day disease: Tetanus neonatorum

> **Key points**
> Koch's Phenomenon: Tuberculosis

> **Key points**
> National Tuberculosis Institute (NTI): Bangalore

Smallpox Eradication
- *Last case of smallpox in world*^{Q}: 26th October 1977 (Somalia)
- *WHO declared global eradication of smallpox*^{Q}: 8th May 1980
- *Last indigenous case of smallpox in India*: 17th May 1975 (Bihar)
- *Last known case of smallpox in India*: 24th May 1975 (Importation from Bangladesh)
- *India declared smallpox free*: 23rd April, 1977.

Few Important Diseases in Public Health
- *Father of Public Health*: Cholera^Q
- *Barometer of Social Welfare*: Tuberculosis
- *Slims' Disease*: HIV/AIDS^Q
- *Black Sickness*: Kala Azar (Leishmaniasis)^Q
- *Black Death*: Plague^Q
- *Cerebrospinal fever*: Meningococcal meningitis
- *Break-bone fever*: Dengue^Q
- *Monkey fever/disease*: KFD (Kyasanur Forest Disease)^Q
- *5-day fever*: Trench fever
- *8th day disease*: Tetanus neonatorum^Q
- *100-day cough*: Pertussis (Whooping cough)
- *Koch's Phenomenon*: Tuberculosis^Q
- *Hansen's disease*: Leprosy^Q
- *Rubeola*: Measles
- *Rubella*: German measles^Q
- *Rubula*: Mumps

Institutes of Public Health Importance in India

Institute	Location
Central Drug Research Institute (CDRI)^Q	Lucknow
Central Leprosy Training & Research Institute (CLTRI)	Chengalpattu
Central Research Institute	Kasauli
Haffkine Institute	Mumbai
LRS Institute of T.B & allied Diseases	New Delhi
National Tuberculosis Institute (NTI)^Q	Bengaluru
National Environmental Engineering Research Institute (NEERI)^Q	Nagpur
National AIDS Control Organisation (NACO)	New Delhi
National Institue of Communicable Disease (NICD)	New Delhi
National Institue of Virology (NIV)^Q	Pune
National Institute of Nutrition (NIN)^Q	Hyderabad

Contd..

Contd..

Institute	Location
National JALMA Institute for Leprosy	Agra
Tuberculosis Research Institute (TRC)^Q	Chennai
National Institute of Occupational Health (NIOH)^Q	Ahmedabad
National Institute Mental Health and Neurosciences (NIMHANS)	Bengaluru
National Institute of Epidemiology^Q	Chennai
National AIDS Research Institute (NARI)	Pune

PYQs: Quick Review for NEET

History of Medicine	
First Country to Socialize Medicine completely	Russia
Marc Koska discovered	K1 auto-disable syringes
Plasmodium discovered by	CA Laveran
Life cycle of Plasmodium given by	Ronald Ross
Web of causation proposed by	McMohan and Pugh
Spot map was used for study of disease	Cholera
Louis Pasteur (1822-1895) died in	France
Edward Jenner died in	1823
Sushruta Samhita was translated by	Hessler
Cradle of civilization	Mesopotamia
James Lind is related to the discovery of	Prevention of scurvy
"Barometer of Social Welfare"	Tuberculosis
Free medical care by Government of a country is	State medicine
Honours in Medicine	
Father of Medicine/First True Epidemiologist	Hippocrates
Father of Public Health	Cholera
Father of Modern Anatomy	Andreas Vesalius
Father of Obstetric Ultrasound	Ian Donald
Father of Modern Toxicology	Mathieu Orfila
Father of Modern Microbiology	Louis Pasteur
Father of Indian Surgery	Sushruta

Multiple Choice Questions

PRIMITIVE MEDICINE

1. **Samuel Hahnemann is referred to as Founding Father of:**
   (a) Ayurveda *[AIIMS Nov 1993]*
   (b) Allopathy
   (c) Homeopathy
   (d) Yoga

2. **Match the following authors and their books:**
   A. Sushruta, I-Airs, Water and Places
   B. Avicenna, II-Sushruta Samhita
   C. Hippocrates, III-Canon of Medicine
   (a) A-III, B-I, C-II *[AIIMS May 1995]*
   (b) A-III, B-II, C-I
   (c) A-II, B-I, C-III
   (d) A-II, B-III, C-I

3. **Who is known as 'First True Epidemiologist' in history of medicine?** *[AIIMS Sep 1996]*
   (a) John Snow
   (b) Hippocrates
   (c) James Lind
   (d) Joseph Lister

4. **Match the following:** *[AIPGME 1994]*
   A. Sushruta, I-Hindu God of Medicine
   B. Dhanvantari, II-Father of Public Health
   C. Hippocrates, III-Father of Medicine
   D. Cholera, IV-Father of Indian Surgery
   (a) A-III, B-IV, C-II, D-I
   (b) A-IV, B-III, C-II, D-I
   (c) A-IV, B-I, C-III, D-II
   (d) A-I, B-IV, C-II, D-III

Review Question

5. **Which medicine claims to be the World's first organized body of medical knowledge?** *[PGMCET 2015]*
   (a) Indian
   (b) Chinese
   (c) Egyptian
   (d) Mesopotamian

SCIENTIFIC MEDICINE

6. **Match the following scientists with their discoveries:** *[INICET Nov 2022]*

1-Walter Reed	a-Prevention of scurvy by citrus fruits
2-Edward Jenner	b-Yellow fever
3-James Lind	c-Smallpox vaccination

   (a) 1-a, 2-b, 3-a
   (b) 1-b, 2-a, 3-c
   (c) 1-c, 2-b, 3-a
   (d) 1-b, 2-c, 3-a

7. **Match the following:** *[AIIMS Nov 1993]*
   A. Pattenkofer, I-Spontaneous Generation Theory
   B. Louis Pasteur, II-Germ Theory of Disease
   C. Aristotle, III-Multifactorial Causation of Disease
   (a) A-III, B-I, C-II
   (b) A-III, B-II, C-I
   (c) A-II, B-I, C-III
   (d) A-II, B-III, C-I

8. **Match the following Pioneers of Preventive Medicine and their achievements:** *[AIPGME 1996]*
   A. Edward Jenner, I-Transmission of Yellow Fever
   B. James Lind, II-Vaccination against Smallpox
   C. Walter Reed, III-Prevention of Scurvy
   (a) A-III, B-I, C-II
   (b) A-III, B-II, C-I
   (c) A-II, B-I, C-III
   (d) A-II, B-III, C-I

9. **Which of the following is known as "Father of Public Health"?** *[AIIMS Feb 1997] [DNB June 2011]*
   [NEET Pattern 2013, 2014]
   (a) Tuberculosis
   (b) Cholera
   (c) John Snow
   (d) Louis Pasteur

10. **Smallpox vaccine was introduced by:** *[AIIMS Dec 1992]*
    (a) Paul Ehrlich *[DNB 2011, MP 2003]*
    (b) Robert Koch *[NEET Pattern 2015]*
    (c) Louis Pasteur
    (d) Edward Jenner

11. **Malarial parasite was discovered by:**
    (a) Robert Koch *[NEET Pattern 2013]*
    (b) Louis Pasteur
    (c) Charles Alphonse Laveran
    (d) Ronald Ross

12. **Theory of web of causation was given by:**
    [NEET Pattern 2013] [DNB Dec 2010]
    (a) McMohan and Pugh
    (b) Pettenkofer
    (c) John Snow
    (d) Louis Pasteur

13. **Pioneer in concept of 'Specific protection by vaccine':**
    (a) Chinese medicine *[NEET Pattern 2016]*
    (b) Robert Koch
    (c) Ambroise Pare
    (d) Louis Pasteur

Review Questions

14. Who discovered the transmission of malaria by Anopheline mosquitoes? [TN 2003]
    (a) Ronald Ross   [NEET Pattern 2013]
    (b) Laveran
    (c) Muller
    (d) Pampana

MODERN MEDICINE

15. Yoga is considered a part of Modern medicine. It will be a part of: [AIPGME 2012]
    (a) Physiotherapy
    (b) Preventive medicine
    (c) Therapeutic medicine
    (d) Caloric usurper

16. The lawyer who designed the Public Health Act 1848 was: [NEET Pattern 2013]
    (a) John Snow
    (b) Edwin Chadwick
    (c) Joseph Lister
    (d) William Farr

17. Term 'Social Medicine' was introduced by:
    (a) Jules Guerin   [NEET Pattern 2015]
    (b) Crew
    (c) John Ryle
    (d) Alfred Grotjahn

18. Who among the following introduced the concept of relationship of Environment with Human health?
    (a) Hippocrates   [NEET Pattern 2016]
    (b) Louis Pasteur
    (c) David Moley
    (d) Ambroise Pare

19. Ministry of AYUSH was formed in 2014 for the development of education and research in the field of:
    (a) Ayurveda and Yoga only   [NEET Pattern 2016]
    (b) Unani and Naturopathy only
    (c) Siddha and Homeopathy only
    (d) All of the above

REVOLUTION IN MEDICINE

20. Socialized medicine is: [AIIMS Nov 2006]
    (a) Health care at people's expense
    (b) Charitable care at government expense
    (c) Free medical care at government expense, regulated by professional groups
    (d) Integration of social medicine with health care

21. All of the following are true about Socialized medicine except: [AIIMS Nov 2011]
    (a) Ensures social equity - universal coverage
    (b) Reduces competition among practitioners
    (c) Use state funds for free medicine
    (d) Increase utilization of health facilities

22. 'Secret of national health lies in the homes of people' statement by: [NEET Pattern 2012]
    (a) Indira Gandhi
    (b) Abraham Lincoln
    (c) Joseph Bhore
    (d) Florence Nightingale

23. First bacterium discovered as cause of a disease was: [NEET Pattern 2014]
    (a) TB bacillus
    (b) Leprosy bacillus
    (c) Anthrax bacillus
    (d) Plague bacillus

MISCELLANEOUS

24. Match the following: [AIIMS May 2001]
    A. Edward Jenner, I- Rabies and Anthrax
    B. Louis Pasteur, II- Small pox
    C. Albert Calmette and Camille Guérin, III- Poliomyelitis
    D. Pierre Lépine, IV- Tuberculosis
    (a) A-II, B-I, C-IV, D-III
    (b) A-II, B-III, C-IV, D-I
    (c) A-IV, B-I, C-III, D-II
    (d) A-I, B-IV, C-II, D-III

25. WHO declared that smallpox has been eradicated in: [AIPGME 1991]
    (a) May 1978
    (b) September 1984
    (c) May 1980
    (d) July 1987

26. Breastfeeding week is celebrated on: [NEET Pattern 2012, 2013, 2014]
    (a) 1st week of March
    (b) 1st week of July
    (c) 1st week of August
    (d) 1st December

27. World Health Day is celebrated on: [DNB June 2011]
    (a) 1st December
    (b) 31st May
    (c) 7th April
    (d) 8th May

28. Who is regarded as Father of Public Health?
    (a) Louis Pasteur   [DNB June 2011]
    (b) Cholera
    (c) John Snow
    (d) Robert Koch

29. **Quarantine of earlier time has now been replaced by:**
    [NEET Pattern 2017]
    (a) Isolation
    (b) Ring immunization
    (c) Active surveillance
    (d) None of the above

Review Questions

30. **Socialization of medicine means:** *[RJ 2007]*
    (a) Study of man as a social being in his total environment
    (b) Provision of medical services and professional education by the state but operated and regulated by the government
    (c) Provision of medical services and professional education by the state but operated and regulated by professional groups rather than by the government
    (d) Study of man as a social being in his whole life

31. **Benefit of socialization of medicine are all *except*:**
    [RJ 2007]
    (a) It eliminate competition among physicians in search of clients
    (b) It ensures social equity and universal coverage
    (c) Medical care becomes free for the patients, which is supported by the state
    (d) Patients can get good quality of treatment without cost

Explanations

PRIMITIVE MEDICINE

1. **Ans. (c) Homeopathy** *[Ref. Park 27/e p2]*
   - *Founding Father of Homeopathy:* Samuel Hahnemann (Germany)

ALSO REMEMBER
HOMEOPATHY:
- *Principle of Homeopathy system of medicine:*
  - First principle – 'similia similibus curenter': In healthy persons, produces symptoms similar to those of the disease being treated (known as 'Human drug pathogenicity study').
  - Second principle: Single medicine at the time of treatment
  - Third principle: Minimum dose to be used
- ISM and H (Indigenous Systems of Medicine and Homeopathy) have been now re-designated as 'AYUSH system' of medicine
  - Ayurveda
  - Yoga and Naturopathy
  - Unani
  - Siddha
  - Homeopathy

2. **Ans. (d) A-II, B-III, C-I** *[Ref. Park 27/e p2-4]*
   - *Authors of important books in Public Health:*
     - The Canon of Medicine: Avicenna
     - The Book on Healing: Avicenna
     - Antiseptic Principle of the Practice of Surgery: Joseph Lister
     - Air, Water and Places: Hippocrates
     - Ayurvedic Text Nidana: Madhav
     - Charaka Samhita: Charaka
     - Sushruta Samhita: Susruta

3. **Ans. (b) Hippocrates** *[Ref. Park 27/e p3]*
   HIPPOCRATES:
   - Also known as: *Father of Medicine, First True Epidemiologist*
   - Wrote book: *Air, Water and Places*

ALSO REMEMBER
- James Lind gave the concept that Citrus fruits can prevent/cure Scurvy (Later found to be due to deficiency of Vitamin-C/Ascorbic Acid)
- Joseph Lister is also known as 'Father of Anti-sepsis'

4. **Ans. (c) A-IV, B-I, C-III, D-II** *[Ref. Park 27/e p2-3]*

ALSO REMEMBER
- *Sushruta:*
  - Wrote *'Sushruta Samhita'*
  - Is also known as *'Father of Plastic Surgery and Cosmetic Surgery'*
  - Father of Surgery: *Ambroise Pare*
- *Hippocrates:*
  - Is also known as *'First true epidemiologist'*
  - Wrote book *'Airs, Waters and Places'*

Review Question

5. **Ans. (b) Chinese** *[Ref. Park 27/e p2]*
   - Chinese medicine claims to be the World's first organized body of medical knowledge, dating back to 2700 BC
   - Based on 2 principles: Yang and Yin

SCIENTIFIC MEDICINE

6. **Ans. (d) 1-b, 2-c, 3-a** *[Ref. Park 27/e p6]*
   - Walter Reed showed that yellow fever is transmitted by the Aedes mosquito.
   - Edward Jenner discovered first vaccine – Small pox vaccine
   - James Lind established that prevention of scurvy is possible by intake of citrus fruits

7. **Ans. (b) A-III, B-II, C-I** *[Ref. Park 27/e p6, 40]*
   - *Profounder of theories in Public Health:*
     - Germ theory of disease: Louis Pasteur
     - Multi-factorial causation of disease: Pattenkoffer
     - Spontaneous generation theory: Aristotle

ALSO REMEMBER
- Order of appearance/acceptance of theories in Public Health: Spontaneous Generation Theory, Germ Theory of Disease, Multifactorial Causation of Disease

8. **Ans. (d) A-II, B-III, C-I** *[Ref. Park 27/e p6]*

9. **Ans. (b) Cholera** *[Ref. Park 27/e p5]*
   - *Father of Public Health* is cholera disease, not a person

10. **Ans. (d) Edward Jenner** *[Ref. Park 27/e p6]*
    - Edward Jenner discovered Smallpox vaccine in 1796
      - Smallpox vaccine was the 'First Vaccine' to be discovered
      - Smallpox is the 'First and Only' disease to be eradicated [Poliovirus 2 eradicated on 20 Sep 2015]
      - Term 'Vaccination' was coined by Edward Jenner

ALSO REMEMBER
- Paul Ehrlich coined terms 'Chemotherapy' and 'Auto-immunity' and giving 'Magic Bullet for Syphilis- Salvarsan'

11. **Ans. (c) Charles Alphonse Laveran**
    [Ref. Physiology of Medicine 1901-21 by J Lindsten, 1/e p261]

12. **Ans. (a) McMohan and Pugh** *[Ref. Park 27/e p39, 41]*

13. **Ans. (a) Chinese medicine** *[Ref. Park 27/e p2]*
    - Chinese were early pioneers of immunization
    - They practiced variolation to prevent smallpox

> **ALSO REMEMBER**
>
> **Chinese Barefoot Doctors**
> - Farmers who received minimal basic medical and paramedical training and worked in rural villages of China
> - Name comes from southern farmers, who would often work barefoot in the rice paddies promoted basic hygiene, preventive health care, family planning and treated common illnesses
> - Purpose: To bring health care to rural areas where urban-trained doctors would not settle

Review Question

14. Ans. (a) Ronald Ross   [Ref. Park 27/e p6]

MODERN MEDICINE

15. Ans. (b) Preventive medicine   [Logical reasoning]
16. Ans. (b) Edwin Chadwick   [Ref. Park 27/e p5]
17. Ans. (a) Jules Guerin
    [Ref. Dictionary of Medical Sociology by Joseph, 1/e p119]
    - Alfred Grotjahn gave concept of Social pathology
18. Ans. (a) Hippocrates   [Ref. Park 27/e p3]
    - Hippocratic concept of health and disease:
      – Introduced the concept of relationship of Environment with Human health
      – Wrote book: 'Airs, Waters, and Places' (400 BC)
19. Ans. (d) All of the above   [Ref. Park 25/e p54, AYUSH Website, MOHFW, GOI]
    - The Ministry of AYUSH was formed on 9th November 2014 to ensure the optimal development and propagation of AYUSH systems of health care
    - Earlier it was known as the Department of Indian System of Medicine and Homeopathy (ISM&H)
    - Renamed as Department of Ayurveda, Yoga and Naturopathy, Unani, Siddha and Homoeopathy (AYUSH) in November 2003
    - Focused attention for development of Education and Research in Ayurveda, Yoga and Naturopathy, Unani, Siddha and Homoeopathy

REVOLUTION IN MEDICINE

20. Ans. (c) Free medical care at government expense, regulated by professional groups   [Ref. Park 27/e p9]
    - *State Medicine*: Provision of free medical services to the people at government expense
    - *Socialized Medicine:* Provision of medical service and professional education by the State (as in state medicine), but the programme is operated and regulated by professional groups rather than by government
      – Prevents competition between practitioners and clients
      – Provision of medical services supported by state government
      – Ensures social equity that is universally operated by professional health services
    - *Social Medicine:* Study of the social, economical, environmental, cultural, psychological and genetic factors, which have a bearing on health

> **ALSO REMEMBER**
> - First country to socialize medicine completely: Russia

21. Ans. (d) Increase utilization of health facilitie
                                            [Ref. Park 27/e p9]
    - Socialized medicine cannot ensure increased utilization of health services alone; it requires 'Community participation (Health by the people)' also
22. Ans. (d) Florence Nightingale   [Ref. Recent Advances in Public Health by JL Burn, 1/e p203]
23. Ans. (c) Anthrax bacillus   [Ref. Living in a Microbial World by Bruce V Hopkin, 1/e p126]

MISCELLANEOUS

24. Ans. (a) A-II, B-I, C-IV, D-III   [Ref. Park 27/e p6]

> **ALSO REMEMBER**
> - Louis Pasteur:
>   – Gave the 'Germ theory of disease'
>   – Coined term 'Vaccine'
>   – Developed 'vaccines for Rabies and Chicken cholera'
>   – Techniques of 'Sterilization' and 'Pasteurization'

25. Ans. (c) May 1980   [Ref. Park 27/e p159]
    - WHO declared global eradication of smallpox: 8th May 1980

> **ALSO REMEMBER**
> - Eradication is defined as 'termination of transmission of infection completely by extermination of the infectious agent'
>   – Globally only one disease (Smallpox) has been eradicated till date [Poliovirus 2 eradicated on 20 Sep 2015]
> - Few important dates in Public Health:
>   – 7th April 1948: Constitution of WHO came into force
>   – 8th May 1980: WHO declared eradication of Smallpox

26. Ans. (c) 1st week of August
    [Ref. Disaster Nursing and Emergency Preparedness by TG Veenema, 3/e p2]
    - Theme for WBFW 2014: Breastfeeding - A winning goal for life!
27. Ans. (c) 7th April   [Ref. Park 27/e p1026]
28. Ans. (b) Cholera   [Ref. Park 27/e p5]
29. Ans. (c) Active surveillance   [Ref. Park 27/e p133]
    - With availability of better methods of prevention, diagnosis and treatment of a disease, Quarantine use has declined.
    - Quarantine has been nowadays replaced by Active surveillance.

Review Questions

30. Ans. (c) Provision of medical services and professional education by the state but operated and regulated by professional groups rather than by the government
                                            [Ref. Park 27/e p9]
31. Ans. (d) Patients can get good quality of treatment without cost   [Ref. Park 27/e p9]

CHAPTER 2

Concepts of Health and Disease

HEALTH AND WELL-BEING

WHO Definition of Health^Q
- *WHO [1948] definition of Health*: Health is a state of complete physical, mental and social well-being, and not merely an absence of disease or infirmity; *[recently amplified to include –]* and an ability to lead a socially and economically productive life
  - Is an *'idealistic goal rather than a realistic proposition'*
  - It does not regard health as a dynamic concept (but as a state)

Standard of Living
- *Standard of Living*: Refers to the usual scale of our expenditure, goods we consume and services we enjoy
- *Standard of living [WHO] includes*:^Q
  - Income and Occupation
  - Standards of housing, sanitation and nutrition
  - Level of provision of health, educational, recreational and other services
- Standard of living depends on *'Per capita GNP'*

> **Key points**
> Standard of living depends on 'Per capita GNP'

HDI & PQLI

Human Development Index (HDI)
- *HDI values range*^Q: 0 to + 1
  - **HDI India is 0.633** (Rank 132 out of 189 countries) [2022]
- *Human poverty index [HPI] is complementary to HDI* ^Q

> **Key points**
> HDI is a composite index comprising of 3 dimensions^Q:
> - Knowledge
> - Income
> - Longevity

Estimation of HDI by New Method (2010 Onwards)
- *Goalposts to construct HDI index: [New Guidelines for calculation, 2018]*:

Dimension	Indicator	Minimum value	Maximum value
Health	Life expectancy at birth/LE_0 (years)	20	85

Education	Education Index
	    Mean years of schooling
	    Expected years of schooling
		
		0
		0
			
			15
			18

Standard of Living	Real GNI per capita (2011 $ PPP)	100	75,000

- Calculation of each dimension index:

$$= \frac{\text{Actual value - Minimum value}}{\text{Maximum value - Minimum value}}$$

- HDI is Geometric mean of 3 dimension indices = $I_{Life}^{1/3} \times I_{Education}^{1/3} \times I_{Income}^{1/3}$

Human Development Index vs Physical Quality of Life Index [PQLI]^Q

	HDI	PQLI
Components	1. Longevity – Life expectancy at birth (LE_B/LE_0) 2. Income (Real GDP per capita in PPP US$) 3. Knowledge (Mean years of schooling – Gross enrolment ratio & Literacy rate)	1. Life expectancy at 1 year age (LE_1) 2. Infant mortality rate (IMR) 3. Literacy rate
Range	0 to +1	0 to 100
Value of India	0.633	65

Key points

HDI values range^Q: 0 to + 1

Multi-dimensional Poverty Index (MDPI)

- International measure of acute poverty covering over 100 developing countries
- MDPI has replaced HPI: MDPI is not over-dependent on Income per capita
- MDPI uses 3 dimensions measured using 10 indicators^Q

Dimensions	Indicator	Deprived if living in the household where…	Weight
Health	Nutrition	An adult <70 years age Or a child is undernourished	1/6
	Child mortality	Any child has died in the family in last 5-year period	1/6
Education	Years of schooling	No member aged ≥10 years has completed 6 years of schooling	1/6
	School attendance	Any child is not attending school upto age at which would complete class 8	1/6
Standard of living	Cooking Fuel	Household cooks with dung, wood, charcoal or coal	1/18
	Sanitation	Sanitation facility is not improved Or is improved but shared with others	1/18
	Drinking Water	No access to improved drinking water Or >30-minute walk round trip	1/18
	Electricity	No electricity	1/18
	Housing	Housing materials for at least one of roof, walls and floor are inadequate*	1/18
	Assets	Household does not own more than one of the assets#	1/18

(*The floor is of natural materials and/or the roof and/or walls are of natural or rudimentary materials) (#Radio, TV, telephone, computer, animal cart, bicycle, motorbike or refrigerator, and does not own a car or truck)

(Child mortality: Any death in last 5 years; Nutrition: Stunting; Years of schooling: Minimum 6 years; School attendance: Up to 8th class)
- **Range of MDPI^Q:** 0 < MDPI < +1
- **MDPI India: 0.069** (2022); 16.4% Poor population
- Interpretation of MDPI: Poor if deprivation in more than 1/3rd of indicators^Q

Deprivation in Indicators	Interpretation
20–33.3%	Vulnerable to poverty
>33%	**Poverty**
>50%	Severe poverty

Key points

Life Expectancy is a 'Positive mortality indicator'

INDICATORS OF HEALTH

Mortality and Morbidity Indicators

Mortality indicators	Morbidity indicators
Crude Death Rate	Incidence & Prevalence
Expectation of Life^Q	Notification Rates
Infant Mortality Rate	Attendance Rates at hospitals, etc.

Contd…

Contd...

Mortality indicators	Morbidity indicators
Child Mortality Rate	Admission, readmission and discharge rates
Under-5 proportionate mortality rate	Duration of hospital stay
Maternal Mortality Rate	Spells of sickness
Proportional Mortality Rate	
Disease-specific Mortality Rate	

- Life Expectancy is a *'Positive mortality indicator'*^{Q}

Sullivan's Index

- *Sullivan's Index* = Life Expectancy MINUS Duration of disability (bed disability and inability to perform major activities)^Q
    - Is known as *'Disability free life expectancy (DFLE^Q)'*

Key points

'Disability free life expectancy', DFLE = Sullivan's Index

Disability Adjusted Life Years [DALYs]

- Is BEST measure of burden of disease in a defined population and the effectiveness of interventions^Q
- It expresses years lost to premature death and years lived with disability (adjusted for its' severity)
- DALYs can measure *'both mortality and disability together'*
- DALY = YLL (Years of lost life) + YLD (Years lost to disability)
- **One DALY = One year of healthy life lost**
- Standards of Life expectancy used: Japan life expectancy statistics.

Key points

DALY is BEST measure of burden of disease in a defined population

Quality Adjusted Life Years (QALYs)

- QALY is a measure of both quality and quantity of life lived
- QALY is years of life lived in perfect health
- QALY is used in assessing the value of money of a medical intervention

Years of Potential Life Lost (YPLL)

- *Definition*: YPLL is based on Years of life lost through premature death
- *Importance*:
    - YPLL occurs before the age to which a dying person could have expected to survive
    - YPLL is a type of mortality indicator

Health Adjusted Life Expectancy (HALE)

- Equivalent number of years in full-health a newborn is expected to live based on current rates of ill-health and mortality in a country
- Based on Life expectancy at birth but adjusted for time spent in poor health
- HALE has replaced DALE (Disability adjusted life expectancy)^Q

Socio-economic Indicators [Mnemonic: He FLAGGED]^Q

- **H**ousing
- **F**amily size
- **L**iteracy rate
- **A**vailability per capita calorie
- **G**NP per capita
- **G**rowth rate
- Un**E**mployment level
- **D**ependency ratio

Case Fatality Rate (CFR)

- CFR represents *'killing power of a disease*$^{Q'}$
- It is *'closely related to virulence of organism*$^{Q'}$

Key points

- CFR represents 'killing power of a disease^Q'
- It is 'closely related to virulence of organism^Q'

- CFR = Total no. of deaths due to a disease/Total no. of cases due to a disease × 100
- *CFR is a Proportion^Q*: Always expressed in percentage
- CFR is the *'complement of Survival Rate'*, thus CFR = 1 – Survival Rate
- CFR of few important diseases:

Diseases	Case fatality rate
Rabies	100%
Yellow fever	80%
Japanese encephalitis	30–35% (median 35%)
Chicken pox	< 1%

- Limitations of CFR^Q:
  - *Time interval is not specified*
  - *Usefulness is limited for chronic diseases (CFR typically used in acute infections)*
  - *CFR for the same disease may vary in different epidemics* due to changes in agent, host and environmental factors

NATURAL HISTORY OF DISEASE

Iceberg Phenomenon of Disease

- *Iceberg Phenomenon of disease*: Disease in a community may be compared to an iceberg
  - *Floating tip*: What physician sees in community (Clinical cases)
  - *Vast submerged portion^Q*: Hidden mass of disease (Latent, inapparent, pre-symptomatic and undiagnosed cases and carriers)
  - *Line of demarcation (water surface)*: Is between apparent and inapparent infections^Q
- *'Epidemiologist is concerned with Hidden portion of iceberg'* whereas Clinician is concerned with Tip of iceberg^Q
- *'Screening is done for Hidden portion of Iceberg'* whereas diagnosis is done for tip of iceberg^Q
- *Iceberg phenomenon of disease is not shown by^Q*:
  - Rabies
  - Tetanus
  - Measles
  - Rubella

Key points

Line of demarcation (water surface): Is between apparent and inapparent infections

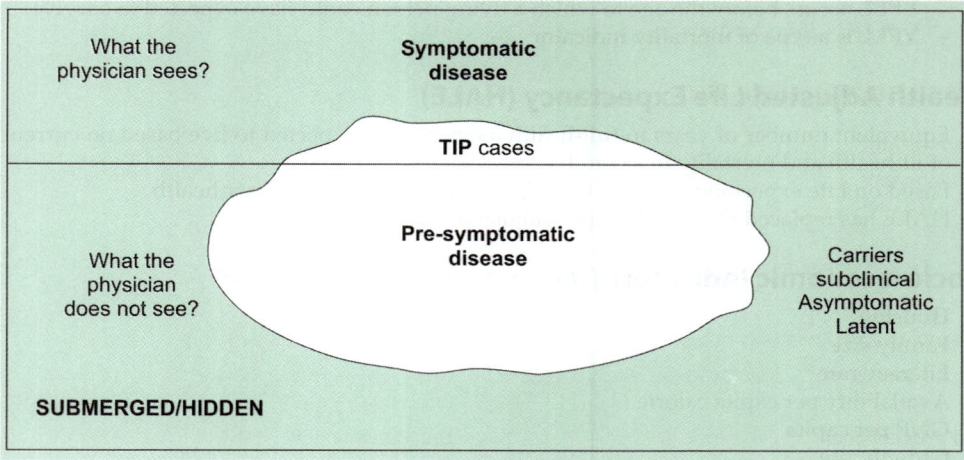

The iceberg of disease

Prepathogenesis Phase of Disease

- Is period before onset of disease in man (man at risk)
- *Epidemiological triad*: Interaction between agent, host and environment^Q
- Primary level of prevention is possible^Q

Key points

Epidemiological triad: Interaction between agent, host and environment

Pathogenesis Phase of Disease

- Begins with: 'Entry of organism' in susceptible host
- Multiplication of organism, disease initiation and progression
- Final outcome may be recovery, disability or death
- Host may become a clinical case, subclinical case or carrier
- Secondary and tertiary levels of prevention are possible^Q
- Screening of disease may improve prognosis and increase survival

CONTROL OF DISEASE

Surveillance

- *Surveillance*: Is the ongoing systematic collection and analysis of data and the provision of information which leads to action being taken to prevent and control a disease, usually one of an infectious nature^Q
- *Surveillance is of many types*:
    1. *Passive Surveillance*: Data is itself reported to the health system
        - Example: A patient with fever coming on his own to the PHC, CHC, Dispensary, Private Practitioner, Hospital
            - Most of the national health programmes in India rely on Passive Surveillance for morbidity and mortality data collection
    2. *Active Surveillance*: Health system seeks out 'actively' the collection of data, i.e., goes out to community to collect data
        - Example: Health worker goes house to house every fortnight to detect fever cases, collect blood slides (under malaria component of National Vector Borne Disease Control Program^Q)
        - *Active Surveillance in National Health Programmes of India*: Is seen in NVBDCP (Health worker goes house to house every fortnight to detect fever cases, collect blood slides and provide presumptive treatment under malaria component), NVBDCP (Kala Azar) and National Leprosy Elimination Programme (Modified Leprosy Elimination Campaigns). NPEP and RNTCP
    3. *Sentinel Surveillance*: Monitoring of rate of occurrence of specific conditions to assess the stability or change in health levels of a population, It is also the study of disease rates in a specific population to estimate trends in larger population
        - Example: Use of health practitioners to monitor trends of a health event in a population
        - Helps in *'identifying missing cases'* and *'supplementing notified cases*^Q*'*
        - Sentinel Surveillance is done in National AIDS Control Program wherein STD Clinics, ANC Clinics are sentinel sites to monitor trends^Q

> **Key points**
> **Sentinel Surveillance**
> Helps in *'identifying missing cases'* and *'supplementing notified cases'*

Monitoring versus Surveillance^Q

Monitoring	Surveillance
Performance and analysis of routine measurements aimed at detecting changes in environment or health status of a population	Continuous scrutiny of the factors that determine the occurrence and distribution of disease and other conditions of ill-health
One Time linear activity	Continuous cycle
No feedback present	Feedback present
No inbuilt action component present	Inbuilt action component present
Stops once disease is eliminated/eradicated	Continues even after disease is eliminated/eradicated
Smaller concept	Broader concept

Disease Control

- Disease control primarily refers to *'Primary and Secondary Levels'* of prevention
- *Sequence of Disease Control*:
    - Disease Control
    - Disease Elimination
    - Disease Eradication

> **Key points**
>
> **Disease elimination:** Is complete interruption of transmission but organism persist in environment

Concepts of Control of Disease

- *Disease control*: Is reducing the transmission of disease agent to such a low level that it ceases to be a public health problem
    - It aims at reducing[Q]:
        - Incidence of the disease
        - Duration of the disease
        - Effects of infection (complications)
        - Financial burden to the community
- *Disease elimination*: Is complete interruption of transmission of disease in a defined geographical area, but the causative organism may be persisting in environment[Q]
    - Disease elimination is a *'geographical term'*, i.e. can be used only for a country or a region
    - **India has eliminated 4 diseases till date:**
        - Guinea worm (Dracunculiasis): February 2000
        - Leprosy: December 2005 (Elimination criterion[Q]: <1/10,000)
        - Yaws: 14 July 2016
        - MT and NNT: 14 July 2016
    - *Next diseases likely to be eliminated from India*: Poliomyelitis, Kala azar, Lymphatic filariasis
- *Disease eradication*: Is complete *'extermination'* of organism[Q]
    - Is *'tearing out by roots'* of a disease[Q]
    - Exhibits *'All or none phenomenon'*[Q]
    - Disease eradication is a *'global term'*, i.e. can be used only for whole planet
        - **World has eradicated ONLY 1 disease till date**: Small pox (declared eradicated on 8 May, 1980[Q])
    - *3 next target diseases for eradication, globally*: Polio, Measles, Guineaworm
    - *Poliovirus 2 was declared eradicated on 20 Sep 2015*

> **Key points**
>
> **Disease eradication:** Is complete *'extermination'* of organism

PREVENTION OF DISEASE

Levels of Prevention

Level	Phase of disease	Objective	Interventions	Targets
Primordial	Underlying conditions lead to causation	Minimize hazards to health	Inhibit emergence of risk conditions	Total population or selected groups
Primary	Specific causal factors	Reduce incidence	Personal and community efforts	Total population, selected groups, individuals
Secondary	Early stages of disease	Shorten duration, Reduce prevalence	Early detection and prompt intervention	Individuals with established disease
Tertiary	Late stages of disease	Reduce no./impact of complications	Lessen impact of long-term disease/disability, minimize suffering	Patients

Primordial Level of Prevention

- It is the *prevention of the emergence or development of risk factors* in countries or population groups in which they have not yet appeared[Q]
- *Modes of Intervention*:
    - **Individual Education**
    - **Mass Education**
- Is primary prevention (see below) in purest sense
- Primordial Level is *Best level of prevention for Non-communicable diseases*[Q]

> **Key points**
>
> **Primordial prevention**
> It is the *prevention of the emergence or development of risk factors*

Primary Level of Prevention

- It is the *action taken prior to onset of disease*, which removes the possibility that a disease will ever occur[Q]
- *Modes of Intervention*[Q]:
    - **Health Promotion**: Is targeted at strengthening the host through a variety of approaches/ interventions
    - Example: Health Education, Environmental modifications, Nutritional interventions, Lifestyle and behavioral changes

> **Key points**
>
> **Primary level of prevention** is applied when *'risk factors are present but disease has not yet taken place'*

- *Specific Protection*: Is targeting the prevention of disease through a specific intervention
- Example: Contraception, Vaccines
• Primary level of prevention is applied when *'risk factors are present but disease has not yet taken place'*
• It signifies *'intervention in the Pre-pathogenesis Phase of a disease/health problem^Q'*

Secondary Level of Prevention

• It *halts the progress of disease at its' incipient stage and prevents complications^Q*
• Modes of Intervention^Q:
  - **Early Diagnosis**: Detection of disturbances while biochemical, functional and morphological changes are still reversible or prior to occurrence of manifest signs and symptoms
    ▪ Examples: Sputum smear exam for AFB, P/S for MP
  - **Treatment**: Shortens period of communicability, reduces mortality and prevents occurrence of further cases (secondary cases) or any long term disability
    ▪ Example: DOTS, MDT
• *Secondary level of prevention is applied when disease has possibly set in*: It attempts to arrest the disease process, seek unrecognized disease and treat it before irreversibility and reverse communicability of infectious diseases
• National Health Programmes by Govt. of India mostly operate at Secondary level of prevention^Q
• *Secondary prevention is an imperfect tool in control of transmission of disease*: It is more expensive and less effective than primary prevention
• It is an important level of prevention for diseases like Tuberculosis, Leprosy and STDs

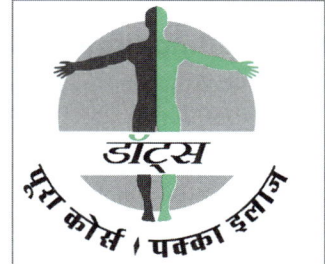
DOTS Secondary level

> **Key points**
>
> **Secondary prevention**
> It *halts the progress of disease at its' incipient stage and prevents complications*

> **Key points**
>
> **Tertiary level of prevention** signifies *'intervention in late pathogenesis phase'*

Tertiary Level of Prevention

• Is applied when *disease has advanced beyond early stages*: It aims to reduce or limit impairments and disabilities, minimize suffering caused by existing departures from good health
• Modes of Intervention^Q:
  - **Disability Limitation**: It *'prevents the transition of disease from impairment to handicap'*
    ▪ Example: Physiotherapy in Poliomyelitis
  - **Rehabilitation**: Training and retraining of an individual to the highest possible level of functional ability; it can be medical, vocational, social or psychological
    ▪ *Example*: Crutches in Poliomyelitis
• Tertiary level of prevention signifies *'intervention in late pathogenesis phase'*

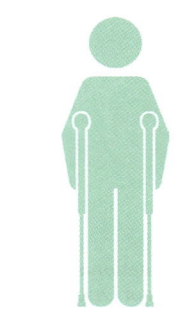
Crutches-Tertiary level

Examples of Levels of Prevention^Q

• *A patient with fever and cough >3 weeks comes to DOTS Clinic for 'Sputum for AFB'*: Early diagnosis mode of intervention, *Secondary Level* of Prevention (as disease has possibly set in and sputum for AFB is used to confirm it as a case of tuberculosis)
• *A patient with Sputum +ve for AFB was categorized as Category I under RNTCP and started with Intensive Phase drugs*: Treatment mode of intervention, *Secondary Level* of prevention (as disease has been diagnosed and now treatment has been started)
• *A patient with fever and chills comes to Malaria Clinic for 'Peripheral Smear for MP'*: Early diagnosis mode of intervention, *Secondary Level* of prevention (as disease has possibly set in and peripheral smear for malarial parasite is used to confirm it as a case of Malaria)
• *A patient with fever and chills comes to Malaria Clinic and was given Presumptive Treatment/Radical Treatment*: Treatment mode of intervention, *Secondary Level* of prevention (as disease has possibly set in and now treatment has been started)
• *A person sleeps inside a bednet*: Specific Protection mode of intervention, *Primary Level* of prevention (risk factors, i.e., mosquitoes are already present, disease has not yet taken place)
• *A child coming to Immunization clinic for OPV Vaccine*: Specific Protection mode of intervention, *Primary Level* of prevention (risk factors, i.e., polio infection already present, disease has not yet taken place)
• *A Urine strip for sugar detection was employed to screen diabetics in a community*: Early diagnosis mode of intervention, *Secondary Level* of prevention (screening is meant for early diagnosis of a disease)

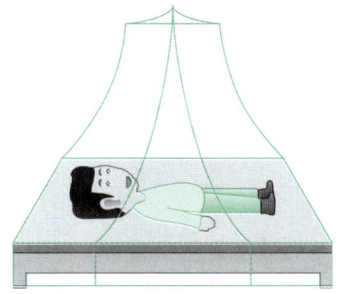
Mosquito nets–Primary level

- *A village community was given health education to prevent spread of malaria*: *Health Promotion* mode of intervention, *Primary Level* of prevention (to enable/strengthen the host)
- *A 20-year-old male takes chemoprophylaxis during an epidemic of Meningococcal meningitis*: *Specific Protection* mode of intervention, *Primary Level* of prevention (risk factors, i.e., epidemic of meningococcal meningitis is already present; disease has not yet taken place in that male)
- *A class of 5-year-old children is discouraged from adopting harmful lifestyles, smoking, etc.*: *Primordial Level* of prevention (intervention before emergence of risk factors)
- *A child afflicted with poliomyelitis is given crutches to walk*: *Rehabilitation* mode of intervention, *Tertiary Level* of prevention

Disease-Impairment-Disability-Handicap

- *Disease*: Any abnormal condition of an organism that impairs function
- *Impairment*: Any loss or abnormality of psychological, physiological or anatomical structure or function
- *Disability*: (Because of impairment,) any restriction or inability to perform an activity in a range considered normal for a human being
- *Handicap*: A disadvantage for a given individual, resulting from an impairment/disability, that limits/prevents fulfillment of a role considered normal (depending on age, sex, social, cultural factors) for that individual

For Example,

Event	Classification	Interpretation^Q
Accident	*Disease*	Impairs function of a person
Loss of foot	*Impairment*	Loss of anatomical structure in the form of foot
Cannot Walk	*Disability*	Walking is a normal routine daily activity of a human being
Unemployed	*Handicap*	Loses out his job because he cannot walk, so cannot fulfill his role in the society, i.e., earning for his family members

ICD-10, ICD-11

International Classification of Diseases, 10th Revision/Edition [ICD-10]^Q

> **Key points**
> **ICD-10**: International Statistical Classification of Disease

- ICD-10 is an abbreviation for the International Statistical Classification of Disease and Related Health Problems (10th revision)
  - Uniform classification for morbidity and mortality data in world
  - International standard diagnostic classification for all general epidemiological and many health management purposes
  - ICD is revised every 10 years
- *ICD-10 came in 1993*: It covers disease, illnesses and injuries
- ICD-10 is arranged in 22 chapters^Q (ICD-10-CM has 21 chapters)

International Classification of Diseases, 11th Revision/Edition [ICD-11]

- Released: June 2018 (WHO)
- Composition: **3 Volumes, 26 Chapters** with V, X^Q
- Three volumes:
- Tabular List (Volume 1)
  - Reference Guide (Volume 2)
  - Alphabetical Index (Volume 3)
- 26 Chapters:
  - 01 Certain infectious or parasitic diseases
  - 02 Neoplasms
  - 03 Diseases of the blood or blood-forming organs
  - 04 Diseases of the immune system
  - 05 Endocrine, nutritional or metabolic diseases
  - **06 Mental, behavioural or neurodevelopmental disorders**^Q
  - 07 Sleep-wake disorders

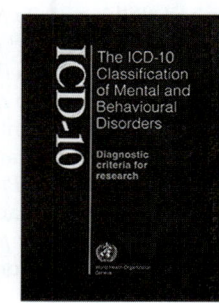
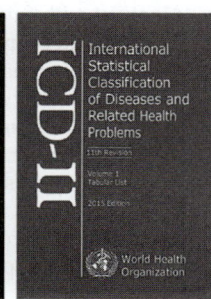

- 08 Diseases of the nervous system
- 09 Diseases of the visual system
- 10 Diseases of the ear or mastoid process
- 11 Diseases of the circulatory system
- 12 Diseases of the respiratory system
- 13 Diseases of the digestive system
- 14 Diseases of the skin
- 15 Diseases of the musculoskeletal system or connective tissue
- 16 Diseases of the genitourinary system
- 17 Conditions related to sexual health
- 18 Pregnancy, childbirth or the puerperium
- 19 Certain conditions originating in the perinatal period
- 20 Developmental anomalies
- 21 Symptoms, signs or clinical findings, not elsewhere classified^Q
- 22 Injury, poisoning or certain other consequences of external causes
- 23 External causes of morbidity or mortality
- 24 Factors influencing health status or contact with health services
- 25 Codes for special purposes
- **26 Traditional Medicine conditions - Module I**^{Q}
- **V Supplementary section for functioning assessment**^{Q}
- **X Extension Codes**^{Q}
- Advantages over ICD-10:
  - Reflects current medical terminology and information needs
  - Functions in digital and electronic health record (EHR) environments
  - More comprehensive for use in broader clinical settings and enables greater international comparability, with no country-specific versions
- ICD-11 Linkage to other data standards
  - International Classification of Functioning, Disability and Health (ICF)
  - International Classification of Health Interventions (ICHI)
  - SNOMED-CT

MISCELLANEOUS

Time Distribution of Disease
- Short term fluctuations
- Long term fluctuations
- Periodic fluctuations

> **Key points**
> *Epidemic*: Occurrence of no. of cases of a disease '*clearly in excess of normal expectancy*'.

Short-term Fluctuations (Epidemic)
- *Definitions*:
  - Occurrence of no. of cases of a disease 'clearly in excess of normal expectancy [NE]$^{Q'}$

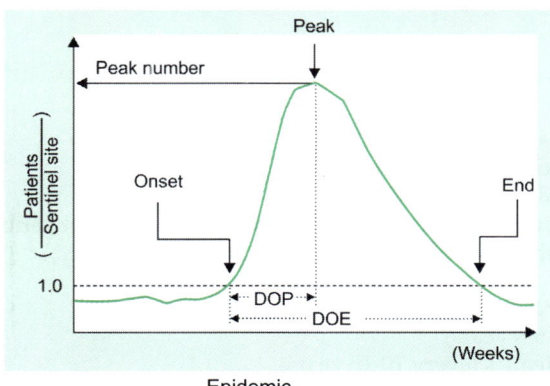

Epidemic

- Normal expectancy is derived by looking at average of no. of cases of the disease in previous 3-5 years in that geographical area

- If NE = zero, 'even one case is considered epidemic'
- Statistically speaking, epidemic is when no. of cases *'exceed twice the standard deviation'*
  - No. of cases > Mean + 2SD^Q
- Occurrence of a new disease in a population (as NE = Zero)
- Reoccurrence of an eliminated/eradicated disease in a population (as NE = Zero)
- *Types of epidemics*:
  - *Common-source epidemics*:
    - Single exposure or 'Point source' epidemics
    - Continuous or multiple exposure epidemics
  - *Propagated epidemics*:
    - Person-to-person
    - Arthropod vector
    - Animal reservoir
  - Slow (modern) epidemics

Periodic Fluctuations

> **Key points**
> *Seasonal trends:* Is due to vector variation, environmental factors and change in herd immunity

- *Seasonal trends*: Is seasonal variation/fluctuation in occurrence of a disease:
  - Is due to vector variation, environmental factors and change in herd immunity^Q

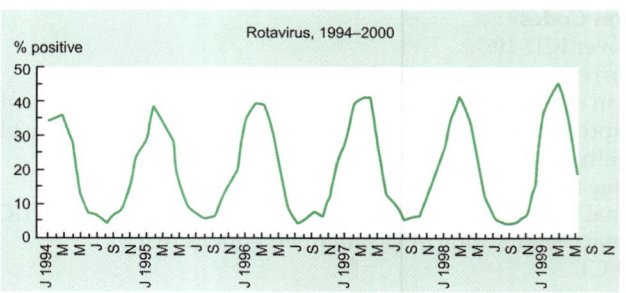

Seasonal trend

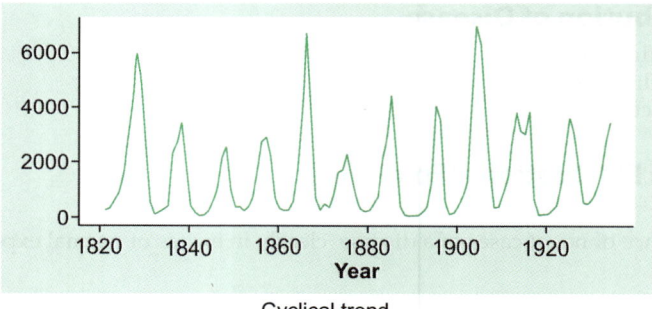

Cyclical trend

> **Key points**
> *Cyclical trends:*
> - Measles (every 2-3 years)
> - Rubella (every 6-9 years)

  - Examples:
    - Measles (early spring)
    - Upper respiratory infections (winters)
    - Gastrointestinal infections (summers)
- *Cyclical trends*: Is occurrence of a disease in cycles spread over short periods of time, which may be days, weeks, months or years:
  - Examples^Q:
    - Measles (every 2-3 years)
    - Rubella (every 6-9 years)
    - Influenza pandemics (every 10-15 years)

Long-term Fluctuations [Secular Trends]

- Implies changes in occurrence of a disease (progressive increase or decrease) over a long period of time, generally several years or decades^Q
  - Is the consistent tendency to change in a particular direction or a definite movement in one direction^Q
- *Examples:*
  - Communicable diseases (Poliomyelitis, Diphtheria, Pertussis) are reducing in India in past few decades
  - Non-communicable diseases (Diabetes, Hypertension, Obesity) are increasing in India in past few decades.

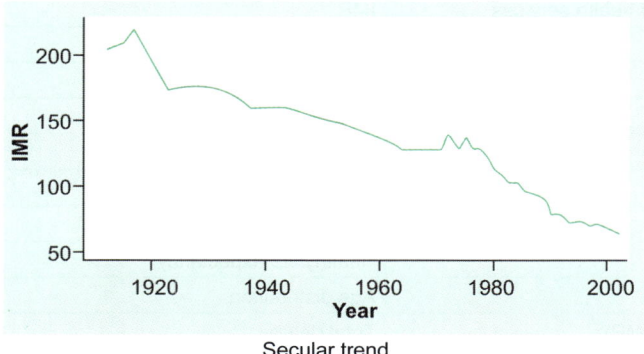

Secular trend

PYQs: Quick Review for NEET

Health & Disease	
Health - "State of complete physical, social & mental wellbeing" defined by	WHO
"Epidemiological Triad" comprises of	Agent, Host and Environment
Extermination of organism is	Eradication
Missing cases of a disease are detected by	Sentinel surveillance
Routine surveillance is supplemented by	Sentinel surveillance
Watching with attention, authority, suspicion is	Surveillance
Ivory Towers of Disease	Large Hospitals
A child 'lost' his hands, unable to do routine work is called	Disability
Disease elimination is	Interruption of transmission from large areas
Bhopal gas tragedy is _____ type of Epidemic	Single exposure Point source epidemic
Millennium development goals aim to reduce MMR by	3/4th
Limit for registration of birth is	21 days
In India death has to be registered with in	21 days
Only disease which is eradicated worldwide	Small pox
Incubation period is defined as	From receipt of infection to clinical feature
Infected person harbouring infectious agent without clinical features	Carrier
Line in Death certificate representing Direct cause of death	Line Ia
Epidemic is	Short term fluctuation
Cyclical trend is shown by	Measles, Rubella, Influenza

Contd...

Contd...

Indicators & Indices	
HDI comprises	Knowledge (Literacy and Mean years of schooling), Income and Longevity (Life Expectancy at Birth)
HDI of India is	0.640 (Rank 130)
PQLI stands for	Physical quality of life index
PQLI lies between	0-100
Gender developmental index is	Corrected development index as per gender inequalities
Life Expectancy is a type of _____ Indicator	Mortality Indicator (Positive Health Indicator)
Best indicator of availability, utilization, effectiveness of health services	IMR
Most important health status indicator of a country	Infant mortality rate
One DALY signifies	One lost year of healthy life
DALY is	Disability Adjusted Life year
DALE has been replaced by	HALE
Bed: Population ratio in India is	0.5 per 1000
Disability free life expectancy is measured by	Sullivan's index
HALE is used to measure	Healthy life expectancy
Standardization is most important for	Age distribution
Denominator in Under 5 proportional mortality rate (U5MR)	Total deaths
Levels of Prevention	
Following traditional lifestyles for CHD _____ level of prevention	Primordial level
Disability limitation is a type of	Tertiary level of prevention
Psychotherapy is _____ level of prevention	Secondary
Screening of the diseases is _____ prevention	Secondary
Health promotion is prevention level	Primary level
Preventive action taken prior to onset of disease is	Primary Prevention
Early Diagnosis and Treatment are _____ level of prevention	Secondary Prevention
Halts disease in incipient stage & prevent complications	Secondary level of prevention
Prevention of emergence of risk factor is	Primordial prevention
School health checkup comes under	Secondary level of prevention
Immunize a child for measles is	Primary level (Specific protection)
Level of prevention that includes Specific protection	Primary
Not performing anatomical/physiological/psychological function	Impairment
Target group in Secondary prevention	Individuals with established disease
Pasteurization of milk is a type of ____ prevention	Primary prevention
ICD-10	
ICD-10 Classification is for classification of	Diseases
ICD-10 classification is revised every	10 years
ICD-10 is a	Multiaxial system
Number of chapters in ICD-10	22
Chapter-14 in ICD-10 is related to	Disease of Genitourinary system

Concepts of Health and Disease 99

Multiple Choice Questions

HEALTH AND WELL-BEING

1. Definition of health given by WHO includes which of the following dimensions? *[PGI Dec 01]*
   (a) Social *[NEET Pattern 2017]*
   (b) Physical
   (c) Mental
   (d) Emotional
   (e) Economic

2. Standard of Living (WHO) includes all *except*:
   (a) Income *[AIPGME 2006]*
   (b) Sanitation and nutrition
   (c) Level of provision of health
   (d) Human rights

3. Ottawa Charter of health promotion incorporates all of the following key action areas *except*: *[PGMCET 2015]*
   (a) Build healthy public policy
   (b) Strengthen community action for health
   (c) Build social security system
   (d) Reorient health services

4. Biomedical concept of health is based on:
   (a) Germ theory of disease *[NEET Pattern 2016]*
   (b) Absence of pain
   (c) Social and psychological factors
   (d) Equilibrium between man and environment

5. All are true of 'Positive health' in today's world *except*:
   [NEET Pattern 2015]
   (a) Dependent on social, economic and culture
   (b) Mirage because of changing environment
   (c) Body and mind at peace
   (d) Changing behavior with respect to change in future

HDI AND PQLI

6. Human development index includes:
   [INICET November 2021]
   (a) LE at 1 year, Income, Literacy rate
   (b) LE at birth, Decent living standard, Knowledge
   (c) LE at 1 year, Income, Decent living standard
   (d) IMR, Decent living standard, Knowledge

7. Human developmental index includes all *except*:
   [JIPMER May 2019]
   (a) Adult literacy rate
   (b) Per capita income
   (c) Life expectancy
   (d) Infant mortality rate

8. Human Development Index does not include:
   [AIPGME 2011, DNB 2003, Kolkata 2004, Karnataka 2007, MP 2005, AI 2000, MH 2007, MH 2002, MH 2006, AP 2008, JIPMER 2001, NEET Pattern 2017]
   (a) Mean years of schooling *[AIPGME 1999]*
   (b) Life expectancy at age 1 *[AIIMS May 01, May 05]*
   (c) Real GDP per capita *[NEET Patterns 2014]*
   (d) Adult literacy rate

9. The Physical Quality of the Life Index considers:
   [AIIMS May 2006, AIIMS Nov 2006, AIPGME 2000, 06, 07, AIIMS Nov 06, Karnataka 2011, NEET Pattern 2013, Karnataka 2006, 2008, PGI 2008, 2001, DNB 2002, 2005, Bihar 2003, UP 2004, AP 1996, 2005, MP 2000, RJ 2005]
   I. Expectancy of life at birth
   II. Expectancy of life at age one
   III. Infant mortality rate
   IV. Literacy rate
   Of these components:
   (a) I alone is correct
   (b) I, III and IV are correct
   (c) I, II and III are correct
   (d) II, III and IV are correct

10. Minimum and Maximum Values established for calculation of Life Expectancy index in HDI are:
    (a) 0 years and 65 years *[AIPGME 2007]*
    (b) 0 years and 85 years *[NEET Pattern 2013]*
    (c) 25 years and 85 years
    (d) 0 years and 100 years

11. Human Development Index values range between:
    [AIIMS Jan 2003]
    (a) –1 to +1   (b) 0 to 1
    (c) 0 to 3   (d) 1 to 3

12. Poverty index does not include deprivation of
    (a) Health *[DNB June 2010]*
    (b) Knowledge
    (c) Standard of living
    (d) Income

13. PQLI lies between: *[NEET Patterns 2014, 2017]*
    (a) 0 and 1   (b) 0 and 10
    (c) 0 and 100   (d) 1 and 10

14. PQLI is: *[NEET Pattern 2017]*
    (a) Objective component of level of living
    (b) Subjective component of level of living
    (c) Objective component of quality of life
    (d) Subjective component of quality of life

INDICATORS OF HEALTH

15. Best indicator used to assess health status of a given community, and for assessment of availability and utilization of health services is: *[NEET PG Pattern 2023]*
    - (a) DALY
    - (b) IMR
    - (c) MMR
    - (d) U5MR

16. Life span of Japanese women is 84.3 years. As Japanese have longest life expectancy, their life expectancy statistics are used as a standard for measuring premature death in: *[NEET PG Pattern 2022]*
    - (a) HALE
    - (b) QALY
    - (c) DFLE
    - (d) DALY

17. Which of the following is a Mortality Indicator?
    - (a) Life Expectancy *[AIIMS May 1993]*
    - (b) Notification Rate
    - (c) DALY
    - (d) Bed turn-over ratio

18. Expectation of life, free of disability is known as:
    - (a) Park's index *[AIPGME 2006]*
    - (b) Smith's index *[UP 2005]*
    - (c) Sullivan's index *[DNB 2008]*
    - (d) Life index

19. Which is the best index for burden of disease and effectivenss of interventions? *[AIIMS June 1997]*
    - (a) Case fatality rate *[AIIMS Nov 2001]*
    - (b) Disability adjusted life years
    - (c) Dependency ratio
    - (d) Morbidity data

20. Which one of the following is NOT a socioeconomic indicator? *[AIIMS Dec 1997]*
    - (a) Literacy rate
    - (b) Family size
    - (c) Housing
    - (d) Life expectancy at birth

21. Most universally accepted indicator of health status of whole population and their socioeconomic conditions among the following is: *[AIIMS Nov 2001]*
    - (a) MMR
    - (b) IMR
    - (c) Life expectancy
    - (d) Disease notification rates

22. Sullivan index indicates: *[AIIMS Dec 1994]*
    - (a) Life free of disability
    - (b) Hookworm eggs/gm of stool
    - (c) Standard of living
    - (d) Pregnancy rate per HWY

23. Which of the following is true about DALYs?
    - (a) Life is adjusted for disease *[AIPGME 2012]*
    - (b) Premature death is adjusted for disability *[NEET Pattern 2012]*
    - (c) Life expectancy free of disability
    - (d) Years lost to premature death and years lived with disability adjusted for severity of disability

24. In a village with population of 5000, 50 people have a disease and 10 of them died. What is case fatality rate?
    - (a) 1% *[NEET Patterns 2013, 2017]*
    - (b) 2% *[DNB December 2009]*
    - (c) 0.5%
    - (d) 20%

25. For optimum utilization of health services in a hospital, Bed turnover interval should always be *[JIPMER 2014]*
    - (a) Slightly positive
    - (b) Largely positive
    - (c) Slightly negative
    - (d) Largely negative

26. All of the following are Utilization rates *except*: *[NEET Patterns 2016, 2017]*
    - (a) Population bed ratio
    - (b) Bed occupancy rate
    - (c) Bed turnover ratio
    - (d) Average length of stay

27. Which is not a mortality indicator? *[NEET Pattern 2015]*
    - (a) Years of potential life lost
    - (b) Life expectancy
    - (c) IMR
    - (d) Prevalence

28. Health indicator characteristics include all *except*: *[NEET Pattern 2017]*
    - (a) Alidity
    - (b) Reliability
    - (c) Affordability
    - (d) Feasibility

29. DALY measures: *[NEET Pattern 2017]*
    - (a) Morbidity & mortality
    - (b) Morbidity & disability
    - (c) Mortality & disability
    - (d) None of the above

30. A city with 800 deaths per year. Mortuary, body stored for average duration of 8 days with 80% occupancy in a year. What number of mortuary beds needed? *[JIPMER November 2017]*
    - (a) 22
    - (b) 17
    - (c) 7
    - (d) 34

Review Questions

31. Which of the following is best to compare the vital statistics of countries? *[MH 2007]*
    - (a) Crude death and birth rates
    - (b) Age standardized death rate
    - (c) Age specific death rate
    - (d) Proportional mortality rate

32. **Disability adjusted life year (DALY) Expresses the:**
    [NEET Pattern 2017] [R] 2006]
    (a) Extent of disability in the population
    (b) Expectation of life free of disability
    (c) Years of life lost to premature death
    (d) Lost year of life due to premature death and disability

NATURAL HISTORY OF DISEASE

33. **Match the following stages with their relevant descriptions:** [INICET November 2022]

1. Pre-pathogenesis	A.	Normal course without any intervention
2. Pathogenesis	B.	Appearance of clinical signs and symptoms
3. Natural history of a disease	C.	Reaching normalcy to best functional ability
4. Rehabilitation	D.	Period before the onset of the disease

    (a) 1-C, 2-D, 3-A, 4-D
    (b) 1-D, 2-B, 3-A, 4-C
    (c) 1-B, 2-D, 3-C, 4-D
    (d) 1-A, 2-C, 3-D, 4-B

34. **'Silent epidemic' of the century is:** [AIPGME 02]
    (a) Coronary artery disease
    (b) Chronic liver disease
    (c) Chronic obstructive lung disease
    (d) Alzheimer's disease

35. **Which one of the following does not represent the submerged portion of the iceberg?**
    (a) Diagnosed cases under treatment
    (b) Undiagnosed cases [AIIMS Jan 1999, Feb 1997]
    (c) Pre-symptomatic cases
    (d) Carriers sub clinical cases
    (e) Latent & Healthy population

36. **Which of the following is NOT true regarding pathogenesis of a disease?** [AIPGME 2012]
    (a) Screening is of no use in changing course of disease
    (b) Tertiary prevention is possible
    (c) Entry of organism occurs
    (d) Includes subclinical cases

37. **Web of causation of disease, which statement is most appropriate?** [NEET Pattern 2013]
    (a) Mostly applicable for common diseases
    (b) Requires complete understanding of all factors associated with causation of disease
    (c) Epidemiological ratio
    (d) Helps to suggest ways to interrupt the risk of transmission

38. **Transition from increased prevalence of infectious pandemic diseases to manmade disease is known as:**
    (a) Paradoxical transition [AIIMS November 2012]
    (b) Reversal of transition
    (c) Epidemiological transition
    (d) Demographic transition

39. **Triangle of Epidemiology stands for:** [NEET Pattern 2017]
    (a) Interaction of agent, host & environment
    (b) Interaction of agent, host, environment & time
    (c) Interaction & interdependence of agent, host, environment & time
    (d) None of the above

Review Questions

40. **Epidemiological triad are all included *except*:**
    [UP 2000], [NEET Patterns 2014], [R] 2000]
    (a) Host   (b) Environmental factors
    (c) Agent   (d) Investigator

41. **The period preliminary to the onset of disease in man, when the disease agent has not yet entered man but the factors favouring its interaction with human host exist in the environment is known as:** [MP 2006]
    (a) Incubation period
    (b) Pre-pathogenesis period
    (c) Pathogenesis period
    (d) Pre-symptomatic period

CONTROL OF DISEASE

42. **Measures involved in sentinel surveillance includes all of the following *except*:**
    [DNB 2008, AIPGME 2001, AIIMS Nov 1999]
    (a) Identifying missing cases in notification of diseases
    (b) Identifying new cases of infection
    (c) Identifying old and new cases
    (d) Identifying cases free of disability

43. **Consider the following statements:**
    The term 'disease control' describes ongoing operations aimed at reducing the [AIIMS November 2014]
    1. Incidence of disease [AIPGME 2002]
    2. Financial burden to the community
    3. Effects of infection including both physical and psychological complications
    4. Duration of disease and its transmission **of these statements,**
    (a) 1, 2 and 3 are correct
    (b) 1, 3 and 4 are correct
    (c) 1, 2 and 4 are correct
    (d) 1, 2, 3 and 4 are correct

44. **All of the following statements about eradication programme are true *except*:** [AIPGME 1995]
    (a) There is complete interruption of disease transmission in the entire area of the community
    (b) Eradication programme is over once the disease has been certified as having been eradicated

(c) Case finding is of secondary importance
(d) The objective is to eliminate the disease to the extent that no new case occurs in the future

45. Continuous scrutiny of factors that determine the occurrence and distribution of disease and other condition of ill health is the definition of: [AIPGME 1996]
    (a) Monitoring   (b) Surveillance
    (c) Disease control (d) System analysis

46. Disease eliminated from India is/are: [PGI June 08]
    (a) Small pox
    (b) Guinea worm disease
    (c) Yaws, Leprosy and Neonatal Tetanus
    (d) Measles
    (e) Polio

47. Candidate(s) for global eradication by WHO:
    (a) Malaria [PGI June 01]
    (b) Dracunculiasis
    (c) Polio
    (d) Measles
    (e) Chicken pox

48. Disease eradicated from world: [PGI June 03]
    (a) Small pox   (b) Guineworm
    (c) Polio   (d) Diphtheria
    (e) Measles

49. Causative agent is present but there is no transmission is known as: [AIPGME 2012]
    (a) Elimination   (b) Control
    (c) Eradication   (d) Holoendemic

50. Disease elimination is helped by: [NEET Pattern 2013]
    (a) Herd immunity   (b) Isolation
    (c) Quarantine   (d) None

51. Analysis of routine measurement is aimed at detecting changes in environment: [NEET Pattern 2012] [NEET Pattern 2013]
    (a) Monitoring   (b) Surveillance
    (c) Isolation   (d) Evaluation

52. All of the following are eradicable diseases except:
    (a) Tuberculosis   (b) Guineaworm
    (c) Poliomyelitis   (d) Measles

53. Surveillance actual targets: [NEET Pattern 2015]
    (a) Prevent disease (b) Health planning
    (c) Disease eradication (d) Disease monitoring

Review Questions

54. Disease elimination refers to: [MP 2007]
    (a) Extinction of disease agent
    (b) Termination of all disease
    (c) Global removal of disease agent
    (d) Regional removal of disease agent

55. In India which disease is near to elimination: [RJ 2003]
    (a) Tetanus   (b) Rabies
    (c) Polio   (d) Mumps

PREVENTION OF DISEASE

56. Which of the following does not include Specific protection under Primary prevention? [AIIMS November 2019]
    (a) Tab Rifampicin to those in contact with meningitis
    (b) Health education
    (c) Pentavalent vaccination
    (d) Wheat flour fortified with added iron

57. All of the following represent Specific protection mode of Disease prevention except: [AIPGME 2000]
    (a) Chemoprophylaxis for meningococcal meningitis
    (b) Personal hygiene and Environmental sanitation
    (c) Usage of condoms
    (d) Iodisation of salt

58. Secondary level of prevention include all of the following except: [AIIMS Jan 2000]
    (a) Health screening for Diabetes Mellitus
    (b) Case finding for Falciparum Malaria
    (c) Contact tracing for STIs
    (d) Reconstructive Surgery in Leprosy

59. In a population to prevent coronary artery disease changing harmful lifestyles by education is referred to as: [AIIMS May 2001]
    (a) High risk strategy (b) Primary prevention
    (c) Secondary prevention (d) Tertiary prevention

60. In an area with fluoride rich water, the defluoridation of water is which level of prevention? [AIIMS May 1994]
    (a) Primary   (b) Secondary
    (c) Tertiary   (d) Primordial

61. Which of the following is primordial prevention? [AIIMS May 1994]
    (a) Action taken prior to the onset of disease
    (b) Prevention of emergence of development of risk factors
    (c) Action taken to remove the possibility that a disease will ever occur
    (d) Action that halts the progress of a disease

62. 'Disability Limitation' is mode of intervention for:
    (a) Primordial Prevention [AIIMS May 2008]
    (b) Primary Prevention [NEET Pattern 2013]
    (c) Secondary Prevention
    (d) Tertiary Prevention

63. Which of the following is the most logical sequence? [AIIMS Nov 2006] [NEET Pattern 2013]
    (a) Impairment-Disease-Disability-Handicap
    (b) Disease-Impairment-Disability-Handicap
    (c) Disease-Impairment-Handicap-Disability
    (d) Disease-Handicap-Impairment-Disability

64. **Pap smear test for detection of carcinoma of cervix is which level of prevention?** *[Karnataka 2007] [NEET Patterns 2014]*
    (a) Primordial (b) Primary
    (c) Secondary (d) Tertiary

65. **A person who has lost his foot in an accident and is not able to walk is an example of:** *[Karnataka 2007]*
    (a) Disease (b) Disability
    (c) Impairment (d) Handicap

66. **Primary prevention of obesity:** *[DPG 1998]*
    (a) Low fiber diet (b) High fiber diet
    (c) High cholesterol diet (d) High intake of protein

67. **Primordial prevention in coronary heart disease:**
    (a) Exercise in high risk area *[PGI Dec 1997]*
    (b) BP monitoring
    (c) Salt restriction
    (d) Statins
    (e) TMT

68. **Primary prevention of dental caries includes:**
    (a) Fluoridation *[PGI June 03, [PGI Dec 03]*
    (b) Dental health education
    (c) Mass screening
    (d) Dental fitting
    (e) Teeth extraction

69. **Primary prevention:** *[PGI June 05]*
    (a) Marriage counseling
    (b) Early diagnosis and treatment
    (c) Pap smear
    (d) Self breast examination
    (e) Immunization

70. **Vitamin A prophylaxis to a child is:** *[AIIMS May 2010] [NEET Pattern 2017]*
    (a) Health promotion
    (b) Specific protection
    (c) Primordial prevention
    (d) Secondary prevention

71. **Which of the following is not a primary prevention strategy?** *[DNB December 2011]*
    (a) Breast self examination
    (b) Control of tobacco
    (c) Radiation protection
    (d) Cancer education

72. **CAD primordial prevention is by:** *[NEET Pattern 2013]*
    (a) Lifestyle change (b) Coronary bypass
    (c) Treatment of CAD (d) None

73. **Immunization is:** *[NEET Pattern 2013, 2014]*
    (a) Primary prevention (b) Secondary prevention
    (c) Tertiary prevention (d) Disability limitation

74. **Iodized salt in iodine deficiency control programme is:**
    (a) Primary prevention *[NEET Pattern 2012]*
    (b) Secondary prevention
    (c) Tertiary prevention
    (d) Primordial prevention

75. **Target group in Secondary prevention:** *[NEET Pattern 2012]*
    (a) Healthy individuals (b) Patients
    (c) Animals (d) Children

76. **Desks provided with table top to prevent neck problems is an example of:** *[DNB December 2010] [NEET Pattern 2014]*
    (a) Primordial prevention
    (b) Primary prevention
    (c) Specific protection
    (d) Disability limitation

77. **Monitoring of blood pressure which type of prevention:** *[NEET Pattern 2014]*
    (a) Primordial (b) Primary
    (c) Secondary (d) Tertiary

78. **All of the following comes under primary prevention except:** *[NEET Pattern 2014]*
    (a) Pap smear (b) Helmets
    (c) Contraception (d) Vaccines

79. **Which of the following is an example of primary prevention?** *[PGMCET 2015]*
    (a) Measles immunization
    (b) Cervical cytology screening
    (c) Smoking cessation after a heart attack
    (d) Self examination of breast for lumps

80. **Consider the following**
    1. Health Education
    2. Treatment of hypertension
    3. Screening for cervical cancer
    4. Changing lifestyles to prevent stress
    Which are the examples of primary prevention? *[UPSC CMS 2015]*
    (a) 1 and 4 (b) 2 and 3
    (c) 1 and 3 (d) 2 and 4

81. **Example of disability limitation:** *[NEET Pattern 2015]*
    (a) DOTS
    (b) Quit smoking
    (c) BCG vaccine
    (d) Spectacles for refractory error

82. **National Iron Plus Initiative is an example of:**
    (a) Primordial prevention *[NEET Pattern 2016]*
    (b) Primary prevention
    (c) Secondary prevention
    (d) Tertiary prevention

83. **Primordial prevention in Myocardial infarction are all except:** *[NEET Pattern 2017]*
    (a) Maintenance of normal body weight
    (b) Preservation of life style
    (c) Primitive nutritional habits
    (d) Screening for hypertension

84. Primary prevention of Hypertension includes?
    (a) Weight reduction   [PGI May 2018]
    (b) Dietary salt reduction
    (c) Exercise promotion
    (d) Early diagnosis
    (e) Antihypertensive drugs

85. Installation and usage of Sanitary latrines by General public constitutes which level of prevention
                                            [NEET Pattern 2018]
    (a) Health promotion
    (b) Specific protection
    (c) Early diagnosis and treatment
    (d) Disability limitation and rehabilitation

86. Best level of prevention for Breast cancer
                                            [NEET Pattern 2019]
    (a) Specific protection
    (b) Early diagnosis and treatment
    (c) Disability limitation
    (d) Rehabilitation

Review Questions

87. All are health promotion strategies *except*:
    (a) Insecticides spray   [Kerala 2001] [UP 2004]
    (b) Potable safe water supply
    (c) Life style modification
    (d) Chemoprophylaxis

88. One of the following is an example for tertiary prevention: [AP 2000]
    (a) Vaccination
    (b) Immediate diagnosis and treatment
    (c) Rehabilitation
    (d) Health education

89. Action which halts the progress of a disease at its incipient stage and prevents complications: [AP 2004]
    (a) Primary prevention
    (b) Primordial prevention
    (c) Secondary prevention
    (d) Tertiary prevention

90. The following does not determine specific protection:
    (a) Pap smear for early detection of carcinoma cervix in community   [AP 2005]
    (b) Wearing of goggles by welders
    (c) Wearing of seat belts by car drivers
    (d) Vitamin A for children prophylaxis

91. Health promotion includes all *except*:   [Kolkata 2007]
    (a) Specific protection
    (b) Health education
    (c) Food fortification
    (d) Environment modification

92. Which of the following is a primary prevention in polio?
                                                    [MP 2002]
    (a) Good sanitary measures
    (b) Rehabilitation
    (c) Provision of 3 doses of OPV in early infancy
    (d) Collection of stool sample for diagnosis

93. First in sequence: [MH 2002]
    (a) Impairment   (b) Disease
    (c) Disability   (d) Rehabilitation

94. Chemoprophylaxis is prevention type: [RJ 2000, RJ 2004]
    (a) Primary   (b) Secondary
    (c) Tertiary   (d) Quaternary

ICD–10

95. ICD-10 stands for: [AIIMS June 1997]
    (a) International Classification of Drugs, 10th revision
    (b) International Classification of Disabilities, 10th revision
    (c) International Classification of Diseases, 10th revision
    (d) International Classification of Disasters, 10th revision

96. ICD-10 true is: [NEET Pattern 2013]
    (a) Revised every 5 years   [AP 2004]
    (b) Consists of 10 chapters
    (c) Arranged in 3 volumes
    (d) Was produced by UNICEF

Review Question

97. Regarding International classification of disease untrue is: [MH 2007]
    (a) Revised every 10 years
    (b) 10th revision has 15 major chapters
    (c) Is base for use in other health fields
    (d) Coding system in 10th revision is alphanumerical

MISCELLANEOUS

98. Isolation for which air borne disease(s) is done?
                                            [INICET May 2022]
    (a) Measles   (b) NIPAH
    (c) Aseptic meningitis (d) Rabies

99. In recent years, incidence of noncommunicable diseases like diabetes and hypertension have increased. This is an example of: [INICET November 2021]
    (a) Cyclical trend
    (b) Seasonal trend
    (c) Periodic trend
    (d) Secular trend

100. Iceberg phenomenon differentiates: [AIPGME 08]
    (a) Apparent and Inapparent
    (b) Symptomatic and Asymptomatic
    (c) Cases and Carriers
    (d) Diagnosed and Undiagnosed

101. **Seasonal trend is due to:** [AIPGME 01]
    - (a) Vector variation
    - (b) Environmental factors
    - (c) Change in herd immunity
    - (d) All of the above

102. **Intraspecies competition is the competition among:** [AIIMS Dec 1994]
    - (a) Species
    - (b) Individuals of a population
    - (c) Individuals of a community
    - (d) Populations and their regulatory factors

103. **Which of the following is characteristic of a single exposure common vehicle outbreak?** [AIIMS May 05]
    - (a) Frequent secondary cases
    - (b) Severity increases with increasing age
    - (c) Explosive
    - (d) Cases occur continuously beyond the longest incubation period

104. **Global eradication of small pox was done on:** [AIIMS Jan 1998]
    - (a) 26th Oct 1977
    - (b) 8th May 1980
    - (c) 17th March 1980
    - (d) 17th April 1977

105. **Direct standardisation is used to compare mortality data of two countries. This is done because of difference in:** [NEET Pattern 2017]
    - (a) Causes of deaths [AIPGME 2011]
    - (b) Numerators
    - (c) Denominators
    - (d) Age distribution

106. **True about single exposure, point source epidemic is:** [DNB June 2011]
    - (a) Occurs in more than 1 incubation period
    - (b) Occurs in one incubation period
    - (c) The exposure is continuous [NEET Pattern 2017]
    - (d) Epidemic curve falls very slowly

107. **Long term fluctuation is seen with:** [DNB December 2011]
    - (a) Cyclic trends
    - (b) Epidemics
    - (c) Secular trends
    - (d) Seasonal trends

108. **True about continuous common source epidemics:**
    - (a) High secondary attack rate [NEET Pattern 2012]
    - (b) Duration more than one incubation period
    - (c) Rapid rise and fall of epidemic curve
    - (d) Brief and simultaneous exposure

109. **Cyclic trend is:** [DNB December 2011]
    - (a) Variations in herd immunity
    - (b) Environmental
    - (c) Nutritional
    - (d) Short term

110. **An epidemic of Hepatitis A is an example of:** [AP 2014]
    - (a) Common source, single exposure epidemic
    - (b) Common source, continuous exposure epidemic
    - (c) Propagated epidemic
    - (d) Slow epidemic

111. **Observation under nursing care for more than 24 hours in a hospital is defined as:** [NEET Pattern 2016]
    - (a) Inpatient
    - (b) Outpatient
    - (c) Observation status patient
    - (d) Urgent care patient

112. **Personal services rendered by doctors to patients in hospital, nursing home and at home is:** [NEET Pattern 2015]
    - (a) Health care
    - (b) Medical care
    - (c) Domiciliary care
    - (d) Nursing care

Review Questions

113. **Surveillance is:** [DNB 2001]
    - (a) Scrutiny of factors [NEET Pattern 2017]
    - (b) Treatment of contacts
    - (c) Prevention of disease
    - (d) Chemoprophylaxis of disease

114. **True morbidity is measured by:** [UP 2000]
    - (a) Active surveillance
    - (b) Passive surveillance
    - (c) Sentinel surveillance
    - (d) Continuous surveillance

115. **Tip of iceberg phenomenon is mostly appropriately represented by:** [Kolkata 2002]
    - (a) Malaria
    - (b) Measles
    - (c) PEM
    - (d) Rabies

116. **Quarantine is seperation of healthy individual:** [MP 2000]
    - (a) For longest incubation period of disease
    - (b) For shortest incubation period of disease
    - (c) For twice the incubation period of disease
    - (d) For period of generation time [Kolkata 2008]

117. **Part I of the 'death certificate' deals with:** [MH 2006]
    - (a) Immediate cause, and the direct underlying cause which started the whole trend of events leading to death
    - (b) Any significant associated diases that contributed to the death but did not directly lead to it
    - (c) Approximate interval between onset and cause of death
    - (d) The mode of death

Explanations

HEALTH AND WELL-BEING

1. **Ans. (a) Social; (b) Physical; (c) Mental; (e) Economic**
   [Ref. Park 27/e p14]
   - WHO [1948] definition of Health: Health is a state of complete physical, mental and social well-being, and not merely an absence of disease or infirmity; [recently amplified to include –] and an ability to lead a socially and economically productive life.
     – Is an 'idealistic goal rather than a realistic proposition'
     – It does not regard health as a dynamic concept (but as a state)

2. **Ans. (d) Human rights** [Ref. Park 27/e p16]
   - *Standard of Living:* Refers to the usual scale of our expenditure, goods we consume and services we enjoy
   - *Standard of living [WHO] includes:*
     – Income and Occupation
     – Standards of housing, sanitation and nutrition
     – Level of provision of health, educational, recreational and other services

   > **ALSO REMEMBER**
   > - Standard of living depends on 'Per capita GNP'

3. **Ans. (c) Build social security system** [Ref. Park 27/e p37]

   OTTAWA CHARTER FOR HEALTH PROMOTION

Five Key action areas	Basic strategies
Public Health **P**olicy Strengthen **C**ommunity action for health **R**eorientation of health services Personal **S**kills development Supportive **E**nvironment for health [*Mnemonic*: Promotion **C**an **R**eorient **S**killed **E**nvironment]	Advocate Enable Mediate
	Health Promotion Logo
	Circle with 3 wings Incorporates 5 key action areas Incorporates 3 basic strategies

   > **ALSO REMEMBER**
   > **JAKARTA DECLARATION OF HEALTH PROMOTION**
   > - Vision and focus on Health Promotion in 21st Century
   > - Focus areas:
   >   – Determinants of health
   >   – New challenges in 21st century
   >   – Fundamental conditions/resources for health: Peace, shelter, education, social security, social relations, food, income, women-empowerment, stable ecosystem, sustainable resource use, social justice, respect for human rights, poverty

4. **Ans. (a) Germ theory of disease** [Ref. Park 27/e p13]

   BIOMEDICAL CONCEPT OF HEALTH
   - Healthy is being 'Free from disease'
   - Based on 'Germ theory of disease'
   - Limitation of concept: Minimal role of environmental, social, psychological and cultural determinants of health

5. **Ans. (d) Changing behavior with respect to change in future** [Ref. Park 27/e p16]

   CONCEPT OF POSITIVE HEALTH
   - Perfect functioning of health and mind
   - Conceptualize health biologically, psychologically and socially
   - Depends on economic, social and cultural factors
   - Positive health remains a mirage due to constant change

HDI and PQLI

6. **Ans. (b) LE at birth, Decent living standard, Knowledge** [Ref. Park 26/e p17]
   - HDI is calculated based on Health (Life expectancy at birth), Education (Knowledge) and Standard of Living (Real GNI per capita)

7. **Ans. (d) Infant mortality rate** [Ref. Park 25/e p17]
   - **Components of HDI** include Longevity (Life expectancy at birth LEB/LE0), Income (Real GDP per capita in PPP US$) and Knowledge (Mean years of schooling – Gross enrolment ratio & Literacy rate)

8. **Ans. (b) Life expectancy at age 1** [Ref. Park 27/e p17]

   > **ALSO REMEMBER**
   > - Human poverty index is complementary to HDI
   > - *Human development index Vs Physical quality of life index:*
   >
   > | | HDI | PQLI |
   > |---|---|---|
   > | Indicator components | 1. Longevity – Life expectancy at birth (LE_B/LEo)
2. Income (Real GDP per capita in PPP US$)
3. Knowledge (Mean years of schooling – Gross enrolment ratio and Literacy rate) | 1. Life expectancy at 1 year age (LE_1)
2. Infant mortality rate (IMR)
3. Literacy rate |
   > | Range
India | 0 to +1
0.633 | 0 to 100
65 |

   > **ALSO REMEMBER**
   > **Human Poverty Index: Used earlier**
   > - *HPI measures:* Deprivation in basic dimensions of human development
   >   – HPI is complimentary to Human Development Index

Contd...

Contd...

Components of HPI – I: (Used for developing countries)	Components of HPI – II: (Used for developed countries)

• Probability at birth of not surviving to age 40
• Adult Illiteracy Rate
• Un-weighted average of two indicators:
  1. % population not using an improved water source
  2. % children underweight-for-age
	• Probability at birth of not surviving to age 60
	• % adults (aged 16-65 years) lacking functional literacy skills
	• % people living below poverty line (BPL)
	• Rate of long term unemployment (12 months or more)

9. **Ans. (d) II, III and IV are correct** [Ref. Park 27/e p17]
10. **Ans. None** [Ref. Park 27/e p18] [Now 20 and 85 years]
11. **Ans. (b) 0 to 1** [Ref. Park 27/e p17]

> **ALSO REMEMBER**
> *Few important ranges in Public Health:*
>
> | Parameter | Range (Lies between) |
> |---|---|
> | Correlation coefficient [r] | −1 to +1 (−1 < r < +1) |
> | Coefficient of determination [r²] | 0 to +1 (0 < r² < +1) |
> | Physical quality of life index | 0 to +100 (0 < PQLI < +100) |
> | Human development index | 0 to +1 (0 < HDI < +1) |
> | Probability | 0 to +1 (0% < Prob. < 100%) |
> | Sensitivity [screening test] | 0% < Sensitivity < 100% |
> | Specificity [screening test] | 0% < Specificity < 100% |
> | PPV (screening test) | 0% < PPV < 100% |
> | NPV (screening test) | 0% < NPV < 100% |

12. **Ans. (d) Income** [Ref. Park 23/e p18]
13. **Ans. (c) 0 and 100** [Ref. Park 27/e p17]
14. **Ans. (d) Subjective component of quality of life**
    [Ref. Vital's Homoeopathic MCQ Companion, 2/e p220]
    WHO Concept of Well-being
    • Objective component: Standard of living, Level of living
    • Subjective component: Quality of life

INDICATORS OF HEALTH

15. **Ans. (b) IMR** [Ref. Park 27/e p25]
    • IMR is a sensitive indicator of availability, utilization and effectiveness of health care, particularly perinatal care
16. **Ans. (d) DALY** [Ref. Park 26/e p26]
    DALY Calculation = YLL + YLD
    • Years of Life Lost (YLL): No of deaths X Expected remaining years of life (As per Global standard life expectancy – Japan)
    • Years Lost to Disability (YLD): No of incident cases injury/illness X Average duration of disease X Weighting factor (0 Perfect health to 1 Death)
17. **Ans. (a) Life Expectancy** [Ref. Park 27/e p25]
    • Life Expectancy is a 'Positive mortality indicator'

> **ALSO REMEMBER**
> • DALY is a type of disability rate
> • Bed turn-over ratio is a type of heath care utilization rate

18. **Ans. (c) Sullivan's index** [Ref. Park 27/e p26]
    • Sullivan's Index = Life Expectancy MINUS Duration of disability (bed disability and inability to perform major activities)
      – It is one of the most advanced indicators currently available
19. **Ans. (b) Disability adjusted life years** [Ref. Park 27/e p26]
    • *Disability adjusted life years [DALYs]*: Is a measure of the burden of disease in a defined population and the effectiveness of interventions; It expresses years lost to premature death and years lived with disability adjusted for its' severity

> **ALSO REMEMBER**
> • DALYs can measure *'both mortality and disability together'*
> • Case fatality rate measures *'virulence of an organism'* or *'killing power of a disease'*
> • Dependency ratio measures the *'need for society to provide for its' younger and older groups'*
> • Morbidity data measures *'any departure from health'*

20. **Ans. (d) Life expectancy at birth** [Ref. Park 27/e p27]
    • *Socio-economic indicators:* [**Mnemonic: He FLAGGED**]
      – Housing
      – Family size
      – Literacy rate
      – Availability per capita calorie
      – Per capita GNP
      – Growth rate
      – Level of unEmployment
      – Dependency ratio
21. **Ans. (b) IMR** [Ref. Park 27/e p25]
    • *Infant Mortality Rate [IMR]*: Is one of the most universally accepted indicators of health status not only of infants, but also of the whole population and the socio-economic conditions under which they live
    • IMR is a sensitive indicator of availability, utilization and effectiveness of health care, particularly perinatal care
    • IMR:
      – IMR is a rate
      – Is the second best indicator of socio-economic development of a country: Ultimate solution for lowering IMR lies in socio-economic development [Best indicator is U5MR]
      – Is most important indicator of health status of a community, level of living and effectiveness of MCH services in general
      – IMR is among 'the best predictors of state failure'

> **ALSO REMEMBER**
> - UNICEF considers U5MR or CMR as 'single best indicator of socio-economic development and well-being' (even better than IMR)

22. Ans. (a) Life free of disability [Ref. Park 27/e p26]
- The simplest index of health which incorporates morbidity as well as mortality is Sullivan's Index of Disability-Free Life Expectancy (DFLE)

> **ALSO REMEMBER**
> - *Chandler's Index:* Hookworm eggs/gm of stool
> - *Standard of living [WHO]:* Income and occupation, standards of housing, sanitation and nutrition, level of provision of health, educational, recreational and other services
> - *Pregnancy rate per HWY:* Pearl Index (Failure rate of Contraceptives)

23. Ans. (d) Years lost to premature death and years lived with disability adjusted for severity of disability [Ref. Park 27/e p25]

24. Ans. (d) 20% [Ref. Park 27/e p66]

25. Ans. (a) Slightly positive
[Ref. Financial and Business Management for the Doctor of Nursing Practice, KT Waxman, 1/e p61]
- Bed turn over interval: Amount of time beds at hospital are unoccupied until next patients' admission following a patients' discharge
  - Negative values: Indicate over 100% occupancy, scarcity of beds, over-utilization of services
  - Positive values: Indicate vacant beds, underutilization of services due to defective admission process or poor quality medical care
  - Slight positive values: Indicate optimum utilization of services

26. Ans. (a) Population bed ratio [Ref. Park 27/e p27]

Health care delivery indicators	Health care utilization indicators
Doctor-population ratio	% Fully immunized infants
Doctor-nurse ratio	% Pregnant women received ANC
Population-bed ratio	% Population using contraceptives
Population per health centre	Bed occupancy rate
Population per birth attendant	Average length of stay
	Bed turnover ratio

27. Ans. (d) Prevalence [Ref. Park 27/e p24–25]

MORTALITY INDICATORS
- Crude Death Rate, Age specific death rates, Disease-specific Mortality Rate
- Expectation of Life
- IMR, MMR, U5MR, Child Mortality Rate
- Case fatality rate, Proportional Mortality Rate
- Years of potential life years lost

28. Ans. (c) Affordability [Ref. Park 27/e p24]
Characteristics of Ideal Health Indicator
- Validity: Actually measures what it is supposed to measure
- Reliability: Reproducible results if measured by different persons
- Objectivity: Independent of subjects perception
- Sensitivity: Sensitive to change in situations
- Specificity: Reflect changes only in the situation concerned with that indicator
- Feasibility: Practical possibility of obtaining the necessary data
- Relevancy: Contribution to understanding the phenomenon of interest

29. Ans. (c) Mortality & disability [Ref. Park 27/e p26]

30. Ans. (a) 22 [Ref. District Health Facilities: Guidelines for Development & Operations by WHO p8]
In the given question,
- Total Bed-days required per year = Total number of admissions per year × average length of stay in hospital = 800 × 8 = 6400
- Total number of beds required when occupancy is 100% = Bed-days per year/ 365 days = 6400/365 = 17.5 = 18 beds
- Total number of beds required when occupancy is 80% = Bed-days per year/ (365 × 80%) = 6400/(365 × 80%) = 21.9 beds = 22 beds

Review Questions

31. Ans. (b) Age standardized death rate [Ref. Park 27/e p66]

32. Ans. (d) Lost year of life due to premature death and disability [Ref. Park 27/e p26]

NATURAL HISTORY OF DISEASE

33. Ans. (b) 1-d, 2-b, 3-a, 4-c [Ref. Park 27/e p41]
- Natural history of disease refers to the progression of a disease in an individual over time, in the absence of treatment. It has two phases, a period of pre-pathogenesis and a period of pathogenesis.
- The period of pre-pathogenesis is before the onset of disease in humans where an interaction between the agent, host and the environment occurs in this phase before the pathogenesis
- The period of pathogenesis starts after the disease process has been triggered and pathological changes occur without the individual being aware of it. It begins with the entry of the organism till recovery, death, or disability
- Rehabilitation has been defined as the use of medical, social, educational, and vocational measures for training the individual to the highest possible level of functional ability

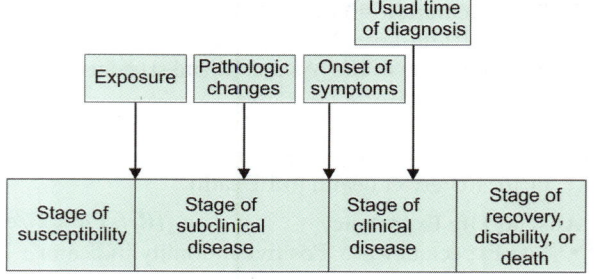

34. **Ans. (d) Alzheimer's disease** [Ref. Park 27/e p52]
    - *'Silent epidemic' of last century:* Alzheimer's disease

> **ALSO REMEMBER**
> - *Modern epidemic:* Coronary heart disease
> - *Most important discovery of 20th century:* ORS

35. **Ans. (a) Diagnosed cases under treatment** [Ref. Park 27/e p46]
    - *Iceberg Phenomenon of disease:* Disease in a community may be compared to an iceberg
      - Floating tip is what physician sees in community, i.e., clinical cases
      - Vast submerged portion of iceberg represents hidden mass of disease, i.e., latent, inapparent, pre-symptomatic and undiagnosed cases and carriers in community
      - Line of demarcation (water surface): Is between apparent and inapparent infections
      - Water surrounding iceberg: Healthy population

> **ALSO REMEMBER**
> - *'Epidemiologist is concerned with Hidden portion of iceberg'* whereas Clinician is concerned with Tip of iceberg
> - *'Screening is done for Hidden portion of Iceberg'* whereas diagnosis is done for tip of iceberg
> - *Iceberg phenomenon of disease is not shown by:*
>   - Rabies
>   - Tetanus
>   - Measles
>   - Rubella

36. **Ans. (a) Screening is of no use in changing course of disease** [Ref. Park 27/e p42]

Prepathogenesis Phase of Disease
- Is period before onset of disease in man (man at risk)
- Epidemiological triad: Interaction between agent, host and environment
- Primary level of prevention is possible

Pathogenesis Phase of Disease
- Begins with 'Entry of organism' in susceptible host
- Multiplication of organism, disease initiation and progression
- Final outcome may be recovery, disability or death
- Host may become a clinical case, subclinical case or carrier
- Secondary and tertiary levels of prevention are possible
- Screening of disease may improve prognosis and increase survival

37. **Ans. (d) Helps to suggest ways to interrupt the risk of transmission** [Ref. Park 27/e p41]

38. **Ans. (c) Epidemiological transition** [Ref. Health and Lifestyle Change, Volume 9, p8]

> **ALSO REMEMBER**
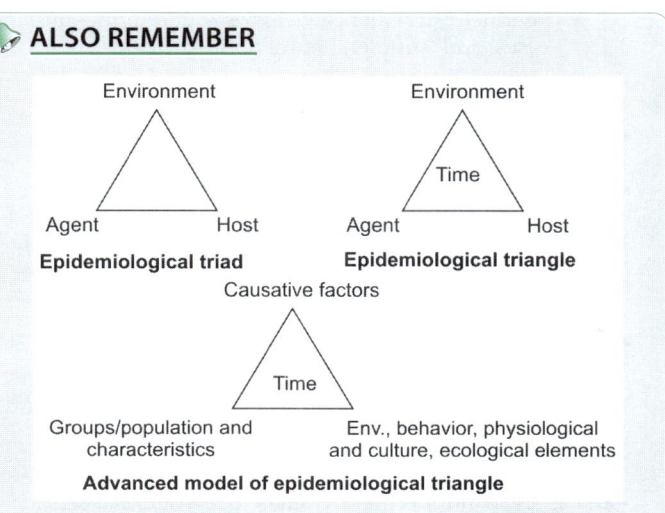

39. **Ans. (c) Interaction & interdependence of agent, host, environment & time** [Ref. Park 27/e p39-40]

Epidemiological triad	Triangle of epidemiology	Advanced model of triangle of epidemiology
1. Agent 2. Host 3. Environment	1. Agent 2. Host 3. Environment 4. Time	1. Causative factors 2. Groups/population & characteristics 3. Environmental, behavioral, cultural, psychological, Ecological factors 4. Time

Review Questions

40. **Ans. (d) Investigator** [Ref. Park 27/e p39-40]
41. **Ans. (b) Pre-pathogenesis period** [Ref. Park 27/e p42]

CONTROL OF DISEASE

42. **Ans. (d) Identifying cases free of disability** [Ref. Park 27/e p47]
    - *Surveillance:* Is the ongoing systematic collection and analysis of data and the provision of information which leads to action being taken to prevent and control a disease, usually one of an infectious nature
    - *Surveillance is of many types:*
      - Passive Surveillance: Data is itself reported to the health system; For example, A patient with fever coming on his own to the PHC, CHC, Dispensary, Private Practitioner, Hospital.
      - Active Surveillance: Health system seeks out 'actively' the collection of data, i.e., goes out to community to collect data; For example, Stool sample collection from home in Polio Program.
      - Sentinel Surveillance: Monitoring of rate of occurrence of specific conditions to assess the stability or change in health levels of a population, It is also the study of disease rates in a specific cohort, geographic area, population subgroup, etc. to estimate trends in larger population; For example, Use of health practitioners to monitor trends of a health event in a population.

– Sentinel Surveillance helps in 'identifying missing cases' and 'supplementing notified cases'

> **ALSO REMEMBER**
> - Most of the national health programmes in India rely on Passive Surveillance for morbidity and mortality data collection.
> - *Active Surveillance*: Is seen in NVBDCP (Health worker goes house to house every fortnight to detect fever cases, collect blood slides and provide presumptive treatment under malaria component) and National Leprosy Elimination Programme (Modified Leprosy Elimination Campaigns)
> - **Sentinel Surveillance** is done in National AIDS Control Programme wherein STD Clinics, ANC Clinics have been identified as sentinel sites to monitor trends of HIV/AIDS in the country

43. Ans. (d) 1, 2, 3 and 4 are correct [Ref. Park 27/e p46]
    - Disease control primarily refers to *'Primary and Secondary Levels'* of prevention
    - Sequence of Disease Control:
      – Disease Control
      – Disease Elimination
      – Disease Eradication

> **ALSO REMEMBER**
> - Concepts of control of disease:
>   – *Disease control:* Is reducing the transmission of disease agent to such a low level that it ceases to be a public health problem; it aims at reducing,
>   1. Incidence of the disease
>   2. Duration of the disease
>   3. Effects of infection
>   4. Financial burden to the community
>   – *Disease elimination:* Is complete interruption of transmission of disease in a defined geographical area, but the causative organism may be persisting somewhere
>   1. Disease elimination is a 'geographical term', i.e. can be used only for a country or a region
>   2. India has eliminated 4 diseases till date:
>   i. Guinea worm (Dracunculiasis): February 2000
>   ii. Leprosy: December 2005 (Elimination criterion: <1/10,000)
>   iii. Yaws: July 2016
>   iv. Maternal & Neonatal Tetanus July 2016
>   3. Next diseases likely to be eliminated from India: Poliomyelitis, Kala azar, Lymphatic filariasis
>   4. India declared 'Trachoma-Free' in December 2017. 'Polio free in March' 2014
>   – *Disease eradication*: Is complete 'extermination' of organism
>   1. Is *'tearing out by roots'* of a disease
>   2. Exhibits *'All or none phenomenon'*
>   3. Disease eradication is a *'global term'*, i.e. can be used only for whole planet
>   4. *World has eradicated ONLY 1 disease till date:* Small pox (declared eradicated on 8 May, 1980)

Contd...

> 5. 3 next target diseases for eradication, globally:
>   i. Poliomyelitis (Poliovirus 2 was eradicated on 20 September 2015)
>   ii. Measles
>   iii. Guinea worm

44. Ans. (c) Case finding is of secondary importance [Ref. Park 27/e p46]
    - *Disease eradication:*
      – In eradication, there is complete interruption of disease transmission in the entire area of the community
      – Eradication programme is over once the disease has been certified as having been eradicated
      – Case finding is of primary importance
      – Objective of eradication: Is to eliminate the disease to the extent that no new case occurs in the future

45. Ans. (b) Surveillance [Ref. Park 27/e p47]

> **ALSO REMEMBER**
> - *Diseases under International Surveillance [WHO]:*
>   – Louse borne typhus fever
>   – Relapsing fever
>   – Poliomyelitis
>   – Malaria
>   – Human Influenza
>   – Rabies
>   – Salmonellosis
> - *Monitoring versus surveillance:*

Monitoring	Surveillance
– Performance and analysis of routine measurements aimed at detecting changes in environment or health status of a population	– Continuous scrutiny of the factors that determine the occurrence and distribution of disease and other conditions of ill-health
– One Time linear activity	– Continuous Cycle
– No feedback present	– Feedback present
– No inbuilt action component present	– Inbuilt action component present
– Stops once disease is eliminated/eradicated	– Continues even after disease is eliminated/eradicated
– Smaller concept	– Broader concept

46. Ans. (a) Small pox; (b) Guinea worm disease; (c) Yaws; Leprosy and Neonatal Tetanus [Ref. Park 27/e p159]

47. Ans. (b) Dracunculiasis; (c) Polio; (d) Measles [Ref. Park 27/e p46]

48. Ans. (a) Small pox [Ref. Park 27/e p159]

49. Ans. (a) Elimination [Ref. Park 27/e p46]

50. Ans. (a) Herd immunity [Ref. Park 27/e p110]

51. Ans. (a) Monitoring [Ref. Park 27/e p46–47]

52. Ans. (a) Tuberculosis [Ref. Park 27/e p46]

53. Ans. (b) Health planning [Ref. Park 27/e p47]

Contd...

PUBLIC HEALTH SURVEILLANCE

- Ongoing systematic collection, analysis and interpretation of outcome-specific data, closely integrated with the timely dissemination of these data to those responsible for taking public health action to prevent and control disease or injury
- Results used for national health planning, policy-setting and targeted outcomes
- Provides essential information for defining problems and taking action
- Health authorities use the information to set priorities, plan interventions, allocate resources, detect outbreaks promptly, and recognize problems during the routine analysis of data from ongoing public health programs
- Requires professional analysis and sophisticated judgement of data leading to recommendations for control activities

Review Questions

54. Ans. (d) Regional removal of disease agent
 [Ref. Park 27/e p46]

55. Ans. (c) Polio [Ref. Park 27/e p46]

PREVENTION OF DISEASE

56. Ans. (b) Health education [Ref. Park 25/e p50]
    - Health education is Health promotion (Primary level of prevention)

57. Ans. (b) Personal hygiene and Environmental sanitation
 [Ref. Park 27/e p48-49]
    - Specific protection mode of disease prevention: Is a Primary level of disease prevention (applied when risk factors are present in environment but disease has not yet taken place). Risk factors are already present but disease is prevented from occurring by using a specific modality. E.g., Chemoprophylaxis to prevent meningococcal meningitis, Usage of condoms to prevent pregnancy/STIs, Iodisation of salt to prevent Iodine Deficiency Disorders.
    - Personal hygiene and Environmental sanitation is Health Promotion mode of intervention, also a type of Primary level of prevention

58. Ans. (d) Reconstructive Surgery in Leprosy
 [Ref. Park 27/e p48-49]
    - *Health screening for Diabetes Mellitus, Case finding for Falciparum malaria and Contact tracing for STIs represent Secondary level of prevention:* as disease has possibly set in and we want to diagnose early and provide treatment
    - *Reconstructive Surgery in Leprosy:* Disease (leprosy) with possible deformities have already taken place and we are now aiming to rehabilitate the patient through reconstructive surgery; thus it is a form of Tertiary level of prevention

59. Ans. (b) Primary prevention [Ref. Park 27/e p48-49]

LEVELS OF PREVENTION

- *Primordial Level of Prevention:* Is primary prevention (see below) in purest sense
  - It is the prevention of the emergence or development of risk factors in countries or population groups in which they have not yet appeared
  - **Modes of Intervention:**
    1. Individual Education
    2. Mass Education
  - Primordial Level is Best level of prevention for Non-communicable diseases
- *Primary Level of Prevention:*
  - It is the action taken prior to onset of disease, which removes the possibility that a disease will ever occur
  - **Modes of Intervention:**
    1. *Health Promotion:* Is targeted at strengthening the host through a variety of approaches/interventions, e.g. Health Education, Environmental modifications, Nutritional interventions, Lifestyle and behavioural changes
    2. *Specific Protection:* Is targeting the prevention of disease through a specific intervention
  - Primary level of prevention is applied when 'risk factors are present but disease has not yet taken place'
  - It signifies 'intervention in the Pre-pathogenesis Phase of a disease/health problem'
- *Secondary Level of Prevention:*
  - It halts the progress of disease at its' incipient stage and prevents complications
  - **Modes of Intervention:**
    1. *Early Diagnosis:* Detection of disturbances while biochemical, functional and morphological changes are still reversible or prior to occurrence of manifest signs and symptoms
    2. *Treatment:* Shortens period of communicability, reduces mortality and prevents occurrence of further cases (secondary cases) or any long term disability
  - *Secondary level of prevention is applied when disease has possibly set in*: It attempts to arrest the disease process, seek unrecognized disease and treat it before irreversibility and reverse communicability of infectious diseases
  - National Health Programmes by Govt. of India mostly operate at Secondary level of prevention
  - Secondary prevention is an imperfect tool in control of transmission of disease: It is more expensive and less effective than primary prevention
  - It is an important level of prevention for diseases like Tuberculosis, Leprosy and STDs
- *Tertiary Level of Prevention:*
  - Is applied when disease has advanced beyond early stages: It aims to reduce or limit impairments and disabilities, minimize suffering caused by existing departures from good health
  - **Modes of Intervention:**
    1. *Disability Limitation:* It 'prevents the transition of disease from impairment to handicap'
    2. *Rehabilitation:* Training and retraining of an individual to the highest possible level of functional ability; It can be medical, vocational, social or psychological
  - Tertiary level of prevention signifies 'intervention in late pathogenesis phase'

> **ALSO REMEMBER**
> - All Vaccines (including Anti-rabies vaccine): *Specific Protection* mode of intervention, *Primary Level of prevention*
> - Screening is predominantly Secondary Level of Prevention with some component of *Primary Prevention* also

60. Ans. (a) Primary [Ref. Park 27/e p48]
    In the given question, risk factor (fluoride rich water) is already present in the environment and step is taken (defluoridation of water) to prevent occurrence of disease (Fluorosis): Thus it is an example of Primary level of prevention (Mode of Intervention: Specific Protection)

61. Ans. (b) Prevention of emergence of development of risk factors [Ref. Park 27/e p48]

> **ALSO REMEMBER**
> - Action taken prior to the onset of disease: Primary Prevention
> - Action taken to remove the possibility that a disease will ever occur: Primary Prevention
> - Action which halts the progress of a disease: Secondary Prevention

62. Ans. (d) Tertiary Prevention [Ref. Park 27/e p48–49]

Levels of prevention	Modes of intervention
Primary Level	Health Promotion and Specific Protection
Secondary Level	Early Diagnosis and Treatment
Tertiary Level	Disability Limitation and Rehabilitation

63. Ans. (b) Disease-Impairment-Disability-Handicap [Ref. Park 27/e p50]
    - According to WHO definitions,
      – Disease: Any abnormal condition of an organism that impairs function
      – Impairment: Any loss or abnormality of psychological, physiological or anatomical structure or function
      – Disability: (Because of impairment,) any restriction or inability to perform an activity in a range considered normal for a human being
      – Handicap: A disadvantage for a given individual, resulting from an impairment/disability, that limits/prevents fulfillment of a role considered normal (depending on age, sex, social, cultural factors) for that individual.

> **ALSO REMEMBER**
> - *Continuum of disease-handicap:*
>   – Disease: Intrinsic pathology
>   – Impairment: Anatomical and functional abnormality
>   – Disability: Activity restriction
>   – Handicap: Psychosocial disadvantage

64. Ans. (c) Secondary [Ref. Park 27/e p50]

65. Ans. (b) Disability [Ref. Park 27/e p50]
66. Ans. (b) High fiber diet [Ref. Park 27/e p48]
67. Ans. (c) Salt restriction [Ref. Park 27/e p48]
68. Ans. (a) Fluoridation; (b) Dental health education [Ref. Park 27/e p50]
    - Most effective means to prevent dental caries: Use of fluoride
69. Ans. (a) Marriage counselling; (e) Immunization [Ref. Park 27/e p50]
70. Ans. (b) Specific protection [Ref. Park 27/e p50]
71. Ans. (a) Breast self examination [Ref. Park 27/e p50]
72. Ans. (d) None [Ref. Park 27/e p50]
73. Ans. (a) Primary prevention [Ref. Park 27/e p50]
74. Ans. (a) Primary prevention [Ref. Park 27/e p50]
75. Ans. (b) Patients [Ref. Park 27/e p50]
76. Ans. (b) Primary prevention; (c) Specific protection [Ref. Park 27/e p50]
77. Ans. (c) Secondary [Ref. Park 27/e p48]
78. Ans. (a) Pap smear [Ref. Park 27/e p50]
79. Ans. (a) Measles immunization [Ref. Park 27/e p50]
80. Ans. (a) 1 and 4 [Ref. Park 27/e p48]
81. Ans. (d) Spectacles for refractory error [Ref. Park 27/e p50–51]

Disability Limitation

- Tertiary level of prevention when patient reports late in Pathogenesis phase
- Prevent transition if disease from impairment to handicap
- Spectacles in refractive error stabilizes visual acuity (Disability limitation) and provides visual clarity (Rehabilitation) too

82. Ans. (b) Primary prevention [Ref. Park 27/e p50]
    - National Iron PLUS Initiative is an attempt to look at Iron Deficiency Anaemia in which beneficiaries will receive iron and folic acid supplementation irrespective of their Iron/hemoglobin status
    - Thus its Primary level of prevention (Specific protection)
83. Ans. (d) Screening for hypertension [Ref. Park 27/e p50]
    - Screening for HT is Secondary level of prevention
84. Ans. (a) Weight reduction; (b) Dietary salt reduction; (c) Exercise promotion [Ref. Park 27/e p428]
    - Early diagnosis, Antihypertensive drugs are Secondary level of prevention for Hypertension
85. Ans. (a) Health promotion [Ref. Park 27/e p47]
    - Environmental modifications, viz., Safe water provision, Installation of Sanitary latrines, Improvement of housing conditions, Rodent/insect control constitute Health promotion
86. Ans. (b) Early diagnosis and treatment [Ref. Park 27/e p443]

Screening of Breast Cancer
- Tests: Mammography, USG, Thermography, Breast self-examination (BSE), Palpation by Physician/Surgeon, MRI
- Level of prevention: Secondary (Early diagnosis)

Review Questions

87. Ans. (d) Chemoprophylaxis　　*[Ref. Park 27/e p50]*
88. Ans. (c) Rehabilitation　　*[Ref. Park 27/e p50-51]*
89. Ans. (c) Secondary prevention　　*[Ref. Park 27/e p47-50]*
90. Ans. (a) Pap smear for early detection of carcinoma cervix in community　　*[Ref. Park 27/e p50]*
91. Ans. (a) Specific protection　　*[Ref. Park 27/e p50]*
92. Ans. (c) Provision of 3 doses of OPV in early infancy　　*[Ref. Park 27/e p50]*
93. Ans. (b) Disease　　*[Ref. Park 27/e p50]*
94. Ans. (a) Primary　　*[Ref. Park 27/e p50]*

ICD-10

95. Ans. (c) International Classification of Diseases, 10th revision　　*[Ref. Park 25/e p56-57]*
    Refer to Theory

> **ALSO REMEMBER**
> - ICF Classification (WHO): International Classification of Functioning, Disability and Health

96. Ans. (c) Arranged in 3 volumes　　*[Ref. Park 25/e p56-57]*

Review Question

97. Ans. (b) 10th revision has 15 major chapters　　*[Ref. Park 25/e p56-57]*

MISCELLANEOUS

98. Ans. (a) Measles　　*[Ref. Park 26/e p 132]*
    - Isolation is done for Chicken pox, Herpes zoster, Measles, Mumps, Rubella, Diphtheria, Pertussis, Influenza, TB (Sputum smear positive), Meningococcal meningitis, Streptococcal pharyngitis, Poliomyelitis, Cholera, Shigellosis, Salmonellosis, Hepatitis A

99. Ans. (d) Secular trend　　*[Ref. Park 26/e p74]*
    Long-term Fluctuations [Secular Trends]
    - Implies changes in occurrence of a disease (progressive increase or decrease) over a long period of time, generally several years or decades
    - Communicable diseases (Poliomyelitis, Diphtheria, Pertussis) are reducing in India in past few decades
    - Non-communicable diseases (Diabetes, Hypertension, Obesity) are increasing in India in past few decades.

100. Ans. (a) Apparent and Inapparent　　*[Ref. Park 27/e p46]*

> **ALSO REMEMBER**
> - Iceberg Phenomenon of disease is also sometimes known as *'Biological spectrum of a disease'*
> - CLINICIAN'S FALLACY: The iceberg phenomenon thwarts attempts to assess the burden of disease and the need for services, as well as the selection of representative cases for study; this leads to what has been called the 'clinician's fallacy' in which an inaccurate view of the nature and causes of a disease results from studying the minority of cases of the disease that are seen in clinical treatment

101. Ans. (d) All of the above　　*[Ref. Textbook of Community Medicine by Sunder Lal, 2/e p305, Park 27/e p73]*
     - *Periodic fluctuations:*
     Seasonal trends:
     1. Is seasonal variation/fluctuation in occurrence of a disease
     2. Is due to vector variation, environmental factors and change in herd immunity
     3. Examples:
        i. Measles (early spring)
        ii. Upper respiratory infections (winters)
        iii. Gastrointestinal infections (summers)
     Cyclical trends:
     1. Is occurrence of a disease in cycles spread over short periods of time, which may be days, weeks, months or years
     2. Examples:
        i. Measles (every 2-3 years)
        ii. Rubella (every 6-9 years)
        iii. Influenza pandemics (every 10-15 years)

102. Ans. (b) Individuals of a population　　*[Ref. Internet]*
     - *Intraspecies/Intraspecific competition:* Competition between individuals of a same species
     - *Interspecies/Interspecific competition:* Competition between individuals of two different species.

103. Ans. (c) Explosive　　*[Ref. Park 27/e p72]*
     - *Single exposure common vehicle outbreak:* Also known as *'Point Source Epidemic'*, where exposure to disease agent is brief and essentially simultaneous
       – Epidemic Curve rises and falls rapidly, with no secondary waves
       – Explosive: Clustering of cases within a narrow interval of time
       – All cases develop within one incubation period of disease

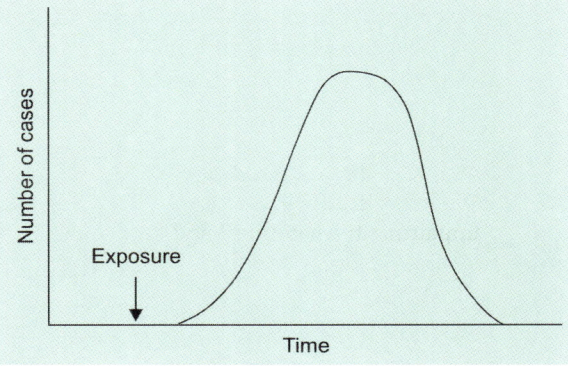

Epidemic curve

104. **Ans. (b) 8th May 1980** *[Ref. Park 27/e p159]*
    - *Last indigenous case of Small pox in India:* 17th May 1975
    - *Last [importation] case of Small pox in India:* 24th May 1975
    - *India declared Small pox-free:* 23 April, 1977
    - *Last case of Small pox globally:* 26th October 1977 (Somalia)
    - *Actual last case of small pox [Laboratory accident]:* 1978
    - *Global eradication of Small pox:* 8th May 1980

105. **Ans. (d) Age distribution** *[Ref. Park 27/e p66]*
106. **Ans. (b) Occurs in one incubation period** *[Ref. Park 27/e p72]*
107. **Ans. (c) Secular trends** *[Ref. Park 27/e p74]*
108. **Ans. (b) Duration more than one incubation period** *[Ref. Park 27/e p72]*
109. **Ans. (a) Variations in herd immunity** *[Ref. Park 27/e p73]*
110. **Ans. (c) Propagated epidemic** *[Ref. Park 27/e p73]*
111. **Ans. (a) Inpatient**
    [Ref. Understanding Health Insurance by Green 11/e p764]
    - Inpatient: If duration of observation care of patient is expected to be 24 hours or more
    - Outpatient: Patient receiving care in hospital's clinic or emergency or same-day surgicentre, where patient is released within 23 hours
    - Observation status patient: Active treatment is required to determine of patient requires hospitalization or discharge the same day
    - Urgent care patient: Patient who requires stabilization due to emergency situation

112. **Ans. (c) Domiciliary care**
    [Ref. Master Facility Inventory Survey 1967 p28]
    - Domiciliary care: Personal services rendered by doctors to patients in hospital, nursing home and at home

Review Questions

113. **Ans. (a) Scrutiny of factors** *[Ref. Park 27/e p47]*
114. **Ans. (c) Sentinel surveillance** *[Ref. Park 27/e p47]*
115. **Ans. (c) PEM** *[Ref. Park 27/e p47]*
116. **Ans. (a) For longest incubation period of disease** *[Ref. Park 27/e p133]*
117. **Ans. (a) Immediate cause, and the direct underlying cause which started the whole trend of events leading to death** *[Ref. Park 27/e p64]*

CHAPTER 3

Epidemiology and Vaccines

DEFINITION AND EPIDEMIOLOGICAL METHODS

Types of Epidemiological Studies

- *Types of epidemiological studies:*

Type of epidemiological study	Unit of study[a]
1. Observational studies[a]	
a. Descriptive studies (Hypothesis formulation[a])	
b. Analytical studies (Hypothesis testing[a])	
i. Cohort study	Individual
ii. Case control study	Individual
iii. Cross-sectional study	Individual
iv. Ecological study	Population[a]
2. Experimental studies (Hypothesis confirmation)[a]	
a. Randomized controlled trial	Patients[a]
b. Field trial	Healthy people
c. Community trial	Community
d. Clinical trial	Patients

Key points

Evidence Based Medicine/Practice is considered 'Gold standard for clinical practice'.

- *Synonyms of names of epidemiological studies[Q]:*

Type of epidemiological study	Unit of study[a]
Cohort study Prospective study Forward looking study Cause to effect study Risk factor to disease study Exposure to outcome study Follow-up study Incidence study	**Case control study** Retrospective study Backward looking study Effect to cause study Disease to risk factor study Outcome to exposure study TROHOC study
Cross-sectional study Prevalence study SNAPSHOT of population study	**Ecological study** Correlational study

Evidence Based Medicine/Practice

- Is considered 'Gold standard for clinical practice'[Q]
- Aims to apply best available evidence gained from scientific method to clinical decision making
- *Highest importance is given to strongest epidemiological studies*:
  - *Most important*: Meta-analyses, Systematic reviews, Blinded trials
  - *Least importance*: Opinions and conventional wisdom of researchers and experts
- *Statistical parameters used*:
  - Likelihood ratios
  - Receiver operator characteristic curve

Key points

EBM: Highest importance is given to Meta-analyses

> **Key points**
>
> EBM: In-vitro (test-tube) research (Lowest clinical relevance)

Evidence-Pyramid in Research [From top to bottom]^Q

- Meta-analysis (Highest clinical relevance: GOLD STANDARD^Q)
- Systematic review
- Cohort study
- Case control study
- Case series
- Case report^Q
- Ideas, Editorials, Opinions^Q
- Animal research
- In-vitro (test-tube) research (Lowest clinical relevance^Q)

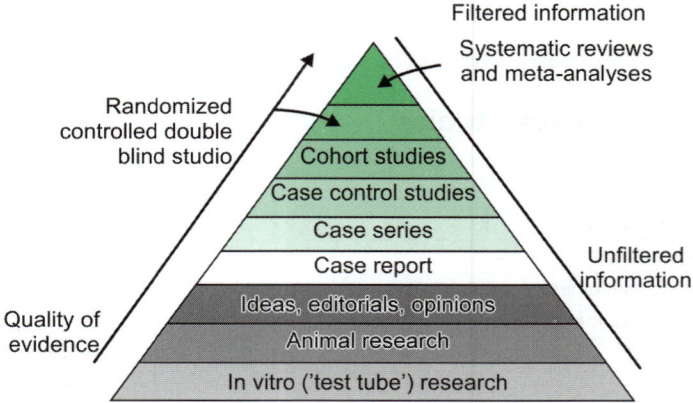

MEASUREMENTS IN EPIDEMIOLOGY

Tools of Measurement in Epidemiology

- *Rate*: Numerator (a) is a part of denominator (b) and multiplier is 1000 or 10,000 or 100,000 or so on...
- *Ratio*: Numerator (a) is not a part of denominator (b) and BOTH numerator and denominator are unrelated
- *Proportion*: Numerator (a) is a part of denominator (b) and multiplier is 100
  – Proportion is always expressed in percentage (%)

Examples of Tools of Measurement in Epidemiology

Parameter	Formula	Numerator (N) & Denominator (D)	Conclusion
Infant mortality rate (IMR)	$\frac{\text{No. of infant deaths}}{\text{No. of Live births}} \times 1000$	N is a part of D; multiplier NOT 100	Rate
Maternal mortality ratio (MMR)^Q	$\frac{\text{No. of maternal deaths}}{\text{No. of Live births}} \times 100000$	N is NOT a part of D; both unrelated	Ratio
Sex ratio (SR)	$\frac{\text{No. of females}}{\text{No. of males}} \times 1000$	N is NOT a part of D; both unrelated	Ratio
Incidence^Q	$\frac{\text{No. of new case}}{\text{Total population at risk}} \times 1000$	N is a part of D; multiplier NOT 100	Rate
Prevalence^Q	$\frac{\text{No. of new + old cases}}{\text{Total population}} \times 100$	N is a part of D; multiplier 100	Proportion
Case fatality rate^Q (CFR)	$\frac{\text{No. of deaths}}{\text{No. of cases}} \times 100$	N is a part of D; multiplier 100	Proportion
Relative risk (RR^Q)	$\frac{\text{Incidence among exposed}}{\text{Incidence among non-exposed}}$	N is NOT a part of D; both unrelated	Ratio

Indicators of Health

- *Mortality indicators*[Q]:
    - Crude death rate (CDR)
    - Life expectancy (LE[Q])
    - Infant mortality rate (IMR)
    - Child mortality rate (CMR)
    - Under 5 proportional mortality rate (U5MR)
    - Maternal mortality rate (MMR)
    - Disease specific mortality
    - Proportional mortality rate
- *Morbidity indicators*[Q]:
    - Incidence and prevalence
    - Notification rates
    - Attendance rates at OPD, health centres
    - Admission, re-admission and discharge rates
    - Duration of stay in hospital
    - Spells of sickness or absence from work/school
- *Disability rates*:

Event type indicators[a]	Person type indicators[a]
• No. of days of restricted activity • Bed disability days • Work-loss days	*Limitation of mobility*: • Confined to bed/house • Special aid in getting around *Limitation of activity*: • Limitation to perform ADL • Limitation in major activity

- *Nutritional status indicators*:
    - Anthropometric measurements of preschool children
    - Heights of children at school entry
    - Prevalence of Low birth weight
- *Health care delivery indicators*[Q]:
    - Doctor – population ratio
    - Doctor – nurse ratio
    - Population – bed ratio
    - Population per health centre
    - Population per traditional birth attendant
- *Utilization rates*[Q]:
    - Proportion of infants fully immunized against 6 EPI diseases
    - Proportion of pregnant women who receive antenatal care
    - Percentage of population using various methods of family planning
    - Bed-occupancy rate
    - Average length of stay in a hospital
    - Bed turn over ratio
- *Indicators of social and mental health*: Suicide/homicide/acts of violence/road traffic accidents/alcohol or tobacco use rates
- *Environmental indicators*: Air or water pollution indicators, Proportion of population having access to safe water supply and sanitation
- *Socioeconomic indicators*: Per capita GNP, Level of unemployment, Dependency ratio, Literacy rates
- *Health policy indicators*: Proportion of GNP spent on health services, Proportion of GNP spent on health related activities
- *Indicators for quality of life*: Physical quality of life index (PQLI)
- *Other indicators*: Social indicators, HFA indicators, SDGs indicators

INTERNATIONAL DEATH CERTIFICATE (IDC)

NEW WHO Recommended Death Certificate (For International Use: IDC)

> **Key points**
> **Death Certificate**
> *Consist of four lines*

> **Key points**
> **Line Ic/Line Id:** Main Underlying Cause

> **Key points**
> **Line Ic/Line Id:**
> *'Essence of Death Certificate^Q'*

- Consists of Five lines:
  - Line Ia: Disease or condition directly leading to death
  - Line Ib: Antecedent/underlying cause
  - Line Ic/Line Id: Main Antecedent/Underlying Cause (If line Id could be filled up, it becomes the Main Antecedent/Underlying cause)
  - Line II: Other significant conditions contributing to death BUT not related to disease/condition causing it
- Example of a Death certificate:

Example 1	Example 2
Line Ia: Renal failure	Line Ia: Intraperitoneal hemorrhage
Line Ib: Diabetic nephropathy	Line Ib: Ruptured metastatic deposit in liver
Line Ic: Diabetes Mellitus	Line Ic: Metastatic deposit in liver
Line Id: …………………………..	**Line Id: Primary adenocarcinoma of ascending colon**
Line II: Hypertension	Line II: Hypertension

- Concept of Underlying cause: Line Ic (or if Line Id could be filled up) is the MOST IMPORTANT line in death certificate, thus also known as 'Essence of Death Certificate'.

MORTALITY MEASUREMENTS

Crude Death Rate (CDR) [& Crude Birth Rate CBR]

- *Crude birth rate (CBR):* Annual number of live births per 1000 mid-year population

$$CBR = \frac{\text{No. of births in an area in a year}}{\text{Total Mid-year population}^Q} \times 1000$$

- *Crude death rate (CDR):* Annual number of deaths per 1000 mid-year population

$$CDR = \frac{\text{No. of deaths in an area in a year}}{\text{Total Mid-year population}^Q} \times 1000$$

> **Key points**
> *Crude death rate (CDR):* Annual number of deaths per 1000 mid-year population

- *Findings of SRS Bulletin:* [2017]
  - Crude Birth Rate (CBR): 20.4 per 1000 mid-year population
  - Crude Death Rate (CDR): 6.4 per 1000 mid-year population

Specific Death Rate (SDR)

- May be cause/disease-specific or group specific (age-specific, sex-specific, age-sex specific)
- Help identify particular 'at risk' group(s) for preventive action
- Permit comparison between different causes within same population

$$SDR = \frac{\text{No. of deaths from a specific cause in a year}}{\text{Mid-year population}} \times 1000$$

Proportional Mortality Rate (PMR)

- PMR is number of deaths due to a particular cause (or in a specific age group) per 100 (or 1000) total deaths
- *Advantages of PMR*:
  - Is 'simplest measure of estimating the burden of a disease' in the community^Q
  - *Is a useful health status indicator*: Indicates magnitude of preventable mortality
  - Is used when population data is not available
- *Disadvantages of PMR*:
  - Is of limited value in making comparisons between population groups or different time periods
  - Does not indicate the risk of members of population contracting or dying from the disease
- Leading causes of Deaths in World (2016) expressed as PMR: **Ischemic heart disease** (16.6%) > Stroke (10%) > COPD (5.4%) > LRI (5.2%) > Dementias (3.5%) > Trachea/Bronchus/Lung cancers > DM > RTA > Diarrheal diseases > TB > Others.

> **Key points**
> **PMR**
> Is 'simplest measure of estimating the burden of a disease'

Case Fatality Rate (CFR)

- CFR represents *'killing power of a disease'*
  - It is *'closely related to virulence of organism*^Q*'*
- *CFR is a Proportion*: Always expressed in percentage
- CFR is the *'complement of Survival Rate'*
  - CFR = 1 – Survival Rate
- *Limitations of CFR*:
  - *Time interval is not specified*^Q
  - Usefulness of CFR is limited for chronic diseases

$$\text{CFR} = \frac{\text{Total no. of deaths due to a disease}}{\text{Total no. of cases due to a disease}} \times 100$$

> **Key points**
> CFR = 1 – Survival Rate

Survival Rate (SR)

- *Survival rate*: Is the proportion of survivors in a group (e.g. of patients), studied and followed over a period of time (e.g. over a period of 5 years)
- Is used to *'describe prognosis'* in certain disease conditions
- Quite useful in cancer studies
- Can be used as a *'yardstick for the assessment of standards of therapy'*
- Survival period is usually reckoned from date of diagnosis or start of treatment^Q

$$\text{SR} = \frac{\text{Total no. of patients alive after 5 years}}{\text{Total no. of patients diagnosed/treated}} \times 100$$

Standardization of Death Rates

- *Adjusted or standardized rates*:
  - While comparison of death rates of two populations, *'crude death rate is not the right yardstick'*, as age-compositions are different^Q
  - Age-adjustment or age-standardization removes confounding effect of different age structures
  - Standardization may be direct or indirect
  - Standardization is carried out beginning by using a *'Standard Population'*
- *Standard population*: Is a population where numbers in each age and sex group are known
  - *Two frequently used standard populations are*:
    - Segi world population
    - European standard population
  - *Choice of standard population is arbitrary*:^Q
    - Available standard populations may be used
    - Standard population may also be created using 2 populations
    - National population need not always be taken as Standard population
    - Is commonly used in occupational studies: Comparison of mortality in an industry and general population
    - Can be used for occurrence of disease (rather than death)

> **Key points**
> National population need not always be taken as Standard population

> **Key points**
> *Direct standardization:*
> *Feasibility:*
> Availability of age-specific death rates (ASDR^Q)

Types of Standardized Death Rates

- *Direct standardization*:
  - *Method*:
    - Age-specific rates of the population (whose crude death rate is to be standardized) is *applied on a standard population*
    - Total expected deaths calculated
    - Total expected deaths divided by total standard population to yield standardized death rate
  - *Feasibility*:
    - Availability of age-specific death rates (ASDR)^Q
    - Availability of population in each age group
- *Indirect standardization*: Standardized mortality ratio (SMR): Is simplest and most useful form
  - *Method*: Calculate expected deaths, assuming that study group experiences the death rates of a standard population
  - *Feasibility*: Permits adjustment where age-specific rates are not available or are unstable because of small numbers
  - *Examples of indirect Standardization^Q*:
    - *Standardized mortality ratio (SMR)^Q*: SMR = Observed deaths/Expected deaths × 100
    - Life Table Analysis
    - Survival Analysis
    - Regression Analysis
    - Multivariate Analysis

	Direct Standardization	Indirect Standardization
Method	Use actual ASDRs* on the standard age structure	Use standard ASDRs* on the actual age structures
No. of deaths in each age group Population in each age group	Both are available	Both are unavailable

(ASDR* = Age Specific Death Rates)

MORBIDITY MEASUREMENTS

Incidence

> **Key points**
> *Incidence can be determined from:* Cohort study

- *Incidence*: Is defined as the '*no. of new cases*' occurring in a defined population during a specified period of time
- *For a given period,*

$$\text{Incidence} = \frac{\text{No. of new cases of a disease in a year}}{\text{Total population at risk}} \times 1000$$

> **Key points**
> PREVALENCE IS A PROPORTION

  - Incidence is a RATE, expressed per 1000
- *Special types of incidence rates*:
  - *Attack rate^Q*: Incidence rate used when population is exposed for a small interval of time, e.g. epidemic
  - *Secondary Attack Rate (SAR)*: Is no. of exposed persons developing the disease within range of incubation period, following exposure to the primary case
- Incidence is the best measure of disease frequency in etiological studies
  - *Incidence can be determined from*: Cohort study^Q

Prevalence

- *Prevalence*: Is total current (Old + New) cases in a given population over a point or period of time

- *Types of prevalence*:
  - A point of time (*Point Prevalence*)
  - A period of time (*Period Prevalence*)

$$\text{Prevalence} = \frac{\text{No. of total (new + old) cases of a disease in a year}}{\text{Total population}} \times 100$$

  - PREVALENCE IS A PROPORTION (Prevalence IS NOT A RATIO): Numerator is a part of denominator, and is always expressed in percentage[Q]
- *Prevalence can be determined from*: Cross-Sectional Study[Q]
- *Relationship between Incidence and Prevalence*: Given the assumption that population is stable AND incidence & duration are unchanging[Q],
  - Prevalence = Incidence × Mean duration of the disease P = I × d
  - Prevalence describes balance between incidence, mortality and recovery
  - Incidence reflects causal factors
  - Duration reflects the prognostic factors

> **Key points**
> *Prevalence can be determined from*: Cross-Sectional Study

> **Key points**
> P = I × d

DESCRIPTIVE EPIDEMIOLOGY

Time Distribution of Disease
Please Refer to Chapter 2

Types of Epidemics
- *Single exposure or 'Point source' epidemics*:
  - 'Sharp rise and sharp fall' in no. of cases[Q]
  - 'Clustering of cases' in a narrow interval of time[Q]
  - All 'cases develop within one incubation period' of the disease[Q]
  - Examples: Food poisoning, Measles, Chicken pox, Cholera, BHOPAL GAS TRAGEDY
- *'Common source', continuous or repeated exposure epidemics*:
  - 'Sharp rise' in no. of cases
  - Fall in no. of cases is interrupted by 'Secondary waves/peaks'[Q]
  - Examples: Contaminated well in a village, nationally distributed brand vaccine or food, prostitute in a gonorrhoea outbreak, LEGIONNAIRE'S DISEASE outbreak in Philadelphia (1976)
- *Propagated epidemics*:
  - 'Gradual rise and gradual fall' over a long time (Tail off)
  - Results from *'person-to-person transmission*[Q]*'*
  - Transmission continues till no. of susceptibles is depleted or susceptibles are no longer exposed to infected individuals
  - Speed of spread depends upon herd immunity, secondary attack rate, opportunities for contact
  - Examples: HIV, tuberculosis

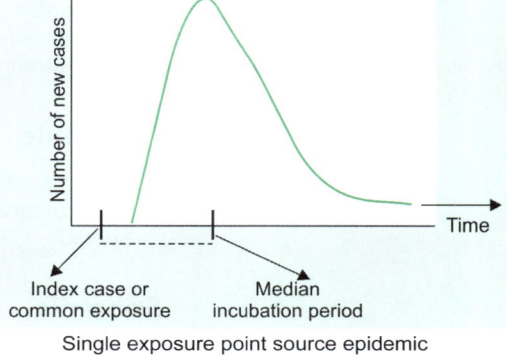
Single exposure point source epidemic

> **Key points**
> *Single exposure or 'Point source' epidemics:*
> All 'cases develop within one incubation period'

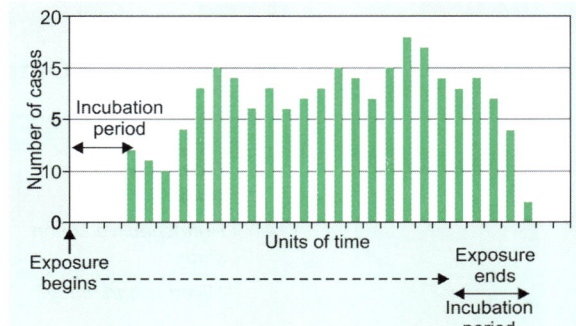
Multiple exposure point source epidemic

> **Key points**
> *Continuous or repeated exposure epidemics:*
> 'Secondary waves/peaks'

> **Key points**
> *Propagated epidemics:*
> Results from *'person-to-person transmission'*

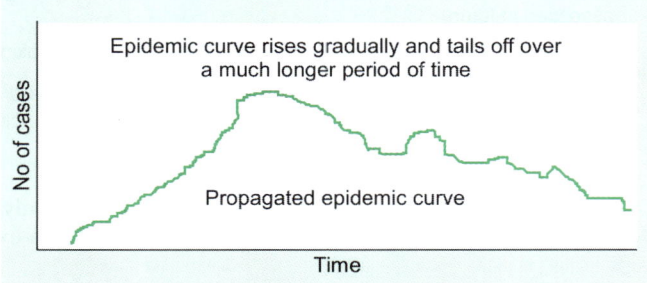
Propagated epidemic

> **Key points**
>
> *Endemic:* Is the 'usual or expected frequency' of a disease in a population

Endemic

- *Endemic:* Constant presence of a disease or infectious agent in a defined geographical area
  - Is the 'usual or expected frequency' of a disease in a population[Q]
- *Types of Endemic:*
  - *Hyper-endemic:* Constant presence of a disease or infectious agent at high incidence/prevalence AND affects all age groups equally
  - *Holo-endemic:* A high level of infection beginning early in life AND affecting most of the children population

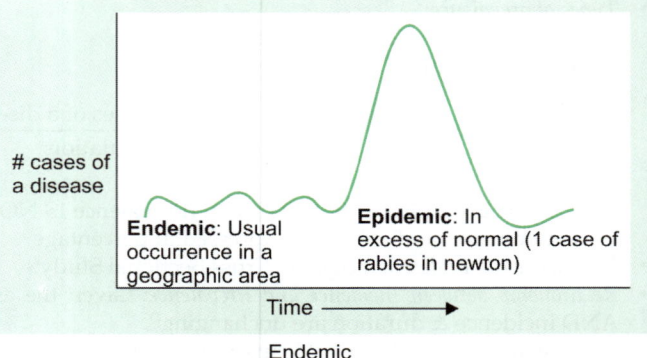

Pandemic

- *Pandemic:* An epidemic usually affecting a large proportion of the population, occurring over a large geographical area such as part of a nation, nation, continent or world (Country-to-country spread)

Sporadic

- *Sporadic:* Cases which are *'scattered about[Q]'*
  - Cases are widely separated in space and time
  - Show little or no connection with each other
  - There is no recognizable source of infection

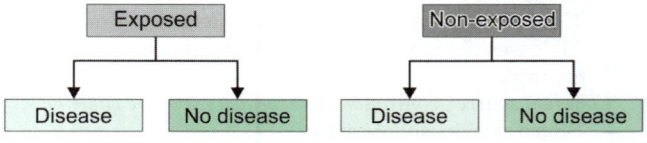

Prospective cohort study

ANALYTICAL EPIDEMIOLOGY

Exposure & Outcome in Analytical Studies[Q]

	Exposure	Outcome	Remarks	Direction
Prospective cohort study	Occurred	Followed-up	Start with exposure	Forward looking
Retrospective cohort study	Occurred	Occurred	Start with exposure	Forward looking
Mixed cohort study	Occurred	Occurred; further assessed in future	Start with exposure	Forward looking
Case control study	Occurred	Occurred	Start with outcome	Backward looking
Cross-sectional study	Occurred	Occurred	Both exposure and outcome assessed at a point of time	Neither forward looking nor backward looking

- *In a Prospective cohort study, Outcome has not yet occurred when the study has begun:* Only exposure has occurred; we look for development of same disease in both exposed and non-exposed groups
- *In a Retrospective cohort study, both exposure as well as outcome have occurred when the study has begun:* First we go back in time and take only exposure into consideration (cohorts identified from past hospital/college records), then look for development of same disease in both exposed and non-exposed groups

- *In a Combined prospective-retrospective cohort study, both exposure as well as outcome have occurred when the study has begun*: First we go back in time and take only exposure into consideration (cohorts identified from past hospital/college records), then look for development of same disease in both exposed and non-exposed groups; later cohort is followed prospectively into future for outcome
- *In a Case control study, both exposure as well as outcome have occurred when the study has begun*: First we take outcome into consideration, and then go back in time taking exposure into consideration; then compare exposure in both diseased (cases) and non-diseased (controls)
- *In a nested case control study*, only exposure has occurred when the study begins; when the disease develops in a population, then 2 groups of cases (diseased) and controls (non-diseased) are formed and their exposure status is compared
- *In a case-series study, both exposure as well as outcome have occurred when the study has begun*: First we take outcome into consideration, and then go back in time taking exposure into consideration; there is NO COMPARISON with non-diseased (controls)
- *In a prevalence survey (cross-sectional study)*, exposure as well as outcome may co-exist at the time of study (there is no longitudinal direction)

Cohort Study

- Is a type of analytical (observational) study used for 'hypothesis testing'
- *Is known by several synonyms*^Q:
  - Prospective study
  - Forward looking study
  - Cause to effect study
  - Exposure to outcome study
  - Risk factor to disease study
  - *Incidence study*
  - Follow-up study
- *Types of cohort studies*:
  - **Prospective cohort study**^Q:
    - Known as *'Current cohort study'* or *'Concurrent cohort study'*
    - *Outcome has not yet occurred when the study has begun*: Only exposure has occurred; we look for development of same disease in both exposed and non-exposed groups
    - Examples:
      1. Framingham heart study
      2. Doll & Hills prospective study on smoking and lung cancer
  - **Retrospective cohort study**^Q:
    - Known as 'Historical cohort study' or 'Non-concurrent cohort study'
    - Combines advantages of both Cohort study and Case control study
    - Both exposure as well as outcome have occurred when the study has begun: First we go back in time and take only exposure into consideration (cohorts identified from past hospital/college records), then look for development of same disease in both exposed and non-exposed groups
    - *Sample size required is same as that of prospective cohort study*
    - Examples:
      1. Effect of fetal monitoring on neonatal deaths
      2. PVC exposure and angiosarcoma of liver
  - **Combined prospective-retrospective cohort study**^Q:
    - Known as *'Mixed cohort study'*
    - Combines designs of both prospective cohort study and retrospective cohort study
    - *Both exposure as well as outcome have occurred when the study has begun*: First we go back in time and take only exposure into consideration (cohorts identified from past hospital/college records), then look for development of same disease in both exposed and non-exposed groups; later cohort is followed prospectively into future for outcome
    - Examples: Court-Brown & Doll study on effects of radiation therapy

> **Key points**
>
> **Cohort Study**
> Is a type of analytical (observational) study used for 'hypothesis testing'

Strength of Association in Cohort Study

- Strength of association in a cohort study is evaluated by^Q:
  - Relative risk (RR)
  - Attributable risk (AR)
  - Population attributable risk (PAR)
- *Relative risk (RR)* = Incidence among exposed/Incidence among non-exposed^Q
  - RR = $I_{exposed}/I_{non-exposed}$
  - *Interpretation of RR*^{Q}: Incidence of lung disease among exposed IS SO MANY TIMES HIGHER as compared to that among non-exposed
- *Attributable risk (AR)* = (Incidence among exposed – Incidence among non-exposed)/Incidence among exposed × 100

  AR = $(I_{exposed} - I_{non-exposed})/I_{exposed} \times 100$

  - *Interpretation of AR*^{Q}: So much disease can be attributed to exposure
- *Population attributable risk (PAR)* = (Incidence among total – Incidence among non-exposed)/Incidence among total × 100

  PAR = $(I_{total} - I_{non-exposed})/I_{tot} \times 100$

  - *Interpretation of PAR*^{Q}: If risk factor is modified or eliminated, there will be so much annual reduction in incidence of disease in the given population

> **Key points**
>
> **Strength of association in a cohort study**
> - Relative risk (RR)
> - Attributable risk (AR)
> - Population attributable risk (PAR)

> **Key points**
>
> RR = $I_{exposed}/I_{non-exposed}$

Interpretation of Relative Risk (RR)

RR	Interpretation^Q		Example	
			Risk Factor	Disease
RR > 1	$I_{exp} > I_{nonexp}$	So many times chances/incidence of disease development is more among exposed as compared to non-exposed **(Positive Association)**	Smoking	Lung Cancer
RR = 1	$I_{exp} = I_{nonexp}$	Chances/incidence of disease development is same among exposed as compared to non-exposed **(No Association)**	Smoking	HIV/AIDS
RR < 1	$I_{exp} < I_{nonexp}$	Chances/incidence of disease development is less among exposed as compared to non-exposed **(Negative Association)**	Vitamin-A intake	Epithelial cancers

> **Key points**
>
> RR = 1 (No Association)

Framingham Heart Study^Q

- *Is a classical example of cohort study*
  - Initiated in 1948 by US Public Health Service at Framingham, a town in Massachusetts, USA
- *Aim*: To study the relationship of risk factors (serum cholesterol, blood pressure, weight, smoking) to the subsequent development of cardiovascular diseases
  - **Age group: 30–62 years**
  - *Sample size*: 5127 (4469 – 69% of the sample actually underwent first examination)
- *Method*: Multiple exposure were studied, as well as complex interactions among the exposures using multivariate techniques
  - *Follow-up*:
    - Study population was examined **every 2 years for 20 years**
    - Daily surveillance of hospitalizations at only hospital at Framingham
- *Findings of study*:
  - Increasing risk of CHD with increasing age & more seen in males
  - Hypertensive have a greater risk of CHD
  - Elevated blood cholesterol level is associated with CHD
  - Tobacco smoking and habitual use of alcohol increase risk of CHD
  - Increased physical activity decrease CHD development
  - Increase in body weight is associated predisposes to CHD
  - Diabetes mellitus increases risk of CHD

> **Key points**
>
> **Framingham Heart Study**
> *Is a classical example of cohort study*

Cohort Studies versus Case Control Studies^Q

	Cohort Studies	Case Control Studies
Before start	Only exposure has occurred	Both exposure as well as outcome have occurred
Synonyms	Prospective study Forward looking study Cause to effect study Exposure to outcome study Risk factor to disease study Incidence study Follow up study	Retrospective study Backward looking study Effect to cause to study Outcome to exposure study Disease to risk factor study TROHOC study
Advantages^Q	Provides Incidence, Relative risk Allows study of several etiological factors simultaneously No Recall bias	Easy to carry out Rapid & Inexpensive No risk to subjects Minimal ethical problems No loss to follow up/Attrition *'Particularly suitable to investigate rare diseases'*
Disadvantages^Q	Ethical problems Loss to follow up (attrition) Time consuming Expensive Not suitable to investigate rare diseases	Selection of an appropriate control group may be difficult Cannot measure incidence: can only estimate Odds ratio Recall bias
Strength of association	Relative risk (RR) AR PAR	Odds ratio (OR)

Controls in a Case Control Study

- In a case control study, selection of controls is a prerequisite
- If the study group is small, choose up to 4 controls per case (In larger studies with equal cost to collect cases and controls 1 : 1 is sufficient^Q)
- Cases are diseased individuals, Controls are those free from the disease under study
- Controls must be similar to cases, as much as possible except for the absence of disease under study
- Sources of controls^Q:
  - Hospital controls: are often a 'source of selection bias'
  - Neighbourhood controls: provide similar socio-economic and living conditions
  - Relatives: Sibling controls are unsuitable in genetic studies^Q
  - General population: by choosing a random sample
  - Best friends controls

> **Key points**
> Sibling controls are unsuitable in genetic studies

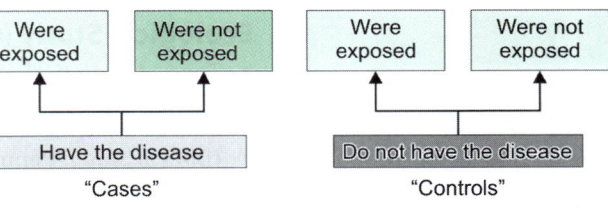

Case control study

Strength of Association in a Case Control Study

- *Strength of association in a case control study*^Q: Case Control Study cannot provide with incidences, so Relative Risk cannot be calculated; so in a Case Control Study, we calculate *'an estimate of Relative Risk'*, known as *'Odds Ratio'* (CROSS PRODUCT RATIO)
- CORRECT TABLE CONSTRUCTION in a case control study: Table will have disease at the top (row) and history of exposure/risk factor on the left (column)
- Odds Ratio In a 2 × 2 table for a case control study:

> **Key points**
> Strength of association in a case control study^Q: 'Odds Ratio'

	Disease Present (cases)	Disease Absent (controls)
Exposure present	a	b
Exposure absent	c	d

Odds Ratio (Cross Product Ratio) = ad/bc

> **Key points**
> **Odds Ratio** (Cross Product Ratio) = ad/bc

Relative Risk (RR) versus Odds Ratio (OR)^Q

> **Key points**
> Cross-Sectional Study Provides *'Prevalence of the disease'*

	Relative risk (RR)	Odds ratio (OR)
Synonyms	Risk ratio	Cross product ratio
Utility	Estimates strength of association in a cohort study	Estimates strength of association in a case control study
Measure of strength of association	More accurate estimate	Less accurate (only an estimate of RR)
Calculation	exposed/non-exposed	ad/bc

Cross-Sectional Study

- Is based on the single examination of a cross-section of a population *'at one point of time'*, results of sample are then projected to whole population
- Is simplest form of observational epidemiological study^Q
- *Advantages*:
  - Provides *'Prevalence of the disease'* under study^Q
  - Gives *'Snapshot of a population'*
  - More useful for chronic diseases
- *Disadvantages*:
  - Tells about distribution of a disease, *'rather than its etiology'*
  - **Cannot establish causality as *'does not establish time sequence^Q'***
  - Provides little information about natural history of disease or incidence

Cross sectional study: Defined population → Gather data on exposure and disease → Exposed and have disease | Exposed and do not have | Not exposed have | Not exposed and do

Ecological Study (Correlational Study)

> **Key points**
> Ecological Study *Units of Study*: Population

- Type of analytical (observational) epidemiological study which provide the *'least satisfactory type of evidence on causality'*
- Is the least preferable observational/analytical study design^Q
- **Units of study: Population^Q**
- *Done in a small time frame*: Inexpensive; use data that is already available
- *Advantage*: Data can be used from populations with different characteristics
- *Disadvantages*:
  - *Potential problem*: Socio-economic confounding
  - *Ecological fallacy^Q*: Is an error of interpretation of statistical data in an ecological study, whereby characteristics are ascribed to a group of individuals which they may not possess as individuals

Utilities of Epidemiological Studies

> **Key points**
> Preference of epidemiological studies for establishing causality^Q: 1st preference: Meta-analysis

- *Preference of epidemiological studies for establishing causality^Q*:
  - **1st preference: Meta-analysis**
  - 2nd preference: Randomised controlled trials (RCTs)
  - 3rd preference: Retrospective (Non-concurrent/Historical) cohort study
  - 4th preference: Prospective cohort study (Concurrent cohort study)
  - 5th preference: Case control study
  - 6th preference: Cross-sectional study
  - 7th preference: Ecological study

- *Useful Parameter(s) obtained by epidemiological studies^Q*:

Epidemiological studies	Useful parameter(s) obtained
Cohort study	Incidence, Relative risk, Attributable risk (AR), Population AR
Case control study	Odds ratio
Cross sectional study	Prevalence
Ecological study	Group characteristics

- *Abilities of epidemiological studies to prove causation^Q*:

Type of study	Ability to prove causation
Randomised controlled trial	Strong
Cohort study	Moderate
Case control study	Moderate
Cross sectional study	Weak
Ecological study	Weak

- *Applications of various study designs^Q*:

Application	Utility of study			
	Cohort	Case-control	Cross-sectional	Ecological
Investigation of rare disease	–	+++++	–	++++
Investigation of rare cause	+++++	–	–	++
Testing multiple effects	+++++	–	++	+
Study of multiple exposure	+++	++++	++	++
Measurement of time relationship	+++++	+	–	++
Direct incidence measurement	+++++	+	–	–
Investigation of long latent periods	+	+++	–	–

Potential Errors in Epidemiological Studies

- *Random errors*: SAMPLING ERRORS
  - Is *'divergence due to chance alone'* of an observation on a sample from true population value, leading to *'lack of precision'* in measurement
  - Random error *'cannot be completely eliminated'*
  - Random errors can be reduced by: careful measurement of exposure and outcome, thus making individual measurements precise
  - Best way of reducing sampling errors (increasing precision): Increase the sample size in the study
- *Systematic errors*: BIASES
  - Occur whenever there is a tendency to produce results that differ in systematic manner from the true values
  - Bias is any *'systematic error'* in an epidemiological study, occurring during data collection, compilation, analysis and interpretation

Bias

- *Bias*: Is any *'systematic error'* in an epidemiological study, occurring during data collection, compilation, analysis and interpretation^Q
- *Predominantly biases are of 3 types*:
  - *Subject bias*: Error introduced by study subjects. Examples:
    - Hawthorne effect^Q
    - Recall bias^Q
  - *Investigator bias*: Error introduced by investigator
    - Selection bias^Q
  - *Analyzer bias*: Error introduced by analyzer

> **Key points**
>
> **Bias** is any *'systematic error'* in an epidemiological study

Some Important Types of Biases in Epidemiological Studies

- *Apprehension bias*: Certain levels (pulse, blood pressure) may alter systematically from their usual levels when the subject is apprehensive
- *Attention bias (Hawthorne effect)*: Study subjects may systematically alter their behaviour when they know they are being observed^Q
- *Berksonian bias (Admission rate bias)*: Bias due to hospital cases and controls being systematically different from each other^Q
- *Interviewer bias*: Interviewer devotes more time of interview with cases as compared to controls^Q
- *Lead time bias (Zero time shift bias)*: Bias of over-estimation of survival time, due to backward shift in starting point, as by screening procedures^Q
- *Memory/Recall bias*: Cases are more likely to remember exposure more correctly than controls^Q
- *Neyman bias (Prevalence-incidence bias)*: Bias due to missing of fatal cases, mild/silent cases and cases of short duration of episodes from the study^Q
- *Selection bias (Susceptibility bias)*: Groups to be compared are differentially susceptible to the outcome of interest, even before the experimental maneuver is performed^Q

Minimization of Biases in Epidemiological Studies

- *Blinding*:

Type	Method^Q	Minimizes^Q
Single blinding	Study subjects are not aware of the treatment they are receiving	Subject bias
Double blinding	Study subjects as well as investigator are not aware of the treatment study subjects are receiving	Subject bias + Investigator bias
Triple blinding	Study subjects, investigator as well as analyzer are not aware of the treatment study subjects are receiving	Subject bias + Investigator bias + Analyzer bias

Confounding

- *Confounding*: Any factor associated with both exposure and outcome, and has an independent effect in causation of outcome is a confounder^Q
    - It is found unequally distributed between the study and control groups
    - Is associated with both exposure and outcome
    - Has an independent effect in causation of outcome (thus is a risk factor itself)

Methods Used to Control Confounding

Method	Utility to control confounding^Q
Randomization	Most ideal method^Q
Restriction	Limiting study to people who have particular characteristics
Matching	Mostly useful in case control studies
Stratification	Useful for larger studies
Statistical modeling	When many confounding variables exist simultaneously

Matching

- *Matching*: Process of selecting controls in such a way that they are similar to cases (with regard to certain pertinent selected variables which may influence the outcome of disease, thereby distorting the results)
    - *Matching eliminates confounding*: Matching distributes known confounding factors equally in two groups^Q
- *Types of matching*:
    - *Caliper matching*: Process of matching comparison group subjects to study group subjects within a specified distance for a continuous variable (matching age to within 2 years)
    - *Frequency matching*: Frequency distributions of matched variable(s) are similar in study and comparison groups
    - *Category matching*: Process of matching study and control group subjects in broad classes (e.g. occupational groups)

- *Individual matching*: Relies on identifying individual subjects for comparison, each resembling a study subject for matched variable(s)
- *Pair matching*: Individual matching in which study & comparison subjects are paired

Randomization is Superior to BOTH Matching and Blinding

	Blinding	Matching	Randomization
Removes	Bias	Known confounding	Selection bias Known confounding Unknown confounding
Types	Single blinding Double blinding Triple blinding	Caliper matching Frequency matching Category matching Individual matching Pair matching	Random number tables Computer software Currency notes Lottery method

Nested Case Control Study

- Is a hybrid design where *'a case control study is nested in a cohort study'*
- Is predominantly a type of Cohort study (due to forward direction)^Q
- Usefulness limited for studies involving *'rare diseases AND whose diagnostic tests are very expensive'*
- *Study design*:
  - A population is identified and baseline data is obtained from interviews, blood or urine tests, etc.
  - Population is then followed up for a period of time (Cohort study) for development for the disease under study
  - A Case control study is then carried out:
    - *Cases:* people who developed the disease
    - *Controls:* Sample from those who did not develop the disease
    - Samples/history collected at baseline are then examined
- *Advantages*:
  - *Elimination of problem of Recall bias*: Interviews are performed at the beginning of the study (at baseline), and data are obtained before the disease has developed
  - *Maintenance of temporal association*^{Q}: If any disease or abnormality in a biological characteristic is noted, it is more likely that it represent risk factors or other pre-morbid characteristics rather than a manifestation of early, subclinical disease
  - *Economical to conduct*: Expensive tests need not be conducted on entire population; only carried out among cases and controls

> **Key points**
> Nested Case Control Study *Is predominantly a type of Cohort study*

EXPERIMENTAL EPIDEMIOLOGY

Randomised Controlled Trials (RCTs)

- Unit of study in RCT: Patient^Q
- RCT is of two types:
  - **Concurrent parallel design**: Comparisons are made between 2 groups:
    - *Experimental group*: Is exposed to specific medication or intervention
    - *Reference group*: Is not exposed to specific medication or intervention
  - **Crossover design**: Comparisons are made between 2 groups:
    - *Experimental group*: Is exposed to specific medication or intervention
    - *Reference group*: Is not exposed to specific medication or intervention
  - Then the groups are crossed-over (exposed group now becomes non-exposed and vice-versa)
  - Cross-over design RCT helps removing ethical concerns^Q
- **Intention to treat trial**: Implies that the results of a RCT are unaffected by attrition (loss to follow up) or change over of study subjects from one group to another^Q

> **Key points**
> Unit of study in RCT: Patient^Q

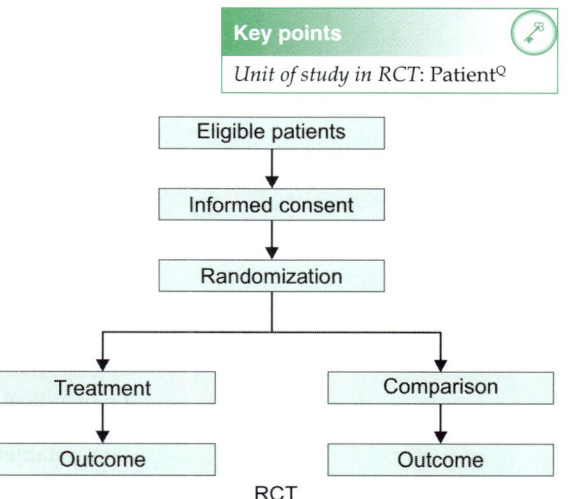

RCT

Randomisation in RCT

- *Randomisation* in Randomized Controlled trial (RCT) is a statistical procedure by which participants are allocated into either of two groups, viz., *'Experimental Group'* (in which intervention is given) and *'Reference Group'* (in which intervention is not given)
- Randomisation is best done by 'Random number tables'
- The essential purposes of randomization in a randomized controlled trial[Q]:
  - Participants have *'Equal and Known Chance'*[Q] of falling into either 'Experimental Group' or 'Reference Group'
  - To *eliminate Selection Bias*[Q]
  - To *ensure comparability* among two groups[Q]
  - To have *'similar prognostic factors'* among two groups[Q]
- Randomisation is known as *'Heart of a trial'*[Q]
- Randomization *'removes both confounding and bias'*
  - *Randomisation IS SUPERIOR to Matching*: Randomization ensures *'both known and unknown'* confounding factors are distributed equally among the two groups, thereby nullifying their effect on result (whereas matching is useful for only known confounding factors)

> **Key points**
> The essential purposes of Randomization:
> To *eliminate Selection Bias*

> **Key points**
> Randomisation is known as 'Heart of a Trial'

Pre-post Clinical Trial

- *Does not have a true control group:* Patient act as his or her own control[Q]
- *Each patient has a pre-test score followed by a post-test:* Difference in scores reflect change attributed to intervention
- *Use:* Is often used in assessing whether knowledge, attitudes or pre-existing risk behaviors change when a subject is assigned to an intervention
- *Limitations:*
  - Difficult to assess if change is due to developmental intercourse
  - Difficult to assess if change is due to regression to mean
  - Not useful in studies involving mortality as post-test won't be available
  - More difficult to interpret than the comparable parallel clinical trial
  - Cannot be randomized

> **Key points**
> *Pre-post Clinical Trial:* Patient act as his or her own control[Q]

Preclinical and Clinical Trials

Phase	Unit of study	Purpose
PRECLINICAL PHASE		
Lab experiments	Animals[Q]	Pretesting
CLINICAL PHASES		
Phase 0	Healthy human volunteers	Micro-dosing[Q]
Phase I	Healthy human volunteers[Q]	Safety and non-toxicity profile[Q]
Phase II	Patients	Efficacy
Phase III	Patients	Comparison with existing drugs[Q]
Phase IV	Patients	Long-term and rare side effects[Q]

> **Key points**
> *Phase III is an RCT*

- *Phase III is an RCT:* Comparison of a new drug with an existing old drug[Q]
- *New drug is launched in market after:* Phase III
- Longest phase of a trial: Phase IV
- *Post-marketing surveillance:* Phase IV[Q]
- Maximum tolerated dose (MTD) of a drug: Phase I[Q]
- Maximum drug failure reported: Phase II

> **Key points**
> *Post-marketing surveillance:* Phase IV

Meta-analysis

- Description:
  - An objective, systematic review that employs statistical methods to combine and summarize the results of several studies[Q]
  - A quantitative synthesis of all unbiased evidence, meant for summarizing large volume of data, establishing and determining the magnitude of an effect, and to increase power and precision of studies

- Results:
  - *Forest plot*^Q: To describe the distribution of your effect sizes
  - *Funnel plot*^Q: To check the existence of publication bias
- *Strengths*^Q:
  - Provides a point estimate of an effect size
  - Commonly report confidence intervals around effect sizes
  - Identify few gaps in a particular field
- *Limitations*^Q:
  - GIGO (Garbage in, garbage out): Results can only be as good as the original data is valid
  - Apples and oranges effect: Tendency to average/mash together different effects
  - File drawer effect: Publication bias
  - Relies on shared subjectivity rather than objectivity

ASSOCIATION AND CAUSATION

Hill's (Surgeon General's) Criteria of Causal Association^Q

- *Temporal association*: Implies *'cause precedes effect'* or *'effect follows cause'*
  - Considers both *'order of appearance'* as well as *'length of interval between exposure and disease'*
  - Is *'most important criterion'* of causal association^Q
  - Is *'best established by a cohort study'* (Especially Concurrent cohort study)^Q
- *Strength of association*:
  - Relative risk (cohort study)
  - Odds ratio (case control study)
- *Specificity of association*: Implies that disease under study is caused only by risk factor under study
  - Is *'most difficult criterion to establish*^Q*'*
  - Is *'weakest criterion'* of causal association
- *Consistency of association*^Q: Implies that results are replicable in different settings and by different methods
- *Biological plausibility*: Implies existence of biological credibility of association (anatomically, physiologically explainable/justifiable)
- *Coherence of association*: Implies that the causal association must be coherent (supported by) with relevant facts/related studies
- *Dose-response relationshipQ*: Implies that increase in dose of cause increases incidence/prevalence of effect
- *Cessation of exposure; Reversibility*: Implies that removal of possible cause reduces the risk of disease
- *Study design*: Implies that if study design is based on a strong study design

Key points

Temporal association:
Is *'most important criterion'* of causal association

EPIDEMIOLOGY OF INFECTIOUS DISEASES

Definitions^Q

- *Infectivity*: Number infected/Number exposed
- *Pathogenicity*: Number of diseased/Number infected
- *Virulence*: Number of serious condition & mortality/Number diseased
- *Case fatality*: Number of deaths/Number of cases
- *Communicability*: Ability of a disease to spread from infective to susceptible hosts

Zoonoses

- *Zoonoses*: An infection or infectious disease transmissible under natural conditions from vertebrate animals to man
- **Classification of Zoonoses based on direction of transmission:**
  - *Anthropozoonoses*: Infections transmitted from animals (zoo) to man (anthro)
    - *Examples*: Rabies^Q, Plague, Anthrax, Hydatid disease, Trichinosis
  - *Zooanthroponoses*: Infections transmitted from man (anthro) to animals (zoo)
    - *Example*: Human TB in cattle

Key points

Anthropozoonoses: Infections transmitted from animals (zoo) to man (anthro)

- *Amphixenosis*: Infections transmitted in either direction between animals and man
  - *Example*: Trypanosoma cruzi, Schistosoma japonicum
- **Classification of Zoonoses based upon life cycle of infecting organism:**
  - *Direct zoonoses*: Transmitted from infected to susceptible vertebrate host by direct contact/fomite/vector. Examples: Rabies, Brucellosis, Trichinosis
  - *Cyclo-zoonoses*: Involve more than one vertebrate species. Examples: Taeniasis, Echinococcosis
  - *Meta-zoonoses*: Transmitted biologically by invertebrate vectors. Examples: Plague^Q, Schistosomiasis, Arboviral infections
  - *Sapro-zoonoses*: Involves non-animal developmental site or reservoir.
    - Examples: Mycoses, Larva migrans
- *Related terminology:*
  - *Reverse Zoonoses*: Is synonymous with Zooanthroponoses
  - *Epizootic*: Outbreak (epidemic) of a disease in animal population. Examples: Anthrax, Brucellosis, Influenza, Rabies, Rift Valley Fever, Q-fever, Japanese encephalitis, Equine encephalitis
  - *Enzootic*: Endemic of disease occurring in animals. Examples: Anthrax, Rabies, Brucellosis, Bovine TB, Endemic typhus, Tick typhus
  - *Epornithic*: Outbreak (epidemic) of a disease in bird population

> **Key points**
> *Meta-zoonoses:* Transmitted biologically by invertebrate vectors. Example: Plague

Endemic

- *Endemic:* Refers to the *'usual or expected frequency of disease'* within a population group; is the *'constant presence of a disease in a defined geographical area'*
  - *Hyperendemic*: When a disease is constantly present at a high incidence and/or prevalence rate and affects all age groups equally.
  - *Holoendemic*: When a disease has a high level of infection beginning early in life and affects most of children population. So, disease is more common among children than adults
  - For the disease to be in an endemic steady state: $R0 \times S = 1$ [where, R0 = Basic reproduction number of an infection (the mean number of secondary cases a typical single infected case will cause in a population with no immunity and in the absence of interventions); S = Proportion of susceptibles in population]
- *Endemic curve:* Is drawn between no. of cases due to a disease and the time
  - *Endemic curve IS NOT a straight line*: As number of cases for the endemic disease in a population will not be fixed throughout a year; it will show a seasonal or other variation
  - *Endemic curve Vs epidemic curve*: In endemic curve, the baseline of the curve NEVER touches zero

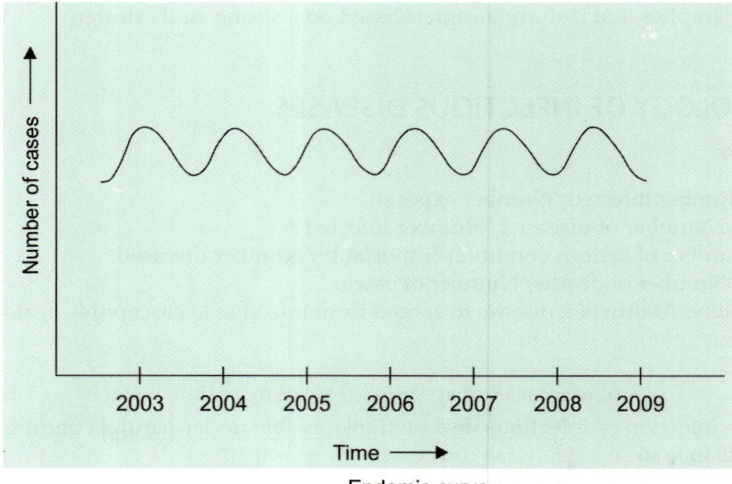

Endemic curve

  - When a disease occurs *'clearly in excess of normal expectancy'*, it becomes an *Epidemic*
- *Ecdemic:* of or relating to a disease that originates outside the geographical area in which it occurs

DISEASE TRANSMISSION

Definitions

- *Incubation period^Q:* Is the time interval between invasion by an infectious agent and appearance of the first sign or symptom of the disease in question
- *Median incubation period^Q:* Is the time required for 50% of cases to occur
- *Generation time^Q:* Is the time taken for a person from receipt of infection to develop maximum infectivity
  - Is roughly equal to the incubation period of the disease
- *Latent period:* Is the period from disease initiation to disease detection, used in non-infectious diseases as equivalent of incubation period
- *Serial interval^Q:* is the gap in onset between primary case (first case in the community) and secondary case (case developing through infection from the primary case)
  - By collecting information on series of secondary cases with serial intervals, one can guess the incubation period of a disease
- *Period of communicability:* Is the time during which an infectious agent may be transferred directly/indirectly from an infected person to another person, from infected animal to man or from an infected person to animal, including arthropods
  - An important measure of communicability is secondary attack rate

Key points

Serial interval^Q: is the gap in onset between primary case (first case in the community) and secondary case

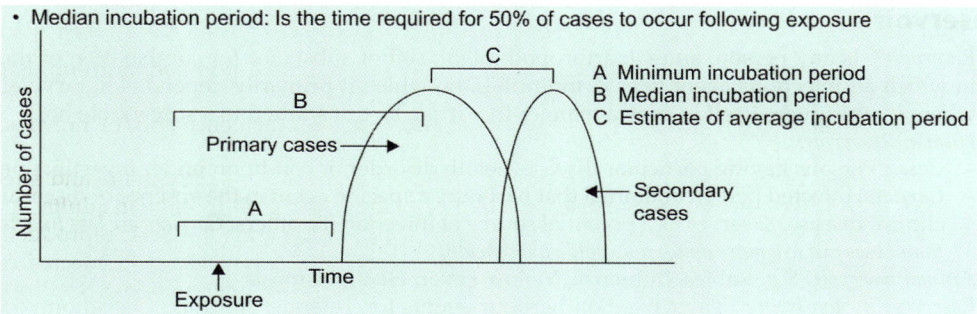

- Median incubation period: Is the time required for 50% of cases to occur following exposure

A Minimum incubation period
B Median incubation period
C Estimate of average incubation period

Incubation period and serial interval

Incubation Period

- Incubation period depends upon^Q:
  - Generation time of the pathogen
  - Infective dose
  - Portal of entry
  - Individual susceptibility
- Incubation period of a disease is useful for^Q:
  - Tracing the source of infection and contacts
  - Determining the period of surveillance
  - Applying immunization principles for prevention of diseases
  - Identification of point source or propagated epidemics
  - Estimating prognosis of a disease

Attack Rate (AR)

- Relates to no. of cases in the population at risk
- Reflects extent of epidemic
- Is used when 'population is exposed to risk for a limited period of time, such as epidemic'

$$AR = \frac{\text{No. of new cases of specified disease in a specified time interval}}{\text{Total population at risk during the same time interval}} \times 100$$

Secondary Attack Rate

- *Secondary Attack Rate (SAR^Q):* Is no. of exposed persons developing the disease within range of incubation period (IP), following exposure to the primary case

$$\text{SAR} = \frac{\text{No. of exposed persons developing disease within range of IP}}{\text{Total no. of exposed 'susceptible' contacts}} \times 100$$

- Denominator includes *only those susceptible in close contact*^{Q}
- *Primary case is always excluded both from numerator and denominator* for SAR calculation
- Secondary Attack Rate (SAR) of few diseases:

Disease	Secondary Attack Rate (SAR)
Small pox	30 – 45%
Measles^Q	> 80%
Chicken pox^Q	~90%
Mumps^Q	~86%
Pertussis	~90%

Source

- *Source:* Is a person, animal, object or substance from which an infectious agent passes or is disseminated to the host
  - Source refers to immediate source of infection & may or may not be part of reservoir

Reservoir

- *Reservoir^Q:* Is any person, animal, arthropod, plant, soil or substance (or combination of these) in which an infectious agent lives & multiplies, on which it primarily depends for survival, & where it reproduces itself in such a manner that it can be transmitted to a susceptible host
- *Human Reservoir:*
  - *Cases*: Persons having particular disease, health disorder or condition under investigation
  - *Carriers*: Infected person or animal that harbours a specific agent in the absence of discernible clinical disease, & serves as a potential source of infection for others; *Carriers are less infectious than cases but are more dangerous epidemiologically*
- *Animal reservoir:* E.g. Rabies, Influenza, Yellow Fever, Histoplasmosis
- *Reservoir in non-living things:* E.g. Soil harbour agents for Tetanus, Anthrax, Coccidiomycosis, Mycetoma

Infection	Source	Reservoir
Hookworm	Soil^Q	Man^Q
Tetanus	Soil^Q	Soil^Q
Typhoid	Feces/urine/Food/Milk/Water	Case/Carrier

Cases

- *Cases:* Persons having particular disease, health disorder or condition under investigation
  - *Clinical cases*: Mild, Moderate, Severe or Fatal
  - *Subclinical cases*: Inapparent, covert, missed or abortive
  - *Latent Infection*: Host does not shed the infectious agent which lies dormant in host without symptoms. (E.g. Herpes simplex, Brill Zinsser Disease, Ancylostomiasis)

Cases in Epidemiology

- *Primary case:* First case of communicable disease introduced into the population unit being studied
- *Secondary cases:* Cases that develop from contact with the primary case
- *Index case^Q:* First case that comes to the notice of the investigator (first case reported to the health system)

Carriers

- *Carriers:* Infected person or animal that harbours a specific agent in the absence of discernible clinical disease, & serves as a potential source of infection for others
  - Carriers are less infectious than cases but are more dangerous epidemiologically^Q
- *Carriers by type:*
  - *Incubatory Carriers*: Shed infectious agent during incubation period of disease, e.g. Measles, Mumps, Polio, Pertussis, Influenza, Diphtheria, Hepatitis-B^Q

> **Key points**
> Primary case is always excluded both from numerator and denominator for SAR calculation

> **Key points**
> *Index case^Q*: First case that comes to the notice of the investigator

- *Convalescent Carriers*: shed the disease agent during the period of Convalescence, e.g. Typhoid, Bacillary Dysentery, Amoebic Dysentery, Cholera, Diphtheria & Pertussis[Q] (*Clinical recovery does not coincide with bacteriological recovery[Q]*)
- *Healthy carriers*: emerge from subclinical cases without suffering from overt disease, e.g. Poliomyelitis, Cholera, Meningococcal Meningitis, Diphtheria & Salmonellosis

- Carriers by duration:
  - *Temporary Carriers*: Shed infectious agent for short periods of time, e.g. Incubatory carriers, Convalescent carriers, Healthy carriers
  - *Chronic Carriers*: Excretes infectious agents for indefinite periods, e.g. Typhoid, Hepatitis-B, Dysentery, Meningococcal Meningitis, Malaria, Gonorrhoea, etc.
- Carriers by portal of exit:
  - Urinary carriers, e.g. typhoid
  - Intestinal carriers, e.g. typhoid, cholera, amoebiasis
  - Nasal carriers, e.g. Diphtheria, staphylococcal food poisoning
  - Respiratory carriers
  - Nasopharyngeal carriers, e.g. Meningococcus

INVESTIGATION OF AN EPIDEMIC

Objectives of Investigation of an Epidemic
- To define magnitude or involvement (time, place, person)
- To determine responsible conditions and factors
- To identify causes, source(s) and modes of transmission
- To make recommendations to prevent reoccurrence

Steps for Investigation of an Epidemic
- *Verification of diagnosis*:
  - Is the '*first step in investigation of an epidemic[Q]*'
  - It is '*not necessary to examine all cases*': take sample
  - Do not wait for laboratory results for epidemiological investigations
- *Confirmation of existence of an epidemic*:
  - Compare with disease frequencies during same period in previous years
  - *Epidemic threshold*: An arbitrary limit of '*2 standard errors from the endemic occurrence*'
- *Defining the population at risk*:
  - Obtaining the map of the area
  - Calculation of '*appropriate denominator of population at risk*'
- *Rapid search for all cases and their characteristics*:
  - Medical survey
  - Epidemiological case sheet
  - Searching for more cases: Search for new cases is carried out everyday, till the area is declared free of epidemic; this period is usually taken as '*twice the incubation period of the disease since the occurrence of last case[Q]*'
- *Data analysis*:
  - Time: Construction of an epidemic curve
  - Place: Preparation of a spot map
  - Person: Analysis by age, sex, occupation and other risk factors
- *Formulation of hypothesis*
- *Testing of hypothesis*
- *Evaluation of ecological factors*
- *Further investigation of population at risk*
- *Writing the report*

Key points

Verification of diagnosis:
Is the '*first step in investigation of an epidemic[Q]*'

Key points

During Epidemic: Search for new cases is carried out everyday, till the area is declared free of epidemic; this period is usually taken as '*twice the incubation period of the disease since the occurrence of last case[Q]*'

IMMUNITY, VACCINES AND COLD CHAIN

Vaccine
- *Vaccine*: Is an immuno-biological substance designed to produce specific protection against a given disease

History of Vaccination

- *Term 'Vaccine' was coined by:* Louis Pasteur[Q]
- *Term 'Vaccination' was coined by:* Edward Jenner[Q]
- *First vaccine to be developed*[Q]: Small pox (1798)
- *First vaccine was developed by:* Edward Jenner
- *Important milestones in vaccination:*

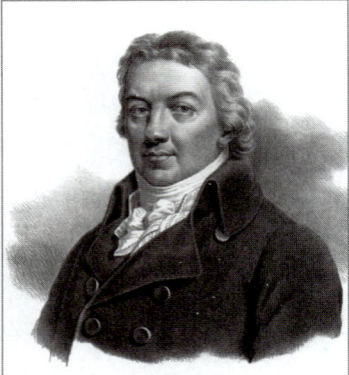

Edward Jenner

Year	Vaccine
1798	Small pox vaccine
1885	Rabies vaccine
1892	Cholera vaccine
1921	BCG vaccine
1923	Diphtheria toxoid
1923	Pertussis vaccine
1927	Tetanus toxoid
1937	Influenza vaccine
1937	Yellow fever vaccine
1949	Mumps vaccine
1954	IPV
1957	OPV
1960	Measles vaccine
1962	Rubella vaccine
1968	Type C meningococcal vaccine
1971	Type A meningococcal vaccine
1976	Hepatitis B vaccine
1986	Recombinant Hepatitis B vaccine
2006	Live Oral Rotavirus vaccine
2007	Human Papilloma virus vaccine
2008	Rotarix (2 dose)
2009	H_1N_1 Influenza A

> **Key points**
> *First vaccine to be developed*[Q]: Small pox (1798)

Types of Vaccines

- *Live 'attenuated' vaccines:*
  - Are prepared from repeated passage of organisms in tissue culture or chick embryos
  - Attenuation implies *'Reduced pathogenicity/virulence; Maintained antigenicity/immunogenicity*[Q]'
- *Inactivated/Killed vaccines:*
  - Organisms killed by heat or chemicals stimulate active immunity, when introduced in body
  - Safe but less efficacious than live vaccines
  - Usually administered by intramuscular or subcutaneous route
- *Toxoids:*
  - Toxins produced by organisms are detoxicated and used for vaccine preparation
  - Highly efficacious and safe
- *Cellular fractions:*
  - Vaccines are prepared from extracted cellular fractions
- *Recombinant (or Mixed) vaccines:*
  - More than one kind of immunizing agents is used in vaccine

> **Key points**
> Attenuation implies *'Reduced pathogenicity/virulence; Maintained antigenicity/immunogenicity*[Q]'

Live 'attenuated' vaccines	Killed 'inactivated' vaccines
BCG	Pertussis
OPV (Sabin – Oral polio vaccine)	IPV (Salk – Inactivated polio vaccine)
Measles vaccine	Rabies vaccine
Mumps vaccine	Cholera vaccine
Rubella vaccine	Meningococcal vaccine

Contd...

Contd...

Yellow fever vaccine Typhoral Live plague vaccine Varicella vaccine Epidemic typhus vaccine Zoster vaccine Cold adapted Influenza Rotavirus reassortants JE Live Vaccine	Killed plague vaccine Killed influenza vaccine JE (Japanese encephalitis) vaccine KFD (Kyasanur forest disease) vaccine Tick-borne encephalitis vaccine Hepatitis A Vaccine Covaxin
Subunit vaccines – Recombinant protein Hepatitis B vaccine Anti-HPV vaccines Lyme disease vaccine Cholera toxin B vaccine	**Subunit vaccines – Proteinaceous** Acellular pertussis vaccine Anthrax vaccine Inactivated influenza subunit vaccine Corbevax
Subunit vaccines – Polysaccharide based Pneumococcal vaccine Meningococcal vaccine HiB vaccine Typhim-Vi vaccine	**Subunit vaccines – Glycoconjugate** Pneumococcal vaccine MenACWY vaccine HiB vaccine
Subunit vaccines – Toxoids Diphtheria toxoid Tetanus toxoid	**Combination vaccines** DPT vaccine, DT vaccine, DPT-Typhoid vaccine MMR vaccine DPTP (DPT+IPV) Pentavalent vaccine (DPT+HepB+HiB)
Viral vector based Covishield Incovacc	

Strains of Commonly Used Vaccines

Vaccine	Strain(s)^a
BCG	Danish-1331 strain (WHO recommended)
OPV/IPV	P1, P2, P3 strains (Monovalent or Trivalent or Bivalent)
Measles vaccine	Edmonston Zagreb strain (MC) Schwartz strain Moraten strain
Mumps vaccine	Jeryll Lynn strain
Rubella vaccine	RA 27/3
Yellow Fever vaccine	17 D strain
Varicella vaccine	OKA strain
Japanese Encephalitis vaccine	Nakayama strain Beijing P3 strain SA 14-14-2 (Used in India)
Swine Flu Vaccine (killed)	A7/California/2009
Malaria vaccine	SPf 66 strain (Lytic Coktail) Pf 25 strain RTS,S/AS01 (Mosquirix)
HIV vaccines	mVA (modified Vaccinia Ankara) strain rAAV (recombinant Adeno associated viral vaccine) strain CTL (Cytotoxic T- lymphocytic) strain AIDSVAX strain Subunit Vaccine strain
Typhoral vaccine	Ty 21 a
Covaxin	Niv-2020-770

> **Key points**
> *Rubella vaccine* RA 27/3
> *Yellow Fever vaccine* 17 D strain

Contraindications to Vaccines

- *Vaccines contraindicated in Pregnancy^Q:* All live vaccines EXCEPT Yellow fever vaccine
- *Vaccines contraindicated in HIV^Q:*
  - Asymptomatic HIV: NONE
  - Symptomatic HIV: All live vaccines EXCEPT MMR, Varicella & Zoster may be given if required
- *Vaccines contraindicated in Immuno-suppression:* All live vaccines
- *Vaccines contraindicated in Corticosteroid therapy:* All live vaccines
- *Vaccines contraindicated in fever:* Typhoid vaccines
  - Typhoral
  - Typhim – Vi
  - TAB
- *Vaccines contraindicated in ARTI/diarrhoea:* NONE
- *Vaccines contraindicated together:* Yellow fever and Cholera vaccine
- *Vaccine contraindicated in Preterm-premature baby with birth weight < 2 kg^Q:* Hepatitis B
- *Vaccines contraindicated in age < 1 year (infants):*
  - Yellow fever vaccine
  - Meningococcal vaccine
  - Pneumococcal vaccine
- *Vaccines contraindicated in age < 2 year (infants):*
  - Meningococcal vaccine
  - Pneumococcal vaccine
  - Typhoid vaccines
- *Vaccine contraindicated in progressive neurological disease:* Pertussis vaccine (Pertussis vaccine IS NOT CONTRAINDICATED IN epilepsy controlled on medications, Cerebral palsy)
- *Only absolute contraindication to killed vaccines:* Severe local or general reaction to a previous dose

> **Key points**
> Vaccines contraindicated in Pregnancy^Q: All live vaccines

Specific Side-effects of Vaccines

- *Guillain Barré Syndrome:* Killed influenza vaccine^Q
- *Vaccine associated paralysis:* OPV (Sabin)^Q
- *Toxic shock syndrome (TSS):* Measles vaccine, MMR^Q
- *Shock:* DPT, Pertussis vaccine^Q
- *Hypersensitivity:* Hep-B, Meningococcal vaccine, DPT, dT^Q

> **Key points**
> Vaccine associated paralysis: OPV (Sabin)^Q

General Rules for Multiple Vaccine Administration

- 2 live vaccines can be given together
- Live and killed vaccines can be given together
- Multiple vaccines can be given together
- Cholera vaccine and Yellow fever vaccine cannot be given together
- OPV is a live vaccine where single dose is not sufficient for immunization

Adjuvants in Vaccines

Name	Class	Components	Vaccine
Alum	Mineral salts	Aluminium hydroxide, Aluminium phosphate	Diphtheria, Pertussis, Pneumococcus, HPV, Anthrax, HAV, HBV, Tick encephalitis, MenC
MF59	Oil-in-water emulsion	Squalene, Tween 80, Span 85	Influenza (Seasonal/Pandemic)
AS03	Oil-in-water emulsion	Squalene, Tween 80, Alpha-tocopherol	Pandemic influenza
AF03	Oil-in-water emulsion	Squalene, Montane 80, Eumulgin B1PH	Pandemic influenza
Virosomes	Liposomes	Phospholipids, Cholesterol, HA	Seasonal influenza, HAV
AS04	Alum-adsorbed TLR4 agent	Aluminium hydroxide, MPL	HBV, HPV
RC529	Alum-adsorbed TLR4 agent	Aluminium hydroxide, Synthetic MPL	HBV

Live Vaccines

- Live vaccines are prepared from live attenuated organisms
  - *Attenuation*: Reduced pathogenicity/virulence BUT maintained antigenicity/immunogenicity^Q
- *Live vaccines are more potent agents than killed vaccines^Q*:
  - Multiply in the host and the resulting antigenic host is larger than what is injected
  - Have all the major and minor antigenic components
  - Engage certain tissues of the body (e.g. intestinal mucosa by OPV)
  - There may be other mechanisms such as persistence of latent virus
- *General properties to Live vaccines:*
  - Immunization is generally achieved with a single dose (EXCEPT OPV^Q)
  - Should not be administered to immuno-deficient/immuno-suppressed
  - 2 live vaccines can be administered simultaneously at different sites (or at an interval of 3 weeks)
- *Examples of Live 'attenuated' vaccines:*
  - BCG – OPV (Sabin – Oral polio vaccine)
  - Measles vaccine – Mumps vaccine
  - Rubella vaccine – Yellow fever vaccine
  - Typhoral – Live plague vaccine
  - LAIV (live attenuated influenza vaccine) – Varicella vaccine
  - Epidemic typhus vaccine

BCG Vaccine

- BCG stands for '*Bacille Calmette Guerin^Q*' – an '*avirulent strain*' produced by 239 subcultures over a period of 13 years
- *Type of vaccine:* Live attenuated vaccine
  - *Liquid (fresh) type vaccine*
  - *Freeze dried (lyophilized) vaccine*: More stable; used currently
- *WHO recommended strain:* **DANISH 1331 strain^Q**
  - *Vaccine strain is derived from 'Mycobacterium bovis'^{Q}*
  - *Prepared at BCG laboratory, Guindy, Chennai in India^Q*
- BCG is a lyophiliosed (freeze dried) vaccine:
  - Is reconstituted with Normal Saline (NaCl) as diluent^Q
  - Must be used within 4 hours of reconstitution
- *Dose:* 0.1 mL (for all ages^Q)
- **Strength: 0.1 mg in 0.1 mL**
- *Route:* Intra-dermal^Q
  - Tuberculin syringe (Omega microstat syringe, 1 cm steel, 26 gauge needle)
- *Site:* Skin over left deltoid muscle^Q
  - Left deltoid muscle is chosen ONLY by convention
- *Age for vaccination:*
  - **Direct BCG^Q:** Is administered up to 1 year age, without Mantoux Test
  - **Indirect BCG:** Beyond age 1 year, it is recommended after prior Mantoux Test
- *Phenomena after vaccination^Q:*
  - After 2–3 weeks: Papule formation
  - 5 weeks: 4–8 mm diameter of papule
  - 6–8 weeks: Breaks into a shallow ulcer, seen covered with a crust
  - 6–12 weeks: Permanent tiny, round scar, typically 4–8 mm diameter
  - 8–14 weeks: Mantoux test becomes positive^Q
- *Protective efficacy:*
  - For pulmonary tuberculosis: 0% (Zero)
  - For severe forms of tuberculosis^Q: 0–80% (median 50%)
  - For Leprosy: 20–40%
- *Protective duration:* 20 years^Q

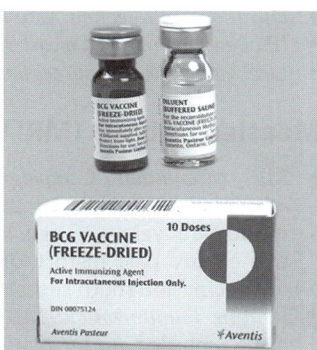

BCG

> **Key points**
> WHO recommended strain: DANISH 1331 strain^Q

> **Key points**
> BCG is a lyophiliosed (freeze dried) vaccine:

> **Key points**
> Strength: 0.1 mg in 0.1 mL

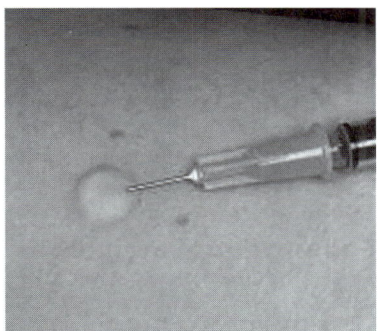

Intradermal Injection

- *Complications:*
  - Prolonged severe ulceration at site of vaccination
  - Suppurative lymphadenitis^Q
  - Osteomyelitis
  - Disseminated BCG infection
  - Death

Measles Vaccine

- *Type:* Live attenuated, lyophilized (Freeze dried^Q) vaccine (Tissue culture vaccines – Chick embryo or Human diploid cell line)
- *Strains used:*
  - Edmonston Zagreb Strain (Most Common^Q)
  - Schwartz Strain
  - Moraten Strain
- *Dose:* 0.5 mL (≥ 1000 viral infective units)
- *Route:* Subcutaneous^Q
- *Site:* Right arm
- *Age of administration in National Immunization schedule (India):* 9 months^Q (can be lowered to 6-9 months in epidemics & malnutrition) & 16–24 months
- *Stabilizers in the vaccine:* Sorbitol, Hydrolysed gelatin
- *Diluent for Reconstitution:* Distilled Water or sterile water^Q
  - Use within 4 hours after reconstitution with diluent
- Measles (& MMR) vaccine can lead to Toxic Shock Syndrome
- Measles vaccine is contraindicated in pregnancy
- *Cold chain Temperature for storage:* +2 to +8°C
- *Protective efficacy^Q:* > 90% (with one dose), > 99% (2 doses)
- *Duration of Protection:* Life long
- *IP of vaccine induced measles:* 7 days^Q
- *Ideal gap between 2 successive doses of Measles vaccine:* 6 months^Q

Key points
Measles Vaccine
Route: Subcutaneous^Q

Key points
IP of vaccine induced measles: 7 days^Q

Measles-Rubella (MR) Vaccine

- *MR vaccination Campaign:* Dose administered to all the children 9 months-15 years of age, irrespective of any past history of disease or vaccination (both sexes)
- *Routine immunization:* MR vaccine to be included under National Immunization Schedule after the completion of MR Campaign
  - Every child who is eligible for either 1st or 2nd dose of measles vaccine in RI schedule will be provided with combined MR vaccine
  - Two doses under NIS: MR-1 at 9 months age, MR-2 at 16-24 months age
  - Delayed immunization: If a child misses the scheduled dose, MR vaccine can be given till 5 years of age

MR Campaign

Poliomyelitis Vaccines^Q

	OPV (Sabin)	IPV (Salk)
Type of vaccine	Live attenuated virus	Killed formolised virus
Mode of administration	Oral	Subcutaneous or i.m.
Type of immunity^Q	Humoral + Intestinal (local)	Humoral
Prevention of	Paralysis + intestinal re-infection	Paralysis

Contd...

Contd...

	OPV (Sabin)	IPV (Salk)
Control of epidemics	Effective	Not useful
Manufacture	Easy	Difficult
Cost	Cheaper	Expensive
Storage & transport	Require sub-zero temperatures	Less stringent conditions
Shelf life	Short	Longer
VAPP	1 per 2.7 million vaccinees	Zero incidence

Inactivated (Salk) Polio Vaccine (IPV)
- Is a type of killed vaccine
- *Schedule:* First 3 doses at 1-2 month interval each and 4th dose after 6-12 months of last dose
- Induces Humoral immunity (IgM, IgG, IgA); NO LOCAL IMMUNITY
- *Composition of IPV:*

Components	Strength
Poliovirus type 1	20 D antigen units
Poliovirus type 2	2 D antigen units
Poliovirus type 3	4 D antigen units

- *Advantages of IPV:*
  - Safe in immunodeficiency disorders
  - Safe in persons on radiation therapy/corticosteroid therapy
  - Useful in those over 50 years age
  - Safe during pregnancy[Q]
  - No risk of Vaccine associated paralytic polio (VAPP[Q])
- *IPV is unsuitable in epidemics:*
  - Immunity is not rapidly achieved as > 1 doses required
  - Injections can precipitate paralysis during epidemics
- *Composition of Improved IPV:*

Components	Strength
Poliovirus type 1	40 D antigen units
Poliovirus type 2	8 D antigen units
Poliovirus type 3	32 D antigen units

IPV vs Fractional Dose IPV

	IPV	f-IPV
Dose	0.5 mL	0.1 mL
Route	IM	ID
Site	Thigh	Upper arm
No. of doses	1	2
Schedule	14 weeks	6 weeks, 14 weeks
Syringe	0.5 mL AD	0.1 mL AD
Immunogenicity	++	++++

Oral (Sabin) Polio Vaccine (OPV)
- *Is a live attenuated 'trivalent' vaccine:* Contains 3 strains of poliovirus
- Schedule for OPV in NIS, India:

Dose	Age
OPV-0 (Zero dose)	At birth
OPV-1	6 weeks
OPV-2	10 weeks
OPV-3	14 weeks
OPV-B (Booster dose)	16-24 months

- *Mechanism of action:*
  - *Primary multiplication*: Intestinal epithelial cells
  - *SECONDARY MULTIPLICATION*^{Q}: Peyer's patches (leads to viraemia)
  - Induces *'both systemic as well as local immunity'* (Nasal & duodenal IgA, Serum IgM, IgG, IgA)
- *Composition of OPV*^{Q}: *(NEW Bivalent composition)*

> **Key points**
> OPV Induces *'both systemic as well as local immunity'*

Components	Strength
Poliovirus type 1	3 lac TCID 50 (NOW 10^6 CCID)
Poliovirus type 2	1 lac TCID 50
Poliovirus type 3^Q	3 lac TCID 50 (NOW $10^{5.8}$ CCID)

- *Dose:* 2 drops (EQUIVALENT TO 0.1 mL^Q)
- *Advantages of OPV*^{Q}:
  - Easy to administer
  - Induces both humoral and systemic immunity
  - Single dose also produces substantial immunity
  - Vaccines spread immunity to others by excretion of virus
  - Relatively inexpensive
  - Useful in controlling epidemics
- *Complication:* Can lead to Vaccine associated paralytic poliomyelitis (VAPP)
  - 1 case per 2.7 million vaccines^Q
- OPV is quite a thermolabile vaccine
- OPV should not be repeatedly freezed and thawed
- *Cold chain temperature for long term storage:* –15°C to –25°C
- *During transportation, OPV should be kept on:*
  - Dry ice (solidified carbon dioxide)^Q
  - A freezing mixture (wet ice + ammonium chloride)
  - *Heat-stabilized OPV vaccine*: Can be kept without loosing potency for 1 year at 4°C and for a month at room temperature

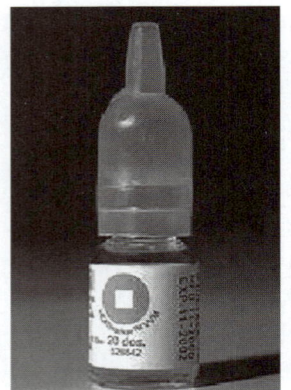

OPV

Vaccine Vial Monitor

- *VVM is a marker of potency:* VVM is a simple tool which enables vaccinator to know if vaccine is potent at the time of administration
  - VVM is a label containing a heat-sensitive material which is placed on a vaccine vial to register cumulative heat exposure over time
- *VVM indicates efficiency of cold chain*^{Q} *(temperature maintenance)*
- *VVM is a mark on OPV vial consisting of:*
  - An outer circle
  - An inner square (made of heat sensitive material)

> **Key points**
> VVM is a marker of potency but measures cumulative heat exposure overtime

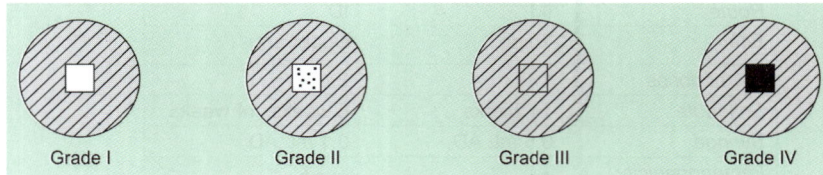

Vaccine vial monitor

- *WHO grading of VVM in OPV:*
  - *Is based on colour changes in VVM*: ONLY INNER SQUARE CHANGES COLOUR, circle always remain blue
  - *Based on VVM, OPV is usable upto Grade II*^{Q}

WHO Grade	Outer Circle	Inner Square	Inference^Q
Grade I	Blue	White	OPV can be used
Grade II	Blue	Light blue	OPV can be used
Grade III	Blue	Blue	OPV CANNOT be used
Grade IV	Blue	Purple/Black	OPV CANNOT be used

  - *(Grade III is Discard point)*

Open Vial Policy 2015

- Applicable for Vaccines: OPV, DPT, Hepatitis B, TT, Liquid Pentavalent
- Not applicable for Vaccines: Measles, BCG, JE
- Opened vaccine vials can be used in subsequent session 'UP TO 4 WEEKS'
- Expiry date should not pass, VVM within usability limits, Cold chain maintenance
- Vaccine vial septum not submerged in water or contaminated, Aseptic technique used to withdraw doses
- Record date and time of each vial opening
- At end of session return all open vials to Cold chain:
  - Reusable open vials: DPT, DT, Hepatitis B, Pentavalent
  - Non-reusable open vials: Measles, BCG, JE (Destroy after 48 hours or Next session whichever earlier)
  - If any AEFI reported: Store all vials in Cold chain till completion of investigation

Vaccine-associated Paralytic Polio (VAPP)

- Approximately 1 in 2.7 million doses of OPV^Q
- **MCC: Poliovirus type 3**^{Q}
- Caused by a strain of poliovirus that has genetically changed in the intestine from the original attenuated vaccine strain contained in OPV
- It is associated with a single dose of OPV administered in a child or can occur in a close unvaccinated or non-immune contact of the vaccine recipient who is excreting the mutated virus
- Risk of VAPP from subsequent doses of vaccine is even lower than from the first dose
- There are no outbreaks associated with VAPP

> **Key points**
> MCC of VAPP: P3
> MCC of VDPV: P2 (cVDPV)

Vaccine Derived Poliovirus (VDPV)

- A VDPV is a very rare strain of poliovirus, genetically changed from the original strain contained in OPV
- **MCC: Poliovirus type 2 (cVDPV type)**^{Q}
- Circulating VPDV (cVDPV): On very rare occasions, under certain conditions, a strain of poliovirus in OPV may change and revert to a form that may be able to cause paralysis (VDPV) in humans and develop the capacity for sustained circulation

"SWITCH" - Replacing Trivalent OPV with Bivalent OPV^Q

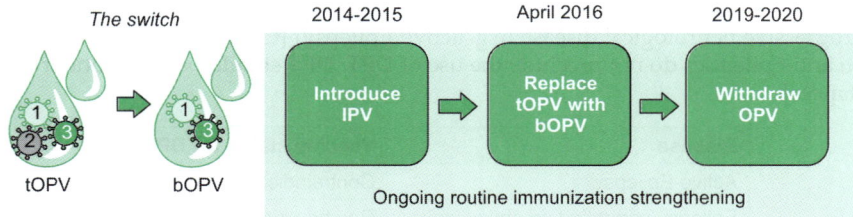

- *Concept*: An important transition in the vaccines used to eradicate polio requires removal of all OPVs in the long-term so as to eliminate rare risks of VAPP and cVDPV
- *Strategy*:
  - Withdrawal of OPVs must occur in a globally synchronized manner, starting in April 2016 with a switch from trivalent OPV (tOPV) to bivalent OPV (bOPV), removing the type 2 component (OPV2) from immunization programs of countries^Q
  - Preparation for the removal of OPVs also includes the introduction of at least one dose of IPV in routine immunization programs in all countries by end of 2015
- *Indian "Switch"*:
  - National Switch Date: April 25, 2016^Q
  - National Validation Day: May 09, 2016 (India to be declared free of tOPV^Q)
  - Destroy all tOPV on/after 25th April 2016
  - IPV in 6 states (UP, Bihar, Madhya Pradesh, Gujarat, Punjab, Assam): One Intramuscular dose given along with 3rd dose of DTP at 14 weeks
  - IPV in other states (Orissa, Andhra Pradesh, Telangana, Tamil Nadu, Kerala, Karnataka, Maharashtra, Puducherry): Fractional dose (0.1 mL instead of 0.5 mL) by intradermal route at 6 and 14 weeks from April, 2016 (Right deltoid upper arm)

DPT Vaccine

- *Type:* Combined TRIPLE vaccine for Diphtheria, Pertussis & Tetanus; D & T are Toxoids, P is killed acellular bacilli
- *Dose:* 0.5 mL
- *Route:* Intramuscular^Q
- *Site:* Antero-lateral aspect of thigh, middle 1/3 (earlier it was administered at gluteal region, but presence of fat in buttocks breaks the adjuvant & reduces absorption of DPT vaccine)
- *Composition of DPT Vaccine:*

Contents	Amount per dose (0.5 mL)	
	Glaxo	Kasauli
Diphtheria Toxoid	25 Lf^Q	30 Lf
Tetanus Toxoid	5 Lf	10 Lf
Pertussis killed acellular bacilli	20,000 million	32,000 million
Aluminium phosphate	2.5 mg	3.0 mg
Thiomersal	0.01%	0.01%

> **Key points**
> *Aluminium phosphate or aluminium hydroxide is used as adjuvant in DPT vaccine:* It increases immunogenicity of vaccine^Q

  - *Aluminium phosphate or aluminium hydroxide is used as adjuvant in DPT vaccine:* It increases immunogenicity of vaccine^Q
  - *Thiomersal is used as preservative* in DPT Vaccine^Q
- *Age for immunization in National Immunization schedule (NIS, India):*

Dose	Age
DPT$_1$	6 weeks of age
DPT$_2$	10 weeks of age
DPT$_3$	14 weeks of age
DPT$_{Booster}$	16-24 months of age
DPT$_{Booster}$	5 years of age

  - *Recommended interval between 3 successive doses:* 1 month
  - 2 months gap between 2 successive doses of DPT do not offer any advantage over one-month interval
- *Absolute Contraindications to DPT vaccine:*
  - Severe hypersensitivity reaction to previous dose
  - Progressive neurological disease (e.g. active Epilepsy) [Cerebral palsy & seizures controlled on anti-epileptics do not preclude the use of DPT; DPT should be given under these circumstances]

Disease	Vaccine status for DPT
Active Epilepsy	Contraindicated
Epilepsy controlled on antiepileptic	Can be given
Cerebral Palsy	Can be given

- *DPT vaccine (& Measles vaccine) can result in fever:* Antipyretic is given with DPT vaccine as 'take home, need based' medication
- *Cold Chain Temperature of DPT:* +2° to +8°C
  - *If DPT vaccine gets frozen accidentally:* discard the vaccine
- *Adult type of Diphtheria – tetanus vaccine (dT):* contains up to 2 Lf of diphtheria toxoid per dose; given 2 doses 4-6 weeks apart, followed by a booster after 6–12 months; is useful for immunizing children over 12 yrs of age & adults

CERVAVAC

- India's first indigenously developed vaccine to prevent cervical cancer
- *Expected cost:* ₹200-400 a shot
- *Effectivity:* CERVAVAC will be effective against at least 4 variants of HPV (HPV 16,18,6,11)

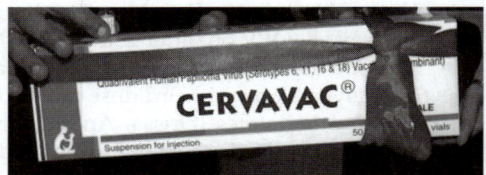

- *Doses:*
  - 2-dose regimen: 6 months apart (9-14 years age group)
  - 3-dose regimen: 0, 1-2, 6 months (15-26 years age group)
- *Manufacturer:* Serum Institute of India

ThRabis (THRABIS)

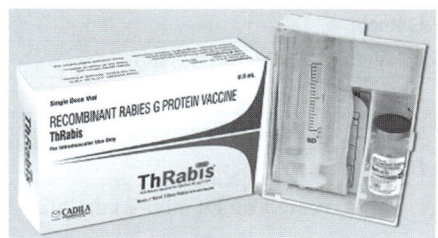

- World's First 3-dose Rabies vaccine is a part of National Action Plan for dog-Mediated Rabies Elimination (NAPRE) by 2030 (Launched October 2021)
- *Campaign:* "One, Two, Three. Rabies Free".
- *Type of vaccine:* Recombinant nano particle-based rabies G protein vaccine
- *Mechanism of action:* Vaccine generates antibodies against rabies G protein, which leads to virus neutralisation, as well as prevents virus attachment to the cell to confer protection against rabies.
- *Doses:* Three doses over a 7-day period (Day 0, 3, 7)
- *Cost:* Rs 715/- per dose
- *Manufacturers:* Cadila Pharmaceuticals

COVID-19 VACCINES

Introduction

- Number of Vaccines Under Clinical Development Phase: 126
  - *Types of vaccines:* Protein subunit (34%), Inactivated (14%), Viral vector – non-replicating (14%), RNA (17%), DNA (11%), Others
- Number of Vaccines Under Pre-clinical Development Phase: 194

Classification of Major COVID-19 Vaccines

RNA-based Vaccines • Pfizer-BioNTech (Comirnaty) • Moderna (SpikeVax)	Protein Subunit Vaccines • NovaVax (Covovax) • Sanofi Pasteur & GSK (VAT00008)) • Chinese AOS • Medigen Biologics (Medigen)
Viral Vector Based • Oxford-AstraZeneca (Covishield) • Cansino Biologics (Convidecia) • Johnson & Johnson (Janssen) • Gamaleya RI (SputnikV)	Whole Virion Inactivated • SinoVac Biotech (CoronaVac) • Bharat Biotech (Covaxin) • Sinopharm (BBIBP CorV) • Sinopharm (WIBP CorV) • Chumakov (CoviVac)

(© Table created by Dr Vivek Jain 2022-23)

COVID-19 Vaccination Update [As on 01 June 2023]

- India: 2206 million doses administered
  - Covid Vaccination started: 16 January 2021
  - 100 Crore vaccination doses: 21 October 2021
  - 200 Crore vaccination doses: 17 July 2022
  - Total doses given till date: 220 Crore vaccination doses

COVID-19 VACCINES IN INDIA

COVID-19 Vaccines Approved in India [As on 01 June 2023]: Twelve

Biologicals	Vaccine	Type
Serum Institute of India	COVOVAX	Protein Subunit
Zydus Cadilla	ZyCoV-D	DNA based
Biological E Limited	Corbevax	Protein Subunit
Gennova Biopharmaceuticals Ltd	GEMCOVAC-19	RNA based

Contd...

Contd...

Biologicals	Vaccine	Type
Moderna	Spikevax	RNA based
Bharat Biotech	iNCOVACC	Non-replicating Viral Vector
Gameleya	Sputnik V	Non-replicating Viral Vector
Gameleya	Sputnik Light	Non-replicating Viral Vector
Johnson & Johnson – Janssen	Jcovden	Non-replicating Viral Vector
Oxford/AstraZeneca	Vaxzevria	Non-replicating Viral Vector
Oxford/AstraZeneca/Serum Institute	Covishield	Non-replicating Viral Vector
Bharat Biotech	Covaxin	Inactivated

(© Table created by Dr Vivek Jain 2022-23)

COVID-19 Vaccines under Clinical Trials in India [As on 01 June 2023]: Sixteen

Biologicals	Vaccine	Type
Biological E Limited	BECOV2B	Protein Subunit
Biological E Limited	BECOV2C	Protein Subunit
Biological E Limited	BECOV2D	Protein Subunit
Gennova Biopharmaceuticals	HCGO19	RNA based
Bharat Biotech	Covaxin	Inactivated
Serum Institute of India	Covishield	Non-replicating Viral Vector
Oxford/AstraZeneca	Vaxzevria	Non-replicating Viral Vector
Bharat Biotech	iNCOVACC	Non-replicating Viral Vector
Gameleya	Sputnik V	Non-replicating Viral Vector
Gameleya	Sputnik Light	Non-replicating Viral Vector
Gennova Biopharmaceuticals Ltd	GEMCOVAC-19	RNA based
Zydus Cadilla	ZyCoV-D	DNA based
University Medical Center Groningen	AKS-452	Protein Subunit
Novavax	Nuvaxovid	Protein Subunit
Serum Institute of India	COVOVAX	Protein Subunit
Biological E Limited	Corbevax	Protein Subunit

(© Table created by Dr Vivek Jain 2022-23)

COVAXIN Vaccine (BB152)

- *Type of Vaccine:* Whole-virion Inactivated SARS-CoV-2 Vaccine
- *Manufactured by:* Manufactured by Bharat Biotech BSL-3 facility & ICMR & NIV (100% Indigenous vaccine of India)
- *Strain:* NIV-2020-770
- *Strength:* 6 mcg per 0.5 mL dose
- *Vaccine Excipients:* Inactivated Coronavirus, Aluminium Hydroxide Gel, TLR 7/8 Agonist, 2-Phenoxyethanol, Phosphate Buffered Saline [NKA1]
- *Cold chain temperature:* +2 to +8° C (Use ASAP, Maximum < 6 hours)
- *Vaccination Guidelines:* Age group Individuals ≥18 years old, 2 doses (0.5 mL each) 4-6 weeks apart, Route Intramuscular "ONLY", Site Deltoid muscle, Duration & Level of protection unknown
- *Protective efficacy:* 86-96%.

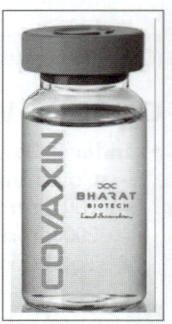

COVISHIELD Vaccine (AZD1222)

- *Type of Vaccine:* ChAdOx1 nCoV- 19 Corona Virus Vaccine (Recombinant) - Monovalent vaccine, Single recombinant, replication-deficient chimpanzee adenovirus (ChAdOx1) vector encoding the S glycoprotein of SARS-CoV-2, produced by Genetically modified Human embryonic kidney (HEK) 293 cells
- *Mechanism of action:* Following administration, the S glycoprotein of SARS-CoV-2 is expressed locally stimulating neutralizing antibody and cellular immune response

- *Manufactured by:* Serum Institute of India Pvt Ltd (With AstraZanaca)
- *Vaccine excipients:* L-Histidine, L-Histidine hydrochloride monohydrate, Magnesium chloride hexahydrate, Polysorbate 80, Ethanol, Sucrose, Sodium chloride, Disodium edetate dihydrate (EDTA)
- *Cold chain temperature:* +2 to +8° C (Use ASAP, Maximum < 6 hours when kept between +2° to +25°C)
- *Vaccination Guidelines:* Age group Individuals ≥18 years old, 2 doses (0.5 mL each) 12-16 weeks apart, Route Intramuscular, Site Deltoid muscle, Duration & Level of protection unknown
- *Protective efficacy:* 70.42% overall
- *Contraindications:*
  - People with hypersensitivity to the active substance or to any of the excipients
  - Patients who have experienced major blood clotting (venous and/or arterial thrombosis) in combination with low platelet count (thrombocytopenia) following any COVID-19 vaccine

CORBEVAX

- *Type of vaccine:* India's first indigenously developed RBD (receptor binding domain) protein subunit vaccine
- *Age group recommended:*
  - 12-14 years children
  - As a precaution dose after 6 months of Primary immunization with Covaxin/Covishield
- *Doses:* Two doses 0.5 mL each, 4 weeks apart, Intramuscular
- *Cold chain temperature:* +2 to +8 degrees C
- *Manufacturers:* Biologicals E Ltd

iNCOVACC (BBV154)

- *Type of vaccine:* ChAd36-SARS-CoV-S COVID-19 (Chimpanzee Adenovirus Vectored) recombinant nasal vaccine
- *Mechanism:* Recombinant replication deficient adenovirus vectored vaccine vectored vaccine with a pre-fusion stabilized spike protein
- India's first intranasal Covid vaccine
- *Age group:* Age more than 18 years
- *Doses:* Two doses for primary immunization
- *Cold chain temperature:* +2 to +8 degrees C
- *Manufacturers:* Bharat Biotech

Must Know Facts about COVID-19 Vaccines in India

- *Procedure for Vaccination:*
  - Register on the Co-WIN Portal and schedule your vaccination appointment
  - Vaccines are available from Government and Private Health Facilities as notified, known as COVID Vaccination Centres (CVCs)
  - Photo ID is a must for both registration and verification at session site
- *AEFI Observation Period:* 30 minutes
- Status in Pregnancy & Lactation: Permitted by MoHFW, Govt of India
- *Status in Children:*
  - Covaxin permitted in 2-18 years age by MoHFW, Govt of India
  - Approval given for use in 12-18 years age
- *Boosters drive started:* Frontline health workers and older population with comorbidity to be given priority
- Interchangeability of vaccine is not permitted yet (Studies going on).

For Other Vaccines

Refer to Chapter 5, Theory

NEW National Immunization Schedule (NIS) 2023-24

Age	Vaccine dose(s)
At birth	BCG, OPV-0, HepB
6 weeks	DPT-1, OPV-1, HepB-1, HiB-1, RotaV-1, fIPV-1, PCV-1
10 weeks	DPT-2, OPV-2, HepB-2, HiB-2, RotaV-2
14 weeks	DPT-3, OPV-3, HepB-3, HiB-3, RotaV-3, fIPV-2, PCV-2
9 months (completed)	Measles-1 **or** MR-1, JE Live-1, PCV-B, fIPV-3, Vitamin A (1 Lac IU)
Every 6 months: Vitamin A (2 Lac IU each dose) till 5 years age of the child	
16-24 months	DPT-B, OPV-B, Measles-2 **or** MR-2, JE Live-2
5-6 years	DPT-B
10 years	Td
16 years	Td
For Pregnant women	Td-1 and Td-2 (1 month apart) Td-B (If 2 doses TT received in last 3 years)

(JE vaccine only in Endemic districts) (HiB Vaccine introduced as Pentavalent vaccine – DPT + HepB + HiB vaccine in 16 states) (fIPV is fractionated intradermal at 6 weeks & 14 weeks or IPV Intramuscular only at 14 weeks) (Rotaviral vaccine introduced in 9 States – Andhra Pradesh, Haryana, Himachal Pradesh, Odisha, Madhya Pradesh, Assam, Rajasthan, Tamil Nadu and Tripura) (Measles-Rubella MR vaccine started from 5 States/UTs - Karnataka, Tamil Nadu, Goa, Lakshadweep and Puducherry) (Pneumococcal conjugate PCV vaccine introduced in all 12 districts of Himachal Pradesh, 6 districts of Uttar Pradesh and 17 districts of Bihar) (Adult JE Vaccine introduced in 31 high burden districts from Assam, Uttar Pradesh and West Bengal for adult JE vaccination in the age-group of 15-65 years).

Td Vaccine under NIS, India (NEW Guidelines 2018-19)

- WHO (1998): To avoid the threat of diphtheria outbreaks, all countries must replace TT (Tetanus toxoid) with Td (Tetanus-Adult diphtheria) for vaccination of women of reproductive age (and/or pregnant women as per national immunization target), older children and adolescents to improve protection against diphtheria
- Joint communiqué of the WHO/UNICEF (June 2018): All countries that have not yet replaced TT with Td, do so immediately, and achieve complete replacement by January 2020
- **MoHFW-GOI (August 2018): TT be replaced by Td**; Replacement for TT booster doses given at 10 years, 16 years age and Pregnant women (booster dose)

Important Practical Considerations under NIS

- *Vitamin-A* is given at 9th, 18th, 24th, 30th, 36th, 42th, 48th, 54th, 60th months (A total of 1 Lac + 2 Lac + 2 Lac + 2 Lac + 2 Lac + 2 Lac + 2 Lac + 2 Lac + 2 Lac = 17 Lac IU is given to a completely immunized child by 5 years of age[Q])
- *OPV:* Minimum 5 doses are required for development of immunity[Q]
- *DPT:* Minimum 3 doses are given a month apart with booster after 1 year of the 3rd dose (and another booster at 5-6 years age)
- *TT:* A fully immunized adult (excluding pregnancy in females) would have received 7 doses of TT

Guidelines on Td in Pregnancy

- Primigravida: 2 doses 1 month apart, As soon as possible (New Guideline)
  - OR Td1 (16-20 weeks) & Td2 (20-24 weeks) (Older Guideline)
  - *Duration of protection with 2 doses*: All subsequent pregnancies in next 3 years[Q]
- *Multigravida (completely immunized in last 3 years):* 1 booster dose[Q]
- *Multigravida (partially immunized in previous pregnancy in last 3 years):* 2 doses, 1 month apart
- *Multigravida (unimmunized in previous pregnancy in last 3 years):* 2 doses, 1 month apart
- *Multigravida (completely immunized in previous pregnancy earlier than 3 years):* 2 doses, 1 month apart
- *RULE FOR Delayed immunization of Td in pregnancy (as per Period of gestation – POG):* Give 2 doses of TT, 1 month apart, anytime in pregnancy, IRRESPECTIVE OF TIME OF DELIVERY (so as to provide protection for atleast next 3 years)

Situations (pregnant female reporting for the 1st time at)	Recommendation	Status of patient
4½ month POG	2 doses; 1 each at 4½ m & 5½ m POG	Completely immunized for current pregnancy; subsequent half protection for next 3 years
5th month POG	2 doses; 1 each at 5th m & 6th m POG	
6th month POG	2 doses; 1 each at 6th m & 7th m POG	
7th month POG	2 doses; 1 each at 7th m & 8th m POG	
8th month POG	2 doses; 1 each at 8th m & 9th m POG	Partially immunized for current pregnancy; subsequent half protection for next 3 years
9th month POG	2 doses; 1st at 9th m POG & 2nd 1 m after (post-delivery)	
Just before delivery	2 doses; 1st before delivery & 2nd 1 m after	Unimmunized for current pregnancy; subsequent half protection for next 3 years
Post delivery	2 doses; 1 each at just after delivery & 1 m later (post-delivery)	

- *A child born to unimmunised/partially-immunized mother must be given protection*: Give 750 IU of antitoxin (heterologous serum) within 6 hours of birth

Age Limits for Delayed Immunization in NIS, India^Q

Vaccine	Age limit (Under NIS)
BCG	Upto 1 year age (Direct BCG)
bOPV-0	Within 15 days of life
bOPV-1/2/3	Upto 5 years age
Hepatitis B	Upto 1 years age
Pentavalent vaccine	Upto 1 year age
Fractionated IPV (fIPV)	Upto 1 year age
Rotavirus vaccine	Upto 1 year age
Pneumococcal conjugate (PCV)	Upto 1 year age
Measles	Upto 5 years age
Measles-Rubella (MR)	Upto 5 years age
JE vaccine	Upto 15 years age
Vitamin A	Upto 5 years age
DPT Booster-1/2	Upto 7 years age
Tetanus toxoid (TT)	Upto 16 years age

Cases of Delayed Immunization

- **A completely unimmunized child 9 months of age should receive**^{Q}: BCG, DPT-1 *(next two doses one month apart each and booster after 1 year of 3rd dose)*, OPV-1 *(next two doses one month apart each and booster after 1 year of 3rd dose)*, HepB -1 *(next two doses one month apart each)*, Measles-1 or MR-1, JE-1, PCV-1, Pentavalent-1 *(2 doses 1 m apart)*, FIPV-1, Rotav-1 and Vitamin A *(1 Lac IU)* and Hib-1 *(1 dose one month later)*
- **A completely unimmunized child 18 months of age should receive:** BCG *(Only after Mantoux Test: Indirect BCG)*, DPT-1 *(next two doses one month apart each and booster after 1 year of 3rd dose)*, OPV-1 *(next two doses one month apart each and booster after 1 year of 3rd dose)*, Measles-1 or MR-1, JE-1, and Vitamin A *(2 Lac IU)*, HiB, JE-1
- **A completely unimmunized child 30 months of age should receive:** BCG *(Only after Mantoux Test: Indirect BCG)*, DPT-1, OPV-1 *(next two doses one month apart each and booster after 1 year of 3rd dose)*, Measles-1 or MR-1 *(if not suffered from measles disease previously)*, and Vitamin A *(2 Lac IU)*, JE-1
- **A completely unimmunized child 4 years of age should receive**^{Q}: BCG *(Only after Mantoux Test: Indirect BCG)*, DPT-1, OPV-1 *(next two doses one month apart each and booster after 1 year of 3rd dose)*, Measles-1 or MR-1 *(if not suffered from measles disease previously)*, Vitamin A *(2 lac IU)*, JE-1

Mission Indradhanush 2014

Launch: 25 December 2014^Q

Description: Indradhanush depicting seven colors of the rainbow, aims to cover all those children by 2020^Q who are either unvaccinated, or are partially vaccinated against 7 vaccine preventable diseases (7 VPD's)^Q

- Diphtheria
- Pertussis
- Tetanus
- Childhood Tuberculosis
- Poliomyelitis
- Hepatitis B
- Measles

Strategy:
- *Focused and systematic immunization drive*: "Catch-up" campaign mode to cover all the children who have been left missed out[Q]
- *Four special vaccination campaigns*: January-June 2015 with intensive planning and monitoring
- *Learning of Polio program*: Apply in planning and implementation
- *Coverage*:
  - First phase: 201 districts
  - Second phase: 297 districts
  - 82 districts in 4 states of UP, Bihar, Madhya Pradesh and Rajasthan

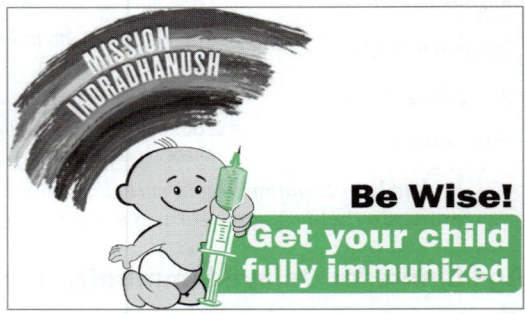

Mission Indradhanush

Six new vaccines added to MI: (MI may be renamed soon)
- Rotavirus
- Measles rubella
- Inactivated polio vaccine (IPV) bivalent
- Japanese Encephalitis
- HiB vaccine
- PCV

Intensified Mission Indradhanush

- Launched in select districts and urban areas of the country in October 2017: 121 districts in 16 States, 52 districts in the North Eastern States and 17 urban areas where immunization coverage has been very low
- *Strategy:* To cover all left-outs and drop-outs with low routine immunization coverage
- *Target:* **To achieve >90% immunization coverage by December 2018**
- *Focus on:* Children up to 2 years of age, Pregnant women who have missed out on routine immunization (with Vaccination-on-demand for children <5 years of age)
- *Immunization drive:* Spread over 7 working days starting from 7th date of every month
- *Areas identified:*
  - Areas with vacant Subcenters (ANM not posted or absent for >3 months)
  - Unserved/low coverage pockets due to vaccine hesitancy, Subcenter/ANM catering to populations much higher than norms
  - Villages/areas with >3 consecutive missed routine immunization sessions
  - High risk areas
    1. Urban slums with migratory population
    2. Nomadic sites - brick kilns/construction sites
    3. Other migrant settlements - fisherman villages/riverine areas with shifting populations/ underserved and hard-to-reach populations-forested and tribal populations, hilly areas
    4. Areas with low routine immunization coverage identified through measles outbreaks, cases of diphtheria and neonatal tetanus in the last two years.

Global Vaccine Action Plan 2011–2020 (Targets by 2020)

- Achieve a world free of poliomyelitis: Certification of poliomyelitis eradication (by 2018)
- Measles and rubella eliminated in at least five WHO regions
- Reach 90% national coverage and 80% in every district or equivalent administrative unit
- All low-income and middle-income countries have introduced one or more new or underutilized vaccines
- Exceed the Millennium Development Goal 4 Target of reduction by 2/3rd for child mortality

Cold Chain

- *Cold chain:* Is a system of storage and transportation of vaccines from the point of manufacture to the point of administration (actual vaccination site)
- *Cold chain temperature of vaccines available in India:*
- *OPV (Sabin):*
  - Routine storage: +2°C to +8°C
  - Long term storage: −15°C to −25°C
- *Yellow fever vaccine:* −30°C to +5°C
- **All other vaccines: +2°C to +8°C** (Also known as the 'cold chain temperature of vaccines in India^Q')
- *Diluents:* Can be stored in +2°C to +8°C **OR** can be kept outside cold chain (at room temperature)
- *Vitamin A:* Is stored outside cold chain (at room temperature)

> **Key points**
> +2°C to +8°C 'cold chain temperature of vaccines in India^Q'

Cold Chain Components (Equipments) & Levels in India

Level	Component	Temperature	Storage duration
State/Regional level	Walk-in-cold rooms (WIC)	+2°C to +8°C	3 months
	Walk-in-freezers (WIF)	−15°C to −25°C	
District level	Large ILRs (Ice-lined refrigerator)	+2°C to +8°C	1 month
	Large DFs (Deep freezers)	−15°C to −25°C	
PHC level	Small ILRs	+2°C to +8°C	1 month^a
	Small DFs	−15°C to −25°C	
Sub-centre level	Vaccine carriers	+2°C to +8°C	48–72 hours
	Day carriers		
Session level	Fully frozen icepack	+2°C to +8°C	1–3 hours

- Most important component of cold chain in India: ILR^Q
- Temperature of cold chain in India: +2°C to +8°C^Q
- Minimum level of vaccine storage (in cold chain) in India^Q: Primary health centre (below PHC level, vaccines are 'transported *to sub-centres on immunization days*' in vaccine carriers and day carriers)
- Maximum chance of cold chain failure in India: Sub-centre and village level^Q
- Instrument used to monitor the temperature of cold chain at PHC: Dial Thermometer^Q

> **Key points**
> *Most important component of cold chain in India:* ILR^Q

Ice-lined Refrigerator (ILR)

- Is '*most important component of cold chain*' in India
- *Temperature of ILR (Cold chain) in India:* +2°C to +8°C
- *Temperature monitoring of ILR:* Dial thermometer (Twice daily)
- *ILR is used for storage of:* All vaccines
- 300/240 litres ILRs are supplied to districts and 140 litres ILR is supplied to PHCs
- ILRs must be kept on a horizontal leveled surface, at least 10 cms away from walls
- ILRs can maintain temperature of vaccines if provided '*with even 8 hours of uninterrupted electricity per day*'

> **Key points**
> *Instrument used to monitor the temperature of cold chain at PHC:* Dial Thermometer^Q

ILR

Ice-pack

- Is prepared by keeping in a Deep freezer
- *Is used for:*
  - Temperature maintenance during vaccine transportation, in a vaccine carrier
  - Temperature maintenance during an immunization session
- Is of total 320–340 mL capacity
- Has a 'horizontal mark' – water fill level (as water expands on freezing)
  - NOTHING should be added to water for freezing in an ice-pack
- Has generally 2 holes – MEANT FOR keeping vaccines^Q

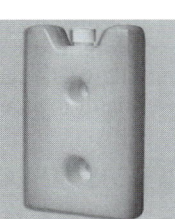

Ice pack

Dial Thermometer

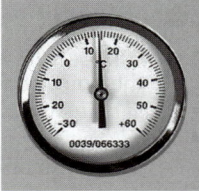
Dial thermometer

- Is the instrument used to monitor the temperature of cold chain at PHC
- Is kept in ILR (Ice-lined refrigerator- component of cold chain) at PHC
- Is *'based on principle of thermocouple*^{Q}*'*
- *Recommended temperature monitoring at PHC level is:* Twice daily^Q

Immunoglobulins

> **Key points**
>
> **IgG:** *'only class of immunoglobulins to cross placenta'*

- Types of immunoglobulins:
  - IgG: Comprises 85% of total serum immunoglobulins, largely extravascular, *'only class of immunoglobulins to cross placenta'*
  - IgM: Comprises 10% of total serum immunoglobulins, *'indicative of recent infection'*, has high agglutinating and complement-fixing ability
  - IgA: Comprises 15% of total serum immunoglobulins, predominantly found in secretions, *'primary defence mechanism at mucous membranes'*
  - IgD: Exact function not known
  - IgE: concentrated in submucous tissues, *'responsible for immediate allergic anaphylaxis reaction'*
- Preparations of immunoglobulins:

	Human normal Ig's	Human specific Ig's
Source	Antibody-rich fraction obtained from a pool of > 1000 donors	Plasma of recovered patients or immunized individuals
Composition	> 90% IgG; less IgA	5 times antibody potential of standard preparation
Examples	Hepatitis A Measles Mumps Rabies Tetanus	Hepatitis B Varicella Diphtheria

Mycobacterium Indicus Pranii (MIP) Vaccine^Q

- Made-in-India leprosy vaccine to be launched^Q
- Pilot basis in five districts in Bihar and Gujarat
- Preventive measure to people living in close contact with those infected
- **To be given along with a dose of Rifampicin**^{Q}
- Developed by GP Talwar, Founder-Director, **National Institute of Immunology, Delhi**
- Approved by the Drug Controller General of India and the FDA in the U.S.
- Cases can be brought down by 60% in three years

Rotavirus Vaccines

- **Rotarix:**
  - Monovalent human strain
  - Live attenuated oral vaccine
  - Schedule: 2 doses, at 2 months and 4 months age (must be completed by 16 weeks age, no later than 24 weeks age)
- **RotaTeq:**
  - Pentavalent bovine-human reassortant strain
  - Live attenuated oral vaccine
  - Schedule: 3 doses at 2, 4, 6 months age (must be completed by 32 weeks age; Not to be initiated for age >12 weeks)
- **Potential complication of Rotavirus vaccines: Intussusception** (when first dose given after 12 weeks age), so preferably avoided in catch-up campaigns where exact age of vaccine is difficult to ascertain

DISINFECTION

Definitions in Disinfection

- *Asepsis:* Prevention of contact with microorganisms

- *Cleaning*: Removal of adherent visible blood/soil/proteinaceous substances/microorganisms/debris from surfaces, crevices, serrations, joints, lumens of instruments/devices/equipment by manual/mechanical process for handling or further decontamination
- *Detergent:* Surface cleaning agent (hydrophilic and lipophilic component) that acts by lowering surface tension
- *Disinfection:* Thermal or chemical destruction of most of the pathogens
- *Germicide:* Agent that destroys microorganisms, especially pathogens
- *Hospital disinfectant:* Disinfectant registered for use in any medical facility; efficacy is demonstrated against Salmonella choleraesuis, Staphylococcus aureus, Pseudomonas aeruginosa
- *Sanitizer:* Agent that reduces number of bacterial contaminants to safe levels as per public health requirements (mainly used for inanimate objects)
- *Sterile:* State of being free from all living microorganisms

Properties of Ideal Disinfectant [Mnemonic: SOURCES BEEN Fully Sterile]
- **S**oluble in water
- **O**dourless
- **U**naffected environmentally (active with organic matter; compatible with chemicals)
- **R**esidual effect
- **C**leaner
- **E**nvironmental friendly
- **S**table in concentration and use-dilution
- **B**road antimicrobial spectrum
- **E**asy to use
- **E**conomical
- **N**ontoxic
- **F**ast acting
- **S**urface compatible (non corrosive, no deterioration)

Chemical Disinfectants: Oxidizing Agents
- *Potassium permanganate:*
  - Aquariums
  - Feet before entering swimming pools
  - Fruits and vegetables
- *Hydrogen peroxide:* Bactericidal, virucidal, fungicidal, Sporicidal
  - Surfaces in hospital settings
  - Antiseptic
  - Cleaning wounds and discharging ulcers
- *Paracetic acid:*
  - Gram-positive, gram-negative bacteria
  - Fungi, yeasts, viruses

Chemical Disinfectants: Metals as Microbicides
- Silver (Prophylaxis of conjunctivitis, Topical therapy for burns, Bonding to indwelling catheters)
- Iron, Copper, Zinc

Chemical Disinfectants: Miscellaneous
- *Pasteurization:* 70° Celsius for 30 minutes for pathogenic microorganisms except spores
- *Microwaves:* Disinfect contact lenses, dental instruments, dentures, milk, urinary catheters, cultures
- *Flushing and Water Disinfectors:* Disinfect bedpans, urinals, washbowls, surgical instruments and anaesthesia tubes
- *Ultraviolet radiation:* Disinfect drinking water, air, titanium implants, contact lenses
- *Ozone*

Factors affecting Efficacy of Sterilization
- Cleaning
- Pathogen type
- Biofilm accumulation
- Lumen length, diameter
- Restricted flow
- Device design, construction

PYQs: Quick Review for NEET

Infectious disease Epidemiology

Occurrence of a Disease Clearly in excess of normal expectancy	Epidemic
Disease imported in a country where it doesn't occur	Exotic
Iatrogenic Disease is	Physician-induced
First case to come to notice of investigator	Index Case
Pseudo-Carriers are	Carriers of avirulent Organisms
Transmission type of Malaria parasite in Mosquito	Cyclo-propagative Transmission
Gap between Primary case and Secondary Case is	Serial Interval
Quarantine is used for group of	Healthy Contacts
Search for cases in epidemic is done till	Twice the Incubation period since last case
Point source epidemic characterized by	Sharp rise/fall, all cases in 1 Incubation period
Disease imported to a country for first time	Exotic Disease
Secular trend refers to	Long term changes
Bhopal gas tragedy is type of epidemic	Single exposure point source epidemic
Rapid rise & fall in epidemic curve, no secondary waves	Point source epidemic, single exposure
Secular trend of disease refers to occurrence of	Consistent change in one direction
Human/animal/fomite/objects from which infective organism enters host	Source
Person/animal/substance in which infectious agent lives and multiplies	Reservoir
Anthropozoonses is the transmission of infection from	Animal to man
MC Nosocomial infection is	Urinary tract infections (UTI)
Not a type of Direct transmission	Droplet nuclei
Point Prevalence is defined as	Number of total cases at a given point of time
Period prevalence is defined by	Number of total cases in a given year
Relationship between Incidence and Prevalence	Prevalence = Incidence × Duration

General Epidemiology

First Distinguished Epidemiologist	Syndenham
Incidence rate refers to	Only new cases
Cross-product ratio is used in	Case control study
Prevalence is a Rate/Ratio/Proportion	Proportion (Total=New + Old Cases)
Total no. of deaths/Total no. of cases is	Case Fatality Rate
Observed Deaths/Expected Deaths is	Standardized Mortality Ratio (SMR)
Prevalence/Duration is	Incidence
For calculation of incidence denominator is taken as	Population at risk
MMR is a Rate/Ratio/Proportion	Ratio
Case fatality rate represents	Killing power of a disease
Denominator of incidence	1000 total population at risk
Measure of killing power of a disease	Case fatality rate
Maximum power of destruction of a disease is measured by	Case fatality rate
Usefulness for "Case Fatality Rate" is very limited in	Chronic illness
Direct standardization is done because there are differences in	Age distributions
Health status of two populations is best compared by	Standardized mortality

Contd...

Contd...

Study Designs	
Forward Looking/Prospective Study is	Cohort Study
Both exposure and outcome have occurred before study starts in	Case Control Study
Strength of association in Case control study	Odds ratio
Odds ratio formula is	ad/bc
Prevalence of cataract at one point of time can be determined by	Cross-sectional study
Incidence rate can be calculated from	Cohort study
Purpose of Matching	Removes confounding, ensures Comparability
Bias due to different hospital admission rates	Berkesonian bias
Framingham Heart Study is type of	Cohort Study
Relative Risk is	Incidence in Exposed/Incidence in non-exposed
Natural history of disease is best studied by	Cohort study
Heart of RCT is	Randomization
Unit of study in Phase I clinical trial	Health volunteers
Phase I clinical trial of drugs done on	Healthy volunteers
Phase IV clinical trial is done	After marketing drug
For a community physician, important strength of association	Attributable risk
Nested case control study is a type of	Prospective study
Recall bias is most commonly associated with study design	Case control study
Analytical study with population as unit of study	Ecological
30/50 smokers & 10/50 non-smokers developed disease, Odds ratio is	6
Relative risk studied for disease and cause was One, it means	No association
Healthy worker effect is bias of which type	Selection bias
MC used strength of association is	Relative risk
Selection bias in RCT can be eliminated by	Randomization
Communicability of a disease is determined by	Secondary attack rate
Serial Interval almost gives	Incubation period
Type of study used for discovery of cholera by John Snow	Natural experiment study
Incidence of disease in exposed divided by incidence among non-exposed is	Risk ratio
Study that gives prevalence of delusion in elderly at a given paint of time	Cross-sectional study
Cohort study is which type of study	Analytic observational
Recall bias is most commonly associated with _____ study	Case-control study
Epidemiological study with population as a unit of study is	Ecological study
Heart of Randomised controlled trial is	Randomization
Berkesonian bias is a type of	Admission rate bias
Natural history of disease can be studied by	Longitudinal study
Selection bias is due to	Procedure used to select subjects
Dose response relationship is a measure of	Strength of association
Relative risk of 5 means	Incidence of disease is 5 times higher in exposed group
Unit of study in Ecological study	Population
Study used to study more than one possible outcomes	Cohort study
Case series study is type of	Observational study

Contd...

Contd...

Vaccines	
Marc Koska developed	Disposable K1-syringe (auto-disabled)
Measles vaccine stored at	+ 2° to + 8° C
BCG is diluted with	Normal saline
Rubella vaccine is	Live vaccine and C/I in pregnancy
Period of infectivity of Measles	4 days before to 5 days after rash appearance
Yellow fever Vaccine (17 D) type of vaccine	Live vaccine
Lyophilized (freeze dried) Vaccines	BCG, Yellow Fever, Measles, MMR, HiB, JE Live
Cold Chain Temperature of vaccines	+ 2° to + 8° C
Yellow Fever/BCG/Measles vaccines are types of	Live Vaccines/Lyophilized vaccines
First Vaccine to be discovered	Smallpox Vaccine (Edward Jenner)
Risk of Cold Chain failure is greatest at level of	Sub-centre and Village level
Hepatitis B vaccine is a type of	Killed vaccine
Vaccine strain for Swine flu vaccine in India	A7/California/2009
Vaccine given at 9 months age is	Measles vaccine
OPV vaccine doses in immunization program	5
Intradermal schedule for Rabies vaccine	Thai Updated Cross Regimen 2-2-2-0-2
Virus used to prepare Rabies vaccine	Fixed virus
Validity of YF vaccine	Lifelong
Toxoids are prepared from	Exotoxins
Strain of Varicella vaccine	OKA strain
Number of vaccine vials in Day carrier box	6–8 vials
Number of vaccine vials in Vaccine carrier	16–20 vials
Pre-exposure i/m schedule of Rabies vaccine	Day 0, 7, 28
Activation of Yellow fever vaccine after	10 days
Strain for Measles Vaccine is	Edmonston Zagreb
Strain for Rubella Vaccine	RA 27/3
BCG vaccination is given by route	Intradermally
At PHC level vaccine storage is by using	Ice Lined Refrigerator (ILR)
MMR vaccine is a type of	Live attenuated vaccine
Immunization with 3 doses of tetanus toxoid, confers protection for	10 years
Rabies vaccine for pre exposure prophylaxis is given at	0, 7, 21/28 days
Hepatitis B vaccine, dose schedule in adult (months)	0, 1, 6 months
OPV Bivalent vaccine contains Polio viruses	P1 & P3
Yellow fever vaccine starts protection after gap of	10 days
DPT vaccine stored at temperature of	+2 to +8 degrees Celsius
Immunoglobulins found maximum is secretions	IgA
Vaccine preventable neonatal disease is	Tetanus
Under UIP program, vaccine administered at 9 months of age	Measles
Salk vaccine is type of	Killed vaccine
Route of administration of Measles vaccine	Subcutaneous
Besides OPV, highest coverage of vaccine in India	BCG vaccine

Contd...

Contd...

DPT vaccine route is	Intramuscular
Dose of Rabies Immunoglobulin	20 IU/kg (Human Ig), 40 IU/kg (Equine Ig)
Dose of Varicella Immunoglobulin	15-25 units/kg BW
Bivalent oral polio vaccine contains _____ strains of polio virus	P1 & P3
Chicken pox vaccine is a type of	Live vaccine
Rotavirus vaccine is type of	Live oral
Post-exposure prophylaxis intramuscular schedule for rabies vaccination	1-1-1-1-1
Role of magnesium [Mg] in OPV	Stabilizer
Vaccine used to prevent death from pneumonia in children	Measles vaccine
Live influenza vaccine is given by _____ route	Intranasal
Protective efficacy of Measles vaccine	90-95%
Route for BCG vaccine	Intradermal
Disinfection	
Most effective sterilizing agent	Autoclaving (Steam under pressure)
Beaching Powder contains _____ available chlorine	33% available chlorine
Best method to prevent Nosocomial infection	Hand washing
Biosafety cabinets are disinfected by	40% Formaldehyde
Sterilization and disinfection of blood spills is done by	Sodium hypochlorite
Syringes and glassware are sterilized by	Hot air oven

Multiple Choice Questions

DEFINITION AND EPIDEMIOLOGICAL Methods

1. Residence of three villages with three different types of water supply were asked to participate in a study to identify cholera carriers. Because several cholera deaths had occurred in the recent past, virtually everyone present at the time submitted to examination. The proportion of residents in each village who were carriers was computed and compared. This study is a:
   (a) Cross-sectional study [AIIMS May 03]
   (b) Case-control study [NEET Pattern 2017]
   (c) Concurrent cohort study
   (d) Non-concurrent

2. The analytical study where population is the unit of study is: [AIPGME 1996]
   (a) Cross-sectional (b) Ecological
   (c) Case-control (d) Cohort

3. Natural history of disease is studied with:
   (a) Longitudinal studies [NEET Pattern 2013, 2015]
   (b) Cross-sectional studies [WBPG 2014]
   (c) Trials
   (d) None

4. Cause to effect progression is seen in all *except*:
   [DNB June 2010] [DNB December 2011]
   (a) Case control study
   (b) Ecological study
   (c) Cohort study
   (d) Randomized control trial

5. Father of Evidence Based Medicine is: [AIIMS May 2014]
   (a) Sackett (b) Da vinci
   (c) Hippocrates (d) Tolstoy

6. Evidence-based medicine refers to: [NEET Pattern 2016]
   (a) Clinical trials to prove adverse effects of drugs
   (b) Clinical trials to prove safety of drugs
   (c) Use of various research finding for taking decisions about best patients care
   (d) All of the above

7. Spot maps are used for a disease in Epidemiology for depiction of: [NEET Pattern 2016]
   (a) Local distributions
   (b) Rural-urban variations
   (c) National variations
   (d) International variations

8. The difference between Descriptive and Analytic studies: [NEET Pattern 2017]
   (a) Descriptive studies are used to test hypothesis
   (b) Analytic studies are used to formulate a hypothesis
   (c) Descriptive studies are first phase in epidemiology
   (d) Analytic studies observe distribution of disease

9. Evidence-based medicine refers to: [NEET Pattern 2017]
   (a) Clinical trials to prove adverse effects of drugs
   (b) Clinical trials to prove safety of drugs
   (c) Use of various research finding for taking decisions about best patients care
   (d) All of the above

10. Unit of study in Ecological study is [NEET Pattern 2018]
    (a) Individual (b) Population
    (c) Community (d) Patient/Case

Review Questions

11. Hypothesis is a: [MP 2000]
    (a) Axiom (b) Verified variable
    (c) Established document (d) Variable to be tested

12. Best study of first choice for assessment of UNKNOWN or New disease with no etiological hypothesis:
    (a) Cohort study [MH 2007]
    (b) Case-control study
    (c) Cross-sectional study
    (d) Descriptive epidemiology

MEASUREMENTS IN EPIDEMIOLOGY

13. The following is true about prevalence and incidence:
    (a) Both are rates [AIIMS Nov 03, AIIMS May 05]
    (b) Prevalence is a rate but incidence is not
    (c) Incidence is a rate but prevalence is not
    (d) Both are not rates

14. Which of the following is 'Event-type' disability indicator? [NEET Pattern 2017]
    (a) Notification rate
    (b) Bed disability days
    (c) Limitation of activity
    (d) Limitation of mobility

Review Questions

15. All of the following are true regarding the Ratio *except*: [AP 2001]
    (a) Numerator is component of denominator
    (b) Numerator is not a component of denominator
    (c) Numerator & denominator are not related values
    (d) It is expressed as a number

Epidemiology and Vaccines 159

16. True about prevalence: [MP 2002]
    (a) It is a ratio
    (b) Prevalence rate is the ideal measure for studying disease etiology or causation
    (c) Increases with increase in duration of disease
    (d) Decreases with decrease in case fatality

17. In the Death Certificate given below, Main underlying cause of death is [NEET Pattern 2019]

    (a) Pulmonary embolism
    (b) Secondary carcinoma shaft of femur
    (c) Fracture of femur
    (d) Malignant neoplasm of breast

IDC

18. In WHO recommended Death Certificate, Main Underlying Cause of Death is recorded on: [AIIMS Nov 1999]
    (a) Line Ia
    (b) Line Ib
    (c) Line Ic
    (d) Line II

MORTALITY MEASUREMENTS

19. Standardized age mortality ratio is an indicator for: [INICET November 2021]
    (a) Death rate of a population adjusted to a Standard age distribution
    (b) Death rate of a population adjusted to a Standard sex distribution
    (c) To eliminate age structure of different countries
    (d) To remove bias due to different age group population in different regions

20. Following can be used as a yardstick for the assessment of standards of therapy: [AIPGME 1996]
    (a) Specific death rate
    (b) Case fatality rate
    (c) Proportional mortality rate
    (d) Survival rate

21. About direct standardization all are true except: [AIPGME 00, 02]
    (a) Age specific death rate is not needed
    (b) A standard population is needed [UP 2002]
    (c) Population should be comparable
    (d) Two populations are compared

22. The rate adjusted to allow for the age distribution of the population is: [AIIMS Nov 03, AIIMS May 05]
    (a) Perinatal mortality rate
    (b) Crude mortality rate
    (c) Fertility rate
    (d) Age-standardized mortality rate

23. Which is best in order to make a comparison between Health status of 2 populations? [AIIMS Nov 2001]
    (a) Standardized mortality rate [RJ 2001]
    (b) Disease specific death rate
    (c) Proportional mortality rate
    (d) Age specific death rate

24. At what point in time is the population assessed for calculation of the crude death rate? [AIIMS May 01]
    (a) 1st Jan
    (b) 1st May
    (c) 1st July
    (d) 31st Dec

25. All are indicators of mortality except: [AIIMS May 1994]
    (a) Case fatality rate
    (b) Life expectancy
    (c) Duration of sickness
    (d) Standardised death rate

26. In an outbreak of cholera in a village of 2000 population 20 cases have occurred and 5 have died. Case fatality rate is: [AIPGME 1991]
    (a) 1%
    (b) 0.25%
    (c) 5%
    (d) 25%

27. Which one of the following is a better indicator of the severity of an acute disease? [AIIMS May 1995, 04, AIPGME 2005, AIIMS Nov 1999]
    (a) Cause specific death rate
    (b) Case fatality rate
    (c) Standardized mortality ratio
    (d) Five year survival rate

28. Estimating the burden of particular disease in a community is measured by: [Karnataka 2005]
    (a) Proportional mortality rate [UP 2007]
    (b) Disease specific mortality
    (c) Crude death rate
    (d) Incidence of disease

29. Case fatality rate is a method measuring: [Karnataka 2005]
    (a) Infectivity
    (b) Pathogenicity
    (c) Virulence
    (d) Average duration of disease

30. Which one is not true of case fatality rate?
    (a) It is a ratio [Karnataka 2006, 2009]
    (b) Time interval is non-specified
    (c) It may vary from the same disease in different epidemics
    (d) It is useful in chronic diseases

31. Most useful parameter to predict the virulence of acute illness is: [AIPGME 2011]
    (a) Standardised mortality ratio (SMR)
    (b) Case fatality rate (CFR)
    (c) Secondary attack rate (SAR)
    (d) Incidence

32. Standardised mortality rate is standardised for:
    (a) Age [DPG 2011]
    (b) Disease
    (c) Region
    (d) A particular time period

33. Proportional mortality rate is: [NEET Pattern 2012]
    (a) Rate
    (b) Ratio
    (c) Proportion
    (d) None

34. Denominator for calculating proportional mortality rate from a specific disease is: [NEET Pattern 2017] [UPSC CMS 2015]
    (a) Mid-year population during that year
    (b) Population at risk in that particular area
    (c) Total deaths in that year
    (d) Attributable deaths of a particular disease

35. A community of 500000 people had 100 deaths in a year. Out of those 100 deaths 10 individuals died due to pulmonary TB. What is the proportional mortality rate from TB? [NEET Pattern 2017]
    (a) 10%
    (b) 50%
    (c) 75%
    (d) None

36. Standardized death rates are used because health. [NEET Pattern 2017]
    (a) For valid comparison of two groups of different health determinants
    (b) Calculations are more accurate
    (c) To avoid selection bias
    (d) All of the above

37. Denominator in calculation of Case fatality rate is [NEET Pattern 2018]
    (a) Total number of deaths due to all causes
    (b) Total number of hospital admissions
    (c) Total number of cases due to the disease concerned
    (d) Total number of deaths due to the disease concerned

Review Questions

38. Sullivan's Index: [DNB 2008]
    (a) Measures disability
    (b) Measures life years adjusted with death
    (c) Measures life expectancy free of disability
    (d) Measures life expectancy

39. True statement regarding specific death rates:
    (a) Specific for age and sex [UP 2005]
    (b) Identify particular group or group "at risk for preventive action"
    (c) Maybe cause or disease specific
    (d) All of the above

40. Case fatality rate is: [MH 2002] [AIIMS 1997] [MP 2001] [AP 2014] [AP 2001] [NEET Pattern 2017]
    (a) Spreading power of a disease
    (b) Killing power of a disease in a time
    (c) Killing power of a disease with no time interval
    (d) Resistance of disease

MORBIDITY MEASUREMENTS

41. A drug reduces mortality but don't cure the disease. True statement from the following: [INICET November 2021]
    (a) Prevalence of disease increases
    (b) Prevalence of disease decreases
    (c) Incidence of disease increase
    (d) Incidence of disease decrease

42. If a new effective treatment is initiated and all other factors remain the same; which of the following is most likely to happen? [AIIMS May 04]
    (a) Incidence will not change
    (b) Prevalence will not change
    (c) Neither incidence nor prevalence will change
    (d) Incidence and prevalence will change

43. Improved prevention of an acute, nonfatal disease is likely to: [NEET Pattern 2017] [AIPGME 1996]
    (a) Decrease the prevalence of the disease
    (b) Increase the prevalence of the disease
    (c) Decrease the incidence of the disease
    (d) Increase the incidence of the disease

44. A diagnostic test has been introduced that will detect a certain disease 1 yrs earlier than it is usually detected. Which of the following is most likely to happen to the disease within the 10 yrs after the test its introduced? (Assumed that early detection has no effect on the natural history of the disease. Also assume that no changes in death certification practices occur during the 10 yrs.): [AIPGME 1998]
    (a) The period prevalence rate will decrease
    (b) The apparent 5-year survival rate will increase
    (c) The age adjusted mortality rate will decrease
    (d) The incidence rate will decrease

45. The incidence rate of a disease is 5 times greater in women than in men, but the prevalence rates show no sex difference. The best explanation is that: [AIIMS June 1999]
    (a) The case fatality rate for this disease is lower in women
    (b) The case fatality rate for this disease is higher for women
    (c) The duration of disease is shorter in men
    (d) Risk factors for developing the disease are more common in women

46. Prevalence of a disease: [AIIMS Nov 2002]
    (a) Is the best measure of disease frequency in etiological studies
    (b) Can only be determined by a cohort study
    (c) Is the number of new cases in a defined population
    (d) Describes the balance between incidence, mortality and recovery

47. In a village having population of 1000, we found patients with certain disease. The results of as new diagnostic test on that disease are as follows:

Test result	Disease	
	Present	Absent
+	180	400
–	20	400

    What is the percent prevalence of disease? [AIPGME 2005]
    (a) 0.20
    (b) 2
    (c) 18
    (d) 20

48. The relationship between incidence and prevalence can be expresses as: [Karnataka 2005]
    (a) The product of incidence and mean duration of disease
    (b) The dividend of incidence and mean duration of disease
    (c) The sum of incidence and mean duration of disease
    (d) The difference of incidence of mean duration of disease

49. A district has total population 10 lacs, with under-16 population being 30%. The prevalence of blindness is 0.8/1000 among under-16 population. Calculate total number of blind among under-16 population in the district: [AIIMS November 2012]
    (a) 240
    (b) 2400
    (c) 24000
    (d) 240000

50. In a town of population 5000, 500 are already myopic on January 1, 2011. Number of new myopia cases is 90 till December 31, 2011. Calculate incidence of Myopia in the town in 2011: [AIIMS November 2012]
    (a) 0.018
    (b) 0.02
    (c) 0.05
    (d) 18

51. In a population of 5000 number of new cases of TB is 500; old cases in the same population are 150. What is the prevalence of TB? [NEET Pattern 2014]
    (a) 9%
    (b) 12%
    (c) 13%
    (d) 18%

52. Which of the following is a better indicator of efficacy of hospital services and health programs?
    (a) Case fatality rate [NEET Pattern 2015]
    (b) Prevalence
    (c) Secondary attack rate
    (d) Incidence

53. When the prevalence rate is used without any qualification, it is taken to mean as? [UPSC CMS 2015]
    (a) Point prevalence rate
    (b) Period prevalence rate
    (c) Annual prevalence rate
    (d) Mean duration prevalence rate

54. A drug which reduces mortality but does not cure a disease, will gradually lead to: [AIIMS November 2015]
    (a) Incidence and prevalence both increase
    (b) Incidence and prevalence both decrease
    (c) Incidence increases while prevalence decreases
    (d) Incidence same, prevalence increases

55. A couple has 4 children, all unvaccinated for Measles. A child got Measles on 5 August 2015. Two other children developed Measles by 15 August 2015. Secondary attack rate is: [NEET Pattern 2015]
    (a) 0%
    (b) 33%
    (c) 66%
    (d) 75%

56. A party was attended by 110 people out which 40 didn't eat fruit salad. From the rest who ate fruit salad, 55 developed food poisoning. What is the attack rate? [NEET Pattern 2016]
    (a) 46
    (b) 56
    (c) 78
    (d) 50

57. All the statements are true about the disease *except*: [AIIMS May 2016]
    (a) Incidence is a probability that a healthy individual will develop the disease during specified period
    (b) Incidence will decrease if a new drug is effective in reducing deaths from the disease
    (c) Incidence measures the absolute risk of developing the disease
    (d) Incidence decreases if a particular prevention program is effective

Review Questions

58. Incidence rate is calculated from: [AP 2007]
    (a) Case-control [Kolkata 2005]
    (b) Prospective study
    (c) Retrospective study
    (d) RCT

59. Which one of the following is an Index of communicability of an Infection? [RJ 2007]
    (a) Carrier rate [NEET Pattern 2018]
    (b) Prevalence rate
    (c) Secondary attack rate
    (d) Primary attack rate

60. High prevalence associated with: [RJ 2008]
    (a) High cure rate
    (b) Immigration of healthy people

(c) longer duration of disease
(d) Less Incidence of disease

DESCRIPTIVE EPIDEMIOLOGY

61. All are true for Point source epidemic *except*:
    (a) Epidemic curve rises and falls sharply
    (b) Clustering of cases within a short period of time
    (c) Person-to-person transmission
    (d) All cases usually develop within one incubation period [JIPMER 2014] [AIIMS Nov 06]

62. True regarding point source epidemic is: [AIIMS Sep 1996] [AIPGME 2000]
    (a) Secondary waves occur
    (b) There is a rapid rise in the wave which flattens (Plateau)
    (c) All cases occur in a single incubation period of the disease
    (d) It is propagative

63. Regarding point source epidemic true:
    (a) Rapid rise and fall [MP 2001] [PGI Dec 08]
    (b) Only infectious cause [PGI June 02]
    (c) Explosive [AP 2008]
    (d) ↑secondary attack rate
    (e) No secondary wave

64. Migration study is used to study: [NEET Pattern 2015]
    (a) Sociodemographic reasons for migration of a population
    (b) Prevalence of disease in a population
    (c) Environmental and genetic factors in a disease in population
    (d) Diseases with Long Incubation period

65. An outbreak of Viral hepatitis A was reported from a town between June and August of a particular year. Of total cases, 60% occurred in July. Exposure of the community to infection is from: [UPSC CMS 2015]
    (a) Common single source for a short period
    (b) Common single source for a prolonged period
    (c) Multiple sources for a short period
    (d) Multiple sources for a prolonged period

66. A well of contaminated water resulting in an epidemic of acute watery diarrhea is a typical example for [NEET Pattern 2018]
    (a) Common source, single exposure epidemic
    (b) Common source, continuous exposure epidemic
    (c) Slow epidemic
    (d) Propagated epidemic

67. A primary health center (PHC) reports 40-50 cases in a week in the community. This week there are 48 cases normally, based on previous records. This is called
    (a) Epidemic [AIIMS November 2018]
    (b) Sporadic
    (c) Endemic
    (d) Outbreak

Review Questions

68. Seasonal trend is: [UP 2002]
    (a) Seasonal variation of disease occurrence may be related to environmental conditions
    (b) Some diseases occurs in cyclic spread over short periods of time
    (c) Some disease occurs in cyclic changes over long period of time
    (d) Non-infectious conditions never show periodic fluctuations

69. Descriptive epidemiology includes all *except*:
    (a) Retrospective and prospective study
    (b) Disease [UP 2003]
    (c) Time
    (d) Place

70. A graph shows an uniform curve with no secondary curves the following statement is correct: [AP 2000]
    (a) Multiple exposure
    (b) Pointed epidemic
    (c) Sporadic
    (d) Pandemic

71. Food poisoning is an example of: [NEET Pattern 2018] [TN 2005]
    (a) Common source, single exposure epidemic
    (b) Common source, continuous exposure epidemic
    (c) Propagated epidemic
    (d) Modern epidemic

ANALYTICAL EPIDEMIOLOGY

72. In a study, 30000 women were followed up for 20 years and 1500 out of them developed Breast cancer. Now additional 2000 healthy women were taken as controls. Risk factors were compared from the baseline data at the start of the study by giving questionnaires to both the groups. This study design is: [INICET May 2023]
    (a) Retrospective cohort study
    (b) Nested case control study
    (c) Case control study
    (d) Cross sectional study

73. A study among factory workers, of 20 years duration, is conducted to study the relation between aniline dye exposure and bladder cancer. One group was people working in the aniline dye factory and other group of people working in the factory office as clerical staff. The duration of exposure was obtained from past records of employment. What is this study? [NEET PG Pattern 2023]
    (a) Prospective cohort study
    (b) Retrospective cohort study
    (c) Case control study
    (d) Ecological study

74. Attributable risk calculated to understand the relation between smoking and lung cancer is 90%. Which of the following is true? **[INICET November 2022]**
    (a) 10% of lung cancers in smokers is not associated with smoking
    (b) 90% cases of lung cancer can be eliminated in population if smoking is eliminated
    (c) 90% cases of lung cancer can be eliminated in smokers if smoking is eliminated
    (d) 10% cases of lung cancer can be eliminated in population if smoking is eliminated

75. Many children from a particular community coming to a hospital were detected as having ALL. The hospital said that it is due to a chemical in the water of that community. If a case control study has to be done to find whether that chemical and ALL are associated, children introduced to chemicals having ALL are taken as cases. Then what will be taken as controls? **[NEET PG Pattern 2022]**
    (a) Children in same community with ALL getting exposed to chemicals
    (b) Children in same community without ALL not getting exposed to chemicals
    (c) Children from hospital with ALL getting exposed to chemicals
    (d) Children from hospital without ALL not getting exposed to chemicals

76. A Cohort study is undertaken to study association between Green tea intake and Diabetes mellitus. Relative risk was found to be '0.85'. Which of the following is correct regarding association between green tea and DM? **[NEET PG Pattern 2022]**
    (a) Green tea consumption increases the risk of DM
    (b) Green tea consumption decreases the risk of DM
    (c) Green tea consumption has no effect on the risk of DM
    (d) Cannot be determined

77. Steps in Case control studies includes (Multiple response type): **[INICET November 2021]**
    1. Follow up
    2. Matching
    3. Selection/Allocation
    4. Inference of result data
    (a) 2, 3
    (b) 1, 2, 3, 4
    (c) 1, 2
    (d) 2, 3, 4

78. Best study to find out strength of association i.e. relation between exposure and outcome? **[INICET November 2021]**
    (a) Cohort study
    (b) Case control
    (c) Cross sectional
    (d) Ecological study

79. Difference between the Incidence in exposed and non-exposed group is best given by: **[NEET PG Pattern January 2020]**
    (a) Attributable risk
    (b) Odd ratio
    (c) Relative risk
    (d) Population attributable risk

80. A study was undertaken to find the relation between COPD and smoking. Patients' data was collected through records from Government hospital and record of cigarettes sale from finance and taxation departments. Study design? **[NEET PG Pattern January 2020]**
    (a) Cross sectional
    (b) Pesological study
    (c) Ecological study
    (d) Operational study

81. All of the following are done to remove Confounding except: **[AIIMS May 2019]**
    (a) Randomization
    (b) Random Selection
    (c) Matching
    (d) Blinding

82. Study design of choice for finding out Diurnal variation of fat in Expressed breast milk (EBM) for Preterm babies: **[AIIMS May 2019]**
    (a) Prospective cohort
    (b) Ambispective cohort
    (c) Case control
    (d) Cross sectional

83. The systematic distortion of retrospective studies that can be eliminated by a prospective design is:
    (a) Confounding **[AIIMS May 04]**
    (b) Effect modification
    (c) Recall bias
    (d) Measurement bias

84. The ratio between the incidence of disease among exposed and non-exposed is called: **[AIIMS Nov 1993]**
    (a) Causal risk
    (b) Relative risk
    (c) Attributable risk
    (d) Odds ratio

85. Hawthorne effect is seen in: **[AIPGME 1996]**
    (a) Case-control study
    (b) Cohort study
    (c) Cross-sectional study
    (d) Retrospective cohort study

86. A study compared 150 children with a particular disease with 300 disease free children to examine past experiences that may contribute to the development of the illness. What kind of study is this? **[AIPGME 2002]**
    (a) Cohort
    (b) Controlled clinical trial

Epidemiology and Vaccines 163

(c) Case series
(d) Case control

87. Which of the following is not a cause of bias?
[AIPGME 1993]
   (a) Confounding
   (b) Selection
   (c) Misclassification
   (d) Random error

88. The table given below shows cases of breast cancer occurring in a randomized clinical trial of a new drug designed to prevent the disease. In this study, 1000 healthy women between the ages of 60 and 65 were given the drug and 1000 were given the placebo for 5 years.
[AIIMS Sep 1996]

	Breast Cancer	No Breast Cancer	Total
Placebo	40	960	1000
New Drug	10	990	1000

What is the relative risk of breast cancer in patients exposed to drug?
   (a) 25%
   (b) 50%
   (c) 75%
   (d) 100%

89. A study began in 1970 with a group of 5000 adults in Delhi who were asked about their alcohol consumption. The occurrence of cancer was studied in this group between 1990 and 1995. This is an example of:
   (a) Cross-sectional study [AIPGME 2000]
   (b) Retrospective cohort study
   (c) Concurrent cohort study
   (d) Case-control study

90. TATA memorial hospital conducted a cohort study on 7000 subjects who were smokers over a ten-year period & found 70 subjects developed lung cancer. Concurrent evaluation of general population in the catchment area of hospital, out of 7000 non-smoker subjects only 7 developed lung cancer. The RR for developing lung cancer is:
[AIPGME 1996]
   (a) 1
   (b) 10
   (c) 100
   (d) 0.1

91. In an investigation to study the effect of smoking on renal cell cancer, it is observed that 30 of the 50 patients were smokers as compared to 10 out of 50 control subjects. The odd ratio of renal cancer associated with smoking will be:
[AIIMS Nov 05]
   (a) 3.0
   (b) 0.33
   (c) 6.0
   (d) 0.16

92. In a study of 200 smokers & 300 non-smokers were followed up over a period of 10 years to find out incidence of hypertension. Out of 200 smokers, 60 developed hypertension, as compared to 600 non-smokers of which 30 developed hypertension. The risk ratio of the study:
[AIIMS Nov 2001]
   (a) 3
   (b) 30
   (c) 1/3
   (d) 6

93. In a study begun in 1965, a group of 3000 adults in Baltimore were asked about alcohol consumption. The occurrence of cancer was studied in the group between 1981 and 1995. This is an example of: [AIPGME 2004]
   (a) Cross-sectional study
   (b) Concurrent cohort
   (c) Retrospective cohort
   (d) Clinical trial

94. The physical examination records of the entire incoming freshman class of 1935 at the University of Minnesota were examined in 1977 to see if their recorded height and weight at the time of admission to university was related to their chance of developing CHD. This is an example of: [AIIMS Dec 1997]
   (a) Cross-sectional study
   (b) Concurrent cohort
   (c) Retrospective cohort
   (d) Clinical trial

95. Retrospective cohort studies are characterized by all the following except: [AIIMS May 1995]
   (a) The study groups are exposed and non-exposed
   (b) Incidence rates are compared
   (c) The required sample size is smaller than that needed for a concurrent cohort study
   (d) The required sample size is similar to that needed for a concurrent cohort study

96. At an initial examination in Oxford, Migraine head ache was found in 5 of 1000 men aged 30–35 years and in 10 of 1000 women aged 30 to 35 years. The inference that women have a two times greater risk of developing migraine headache than men in this age group is: [AIIMS Feb 1997]
   (a) Correct
   (b) Incorrect, because a ratio has been used to compare male and female rates
   (c) Incorrect, because of failure to recognize the cohort effect of age in the two groups
   (d) Incorrect, because of failure to distinguish between incidence and prevalence

97. All the following are advantages of case control studies except: [NEET Pattern 2013] [AIPGME 1996- 02]
   (a) Useful in rare diseases [AIIMS June 2000]
   (b) Relative risk can be calculated
   (c) Odds ratio can be calculated
   (d) Cost-effective and inexpensive

98. A one day census of inpatients in a mental hospital could: [AIIMS May 2005]
   (a) Give good information about the patients in that hospital at that time
   (b) Give reliable estimates of seasonal factors in admissions

(c) Enable us to draw conclusions about the mental hospitals of India
(d) Enable us to estimate the distribution of different diagnosis in mental illness in the local area

99. The incidence of carcinoma cervix in women with multiple sexual partners is 5 times the incidence seen in those with a single partner. Based on this, what is the attributable risk? *[AIIMS May 2001]*
   (a) 20%
   (b) 40%
   (c) 50%
   (d) 80%

100. In a study 400 smokers and 600 non-smokers were followed up over a period of 10 years to find out the incidence of hypertension. The following table summarizes the data at the end of the study:

		Hypertension		
		Yes	No	Total
Smoking	Yes	120	280	400
	No	30	570	600
	Total	150	850	1000

   The risk ratio in this study is: *[AIIMS Nov 05] [DPG 2011]*
   (a) 0.06
   (b) 0.60
   (c) 6.0
   (d) 60.0

101. Several studies have shown that 85% of cases of lung cancer are due to cigarette smoking. It is a measure of: *[AIIMS Nov 05, AIPGME 07]*
   (a) Incidence rate
   (b) Relative risk
   (c) Attributable risk
   (d) Population attributable risk

102. It is probable that physician have a higher index of suspicion for tuberculosis in children without BCG scar than those with BCG scar. This is so and an association is found between Tuberculosis and not having BCG scar, the association may be due to: *[AIIMS Nov 2005]*
   (a) Selection bias
   (b) Interviewer bias
   (c) Surveillance bias
   (d) Non-response bias

103. Framingham Heart Study is an example of:
   (a) Case-control study *[AIIMS Sep 1996]*
   (b) Cohort study *[PGMCET 2015]*
   (c) Cross-sectional study *[NEET Pattern 2017]*
   (d) Interventional study

104. Which of the following statements is not correct? *[AIIMS Nov 2001] [AIPGME 1994]*
   (a) A cohort study is more expensive in comparison to case control study
   (b) A cohort study starts with people exposed to risk factor or suspected cause while case control study starts with disease
   (c) A long follow-up period often needed with delayed results in a cohort study whereas a case control study yields relatively quick results
   (d) A cohort study is more appropriate when the disease or exposure under investigation is rare, in comparison to case control study

105. Which of the following research methods studies have only people who are initially free of the disease of interest? *[AIIMS Dec 1994]*
   (a) A case–control study
   (b) A case series study
   (c) A prevalence survey
   (d) A cohort study

106. An Odds ratio = 1 indicates that the association between the two factors is: *[AIIMS June 1992]*
   (a) Is perfect
   (b) Is low
   (c) Is high
   (d) Does not exist

107. Which of the following bias can be reduced by allowing equal interview time? *[AIPGME 08]*
   (a) Berkesonian bias
   (b) Recall bias
   (c) Selection bias
   (d) Interviewer bias

108. Which of the following is ideal to ensure similarity between experimental & control groups?
   (a) Randomization *[AIIMS May 2001]*
   (b) Matching
   (c) Stratified randomization
   (d) Cross over study

109. All can be used as controls in a study of genetic condition *except*: *[AIPGME 1998]*
   (a) Hospital Controls
   (b) Sibling Controls
   (c) Neighbourhood Controls
   (d) General Population

110. True about case control studies is: *[AIIMS Nov 95]*
   (a) Minimal problems of bias *[AIPGME 1994]*
   (b) Time consuming & expensive to carry out
   (c) Easy to measure incidence
   (d) Suitable to investigate rare diseases

111. A study was carried out to find out safety of OCPs. Relative risk (or Odds Ratio) of thromboembolism among OCP users to non-users in the given case control study is:

	Number	%who used OCPs
Cases of thromboembolism	84	50
Controls	168	14

   (a) 0.14 *[AIPGME 1996]*
   (b) 6
   (c) 1
   (d) Insufficient data to calculate

112. Incidence rate of lung cancer among smokers is 10 per 1000 and among Non-smokers is 1 per 1000. The

extent to which lung cancer can be attributed to smoking is: [AIIMS June 1997]
(a) 10%
(b) 90%
(c) 1%
(d) 100%

113. Match the following: [AIIMS Nov 1993]

Type of study	Unit of study
A. Cohort study	I. Healthy volunteers
B. Ecological study	II. Population
C. RCT	III. Individual
D. Field trials	IV. Patient

(a) A – I, B – III, C – IV, D – II
(b) A – III, B – II, C – IV, D – I
(c) A – III, B – II, C – I, D – IV
(d) A – I, B – III, C – II, D – IV

114. In a case-control study of a suspected association between breast cancer and the contraceptive pill, all of the following are true statements *except*: [AIIMS Nov 2002]
(a) The control should come from a population that has the same potential for breast cancer as the cases
(b) The control should exclude women known to be taking the pill at the time of the survey
(c) All the controls need to be healthy
(d) The attributable risk of breast cancer resulting from the pill may be directly measured

115. Which of the following statements is not true about 'cohort study'? [AIIMS Nov 95, AIIMS Dec 94]
(a) Provides incidence of disease
(b) Indicated when there is good evidence of association between exposure and disease
(c) Done when incidence of disease is very low among exposed
(d) Done when ample funds are available

116. The association between coronary artery disease (CAD) and smoking was found to be as follows:

	CAD	No CAD
Smokers	30	20
Nonsmokers	20	30

The Odds ratio can be estimated as: [AIPGME 02]
(a) 0.65
(b) 0.8
(c) 1.3
(d) 2.25

117. In a prospective study comprising 10000 subjects, 6000 subjects were put on beta carotene and 4000 were not. 3 out of the first 6000 developed lung cancer and 2 out of the second 4000 developed lung cancer. What is the interpretation of the above? [AIPGME 01, 02]
(a) Beta carotene is protective in lung cancer
(b) Beta carotene is not protective in lung cancer
(c) The study design is not sufficient to draw any meaningful conclusions
(d) Beta carotene is carcinogenic

118. Relative risk is the measure of the strength of the association between the suspected cause & event. Relative risk of one indicates: [AIIMS Dec 1991]
(a) Positive association exposure & disease
(b) 2 times high association
(c) No association at all
(d) 4 times higher association

119. The association between low birth weight and maternal smoking during pregnancy can be studied by obtaining smoking histories of women at the time of their visit and then subsequently correlating birth weight with smoking histories. What type of study is this?
(a) Clinical trial [Karnataka 2007]
(b) Cross-sectional
(c) Prospective
(d) Case-control

120. False about Randomised Control Trials is:
(a) Results of attrition are included in the analysis
(b) Randomisation is done while selecting subjects for the study [AIPGME 1994]
(c) Double blinding is the most common form of blinding observed
(d) Cross-over design helps removing ethical concerns

121. True about case control study is: [PGI June 01]
(a) Helpful for evaluation of rare disease [PGI 2005]
(b) Expensive [AP 1999, 2003]
(c) Incidence can be measured
(d) Rare causes studied
(e) Selection bias common

122. True about confounding factor: [AIIMS May 2009]
(a) It is found equally between the study and the control groups
(b) It is itself a risk factor for the disease
(c) Confounding can be eliminated by selecting a small group
(d) It is associated either with the exposure or the disease

123. Incidence can be calculated in: [AIIMS May 2010]
(a) Case-control study [AIIMS May 2011]
(b) Prospective study [UP 2000, RJ 2000, 2001]
(c) Retrospective study [Kolkata 2005]
(d) Cross-sectional study

124. A person wants to study a disease 'X' and fat consumption. He collected data for a number of people affected with 'X' from the government hospital and details of fat consumption from food industry. This type of study is known as: [AIIMS May 2012] [AIIMS Nov 2010]
(a) Experimental study
(b) Ecological study
(c) Pesiological study
(d) Cross-sectional study

125. A study revealed that in a study group, intake of beta-carotene decreases carcinoma of colon but it actually may be due to increased intake of dietary fibre. This is due to:
    [AIIMS Nov 2010]
    (a) Confounding factor
    (b) Misclassification bias
    (c) Randomisation
    (d) Sampling error

126. Case control study is used for study of: [DPG 2011]
    (a) Common diseases   (b) Uncommon diseases
    (c) Rare diseases   (d) Unknown diseases

127. In a UK study, it was found that there were more deaths from Asthma than the sale of Anti-asthma drugs. This is an example of: [AIIMS November 2011]
    (a) Cohort study
    (b) Case reference study
    (c) Ecological study
    (d) Experimental study

128. Which of the following is not a true difference between Case control and Cohort study? [AIPGME 2012]
    (a) Case control study requires more time than cohort study
    (b) Cohorts are chosen based on exposure in a cohort study
    (c) Cohort study is generally prospective in direction
    (d) Case control study must be used for rare diseases

129. Case-control study is a type of: [DNB 2008]
    (a) Descriptive epidemiological study
    (b) Analytical study
    (c) Longitudinal study
    (d) Experimental epidemiological study

130. A study revealed lesser incidence of carcinoma colon in pure vegetarians than non vegetarians by which it was concluded that beta-carotene is protective against cancer. This may not be true because the vegetarian subjects may be consuming high fibre diet which is protective against cancer. This is an example of: [AIIMS May 2012]
    (a) Multifactorial causation
    (b) Causal association
    (c) Confounding factor
    (d) Common association

131. Berksonian bias is a type of:
    [NEET Pattern 2012] [NEET Pattern 2013]
    (a) Selection bias
    (b) Interviewer bias
    (c) Information bias
    (d) Recall bias

132. Confounding can be removed by: [DNB June 2011]
    (a) Assign confounders equally to both cases and controls
    (b) Stratification
    (c) Matching
    (d) All of the above

133. Attributable risk means: [NEET Pattern 2012]
    (a) Fatality of a disease
    (b) Disease risk ratio between exposed and non-exposed
    (c) Risk difference between exposed and non-exposed
    (d) Communicability of a disease

134. Berksonian bias is due to: [DNB December 2010]
    (a) Presence of confounding factors in both cases and controls
    (b) Questioning the cases more thoroughly ac compared to controls
    (c) Different rates of admission to hospital due to different diseases
    (d) Better recall by the cases as compared to controls

135. Which of the following is true about cohort study?
    (a) Disease to risk factor study [NEET Pattern 2014]
    (b) Effect to cause study
    (c) NOT associated with attributable risk
    (d) Associated with antecedent causation

136. Researcher wants to study the Blood levels of Lipids among people who smoke and those do not. But he is now concerned that the Smokers might differ from Non-smokers in their diet, exercise, etc. as well. This concern is known as: [AIIMS May 2015]
    (a) Recall bias
    (b) Information bias
    (c) Hawthorne bias
    (d) Selection bias

137. A study has been done to establish relationship between Smoking and Lung cancer. It was found that association was more in people who exercise less and less in people who exercise more. In this situation, Exercise is a:
    [AIIMS May 2015]
    (a) Bias
    (b) Effect modifier
    (c) Confounding factor
    (d) Collinear factor

138. Analytical studies include the following methods of studies except: [UPSC CMS 2015]
    (a) Case-control studies
    (b) Randomised controlled trials
    (c) Cohort studies [DNB 2008, 2011]
    (d) Cross-sectional studies

139. A study was done in 3 states to see the mean blood pressure in each community. Health workers were assigned and they visited each house in the three communities. Mean blood pressure in each community was found and compared. What type of study design is represented here?
    [AIIMS November 2016]
    (a) Cohort study
    (b) Cross-sectional study
    (c) Case control study
    (d) Field trial

140. A study was done to identify the number of Typhoid cases due to exposure from a common well in the village. Groups were formed of carriers and diseased people. What type of study design is represented here?
    [AIIMS November 2016]
    (a) Cohort study
    (b) Cross-sectional study
    (c) Case-control study
    (d) Field trial

141. In a population of 9000, 2100 were alcoholic. 70 alcoholics among these developed cirrhosis and 23 non-alcoholic developed cirrhosis. What is Attributable risk?
    [NEET Pattern 2016]
    (a) 40%
    (b) 60%
    (c) 70%
    (d) 90%

142. Attributable risk is defined as:
    [NEET Pattern 2015, 2017]
    (a) Incidence among exposed minus incidence among non-exposed
    (b) Incidence among exposed divided by incidence among non-exposed
    (c) Incidence among non-exposed minus incidence among exposed
    (d) Incidence among non-exposed divided by incidence among exposed

143. Population attributable risk is: [NEET Pattern 2016]
    (a) Incidence among exposed minus incidence among non-exposed
    (b) Incidence among exposed divided by incidence among non-exposed
    (c) Incidence in total population minus incidence in non-exposed
    (d) Incidence in total population divided by incidence in non-exposed

144. Selection bias occurs during: [NEET Pattern 2016]
    (a) Recruitment
    (b) Treatment
    (c) Analysis
    (d) Observation

145. A PhD scholar want to do a Prospective cohort study for H. pylori and IBD from gastroenterology wards. What is correct? [NEET Pattern 2016]
    (a) Enroll all patients taking proton pump inhibitor
    (b) Enroll all patients on whom endoscopy done
    (c) Exclude patient who are positive for urea breath test for H. pylori
    (d) Exclude all patients diagnosed as inflammatory bowel disease

146. In a cohort study to study association between factor and disease, the risk ratio was calculated to be equal to 1. What does this signify? [AIIMS November 2016]
    (a) There is no association present between the factor and the disease
    (b) There is positive association between the factor and the disease
    (c) There is negative association between the factor and the disease
    (d) Data insufficient to comment

147. Strength of association between a Putative risk factor and a disease is measured by: [AIIMS November 2016]
    [NEET Pattern 2017]
    (a) Absolute risk
    (b) Attributable risk
    (c) Relative risk
    (d) Magnitude of p-value

148. Which of the following is the least time consuming study design to see relation between Lung cancer and Smoking? [AIIMS November 2016]
    (a) Cohort study
    (b) Case-control study
    (c) Cross-sectional study
    (d) RCT

149. Natural history of disease is best studied by:
    (a) Cohort study [NEET Pattern 2017]
    (b) Case control study
    (c) Cross sectional study
    (d) Ecological study

150. In a study a patient does not know the nature of drug [whether a placebo or curative drug] he is taking. The researcher knows the drug type to be given to the individuals in study. Types of blinding in this study is:
    (a) Single blinding [NEET Pattern 2017]
    (b) Double blinding
    (c) Triple blinding
    (d) Combined double/triple blinding

151. Important measure for National health policy:
    (a) Relative risk [NEET Pattern 2017]
    (b) Odds ratio
    (c) Population attributable risk
    (d) Attributable risk

152. In a study there were 35 cases of lung carcinoma and 82 controls were there. On taking history, 33 cases had positive history of smoking and 55 individuals among controls had positive history of smoking. What is the odds ratio? [NEET Pattern 2017]
    (a) 8
    (b) 20
    (c) 50
    (d) 100

153. 100 individuals are diagnosed with lung cancer in a population of 100000. Out of 100 patients, 80 were smokers and 20000 were smokers in total population. What is PAR?
    [NEET Pattern 2017]
    (a) 60
    (b) 75
    (c) 80
    (d) 90

154. True about Case control study for association between carcinoma breast and oral contraceptive use:
    [NEET Pattern 2017]
    (a) Study can confirm OCP as a cause of breast cancer or disprove it
    (b) Study can hypothesize OCP as a cause of breast cancer
    (c) Both are correct
    (d) None of the above correct

155. A cohort of nurses with control group is studied for use of IUD and abdominal pain as side effect, in case-control manner. This type of study is:
    (a) Current Cohort Study [NEET Pattern 2017]
    (b) Non-concurrent Cohort Study
    (c) Concurrent Cohort Study
    (d) Mixed Cohort Study

156. Number of adverse outcomes with a New drug 'A' in comparison to a Placebo drug 'B', were seen in a trial. Data is given below.

	Total patients	Adverse outcomes
Drug 'A'	15225	1605
Placebo 'B'	15225	1804

    Calculate Relative risk reduction (RRR) and Absolute risk reduction (ARR). [AIIMS November 2017]
    (a) RRR 11%, ARR 11% (b) RRR 11%, ARR 1%
    (c) RRR 1%, ARR 11%   (d) RRR 1%, ARR 1%

157. True statement about Epidemiological studies is/are [PGI November 2017]
    (a) Cross sectional study: Concept of causality can be deducted
    (b) Case control study: Suitable for study of rare disease
    (c) Cohort study: Help in assessing concept of causality
    (d) Cohort study: Groups are allocated by randomization
    (e) Case control study: Estimates only Odds ratio

158. A study found Odds ratio of maternal hypertension to have IUGR fetus to be 1:5. What is the interpretation? [JIPMER November 2017]
    (a) Positive association
    (b) Common association
    (c) Inverse association
    (d) Rare outcome

159. In a study, group of smokers followed up for 10 years to find incidence of a cancer. What type of study design is this? [JIPMER November 2017]
    (a) Retrospective cohort
    (b) Prospective cohort
    (c) Case control study
    (d) Randomized control trials

160. What is the study design used for Consanguineous marriage and Genetic abnormalities? [NEET Pattern 2018]
    (a) Twin study
    (b) Family study
    (c) Case control study
    (d) Nested case control study

161. Which one of the following is FALSE regarding Confounding factor in epidemiological studies? [NEET Pattern 2018]
    (a) Associated both with exposure and disease
    (b) Distributed equally between study and control groups
    (c) Independent risk factor for disease in question
    (d) Source of bias is interpretation

162. True regarding Odds ratio is/are: [PGI May 2018]
    (a) Indicator of increased risk of disease in pre-disposed population
    (b) It is cross productivity ratio
    (c) Used in cohort study
    (d) Used in case control study
    (e) It is Similar to relative risk

163. Cross product ratio is calculated from: [NEET Pattern 2019]
    (a) Cohort study
    (b) Case control study
    (c) Cross sectional study
    (d) Ecological study

164. In an epidemiological study, Confounding factor has [NEET Pattern 2019]
    (a) No association with risk factor and disease
    (b) Only association with risk factor
    (c) Independent association with risk factor and disease
    (d) Only association with disease

Review Questions

165. Cohort study does not include: [UP 2003]
    (a) Expensive [NEET Pattern 2015]
    (b) Study for chronic disease
    (c) Incidence rate calculated
    (d) Starts with the disease

166. Case control study- estimate: [UP 2008]
    (a) Only odd's ratio
    (b) Odds ratio and attributable risk
    (c) Relative risk, attributable risk, population attributable risk
    (d) Incidence, Relative risk, and attributable risk

167. All are advantages of case control study *except*:
    (a) Cheap and easy [AP 2004]
    (b) Fast and effective
    (c) No ethical problem and several factors identified
    (d) Distinguishing between causes and associated factors

168. All are true regarding confounding factor *except*: [AP 2006]
    (a) It is associated with exposure under investigation
    (b) It is distributed equally in study & control groups
    (c) It is associated both with exposure and disease
    (d) It is removed by matching in case-control study

169. Most appropriate method to know about contribution of risk factor to disease: [AP 2007]
    (a) Relative risk   (b) Attributable risk
    (c) Absolute risk   (d) Odds ratio

170. What is not true about cross-sectional study?
    (a) Also called prevalence study [AP 2008]
    (b) Tells etiology
    (c) Shows pattern of disease
    (d) Snapshot of a population

171. Odds' ratio is an estimate of: [MP 2000]
  (a) Relative risk [RJ 2006]
  (b) Attributable risk [DNB 2009]
  (c) Prevalences
  (d) Incidence rates

172. Attribute risk gives a better idea of: [MP 2007]
  (a) Strength of association between cause and effect
  (b) Impact of successful preventive health programme
  (c) Assessing aetiological role or factor in disease
  (d) Potential public health importance of disease

173. True about cross-sectional epidemiological study is:
  (a) Suitable for study of rare diseases
  (b) Chronic diseases can be studied [MH 2005]
  (c) Involves few number of subjects
  (d) Relatively inexpensive study

174. Bias due to wrong interpretation of laboratory test results and inter-observer variation is: [MH 2005]
  (a) Selection bias (b) Sampling bias
  (c) Observation bias (d) Recall bias

175. What will be the Odds ratio if the diseased with risk factor =a; diseased without risk factor=c; not diseased but with risk factor=b; a not diseased as well as not with risk factor=d? [MH-SS-ET 2007, MH 2008]
  (a) ad/bc (b) ab/cd
  (c) ac/bd (d) bc/ad

176. Attributable risk is measured by: [RJ 2002]
  (a) Cohort study (b) Case-control study
  (c) Cross-sectional study (d) None

177. Study of alcohol intake for 10 years and occurring of hepatic disease type of study is: [RJ 2007]
  (a) Cohort (b) Case-control
  (c) Random (d) Cross-sectional

EXPERIMENTAL EPIDEMIOLOGY

178. For the guidelines used for research studies, find the incorrect match: [INICET May 2023]
  (a) CONSORT – RCT
  (b) MOOSE – Meta-analysis of Observational studies
  (c) CARE – RCT
  (d) PRISMA – Systematic review and Meta-analysis

179. Meta analysis includes all *except*: [INICET November 2021]
  (a) Selection
  (b) Abstraction
  (c) Randomization
  (d) Analysis

180. Best quantitative method to study previous research studies is: [INICET November 2020]
  (a) Systematic reviews
  (b) Meta-analysis
  (c) Surveys
  (d) Group interviews

181. In a Prospective study, 1200 patients were randomly selected to study the effect of a New drug. The drug will be given for 5 years and its association with cataract will be studied. What type of study is this? [JIPMER May 2019]
  (a) Case control study
  (b) Cohort study
  (c) Randomized clinical trial
  (d) Cross sectional study

182. In a double blind clinical drug trial:
  (a) Each patient receives a placebo
  (b) Each patient receives both (double) treatments
  (c) The patients do not know which treatment they are receiving [AIIMS Nov 03, AIPGME 06]
  (d) The patients do not know that they are in a drug trial

183. What is the purpose of a control group in an experimental study? [AIPGME 1997]
  (a) Its permits an ethical alternative for patients who do not wish to be subjected to an experimental treatment
  (b) It allows larger numbers of patients to be used, thus increasing the power of the statistical techniques used
  (c) It helps to eliminate alternative explanations for the results of the study
  (d) It reduces the likelihood of making a type II error in hypothesis testing

184. What is the purpose of randomization in a clinical trial? [AIPGME 2007]
  (a) To equalize the effects of extraneous variables, thus guarding against bias
  (b) To allow inferential statistics to be used
  (c) To guard against placebo effects
  (d) To guard against ethical problems in the allocation of patients to experimental and control groups

185. A pharmaceutical company develops a new anti-hypertensive drug. Samples of 24 hypertensive patients, randomly selected from a large population of hypertensive people, are randomly divided into 2 groups of 12. One group is given the new drug over a period of 1 month; the other group is given a placebo according to the same schedule. Neither the patients nor the treating physicians are aware of which patients are in which group. At the end of the month, measurements are made of the patient's blood pressures. This study:
  (a) Is a randomized controlled clinical trial
  (b) Uses a crossover design [AIIMS Nov 2000]
  (c) Is a single blind experiment
  (d) Is a prospective study

186. Intention-to-treat analysis is done in:
  (a) Cohort study [AIPGME 2002]
  (b) Survival analysis studies
  (c) Randomized control trials
  (d) Multiple time series studies

187. **Random in Randomization in a clinical trial means:**
    (a) Equal but unknown chance [AIIMS Nov 1992]
    (b) Unequal and unknown chance
    (c) Unequal but known chance
    (d) Equal and known chance

188. **The major purpose of random assignment in a clinical trial is to:** [AIPGME 1996]
    (a) Help ensure that study subjects are representative of the general population
    (b) Facilitate double blinding
    (c) Facilitate measurement of outcome variables
    (d) Ensure that the study groups are comparable on base line characteristics

189. **Which one of the following statements regarding pre-post clinical trial is most appropriate?**
    (a) They cannot be randomized [AIIMS May 05]
    (b) They are useful in studies involving mortality
    (c) They use the patient as his or her own control
    (d) They are usually easier to interpret than the comparable parallel clinical trial

190. **The heart of randomized controlled trail is:**
    (a) Protocol [Karnataka 2008]
    (b) Intervention
    (c) Randomization
    (d) None of the above

191. **In a controlled trial to compare two treatments, the main purpose of randomization is to ensure that:**
    (a) The two groups will be similar in prognostic factors [AIIMS Nov 2002]
    (b) The clinician does not know which treatment the subjects will receive
    (c) The sample may be referred to a known population
    (d) The clinician can predict in advance which treatment the subjects will receive

192. **In a randomized controlled trial, the essential purpose of randomization is:** [AIPGME 06]
    (a) To produce double blinding [DNB December 2011]
    (b) To decrease the follow-up period [AP 2000]
    (c) To eliminate the selection bias [MP 2001]
    (d) To decrease the sample size [NEET Pattern 2017]

193. **All are true about Experimental trials except:**
    (a) Can't double blind in animal trials
    (b) All animal trials are unethical
    (c) Can't do interim analysis
    (d) Are always prospective

194. **Efficacy of a new drug A is compared with an existing drug B in:** [AIPGME 2012]
    (a) Clinical trial phase I
    (b) Clinical trial phase II
    (c) Clinical trial phase III
    (d) Clinical trial phase IV

195. **Gold standard study for Clinical research is:**
    (a) Randomised controlled trial
    (b) Systematic meta-analysis
    (c) Ecological study [AIIMS November 2011]
    (d) Retrospective cohort study

196. **About RCT all are true except:** [AIIMS May 2011]
    (a) Baseline characteristics are comparable
    (b) Bias eliminated by double blinding
    (c) Sample size depends on type of study
    (d) Dropouts are excluded from the study

197. **Maximum tolerated dose of a new drug is evaluated in:**
    (a) Phase 1 [AIIMS May 2013]
    (b) Phase 2
    (c) Phase 3
    (d) Phase 4

198. **Maximum Rate of Drug failure is seen in ……… Phase of Clinical trial:** [NEET Pattern 2015]
    (a) 1   (b) 2
    (c) 3   (d) 4

199. **All are True regarding Meta-analysis except:**
     [NEET Pattern 2015]
    (a) Statistical technique for combing the finding from several independent studies on special topic
    (b) Its purpose is not to identify risk factors
    (c) Its purpose is to increase statistical power by increasing the sample size
    (d) The validity does not depend on quality of systemic review

200. **Not a feature of Systematic Review:**
     [NEET Pattern 2015]
    (a) Meta-analysis always performed
    (b) Search for literature is compulsory using explicit search strategy
    (c) Critical appraisal is always criterion based
    (d) Research question always focused

201. **Following is NOT a benefit of Randomization:**
     [AIIMS November 2015]
    (a) Reduction of bias in selection of groups
    (b) Ensure comparability of both groups
    (c) Facilitates blinding of treatment
    (d) Increases external validity of study

202. **All are true about Natural experiments, except:**
    (a) Researcher has no control over the allocation of subjects [NEET Pattern 2017]
    (b) James Snow's experiment is an example
    (c) Includes Randomized controlled trials
    (d) Done when experimental studies not possible in human populations

203. Type of Randomized control trial, in which both groups [experiment and reference] act as exposed group as well as non-exposed group?
    (a) Uncontrolled trial [NEET Pattern 2017]
    (b) Concurrent parallel trial
    (c) Cross over trial
    (d) Natural experiment

204. Case acts as its own control in which of the following study? [JIPMER November 2017]
    (a) Cross-over study
    (b) Retrospective study
    (c) Prospective study
    (d) Case control study

205. Which of the following statements about Clinical trials is true? [NEET Pattern 2019]
    (a) Post-marketing surveillance is done in Phase 3
    (b) Safety and no-toxicity is evaluated in Phase 2
    (c) Randomized controlled trial in patients is done in Phase 3
    (d) Unit of study in Phase 1 is Patients

Review Questions

206. Randomized controlled trials are all *except*:
    (a) Clinical trials [DNB 2002]
    (b) Preventive trials
    (c) Before and after comparison studies
    (d) Evaluation of Health Services

207. Double blind study means: [RJ 2006]
    (a) Observer is blind about the study
    (b) Person or group being observed is blind about the study
    (c) Both observer and person or group being observed is blind about the study
    (d) Interpreters and analyzer are blind about the study

ASSOCIATION AND CAUSATION

208. Most difficult criterion to establish Causal Association in aetiology of a disease is: [AIPGME 2008]
    (a) Temporality
    (b) Strength of association
    (c) Specificity of association
    (d) Biological plausibility

209. Which of the following studies is best for establishing causation? [AIIMS Feb 1997]
    (a) Case-control study
    (b) Cohort study
    (c) Randomized control trials
    (d) Case-series study

210. An advertisement in a medical journal stated that 2000 subjects with sore throat were treated with our new medicine. With in 4 days, 94% were asymptomatic. The advertisement claims that the medicine was effective. Based on the evidence given above, the claim:
    (a) Is correct [AIIMS June 1998]
    (b) May be incorrect as the conclusion is not based on a rate
    (c) May be incorrect because of failure to recognize a long-term cohort effect
    (d) Incorrect because as no control or comparison group was involved

211. To test the association between risk factor and disease, which of the following is the weakest study design?
    (a) Case-control study [AIIMS Nov 04]
    (b) Ecological study
    (c) Cohort study
    (d) Cross-sectional study

212. Of the different epidemiological study designs available to test the association between risk factor and disease, the best design is of: [AIIMS Nov 2005]
    (a) Case-control study
    (b) Ecological study
    (c) Cohort study
    (d) Cross-sectional study

213. In establishing Causal Association, most essential criterion is: [AIIMS Nov 1999]
    (a) Consistency of relationship [AIIMS June 1999]
    (b) Temporal relationship
    (c) Duration of relationship
    (d) Strength of relationship

214. Suspected cause preceding the observed effect is an example for: [NEET Pattern 2012]
    (a) Coherence (b) Temporality
    (c) Biological plausibility (d) Specificity

215. Best study design used for Exposure and Outcome association is: [AIIMS November 2015]
    (a) RCT (b) Cohort study
    (c) Ecological (d) Cross-sectional study

Review Questions

216. Current smokers are at higher risk of developing lung cancer as compared to ex-smokers, criticality of casualty satisfied here is: [MH 2003]
    (a) Temporal relationship
    (b) Consistency
    (c) Strength of association
    (d) Reversibility or reversible association

217. Association of high altitude areas with goiter is example of: [MH 2007]
    (a) Causal association
    (b) Direct association
    (c) Temporal association
    (d) Indirect association

EPIDEMIOLOGY OF INFECTIOUS DISEASES

218. Nosocomial infections are diagnosed after how many hours of hospitalization/ admission?
 [NEET PG Pattern January 2020]
 (a) 24 hours
 (b) 48 hours
 (c) 72 hours
 (d) 96 hours

219. Infections transmitted to man from vertebrate animals are known as: *[AIPGME 1995]*
 (a) Exotic
 (b) Anthropozoonoses
 (c) Zooanthroponoses
 (d) Epizootic

220. 'Endemic Disease' means that a disease:
 [NEET Pattern 2017] [AIPGME 05]
 (a) Occurs clearly in excess of normal expectancy
 (b) Is constantly present in a given population group
 (c) Exhibits seasonal pattern
 (d) Is prevalent among animals

221. Occurrence of a disease in a haphazard and irregular pattern is known as: *[DPG 2004]*
 (a) Endemic
 (b) Epidemic
 (c) Sporadic
 (d) Pandemic

222. Following is part of "Sentinel Surveillance" *except*:
 [Karnataka 2009]
 (a) Method for identifying the missing cases
 (b) Supplementing the notified cases
 (c) To estimate the disease prevalence in total population
 (d) To estimate the fatality of the disease

223. The ability of an infectious agent to invade and multiply in a host is called: *[Karnataka 2009]*
 (a) Pathogenicity
 (b) Infectivity
 (c) Virulence
 (d) Communicability

224. Pandemics are caused by: *[PGI Dec 2K]*
 (a) Hepatitis B
 (b) Influenza – A
 (c) Influenza – B
 (d) Influenza – C

225. Post exposure vaccination is given in:
 (a) Typhoid *[NEET Pattern 2013]*
 (b) Rabies
 (c) Mumps
 (d) Rubella

226. Disease(s) infectious before onset of symptoms is/are:
 (a) Measles *[PGI May 2012]*
 (b) Mumps
 (c) Cholera
 (d) Hepatitis B
 (e) Poliomyelitis

227. MC route of Nosocomial infection (Hospital-acquired infection): *[NEET Pattern 2015]*
 (a) Droplet transmission
 (b) Direct contact
 (c) Indirect contact
 (d) Vehicle transmission

Review Questions

228. Hospital acquired infection of surgical wound is mostly by: *[AP 2005]*
 (a) Doctor
 (b) Patient
 (c) Air borne
 (d) Instruments

229. Hospital Acquired infections are called as:
 (a) Emporiatric infections *[MP 2007]*
 (b) Nosocomial infections
 (c) Iatrogenic infections
 (d) Epomithic infections

230. Disease imported in a country, which was not otherwise present? *[MH 2007]*
 (a) Epornithic disease *[NEET Pattern 2018]*
 (b) Zoonotic disease
 (c) Exotic disease
 (d) Epizootic disease

DISEASE TRANSMISSION

231. Median incubation period means: *[JIPMER May 2019]*
 (a) Time taken for 50% cases to occur
 (b) Time between primary case and secondary case
 (c) Time between onset of infection and period of maximum infectivity
 (d) Median of several incubation periods

232. Which of the following infections necessitate airborne restrictions to stop the spread of airborne droplet nuclei?
 [AIIMS June 2020]
 (a) Measles
 (b) Influenza A (H1N1)
 (c) Diphtheria
 (d) Pertussis

233. Soil is an important reservoir for all *except*:
 (a) Brucellosis *[AIPGME 2008]*
 (b) Coccidiomycosis
 (c) Anthrax
 (d) Tetanus

234. The time taken for 50% of patients to develop the disease following exposure to the disease is known as:
 [JIPMER 2003] [AIIMS June 1999]
 (a) Incubation period *[NEET Pattern 2017,18]*
 (b) Median incubation period
 (c) Generation time
 (d) Secondary Attack rate

235. In a 6-membered family, there are two parents and four children all aged between 2 and 6 years. One of the children (3 years old) is completely immunized for his age, whereas other 3 siblings are totally unimmunised. On 12 August 2006, one of the latter got measles. 2 other siblings also got measles by 18 August 2006. Secondary attack rate is: [AIIMS May 1995]
    (a) Zero
    (b) 33%
    (c) 66%
    (d) 100%

236. A village has 100 under five children. The coverage of measles vaccine is 60%. Following a measles case 26 children developed measles. The secondary attack rate is:
    (a) 25%
    (b) 40%   [AIIMS May 1999]
    (c) 50%
    (d) 65%

237. Generation time in epidemiology is defined as:
    [AIIMS May 1995, DPG 2008, MP 2003, DNB 2011, Karnataka 2004, NEET Pattern 2013, 2017]
    (a) The interval between marriage and the birth of first child
    (b) The interval of time between the receipt of infection by host and maximal infectivity of the host
    (c) The interval of time between primary case and secondary cases
    (d) Interval of time between invasion by infectious agent and appearance of first sign or symptom of the disease/in question

238. All of the following are used as proxy measures for incubation period in disease except:
    (a) Latent period   [AIIMS Nov 1993 & Sep 1996]
    (b) Period of communicability   [DNB 2007]
    (c) Serial interval
    (d) Generation time

239. A family consists of 2 parents & 6 children susceptible to measles. There occurs a primary case of measles and 3 secondary cases within a short period of time. Secondary attack rate is: [AIIMS June 2000]
    (a) 60%
    (b) 38%
    (c) 67%
    (d) 50%

240. Denominator while calculating the secondary attack rate includes: [Bihar, 2004, AIPGME 03]
    (a) All the people living in next fifty houses
    (b) All the close contacts
    (c) All susceptibles amongst close contact
    (d) All susceptibles in the whole village

241. Serial interval is: [Karnataka 2009, NEET Pattern 2013, 2017, UPSC 1993, DPG 2005, AIPGME-2000- 02, [NEET Pattern 2018] AIIMS June 99 & 2000 May 02, DNB 2009, 2011, RJ 2002, 07, WB 2005]
    (a) Time gap between primary and secondary case
    (b) Time gap between index and primary case
    (c) Time taken for a person from receipt of infection to develop maximum infectivity
    (d) The time taken from infection till a person infects another person

242. Which of the following is not spread by fomites?
    (a) AIDS   [DPG 2007]
    (b) Typhoid
    (c) Diarrhea
    (d) Hepatitis A

243. The transmission of filariasis is an example of:
    (a) Propagative transmission   [Karnataka 2005]
    (b) Cyclical transmission
    (c) Cyclo-developmental transmission
    (d) Cyclo-propagative transmission

244. The following diseases are communicable during later part of incubation period except: [Karnataka 2009]
    (a) Measles
    (b) Whooping Cough
    (c) Hepatitis A
    (d) Typhoid

245. Which of the following statement about "Reservoir" of an infection is NOT correct?   [Karnataka 2009]
    (a) Reservoir can transmit infection to a susceptible host
    (b) "Reservoir" and "Source" of infection are synonymous
    (c) Non-living thing can be Reservoir
    (d) Reservoir can be an animal

246. Which of the following statement about "Incubation Period" (IP) is NOT correct?   [Karnataka 2009]
    (a) It is the time interval between invasion by an infectious agent and appearance of the first sign or symptom
    (b) During IP, the infectious agent undergoes multiplication in the host
    (c) The factors such as infective dose of pathogens and portal of entry determines IP
    (d) Infectious disease are not communicable during IP

247. Disease highly transmitted during incubation period is/are: [PGI June 08]
    (a) Pertussis
    (b) Cholera
    (c) Measles
    (d) Brucellosis
    (e) Chicken-pox

248. Incubatory carriers seen in: [PGI June 08]
    (a) Cholera
    (b) Bubonic plague
    (c) Mumps
    (d) Measles
    (e) Influenza

249. Isolation is needed in which of the following diseases?
    (a) Diphtheria   [PGI Dec 06]
    (b) TB   [PGI 2007]
    (c) Cholera   [PGI 2012]
    (d) Herpes zoster
    (e) Streptococcal pharyngitis

250. Isolation is advised in: [PGI June 06]
    (a) Polio
    (b) Diphtheria
    (c) Leprosy
    (d) Pneumonic plague
    (e) HIV

251. Carrier stage seen in: [PGI June 05]
    (a) Polio
    (b) Cholera
    (c) Pertussis
    (d) Plague
    (e) Tetanus

252. Which of the following diseases have incubation period <10 days? [PGI June 06]
    (a) Cholera
    (b) Influenza
    (c) Plague
    (d) Measles
    (e) Rubella

253. Healthy carrier seen in: [PGI Dec 04]
    [PGI 2003]
    (a) T.B.
    (b) Diphtheria
    (c) Cholera
    (d) Typhoid
    (e) Tetanus

254. Quarantine period should be: [NEET Pattern 2012]
    (a) Minimum incubation period
    (b) Maximum incubation period
    (c) Period of communicability
    (d) Median incubation period

255. First case that comes to notice of physician is:
    (a) Primary case [DNB June 2011]
    (b) Secondary case [NEET Patterns 2014, 2015]
    (c) Index case [MP 2003]
    (d) Refer case

256. Application of incubation period is all *except*:
    (a) To differentiate primary case from secondary cases
    (b) To find out time for isolation [AIIMS May 2012]
    (c) To find out time for quarantine
    (d) To prevent infection to the contacts of the infected person

257. Chronic carrier state is seen in: [NEET Pattern 2013]
    (a) Poliomyelitis   (b) Measles
    (c) Malaria   (d) Tetanus

258. All of the following are correct regarding Period of isolation *except*: [AIIMS May 2014]
    (a) Measles – Up to 3 days of onset of rash
    (b) Chicken pox – Up to 6 days of onset of rash
    (c) Herpes zoster – Up to 6 days of onset of rash
    (d) Rubella – Until 7 days after appearance of rash

259. Window period is defined as time taken from: [AIIMS PG May 2015]
    (a) Entry in cell to expulsion of first viral particle
    (b) Entry of pathogen to appearance of first clinical symptom
    (c) Exposure to laboratory detection of disease
    (d) Entry of organism to maximum communicability

260. Healthy carrier are seen in: [NEET Pattern 2017]
    (a) Measles
    (b) Rubella
    (c) Meningococcal meningitis
    (d) Influenza

261. Secondary attack rate is defined as: [NEET Pattern 2017]
    (a) Number of total cases developing disease within maximum incubation period
    (b) Number of cases developing disease within incubation period following exposure to primary care
    (c) Number of cases developing disease after exposure to primary case in any period of time
    (d) Number of cases developing after exposure to secondary case

262. A population of 50 children is having 10 immunized against chickenpox. 5 children developed chickenpox on 1st March 2017. Other 28 children developed chickenpox within next 2 week. What is the SAR of Chickenpox? [NEET Pattern 2017]
    (a) 60%   (b) 70%
    (c) 80%   (d) 90%

263. Number of exposed persons developing a disease within 1 incubation period following exposure to Primary case is known as [NEET Pattern 2018]
    (a) Attack rate
    (b) Secondary attack rate
    (c) Case fatality rate
    (d) Incidence rate

264. Tuberculosis has a Droplet mode of transmission. Which of the following diseases also has a droplet mode of transmission and requires isolation? [AIIMS November 2018]
    (a) Hepatitis B
    (b) Pertussis
    (c) Faucial Diphtheria
    (d) Atypical pneumonia

265. Paradoxical carrier is [NEET Pattern 2019]
    (a) who sheds organism even during Recovery
    (b) who sheds organism even during Incubation period
    (c) who gets infected from a case
    (d) who gets infected from another carrier

Review Questions

266. Man is dead end for: [DNB 2006]
    (a) Tetanus, measles [Bihar 2003]
    (b) Measles, yellow fever
    (c) Tetanus, yellow fever
    (d) Rabies, tetanus

267. Droplet nuclei are seen in all *except*: [MP 2000]
    (a) Typhoid
    (b) Measles
    (c) Diphtheria
    (d) Pertussis

268. Which of the following is not a method of transmission of infection through direct contact?
    (a) Transplacental [MP 2006]
    (b) Kissing
    (c) Sexual intercourse
    (d) Syringe and needle

269. Organism multiplying and developing in the hosts is called as: [All India 2000] [MH 2000] [MH 2000]
    (a) Cyclopropagative [AP 2014]
    (b) Cyclodevelopmental
    (c) Developmental
    (d) Propagative

270. Man is secondary host in: [RJ 2006]
    (a) Malaria   (b) Hydatid disease
    (c) Both   (d) Filariasis only

INVESTIGATION OF AN EPIDEMIC

271. The area is declared free of epidemic: [AIIMS Nov 2007] [NEET Pattern 2017]
    (a) Till last secondary case recovers
    (b) No new case reported for the incubation period of disease since the last case
    (c) No new case reported for twice the incubation period of disease since the last case
    (d) No new case reported for 6 months since the last case

272. Which of the following is the initial-most step in investigation of an epidemic? [AIIMS Dec 1994]
    (a) Defining the population at risk [DNB 2001, 05, 06]
    (b) Confirmation of existence of an epidemic [WB 2007]
    (c) Verification of diagnosis
    (d) Rapid search for all cases and their characteristics

IMMUNITY, VACCINES AND COLD CHAIN

273. Vaccination is not contraindicated in: [INICET May 2023]
    (a) Complement deficiency
    (b) Wiskott-Aldrich syndrome
    (c) Ataxia telangiectasia
    (d) DiGeorge syndrome

274. An infant received DPT-1 dose at 6 weeks age at a PHC. Then he developed a fever of 40 degree C and inconsolable crying. What should be done at 10 weeks age? [INICET May 2023]
    (a) Give DPT next dose as per schedule
    (b) Give DT only at next visit
    (c) Delay vaccination by 2 weeks
    (d) Delay vaccination for 1 month

275. A 10 years old male child presented to your OPD at a PHC. Vaccine advisable to this child as per the National Immunization Schedule of India is: [NEET PG Pattern 2023]
    (a) BCG vaccine   (b) DPT vaccine
    (c) Td Vaccine   (d) Typhoid vaccine

276. Which of the following is True regarding the vaccine vial monitor (VVM)? [INICET November 2022]
    1. It is used for monitoring heat exposure of the vaccine by healthcare workers in primary healthcare.
    2. It shows cumulative exposure of the vaccine to the heat.
    3. It can be used to assess the potential efficacy of the vaccine.
    4. Calculation of the expiry date can be done using VVM.
    5. The expiry date of the vaccine can be relaxed if VVM is in an acceptable range.
    6. If the square and the circle are the same in color, then the vaccine can be safely used.
    (a) 3, 4
    (b) 1, 2
    (c) 1, 2, 3, 4, 5
    (d) 5, 6

277. True about WHO-SAGE criteria for HPV vaccination in 9-14 years age: [INICET May 2022]
    (a) 1-2 dose
    (b) Single dose
    (c) 2 doses
    (d) 3 dose

278. Which of the following immunization is done in elderly? [INICET May 2022]
    (a) Rota virus vaccine
    (b) Meningococcal vaccine
    (c) Diphtheria toxoid
    (d) Varicella Zoster vaccine

279. A 1-year-old child presented to OPD for vaccination. He had 1 dose of DPT at 6 weeks after birth. After that other dose were not administered. What should be the next step? [INICET May 2022]
    (a) Restart DPT
    (b) Give only DT
    (c) Give 2nd dose
    (d) Not to give anything

280. At an urban PHC, you are given 1 vial of Pentavalent vaccine, and 2 vials of MR vaccine. Both were already open from before. Provided that all the cold chain requirements are still intact, will you use them or discard. Mark accordingly. [NEET PG Pattern 2022]
    (a) Use both Pentavalent & MR open vials
    (b) Discard both Pentavalent & MR open vials
    (c) Use Pentavalent vial & discard MR vial
    (d) Use MR vial & discard Pentavalent vial

281. Which of the following vaccines can be administered to a 10 years old boy attending a school? [NEET PG Pattern September 2021]
    (a) BCG   (b) IPV
    (c) TT/Td   (d) Typhoid

282. A female child has history of recurrent yeast and respiratory virus infection since age of 3 months. Immunity status studies are being undertaken. Vaccine contraindicated is: [NEET PG Pattern September 2021]
    (a) TT/Td
    (b) Measles/MMR
    (c) DPT
    (d) Killed IPV

283. Pentavalent vaccine contains: [INI-CET July 2021]
    (a) DPT, Hepatitis B, Pneumococcal
    (b) DPT, Hepatitis B, IPV
    (c) DPT, Hepatitis B, Hemophilus influenzae B
    (d) DPT, Hemophilus influenzae B, IPV

284. Covid vaccine is administered in Deltoid muscle of a beneficiary. After vaccination, there is pain and weakness in the shoulder joint. Possible reason could be injury to: [INI-CET July 2021]
    (a) Deltoid muscle
    (b) Circumflex humeral artery
    (c) Subdeltoid/subacromial bursa
    (d) Radial nerve

285. Intussusception is associated with which vaccine? [INI-CET July 2021]
    (a) Oral polio vaccine
    (b) Adenovirus vaccine
    (c) Rotavirus vaccine
    (d) Influenza vaccine

286. HPV vaccine is based on: [INI-CET November 2020]
    (a) E1, E2
    (b) E6, E7
    (c) E7
    (d) L1, L2

287. A 2 years old child, who is a case of nephrotic syndrome has to be put on steroids. Before starting treatment, which of the following is/are true about vaccination (MULTIPLE RESPONSE)? [INI-CET November 2020]
    (a) Vaccinate as per schedule
    (b) Give Pneumococcal vaccine as per schedule
    (c) Only killed vaccines to be given
    (d) OPV not given to siblings

288. Heat sensitive substance/device present on the vaccine to monitor its viability is: [INI-CET November 2020]
    (a) MMV
    (b) MVM
    (c) VVM
    (d) MVV

289. Diphtheria is which type of Vaccine: [AIIMS June 2020]
    (a) Killed vaccine
    (b) Polysaccharide
    (c) Toxoid
    (d) Live vaccine

290. Mission Indradhanush is for: [NEET PG Pattern January 2020]
    (a) Non-communicable diseases
    (b) Family planning
    (c) Safe water and sanitation
    (d) Universal immunization

291. A 16 years old girl walks into your clinic and asks for Cervical cancer vaccine. Which of the following should be given? [AIIMS November 2019]
    (a) Biovac
    (b) Gardasil
    (c) Tdap
    (d) Rubavac

292. Pneumococcal vaccine PCV 23 polysaccharide has shown the best results in the following people: [AIIMS November 2019]
    (a) Sickle cell anemia
    (b) Cystic fibrosis
    (c) Child less than 2 years age
    (d) Recurrent otitis media and sinusitis

293. Which of the following statements regarding live vaccines is false? [AIPGME 2008]
    (a) Two live vaccines cannot be administered simultaneously
    (b) Booster doses are not required when live vaccines are administered
    (c) Single dose gives life long immunity
    (d) Live vaccine contains both major and minor antigens

294. Which is not true about measles vaccine?
    (a) Egg culture [AIIMS Dec 1995] [AIPGME 1999]
    (b) Freeze dried
    (c) Reconstituted vaccine should be used within one hour
    (d) Given after 9 months of age

295. Most heat sensitive vaccine is: [AIIMS Nov 2008]
    (a) BCG
    (b) Polio
    (c) Measles
    (d) DPT

296. A 10-month-old unimmunised child should be given: [AIPGME 2000]
    (a) DPT-1, OPV-1, Measles, Vitamin-A
    (b) BCG, DPT-1, OPV-1, Measles, Vitamin-A
    (c) BCG, DPT-1, OPV-1
    (d) BCG, DT-1, OPV-1, Measles, Vitamin-A

297. Which of the following statements is true about BCG vaccination? [AIIMS May 05]
    (a) Distilled water is used as diluent for BCG vaccine
    (b) The site for injection should be cleaned thoroughly with spirit
    (c) Mantoux test becomes positive after 48 hours of vaccination
    (d) WHO recommends Danish 1331 strain for vaccine production

298. A 3 years old completely unimmunised child comes to an immunization clinic at PHC for the first time. He should receive: [AIPGME 2004]
    (a) BCG, Measles, Vitamin-A
    (b) DT-1, OPV-1, Measles, Vitamin-A

(c) BCG, DPT-1, OPV-1, Measles, Vitamin-A
(d) DPT-1, OPV-1, Measles, Vitamin-A

299. All of the following are killed vaccines except:
    (a) Salk Polio [AIIMS Dec 1997]
    (b) Japanese encephalitis
    (c) Rabies
    (d) Yellow fever

300. The efficiency of cold chain system for oral polio vaccine as monitored by Vaccine Vial Monitor (VVM) depends on: [AIPGME 2004]
    (a) Change in the colour of vaccine
    (b) Temperature indicator of the system
    (c) Viral potency test
    (d) Change in colour of monitor

301. Which one of the following doses in Loeffler units of Diphtheria Toxoid is incorporated in DPT vaccine per dose? [AIIMS Dec 1997]
    (a) 5
    (b) 15
    (c) 25
    (d) 35

302. Salk vaccine is a: [AIPGME 1994]
    (a) Live vaccine [AIIMS Feb 1997]
    (b) Live attenuated vaccine [JIPMER 2014]
    (c) Killed vaccine
    (d) Toxoid

303. Temperature in an ILR at PHC is recorded using:
    (a) Kata thermometer [AIPGME 1992]
    (b) Sling psychrometer
    (c) Dial thermometer
    (d) Anemometer

304. The risk of cold chain failure is greatest at:
    (a) Regional level [AIPGME 2000]
    (b) District Level
    (c) PHC level
    (d) Subcentre & village level

305. If a 11-month-old child has received two doses of DPT and polio, comes for further immunization after 5 months of the last dose, what should be done?
    (a) Repeat the whole course [AIPGME 1995]
    (b) Repeat the 2nd dose and continue rest of the course
    (c) Give 3rd dose and continue the course
    (d) Give only booster dose

306. In one single visit, a 9-month-old, un-immunized child can be given the following vaccination:
    (a) Only BCG [AIPGME 1995]
    (b) BCG, DPT-1, OPV-1 [DPG 2007]
    (c) DPT-1, OPV-1, Measles
    (d) BCG, DPT-1, OPV-1, Measles

307. All of the following statements are true about DPT vaccine except: [AIIMS Nov 2002]
    (a) It should be stored in deep freezer
    (b) Exposure to direct sunlight when in use should be avoided
    (c) Store stocks are needed for three months at PHC level
    (d) Half used vials should not be put back into the cold chain after the session

308. Which vaccine is contraindicated in pregnancy?
    (a) Rubella [AIIMS Nov 97 & Dec 98;
    (b) Diphtheria AIPGME-1992, 02, 08]
    (c) Tetanus [NEET Patterns 2014]
    (d) Hepatitis B
    (e) Varicella

309. Antisera is obtained from: [DPG 2005]
    (a) Guinea pig (b) Rabbit
    (c) Rat (d) Horse

310. Administration of which vaccine can result in paralysis in children? [DPG 2006]
    (a) Measles vaccine (b) Sabin polio vaccine
    (c) DT vaccine (d) DPT vaccine

311. Which of the following is called 'first immunization' of the baby? [DPG 2007]
    (a) Colostrum
    (b) Handing over the baby to mother
    (c) OPV
    (d) DPT+BCG

312. Which of the following vaccine is not administered at birth? [DPG 2007]
    (a) OPV (b) BCG
    (c) Hepatitis B (d) Hib

313. The following is true for 'Live Vaccines' except:
    (a) Live vaccines engage certain tissues of the body
    (b) Live vaccines should not be administered to a patient of Leukemia [Karnataka 2009]
    (c) Two live vaccines cannot be given simultaneously
    (d) With an exception, immunization is generally achieved with a single dose of live vaccine

314. In which of the following, Herd Immunity cannot protect the individual? [Karnataka 2007]
    (a) Tetanus
    (b) Diphtheria
    (c) Poliomyelitis
    (d) All of the above

315. In vaccines incorrect match is [PGI June 02]
    (a) Measles – Jeryllyn [PGI 2004]
    (b) Rubella – Copenhagen
    (c) Mumps – Schwartz
    (d) Chickenpox – OKA
    (e) Polio – sabin

316. Which of the following is false regarding Oral Polio Vaccine (OPV)? [AIIMS Nov 2009]
    (a) It is a killed vaccine
    (b) Residual neuro-paralysis is a complication
    (c) Requires sub-zero temperature for storage long term
    (d) Induces intestinal and humoral immunity

317. HPV vaccine is: [AIIMS November 2009]
    (a) Monovalent
    (b) Bivalent
    (c) Quadrivalent
    (d) Bivalent & quadrivalent

318. Vaccine with maximum efficacy: [AIIMS May 2010]
    (a) OPV
    (b) Measles
    (c) BCG
    (d) TT

319. Which is true about BCG? [AIIMS May 2011]
    (a) Distilled water is used as diluent
    (b) Site for injection is cleaned with spirit
    (c) Mantoux test positive in 6 weeks
    (d) WHO recommends Danish 1331 for vaccine production

320. False about vaccines: [AIIMS May 2011]
    (a) Thiomersal is used as preservative in DPT vaccine
    (b) Kanamycin is used as preservative in measles vaccine
    (c) Neomycin is used as preservative in BCG vaccine
    (d) Magnesium chloride used to stabilize OPV

321. Vaccine which should not be given to an elderly man is:
    (a) Measles vaccine [AIPGME 2012]
    (b) *H. influenzae* vaccine [NEET Pattern 2015]
    (c) TT vaccine
    (d) Pneumococcal vaccine

322. At Primary Health Centre (PHC) level, vaccines are stored in the [Karnataka 2011]
    (a) Cold box [NEET Pattern 2012]
    (b) Deep freezer [DNB June 2009]
    (c) Ice lined refrigerator
    (d) Walk in cold room

323. Which disease is prevented by giving booster dose to a 5-6 years old child? [DNB December 2011]
    (a) Measles (b) BCG
    (c) DT (d) DPT

324. In measles outbreak, measles vaccine can be given within: [NEET Pattern 2013]
    (a) 2–3 months (b) 3–5 months
    (c) 2–7 months (d) 6–9 months

325. Zero dose of polio vaccine in which given:
    (a) Before giving DPT [DNB 2000, 2001, 2005, 2007]
    (b) At birth
    (c) When child is having diarrhea
    (d) When child is having polio

326. Additional component of UIP PLUS does not include:
    (a) Hepatitis B vaccine [NUPGET 2013]
    (b) Safe motherhood
    (c) Acute respiratory infections
    (d) Diarrhoea

327. Which of the following Human papilloma virus subtypes are not covered by Quadrivalent Anti-cervical cancer vaccine? [PGI May 2013]
    (a) Type 6 (b) Type 7
    (c) Type 11 (d) Type 16
    (e) Type 18

328. According to latest guidelines of vaccination, which of the following is applicable at the age of 5 years?
    (a) DT booster + Vitamin A [AIIMS November 2013]
    (b) DT
    (c) DPT + OPV
    (d) DPT + Vitamin A

329. Protective levels of Tetanus anti-toxin is:
    (a) >0.01 IU/mL [NEET Pattern 2012]
    (b) >0.5 IU/mL
    (c) >1.0 IU/mL
    (d) >5 IU/mL

330. Which of the following is NOT a cholera vaccine?
    (a) Ty21 A [NEET Pattern 2013]
    (b) CVD-103-HgR
    (c) WC-rBS
    (d) mORC-Vax

331. Mass vaccination is ineffective in: [NEET Pattern 2012]
    (a) Measles (b) Poliomyelitis
    (c) Tetanus (d) None of the above

332. True regarding SA-14-14-2 Japanese Encephalitis vaccine: [NEET Pattern 2013, AIIMS November 2013]
    (a) Cell culture derived live attenuated
    (b) Killed vaccine
    (c) Life long immunity
    (d) Primary schedule consist of 2 doses

333. True regarding Cervical cancer vaccine is/are: [PGI November 2013]
    (a) Bivalent and quadrivalent
    (b) Given to married women in 20–45 years age group
    (c) MC subtypes 16, 18
    (d) Two doses given
    (e) Gives 100% protection

334. Which of the following vaccines can result in Thrombocytopenia? [AIIMS May 2014]
    (a) MMR vaccine
    (b) Typhoid vaccine
    (c) Influenza vaccine
    (d) HiB vaccine

335. Which of the following is NOT true about Oral Polio Vaccine? [AIIMS May 2014]
    (a) Induces both local and systemic immunity
    (b) Maternal antibody is completely protective
    (c) Live attenuated vaccine
    (d) Requires sub-zero temperature for long term storage

336. Newborn child with HIV + and symptomatic, which vaccine will NOT be given: [NEET Pattern 2014]
    (a) Measles
    (b) OPV vaccine
    (c) BCG
    (d) Live J.E.

337. Vaccine not given in patient with Egg allergy: [NEET Pattern 2015]
    (a) Measles
    (b) MMR
    (c) Varicella
    (d) Influenza

338. Most common cause of Vaccine failure is: [NEET Pattern 2015]
    (a) Improper storage
    (b) Improper administration
    (c) Inappropriate manufacturing
    (d) Maternally derived antibodies

339. First Recombinant vaccine cloned in yeast is: [PGMCET 2015]
    (a) Hepatitis B vaccine
    (b) Measles vaccine
    (c) Rubella vaccine
    (d) Typhoid vaccine

340. The addition of killed Bordetella pertussis microorganisms to diphtheria toxoid enhances the antibody response of the latter because of: [UPSC CMS 2015]
    (a) Exotoxin of the Bordotella organism
    (b) Additive action of the two antigens
    (c) Formation of local granuloma
    (d) Endotoxin of the Bordotella organism

341. Eight months old child had history of unusual crying and convulsions following previous vaccination after BCG, DPT & OPV (first dose), and Hepatitis B. Now parents have brought child for next doses of vaccination. Which vaccine is contraindicated in this situation?
    (a) Measles [UPSC CMS 2015]
    (b) DPT
    (c) Hepatitis B
    (d) DT

342. VAPP develops after ………. days of OPV administration: [NEET Pattern 2015]
    (a) 7–14
    (b) 20–60
    (c) 60–90
    (d) Immediately

343. Trivalent Influenza Vaccine include all except: [AIIMS November 2015]
    (a) H1N1
    (b) H2N1
    (c) H3N2
    (d) Influenza B

344. Preferred vaccine in a 12 years old child is: [NEET Pattern 2015]
    (a) DPT
    (b) DT
    (c) dT
    (d) DTa

345. A 6-week girl child's parents want to give her vaccine other than National immunization schedule. Which vaccine(s) will be given? [NEET Pattern 2015]
    (a) Typhoid, HiB
    (b) Rota virus, Yellow fever
    (c) Rota virus, Typhoid, MMR
    (d) Rota virus, HiB, Typhoid

346. Regarding Mission Indradhanush all are true except: [NEET Pattern 2016]
    (a) Started on 25th December 2014
    (b) 82 of the 201 focus districts which are initially planned to immunize are located in UP, Bihar, Madhya Pradesh, Rajasthan
    (c) Aim is full immunization for all children by the year 2025
    (d) Receives finances, technical support from other partners

347. Dokoral, Sanchol, mORCVAX are used for production of: [NEET Pattern 2015]
    (a) Typhoid vaccine
    (b) Cholera vaccine
    (c) Influenza vaccine
    (d) Swine flu vaccine

348. Following is Hib conjugate vaccine: [NEET Pattern 2016]
    (a) Capsular polysaccharide
    (b) Cell wall polysaccharide
    (c) Capsular polysaccharide with carrier
    (d) PRP with carrier

349. Ty21a is vaccine for: [NEET Pattern 2015]
    (a) Cholera
    (b) Tuberculosis
    (c) Pertussis
    (d) Typhoid

350. Vaccine derived poliovirus outbreaks are mostly due to: [NEET Pattern 2016, 2017]
    (a) Type-2 virus
    (b) Type-3 virus
    (c) Type-1 virus
    (d) All of the above

351. Dose of Rubella immunoglobulin is: [NEET Pattern 2016]
    (a) 5 mL
    (b) 10 mL
    (c) 20 mL
    (d) 40 mL

352. Which vaccine is not stored in freezer? [NEET Pattern 2017]
    (a) OPV
    (b) Measles
    (c) DPT
    (d) Rubella

353. Passive immunity from mother to child is transferred in: [NEET Pattern 2017]
    (a) Hepatitis B
    (b) Diphtheria
    (c) TB
    (d) Pertussis

354. **NOT True about Pertussis vaccine:** [NEET Pattern 2017]
    (a) Neurological complications are more with Whole cell vaccine
    (b) Efficacy is 85-90%
    (c) Administered as triple vaccine
    (d) Vaccine is live attenuated vaccine

355. **True about Diphtheria vaccine:** [NEET Pattern 2017]
    (a) Is a toxoid
    (b) Can be given as pentavalent vaccine
    (c) For infant DPT is the vaccine of choice
    (d) First dose is given at 6 weeks of age

356. **Which of the following is true?** [NEET Pattern 2017]
    (a) Two live vaccines should not be given together
    (b) Live and killed vaccine should not be given together
    (c) Immunoglobulin should not be given for at least 6 weeks when a live vaccine is administered
    (d) Live vaccine should not be given for 12 weeks if immunoglobulin has been given

357. **True statement about IPV vaccine is/are** [PGI 2017]
    (a) Given through IM route
    (b) Given through Intradermal route
    (c) Does not require stringent conditions
    (d) Dose is 0.1 mL/dose
    (e) Dose is 0.5 mL/dose

358. **9-valent HPV vaccine covers which type(s) HPV strain(s)**
    (a) 6, 11   (b) 16, 18   [PGI 2017]
    (c) 31, 33   (d) 41, 35
    (e) 42, 58

359. **18-months old unvaccinated child comes to PHC for the first time. Vaccines to be given include**
    (a) OPV, DPT   [AIIMS November 2017]
    (b) Pentavalent vaccine
    (c) BCG, OPV
    (d) BCG, OPV, MMR, Pentavalent

360. **Mission Indradhanush does not include**
    (a) Tetanus   [NEET Pattern 2018]
    (b) Measles
    (c) Meningococcal meningitis
    (d) JE

361. **All of the following Live vaccines are contraindicated in pregnancy except:** [NEET Pattern 2017]
    (a) Yellow fever   (b) BCG
    (c) Rubella   (d) OPV

362. **All of the following vaccines are given under Universal immunization Program except:** [AIIMS November 2018]
    (a) Rota virus vaccine
    (b) MR vaccine
    (c) Influenza
    (d) Adult JE vaccine

363. **Which of the following parameters is used to determine the Sensitivity of vaccine due to heat?** [AIIMS May 2018]
    (a) VVM
    (b) VCM
    (c) VMV
    (d) VMM

364. **Which vaccine is not included in Mission Indradhanush?** [NEET Pattern 2018]
    (a) Tuberculosis
    (b) Measles
    (c) Meningococcal meningitis
    (d) Diphtheria

365. **The test used to identify frozen vaccine is**
    (a) Shake test   [AIIMS November 2018]
    (b) Habel test
    (c) Schick test
    (d) Quake Test

366. **Vaccine strains changed every year is**
    (a) Measles   [NEET Pattern 2019]
    (b) Rubella
    (c) BCG
    (d) Influenza

367. **Vaccine contraindicated during Pregnancy is**
    (a) Hepatitis A   [NEET Pattern 2019]
    (b) Hepatitis B
    (c) Rabies
    (d) Varicella

Review Questions

368. **'Ring vaccination' is:** [DNB 2006]
    (a) Given by a ring shaped machine
    (b) Given to produced a ring shaped lesion
    (c) Given around 200 yards of a case detected
    (d) Given around a mile of a case detected

369. **MMR vaccine is given at what age in India:**
    (a) 9–12 months   [Bihar 2004]
    (b) 12–15 months
    (c) 15–18 months
    (d) 18–24 months

370. **For typhoid best vaccine is:** [Bihar 2006]
    (a) Typhoid oral
    (b) Whole cell vaccine
    (c) Vi polysaccharide vaccine
    (d) None

371. **A 5 years male boy having no immunization:**
    (a) OPV + BCG + Measles + DPT   [Bihar 2006]
    (b) BCG + OPV + Measles + DT
    (c) BCG + OPV + TT
    (d) BCG + TT

372. In pulse polio immunization programme, VVM (Vaccine monitoring vial) to maintain the cold chain, which of the following indication to discard the vaccine is: [UP 2002]
    (a) Inner square is white
    (b) Inner square is lighter than outer circle
    (c) Inner square darker than the outer circle
    (d) Outer circle is more dark than inner square

373. Freeze dried vaccine is: [UP 2003]
    (a) BCG (b) Rabies
    (c) DPT (d) Hepatitis-B

374. True about secondary booster response in comparison to that of primary response are all except: [UP 2003]
    (a) Shorter latent period
    (b) Antibody is maximum
    (c) Antibody responses maintained at higher levels for a longer period of time
    (d) Production of antibody more slow

375. Which of the following is inactivated vaccine?
    (a) Salk polio vaccine [Kerala 2001] [UP 2004]
    (b) Ty21 typhoral vaccine
    (c) HDC-Edmonston-Zagreb measles strain
    (d) BCG

376. All are true statement regarding BCG vaccination except:
    (a) Given subcutaneously [UP 2005]
    (b) It can be given in tuberculin negative patients
    (c) Prevent haematogenous spread
    (d) It is prepared from M. bovis

377. The vaccine administered as "Nose drops": [UP 2006]
    (a) Rubella (b) Poliomyelitis
    (c) Influenza (d) Measles

378. Congenital passive immunity is NOT found in:
    (a) Polio (b) Mumps [UP 2008]
    (c) Rubella (d) Measles

379. All are correct regarding Premunition except:
    (a) It is a state of active immunity [AP 2000]
    (b) Protects an individual
    (c) Protects entire community
    (d) Immunity depends on the presence of an inactive infection with the same species in the host

380. Rabies: [AP 2003]
    (a) Cell culture vaccine is cheaper and effective
    (b) BPL vaccine has more number of doses
    (c) Cell culture vaccine is less effective
    (d) None

381. Minimum gap that should be allowed in between to administer two live vaccines: [NEET Pattern 2018] [Kolkata 2004]
    (a) 2 weeks (b) 4 weeks
    (c) 2 months (d) 4 months

382. Mg^{2+} ion is used as an stabilizer in: [Kolkata 2009]
    (a) OPV (b) DPT
    (c) BCG (d) Measles

383. Active and passive immunization is done simultaneously in all except: [MP 2001]
    (a) Hepatitis B (b) Measles
    (c) Rabies (d) Tetanus

384. The strain which is used for production of BCG vaccine at commercial level is: [MP 2003]
    (a) Bacille Calmette-Guerin
    (b) Tween-80
    (c) Danish-1331
    (d) PPD-RT-23

385. Ty 21a is vaccine of: [MP 2005]
    (a) Typhoid (b) Cholera
    (c) Hepatitis (d) Rota virus

386. Recommended dose of anti-rabies serum to be given for passive immunization of adult victim of dog bite is:
    (a) 20 i.u. (b) 40 i.u. [MP 2009]
    (c) 60 i.u. (d) 80 i.u.

387. Toxic shock syndrome is due to which vaccine?
    (a) Mumps (b) Measles [RJ 2001]
    (c) Salk (d) Tetanus

DISINFECTION

388. Which of the following is a disinfectant, but not a sanitizer? [INICET May 2022]
    (a) Bleaching powder
    (b) Penicillin
    (c) Hydrogen peroxide
    (d) Methyl paraben

389. Rideal-Walker Coefficient is employed for the assessment of: [AIIMS June 1991]
    (a) Effect of autoclaving
    (b) Sufficiency of Pasteurisation
    (c) Effect of incineration
    (d) Germicidal power of a disinfectant

390. Standard against which disinfectants are measured is:
    (a) Chlorine [AIIMS Dec 1991]
    (b) Ozone
    (c) Phenol
    (d) UV Radiation

391. Chlorine exerts a disinfectant action in all except:
    (a) Bleaching powder [AIIMS May 2001]
    (b) Cetrimide
    (c) Halozone tablets
    (d) Sodium hypochlorite

392. 'Savlon' contains: [AIIMS Dec 1991]
    (a) Chlorhexidine and chloroxylenol
    (b) Cetavlon and chloroxylenol
    (c) Cetavlon and hibitane
    (d) Hibitane and chloroxylenol

393. Which of the following is not a sporicidal agent?
    (a) Glutaraldehyde [DPG 2007]
    (b) Formaldehyde
    (c) Chlorine dioxide
    (d) Cresol

394. Disinfection of water by routine chlorination can be classified as: [Karnataka 2005, 2007]
    (a) Sterilization
    (b) Concurrent disinfection
    (c) Terminal disinfection
    (d) Pre-current disinfection

395. Sputum can be disinfected by: [DPG 2002]
    (a) Boiling
    (b) Burning
    (c) Drying
    (d) Autoclaving

396. Savlon contains: [AIIMS May 2010]
    (a) Cetrimide + chlorhexidine
    (b) Cetrimide + chlorhexidine + butyl alcohol
    (c) Cetrimide + butyl alcohol
    (d) Cetrimide + Cetavlon

397. There is an outbreak of MRSA infection in a ward of a hospital. What is the best way to control the infection? [AIIMS Nov 2010]
    (a) Vancomycin given empirically to all the patients
    (b) Frequent fumigation of the ward
    (c) Wearing masks before any invasive procedure in ICU
    (d) Washing of hands before and after attending the patients

398. Which of the following is used to test the efficiency of sterilisation of an autoclave? [AIIMS November 2011]
    (a) Bacillus subtilis
    (b) Clostridium tetani
    (c) Bacillus stearothermophilus
    (d) Bacillus pumilus

399. The amount of bleaching powder necessary to disinfect choleric stools, is: [NEET Pattern 2012]
    (a) 50 gm/lit
    (b) 75 gm/lit
    (c) 90 gm/lit
    (d) 100 gm/lit

400. Nosocomial infections are those which develop: [NEET Pattern 2014]
    (a) Within 24 hours after hospitalization
    (b) Within 48 hours of hospitalization
    (c) After 48 hours of hospitalization
    (d) After 7 days of hospitalization

401. Glass can be sterilized by: [NEET Pattern 2015]
    (a) Incineration at 1050 degrees Celsius for 5-10 minutes
    (b) Hot air oven 121 degrees Celsius for 30-60 minutes
    (c) Autoclaving at 121 degrees Celsius for 30-60 minutes
    (d) Hot air oven 160 degrees Celsius for 30-60 minutes

402. Anti-viral agent is: [NEET Pattern 2015]
    (a) Chlorhexidine
    (b) Betapropionolactone
    (c) Hypochlorite
    (d) Phenol

403. All are Methods of sterilization by Dry heat *except*: [ESI IMO 2014]
    (a) Flaming
    (b) Incineration
    (c) Hot air oven
    (d) Autoclaving

404. Disinfection of urine is which type of disinfection?
    (a) Precurrent [NEET Pattern 2016]
    (b) Concurrent
    (c) Preconcurrent
    (d) Terminal

405. Oils and powders are sterilized by: [NEET Pattern 2016]
    (a) Autoclaving
    (b) Microwaving
    (c) Hydroclaving
    (d) Hot air oven

Review Question

406. Fibreoptic scopes are sterilized by:
    (a) Glutaraldehyde [AIIMS Nov 2003 [MH 2002]]
    (b) Ethylene oxide [JIPMER 2014]
    (c) Autoclaving
    (d) Alcohol

MISCELLANEOUS

407. As compared to a routine case control study, nested case control study avoids problems (in study design) related to: [AIIMS Nov 04]
    (a) Temporal association
    (b) Confounding bias
    (c) Need for long follow up
    (d) Randomization

408. When an intervention is applied to community to evaluate its usefulness, it is termed as a trial for:
    (a) Efficacy [AIIMS Nov 05, AIPGME 06]
    (b) Effectiveness
    (c) Efficiency
    (d) Effect modification

409. A total of 5000 patients of glaucoma are identified and surveyed by patient interviews regarding family history of glaucoma. Such a study design is called: [AIIMS Nov 2004]
    (a) Case series report
    (b) Case control study
    (c) Clinical trial
    (d) Cohort study

410. In assessing the association between maternal nutritional status and the birth weight of the newborn, two investigators A and B studied separately and found significant results with P values 0.02 and 0.04 respectively. From this information, what can you infer about the magnitudes of association found by the two investigators? *[AIPGME 2003]*
    (a) The magnitude of association found by investigator A is more than found by B
    (b) The magnitude of association found by investigator B is more than that found by A
    (c) The estimates of association obtained by A and B will be equal, since both are significant
    (d) Nothing can be concluded as the information given is inadequate

411. Which of the following statements is false about nested case control study? *[AIIMS Nov 1992]*
    (a) Is a cohort study nested in a case control study
    (b) It maintains temporal association
    (c) Is useful for rare diseases with expensive diagnostic tests
    (d) Recall bias is not seen

412. A drug company is developing a new pregnancy-test kit for use on an outpatient basis. The company used the pregnancy test on 100 women who are known to be pregnant. Out of 100 women, 99 showed positive test. Upon using the same test on 100 non-pregnant women, 90 showed negative result. What is the sensitivity of the test? *[AIIMS May 03]*
    (a) 90%
    (b) 99%
    (c) Average of 90 & 99
    (d) Can't be calculated from the data

413. The extent to which a specific health care treatment, service, procedure, program, or other intervention does what it is intended to do when used in a community dwelling population is termed its: *[AIPGME 2006]*
    (a) Efficacy
    (b) Effectiveness
    (c) Effect modification
    (d) Efficiency

414. All of the following are true about the Herd Immunity for infectious diseases *except*: *[AIPGME 05, 07]*
    (a) It refers to group protection beyond what is afforded by the protection of immunized individuals
    (b) It is likely to be more for infections that do not have a sub-clinical phase
    (c) It is affected by the presence and distribution of alternative animal hosts
    (d) In the case of tetanus it does not protect the individual

415. Evidence based medicine, which of the following is not useful: *[PGI Dec 07]*
    (a) Personal exposure
    (b) RCT
    (c) Case report
    (d) Meta analysis
    (e) Systematic review

416. Hypothesis is not tested by: *[DNB June 2011]*
    (a) Descriptive studies
    (b) Analytical studies
    (c) Case control studies
    (d) Cohort studies

417. KAP studies were first used in India to study:
    (a) HIV *[NEET Pattern 2015]*
    (b) Malaria
    (c) Family planning
    (d) Carcinoma cervix

418. The resistance of a population to infection and pathogen spread due to the immunity of a large presence of the population is known as: *[NEET Pattern 2017]*
    (a) Resistance effect
    (b) Vicarious immunity
    (c) Herd immunity
    (d) Threshold immunity

Review Questions

419. Reverse cold chain is seen in: *[UP 2000]*
    (a) Expired vaccine from PHC to manufactured
    (b) Carrying vaccine to periphery center
    (c) Testing for potency of vaccine
    (d) Stool specimen of polio send for testing

420. About premunition all are true *except*:
    (a) Good for individual *[MP 2001]*
    (b) Good for community
    (c) Species specificity present
    (d) Prevention from infection

421. In the context of epidemiology-a set of questions is constructed in such a manner that it takes into account all the important epidemiological factors of a given disease:
    (a) Health model *[RJ 2007]*
    (b) Epidemiological triad
    (c) Epidemiological surveillance
    (d) Mathematical model

Explanations

DEFINITION AND EPIDEMIOLOGICAL METHODS

1. **Ans. (a) Cross-sectional study** [Ref. Park 27/e p77]

   CROSS SECTIONAL STUDY:
   - Is based on the single examination of a cross-section of a population *'at one point of time'*, results of sample are then projected to whole population
   - Is simplest form of observational epidemiological study
   - Provides *'Prevalence of the disease'* under study
   - More useful for chronic diseases
   - Tells about distribution of a disease in a population, *'rather than its etiology'*
   - Gives *'Snapshot of a population'*
   - Cannot establish causality as *'does not establish time sequence'*
   - Provides little information about the natural history of disease or incidence

2. **Ans. (b) Ecological** [Ref. Park 27/e p70]

   > **ALSO REMEMBER**
   > - *Types of epidemiological studies*:

Type of epidemiological study		Unit of study
1. Observational studies		
	a. Descriptive studies (Hypothesis formulation)	
	b. Analytical studies (Hypothesis testing)	
	i. Cohort study	Individual
	ii. Case control study	Individual
	iii. Cross sectional study	Individual
	iv. Ecological study	Population
2. Experimental studies (Hypothesis confirmation)		
	a. Randomized controlled trial	Patients
	b. Field trial	Healthy people
	c. Community trial	Community

3. **Ans. (a) Longitudinal studies** [Ref. Park 27/e p41,78]
4. **Ans. (b) Ecological study** [Ref. Park 27/e p70]
5. **Ans. (a) Sackett** [Ref. Encyclopedia of Public Health by W. Kirch, Pg 417]
   - Father of Evidence based medicine (EBM): David Sackett
     - Founded first Department of Clinical Epidemiology in Canada
     - Founded Oxford Centre for EBM
     - Wrote books:
       1. *Clinical Epidemiology*
       2. *Evidence Based Medicine*

6. **Ans. (c) Use of various research finding for taking decisions about best patients care** [Ref. Nursing Research by Fain 4/e p47]

   EVIDENCE BASED MEDICINE (EBM)
   - Integrating individual clinical expertise with the best available external clinical evidence from systematic research
   - Critical appraisal of research findings and decisions regarding whether, and how, to use findings in the care of patients

7. **Ans. (a) Local distributions** [Ref. Park 27/e p74]

   SPOT-MAPS
   - Depict geographical distribution of a disease or health condition in a defined place and time
   - Helps in localizing the source of infection locally in a geographical area
   - Used by John Snow to localize source of Asiatic Cholera in London (1854)

8. **Ans. (c) Descriptive studies are first phase in epidemiology** [Ref. Park 27/e p70-71]
   - Sequence of studies in Epidemiology: Descriptive studies, Analytical studies, Interventional (Experimental) studies
   - Descriptive studies are used to formulate hypothesis, Analytical studies to test hypothesis and Experimental studies to confirm hypothesis
   - Descriptive studies are used to study Distribution of disease in time, place and person

9. **Ans. (c) Use of various research finding for taking decisions about best patients care** [Ref. The Research Process in Nursing by Kate Gerrish, 6/e p489]

   Evidence-based Medicine (EBM)
   - An approach to medical practice intended to optimize decision-making by emphasizing the use of evidence from well-designed and well-conducted research
   - Conscientious, explicit, judicious and reasonable use of modern, best evidence in making decisions about the care of individual patients
   - Integrates clinical experience and patient values with the best available research information
   - It aims to increase the use of high quality clinical research in clinical decision making

10. **Ans. (b) Population** [Ref. Park 27/e p70]

    Unit of Study in Epidemiological Studies
    - Cohort study, Case control study, Cross sectional study: Individual
    - Ecological study: Population
    - Randomized controlled trials (RCTs), Clinical trials: Patients (Cases)
    - Field trials: Healthy people
    - Community trials: Communities

Review Questions

11. **Ans. (d) Variable to be tested**   [Ref. Park 27/e p78]

12. **Ans. (d) Descriptive epidemiology**   [Ref. Park 27/e p71]

MEASUREMENTS IN EPIDEMIOLOGY

13. **Ans. (c) Incidence is a rate but prevalence is not:**
    [Ref. Simple Biostatistics by Indrayan & Indrayan, 1/e p67]

    TOOLS OF MEASUREMENT IN EPIDEMIOLOGY:
    - *Rate*: Numerator (a) is a part of denominator (b) and multiplier is 1000 or 10,000 or 100,000 or so on.
    - *Ratio*: Numerator (a) is not a part of denominator (b) and BOTH numerator and denominator are unrelated
    - *Proportion*: Numerator (a) is a part of denominator (b) and multiplier is 100
      - *Proportion is always expressed in percentage (%)*
    - Incidence is a rate, Prevalence is a proportion

14. **Ans. (b) Bed disability days**   [Ref. Park 27/e p26]

    Disability Rates

Event type indicators	Person type indicators
No. of days of restricted activity Bed disability days Work-loss days	**Limitation of mobility:** Confined to bed/ house Special aid in getting around **Limitation of activity:** Limitation to perform ADL Limitation in major activity

Review Questions

15. **Ans. (a) Numerator is component of denominator**
    [Ref. Park 27/e p63]

16. **Ans. (c) Increases with increase in duration of disease**
    [Ref. Park 27/e p69-70]

17. **Ans. (d) Malignant neoplasm of breast** [Ref. Park 27/e p64]
    Older WHO Recommended Death Certificate (as per the given question)
    - Line Ia: Disease or condition directly leading to death (Pulmonary embolism)
    - Line Ib: Antecedent/underlying cause (Secondary carcinoma shaft of femur with fracture)
    - Line Ic: MAIN ANTECEDENT/ UNDERLYING CAUSE (Malignant neoplasm of central portion of breast)
    - Line II: Other significant conditions contributing to death BUT not related to disease/condition causing it (Nil)

IDC

18. **Ans. (c) Line Ic**   [Ref. Park 27/e p64]
    WHO RECOMMENDED DEATH CERTIFICATE (for International use):
    - *Consist of five lines*:
      - Line Ia: Disease or condition directly leading to death
      - Line Ib: Antecedent/underlying cause
      - Line Ic/Id: MAIN ANTECEDENT/UNDERLYING CAUSE
      - Line II: Other significant conditions contributing to death BUT not related to disease/condition causing it
    - Concept of underlying cause, Line Ic is the MOST IMPORTANT line in death certificate, thus also known as *'Essence of Death Certificate'* (or Id, if it can be filled up)

> **ALSO REMEMBER**
> - *Registration of vital events in India*: 100% registration of 4 vital events by 2010 (under National Population Policy 2000)
>   - *Birth*: Central Births and Deaths Registration Act' 1969 (REGISTER < 21 DAYS)
>   - *Death*: Central Births and Deaths Registration Act' 1969 (REGISTER < 21 DAYS)
>   - *Marriage*: The Hindu Marriage Act, 1955
>   - *Pregnancy*: No legislation yet in India

MORTALITY MEASUREMENTS

19. **Ans. (a) Death rate of a population adjusted to a Standard age distribution**   [Ref. Park 26/e p67]
    - *Indirect standardization*: Standardized mortality ratio (SMR): Is simplest and most useful form
    - *Method*: Calculate expected deaths, assuming that study group experiences the death rates of a standard population.

20. **Ans. (d) Survival rate**   [Ref. Park 27/e p66]
    - *Survival rate*: Is the proportion of survivors in a group (e.g. of patients), studied and followed over a period of time (e.g. over a period of 5 years)
      - Is used to 'describe prognosis' in certain disease conditions
      - Can be used as a 'yardstick for the assessment of standards of therapy'
      - Survival period is usually reckoned from the date of diagnosis or start of the treatment
      - Quite useful in cancer studies
      - Survival rate calculation: SR

    $$= \frac{\text{Total No. of patients alive after 5 years}}{\text{Total No. patients diagnosed or treated}} \times 100$$

> **ALSO REMEMBER**
> - CFR is the *'complement of Survival Rate'*
>   CFR = 1 – Survival Rate
> - Survival analysis is carried out by using *'Kaplan Meier Estimator'* (Product limit estimator)
>   - KME is a non-parametric estimation
>   - *Advantage of KME*: takes into account *'censored data'* (part of sample lost)

Epidemiology and Vaccines   187

21. **Ans. (a) Age specific death rate is not needed**
    [Ref. Park 27/e p63]

	Direct Standardization	Indirect Standardization
Method	Use actual ASDRs* on the standard age structure	Use standard ASDRs* on the actual age structures
Utility when 1. *No. of deaths in each age group* 2. *Population in each age group*	Both are available	Both are unavailable
(ASDR*: Age Specific Death Rate)		

22. **Ans. (d) Age-standardized mortality rate**
    [Ref. Park 27/e p66]
23. **Ans. (a) Standardised mortality rate** *[Ref. Park 27/e p66]*
24. **Ans. (c) 1st July** *[Ref. Park 27/e p65]*
    - *Crude birth rate (CBR)*: Annual number of live births per 1000 mid-year population
    - *Crude death rate (CDR)*: Annual number of deaths per 1000 mid-year population
      – Findings of SRS Bulletin: [2017]
        1. Crude Birth Rate (CBR): 20.4 per 1000 mid-year population
        2. Crude Death Rate (CDR): 6.4 per 1000 mid-year population

25. **Ans. (c) Duration of sickness** *[Ref. Park 27/e p24]*

    INDICATORS OF HEALTH:
    - *Mortality indicators:*
      – *Crude death rate (CDR)*
      – *Life expectancy (LE)*
      – *Infant mortality rate (IMR)*
      – *Child mortality rate (CMR)*
      – *Under 5 proportional mortality rate (U5MR)*
      – *Maternal mortality rate (MMR)*
      – *Disease specific mortality*
      – *Proportional mortality rate*

    > **ALSO REMEMBER**
    > - Best indicators of socio-economic development of a country:
    >   – U5MR (best indicator)
    >   – IMR (2nd best indicator)
    > - Life expectancy (LE):
    >   – LE is a POSITIVE mortality indicator
    >   – LE is used for derivation of:
    >   1. PQLI
    >   2. Human development index (HDI)

26. **Ans. (d) 25%** *[Ref. Park 27/e p66]*
    - **In the given question,** in an outbreak of cholera in a village of 2000 population, 20 cases have occurred and 5 have died,
    - Thus, CFR = Total no. of deaths due to a disease/Total no. of cases due to that disease × 100

    Or, CFR = $\frac{5}{20} \times 100$ = 25% = 25%
    - And, Survival rate = 1 – CFR = 1 – 0.25 = 0.75 (75%)

27. **Ans. (b) Case fatality rate** *[Ref. Park 27/e p66]*
    - CFR is the *'complement of Survival Rate'*
    - CFR = 1 – Survival Rate

    > **ALSO REMEMBER**
    > - *CFR of few important diseases*:
    >
    > | Diseases | Case fatality rate |
    > |---|---|
    > | Rabies | 100% |
    > | Yellow fever | 80% |
    > | Japanese encephalitis | 30 – 35% (median 35%) |
    > | Chicken pox | < 1%. |

28. **Ans. (a) Proportional mortality rate** *[Ref. Park 27/e p66]*
29. **Ans. (c) Virulence** *[Ref. Park 27/e p66]*
30. **Ans. (a) It is a ratio; (d) It is useful in chronic diseases**
    [Ref. Park 27/e p66]
31. **Ans. (b) Case fatality rate (CFR)** *[Ref. Park 27/e p66]*
32. **Ans. (a) Age** *[Ref. Park 27/e p67]*
33. **Ans. (c) Proportion** *[Ref. Park 27/e p66]*
34. **Ans. (c) Total deaths in that year** *[Ref. Park 27/e p66]*
35. **Ans. (a) 10%** *[Ref. Park 27/e p66]*
    - Proportional mortality rate (PMR) = No of deaths from a specific disease/Total deaths from all causes that year × 100

    In the given question,
    - PMR = 10/100 × 100 = 10%

36. **Ans. (a) For valid comparison of two groups of different health determinants** *[Ref. Park 27/e p62-66]*
    - Comparing mortality/morbidity rates help in evaluation of health status in different countries
    - As there is a possibility of having different frequency distributions in different populations, a comparison between Crude rates would be misleading since they are not very informative about the health status of a population
    - Standardization for the characteristic(s) responsible for the differences in comparison is necessary
    - Age and sex are two of the most common variables used for standardization and they are called Standardized rates

37. **Ans. (c) Total number of cases due to the disease concerned** *[Ref. Park 24/e p25, 63]*
    - CFR = No. of deaths due to a disease/No. of cases of that disease × 100

Review Questions

38. **Ans. (c) Measures life expectancy free of disability**
    [Ref. Park 27/e p26]

39. **Ans. (d) All of the above** [Ref. Park 27/e p65]
40. **Ans. (c) Killing power of a disease with no time interval** [Ref. Park 27/e p66]

MORBIDITY MEASUREMENTS

41. **Ans. (a) Prevalence of disease increases** [Ref. Park 27/e p69]
    - A drug reduces mortality but does not cure a disease, so it will lead to accumulation of old cases (cases are not cured so remain cases) while new cases will keep on occurring at same rate
    - Thus Incidence (new cases) remains same while prevalence (new cases + old cases) will increase gradually
    - Examples of such drugs: Anti-retro virals (for HIV/AIDS), Anti-cancer drugs, Anti-hypertensive drugs, Anti-diabetic drugs.

42. **Ans. (a) Incidence will not change** [Ref. Park 25/e p69]
    - *Relationship between Incidence and Prevalence*: **Given the assumption** that population is stable AND incidence & duration are unchanging,
      Prevalence = Incidence × Mean duration of the disease
      $P = I \times d$
      - *Incidence reflects causal factors*
      - *Duration reflects the prognostic factors*

    In the given question, a new effective treatment is initiated and all other factors remain the same,
    Thus new cases will keep on occurring at the same rate,
    So, incidence will not change
    However, effective treatment will cure more cases, so old cases will reduce,
    So, prevalence will reduce
    HOWEVER, OVER LONG PERIOD OF TIME, incidence MAY also reduce if it is an infectious disease (as total case load in the community is reducing)

43. **Ans. (c) Decrease the incidence of the disease** [Ref. Park 27/e p69]

    INCIDENCE:
    - Is defined as the *'no. of new cases'* occurring in a defined population during a specified period of time
    - *For a given period*,
    - Incidence = Number of new cases of disease/Total population at risk × 1000
    - *Incidence is a RATE*, expressed per 1000
    - *Special types of incidence rates*:
      - Attack rate: Incidence rate used when population is exposed for a small interval of time, e.g. epidemic
      - Secondary Attack Rate (SAR): Is no. of exposed persons developing the disease within range of incubation period, following exposure to the primary case

    In the given question, there is an improved prevention of an acute, nonfatal disease,
    Thus, no. of new cases or incidence will reduce

> **ALSO REMEMBER**
> - Incidence rate is also known as *'Incidence density'*
> - Cumulative incidence measures denominator *'only at the beginning of the study'*

44. **Ans. (b) The apparent 5 yr survival rate will increase**
    [Ref. Epidemiology by Leon Gordis 4/e p97, Park 24/e p69-70]
    - *Survival rate*:
      - Survival rate calculation:

      $$SR = \frac{\text{Total No. of patients alive after 5 year}}{\text{Total No. of patients diagnosed or treated}} \times 100$$

      - Survival rate is complement of Case fatality rate (CFR): SR = 1 – CFR
      - WHENEVER screening is performed: Higher 5-year survival rate is observed; THIS IS A POTENTIAL BIAS DUE TO earlier diagnosis being made (and not because people live longer)

    In the given question, a diagnostic test has been introduced that will detect a certain disease 1 yrs earlier than it is usually detected,
    Thus, Incidence rate (new cases) will remain same after 10 years
    Since duration of disease will remain same, the period prevalence rate will remain same after 10 years
    And it will also have no effect on age adjusted mortality rate
    But, since disease is getting detected 1 year earlier than usual (LEAD TIME), treatment can be started 1 year earlier (CFR will be apparently lowered), thus leading to apparent increase in survival rate

> **ALSO REMEMBER**
> - *5-year survival rate*:
>   - Is used as *'an index of success in cancer treatment'*
>   - Is not an appropriate measure to assess therapy that was introduced less than 5 years ago
> - *Life table approach*: Is used for calculating the *'actual observed survival'* overtime
>   - It attempts to predict the onset of events over time from previous patterns for all patients at risk
>   - Cohorts of patients are followed up to determine prognosis
>   - Probabilities are calculated of survival for different lengths of time
>   - Assumptions made in Life table analysis:
>   1. There is no secular (temporal) change in effectiveness of treatment or in survivorship over calendar time
>   2. Survival experience of people who are lost to follow-up is same as experience of those who are followed-up
>   - Kaplan Meier Method:
>   1. Is an approach for Life table analysis
>   2. In KM method, *predetermined intervals (1 month, 1 year, etc.) are not used*
>   3. Exact point in time where death took place is identified; each death terminates previous interval and a new interval is started
>   4. KM method is suited for small studies

- *Median survival time*:
  - Is the length of time that half of the study population survives
  - Advantages over Mean survival:
    1. Median survival time is less affected by extreme values (outliers)
    2. Observation of only half of the deaths in the group is required (not of the whole group)

- Incidence Tuberculosis 2007 = 4/1000 × 1000 = 4 per thousand
- Point Prevalence Tuberculosis January 1, 2007 = 3/1000 × 100 = 0.3%
- Point Prevalence Tuberculosis December 31, 2007 = 4/1000 × 100 = 0.4%
- Period Prevalence Tuberculosis 2007 = 7/1000 × 100 = 0.7%

45. **Ans. (b) The case fatality rate for this disease is higher for women** *[Ref. Park 27/e p69]*
    In the given question, if incidence for a disease is 5 times higher among females but prevalence rate show no sex difference,
    Since P = I × d,
    Thus, d (duration of disease) must be lower among females
    - Either the disease is more fatal among females, or
    - Disease is easily curable among females

46. **Ans. (d) Describes the balance between incidence, mortality and recovery** *[Ref. Park 27/e p69]*
    - Prevalence = Incidence × Mean duration of disease **P = I × d**
      - *Prevalence describes the balance between incidence, mortality and recovery*
    - Incidence is the best measure of disease frequency in etiological studies
    - *Incidence can be determined from*: Cohort study
    - *Prevalence can be determined from*: Cross Sectional Study.

47. **Ans. (d) 20** *[Ref. Park 27/e p69]*
    - *Prevalence* is defined as all current cases (old + new) at a given point of time

    $$\text{Prevalence} = \frac{\text{No. of all current cases of a disease at a time}}{\text{Estimated total population at that time}} \times 100$$

    And *'cases are those persons having the disease'* (Controls are healthy people, without the disease)
    In the given question,

Test result	Disease	
	Present: Cases	Absent: Controls
+	180	400
–	20	400
Total	200	800

    Thus, Prevalence = 200/(200 + 800) × 100 = 20%

ALSO REMEMBER
- PREVALENCE IS A PROPORTION (Prevalence IS NOT A RATIO): Numerator is a part of denominator and is always expressed in percentage.
- *Prevalence of few important infections in India*:

Infection	Prevalence (India)
Tuberculosis infection	40%
HIV infection	0.26%

48. **Ans. (a) The product of incidence and mean duration of disease** *[Ref. Park 27/e p69]*
49. **Ans. (a) 240** *[Ref. Park 27/e p69]*
50. **Ans. (b) 0.02** *[Ref. Park 27/e p69]*
51. **Ans. (c) 13%** *[Ref. Park 27/e p69]*
52. **Ans. (d) Incidence** *[Ref. Park 27/e p68]*
    USES OF INCIDENCE
    - Control of disease
    - Research into etiology & pathogenesis, distribution and efficacy of preventive and therapeutic measures

53. **Ans. (a) Point prevalence rate** *[Ref. Park 27/e p69]*
54. **Ans. (d) Incidence same, prevalence increases** *[Ref. Park 27/e p69]*
    - A drug reduces mortality but does not cure a disease, so it will lead to accumulation of old cases (cases are not cured so remain cases) while new cases will keep on occurring at same rate

ALSO REMEMBER
- Incidence is 'number of new cases occurring in a defined population over a specified period of time'
- *'Prevalence is a Proportion'*
- **Example:** For a city with a population of 1000, following figure represents occurrence of the disease 'Tuberculosis'. Each circle represents one case and length of the horizontal line represents the duration of the disease.

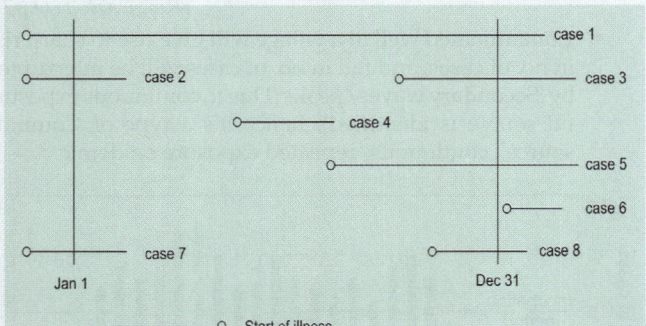

Incidence would include cases	: 3, 4, 5 and 8
Point prevalence (Jan 1) cases	: 1, 2 and 7
Point prevalence (Dec. 31) cases	: 1, 3, 5 and 8
Period prevalence (Jan-Dec) cases	: 1, 2, 3, 4, 5, 7 and 8

Number of cases of a disease beginning, developing and ending during a period of time

- Thus Incidence (new cases) remains same while prevalence (new cases + old cases) will increase gradually
- Examples of such drugs: Anti-retro virals (for HIV/AIDS), Anti-cancer drugs, Anti-hypertensive drugs, Anti-diabetic drugs

55. **Ans. (c) 66%** [Ref. Park 27/e p108]

    In the given question,
    - One primary case gives rise to two secondary cases
    - Total susceptibles = 3 (4 children minus primary case)
    - SAR = No of secondary cases/Total susceptible × 100
    - So, SAR = 2/3 × 100 = 66.6%

56. **Ans. (c) 78** [Ref. Park 27/e p69]
    - Attack rate = No. of new cases of a disease/Total population at risk × 100
    - **In the given question,** No. of new cases = 55
    - Total population at risk = 110-40 = 70 ate fruit salad
    - So AR = 55/70 × 100 = 78.6%

57. **Ans. (b) Incidence will decrease if a new drug is effective in reducing deaths from the disease** [Ref. Park 27/e p69]
    - If a new drug is effective in reducing deaths from the disease BUT not curing: People will continue to suffer from disease and continue transmitting it: Incidence will remain same, Prevalence will increase
    - If a new drug is effective in curing the disease: Both Incidence and prevalence will decrease

Review Questions

58. Ans. (b) Prospective study [Ref. Park 27/e p86]
59. Ans. (c) Secondary attack rate [Ref. Park 27/e p108]
60. Ans. (c) Longer duration of disease [Ref. Park 27/e p69]

DESCRIPTIVE EPIDEMIOLOGY

61. **Ans. (c) Person-to-person transmission** [Ref. Park 27/e p72]

    EPIDEMIC:
    - *Definitions of epidemic*:
      - *Occurrence of no. of cases of a disease 'clearly in excess of normal expectancy (NE)'*
        1. Normal expectancy is derived by looking at average of no. of cases of the disease in previous 3 – 5 years in that geographical area
        2. If NE = zero, 'even one case is considered epidemic'
      - *Statistically speaking, epidemic is when no. of cases 'exceed twice the standard deviation'*
        No. of cases > Mean + 2SD (>μ + 2σ)
      - *Occurrence of a new disease in a population (as NE = Zero)*
      - *Reoccurrence of an eliminated/eradicated disease in a population (as NE = Zero)*
    - Types of Epidemics: Refer to theory.

> **ALSO REMEMBER**
> - *Epidemic curve:* Is drawn between no. of cases in epidemic and time elapsed (time distribution of epidemic cares)

62. **Ans. (c) All cases occur in a single incubation period of the disease** [Ref. Park 27/e p72]

> **ALSO REMEMBER**
> - *Endemic*: Constant presence of a disease or infectious agent in a defined geographical area
> - *Pandemic*: An epidemic usually affecting a large proportion of the population, occurring over a large geographical area such as part of a nation, nation, continent or world
> - *Sporadic*: Cases which are *'scattered about'*
>   - Cases are widely separated in space and time
>   - Show little or no connection with each other
>   - There is no recognizable source of infection

63. **Ans. (a) Rapid rise and fall; (c) Explosive; (e) No secondary wave** [Ref. Park 27/e p72]

64. **Ans. (c) Environmental and genetic factors in a disease in population** [Ref. Park 27/e p75]

    MIGRATION STUDIES
    - Use: Evaluation of role of possible Genetic and Environmental factors in occurrence of a disease in a population
    - Study design: Comparison of Disease rates & Death rates of,
      - *Migrants with Kin who stayed at home*
      - *Migrants with Local population of host country*
    - Limitations:
      - *Non-random assignment to Groups: Migrants are self-selected*
      - *Environmental factors may act at certain age/point only*
      - *Not useful for disease with long incubation period*

65. **Ans. (a) Common single source for a short period** [Ref. Park 27/e p72]

66. **Ans. (b) Common source, continuous exposure epidemic** [Ref. Park 27/e p72]
    - Contaminated well in a village will give rise to sharp rise in no. of cases, and fall in no. of cases will be interrupted by 'Secondary waves/peaks (Due to continuous exposure till source is identified); hence it's a type of Common source', continuous/repeated exposure epidemic

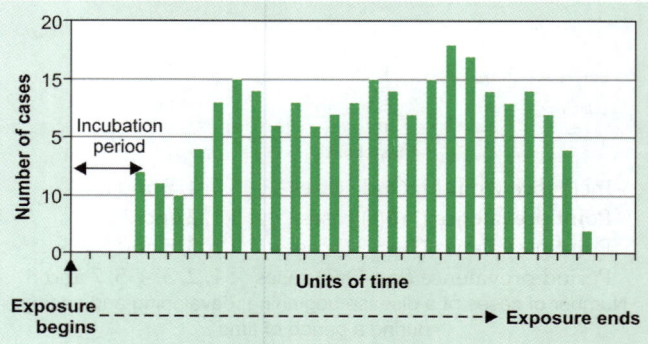

Common source, continuous/ repeated exposure epidemic

67. **Ans. (c) Endemic** [Ref. Park 27/e p101]
    Endemic
    - Constant presence of a disease or infectious agent in a defined geographical area
    - Is the 'usual or expected frequency' of a disease in a population

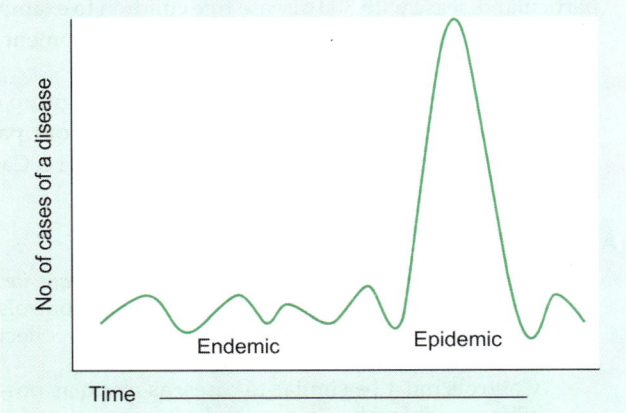

Review Questions

68. **Ans. (a) Seasonal variation of disease occurrence may be related to environmental conditions** [Ref. Park 27/e p73]
69. **Ans. (a) Retrospective and prospective study** [Ref. Park 27/e p70]
70. **Ans. (b) Pointed epidemic** [Ref. Park 27/e p72]
71. **Ans. (a) Common source, single exposure epidemic** [Ref. Park 27/e p72]

ANALYTICAL EPIDEMIOLOGY

72. **Ans. (b) Nested case control study** [Ref. Epidemiology by Gordis, 4/e p172]
    - In a Nested case control study, only exposure has occurred when the study begins; when the disease develops in a population, then 2 groups of cases (diseased) and controls (non-diseased) are formed and their exposure status is compared (baseline data is obtained from interviews, blood or urine tests)
    - Population is then followed up for a period of time (Cohort study) for development for the disease under study
    - A case control study is then carried out through questionnaires or sample testing

73. **Ans. (b) Retrospective cohort study** [Ref. Park 27/e p84]
    - In the given question, both exposure (aniline dye exposure) as well as outcome (bladder cancer) have occurred when the study has begun: First we go back in time and take only exposure into consideration (cohorts identified from past hospital/college records – here duration of exposure was obtained from past records of employment), then look for development of same disease in both exposed and non-exposed groups

74. **Ans. (a) 10% of lung cancers in smokers is not associated with smoking** [Ref. Park 27/e p86]
    - AR is indicative of the extent of the disease attributed to the exposure
    - **In the given question,** the attributable risk of cigarette smoking to lung cancer is 90%; hence, 90% cases of lung cancer can be attributed to smoking as an exposure
    - Remaining 10% can be attributed to other factors

75. **Ans. (b) Children in same community without ALL not getting exposed to chemicals** [Ref. Park 26/e p79]
    - *Case control study:* A study that compares patients who have a disease or outcome of interest (cases) with patients who do not have the disease or outcome (controls), and looks back retrospectively to compare how frequently the exposure to a risk factor is present in each group to determine the relationship between the risk factor and the disease
    - In a case control study, we never try to match the actual risk factor under study

76. **Ans. (b) Green tea consumption decreases the risk of DM** [Ref. Park 26/e p86]
    - Relative risk <1 implies negative/inverse association, i.e., risk factor is rather protective for the disease

77. **Ans. (d) 2,3,4** [Ref. Park 26/e p79-80]
    Steps in Case control studies
    - Selection/Allocation of cases and controls
    - Matching
    - Measurement of exposure
    - Inference of result data (Analysis)

78. **Ans. (a) Cohort study** [Ref. Basic Epidemiology by Beaglehole, WHO; p41]
    - Best study to find out strength of association i.e. relation between exposure and outcome is Cohort study
    - Relative risk (Cohort study) is more accurate measure of Strength of association as compared to Odds ratio (Case control study)

79. **Ans. (a) Attributable risk** [Ref. Park 25/e p86]
    - Attributable risk (AR) = (Incidence among exposed – Incidence among non-exposed)/ Incidence among exposed × 100
    - Interpretation of AR: How much disease can be attributed to given exposure

80. **Ans. (c) Ecological study** [Ref. Park 25/e p70]
    - Secondary data collection (Government hospital records, Finance and taxation departments' records) at a point of time indicates Ecological study
    - Hence difficult to establish association effectively between COPD and smoking

81. **Ans. (b) Random Selection** [Ref. Park 25/e p80]
    - Confounding can be removed by Matching, Randomization, Stratified randomization (Best method), Restriction, Stratification, Statistical modelling (Multivariate analysis)

82. **Ans. (d) Cross sectional** [Ref. Park 25/e p77]
    - Cross-sectional study is the simplest form of an Observational study based on single examination of a cross-section of the population at a given time

83. **Ans. (c) Recall bias** [Ref. Park 27/e p81]

- In a Nested case control study, interviews are performed at the beginning of the study (at baseline), and data are obtained before the disease has developed, thereby eliminating the problem of Recall bias

84. **Ans. (b) Relative risk** [Ref. Park 27/e p86]
    - Strength of association in a cohort study is evaluated by:
      - Relative risk (RR)
      - Attributable risk (AR)
      - Population attributable risk (PAR)

    $$\text{Relative risk (RR)} = \frac{\text{Incidence among exposed}}{\text{Incidence among non-exposed}}$$

    $$RR = \frac{I_{exp}}{I_{nonexp}}$$

    - Interpretation of RR: Incidence of disease among exposed IS SO MANY TIMES HIGHER as compared to that among non-exposed
    - Attributable risk (AR) =

    $$\frac{\text{Incidence among exposed} - \text{Incidence among non-exposed}}{\text{Incidence among exposed}}$$

    $$AR = \frac{I_{exp} - I_{nonexp}}{I_{exp}} \times 100$$

    - Interpretation of AR: So much disease can be attributed to exposure
    - Population attributable risk (PAR) =

    $$\frac{\text{Incidence among total} - \text{Incidence among non-exposed}}{\text{Incidence among total}}$$

    $$PAR = \frac{I_{tot} - I_{nonexp}}{I_{tot}} \times 100$$

    - Interpretation of PAR: If risk factor is modified or eliminated, there will be so much reduction in incidence of disease in the given population

> **ALSO REMEMBER**
> - Relative risk (RR) is of importance to clinician, whereas Population attributable risk (PAR) is of importance to public health programme manager/epidemiologist
> - Relative risk (RR) Versus Odds Ratio (OR):
>
> | | Relative risk (RR) | Odds Ratio (OR) |
> | --- | --- | --- |
> | Synonyms | Risk ratio | Cross product ratio |
> | Utility | Estimates strength of association in a cohort study | Estimates strength of association in a case control study |
> | Measure of strength of association | More accurate estimate | Less accurate (only an estimate of RR) |
> | Calculation | Iexposed Inon-exposed | ad bc |

85. **Ans. (b) Cohort study** [Ref. Textbook in Psychiatric Epidemiology; p10 and A Dictionary of Public Health, Dr. Jugal Kishore; p423-24]

- ATTENTION BIAS (HAWTHORNE EFFECT):
  - Is a type of subject bias
  - Study subjects systematically alter their behaviour when they know they are being observed

86. **Ans. (d) Case control** [Ref. Park 27/e p79]
    In the given question, a study compared 150 children with a particular disease with 300 disease free children to examine past experiences that may contribute to the development of the illness,
    Since two groups, one diseased (cases) and one group of disease-free children (controls) are examined about past experiences (exposure), it is a retrospective design, i.e. Case control study.

> **ALSO REMEMBER**
> - In a case control study, selection of controls is a prerequisite:
>   - If the study group is small, choose up to 4 controls per case (In larger studies with equal cost to collect cases and controls 1 : 1 is sufficient)
>   - Controls must be similar to cases, as much as possible except for the absence of disease under study
>   - Choice of cases and controls must not be influenced by exposure status
>   - Failure to select comparable controls can lead to biases

87. **Ans. (d) Random error** [Ref. Basic Epidemiology by Beaglehole, WHO; p46-52, Park 27/e p81]

    POTENTIAL ERRORS IN EPIDEMIOLOGICAL STUDIES:
    - Random errors:
      - Also known as 'Sampling errors': Is 'divergence due to chance alone' of an observation on a sample from the true population value, leading to 'lack of precision' in the measurement of association
      - Random error 'cannot be completely eliminated'
      - Random errors can be reduced by: careful measurement of exposure and outcome, thus making the individual measurements as precise as possible
      - Best way of reducing sampling errors (increasing precision): Increase the sample size in the study
    - Systematic errors:
      - Also known as 'Biases': occur whenever there is a tendency to produce results that differ in systematic manner from the true values (Bias is any systematic error in an epidemiological study, occurring during data collection, compilation, analysis and interpretation)

88. **Ans. (a) 25%** [Ref. Park 27/e p86]
    - Relative Risk (RISK RATIO) is used to estimate risk of disease (calculated as incidence of that disease) with exposure to a factor
    - Relative Risk (RR) = Incidence among exposed/ Incidence among non-exposed

    In the given question,

	Breast Cancer	No Breast Cancer	Total
Placebo	40	960	1000
New Drug	10	960	1000

Thus, considering new drug as exposure (placebo as non-exposure) and development of breast cancer as disease,
I_{exp} = × 1000 = 10 per 1000
$I_{non-exp}$ = × 1000 = 40 per 1000
Thus, RR = $I_{exp}/I_{non-exp}$ = 0.25
(25%; ideally RR is a ratio – MUST NOT be expressed as percentage)
Interpretation: New drug is efficacious in prevention of breast cancer; new drug is protective for breast cancer

89. **Ans. (c) Concurrent cohort study** [Ref. Park 27/e p84]
    - *Prospective cohort study*:
      1. Known as 'Current cohort study' or 'Concurrent cohort study'
      2. Outcome has not yet occurred when the study has begun: Only exposure has occurred; we look for development of same disease in both exposed and non-exposed groups
      3. Examples:
         i. Framingham heart study
         ii. Doll & Hills prospective study on smoking and lung cancer

ALSO REMEMBER
- Exposure and outcome in analytical studies:

	Exposure	Outcome	Remarks	Direction
Prospective cohort study	Occurred	Followed-up	Start with exposure	Forward looking
Retrospective cohort study	Occurred	Occurred	Start with exposure	Forward looking
Mixed cohort study	Occurred	Occurred; further assessed in future	Start with exposure	Forward looking
Case control study	Occurred	Occurred	Start with outcome	Backward looking
Cross sectional study	Occurred	Occurred	Both exposure and outcome assessed at a point of time	Neither forward looking nor backward looking

90. **Ans. (b) 10** [Ref. Park 27/e p86]
    - *Relative Risk* (RISK RATIO) is used to estimate risk of disease (calculated as incidence of that disease) with exposure to a factor
    - Relative Risk (RR) = Incidence among exposed/Incidence among non-exposed
      RR = $I_{exp}/I_{non-exp}$

    In the given question, TATA memorial hospital conducted a cohort study on 7000 subjects who were smokers over a ten-year period & found 70 subjects developed lung cancer,
    Thus, I_{exp} = × 1000 = 10 per thousand
    Also, concurrent evaluation of general population in the catchment area of hospital, out of 7000 non-smoker subjects only 7 developed lung cancer,

Thus, $I_{non-exp}$ = × 1000 = 1 per 1000
Therefore, RR = = 10 per 1000/1 per 1000 = 10
Interpretation: Strength of association between smoking and lung cancer is 10 (Lung cancer is 10 times more common among smokers as compared to non-smokers)
HAD RR BEING 1, it would have implied that exposure (smoking) and disease under study (lung cancer) are not associated at all (Smoking is neither causative nor protective for lung cancer)
HAD RR BEING < 1, it would have implied that exposure (smoking) is protective for the disease under study (lung cancer)

ALSO REMEMBER
- Attributable risk (AR):
  – Is a good measure of extent of public health problem caused by the exposure
  – Is a useful tool for assessing priorities for health action
  – Is also known as 'Absolute risk' or 'excess risk' or 'risk difference'

91. **Ans. (c) 6.0** [Ref. Park 27/e p81]
    - *Strength of association in a case control study*: Case Control Study cannot provide with incidences, so Relative Risk cannot be calculated; so in a Case Control Study, we calculate 'an estimate of Relative Risk', known as 'Odds Ratio' (CROSS PRODUCT RATIO)
    - *CORRECT TABLE CONSTRUCTION in a case control study*: Table will have disease at the top (row) and history of exposure/risk factor on the left (column)
    - *Odds Ratio In a 2 × 2 table for a case control study*:

	Disease Present	Disease Absent
Exposure present	a	b
Exposure absent	c	d

Odds Ratio (Cross Product Ratio) = ad/bc
- **Thus in the given question**, correct table IS TO BE CONSTRUCTED FIRST:

	Renal cell cancer Present (cases)	Renal cell cancer Absent (controls)
Exposure to smoking present	a	b
Exposure to smoking absent	c	d
Total	a + c	b + d

Now, total cases of renal cell cancer (a + c) = 50, smoking exposure present (a) = 30
Total controls (b + d) = 50, smoking exposure present (b) = 10
Therefore, c = [(a + c) – (a)] = [50 – 30] = 20 and,
d = [(b + d) – (b)] = [50 – 10] = 40

Table construction,

	Renal cell cancer Present (cases)	Renal cell cancer Absent (controls)
Exposure to smoking present	30	10
Exposure to smoking absent	20	40
Total	50	50

Odds ratio = ad/bc = 30 × 40/20 × 10 = 6

Interpretation of Odds ratio = 6: Renal cell cancer cases have 6 times higher odds than controls of having had the history of exposure to smoking

> **ALSO REMEMBER**
> - *Interpretation of Odds ratios (OR):* Is similar to Relative risk (RR) in cohort study (as OR is an estimate of RR)
>   - **OR > 1:** Cases have so-many times higher odds than controls of having had the history of exposure under study
>   - **OR = 1:** Cases have equal odds as controls of having had the history of exposure under study; thus exposure IS NOT ASSOCIATED with disease under study
>   - **OR < 1:** Cases have so-many times lesser odds as controls of having had the history of exposure under study; thus exposure IS PROTECTIVE for the disease under study

92. Ans. (d) 6 [Ref. Park 27/e p86]

- *Relative Risk* (RISK RATIO) is used to estimate risk of disease (calculated as incidence of that disease) with exposure to a factor
- Relative Risk (RR) = Incidence among exposed/Incidence among non-exposed

In the given question, 200 smokers & 300 non-smokers were followed up over a period of 10 yrs to find out incidence of hypertension,

Out of 200 smokers, 60 developed hypertension, thus Iexp = 60/200 × 1000 = 300

And, out of 600 non-smokers, 30 developed hypertension, thus Inon-exp = 30/600 × 1000 = 50

Thus, Risk ratio = $I_{exp}/I_{non-exp}$ = 300/50 = 6

Interpretation: Strength of association between smoking and hypertension is 6 (Hypertension is 6 times more common among smokers as compared to non-smokers)

93. Ans. (b) Concurrent cohort [Ref. Epidemiology by Leon Gordis, 4/e p152 and Park 27/e p84]

In the given question, a study began in 1965, a group of 3000 adults in Baltimore were asked about alcohol consumption and the occurrence of cancer was studied in the group between 1981 and 1995,

Since risk factor/exposure (alcohol consumption) was assessed first (1965) and then development of disease was noted in due course of time (followed-up till 1981-1995),

Thus it is a Concurrent cohort study

> **ALSO REMEMBER**
> - *Preference of epidemiological studies for establishing causality:*
>   - 1st preference: Meta-analysis
>   - 2nd preference: Randomised controlled trials (RCTs)
>   - 3rd preference: Retrospective (Non-concurrent/ Historical) cohort study
>   - 4th preference: Prospective cohort study (Concurrent cohort study)
>   - 5th preference: Case control study
>   - 6th preference: Cross-sectional study
>   - 7th preference: Ecological study
> - *Examples* of concurrent cohort study:
>   - Framingham heart study
>   - Doll & Hills prospective study on smoking and lung cancer

94. Ans. (c) Retrospective cohort [Ref. Epidemiology by Leon Gordis, 4/e p152-53 and Park 27/e p84]

In the given question, the physical examination records of the entire incoming freshman class of 1935 at the university of Minnesota were examined in 1977 to see if their recorded height and weight at the time of admission to university was related to their chance of developing CHD.

Since both exposure (Weight and height) as well as outcome (CHD) have occurred when the study has begun AND first they went back in time and take only exposure into consideration (height, weight from past hospital/college records), then looked for development of same disease (CHD) in both exposed and non-exposed groups.

Thus it is a Retrospective cohort study.

95. Ans. (c) The required sample size is smaller than that needed for a concurrent cohort study
[Ref. Epidemiology by Leon Gordis, 4/e p152-53]

96. Ans. (d) Incorrect, because of failure to distinguish between incidence and prevalence [Ref. Park 27/e p77]

In the given question, during an initial examination in Oxford, Migraine head ache was found in 5 of 1000 men aged 30-35 yrs and in 10 of 1000 women aged 30 to 35 yrs Thus, information provided does not distinguish between incidence and prevalence of migraine headache,

Therefore, we cannot infer that women have a two times greater risk of developing migraine headache than men in this age group [for drawing that condusion, a cohort study must be undertaken]

> **ALSO REMEMBER**
> - *Incidence is the best measure of disease frequency in etiological studies*
> - *Incidence can be determined from*: Cohort study
> - *Prevalence can be determined from*: Cross Sectional Study

97. Ans. (b) Relative risk can be calculated [Ref. Park 27/e p82]
- Relative risk calculation requires incidences, which can be found only through cohort studies
- In Case Control Studies, we calculate *'an estimate of relative risk: Odds Ratio'*

> **ALSO REMEMBER**
> - *Cohort studies versus Case control studies*:

	Cohort Studies	**Case Control Studies**
Before start Synonyms	Only exposure has occurred Prospective study Forward looking study Cause to effect study Exposure to outcome study Risk factor to disease study Incidence study Follow up study	Both exposure as well as outcome have occurred Retrospective study Backward looking study Effect to cause to study Outcome to exposure study Disease to risk factor study TROHOC study
Advantages	Provides Incidence, Relative risk Allows study of several etiological factors simultaneously	Easy to carry out Inexpensive Rapid No risk to subjects Minimal ethical problems No loss to follow up (No Attrition) Particularly suitable to investigate rare diseases
Disadvantages	Ethical problems Loss to follow up (attrition) Time consuming Expensive Not suitable to investigate rare diseases	Selection of an appropriate control-group may be difficult Cannot measure incidence Can only estimate Odds ratio

- Maximum allowable attrition rate in a cohort study for valid results: 5% (Thus Ideal retention rate in a Cohort study: > 95%)
- COHORT STUDY IS BETTER THAN A CASE CONTROL STUDY (despite problems of ethics, attrition, expensive & time-consuming): As Relative risk (RR) is a better estimate of strength of association than Odds ratio (OR)

98. Ans. (a) Give good information about the patients in that hospital at that time [Ref. Park 27/e p77]

In the given question, a one day census of inpatients in a mental hospital is carried out AT A POINT OF TIME,

Thus it is a cross-sectional study (neither forward looking, nor backward looking

Being a cross-sectional study, it can provide good information about the patients in that hospital at that time (Is a snapshot of the population, provides prevalence BUT cannot establish causality)

It cannot give reliable estimates of seasonal factors in admissions (since it is done only in a day), for which a longitudinal study design is preferable (as latter can cover all seasons)

It would not enable us to draw conclusions about the mental hospitals of India, as it is being done in only one hospital for only one day

It also would not enable us to estimate the distribution of different diagnosis in mental illness in the local area, as it is being done for only inpatients (Not OPD patients) and only for a day

99. Ans. (d) 80% [Ref. Park 27/e p86]
- AR calculation requires incidence which can be obtained from only a cohort study (Not from a case control study).
- *Is a good measure of extent of public health problem caused by the exposure*
- Is a useful tool for assessing priorities for health action
- Is also known as *'Absolute risk'* or *'excess risk'* or *'risk difference'*

In the given question,

Exposure is multiple sexual partners (and non-exposure is a single sex partner)

If incidence of carcinoma cervix (disease) among non-exposed (single sex partner) is 'x',

Then, incidence of carcinoma cervix (disease) among exposed (multiple sex partners) is '5x',

Thus, AR = (5x – x)/5x × 100 = 80%

Interpretation of AR = 80%: 80% of carcinoma cervix (disease) can be attributed to exposure (multiple sex partners)

100. **Ans. (c) 6.0** *[Ref. Park 27/e p86]*
- *Relative Risk* (RISK RATIO) is used to estimate risk of disease (calculated as incidence of that disease) with exposure to a factor
- Relative Risk (RR)

$$= \frac{\text{Incidence among exposed}}{\text{Incidence among non-exposed}} \quad RR = \frac{I_{exp}}{I_{non\,exp}}$$

In the given question,

	Hypertension		
	Present	Absent	Total
Smoking present	120	280	400
Smoking absent	30	570	600
Total	150	850	1000

Exposed (smokers) = 400

Non-exposed (non-smokers) = 600

Incidence of hypertension in exposed (smokers)
$= \frac{120}{400} \cdot 1000$

Incidence of hypertension in non-exposed
(non-smokers) $= \frac{30}{600} \cdot 1000$

Thus, RR = $I_{exposed}/I_{non-exposed}$ = $\frac{120/400 \cdot 1000}{30/600 \cdot 1000}$ = 6

Interpretation of RR = 6: Smokers (exposed) have SIX times higher chances of development of Hypertension (disease) as compared to non-smokers (non-exposed)

101. **Ans. (c) Attributable risk** *[Ref. Park 27/e p86]*

In the given question, 85% of cases of lung Cancer are due to cigarette smoking, thus it is a measure of attributable risk.

> **ALSO REMEMBER**
> - *Attributable risk (AR)*:
>   - Is a good measure of extent of public health problem caused by the exposure
>   - Is a useful tool for assessing priorities for health action
>   - Is also known as 'Absolute risk' or 'excess risk' or 'risk difference'
> - Relative risk (RR) IS A BETTER ESTIMATE of strength of association than Attributable risk (AR)
> - **Standardized mortality ration (SMR)**:
>   - Is a special type of risk ratio: Comparison of observed mortality with expected mortality
>   - Is a type of Indirect standardization

102. **Ans. (b) Interviewer bias** *[Ref. A Dictionary of Public Health, Dr. Jugal Kishore; p423-24]*

103. **Ans. (b) Cohort study** *[Ref. Park 27/e p88]*

FRAMINGHAM HEART STUDY:
- *Is a classical example of cohort study*
- Initiated in 1948 by US Public Health Service at Framingham, a town in Massachusetts, USA
- *Aim*: To study the relationship of risk factors (serum cholesterol, blood pressure, weight, smoking) to the subsequent development of cardiovascular diseases
- *Age group*: 30–62 years
- *Sample size*: 5127 (4469 – 69% of the sample actually underwent first examination)
- *Method*: Multiple exposure were studied, as well as complex interactions among the exposures using multivariate techniques
- *Follow-up*:
  - Study population was examined every 2 years for 20 years
  - Daily surveillance of hospitalizations at only hospital at Framingham
- *Findings of study*:
  - Increasing risk of CHD with increasing age & more frequently in males
  - Hypertensive have a greater risk of CHD
  - Elevated blood cholesterol level is associated with CHD
  - Tobacco smoking and habitual use of alcohol are associated with increased risk of CHD
  - Increased physical activity is associated with decrease in CHD development
  - Increase in body weight is associated predisposes to CHD
  - Diabetes mellitus increases risk of CHD

104. **Ans. (d) A cohort study is more appropriate when the disease or exposure under investigation is rare, in comparison to case control study** *[Ref. Park 27/e p80–87]*

> **ALSO REMEMBER**
> - *Potential biases in cohort studies*:
>   - Bias in assessment of outcome
>   - Information bias (esp. in retrospective cohort studies)
>   - Bias from non-response and loss to follow up
>   - Analytic bias
> - *Longitudinal studies*:
>   - Cohort study
>   - Case control study

105. **Ans. (d) A cohort study** *[Ref. Park 27/e p83]*

106. **Ans. (d) Does not exist** *[Ref. Epidemiology by Leon Gordis, 4/e p183-84]*

107. **Ans. (d) Interviewer bias** *[Ref. A Dictionary of Public Health, Dr. Jugal Kishore; p284]*
- **INTERVIEWER BIAS**: Systematic error due to interviewer's subconscious or conscious gathering of selective data
  1. Is a type of information bias
  2. Is a type of investigator bias
  3. Commonly occurs due to interviewer devoting more time of interview with cases as compared to controls

4. Can be eliminated/reduced by devoting equal interview time to cases as well as controls

108. **Ans. (c) Stratified randomization**
    [Ref. Epidemiology by Leon Gordis, 4/e p183-84]
    - *Stratified randomization*: Study population is 'first stratified' by each variable which is considered important, and then randomization is done to each treatment groups within each stratum
        - *Comparison groups become similar as possible as regards participant characteristics that might influence the response to the intervention*
        - *Equal numbers of participants with a characteristic thought to affect prognosis or response to the intervention will be allocated to each comparison group.*
        - *Stratification increase the likelihood that two groups will be more comparable*
        - *Stratified randomization is performed by*
            1. Performing separate randomization for each strata
            2. By using minimization

109. **Ans. (b) Sibling Controls**   *[Ref. Park 27/e p76-79]*

    CONTROLS IN A CASE CONTROL STUDY:
    - In a case control study, selection of controls is a prerequisite
    - If the study group is small, choose up to 4 controls per case (In larger studies with equal cost to collect cases and controls 1 : 1 is sufficient).
    - Cases are diseased individuals, Controls are those free from the disease under study
    - Controls must be similar to cases, as much as possible except for the absence of disease under study
    - **Sources of controls**:
        - *Hospital controls*: are often a 'source of selection bias'
        - *Neighbourhood controls*: provide similar socio-economic and living conditions
        - *Relatives*: Sibling controls are unsuitable in genetic studies
        - *General population*: by choosing a random sample
        - *Best friends controls*

    > **ALSO REMEMBER**
    > - *Historical controls*:
    >   - Used in a study of new therapy; especially when disease is uniformly fatal and a new drug becomes available
    >   - 'Comparison group is selected from the past', usually from records of patients with same disease who were treated before new therapy became available
    >   - Disadvantages:
    >   1. Need meticulous system of data collection of patients
    >   2. Quality of data collected is usually not comparable
    >   3. One is not sure if difference is due to therapy only
    > - *Matching*: Is selection of controls so that they are similar to cases in various respects
    >   - Matching is done to 'eliminate known confounding'
    >   - Cases and controls are matched for every factor 'except risk factor under study'

110. **Ans. (d) Suitable to investigate rare diseases**
    [Ref. Park 27/e p82]
    - If there is a rare disease to be studied, and,
        - Cohort study is done: One may get very few cases or no case at the end of study (as disease is rare); this will be wastage of time and money
        - Case control study is done: Controls are chosen for the few available cases and history of possible/suspected exposure(s) is explored

111. **Ans. (b) 6**   *[Ref. Park 27/e p81]*
    - *Strength of association in a case control study*: Case Control Study cannot provide with incidences, so Relative Risk cannot be calculated; so in a Case Control Study, we calculate 'an estimate of Relative Risk', known as 'Odds Ratio' (CROSS PRODUCT RATIO)
    - *CORRECT TABLE CONSTRUCTION in a case control study*: Table will have disease at the top (row) and history of exposure/risk factor on the left (column)
      Odds Ratio (Cross Product Ratio) = ad/bc
    - **Thus in the given question**, correct table IS NOT GIVEN; correct construction of table is required first

	Thromboembolism Present (cases)	Thromboembolism Absent (controls)
Exposure to OCPs present	a	b
Exposure to OCPs absent	c	d
Total	a + c	b + d

    Now, total cases (a + c) = 84, OCP exposure present (a) = 50% of 84 = 42

    Total controls (b + d) = 168, OCP exposure present (b) = 14% of 168 = 24

    Therefore, c = [(a + c) – (a)] = [84 – 42] = 42 and, d = [(b + d) – (b)] = [168 – 24] = 144

    Table construction,

	Thromboembolism Present (cases)	Thromboembolism Absent (controls)
Exposure to OCPs present	42	24
Exposure to OCPs absent	42	144
Total	84	168

    Odds ratio = ad/bc = 42 × 144/24 × 42 = 6

    Interpretation of Odds ratio = 6: Thromboembolic cases have 6 times higher odds than controls of having had the history of exposure to OCPs.

112. **Ans. (b) 90%**   *[Ref. Park 27/e p86]*
    - **In the given data,**
        - *Incidence among exposed (Iexp) = 10/1000*
        - *Incidence among non-exposed (Inonexp) = 1/1000*
        - *Incidence among total (Itot) = 11/1000*
    - *Relative risk (RR)* = $\dfrac{I_{exp}}{I_{non\,exp}}$ = 10

- *Interpretation of RR*: Incidence of lung cancer (disease) among smokers (exposed) IS TEN TIMES HIGHER as compared to that among non-smokers (non-exposed)
- *Attributable risk (AR)* = $(I_{exp} - I_{nonexp})/I_{exp} \times 100 = 90\%$
  - *Interpretation of AR*: 90% of lung cancer (disease) can be attributed to smoking (exposure)
- *Population attributable risk (PAR)*
  = PAR = $(I_{tot} - I_{nonexp})/I_{tot} \times 100 = 91\%$
  - *Interpretation of PAR*: If smoking (risk factor) is modified or eliminated, there will be 91% reduction in incidence of lung cancer (disease) in the given population
- Relative risk (RR) is of importance to clinician, whereas Population attributable risk (PAR) is of importance to public health programme manager/epidemiologist
- *Absolute risk*: Is 'attributable risk' or 'excess risk' or 'risk difference'
  - Is a useful measure of extent of public health problem caused by an exposure

113. **Ans. (b) A – III, B – II, C – IV, D – I**
     [Ref. Park 21/e p70, Park 22/e p60, and Basic Epidemiology by Beaglehole, WHO; p31]

114. **Ans. (d) The attributable risk of breast cancer resulting from the pill may be directly measured** *[Ref. Park 27/e p81]*
     AR calculation requires incidence which can be obtained from only a cohort study (Not from a case control study)
     - In a Case Control Study, 'Cases' are diseased and 'Controls' are healthy
     - Controls should be similar to Cases in all respects (for ensuring comparability)
     - Cases should be matched with controls for all factors 'EXCEPT for the (risk) factor under study' (otherwise the etiological role of risk factor under study, which we are studying, would be eliminated from the study, since both groups are exactly similar in all respects); So if controls do not exclude women known to be taking the pill at the time of the survey, both groups will become similar in respect to risk factor (contraceptive pill) under study and no relationship can be established with breast cancer

115. **Ans. (c) Done when incidence of disease is very low among exposed** *[Ref. Park 27/e p87]*
     - *Case control study is preferable for rare diseases*: Cohort study IS NOT USEFUL to investigate rare diseases as whole time, and expense may yield little/no disease, thus strength of association may not be calculable
     - COHORT STUDY IS BETTER THAN A CASE CONTROL STUDY (despite problems of ethics, attrition, expensive & time-consuming): As Relative risk (RR) is a better estimate of strength of association than Odds ratio (OR)

116. **Ans. (d) 2.25** *[Ref. Park 27/e p81]*
     Thus in the given question,
     Odds Ratio = $30 \times 30 / 20 \times 20 = 2.25$

117. **Ans. (b) Beta carotene is not protective in lung cancer:** *[Ref. Park 27/e p86]*
     - *Relative Risk* (RISK RATIO) is used to estimate risk of disease (calculated as incidence of that disease) with exposure to a factor
     - Relative Risk (RR) = Iexp/Inonexp

     In the given question,

     Exposure is beta carotene and disease is lung cancer
     Incidence of lung cancer among those exposed to beta carotene (I_{exp}) = 3/6000
     Incidence of lung cancer among those not exposed to beta carotene (I_{nonexp}) = 2/4000
     Therefore, RR = 1 (i.e., I_{exp} IS SAME AS I_{nonexp})
     If RR = 1, it implies 'Incidence among exposed' IS SAME AS 'Incidence among non-exposed'. Therefore, whether the person is exposed or not (to a factor), incidence of disease developing later will remain the same. Thus, exposure (beta carotene) and disease under study (lung cancer) are not associated at all.
     Thus 'Beta carotene is neither causative nor protective for lung cancer'

     > **ALSO REMEMBER**
     > - With a *large sample size* (10000 study subjects) this cohort study is sufficient to draw meaningful conclusions

118. **Ans. (c) No association at all** *[Ref. Park 27/e p86]*
     - *Relative Risk* (RISK RATIO) is used to estimate risk of disease (calculated as incidence of that disease) with exposure to a factor
     - Relative Risk (RR)
       = $\dfrac{\text{Incidence among exposed}}{\text{Incidence among non-exposed RR}} = \dfrac{I_{exp}}{I_{nonexp}}$
     - RR measures 'Strength of Association' between risk factor and disease under study
       - If RR > 1, it implies incidence among exposed is SO MANY TIMES more than incidence among non-exposed. Thus non-exposed also have a risk of disease (Incidence among non-exposed) but risk increases with exposure
       - If RR = 1, it implies 'Incidence among exposed' IS SAME AS 'Incidence among non-exposed'. Therefore, whether the person is exposed or not (to a factor), incidence of disease developing later will remain the same. Thus, exposure and disease under study are not associated at all. For example, Milk consumption and Lung cancer

RELATIVE RISK		INTERPRETATION	EXAMPLE	
			Risk Factor/ Exposure	Disease
RR > 1	I_{exp} > I_{nonexp}	So many times chances/ incidence of disease development is more among exposed as compared to non-exposed (Positive Association)	Smoking	Lung Cancer

Contd...

Contd...

RELATIVE RISK		INTERPRETATION	EXAMPLE	
			Risk Factor/ Exposure	Disease
RR = 1	$I_{exp} = I_{nonexp}$	Chances/incidence of disease development is same among exposed as compared to non-exposed **(No Association)**	Smoking	HIV/ AIDS
RR < 1	$I_{exp} < I_{nonexp}$	Chances/incidence of disease development is less among exposed as compared to non-exposed **(Negative Association)**	Vitamin-A intake	Epithelial cancers

- RR < 1 is possible. It implies, incidence among non-exposed is more than incidence among exposed. Thus factor/exposure is NOT CAUSATIVE, rather protective for the disease. For example, Vitamin-A as exposure and development of Epithelial cancers as disease

ALSO REMEMBER
- Relative risk can ONLY be determined exactly from a Cohort Study
- Case Control Study cannot provide with incidences, so Relative Risk cannot be calculated. So in a Case Control Study, we calculate *'an estimate of Relative Risk'*, known as *'Odds Ratio'* (CROSS PRODUCT RATIO)

119. **Ans. (c) Prospective** *[Ref. Park 27/e p84]*

120. **Ans. (b) Randomisation is done while selecting subjects for the study** *[Ref. Park 27/e p90]*
    - *Randomisation* in Randomized Controlled trial (RCT) is a statistical procedure by which participants are allocated into either of two groups, viz., *'Experimental Group'* (in which intervention is given) and *'Reference Group'* (in which intervention is not given)
    - **The essential purposes of randomization in a randomized controlled trial are:**
      - Participants have *'Equal and Known Chance'* of falling into either *'Experimental Group'* or *'Reference Group'*
      - To eliminate Selection Bias (Selection Bias or *'Susceptibility Bias'* is the bias due to differential susceptibility of two groups to outcome, even before intervention/ experiment is performed; Thus two groups are not comparable)
      - To ensure comparability among two groups
      - To have *'similar prognostic factors'* among two groups
    - *'Randomisation is done while dividing patients into the Experimental (Intervention) Group and the Reference Group'* AND not while selecting patients for RCT
    - Randomisation is known as *'Heart of a trial'*
    - Randomisation IS SUPERIOR to Matching:
      - Randomization ensures *'both known and unknown'* confounding factors are distributed equally among the two groups, thereby nullifying their effect on result (whereas matching is useful for only known confounding factors)
      - Randomization *'removes both confounding and bias'*

	Blinding	Matching	Randomization
Removes	Bias	Known confounding	Selection bias Known confounding Unknown confounding
Types	Single B Double B Triple B	Caliper matching Frequency matching Category matching Individual matching Pair matching	Random no. tables Computer software Lottery Method Currency Method

ALSO REMEMBER
- *Unit of study in RCT*: Patient
- *RCT is of two types*:
  - **Concurrent parallel design:** Comparisons are made between 2 groups:
    1. *Experimental group*: Is exposed to specific medication or intervention
    2. *Reference group*: Is not exposed to specific medication or intervention
  - **Crossover design:** Comparisons are made between 2 groups:
    1. *Experimental group*: Is exposed to specific medication or intervention
    2. *Reference group*: Is not exposed to specific medication or intervention
- Then the groups are crossed-over (exposed group now becomes non-exposed and vice-versa)
- Cross-over design RCT helps removing ethical concerns
- *Intention to treat trial*: Implies that the results of a RCT are unaffected by attrition (loss to follow up) or change over of study subjects from one group to another
- *Randomisation is best done by 'Random number tables'*
- Blinding removes Subject Bias *(Single Blinding)*; Subject Bias & Observer Bias *(Double Blinding)* or Subject Bias, Observer Bias & Analyzer Bias *(Triple Blinding)*
  - Double blinding is the most common form of blinding observed
  - OPEN TRIAL is a trial without blinding

121. **Ans. (a) Helpful for evaluation of rare diseases; (e) Selection bias common** *[Ref. Park 27/e p90]*
    - *Case control study*:
      - Selection of an appropriate control group may be difficult
      - Is prone to several biases:
        1. Selection Bias
        2. Recall bias
        3. Survival bias
        4. Admission bias
        5. Non-response bias

122. **Ans. (b) It is itself a risk factor for the disease**
    [Ref. Park 27/e p80]
    Confounding factor:
    - It is found unequally distributed between the study and control groups
    - Is associated with both exposure and outcome
    - Has an independent effect in causation of outcome (thus is a risk factor itself)

123. **Ans. (b) Prospective study** [Ref. Park 27/e p84]

124. **Ans. (b) Ecological study**
    [Ref. Park 21/e p59, Park 22/e p60]
    ECOLOGICAL (CORRELATIONAL) STUDY:
    - *Unit of study*: Population (results not applicable on individuals – "Ecological fallacy")
    - *Done in a small time frame*: inexpensive; use data that is already available
    - *Inferior to Cohort, Case control studies*: Due to ecological fallacy

125. **Ans. (a) Confounding factor** [Ref. Park 27/e p80]
    In the given question, BOTH exposure (beta-carotene) and outcome (carcinoma of colon) are associated with a third independent factor (dietary fiber). Thus dietary fiber may affect the results through confounding.

126. **Ans. (c) Rare diseases** [Ref. Park 27/e p82]

127. **Ans. (c) Ecological study** [Ref. Park 21/e p59, Park 22/e p60]

128. **Ans. (a) Case control study requires more time than cohort study** [Ref. Park 27/e p87]

129. **Ans. (b) Analytical study** [Ref. Park 27/e p70-76]

130. **Ans. (c) Confounding factor** [Ref. Park 27/e p80]

131. **Ans. (a) Selection bias** [Ref. Park 227/e p81]

132. **Ans. (d) All of the above** [Ref. Park 27/e p80]

133. **Ans. (c) Risk difference between exposed and non-exposed** [Ref. Park 27/e p86]

134. **Ans. (c) Different rates of admission to hospital due to different diseases** [Ref. Park 27/e p81]

135. **Ans. (d) Associated with antecedent causation**
    [Ref. Park 27/e p87]

136. **Ans. (d) Selection bias** [Ref. Park 27/e p81]
    - *Selection bias (Susceptibility bias)*: Groups to be compared are differentially susceptible to the outcome of interest, even before the experimental maneuver is performed
    - **In the given question**, Smokers and Non-smokers (Groups to be compared) may have different diet/exercise habits which may affect their Blood lipid levels (Outcome of interest), thus it'd lead to Selection bias

137. **Ans. (b) Effect modifier**
    [Ref. Physical Activity Epidemiology by Dishman, 2/e p33]
    - *Confounding factor*: Any factor associated with both exposure and outcome, and has an independent effect in causation of outcome is a confounder
        - It is found unequally distributed between the study and control groups
        - Example: Smoking is a confounding factor in a study estimating risk of Coffee consumption for Pancreatic cancer
    - *Mediator*: Third variable (mediator, M) carries the influence of a given risk factor to a given disease/outcome
        - Mediator comes in between the risk factor - disease continuum
        - Example: HPV is a mediator in a study estimating risk of Multiple sex partners for Cervical cancer
    - *Effect modifier* (Interactor): Third variable (Effect modifier) whose level determines the magnitude of effect in a study
        - It modifies Strength of association between exposure and outcome
        - Example: Asbestos is an effect modifier in a study estimating risk of Smoking for Lung cancer
    - *Collinearity*: Two independent factors are so highly correlated that it becomes difficult to distinguish their individual effect on disease/outcome
        - Example: Air pollution and Urban area residence exhibit collinearity for development of Lung cancer

138. **Ans. (b) Randomised controlled trials** [Ref. Park 27/e p70]

139. **Ans. (b) Cross-sectional study** [Ref. Park 27/e p77]

140. **Ans. (b) Cross-sectional study** [Ref. Park 27/e p77]

141. **Ans. (d) 90%** [Ref. Park 27/e p86]
    - Total population 9000
    - Total exposed to alcohol = 2100
    - Total nonexposed to alcohol = 6900
    - Incidence among exposed (Ie) = 70/2100
    - Incidence among non-exposed (Ine) = 23/6900
    - Attributable risk = (Ie-Ine)/Ie × 100 = (70/2100 – 23/6900)/70/2100 × 100 = 90%

142. **Ans. (a) Incidence among exposed minus incidence among non-exposed** [Ref. Park 27/e p86]
    - Attributable risk (AR) = (Iexposed – Inon-exposed)/Iexposed × 100
    - Interpretation of AR: So much disease can be attributed to exposure

143. **Ans. (c) Incidence in total population minus incidence in non-exposed** [Ref. Park 27/e p86]
    - Population attributable risk (PAR) = (Itotal – Inon-exposed)/Itot × 100
    - Interpretation of PAR: If risk factor is modified or eliminated, there will be so much annual reduction in incidence of disease in the given population

144. **Ans. (a) Recruitment** [Ref. Modern Pharmaceutical Industry by Jacobsen 1/e p126]
    SELECTION BIAS
    - Occurs through differential representation of subjects in the exposed and unexposed study group
    - Occurs during recruitment and selection of potential bias
    - Can be removed by Randomization

145. **Ans. (d) Exclude all patients diagnosed as inflammatory bowel disease** [Ref. Park 27/e p84]
    - While assembling Cohorts in a Prospective cohort study, they must be initially free of disease of interest

- Those having disease at start of the Prospective cohort study should be excluded

146. **Ans. (a) There is no association present between the factor and the disease** [Ref. Park 27/e p86]

147. **Ans. (c) Relative risk** [Ref. Park 27/e p86]
     - Relative risk is best used as a measure of association between a risk factor and a specific outcome
     - Attributable risk/Absolute risk measure contribution of a risk factor toward occurrence of a disease
     - p-value gives reliable statistical significance of a result in a study

148. **Ans. (c) Cross-sectional study**
     [Ref. Risk Analysis by Cohrssen 1/e p60]
     - Descriptive studies may use correlational (ecological) approach where rate of disease in a population is compared with spatial/temporal distribution of risk factors
     - This study design will help refine hypothesis BUT fall short of establishing causal relationships
     - In analytical cross-sectional studies, the odds ratio can be used to assess the strength of an association between a risk factor and health outcome of interest, provided that the current exposure accurately reflects the past exposure

149. **Ans. (a) Cohort study**
     [Ref. Research Methods in Physical Activity by Thomas, 6/e p320]
     - In Cohort studies, the temporal sequence between exposure and outcome is clearly defined (Primary strength of Cohort studies)
     - Exposure assessments are obtained before disease onset, so the timing of the exposure in the natural history of the disease is in the correct sequence

150. **Ans. (a) Single blinding** [Ref. Park 27/e p91]
     - Single blinding: Study subjects are not aware of the treatment they are receiving in the trial; it helps in removal of Subject bias

151. **Ans. (c) Population attributable risk** [Ref. Park 27/e p86]
     - Epidemiologic research focuses on the identification and assessment of risk factors, and also is concerned with planning and evaluating public health interventions to control disease in the population
     - Being able to predict the impact of removing a particular exposure on the risk of developing a disease is an important public health consideration; Population attributable risk (PAR) is interpreted as 'If risk factor is modified or eliminated, there will be so much annual reduction in incidence of disease in the given population'
     - PAR allows those who are responsible for protecting the public's health to make decisions about allocating scarce resources (time, energy, money and political capital) where they will have the most impact; PAR is useful for development of National health policies and programs in the community

152. **Ans. (a) 8** [Ref. Park 27/e p81]
     In the given question,
     - Cases (a + c) = 35, Controls (b + d) = 82
     - 33 cases (a) had positive history of smoking and 55 individuals (b) among controls had positive history of smoking
     - Therefore c = 35 − 33 = 2; d = 82 − 55 = 27

     So, 2 × 2 table construction,

	Lung cancer present	Lung cancer absent
History of smoking present	33 (a)	55 (b)
History of smoking absent	2 (c)	27 (d)
	35	82

     Odds Ratio = ad/bc = (33 × 27)/(55 × 2) = 8.1

153. **Ans. (b) 75** [Ref. Park 27/e p86]
     In the given question,
     - Total population: 100,000
     - Total exposed population (smokers) = 20000
     - Total non-exposed population (non-smokers) = 80000
     - Total incidence of lung cancer cases = 100/100000
     - Total incidence of Lung cancer among exposed = 80/20000
     - Total incidence of Lung cancer among non-exposed = 20/80000

     Therefore,
     - PAR = (Itot − Inonexp)/Itot × 100 = (100/100000 − 20/80000)/(100/100000) × 100 = 75%

154. **Ans. (a) Study can confirm OCP as a cause of breast cancer or disprove it** [Ref. Park 27/e p77-79]
     - Case control study is an Analytical observational study which is used to test hypothesis whether latter is true or not
     - Descriptive studies are used to make a hypothesis

155. **Ans. (b) Non-concurrent Cohort Study**
     [Ref. Park 27/e p84]
     - Non-concurrent Cohort Study is Retrospective cohort study
     - In a Retrospective cohort study, both exposure (IUD insertion) as well as outcome Abdominal pain) have occurred when the study has begun: First we go back in time and take only exposure into consideration (Find out nurses who get IUD inserted and those who didn't), then look for development of same outcome (abdominal pain) in both exposed and non-exposed groups currently

156. **Ans. (b) RRR 11%, ARR 1%** [Ref. Oxford Handbook of Epidemiology for Clinicians 1/e p42]
     - Relative risk reduction (RRR): Percentage reduction in one outcome (E.g. Death or Adverse outcome) comparing one group (New drug) with another group (Older drug or Placebo)
     - Absolute risk reduction (ARR): Reduction in outcome (E.g. Death or Adverse outcome) comparing one group (New drug) with another group (Older drug or Placebo)
     - Event is taken as Occurrence of adverse outcome in the given example

     In the given question,
     - Event rate Drug = 1605/15225 × 100 = 10.5% (0.105)
     - Event rate Placebo = 1804/15225 × 100 = 11.8% (0.118)

Hence,
- Relative risk of Event rate = Event rate drug/Event rate Placebo = 0.105/0.118 = 0.9
- Relative risk reduction (RRR) = (Event rate Placebo – Event rate drug)/Event rate placebo = (0.118)–0.105)/0.118 = 0.11 = 11%
- Absolute risk reduction = Event rate Drug – Event rate Placebo = 0.105 – 0.118 = – 0.013 = – 1.3%

157. **Ans. (b) Case control study: Suitable for study of rare disease; (c) Cohort study: Help in assessing concept of causality; (e) Case control study: Estimates only Odds ratio** *[Ref. Park 27/e p68-83]*

158. **Ans. (c) Inverse association** *[Ref. Park 27/e p78]*
In the given question, Odds Ratio OR is 1:5 (= 1/5 = 0.20)
- Whenever OR<1, it implies Protective/inverse association (or risk factor is protective for the outcome in the study)
- Interpretation: Mothers of IUGR fetuses are less likely to report history of Maternal hypertension during pregnancy (or Mothers of healthy fetuses are likely to report history of Maternal hypertension five times higher)

159. **Ans. (b) Prospective cohort** *[Ref. Park 27/e p81]*
- In Prospective (Concurrent) cohort study, Outcome has not yet occurred at the time study investigation begins
- Study is started in current time and continued into future

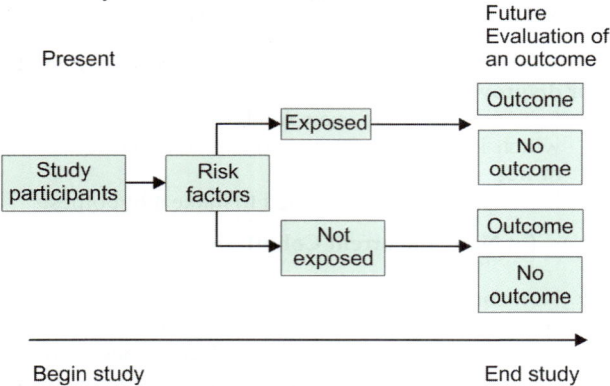

Fig. Prospective Cohort Study

160. **Ans. (d) Nested case control study** *[Ref. Study Design and Statistical Analysis by Katz 1/e p31]*
- Usefulness of Nested case control studies is limited for studies involving 'rare diseases AND whose diagnostic tests are very expensive'

161. **Ans. (b) Distributed equally between study and control groups** *[Ref. Park 27/e p77]*
- Confounding: Any factor associated with both exposure and outcome, and has an independent effect in causation of outcome is a confounder
  - It is found unequally distributed between the study and control groups
  - Is associated with both exposure and outcome
  - Has an independent effect in causation of outcome (thus is a risk factor itself

162. **Ans. (a) Indicator of increased risk of disease in pre-disposed population; (b) It is cross productivity ratio; (d) Used in case control study; (e) It is Similar to relative risk** *[Ref. Park 27/e p78]*

163. **Ans. (b) Case control study** *[Ref. Park 27/e p81]*
- Odds ratio (OR): Ratio of odds that cases were exposed to a risk factor to the odds that the controls were exposed
  – Is used to 'measure strength of association in a case control study'
  – Is also known as 'Cross product ratio' or 'Relative odds'

164. **Ans.** *[Ref. Park 27/e p80]*
Confounding Factor
- Any extraneous variable that is an independent risk factor for the study disease and is also related to the exposure variable
- Such variables may partially or completely account for any apparent association

Review Questions

165. **Ans. (d) Starts with the disease** *[Ref. Park 27/e p83]*
166. **Ans. (a) Only odd's ratio** *[Ref. Park 27/e p81]*
167. **Ans. (d) Distinguishing between causes and associated factors** *[Ref. Park 27/e p82]*
168. **Ans. (b) It is distributed equally in study & control groups** *[Ref. Park 27/e p80]*
169. **Ans. (b) Attributable risk** *[Ref. Park 27/e p86]*
170. **Ans. (b) Tells etiology** *[Ref. Park 27/e p77]*
171. **Ans. (a) Relative risk** *[Ref. Park 27/e p81]*
172. **Ans. (c) Assessing aetiological role or factor in disease** *[Ref. Park 27/e p86]*
173. **Ans. (b) Chronic diseases can be studied** *[Ref. Park 27/e p77]*
174. **Ans. (c) Observation bias** *[Ref. Park 21/e p127, Park 22/e p130, 24/e p151]*
175. **Ans. (a) ad/bc** *[Ref. Park 27/e p81]*
176. **Ans. (a) Cohort study** *[Ref. Park 27/e p86]*
177. **Ans. (a) Cohort** *[Ref. Park 27/e p84-85]*

EXPERIMENTAL EPIDEMIOLOGY

178. **Ans. (c) CARE – RCT** *[Ref. Multiple sources]*

Guidelines for Reporting Medical Research
- CONSORT (Consolidated Standards of Reporting Trials) is a guideline for reporting randomized controlled trials, of which the latest version is from 2010
- MOOSE (Meta-analysis Of Observational Studies in Epidemiology) is a guideline used for reporting meta-analyses of observational studies
- PRISMA (Preferred Reporting Items for Systematic Reviews and Meta-analyses) is developed for the reporting of systematic reviews and meta-analyses
- STROBE (STrengthening the Reporting of OBservational studies in Epidemiology) was developed in 2004 to be used as a guideline for reporting observational studies, specifically cohort, case-control, and cross-sectional studies

- STARD (STAndards for the Reporting of Diagnostic accuracy studies) is intended for reporting studies of diagnostic or prognostic accuracy
- SPIRIT (Standard Protocol Items: Recommendations for Interventional Trials) was created in 2007 for the reporting of scientific trial protocols
- CARE guidelines were developed by an international group of experts to increase the accuracy, transparency, and usefulness of case reports

179. **Ans. (c) Randomization**
[Ref. Evidence-Based Public Health Practice by Fink 1/e]

Four basic steps to any good meta-analysis
- Identification
- Selection
- Abstraction
- Analysis

180. **Ans. (b) Meta-analysis**
[Ref. Doing meta-analysis in research: A systematic approach by Dr Vivek Jain, IJDVL, 2012;78:242-50]
- Meta-analysis is an objective, systematic review that employs statistical methods to combine and summarize the results of several studies
- A quantitative synthesis of all unbiased evidence, meant for summarizing large volume of data, establishing and determining the magnitude of an effect, and to increase power and precision of studies.

181. **Ans. (c) Randomized clinical trial** *[Ref. Park 25/e p89]*
- RCT is a study in which people are allocated at random (by chance alone) to receive one of several clinical interventions (New drug in this question)
- One of these interventions is the standard of comparison or control group.

182. **Ans. (c) The patients do not know which treatment they are receiving** *[Ref. Park 27/e p91]*

183. **Ans. (c) It helps to eliminate alternative explanations for the results of the study** *[Ref. Park 27/e p90]*

184. **Ans. (a) To equalize the effects of extraneous variables, thus guarding against bias** *[Ref. Park 27/e p90]*

> **ALSO REMEMBER**
> - *Inferential statistics*: Includes inference about a population from a random sample drawn from it or, more generally, about a random process from its observed behavior during a finite period of time,
>   – Point estimation
>   – Interval estimation
>   – Hypothesis testing (statistical significance testing)
>   – Prediction
> - *Placebo*: The placebo effect is a phenomenon in which a physiologically inert treatment, or placebo, improves a patient's condition relative to similar patients who receive no treatment
>   – Inert pills and sham surgeries are typical placebos: Do not directly cause any physiological changes to the body, but patients treated with them tend to improve compared to patients who receive no treatment

185. **Ans. (a) Is a randomized controlled clinical trial**
[Ref. Park 27/e p89-90]

In the given question, a pharmaceutical company develops a new anti-hypertensive drug; samples of 24 hypertensive patients, randomly selected from a large population of hypertensive people, are randomly divided into 2 groups of 12, and one group is given the new drug over a period of 1 month & the other group is given a placebo according to the same schedule,

Since a new drug (intervention) is given it is an experimental/interventional study (not a prospective study which is only observational in design)

Also, there are 2 groups, i.e. experimental group (Intervention – new drug is given) and reference group (no intervention is given – only placebo is given) which are compared concurrently, thus it is a *'Concurrent parallel design of RCT'* (there is no cross-over)

Also, neither the patients nor the treating physicians are aware of which patients are in which group, thus it is a *'double blinded RCT'*

186. **Ans. (c) Randomized control trials** *[Ref. The Medical Journal Of Australia. 2003, (79); 438-40]*

187. **Ans. (d) Equal and known chance** *[Ref. The Concise Oxford English Dictionary, 10/e p1185]*

RANDOM: Implies *'Equal and known chance'*

> **ALSO REMEMBER**
> - Randomisation in Random sampling is to ensure every unit of population has equal chance of being selected
>   – Types of random (Probability/Non-purposive sampling):
>   1. Simple random sampling
>   2. Systematic random sampling
>   3. Stratified random sampling
>   4. Multistage random sampling
>   5. Multiphase random sampling
>   6. Cluster random sampling

188. **Ans. (d) Ensure that the study groups are comparable on base line characteristics** *[Ref. Park 22/e p90 and Epidemiology by Leon Gordis, 4/e p116-17]*

189. **Ans. (c) They use the patient as his or her own control**
[Ref. Handbook of Drug Abuse Prevention by Slobada & Bukoski; p534-35]
- *Pre-post clinical trial:*
  – Does not have a true control group: Patient as his or her own control
  – Each patient has a pre-test score followed by a post-test: Difference in scores reflect change attributed to intervention
  – Use: Is often used in assessing whether knowledge, attitudes or pre-existing risk behaviors change when a subject is assigned to an intervention
  – Limitations:
    1. Difficult to assess if change is due to developmental intercourse
    2. Difficult to assess if change is due to regression to mean

3. Cannot be used for studies involving mortality as post-test won't be available
4. More difficult to interpret than the comparable parallel clinical trial
5. Cannot be randomized

190. **Ans. (c) Randomization** *[Ref. Park 27/e p90]*

191. **Ans. (a) The two groups will be similar in prognostic factors** *[Ref. Park 27/e p90]*

192. **Ans. (c) To eliminate the selection bias** *[Ref. Park 27/e p90]*

193. **Ans. (a) Can't double blind in animal trials; (b) All animal trials are unethical; (c) Can't do interin analysis.**
     [Ref. Internet] [Ref. Park 23/e p89-91]
- Double blinding can be performed in animal trials
- Ethical issues in animal trials is under debate
- Interim analysis can be done in experimental trials
- Experimental trials are longitudinal and prospective.

194. **Ans. (c) Clinical trial phase III** *[Ref. Fundamental of Clinical Trials, 1/e p4]*

CLINICAL TRIALS
- *Phases of a Trial*:

Phase	Unit of study	Purpose
PRE-CLINICAL TRIALS/LAB-EXPERIMENTS		
	Animals	Pretesting in animals
CLINICAL TRIALS		
Phase 0	Healthy Human volunteers	Microdosing
Phase I	Healthy human volunteers	Establishment of safety & non-toxicity
Phase II	Patients	Establishment of effectiveness
Phase III	Patients	Comparison with existing drug(s)
Phase IV	Patients	Assessment of long term side effects

- *Phase III is a RCT*: Comparison of a new drug with an existing old drug
- *Longest phase of a trial*: Phase IV
- *New drug is launched in market after*: Phase III
- *Post-marketing surveillance*: Phase IV

195. **Ans. (a) Randomised controlled trial**
     [An introduction to clinical research, 1/e p182]
- RCTs are considered centerpiece of research evidence as they represent the Gold standard for testing new interventions in Clinical research trials
- Systematic reviews and quantitative meta-analyses have been suggested as an even higher level of evidence, because they provide even higher level of evidence in epidemiology

196. **Ans. (d) Dropouts are excluded from the study**
     [Ref. Park 27/e p90-91]

197. **Ans. (a) Phase 1** *[Ref. Prospectives on Cancer Care by Fawcett, 1/e p183]*
- Phase 1 Clinical trials is used to evaluate Maximum tolerated dose (MTD) of a new drug

198. **Ans. (b) 2** *[Ref. Targeted Regulatory Writing Techniques by Foote, 1/e p14]*

199. **Ans. (d) The validity does not depend on quality of systemic review** *[Ref. Doing meta-analysis in research: A systematic approach by Dr Vivek Jain, IJDVL, 2012;78:242-50]*

META-ANALYSIS
- *Description*: Uses a statistical approach to combine the results from multiple studies in an effort to increase power (over individual studies), improve estimates of the size of the effect and/or to resolve uncertainty when reports disagree
  - Meta-analysis is an objective, systematic review that employs statistical methods to combine and summarize the results of several studies
  - It is a quantitative synthesis of all the unbiased evidence, meant for summarizing large volume of data, establishing and determining the magnitude of an effect, and to increase power and precision of studies
- *Strengths of Meta-analysis*:
  - Provides a point estimate of an effect size: It tends to increase power
  - May help to 'Identify few gaps' in a particular field
- *Limitations of Meta-analysis*:
  - 'GIGO principle - Garbage-in, garbage-out procedure': Results can only be as good as the original data is valid, so quality of Systematic review is important
  - 'Apples and oranges effect': Tendency to average/mash together disparate effects which may have resulted from the heterogeneity of the studies
  - 'File drawer effect': Publication bias
  - Meta-analysis 'relies on shared subjectivity' rather than objectivity

200. **Ans. (a) Meta-analysis always performed**
     [Ref. Evidence Based Dermatology by Williams, 2/e p38]

SYSTEMATIC REVIEW
- *Description*: A document related after comprehensively reviewing and combining all the information from both published and unpublished studies (focusing on a particular clinical or health related topic/question) and then summarizing the findings
- *Steps of Systematic Review*:
  - Asking a clear, focused question
  - Explicit through search of literature
  - Data extraction
  - Critical appraisal of quality of primary studies
  - Quantitative pooling of data
  - Interpretation of data, including implications for clinical practice and further research

> **ALSO REMEMBER**
> - Meta-analysis can (and should) be embedded in a systematic review, but this is not always done
> - A single systematic review can contain multiple meta-analyses

201. **Ans. (d) Increases external validity of study**
     [Ref. Experimental Designs by Todmann, 2/e p9]

RANDOMISATION IN RCT
- Reduction of selection

- Ensure comparability of both groups
- Ensure similar prognostic factors in both groups
- Facilitates blinding of treatment
- Increases Internal validity of study

202. **Ans. (c) Includes Randomized controlled trials**
 [Ref. Park 27/e p94]

 Natural Experiments
 - If experimental studies not possible, then natural circumstances can be used in human populations that mimic an experimental study
 - 'Nature' subjects a particular study group to an intervention; the natural experiment can be used to estimate effects of the intervention for that study group
 - Populations that can be used: Migrant populations, Religious groups, Populations affected by nuclear disaster/natural disaster
 - John Snow Cholera study is an experiment of Natural experiment study

203. **Ans. (c) Cross over trial** *[Ref. Park 27/e p91]*

 Types of RCT
 - Concurrent parallel design: Comparisons are made between 2 groups:
   - *Experimental group: Is exposed to specific medication or intervention*
   - *Reference group: Is not exposed to specific medication or intervention*
 - Crossover design: Comparisons are made between 2 groups:
   - *Experimental group: Is exposed to specific medication or intervention*
   - *Reference group: Is not exposed to specific medication or intervention*
   - *Then the groups are crossed-over (exposed group now becomes non-exposed and vice-versa)*
   - *Cross-over design RCT helps removing ethical concerns*

204. **Ans. (a) Cross-over study**
 [Ref. Epidemiology by Talley 1/e p95]

 Crossover Design
 - Cross-over design is a repeated measurements design such that each experimental unit (patient) receives different treatments during the different time periods
 - Cases act as their own controls: Patients cross-over from one treatment arm to another during the course of the trial
 - Advantages: Confounding is reduced, Require fewer study subjects
 - Crossover is in contrast to a Parallel design: Patients are randomized to a treatment and remain on that treatment throughout the duration of the trial

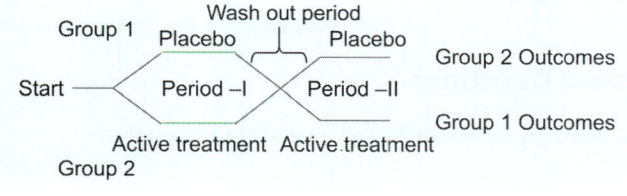

Cross-over Design

205. **Ans. (c) Randomized controlled trial in patients is done in phase 3** *[Ref. Park 27/e p89-92]*

 Clinical Trials

Phase	Purpose
Phase 0 (Healthy human volunteers)	Microdosing
Phase 1 (Healthy human volunteers)	Safety and non-toxicity profile of the drug Maximum tolerated dose of a drug
Phase 2 (Patients)	Efficacy
Phase 3 (Patients)	Comparison with existing drugs (RCT*)
Phase 4 (Patients)	Long term and rare side effects Post-marketing surveillance

(* Phase 3 has a comparison or controlled group)

Review Questions

206. **Ans. (c) Before and after comparison studies**
 [Ref. Park 21/e p79, Park 22/e p80, 27/e p92-93]
207. **Ans. (c) Both observer and person or group being observed is blind about the study** *[Ref. Park 27/e p91]*

ASSOCIATION AND CAUSATION

208. **Ans. (c) Specificity of association** *[Ref. Park 27/e p97-99]*

 HILL'S (Surgeon General's) CRITERIA OF CAUSAL ASSOCIATION:
 - *Temporal association*:
   - Implies 'cause precedes effect' or 'effect follows cause'
   - Considers both 'order of appearance' as well as 'length of interval between exposure and disease'
   - Is 'most important criterion' of causal association
   - Is 'best established by a cohort study' (Especially Concurrent cohort study)
 - *Strength of association*:
   - Relative risk (cohort study)
   - Odds ratio (case control study)
 - *Specificity of association*:
   - Implies that disease under study is caused only by risk factor under study
   - Is 'most difficult criterion to establish'
   - Is 'weakest criterion' of causal association
 - *Consistency of association*:
   - Implies that results are replicable in different settings and by different methods
 - *Biological plausibility*:
   - Implies existence of biological credibility of association (anatomically, physiologically explainable/justifiable)
 - *Coherence of association*:
   - Implies that the causal association must be coherent (supported by) with relevant facts/related studies
 - *Dose-response relationship*:
   - Implies that increase in dose of cause increases incidence/prevalence of effect
 - *Cessation of exposure; Reversibility*:
   - Implies that removal of possible cause reduces the risk of disease

- *Study design*:
  - Implies that if study design is based on a strong study design
  - Abilities of epidemiological study designs to prove causality:

Type of study	Ability to prove causation
Randomised controlled trial	Strong
Cohort study	Moderate
Case control study	Moderate
Cross sectional study	Weak
Ecological study	Ecological study

ALSO REMEMBER

- *Judging the evidence for causal association*:
  - Temporality of association (Highest weight given)
  - Biological plausibility
  - Consistency of association and
  - Dose-response relationship
- Hill's criteria (sometimes also known as *'Surgeon General's Criteria'* of causal association) in epidemiology are ANALOGOUS TO Koch's Postulates (of causal association between a microbe and disease) in Microbiology

209. Ans. (c) Randomized control trials *[Ref. Epidemiology by Leon Gordis, 4/e p221 and Basic Epidemiology by Beaglehole, WHO; p80]*

210. Ans. (d) Incorrect because as no control or comparison group was involved
[Ref. Epidemiology by Leon Gordis, 4/e p 117]
- An epidemiological study is characterized by presence of a *control/comparison group*: Without a comparison group it is difficult to ascribe the causality of risk factor/exposure to a disease
- **COMPARISON GROUPS IN EPIDEMIOLOGICAL STUDIES:**

Type of study	First group	Comparison group
Cohort study	Exposed group (presence of risk factor/exposure)	Non-exposed group (absence of risk factor/exposure)
Case control study	Cases group (diseased persons)	Controls group (non-diseased persons)
Randomized controlled trial	Experimental group (intervention given)	Reference group (no intervention given)

- If no comparison group is chosen in epidemiological studies:
  - In a Cohort study: Strength of association (Relative Risk) between risk factor (exposure) and disease cannot be determined
  - In a case control study: Strength of association (Odds Ratio) between disease and risk factor (exposure) cannot be determined
  - In a Randomized controlled trial: Actual outcome cannot be ascribed to the intervention

In the given question, an advertisement in a medical journal stated that 2000 subjects with sore throat were treated with their new medicine and with in 4 days, 94% were asymptomatic; the advertisement claims that the medicine was effective

Since, no comparison group (Reference group – Patients without new medicine treatment or placebo-treated) was used in the study, there is a possibility that the effect (asymptomatic) could be spontaneous (for e.g. reduction of fever) or due to some other factor (for e.g. environmental) **Thus** the above claim is false/incorrect

211. Ans. (b) Ecological study *[Ref. Epidemiology by Leon Gordis, 4/e p204 and Basic Epidemiology by Beaglehole, WHO; p80]*

212. Ans. (c) Cohort study *[Ref. Basic Epidemiology by Beaglehole, WHO; p41]*
- Most preferable observational/analytical study design: Cohort study
- Least preferable observational/analytical study design: Ecological study
- Useful Parameter(s) obtained by epidemiological studies:

Epidemiological studies	Useful parameter(s) obtained
Cohort study	Incidence, Relative risk, Attributable risk, Population attributable risk
Case control study	Odds ratio
Cross sectional study	Prevalence
Ecological study	Group characteristics

ALSO REMEMBER

- *Applications of various study designs*:

Application	Utility of study			
	Cohort	Case-control	Cross-sectional	Ecological
Investigation of rare disease	–	+++++	–	++++
Investigation of rare cause	+++++	–	–	++
Testing multiple effects	+++++	–	++	+
Study of multiple exposure	+++	++++	++	++
Measurement of time relationship	+++++	+	–	++
Direct incidence measurement	+++++	+	–	–
Investigation of long latent periods	+	+++	–	–

213. Ans. (b) Temporal relationship *[Ref. Park 27/e p97]*
214. Ans. (b) Temporality *[Ref. Park 27/e p97]*
215. Ans. (a) RCT *[Ref. Contemporary Drug Information by Gleason, 1/e p65]*

Review Questions

216. Ans. (d) Reversibility or reversible association *[Ref. Park 27/e p99]*

217. Ans. (d) Indirect association *[Ref. Park 27/e p96]*

Epidemiology and Vaccines | 207

EPIDEMIOLOGY OF INFECTIOUS DISEASES

218. **Ans. (b) 48 hours** *[Ref. Park 25/e p102, 387]*
   - Nosocomial infection is defined as that occurring 48 hours after admission to the hospital and excluding any infection that is present in Incubation period at the time of admission
   - MC subtype: UTI

219. **Ans. (b) Anthropozoonoses** *[Ref. Park 27/e p101-102]*
   - ZOONOSES
     – *Anthropozoonoses*: Infections transmitted from animals (zoo) to man (anthro):
       1. Rabies
       2. Plague
       3. Anthrax
       4. Hydatid disease
       5. Trichinosis
     – *Zooanthroponoses*: Infections transmitted from man (anthro) to animals (zoo):
       1. Human TB in cattle
     – *Amphixenosis*: Infections transmitted in either direction between animals and man:
       1. Trypanosoma cruzi
       2. Schistosoma japonicum

220. **Ans. (b) Is constantly present in a given population group** *[Ref. Park 27/e p101]*
   - *Endemic*: refers to the 'usual or expected frequency of disease' within a population group; is the 'constant presence of a disease in a defined geographical area'
     – *Hyperendemic*: When a disease is constantly present at a high incidence and/or prevalence rate and affects all age groups equally.
     – *Holoendemic*: When a disease has a high level of infection beginning early in life and affects most of children population. So, disease is more common among children than adults
   - *Endemic curve*: Is drawn between no. of cases due to a disease and the time
     – Endemic curve IS NOT a straight line: as number of cases for the endemic disease in a population will not be fixed throughout a year; it will show a seasonal or other variation
     – Endemic curve Vs epidemic curve: In endemic curve, the baseline of the curve NEVER touches zero
   - When a disease occurs 'clearly in excess of normal expectancy', it becomes an *Epidemic*
   - *Endemic*: of or relating to a disease that originates outside the geographical area in which it occurs

221. **Ans. (c) Sporadic** *[Ref. Park 27/e p101]*

222. **Ans. (d) To estimate the fatality of the disease** *[Ref. Park 27/e p47]*

223. **Ans. (b) Infectivity** *[Ref. Internet] [Ref. Park 22/e p100]*
   - *Infectivity*: Number infected/Number exposed
   - *Pathogenicity*: Number of diseased/Number infected
   - *Virulence*: Number of serious condition & mortality/Number diseased
   - *Case fatality*: Number of deaths/Number of cases
   - *Communicability*: Ability of a disease to spread from infective to susceptible hosts

224. **Ans. (b) Influenza-A** *[Ref. Park 26/e p166-167]*
   - Hepatitis B is endemic throughout the world
   - Influenza B and C doesnot cause Pandemics

225. **Ans. (b) Rabies** *[Ref. Park 27/e p322]*

226. **Ans. (a) Measles; (b) Mumps; (d) Hepatitis B; (e) Poliomyelitis** *[Ref. Park 27/e p104]*

227. **Ans. (b) Direct contact** *[Ref. Park 23/e p102, 388]*
   TRANSMISSION OF NOSOCOMIAL INFECTIONS
   - Direct contact: person-to-person transmission
     – Hands of the clinical personnel are MC vehicles for nosocomial infections
   - Indirect contact: Susceptible person comes in contact with contaminated object
   - Droplet transmission
   - Vector borne transmission

Review Questions

228. **Ans. (d) Instruments** *[Ref. Park 27/e p410-412]*
229. **Ans. (b) Nosocomial infections** *[Ref. Park 27/e p322]*
230. **Ans. (c) Exotic disease** *[Ref. Park 21/e p89, Park 22/e p90, 27/e p101]*

DISEASE TRANSMISSION

231. **Ans. (a) Time taken for 50% cases to occur** *[Ref. Park 25/e p107]*
   - Median incubation period means Time taken for 50% cases to occur for a disease in a community in a given time period

232. **Ans. (a) Measles** *[Ref. Transmission-Based Precautions : Infection Control Basics, CDC]*
   Transmission based Precautions
   - *Airborne precautions:* Used for patients infected with pathogens transmitted by the airborne route (Droplet nuclei <5 microns; E.g. TB, Measles, Chickenpox, Disseminated herpes zoster)
   - *Droplet precautions:* Used for patients infected with pathogens transmitted by respiratory droplets that are generated by a patient who is coughing, sneezing, or talking (Droplets >5 microns; E.g. Diphtheria, Mumps, Rubella, Pneumonia, Streptococcal pharyngitis)
   - *Contact precautions:* Used for patients with infections that represent an increased risk for contact transmission (E.g. Shigella, Herpes, Scabies, MDR organisms, Major wound infections)

233. **Ans. (a) Brucellosis** *[Ref. Park 27/e p103]*
   - *Source*: Is a person, animal, object or substance from which an infectious agent passes or is disseminated to the host.
     – Source refers to immediate source of infection & may or may not be part of reservoir

- *Reservoir*: Is any person, animal, arthropod, plant, soil or substance (or combination of these) in which an infectious agent lives & multiplies, on which it primarily depends for survival, & where it reproduces itself in such a manner that it can be transmitted to a susceptible host.

Infection	Source	Reservoir
Hookworm	Soil	Man
Tetanus	Soil	Soil
Typhoid	Feces/urine/Food/Milk/Water	Case/Carrier

- *Human Reservoir*:
  - Cases: Persons having particular disease, health disorder or condition under investigation
  - Carriers: Infected person or animal that harbours a specific agent in the absence of discernible clinical disease, & serves as a potential source of infection for others. Carriers are less infectious than cases but are more dangerous epidemiologically.
- *Animal reservoir*, e.g. Rabies, Influenza, Yellow Fever, Histoplasmosis
- *Reservoir in non-living things*, e.g. Soil harbour agents for Tetanus, Anthrax, Cocciomycosis, Mycetoma

> **ALSO REMEMBER**
> - *Reservoir(s) of important diseases*:
>
> | Disease | Microorganism | Reservoir(s) |
> |---|---|---|
> | Epidemic Typhus | Rickettsia prowazekii | Humans |
> | Endemic Typhus | Rickettsia typhi | Rats |
> | Scrub Typhus | Rickettsia tsutsugamushi | Trombiculid Mite |
> | Indian Tick Typhus | Rickettsia conori | Rodents |
> | RMSF | Rickettsia rickettsii | Rodents |
> | Rickettsial Pox | Rickettsia akari | Mice |
> | Trench fever | Bartonella quintana | Humans |
> | Q fever | Coxiella burnetti | Cattle, sheep, goat |
> | Dracunculiasis | Dracunculus medinensis | Humans |
> | Ascariasis | Ascaris lumbricoides | Humans |
> | Ancylostomiasis | Ancylostoma duodenale | Humans |

- *Secondary Attack Rate (SAR)*: Is no. of exposed persons developing the disease within range of incubation period (IP), following exposure to the primary case

$$SAR = \frac{\text{No. of exposed persons developing disease within range of IP}}{\text{Total no. of exposed 'susceptible' contacts}} \times 100$$

  - Denominator includes only those susceptible to disease
  - Primary case is always excluded both from numerator and denominator for SAR calculation

> **ALSO REMEMBER**
> - *Incubation period depends upon*:
>   - Generation time of the pathogen
>   - Infective dose
>   - Portal of entry
>   - Individual susceptibility
> - *Incubation period of a disease is useful for*:
>   - Tracing the source of infection and contacts
>   - Determining the period of surveillance
>   - Applying immunization principles for prevention of diseases
>   - Identification of point source or propagated epidemics
>   - Estimating prognosis of a disease
> - *Latent period*: Is the period from disease initiation to disease detection, used in non-infectious diseases as equivalent of incubation period
> - *Serial interval*: is the gap in onset between primary case (first case in the community) and secondary case (case developing through infection from the primary case)
>   - By collecting information on series of secondary cases with serial intervals, one can guess the incubation period of a disease
> - *Period of communicability*: is the time during which an infectious agent may be transferred directly/indirectly from an infected person to another person, from infected animal to man or from an infected person to animal, including arthropods
>   - An important measure of communicability is secondary attack rate
> - *Secondary Attack Rate (SAR) of few diseases*:
>
> | Disease | Secondary Attack Rate (SAR) |
> |---|---|
> | Smallpox | 30 – 45% |
> | Measles | > 80% |
> | Chickenpox | ~ 90% |
> | Mumps | ~ 86% |
> | Pertussis | ~ 90% |

234. **Ans. (b) Median incubation period** *[Ref. Park 27/e p107]*
- *Incubation period*: is the time interval between invasion by an infectious agent and appearance of the first sign or symptom of the disease in question
- *Median incubation period*: Is the time required for 50% of cases to occur following exposure
- *Generation time*: is the time taken for a person from receipt of infection to develop maximum infectivity
  - Is roughly equal to the incubation period of the disease

235. **Ans. (d) 100%** *[Ref. Park 27/e p108]*
In the given question,
- There is a 6-membered family, comprising of two parents and four children
- On 12 August 2006, one of the children got measles, so she/he is the primary case by 18 August 2006, 2 other siblings also got measles, so they are the secondary cases
- Parents are *not susceptible* (in a country like India), one of the children (3 yr old) is completely immunized for his

age thus she/he is *not-susceptible*, and primary case is *not included* in numerator or denominator
- Therefore, total no. of susceptibles in the family:
  6 – 2 – 1 – 1 = 2
  So, SAR = 2/2× 100 = 100%

Interpretation: *All of those susceptible develop the disease* from primary case within range of incubation period

236. **Ans. (d) 65%** *[Ref. Park 27/e p108]*
- **In the given question**, a village has 100 under five children and the coverage of measles vaccine is 60%; following a measles case 26 children developed measles,
- Since coverage of Measles vaccine is 60%, 60% of 100 children i.e. 60 children are vaccinated (not susceptible to Measles)
- So only 40 children are susceptible to Measles
- Out of 40 children, 1 child develops Measles (primary case) and then out of rest 39 susceptible (primary case excluded from denominator), 26 develop Measles
- Therefore, SAR = 26/39 × 100 = 66%

Interpretation: *Two-thirds of those susceptible develop the disease* from primary case within range of incubation period.

> **ALSO REMEMBER**
> - *Cases in epidemiology*:
>   - Primary case: First case of communicable disease introduced into the population unit being studied
>   - Index case: First case that comes to the notice of the investigator (first case reported to the health system)
>   - Secondary cases: Cases that develop from contact with the primary case
> - Attack rate (AR):
>   - Relates to no. of cases in the population at risk
>   - Reflects extent of epidemic
>   - Is used when 'population is exposed to risk for a limited period of time, such as epidemic'
>
> $$AR = \frac{\text{No. of new cases of specified disease in a specified time interval}}{\text{Total population at risk during the same time interval}} \times 100$$

237. **Ans. (b) The interval of time between the receipt of infection by host and maximal infectivity of the host**
[Ref. Park 27/e p108]

	Generation time	Incubation period (IP)
Definition	Is the time taken for a person from receipt of infection to develop maximum infectivity	Is time interval between invasion by an infectious agent & appearance of first sign or symptom of disease in question
Remark	Is roughly equal to the IP of the disease	Median IP: Is the time required for 50% of cases to occur following exposure
Applicability	Transmissions of infections whether clinical	Infections that result in manifest disease or subclinical

238. **Ans. (b) Period of communicability**
[Ref. Park 27/e p105-105]

> **ALSO REMEMBER**
> - *Generally communicable disease are not communicable in incubation period EXCEPT*:
>   - Measles
>   - Chickenpox
>   - Whooping cough (Pertussis)
>   - Hepatitis A

239. **Ans. (a) 60%** *[Ref. Park 27/e p108]*
In the given question, A family consists of 2 parents & 6 children susceptible to measles. There occurs a primary case of measles and 3 secondary cases within a short period of time. Thus, **numerator is 3** (*Primary case is excluded from numerator*).
Now denominator includes those susceptible to disease (and in close contact)
Both parents cannot be considered susceptible (*In a country like India, measles infection is quite common in 6 months – 3 years age, virtually affecting everyone. ALSO, like infection, vaccine too provides lifelong immunity*)
There are 6 children, but since one is a primary case, he shall be excluded from the denominator.
Thus 6 MINUS 1 = 5 are only susceptible
Therefore, **Denominator is 5**
So, **SAR** = 3/5 ×100 = **60%**

Interpretation: *Two-fifths of those susceptible develop the disease* from primary case within range of incubation period

240. **Ans. (c) All susceptibles amongst close contact**
[Ref. Park 27/e p108]
- Secondary Attack Rate (SAR): Is no. of exposed persons developing the disease within range of incubation period, following exposure to the primary case
- Denominator includes *only those susceptible* to disease
- Primary case is always excluded both from numerator and denominator for SAR calculation
- **For Example:** In a pre-nursery class of 100 students, 33 students are already immunized for measles and 33 others had suffered from measles previously. Then a student 'Rohit' develops measles one day and 22 other students develop measles subsequently in the next week. What is the SAR?

Solution: 22 other students develop measles within incubation period (IP of Measles: 10-14 days) from primary case 'Rohit'. Thus, **numerator is 22** (*Primary case 'Rohit' is excluded from numerator*).
Now denominator includes those susceptible to disease (and in close contact)
33 students are immunized already, therefore they are not susceptible (*Immunization confers life long immunity to infections like measles*)
33 students have suffered from measles previously, therefore they are not susceptible (*Natural infection confers life long immunity to infections like measles and chickenpox*)

Thus 100 MINUS (33 + 33) = 34 are only susceptible

Therefore, **Denominator is 33** (34 MINUS 1; as *Primary case 'Rohit' is excluded from denominator also*)

So, **SAR** = 22/33 ×100 = **66%**

Interpretation: Two-thirds of those susceptible develop the disease from primary case within range of incubation period.

> **ALSO REMEMBER**
> - In measles disease, both natural infection and vaccination confers life long immunity/protection from infection of measles.

241. Ans. (a) Time gap between primary and secondary case [Ref. Park 25/e p108]
242. Ans. (a) AIDS [Ref. Park 25/e p364]
243. Ans. (c) Cyclo-developmental transmission [Ref. Park 25/e p106]
244. Ans. (d) Typhoid [Ref. Park 21/e p91, Park 22/e p92, 25/e p104]
245. Ans. (b) "Reservoir" and "Source" of infection are synonymous [Ref. Park 25/e p102]
246. Ans. (d) Infectious disease are not communicable during IP [Ref. Park 25/e p104]
247. Ans. (a) Pertussis; (c) Measles [Ref. Park 25/e p104]
248. Ans. (c) Mumps; (d) Measles; (e) Influenza [Ref. Park 25/e p104]
249. Ans. ALL CHOICES [Ref. Park 25/e p132]
    - *Isolation*: Separation for the period of communicability of persons/animals from others to prevent disease transmission

Disease	Duration of isolation
Chicken pox	6 days after onset of rash
Measles	Onset of catarrhal to 3rd day of rash
German Measles	NONE (except Ist trimester of pregnancy)
Cholera, Diphtheria	3 days after tetracyclines started till 48 hours of antibiotics
Shigellosis, Salmonellosis	Until 3 consecutive negative stool cultures
Hepatitis A	3 weeks
Influenza	3 days after onset
Polio	2 weeks adult, 6 weeks paediatric
Tuberculosis	Until 3 weeks of effective chemotherapy
Herpes zoster	6 days after onset of rash
Mumps	Until swelling subsides
Pertussis	4 weeks or until paroxysms cease
Meningococcal meningitis	Until first 6 hours antibiotics completed
Streptococcal pahryngitis	Until first 6 hours antibiotics completed

250. Ans. (a) Polio; (b) Diphtheria; (c) Leprosy; (d) Pneumonic plague [Ref. Park 27/e p133]
251. Ans. (a) Polio; (b) Cholera; (c) Pertussis [Ref. Park 27/e p104]
252. Ans. (a) Cholera; (b) Influenza; (c) Plague [Ref. Park 27/e p172, 270, 339]
253. Ans. (b) Diphtheria; (c) Cholera; (d) Typhoid [Ref. Park 27/e p104]
254. Ans. (b) Maximum incubation period [Ref. Park 27/e p133]
255. Ans. (c) Index case [Ref. Park 27/e p103]
256. Ans. (b) To find out time for isolation [Ref. Park 27/e p133]
257. Ans. (c) Malaria [Ref. Park 27/e p104]
258. Ans. (d) Rubella – Until 7 days after appearance of rash [Ref. Park 27/e p133]
259. Ans. (c) Exposure to laboratory detection of disease [Ref. Practical transfusion Medicine by Murphy, 3/e]

> **ALSO REMEMBER**
> **MODES OF TRANSMISSION**
>
> | Direct transmission | Indirect transmission |
> |---|---|
> | Direct contact | Vehicle-borne |
> | Droplet infection | Vector-borne (Mechanical/biological) |
> | Soil contact | Air-borne (Droplet nuclei/dust) |
> | Inoculation (Skin/mucosa) | Fomite-borne |
> | Vertical/transplacental | Unclean hands/fingers |

260. Ans. (c) Meningococcal meningitis [Ref. Park 27/e p104]
    Healthy carriers
    - Emerge from subclinical cases without suffering from overt disease, but continue to shed the infectious agent
    - Examples: Cholera, Diphtheria, Meningococcal Meningitis, Poliomyelitis, Salmonellosis
261. Ans. (b) Number of cases developing disease within incubation period following exposure to primary care [Ref. Park 27/e p108]
262. Ans. (c) 80% [Ref. Park 27/e p108]
    - SAR = No of secondary cases in one IP/Total susceptible in close contact × 100

    In the given question,
    - Primary cases = 5, Secondary cases developing in one IP = 28
    - Immunization gives immunity against Chicken pox (So, 10 children were already immune)
    - Primary cases are excluded from both numerator and denominator

    So, SAR = 28/(50 – 10 – 5) × 100 = 28/35 × 100 = 80%
263. Ans. (b) Secondary attack rate [Ref. Park 27/e p108]
    Special types of Incidence Rates
    - Attack rate: Incidence rate used when population is exposed for a small interval of time, e.g. epidemic
    - Secondary Attack Rate (SAR): Is no. of exposed persons developing the disease within range of incubation period, following exposure to the primary case

Epidemiology and Vaccines

264. Ans. (b) Pertussis *[Ref. Park 27/e p133]*
- Pertussis bacteria are spread from person to person in airborne droplets or by direct contact with infected throat or nasal discharges
- Period of Isolation for Pertussis: 4 weeks or until paroxysms disease

265. Ans. (d) who gets infected from another carrier
[Ref. Essentials of Microbiology for Nurses by Kannan 1/e p36]
Types of Carriers
- Contact carrier: Carrier who gets infected from a case
- Paradoxical carrier: Carrier who gets infected from another carrier
- Chronic carrier: Carrier who sheds organism for > 6 months duration
- Incubatory carrier: Carrier who sheds organism even during Incubation period
- Convalescent carrier: Carrier who sheds organism even during Recovery
- Pseudo-carrier: Carrier of avirulent organisms

Review Questions

266. Ans. (d) Rabies, tetanus *[Ref. Park 27/e p323, 358]*
267. Ans. (a) Typhoid *[Ref. Park 27/e p105]*
268. Ans. (a) Transplacental *[Ref. Park 27/e p105]*
269. Ans. (a) Cyclopropagative *[Ref. Park 27/e p106]*
270. Ans. (c) Both *[Ref. Park 27/e p302, 350]*

INVESTIGATION OF AN EPIDEMIC

271. Ans. (c) No new case reported for twice the incubation period of disease since the last case
[Ref. Park 22/e p123, 24/e p144]
- Searching for more cases: Search for new cases is carried out everyday, till the area is declared free of epidemic; this period is usually taken as '*twice the incubation period of the disease since the occurrence of last case*'

272. Ans. (c) Verification of diagnosis *[Ref. Park 27/e p147]*
- *Verification of diagnosis*:
  Is the '*first step in investigation of an epidemic*'
  It is '*not necessary to examine all cases*': take sample
  Do not wait for laboratory results for epidemiological investigations

IMMUNITY, VACCINES AND COLD CHAIN

273. Ans. *[Ref. Park 27/e p111]*
- T lymphocyte (cell-mediated and humoral) related disorders with partial defect - Wiskott-Aldrich syndrome, Ataxia telangiectasia, Digeorge syndrome: Live vaccines are contraindicated
- *Complement deficiency*: All routine vaccines effective; Pneumococcal and meningococcal vaccines recommended

274. Ans. (b) Give DT only at next visit *[Ref. Park 27/e p181]*
DPT AEFIs
- Minor illnesses like cough, cold, mild fever are NOT contraindications to next dose of DPT
- Severe reactions (Collapse, shock like state, persistent crying, fever above 40 degrees C, convulsions, neurological symptoms and anaphylaxis): Pertussis is not given in subsequent doses; ONLY DT should be given

275. Ans. (c) Td Vaccine *[Ref. Park 27/e p136]*
- As per National Immunization Schedule (RCH Program, NHM) at the age of 10 years a child is expected to get TT vaccine (now replaced by Td vaccine in India)

276. Ans. (b) 1, 2 *[Ref. Park 27/e p121]*

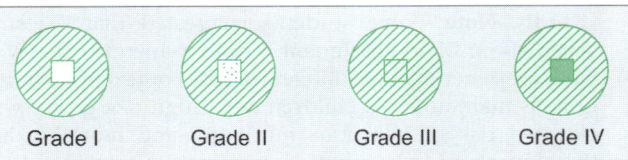

- Vaccine Vial Monitor (VVM) is a marker of potency: VVM is a simple tool which enables vaccinator to know if vaccine is potent at the time of administration
- VVM is a label containing a heat-sensitive material which is placed on a vaccine vial to register cumulative heat exposure over time
- Based on VVM, vaccine is usable only if the inner square is lighter than outer circle

277. Ans. (a) 1-2 dose
[Ref. One-dose HPV vaccine offers solid protection against cervical cancer, 11 April 2022 News release, WHO]

SAGE recommends updating dose schedules for HPV
- One or two-dose schedule for the primary target of girls aged 9-14
- One or two-dose schedule for young women aged 15-20
- Two doses with a 6-month interval for women older than 21

278. Ans. (b) Meningococcal vaccine; (d) Varicella Zoster vaccine *[Ref. Immunization in Older Adults, Issue 21, 2007]*

CDC GUIDELINES FOR IMMUNIZATION OF OLDER PEOPLE
- Influenza intramuscular inactivated vaccine
- Pneumococcal vaccine once
- Tetanus-diphtheria toxoid (Td) booster every 10 years
- In selected patients aged 60 years or more: Herpes zoster (shingles), Hepatitis A, Hepatitis B, Meningococcal disease, Varicella, MMR, Yellow fever vaccine (for travellers)

279. Ans. (c) Give 2nd dose *[Ref. Park 26/e p180]*
- If there is delayed immunization in DPT doses, there is no need to repeat the schedule from start; just continue the schedule

280. Ans. (c) Use Pentavalent vial & discard MR vial
[Ref. Park 26/e p120]
Open Vial Policy
- Opened vaccine vials can be used in subsequent session 'UPTO 4 WEEKS'
- Applicable for Vaccines: OPV, DPT, Hepatitis B, TT, Liquid Pentavalent, IPV, HiB, PCV
- Not applicable for Vaccines: Measles, BCG, JE, Rotavirus, COVID-19 vaccines

281. **Ans. (c) TT/Td** [Ref. Park 26/e p135]
   - As per National Immunization Schedule (RCH Program, NHM) at the age of 10 years a child is expected to get TT vaccine (gradually being replaced by Td vaccine in India
   - In MR (Measles-Rubella campaign), 9 months – 15 years old children are being targeted through schools, community centers and health facilities

282. **Ans. (b) Measles/MMR** [Ref. Park 27/e p164]
   - Live Vaccines (e.g. Measles, MMR) are contraindicated in immunocompromised situations.
   [**Kindly Note:** Some students suggested that Question asked about Malnourishment. Kindly remember that Vaccines are generally immunogenic in the context of malnutrition, as malnourished children are a high-risk group with elevated risk of infectious morbidity and mortality and therefore stand to benefit from vaccination even more than well-nourished children. Malnourished children respond well to DPT, Hepatitis B, HiB, Measles, Pneumococcal, Typhoid killed and Rabies vaccines. Malnourished children response is not clear for Meningococcal and BCG vaccines]

283. **Ans. (c) DPT, Hepatitis B, Hemophilus influenzae B** [Ref. Park 26/e p113]
   Pentavalent Vaccine
   - Vaccine contains five antigens (Diphtheria, Pertussis, Tetanus, Hepatitis B and Haemophilus influenzae type b)
   - The number of injections administered under UIP during the first year of life reduces from nine to six
   - Started for any child aged more than 6 weeks and can be given up to 1 year of age
   - A child whose vaccination schedule has been initiated with DPT/hepatitis B vaccine will continue to receive subsequent doses of DPT/hepatitis B and not Pentavalent Vaccine

284. **Ans. (c) Subdeltoid/subacromial bursa**
   [Ref. Subacromial-subdeltoid bursitis following COVID-19 vaccination: a case of shoulder injury related to vaccine administration (SIRVA) Skeletal Radiol. 2021:1–5. doi: 10.1007/s00256-021-03803-x by Rodrigues et al]

   Shoulder injury related to vaccine administration (SIRVA)
   - Shoulder pain and limited range of motion occurring after the administration of a vaccine intended for intramuscular administration in the upper arm
   - Influenza is the most frequently vaccine reported
   - In such cases, subacromial-subdeltoid bursitis may occur, leading to shoulder dysfunction and ongoing pain

285. **Ans. (c) Rotavirus vaccine** [Ref. Park 26/e p264]
   - Potential complication of Rotavirus vaccines: Intussusception (when first dose given after 12 weeks age), so preferably avoided in catch-up campaigns where exact age of vaccine is difficult to ascertain

286. **Ans. (d) L1, L2**
   [Ref. Human Cancer Viruses by Nicholas 1/e Vol1 p46]

HPV Genome
- Circular double stranded DNA genome containing 800 base pairs
  - Encodes 6 Early genes (E1, E2, E4, E5, E6, E7) and 2 Late genes (L1, L2)
  - Early genes regulate DNA viral replication, Late genes encode Viral capsid
- HPV vaccines target L1, L2 genes: Capsid proteins of L1, L2 act as Target antigens
  - L1 is targeted more by Cervarix, Gardasil
  - L2 based vaccines are cheaper but less immunogenic

287. **Ans. (a), (b), (c), (d)** [Ref. Park 26/e p111]
   Vaccination guidelines of Kid has to be started on Steroids
   - Vaccinate as per schedule UNLESS child is on Prednisolone only for minimum 1 week
   - Live are avoided in immunosuppression, Killed/other vaccines are safe: Give Pneumococcal vaccine as per schedule
   - OPV is not given to close household contacts and siblings when case under study is under high dose steroids
   - Live vaccines CAN BE GIVEN in steroids only if its low dose steroids that too on alternate day regimen

288. **Ans. (c) VVM** [Ref. Park 26/e p121]
   - Vaccine Vial Monitor (VVM) is a marker of potency: VVM is a simple tool which enables vaccinator to know if vaccine is potent at the time of administration
   - VVM is a label containing a heat-sensitive material which is placed on a vaccine vial to register cumulative heat exposure over time

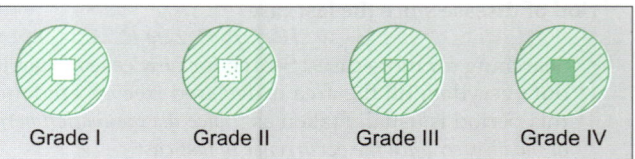

289. **Ans. (c) Toxoid** [Ref. Park 26/e p113]
   - Toxoid vaccines are prepared by detoxification of toxins produced by organisms
   - Highly efficacious and safe
   - Examples: Tetanus, Diphtheria

290. **Ans. (d) Universal immunization** [Ref. Park 25/e p477]
   Mission Indradhanush 2014
   - Indradhanush depicting seven colors of the rainbow, aims to cover all those children by 2020 who are either unvaccinated, or are partially vaccinated against 7 vaccine preventable diseases (7 VPD's)
   - Now it includes 12 diseases to be covered

291. **Ans. (b) Gardasil** [Ref. CDC Website]
   Newer Vaccines
   - Cervarix: Bivalent HPV 16, 18
   - Gardasil: Quadrivalent HPV 16, 18, 6, 11
   - Gardasil-9: Nonavalent HPV 16, 18, 6, 11, 31, 33, 45, 52, 58
   - BioVac: Varicella vaccine

- DTaP used < 7 years age, TDap > 11 years age & 19-64 years age
- RubaVac: Rubella vaccine

292. **Ans. (a) Sickle cell anemia**
     [Ref. ImmunoFacts 2008 by Grabenstein 2008 p158]

   Pneumococcal vaccine PCV 23 polysaccharide
   - Recommended for Older persons >65 years age
   - Recommended for 2-64 years age if Chronic CVD/Chronic pulmonary disease/DM/Alcoholic/Chronic smokers/Chronic liver disease/Liver cirrhosis/Asplenia (Sickle cell disease/Splenectomy)/Immunocompromised (HIV)/Organ transplantation/Renal disease/Renal transplantation.

293. **Ans. (a) Two live vaccines cannot be administered simultaneously**   *[Ref. Park 27/e p111]*
   LIVE VACCINES:
   - Are prepared from live attenuated organisms
   - *Live vaccines are more potent agents than killed vaccines:*
     - *Multiply in the host and the resulting antigenic host is larger than what is injected*
     - *Have all the major and minor antigenic components*
     - *Engage certain tissues of the body (e.g. intestinal mucosa by OPV)*
     - *There may be other mechanisms such as persistence of latent virus*
   - Immunization is generally achieved with a single dose (EXCEPT OPV)
   - Should not be administered to immuno-deficient or immuno-suppressed persons
   - 2 live vaccines can be administered simultaneously at different sites (or at an interval of 3 weeks)

> **ALSO REMEMBER**
> - *Attenuation: Reduced pathogenicity/virulence BUT maintained antigenicity/immunogenicity*
> - *General rules for multiple vaccine administration:*
>   - 2 live vaccines can be given together
>   - Live and killed vaccines can be given together
>   - Cholera vaccine and Yellow fever vaccine cannot be given together
>   - OPV is a live vaccine where single dose is not sufficient for immunization

294. **Ans. (a) Egg culture; (c) Reconstituted vaccine should be used within one hour**
     [Ref. Park 21/e p138, 139, Park 22/e p161-162]
   - **MEASLES VACCINE:**
     - Type: Live attenuated, lyophilized (Freeze dried) vaccine (Tissue culture vaccines – Chick embryo or Human diploid cell line) Strains used:
       1. Edmonston Zagreb Strain (Most Common)
       2. Schwartz Strain
       3. Moraten Strain

> **ALSO REMEMBER**
> - *Measles immunoglobulin*
>   - Type: Human Normal Immunoglobulin
>   - Dose (WHO recommended): 0.25 mL/kg body weight

295. **Ans. (b) Polio**
     [Ref. Combination Vaccines by Ronald W. Ellis; p43]
   - *Thermolability of vaccines*: sensitivity to heat
   - Reconstituted BCG > YF > OPV > Measles & Reconstituted Measles > Hep B > DPT > DT > BCG > TT
     - Most Thermolabile vaccine: Reconstituted BCG
     - Most Thermostable vaccine: TT

296. **Ans. (b) BCG, DPT-1, OPV-1, Measles, Vitamin-A**
     [Ref. IAP Guidebook on Immunization]
   - *Age limits for delayed immunization in NIS, India:*

Vaccine	Age limit	Reason for limit (if any)
BCG	Up to 1 year of age (Direct BCG)	Subclinical immunity develops after 1 yr age
OPV	Up to 5 years of age	Polio cases are MC in < 5 yrs age
HepB	Up to 1 year of age	–
Measles	Up to 5 year of age	Measles cases MC in < 5 yrs age
Vitamin A	Up to 5 year of age*	Xerophthalmia cases MC in < 5 yrs age
DPT	Up to 7 year of age	Diphtheria cases MC in < 7 yrs age
JE	Up to 15 years of age	–
TT	Up to 16 years of age	–

(* Vitamin A was earlier given till the age of 3 years)

> **ALSO REMEMBER**
> - In India, NIS starts at birth; and ends at 16 years (males) and with last pregnancy (females)
> - 'Indirect BCG' is given after 1 year age: After a prior Mantoux test
> - Any number of vaccines (live and/or killed) can be given together
> - There need not be a gap of 1 month between a live and a killed vaccine
> - BCG and Measles vaccine can be given together for a case of delayed immunization
> - Minor fever, diarrhea, ARI or other illness is NOT a contraindication for any of the vaccines
> - Doses and schedule remain same even if baby is premature and/or underweight
> - *In Delhi's Immunization Schedule, there are 2 additional vaccines:*
>   - MMR (single dose at 15 months of age)
>   - Typhoid (single dose between 2-5 years of age)
> - *Guidelines on TT in pregnancy:*
>   - Primigravida: 2 doses 1 month apart, as early as possible in pregnancy
>   - DURATION OF PROTECTION WITH 2 DOSES: ALL SUBSEQUENT PREGNANCIES IN NEXT 3 YEARS
>   - Multigravida (completely immunized in last 3 years): 1 booster dose is sufficient
>   - Multigravida (partially immunized in previous pregnancy in last 3 years): 2 doses, 1 month apart
>   - Multigravida (unimmunized in previous pregnancy in last 3 years): 2 doses, 1 month apart
>   - Multigravida (completely immunized in previous pregnancy earlier than 3 years): 2 doses, 1 month apart

– RULE FOR Delayed immunization of TT in pregnancy (as per Period of gestation – POG): Give 2 doses of TT, 1 month apart, anytime in pregnancy, IRRESPECTIVE OF TIME OF DELIVERY (so as to provide protection for atleast next 3 years).

297. Ans. (d) WHO recommends Danish 1331 strain for vaccine production
[Ref. Park 27/e p231]

- BCG stands for 'Bacille Calmette Guerin' – an 'avirulent strain' produced by 239 subcultures over a period of 13 years
- WHO recommended strain: DANISH 1331 strain
  – Vaccine strain is derived from 'Mycobacterium bovis'
  – Prepared at BCG laboratory, Guindy, Chennai in India

ALSO REMEMBER
- BCG is contraindicated in (Being a live vaccine)
  – Pregnancy
  – Immunosuppressive states
  – During corticosteroid therapy
- WHO recommended policy on BCG vaccination in HIV:
  – Asymptomatic HIV positive infants in high endemic areas: BCG can be given
  – Asymptomatic HIV positive infants in low endemic areas: BCG need not be given

298. Ans. (d) DPT-1, OPV-1 Measles, Vitamin-A
[Ref. IAP Guidebook on Immunization]

- Vaccines to be given in situations of delayed immunizations in India:
  – 9 month old unimmunized child comes for immunization first time:
    1. BCG (Direct)
    2. OPV_1 (3 successive doses 1 month apart, booster after 1 year of 3rd dose)
    3. DPT_1 (3 successive doses 1 month apart, booster after 1 year of 3rd dose)
    4. $HepB_1$ (3 successive doses 1 month apart)
    5. Measles-1/MR-1
    6. Vitamin A (1 Lac IU)
    7. HiB_1 (2 successive doses 1 month apart)
    8. Pentavalent-1
    9. JE-1
    10. Rota V-1
  – 1½ yr old unimmunized child comes for immunization first time:
    1. BCG (Indirect)
    2. OPV_1 (3 successive doses 1 month apart, booster after 1 year of 3rd dose)
    3. DPT_1 (3 successive doses 1 month apart, booster after 1 year of 3rd dose)
    4. Measles-1/MR-1
    5. Vitamin A (2 Lac IU)
    6. Hib (1 dose)
    7. JE-1
  – 3½ yr old unimmunized child comes for immunization first time:
    1. BCG (Indirect)
    2. OPV_1 (3 successive doses 1 month apart, booster after 1 year of 3rd dose)
    3. DPT_1 (3 successive doses 1 month apart, booster after 1 year of 3rd dose)
    4. Measles-1/MR-1
    5. Vitamin A (2 Lac IU)
    6. HiB (1 dose)
    7. JE-1

299. Ans. (d) Yellow fever [Ref. Park 27/e p111]

300. Ans. (d) Change in colour of monitor
[Ref. National Health Programs of India by Dr. J. Kishore 8/e p156, Park 27/e p122]

- WHO grading of VVM in OPV: Marker of pofency
  – Is based on colour changes in VVM: ONLY INNER SQUARE CHANGES COLOUR, circle always remain blue

WHO Grade	Outer Circle	Inner Square	Inference
Grade I	Blue	White	OPV can be used
Grade II	Blue	Light blue	OPV can be used
Grade III	Blue	Blue	OPV CANNOT be used
Grade IV	Blue	Purple/Black	OPV CANNOT be used

ALSO REMEMBER
- VVM has been introduced for almost all vaccines (in NIS) too in India
- In VVM, 'direct relationship exists between the rate of colour change and temperature'
  – The lower the temperature, the slower the colour change
  – The higher the temperature, the faster the colour change
- Rules for VVM use in India:
  – Rule 1: If the inner square is lighter than the outer circle, the vaccine may be used
  – Rule 2: If the inner square is the same colour as, or darker than, the outer circle, the vaccine must not be used
- The VVM inner square start point colour: Is approximately 10% of the outer circle colour
- Validation of VVMs: Optical densitometer (for colour density measurement)
- VVM is best interpreted on a nominal scale: Usable or non-usable

301. Ans. (c) 25 [Ref. Park 27/e p180]
- DPT VACCINE:
  – Composition of DPT Vaccine:

Contents	Amount per dose (0.5 mL)	
	Glaxo	Kasauli
Diphtheria Toxoid	25 Lf	30 Lf
Tetanus Toxoid	5 Lf	10 Lf
Pertussis killed acellular bacilli	20,000 million	32,000 million
Aluminium phosphate	2.5 mg	3.0 mg
Thiomersal	0.01 %	0.01%

302. Ans. (c) Killed vaccine [Ref. Park 27/e p244]

- Vaccines for Poliomyelitis:

	OPV (Sabin)	IPV (Salk)
Type of vaccine	Live attenuated virus	Killed formolised virus
Mode of administration	Oral	Subcutaneous or i.m.
Type of immunity	Humoral + Intestinal (local)	Humoral
Prevention of	Paralysis + intestinal re-infection	Paralysis
Control of epidemics	Effective	Not useful
Manufacture	Easy	Difficult
Cost	Cheaper	Expensive
Storage & transport	Require sub-zero temperatures	Less stringent conditions
Shelf life	Short	Longer
VAPP	1 per 2.7 million vaccinees	Zero incidence

303. Ans. (c) Dial thermometer [Ref. Park 27/e p119]

- *Dial Thermometer*:
  - *Is the instrument used to monitor the temperature of cold chain at PHC*
  - *Is kept in ILR (Ice-lined refrigerator-component of cold chain) at PHC*
  - *Is 'based on principle of thermocouple'*
  - *Recommended temperature monitoring at PHC level is: Twice daily*

304. Ans. (d) Subcentre & village level [Ref. Park 27/e p118-120]

- Cold chain components (equipments) and levels in India:

Level	Component	Temperature	Storage duration
State/ Regional level	Walk-in-cold rooms (WIC) Walk-in-freezers (WIF)	+2°C to +8°C −15°C to −25°C	3 months
District level	Large ILRs (Ice-lined refrigerator) Large DFs (Deep freezers)	+2°C to +8°C −15°C to −25°C	1 month
PHC level	Small ILRs Small DFs	+2°C to +8°C −15°C to −25°C	1 month
Sub-centre level	Vaccine carriers Day carriers	+2°C to +8°C	48–72 hours
Session level	Fully frozen icepack	+2°C to +8°C	1–3 hours

- *Most important component of cold chain in India*: ILR
- *Minimum level of vaccine storage (in cold chain) in India*: Primary health centre (below PHC level, vaccines are 'transported to sub-centres on immunization days' in vaccine carriers and day carriers)
- *Maximum chance of cold chain failure in India*: Sub-centre and village level
- *Instrument used to monitor the temperature of cold chain at PHC*: Dial Thermometer

305. Ans. (c) Give 3rd dose and continue the course [Ref. Park 27/e p180]

- *Interval between doses of DPT*:
  - *Current recommendation: Allow an interval of 4 weeks between 3 doses, followed by a booster at age of 1½ – 2 years, followed by another booster at 5 – 6 years*
  - *2 month intervals DO NOT offer any advantage over 1 – month intervals for protection against Diphtheria and Tetanus, and may not enhance Pertussis protection*
  - *Shorter intervals confer protection at an earlier age which may be particularly important in Pertussis control*

In the given question, a 11-month old child has received two doses of DPT and polio, comes for further immunization after 5 months of the last dose, there is NO NEED to repeat the whole course. Continue form this point onwards, and complete the course.

306. Ans. (d) BCG, DPT-1, OPV-1, Measles [Ref. Park 27/e p136]

> **ALSO REMEMBER**
> **Important Practical Considerations:**
> - *Vitamin-A is given at 9th, 18th, 24th, 30th, 36th, 42nd, 48th, 54th and 60th months (A total of 1 Lac + 2 Lac + 2 Lac + 2 Lac + 2 Lac + 2 Lac + 2 Lac + 2 Lac + 2 Lac = 17 Lac IU is given to a completely immunized child by 5 years of age)*
> - *OPV: Minimum 5 doses are required for development of immunity*
> - *DPT: Minimum 3 doses are given a month apart with booster after 1 year of the 3rd dose*
> - *TT: A fully immunized adult (excluding pregnancy in females) would have received 7 doses of TT*

307. Ans. (a) It should be stored in deep freezer; (c) Store stocks.................. [Ref. Park 27/e p180]

- All vaccines are stored at temperature of +2° to +80° **including OPV** (*OPV vaccine is stored at -15° to -25°C, i.e., Subzero/freezing temperatures only for long term storage*) **but YF vaccine** (*YF vaccine is stored at -30° to +5°C*)
- Vitamin-A and Diluents (Normal Saline for BCG and Distilled/Sterile Water for Measles) need not be stored in cold chain; but they should be brought to temperature of cold chain before reconstitution
- All vaccines opened (partially or totally used) are discarded.

> **ALSO REMEMBER**
> - All unopened/unused vaccines from an immunization session (if maintained in cold chain) can be brought back to ILR at PHC maximum three times
> - *Any vaccine (barring OPV and YF vaccine), if accidently frozen*: DISCARD IT

308. Ans. (a) Rubella; (e) Varicella [Ref. Park 27/e p111]

> **ALSO REMEMBER**
> - *Vaccines contraindicated in Pregnancy*: ALL LIVE VACCINES (barring Yellow Fever Vaccine) and MENINGOCOCCAL VACCINE
>   - BCG
>   - OPV
>   - Yellow fever
>   - Measles vaccine
>   - MMR (Measles, Mumps & Rubella)
>   - Oral Typhoid (Ty 21a)
>   - Varicella
>   - Live Plague vaccine
>   - LAIV (Live attenuated Influenza viral vaccine)
>   - Varicella vaccine
>   - Meningococcal Vaccine
> - *'Live vaccines are usually not given in pregnancy'* due to the potential risk of causing the disease in the immunocompromised mother:
>   - However, when the likelihood of disease exposure is high or when infection would pose a risk to the mother or fetus, then vaccination with a live vaccine is generally recommended in exceptional cases (especially with OPV and Yellow Fever vaccines)
> - *What if a live vaccine is accidentally given during pregnancy? Does this mean that the pregnancy should be terminated?* **No.** This alone would not be considered a medical reason to end a pregnancy because the chance of the fetus being infected is generally very low: Counseling by a knowledgeable healthcare provider would be recommended

309. Ans. (d) Horse [Ref. Park 27/e p116]

- *Antisera (Antitoxins)*: Materials prepared in animals; non-human sources like horses
  - *Provides passive immunization*
  - *Common uses*: Tetanus, Diphtheria, Botulism, Rabies, Gas gangrene, Snake bite

310. Ans. (b) Sabin polio vaccine [Ref. Park 27/e p245]

- *Rare vaccine reactions*:

Vaccine	Reaction
BCG	Suppurative lymphadenitis, Osteitis, Disseminated infection
Hepatitis B	Anaphylaxis
Measles/MMR	Febrile seizures, Thrombocytopenia, Anaphylaxis, Encephalopathy
OPV	Vaccine associated paralytic Poliomyelitis (VAPP)
TT	Brachial neuritis, Anaphylaxis
Pertussis (whole cell)	Persistent screaming, Seizures, Anaphylaxis, Encephalopathy, Hypotonic hyporesponsive episode (HHE)

> **ALSO REMEMBER**
> **ADVERSE EFFECTS FOLLOWING IMMUNIZATION (AEFI):**
> - *Minor Vaccine Reactions*:
>
> | Vaccine | Possible minor reaction | Frequency |
> |---|---|---|
> | DPT | Local reaction (pain, swelling, redness) Fever | Up to 50% Up to 50% |
> | Hepatitis A | Local reaction (pain, swelling, redness) | Up to 50% |
> | Pneumococcal | Local reaction (pain, swelling, redness) | 30-50% |
> | Meningococcal | Mild local reactions | Up to 71% |
>
> - *Rare vaccine reactions*:
>
> | Rare reactions | Vaccine |
> |---|---|
> | Suppurative lymphadenitis BCG osteitis Disseminated BCGiosis | BCG |
> | Anaphylaxis | Hepatitis B |
> | Thrombocytopenia Febrile seizures Anaphylaxis Encephalopathy | Measles/MMR |
> | Arthralgia | Rubella/MMR |
> | Vaccine associated paralytic poliomyelitis | OPV |
> | Anaphylaxis Brachial neuritis | Tetanus/DT |
> | Seizures Anaphylaxis Encephalopathy Persistent (>3 hours) inconsolable screaming Hypotonic hypo-responsive episode (HHE) | Pertussis/DPT-whole cell |

311. Ans. (a) Colostrum [Ref. Park 27/e p609]

COLOSTRUM:

- Is the most suitable food immediately after birth of the baby; Regular milk comes 3 – 6 days after birth
- Also known as *'Beestings'*, *'First milk'* or *'Immune Milk'*
- High in carbohydrates, protein, and antibodies and low in fat
- Contains all five immunoglobulins found in all mammals, IgA, IgD, IgE, IgG and IgM
- Known as *'first immunization'* of newborn

312. Ans. (d) Hib [Ref. Park 27/e p136]

313. Ans. (c) Two live vaccines cannot be given simultaneously [Ref. Park 27/e p111]

[New Guideline: Two live vaccines can be given together except cholera vaccine and Y F vaccine]

314. Ans. (a) Tetanus [Ref. Park 27/e p111]

315. Ans. (a) Measles – Jeryllyn; (b) Rubella - Copenhagen; (c) Mumps - Schwatrz [Ref. Park 23/e p148, 153, 155]

316. **Ans. (a) It is a killed vaccine** [Ref. Park 27/e p111]
317. **Ans. (d) Bivalent & quadrivalent** [Ref. Internet]
    - Currently two Human Papilloma Virus (HPV) vaccines are available in India as a protection against cervical cancer
    - *Gardasil vaccine*: HPV types 6, 11, 16, 18 (Quadrivalent)
    - *Cervarix vaccine*: HPV types 16, 18 (Bivalent)
318. **Ans. (b) Measles** [Ref. Park 27/e p166]
    - Measles vaccine efficacy with single dose: 90%
    - OPV vaccine efficacy with single dose: 65-80%
    - BCG vaccine efficacy with single dose: 50%
    - TT vaccine efficacy with single dose: 70%
    - Rubella vaccine efficacy with single dose: 95% (HIGHEST)
319. **Ans. (d) WHO recommends Donish 1331 for vaccine production** [Ref. Park 27/e p231]
    - New guidelines say that site for BCG vaccine must NOT be cleaned with spirit as it kills the live components of a vaccine
320. **Ans. (c) Neomycin is used as preservative in BCG vaccine** [Ref. Park 23/e p148, 162, 196, 206]
    - DPT vaccine contains Thiomersal (Preservative)
    - OPV contains Magnesium chloride (Thermostabilizer)
    - DPT contains Aluminum hydroxide (Adjuvant)
    - Measles vaccine contain Neomycin and Erythromycin (Preservative)
    - BCG vaccine does not contain preservative
321. **Ans. (b) H. influenzae vaccine**
    [Ref. Immunization in Older Adults, Issue 21, 2007]
    CDC GUIDELINES FOR IMMUNIZATION OF OLDER PEOPLE
    - Influenza intramuscular inactivated vaccine (live intranasal vaccine is contraindicated)
    - Pneumococcal vaccine once
    - Tetanus-diphtheria toxoid (Td) booster every 10 years
    - In selected patients aged 60 years or more
        - Herpes zoster (shingles)
        - Hepatitis A
        - Hepatitis B
        - Meningococcal disease
        - Varicella
        - MMR
        - Yellow fever vaccine (for travellers)

> **ALSO REMEMBER**
> - Haemophilus influenza B vaccine is generally not given after 5-6 years age, unless there is HIV/AIDS, removal of spleen, Sickle cell disease, anti-cancer treatment or bone marrow transplant.

322. **Ans. (c) Ice lined refrigerator** [Ref. Park 27/e p119]
323. **Ans. (d) DPT** [Ref. Park 27/e p136]
324. **Ans. (d) 6-9 months** [Ref. Park 27/e p166]
325. **Ans. (b) At birth** [Ref. Park 27/e p136]

326. **Ans. (a) Hepatitis B vaccine**
    [Ref. Textbook of Paediatric Nursing by Beevi, 1/e p41]
327. **Ans. (b) Type 7** [Ref. Cervical Cancer by TS Kuie, 1/e p90-91]
328. **Ans. (d) DPT + Vitamin A** [Ref. K Park 24/e p135]
    Recent changes in immunization guidelines in India
    - 2 doses of measles vaccine
        - First dose: 9 months
        - Second dose: 16-24 months
    - 1 dose of JE Live vaccine: 16-24 months
    - DPT Booster: 5-6 years age
    - Vitamin A: Every 6 months till age of 5 years age (Starting at 9 months age)
329. **Ans. (a) >0.01 IU/mL** [Ref. Park 27/e p362]
330. **Ans. (a) Ty21 A** [Ref. Park 27/e p275-276]
331. **Ans. (c) Tetanus** [Ref. Park 27/e p360]
332. **Ans. (a) Cell culture derived live attenuated**
    [Ref. Park 27/e p332]
    - SA 14-14-2 vaccine:
        - Live attenuated cell-derived vaccine strain
        - Single dose is sufficient
        - Gives protection for 11 years
    - Killed Mouse-brain derived vaccine:
        - Two primary doses 4weeks apart
        - Booster after 1 year, then at 3-yearly intervals
        - Useful in Inter-epidemic period
333. **Ans. (a) Bivalent and quadrivalent; (c) MC subtypes 16, 18**
334. **Ans. (a) MMR Vaccine** [Ref. K. Park, 23/e p117, 24/e p126]
335. **Ans. (b) Maternal antibody is completely protective**
    [Ref. Park 27/e p245]
336. **Ans. (d) Live J.E.** [Ref. Infectious Diseases in Children and Newer Vaccines by Ghosh, 1/e p142]
337. **Ans. (d) Influenza**
    [Ref. Vaccinophobia by Chatterjee, 1/e p225]
    EGG-ALLERGY IN VACCINEES
    - Underlying reason: Ovalalbumin (main protein in egg white) is responsible for allergic reaction may be found in vaccines cultured on egg
    - Vaccines containing Egg-proteins (Contraindicated in Egg allergy):
        - Rabies vaccine
        - Yellow fever vaccine
        - Herpes simplex vaccine
        - Tick encephalitis vaccine
        - MMR vaccine
        - Influenza vaccine

> **ALSO REMEMBER**
> - MMR vaccine: Propagated on Chick embryo fibroblasts (containing very lesser amounts of protein) so is incapable of causing allergic reaction hence it's NOT contraindicated in egg allergy patients.

338. **Ans. (d) Maternally derived antibodies**
    [*Ref. Microbiology and Infectious Disease by Hagan & Bruner, 8/e p510*]
    - *Primary vaccination failure*: Failure to serologically respond to vaccine
        - *Too young age where Maternal antibodies interfere (MC Cause)*
        - *Vaccine production problems*
        - *Cold chain failure*
        - *Inappropriate administration technique*
        - *Immunodeficiency*
        - *Poor health*
    - *Secondary vaccination failure*: 'Waning immunity' where there is loss of vaccine induced protection in an individual who had previously seroconverted to vaccination
        - *Causes are not well understood*

339. **Ans. (a) Hepatitis B vaccine**
    [*Ref. Viruses, Plagues and History by Oldstone, 1/e p37*]
    - First recombinant vaccine for humans made in yeast: Hepatitis B
    - Hilleman, Merck Sharp & Dohme Inc. developed it in 1984

340. **Ans. (b) Additive action of the two antigens**
    [*Ref. Park 27/e p183*]

341. **Ans. (b) DPT** [*Ref. Park 27/e p183*]

342. **Ans. (a) 7-14** [*Ref. Human Viral Pathogens by Liu, 1/e p79*]
    - *Vaccine associated paralytic poliomyelitis (VAPP)*: Develop Paralytic Polio after 4-30 days (Average 7-14 days) of administration of OPV
    - *Poliomyelitis among Contacts of OPV*: Develop within 7-60 days after exposure to recent OPV-recipient

343. **Ans. (b) H2N1**
    [*Ref. Infectious Diseases by Blaser, 8/e p3534*]

    ## TRIVALENT FLU VACCINE
    - *Type*: Inactivated Influenza vaccine
    - *Protection*:
        - Two influenza A viruses (an H1N1 and an H3N2)
        - An influenza B virus
    - *Types of Trivalent vaccine*:
        - *Standard-dose trivalent shots*: Approved for people of different ages
        - *High-dose trivalent shot*: Approved for people 65 and older.
        - *Trivalent shot*: Approved for people 18 and older
        - *Recombinant trivalent shot*: Approved for people 18 years and older

344. **Ans. (c) dT** [*Ref. Park 27/e p183*]
    ## dT VACCINE
    - Vaccine of choice for children >12 years age and adults
    - Contains < 2 Lf units per dose
    - 2 doses at interval of 4-6 weeks, booster 6-12 months later

345. **Ans. NONE** [*Ref. NIS, GOI Guidelines*]
    - Currently under National Immunization Schedule, DPT, OPV, Hepatitis B, HiB and Rotavirus vaccines are given at 6 weeks age in India

346. **Ans. (c) Aim is full immunization for all children by the year 2025** [*Ref. Park 27/e p508*]
    ## MISSION INDRADHANUSH 2014
    - Launched on 25 December 2014
    - Cover all those children by 2020 who are either unvaccinated, or are partially vaccinated against 7 vaccine preventable diseases (7 VPD's) – Diphtheria, Pertussis, Tetanus, Childhood Tuberculosis, Poliomyelitis, Hepatitis B, Measles

347. **Ans. (b) Cholera vaccine** [*Ref. Park 27/e p275-276*]
    ## CHOLERA ORAL VACCINES
    - **Dukoral (WC-rBS)**: Monovalent, V cholera O1 plus Recombinant toxin B subunit
    - **Sanchol**: Bivalent, Serogroups O1 & O139, No toxin B subunit, No buffer required
    - **mORCVAX**: Bivalent, Serogroups O1 & O139, No toxin B subunit, No buffer required
    - **CVD103-HgR**: Live attenuated, single dose, NOT produced now

348. **Ans. (d) PRP with carrier**
    [*Ref. Clinical Pediatrics by Elzouki 2/e p932*]
    ## HIB CONJUGATED VACCINES
    - Currently available conjugated HiB vaccines are composed of a purified capsular polysaccharide of HiB, known as Polyribosylribitol phosphate (PRP), linked (conjugated) to a protein carrier

Vaccine	Polysaccharide	Protein carrier
PRP-D	Medium	Diphtheria toxoid
PRP-CRM 197	Small	Non-toxic mutant Diphtheria toxin
PRP-OMP	Medium	N. meningitidis outer membrane protein
PRP-T	Large	Tetanus toxoid

349. **Ans. (d) Typhoid** [*Ref. Park 27/e p280*]
    Ty21a VACCINE
    - Orally administered, live attenuated, lyophilized vaccine for Typhoid
    - Strain: 'Ty2 strain' of Salmonella typhi
    - Schedule: Day 1, 3, 5
    - Stop Proguanil and antibacterial drugs 3 days before and until 3 days later of administration

350. **Ans. (a) Type-2 virus** [*Ref. WHO. VAPP and VDPV. Polio Global Eradication Initiative. February 2015*]
    ## VAPP Vs VDPV
    - **Vaccine-associated paralytic polio (VAPP)**:
        - *OPV is made with live attenuated polioviruses that can result in VAPP (1 in 2.7 million doses of OPV)*
        - *VAPP is caused by a strain of poliovirus that has genetically changed in the intestine from the original attenuated vaccine strain contained in OPV*
        - *MC Cause: Polio virus type 3*
    - **Vaccine derived poliovirus (VDPV)**:
        - *VDPV is a very rare strain of poliovirus, genetically changed from the original strain contained in OPV*

- On very rare occasions, under certain conditions, a strain of poliovirus in OPV may change and revert to a form that may be able to cause paralysis (VDPV) in humans and develop the capacity for sustained circulation, latter known as a circulating VPDV (cVDPV)
- MC cause: cVDPV Poliovirus type 2

351. Ans. (c) 20 mL [Ref. Park 27/e p170]

IMMUNOGLOBULIN DOSAGES

Disease/Agent	Dose
Hepatitis A	0.02 mL/kg BW (3.2 mg/kg BW)
Hepatitis B	0.05–0.07 mL/kg BW (8-11 mg/kg BW)
Hepatitis C	0.05 mL/kg BW (3.2-8 mg/kg BW)
Measles	0.25 mL/kg BW
Rubella	20 mL
Varicella	15-25 units/kg BW
Rabies	20 IU/kg BW (HRIg), 40 IU/kg BW (ERIg)
Tetanus	250 units (prophylaxis), 3000–6000 units treatment
Rh isoimmunization	200–300 mcg per 15 mL Rh+ve blood exposure

352. Ans. (b) Measles; (c) DPT; (d) Rubella [Ref. Park 27/e p118-119]
- Under NIS, RCH Program all vaccines are stored in +2° to +8°C
- OPV is also stored in +2° to +8°C Except for long term storage when it's kept in freezer (-15° to -25°C)

353. Ans. (b) Diphtheria [Ref. Immunology by Coico, 7/e p344]

Passive Immunization through Placental Antibody Transfer
- Placental transfer of IgG antibody transfer Passive immunity from mother to child
- *Toxins:* Tetanus, Diphtheria
- *Viruses:* Measles, Poliovirus, Mumps
- *Bacteria:* Hemophilus influenza, Streptococcus agalactiae group B

354. Ans. (d) Vaccine is live attenuated vaccine [Ref. Park 27/e p183]
- Pertussis is a Subunit proteinaceous vaccine

355. ALL CHOICES [Ref. Park 27/e p180]

356. Ans. (d) Live vaccine should not be given for 12 weeks if immunoglobulin has been given [Ref. Microbiology by Surinder Kumar 1/e p731]
- Live vaccines should not normally be given for 12 weeks after an injection of normal human Ig
- If a live vaccine has already been given, NHIg injection should be deferred for 2 weeks

357. Ans. ALL CHOICES ARE CORRECT [Ref. Park 27/e p244]

INJECTABLE POLIO VACCINE (IPV)
- Composition: P1 40 units + P2 8 units + P3 32 units
- Other constituents: Formaldehyde, Streptomycin, Neomycin/Polymyxin B, 0.5% Phenoxyethanol preservative
- Does not contain: Thiomersal or Adjuvants
- Route of administration: Intramuscular or Intradermal (Fractionated dose)
- Dose and schedule: 0.5 mL (I/M at 14 weeks) thigh, 0.1 mL (I/D at 6 weeks and 14 weeks) upper arm
- Advantages:
  - Longer shelf life
  - Does not require stringent storage conditions
  - Safe in Pregnancy, immunodeficiency, corticosteroid therapy, age >50 years

358. Ans. (a) 6, 11; (b) 16, 18; (c) 31, 33 [Ref. Pediatric Infectious Disease by Jackson 1/e p720]

9-valent HPV Vaccine
- Protects against HPV types 6, 11, 16, 18, 31, 33, 45, 52, 58
- Safe and effective
- Will further reduce the incidence of HPV infection, as well as HPV-related cancers

359. Ans. (a) OPV, DPT [Ref. Park 27/e p136]
- 18 month unvaccinated child coming to PHC will get: OPV-1, Measles-1 or MR-1, JE-1, Vitamin A (2 lac IU), DPT-1, HiB-1

360. Ans. (c) Meningococcal meningitis [Ref. Park 27/e p508]

361. Ans. (a) Yellow fever [Ref. Park 27/e p328]
- Yellow fever vaccine can be administered in pregnancy if there is an outbreak and the risk of infection is high

362. Ans. (c) Influenza [Ref. Park 27/e p136]
Vaccines used in India
- Rota virus vaccine: Administered at 6, 10, 14 weeks under National Immunization Schedule (NIS), India
- MR vaccine: Administered at 9 months, 16-24 months under NIS, India
- Adult JE vaccine: Adult JE campaign, covering adults aged 15-65 years, has been completed in 31 districts wherein 33 million adults were vaccinated against JE

363. Ans. (a) VVM [Ref. Park 27/e p122]
Vaccine Vial Monitor (VVM)
- VVM is a marker of potency: VVM is a simple tool which enables vaccinator to know if vaccine is potent at the time of administration
- VVM is a label containing a heat-sensitive material which is placed on a vaccine vial to register cumulative heat exposure over time

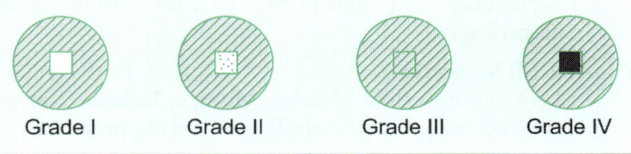
VVM

364. Ans. (c) Meningococcal meningitis [Ref. Park 27/e p508]
Vaccines included in Mission Indradhanush
- Existing 7 vaccines: DPT, BCG, OPV, Hepatitis B, Measles
- Newer 4 vaccines: Rotavirus, MR (Measles rubella), IPV bivalent, Japanese Encephalitis

365. **Ans. (a) Shake test** [Ref. Park 27/e p123]

   SHAKE TEST
   - Utility: Used to check if Freeze sensitive vaccines have been damaged by exposure to freezing temperatures below 0 degrees C; After the test the previously Frozen vaccine shows flakes
   - Method of Shake test:
     - *Test Vial: Vial which is suspected to have been frozen*
     - *Frozen control vial: Take a similar (as Test vial) vaccine vial with same manufacturer, batch number, antigen(s), Label it properly. Freeze it overnight at -20 degrees C, then let it haw (Do not heat)*
     - *Hold the Test vial and Control vials between thumb and forefinger and shake them vigorously (10-15 seconds)*
     - *Place both vials on even flat surface for 30 minutes observation, compare the sedimentation rates (SR)*
   - Interpretation:
     - *If SR in Test vial < Control vial: Vaccine had not been damaged*
     - *If SR in Test vial ≥ Control vial: Vaccine had been damaged, Do not use and Inform the supervisors*

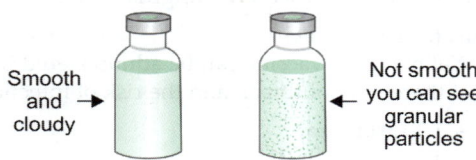

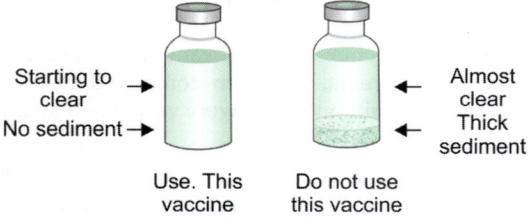

366. **Ans. (d) Influenza** [Ref. IAP Textbook of Pediatrics by Parthasarathy, 6/e p358]
   - Manufacturing flu vaccines is literally a race against the time
   - Every year the circulating virus drifts (Antigenic variations) and hence the vaccine strains change accordingly

367. **Ans. (d) Varicella** [Ref. Park 25/e p111]
   - Live vaccines (like Measles, Mumps, Rubella, Varicella etc. vaccines) are contraindicated during pregnancy

Review Questions

368. **Ans. (c) Given around 200 yards of a case detected**
   [Ref. Refer Dictionary by Dr. J Kishore]

369. **Ans. (c) 15–18 months** [Ref. Park 27/e p166]

370. **Ans. (a) Typhoid oral** [Ref. Park 27/e p280]

371. **Ans. (a) OPV+ BCG + Measles + DPT**
   [Ref. Park 27/e p136]

372. **Ans. (c) Inner square darker than the outer circle**
   [Ref. Park 7/e p122]

373. **Ans. (a) BCG** [Ref. Park 27/e p231]

374. **Ans. (d) Production of antibody more slow**
   [Ref. Park 27/e p109]

375. **Ans. (a) Salk polio vaccine** [Ref. Park 27/e p111]

376. **Ans. (a) Given subcutaneously** [Ref. Park 27/e p231]

377. **Ans. (c) Influenza** [Ref. Park 27/e p176]

378. **Ans. (c) Rubella** [Ref. Park 27/e p169-170]

379. **Ans. (c) Protects entire community** [Ref. Park 27/e p105]

380. **Ans. (b) BPL vaccine has more number of doses**
   [Ref. Park 27/e p324-327]

381. **Ans. (b) 4 weeks** [Ref. Park 27/e p111]

382. **Ans. (a) OPV** [Ref. IAP Guidebook on Immunization]

383. **Ans. (b) Measles** [Ref. Park 27/e p166]

384. **Ans. (c) Danish-1331** [Ref. Park 27/e p231]

385. **Ans. (a) Typhoid** [Ref. Park 27/e p280]

386. **Ans. (b) 40 i.u.; (a) 20 i.u.** [Ref. Park 27/e p326]

387. **Ans. (b) Measles** [Ref. Park 27/e p166]

DISINFECTION

388. **Ans. (a) Bleaching powder** [Ref. Park 26/e p 139-140]
   - Bleach is a strong and effective disinfectant – its active ingredient sodium hypochlorite is effective in killing bacteria, fungi and viruses
   - Sanitizing refers to lowering the number of germs to a safe level by either cleaning or disinfecting, disinfecting itself refers to killing nearly 100 percent of germs on surfaces or objects
   - Disinfectants are used on non-living objects to kill or inactivate pests. Sanitizers reduce, but don't necessarily eliminate, pests from non-living objects to levels considered safe by public health codes or regulations

389. **Ans. (d) Germicidal Power of a disinfectant**
   [Ref. Russell, Hugo and Ayliffe's Principles and Practice of Disinfection; p225]
   - *Rideal Walker Coefficient (RWC):*
     - Also known as *'Carbolic acid coefficient'*
     - Is used to *'represent germicidal power of a disinfectant'*
     - Standard used for comparison: Phenol (RWC = 1)
     - *RWC = 10 implies:* Given disinfectant is 10 times more potent than phenol
     - *Organism used for testing:* Salmonella typhi
     - *In presence of organic matter, RWC is ineffective:* Chic Martin test is employed

> **ALSO REMEMBER**
> - Effect/sufficiency/adequacy of autoclaving is assessed by:
>   - Spores of 'Bacillus stearothermophilus'
>   - Sterigage (chemical indicator strips)
> - Effect/sufficiency/adequacy of pasteurization is assessed by:
>   - Phosphatase test (MC used test)
>   - Standard plate count
>   - Coliform count

390. **Ans. (c) Phenol**   *[Ref. Russell, Hugo and Ayliffe's Principles and Practice of Disinfection; p225]*

391. **Ans. (b) Cetrimide**   *[Ref. Park 27/e p141]*
     - *Chemical agents for disinfection*:

Phenol & related compounds	Quaternary ammonia compounds	Halogens & related compounds
Phenol Crude phenol Cresol Cresol emulsions Chlorhexidine (Hibitane) Hexachlorphane Dettol	Cetrimide Savlon	Bleaching powder Sodium hypochlorite Halozone tablets Iodine Iodophors
Alcohols	Formaldehyde	Miscellaneous
Ethyl alcohol Isopropyl alcohol	Formalin Formaldehyde gas	Lime Ethylene oxide

- *Pure phenol is not an effective disinfectant*
- *Crude phenol*: Phenol + Cresol
- *Cresol emulsions are very powerful disinfectants*:
  - Lysol (50 – 60% cresol)
  - Izal
  - Cyllin
- *Dettol (Chlorxylenol)*: Suitable for disinfection of instruments and plastic equipments
- *Savlon*: Cetavlon (Cetrimide) + Hibitane (Chlorhexidine)
- *Betadine*: Povidone + Iodine
- *Bleaching powder ($CaOCl_2$)*:
  - BP contains '33% available chlorine'
  - Stabilised bleach: Mixing with lime, to stabilize bleaching powder
  - Amount of BP required to disinfect 1000 litres of water: 2.5 grams

> **ALSO REMEMBER**
> - *Most effective skin antiseptics*: Alcoholic solutions of Chlorhexidine (Hibitane) & Iodine
> - *Cresol is known as 'All purpose general disinfectant'*
> - *Cheapest disinfectant*: Lime
> - *Disinfectants recommended*:
>   - For rooms: Formaldehyde
>   - For Lippes loop:
>   1. 1/2500 aqueous solution of Iodine
>   2. Normal strength savlon–
>   - For Handlotions: Hibitane (Chlorhexidine)
>   - For infant feeding bottles: Sodium hypochlorite (containing 100 – 200 ppm of available chlorine)
>   - For sputum: Burning

392. **Ans. (c) Cetavlon and hibitane**   *[Ref. Park 27/e p142]*
     - *Savlon*: Chlorhexidine (*Hibitane*) 0.3% and Cetrimide (*Cetavlon*) 3%.
     - Chlorhexidine is effective against a wide range of Gram-negative and Gram-positive vegetative bacteria, yeasts, dermatophyte fungi and lipophilic viruses; It is inactive against bacterial spores, except at elevated temperatures

> **ALSO REMEMBER**
> - Chlorxylenol/parachlorometaxylenol is the major content of 'Dettol'

393. **Ans. (d) Cresol**   *[Ref. Park 27/e p142]*
     - Cresol has no significant activity against bacterial spores

394. **Ans. (d) Pre-current disinfection**   *[Ref. Park 27/e p140]*

     TYPES OF DISINFECTION:
     - *Concurrent disinfection*: Is application of disinfective measures as soon as possible after discharge of infectious material from body of an infected person
       - *Example: Disinfection of urine, faeces, vomit, contaminated linen, clothes, hands, dressings, gloves, aprons*
     - *Terminal disinfection*: Is application of disinfective measures after the patient has been removed by death or to a hospital or ceased to be a source of infection
       - *Examples: Currently not practices; only cleaning, airing, sunning of rooms, linen, furniture*
     - *Precurrent (Prophylactic) disinfection*: Prior to occurrence of infection
       - *Examples: Chlorination of water, pasteurization of milk, handwashing*

395. **Ans. (a) Boiling; (b) Burning; (d) Autoclaving**   *[Ref. Park 27/e p144]*
     - *Methods recommended for sputum disposal*:
       - Burning (after receiving in gauge/handkerchief)
       - Boiling or Autoclaving at 20 lbs pressure X 20 min (for large volumes, as in TB hospitals) or incineration
       - 5% Cresol in a cup made to stand for 1 hour after spitting sputum in it

396. **Ans. (a) Cetrimide + chlorhexidine**   *[Ref. Park 27/e p142]*

397. **Ans. (d) Washing of hands before and after attending the patients**   *[Ref. Park 27/e p410]*

     MAIN PREVENTIVE MEASURES FOR NOSOCOMIAL INFECTIONS:
     - Isolation of infectious patients
     - Hospital staff infected must be kept away from work till cure; hygiene; aprons
     - "Hand-washing with disinfectants" (not soap and water) as MOST COMMON ROUTE OF INFECTION is hands
     - Dust control: Wet dusting and vaccum cleaning
     - Disinfection: Patient articles and body fluids; instruments
     - Control of droplet infection: Face mask; bed spacing; Lighting; Ventilation
     - Nursing techniques: Barrier nursing; Task nursing
     - Administrative measures: Hospital committee on infection control

398. **Ans. (c) Bacillus stearothermophilus** *[Ref. Modern trends in planning and designing of hospitals, 1/e p189]*
    AUTOCLAVING
    - *Principle*: Steam under pressure
    - *Checking sufficiency of autoclaving*:
      – Spores of Bacillus stearothermophilus
      – Chemical colour indicator strips (Sterigage)

399. **Ans. (a) 50 gm/lit** *[Ref. Park 27/e p142]*

400. **Ans. (c) After 48 hours of hospitalization** *[Ref. Park 27/e p410]*

401. **Ans. (d) Hot air oven 160 degrees Celsius for 30-60 minutes** *[Ref. Microbiology by Fornica, 1/e p89]*

402. **Ans. (c) Hypochlorite** *[Ref. Endodontics by Bakland, 1/e p83]*

403. **Ans. (d) Autoclaving** *[Ref. Microbiology & Immunology by Parija, 2/e p27]*
    STERILIZATION BY HEAT

Sterilization by Dry Heat	Sterilization by Moist Heat
Flaming Hot air oven Incineration	Pasteurization Boiling, Steam sterilizer Autoclaving Tyndallisation

404. **Ans. (b) Concurrent** *[Ref. Park 27/e p140-141]*

405. **Ans. (d) Hot air oven** *[Ref. Park 27/e p140-141]*
    - Hot air oven is used to sterilize glassware, heat resistant material, oils, powders, waxes and other substances that cannot be sterilized by moist heat or don't get sterilized effectively
    - Hot air oven sterilizes by Dry heat, 160 degrees C over 2-4 hours

Review Question

406. **Ans. (a) Glutaraldehyde** *[Ref. Ananthanarayan Microbiology 4/e p32]*

MISCELLANEOUS

407. **Ans. (a) Temporal association** *[Ref. Epidemiology by Leon Gordis, 4/e p172 and Basic Epidemiology by Beaglehole, WHO; p40-41]*
    NESTED CASE CONTROL STUDY:
    - Is a hybrid design where *'a case control study is nested in a cohort study'*
    - *Is predominantly a type of Cohort study* (due to forward direction)
    - Usefulness limited for studies involving *'rare diseases AND whose diagnostic tests are very expensive'*

408. **Ans. (b) Effectiveness** *[Ref. Epidemiology by Leon Gordis, 4/e p267]*
    EVALUATION OF HEALTH SERVICES:
    - *Efficacy*: Is the effect or usefulness of an agent/drug/vaccine under ideal 'controlled laboratory' conditions
    - *Effectiveness*: Is the effect or usefulness of an agent/drug/vaccine in real life community situations
    - *Efficiency*: Is the measure of relationship between the results achieved and the effort expended in terms of money, resources and time
      – Efficiency: Output/Input
      – Evaluation of efficiency:
        1. *Cost-benefit analysis*: Both input as well as output is in monetary terms
        2. *Cost-effectiveness analysis*: Input is in monetary terms whereas output is in terms of 'no. of lives saved'

> **ALSO REMEMBER**
> - Measurement of efficiency requires many assumptions, it is not value-free and can serve only as a general guideline
> - *Cost-effectiveness analysis is expressed as*:
>   – Dollars per life years gained
>   – Dollars per case prevented
>   – Dollars per quality-adjusted life years gained
> - Cost-effectiveness analysis is easier to perform than Cost-benefit analysis

409. **Ans. (a) Case series report** *[Ref. Epidemiology by Leon Gordis, 2/e p102]*
    In the given question, a total of 5000 patients of glaucoma are identified and surveyed by patient interviews regarding family history of glaucoma,
    Since *both exposure as well as outcome have occurred when the study has begun*: First we take outcome into consideration, and then go back in time taking exposure into consideration; and there is NO COMPARISON with non-diseased (controls),
    Therefore, it is a case series report

410. **Ans. (d) Nothing can be concluded as the information given is inadequate** *[Ref. Simple Biostatistics by Indrayan & Indrayan, 1/e p141 and Methods in Biostatistics by Mahajan, 6/e p118]*
    - **In the given question**, In assessing the association between maternal nutritional status and the birth weight of the newborns, two investigators A and B studied separately and found significant results with p values 0.02 and 0.04 respectively
    - Only levels of significance are given, thus we can only conclude that investigator A has 98% chance of being correct whereas investigator B has 96% chance of being correct

411. **Ans. (a) Is a cohort study nested in a case control study** *[Ref. Epidemiology by Leon Gordis, 4/e p172 and Basic Epidemiology by Beaglehole, WHO; p40-41]*

412. **Ans. (b) 99%** *[Ref. Park 25/e p149]*

413. **Ans. (b) Effectiveness** *[Ref. Epidemiology by Leon Gordis, 4/e p267 and Basic Epidemiology by Beaglehole, WHO; p137]*

> **ALSO REMEMBER**
> - COMMUNITY EFFECTIVENESS (CE):
>   CE = Efficacy × Diagnostic accuracy × Patient compliance × Provider compliance × Coverage
>   (E × D × PtC × PrC × C)

414. Ans. (b) It is likely to be more for infections that do not have a sub-clinical phase *[Ref. Park 27/e p110-111]*

HERD IMMUNITY:
- *Herd Immunity* is the level of resistance of a community or group of people to a particular disease. It refers to group protection beyond what is afforded by the protection of immunized individuals
- Elements contributing to herd immunity are:
  - *Occurrence of clinical/subclinical infections in herd*
  - *Immunization of herd*
  - *Structure of herd (hosts, alternative animal hosts, insect vectors, environmental & social factors)*
- It is *'neither possible nor necessary to achieve 100% herd immunity'* to control a disease
- Herd immunity may be determined by *'Serological Surveys'*
- Herd immunity describes a type of immunity that occurs when the vaccination of the a portion of the population (or herd) provides protection to un-vaccinated individuals
- Herd immunity does not protect the individual in the case of tetanus
- *Herd Immunity Threshhold*: Virologists have found that when a certain percentage of a population is vaccinated, the spread of the disease is effectively stopped; This critical percentage (HIT) depends on the disease and the vaccine

Disease	Herd immunity threshold
Diphtheria	85%
Pertussis	92-94%
Measles	83-94%
Mumps	75-86%
Rubella	80-85%
Polio	80-86%
Smallpox	83-85%
Varicella	90%

415. Ans. (a) & (c) Personal Exposure & Case Report *[Ref. BMJ 2004; p1490]*

416. Ans. (a) Descriptive studies *[Ref. Park 27/e p71]*

417. Ans. (c) Family planning *[Ref. India's Population by Mitra, 1/e p631]*

418. Ans. (c) Herd immunity *[Ref. Park 27/e p110-111]*
- Herd immunity is an Immunological barrier to the spread of disease in human community
- With high level of herd immunity, occurrence of epidemic is unlikely

Review Questions

419. Ans. (d) Stool specimen of polio send for testing *[Ref. Park 27/e p242]*

420. Ans. (b) Good for community *[Ref. Dorland's Dictionary 30/e p1502, Jawetz 23/e p681, Park 22/e p98]*

421. Ans. (c) Epidemiological surveillance *[Ref. Park 21/e p90, Park 22/e p102]*

CHAPTER 4: Screening of Disease

CONCEPTS IN SCREENING

Screening of Disease

- *Screening test:* Is used to search for an unrecognized diseases or defect, in apparently healthy individuals, by means of rapidly applied tests, examinations or other procedures
- *Screening versus Diagnosis[Q]:*

	Screening	Diagnosis
Done on	Apparently healthy	Cases (signs/symptoms)
Applied on	Groups, populations	Individuals
Test results	Arbitrary & final	Not final, modifiable
Based on	One criterion (cut-off)	Signs, symptoms, lab findings
Cost	Relatively cheaper	Expensive
Time taken	Relatively rapid	Time-consuming
Accuracy	Relatively inaccurate	Accurate
Basis for treatment	Cannot be used as basis	Useful basis for treatment
Initiative from	Investigator	Case with complaint

- *Examples of important screening tests used[Q]:*

Screening test(s)	Disease screened
Papanicolaou (Pap) smear test, VIA*	Cervical cancer
Breast self examination (BSE)	Breast cancer
Mammography	Breast cancer
Bimanual oral examination	Oral cancer
ELISA, RAPID, SIMPLE	HIV (National AIDS Control Programme)
Urine for Sugar, Random blood sugar	Diabetes mellitus
AFP (alpha feto-protein)	Developmental anomalies in fetus
Digital rectal examination (DRE)	Prostate cancer
Prostate specific antigen (PSA)	Prostate cancer
Fecal occult blood test	Colorectal cancer

(*Visual Inspection with 5% Acetic acid)

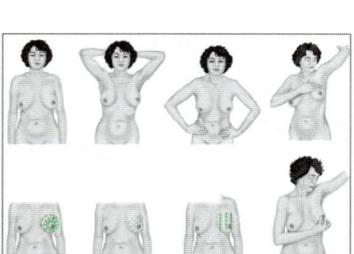

BSE

Principles of Screening (WHO): Suitability of a Disease for Screening (Criteria)[Q]

- The disease should be an important health problem
- There should be an effective treatment available for the disease
- Facilities for diagnosis and treatment should be available
- There should be a latent or early asymptomatic stage of the disease
- There should be a test or examination for the diagnosis of disease
- The test should be acceptable to the population
- The natural history of the disease should be adequately understood

- There should be an agreed policy on who to treat
- The total cost of finding a case should be economically balanced in relation to medical expenditure as a whole
- Case-finding should be a continuous process, not just a 'once and for all' project

TYPES OF SCREENING

Types of Screening^Q

	Prescriptive screening	Prospective screening
Definition	People screened for own's benefit	People screened for other's benefit
Essential purpose	Case detection	Disease control
Request for screening	No specific request	Specific request from authority
Example(s)	Neonatal screening Pap smear Urine for sugar	Screening of immigrants HIV screening among Sex workers

Neonatal Screening (NNS)

- *Neonatal hypothyroidism (NNH):*
  - Most common neonatal disorder to be screened is Neonatal hypothyroidism (NNH)^Q
  - Blood sample of choice: Umbilical cord blood^Q
  - Detection of: TSH, T_4
- *Phenylketonuria (PKU):*
  - *PKU is an autosomal recessive trait* with a frequency of 1 in 10,000 births
  - *Enzyme deficient in PKU:* Phenylalanine hydroxylase^Q
  - *Treatment of PKU:* restricting or eliminating foods high in phenylalanine, such as breast milk, meat, chicken, fish, nuts, cheese, legumes and other dairy products
  - *Guthrie Test^Q:* Is done in neonates for mass screening of Phenylketonuria (PKU)
    - *Guthrie test was the first screening test used in neonates*
    - *Blood sample* is collected by heel prick of the baby 7–10 days after birth^Q
    - *Guthrie Test is negative* in first 0–3 days of life
    - *Guthrie test can detect* PKU, Galactosemia and Maple syrup urine disease
    - *Chemicals detected:* Phenylalanine, Phenylpyruvate and Phenyllactate
    - It is a semi-quantitative test
    - Currently, Guthrie test has been replaced by *Tandem mass Spectrometry* (TMS)

> **Key points**
> Most common neonatal disorder to be screened is Neonatal hypothyroidism

Screening Test for Cervical Cancer

- Screening tests for Cervical cancer include:
  - Visual inspection with 5% acetic acid (VIA)
  - Visual inspection with Lugol's iodine (VILI)
  - Papanicolaou test (Pap test or Pap smear) and
  - HPV DNA testing
- VIA/VILI is recommended for cervical cancer screening in low- and middle-income countries with high incidence of cervical cancer and lack of medical resources
- HPV testing and VIA are more cost-effective screening methods than cytology.

CRITERIA IN SCREENING

Results of Screening Test: Rules for Construction of 2 × 2 Table

- Always disease (present or absent) to be represented on the top-most row of the table
- Always screening test results (positive or negative) to be represented on the left-most column of the table
- Then only all formulae (for evaluation of screening test) can be applied

		Disease	
Results of a screening test for a disease		Present	Absent
Results	Positive	a (TP)	b (FP)
	Negative	c (FN)	d (TN)

- *'a' are known as True positive (TP):* Population having the disease and showing screening test results as positive
- *'d' are known as True negative (TN):* Population not having the disease and showing screening test results as negative
- *'b' are known as False positive (FP):* Population not having the disease but erroneously showing screening test results as positive
- *'c' are known as False negative (FN):* Population having the disease but erroneously showing screening test results as negative
- Total population having the disease, i.e. cases: 'a + c' (True positive + False negative)
- Total population not having the disease, i.e. healthy: 'b + d' (False positive + True negative)

Results of Screening Test: Evaluation/Properties of a Screening Test^Q

- *Sensitivity:* Ability of a screening test to identify correctly all those who have the disease (cases)
- Sensitivity = a/(a + c) × 100 = TP/(TP + FN) × 100
- *Specificity:* Ability of a screening test to identify correctly all those who do not have the disease (healthy)
- Specificity = d/(b + d) × 100 = TN/(TN + FP) × 100
- *Positive predictive value (PPV):* Ability of a screening test to identify correctly all those who have the disease, out of all those who test positive on a screening test
- PPV = a/(a + b) × 100 = TP/(TP + FP) × 100
- *Negative predictive value (NPV):* Ability of a screening test to identify correctly all those who do not have the disease, out of all those who test negative on a screening test
- NPV = d/(c + d) × 100 = TN/(FN + TN) × 100
- Percentage of false positives (FP):
- % FP = b/(b + d) × 100 = FP/(FP + TN) × 100
- Percentage of false negatives (FN):
- % FN = c/(a + c) × 100 = FN/(TP + FN) × 100

> **Key points**
>
> *Sensitivity:* Ability of a screening test to identify correctly all those who have the disease (cases)

Positive Predictive Value (PPV)

- *Definition:* Ability of a screening test to identify correctly all those who have the disease, out of all those who test positive on a screening test
- PPV = a/(a + b) × 100 = TP/(TP + FP) × 100
- *PPV of a screening test depends on^Q:*
  - Sensitivity
  - Specificity
  - Prevalence of disease in the population
- PPV of a screening test is directly proportional to prevalence of disease in the population
  - PPV α Prevalence of disease^Q
  - As the prevalence of a disease increases in a population, PPV increases for the screening test

> **Key points**
>
> *PPV of a screening test depends on^Q:*
> - Sensitivity
> - Specificity
> - Prevalence of disease

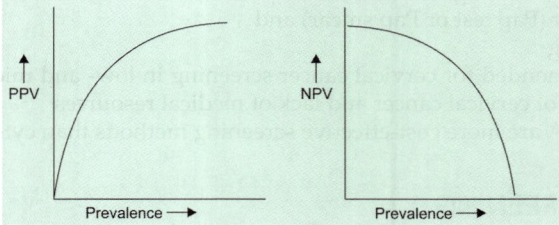

Prevalence and predictive value

Likelihood Ratio^Q

- *Description:* Incorporates both the sensitivity and specificity of the test and provides a direct estimate of how much a test result will change the odds of having a disease
- *Likelihood ratio for a positive result (LR+)* tells you how much the odds of the disease increase when a test is positive
- LR$^+$ = Sensitivity/(1 – Specificity)
- *Likelihood ratio for a negative result (LR-)* tells you how much the odds of the disease decrease when a test is negative
- LR$^-$ = (1 – Sensitivity)/Specificity

> **Key points**
>
> LR$^+$ = Sensitivity/(1 – Specificity)

- Post-test odds (the chances that patient has a disease): Once you have specified the pre-test odds (the likelihood that the patient would have a specific disease prior to testing), you multiply them by the likelihood ratio
- $Odds_{post} = Odds_{pre} \times$ Likelihood ratio

Reliability/Precision/Repeatability/Consistency/Reproducibility^Q

- *Definition:* Test gives consistent results when repeated more than once on the same individual or material, under the same conditions
- *Reliability is measured by:*
  - Pearson product-moment correlation coefficient
  - Cronbach's alpha (internal consistency)
- *Reliability of a test depends on:*
  - Observer variation:
    - *Intra-observer variation:* Same observer taking 2 or more readings give varied results
    - *Inter-observer variation:* Variation between different observers on same subject/material
  - *Biological (subject) variation:* occur due to
    - Changes in parameters observed
    - Variation in perceptions and answers of patients
    - Regression to the mean
  - *Errors relating to technical methods:* occur due to
    - Defective instruments
    - Erroneous calibrations
    - Faulty reagents
    - Inappropriate/unreliable test

Validity/Accuracy

- *Definition:* Refers to what extent the test measures which it purports to measure (adequacy of measurement)
- *Validity has 2 components:*
  - Sensitivity
  - Specificity
- *Types of Validity:*
  - *Conclusion validity:* Defines if there is a relationship between 2 variables
  - *Internal validity:* Assuming relationship between 2 variables, defines if it is causal
    - Is free of bias
    - Valid conclusions can be drawn for individuals in a sample
  - *Construct validity:* Assuming causal relationship between 2 variables, defines if our theory is best to our constructs
  - *External validity:* Assuming causal relationship between 2 variables, defines if our theory can be generalized to the broader population
  - *Concurrent validity:* refers to the degree of correlation with other measures of the same construct measured at the same time
  - *Face (Logical) validity:* Relevance of a measurement appear obvious
  - *Content validity:* Measurement of all variable components
  - *Consensual validity:* If no. of experts agree to a parameter
  - *Criterion validity:* If compared with a reference or gold standard
    - Is best measure of validity^Q
    - Usually expressed as sensitivity & specificity^Q
  - *Discriminant validity:* If not showing strong correlation between 2 variables

> **Key points**
>
> *Criterion validity:* If compared with a reference or gold standard
> - Is best measure of validity^Q
> - Usually expressed as sensitivity & specificity^Q

Precision versus Accuracy

	Precision	Accuracy
Definition	Repeatability, reliability, consistency, reproducibility of a test	Degree of closeness of a measured/ calculated quantity to its actual/ true value, Validity
Test(s)	Range chart R – chart	Mean chart Levy Jennings (LJ) chart^Q Shewhart control chart

Screening Tests in Series & Parallel

- *Screening Tests Used in Series*: A population is subjected to one screening test followed by a second screening test; 2nd screening test is applied on those individuals only who test positive on the 1st screening test
  - *Combined sensitivity of 2 tests A & B in series*:
    = Sensitivity (A) × Sensitivity (B)
  - *Combined specificity of 2 tests A & B in series*:
    = [Specificity (A) + Specificity (B)] − [Specificity (A) × Specificity (B)]
- *Screening Tests Used in Parallel*: A population is subjected to two (or more) screening tests at the same time; each of the individuals is subjected to both (or all) screening tests
  - *Combined sensitivity of 2 tests A & B in parallel*:
    = [Sensitivity (A) + Sensitivity (B)] − [Sensitivity (A) × Sensitivity (B)]
  - *Combined specificity of 2 tests A & B in parallel*:
    = Specificity (A) × Specificity (B)

	Tests in series^Q	Tests in parallel^Q
Combined sensitivity	Decreases	Increases
Combined specificity	Increases	Decreases
Combined PPV	Increases	Decreases
Combined NPV	Decreases	Increases

MISCELLANEOUS

Bayes' Theorem^Q

- *Baye's Theorem*: Gives relationship between PPV of a screening test and Sensitivity, Specificity & Prevalence of disease in a population

$$PPV = \frac{[Sensitivity \times Prevalence]}{[Sensitivity \times Prevalence] + (1 - Specificity)(1 - Prevalence)} \times 100$$

- Actual *Baye's Theorem*: Gives relationship between Post-test probability of a disease in a population (PTP = PPV) and Sensitivity, Specificity & Pre-test probability of a disease in a population (pTP = Prevalence)

$$PTP = \frac{[Sensitivity \times pTP]}{[Sensitivity \times pTP] + [(1 - Specificity)(1 - pTP)]} \times 100$$

  - Post-test probability of a disease in a population (PTP) IS SAME AS PPV
  - Pre-test probability of a disease in a population (pTP) IS SAME AS Prevalence
- NPV is inversely proportional to Prevalence of disease in a population

$$NPV = \frac{[Specificity \times (1 - Prevalence)]}{[Specificity \times (1 - Prevalence)] + [(1 - Sensitivity) \times Prevalence]} \times 100$$

PYQs: Quick Review for NEET

Advantage gained by screening	Lead Time
Sensitivity identifies	True Positives
Usefulness of a screening test is given by	Sensitivity
Sensitivity is given by	True positives
Specificity is given by	True Negatives
PPV is directly proportional to	Prevalence
True positive indicate	Sensitivity
Ability to identify true negatives in screening	Specificity
Best time to do Breast Self-examination screening	One week after menstruation
Screening is _____ level of prevention	Secondary
Screening of cervical cancer at PHC level is done by	Visual inspection of cervix 5% acetic acid (VIA test)
If prevalence of disease increases, predictive value of a positive test will	Increase
Sensitivity is	TP/(TP + FN) X 100
Most important factor for being a good screening test	Sensitivity
Denominator of NPV is	TN + FN
More false positive cases in screening test makes the test	Less specific & more sensitive
Consistency of a screening test depends upon	Reliability

Multiple Choice Questions

CONCEPTS IN SCREENING

1. Which of the following regarding Genetic screening is true? *[INICET May 2022]*
   (a) Screening tests define risk of passing genetic disorder
   (b) Screening tests are more accurate than diagnostic tests
   (c) Screening requires genetic mapping
   (d) Usually involve invasive procedures

2. Study the statement given below for Screening methods. False statement(s) is/are (Multiple response type) *[INICET November 2021]*
   1. For colorectal cancer per rectal exam is used
   2. For breast cancer if mammography is done at 40 years age, females it's prevalence will increase
   3. For Cervical cancer, Pap smear is used
   4. For Oral cancer by examining from outside (visual inspection) is sufficient
   (a) 1 only
   (b) 1, 2
   (c) 1, 4
   (d) 2, 4

3. A woman with Recurrent Trichomoniasis infection was advised Pap smear. She asks you what it is. What would be your answer? *[INICET November 2020]*
   (a) Its screening test for Cervical cancer
   (b) Its diagnostic test for Cervical cancer
   (c) Its screening for cancer of Female genital tract
   (d) Its Diagnostic test for Trichomoniasis infection

4. Screening for Cervical carcinoma done in: *[AIIMS June 2020]*
   (a) More than 60 years age
   (b) Teenagers
   (c) 21 years to 65 years age
   (d) Less than 21 years age

5. There are several points in the course of a disease process: *[AIIMS June 1998]*
   A – Disease onset
   B – Point of first possible detection
   C – Final critical point
   D – Usual time of diagnosis
   E – Final outcome
   For a screening programme to be effective, it should be applied between:
   (a) A and B
   (b) A and C
   (c) B and C
   (d) C and D

6. In "Iceberg Phenomenon" the tip represents what the physician sees in clinical practice and submerged portion of the iceberg represents sub clinical cases, carriers, undiagnosed cases. Essential purpose of screening test for a chronic disease is to identify: *[AIIMS Dec 1995]*
   (a) Tip of the iceberg *[Bihar 2004]*
   (b) Hidden portion of the iceberg
   (c) Both (a) + (b)
   (d) Waterline demarcation

7. The diagnostic power of a test to correctly exclude the disease is reflected by: *[AIIMS Nov 1993]*
   (a) Sensitivity *[NEET Pattern 2017]*
   (b) Specificity
   (c) Positive predictivity
   (d) Negative predictivity

8. 'Lead time' refers to the time between: *[Karnataka 2011] [NEET Pattern 2013, 2017]*
   (a) Disease onset and first critical diagnosis
   (b) Disease onset and first possible point of detection
   (c) First possible point of detection and final critical point
   (d) First possible point of detection and usual time of diagnosis

9. Screening for condition recommended when:
   (a) Low case fatality rate *[NEET Pattern 2012]*
   (b) Diagnostic tools not available
   (c) No effective treatment available
   (d) Early diagnosis can change disease course because of effective treatment

10. Screening is done because of all *except*: *[NEET Pattern 2014]*
    (a) Testing for infection or disease in population or in individuals who are not seeking health care
    (b) It is defined presumptive identification of unrecognized disease
    (c) Search for unrecognized disease or defect by means of rapidly applied test, examinations or other procedures in apparently healthy individuals
    (d) Use of clinical or laboratory tests to detect disease in individual seeking health care for other reasons

11. Which of the following are the characteristic features of screening tests?
    1. Done on healthy people
    2. Done on unhealthy people
    3. More accurate
    4. Less accurate
    5. Less expensive
    6. More expensive

7. Not a basis for treatment
8. Used as a base for treatment

   Select the correct answer using the code given below:
   [UPSC CMS 2015]
   (a) 2, 4, 5 and 8 (b) 1, 3, 5 and 8
   (c) 2, 3, 6 and 7 (d) 1, 4, 5 and 7

12. Ideal screening test should be: *[NEET Pattern 2017]*
    (a) Safe (b) Reliable
    (c) Valid (d) All of the above

13. Screening tests should be? *[PGI May 2018]*
    (a) Costly (b) Easy to perform
    (c) Difficult to perform (d) More specific
    (e) Less sensitive

Review Question

14. Period between the possible time of detection and the actual time of diagnosis is: *[MH 2008]*
    (a) Lead time (b) Screening time
    (c) Generation time (d) Serial interval

TYPES OF SCREENING

15. Prospective screening is done in
    [NEET PG Pattern January 2020]
    (a) Neonate for thyroid disease
    (b) Immigrant screening
    (c) Pap smear for Cervical cancer
    (d) Diabetes mellitus

16. Which of the following is an example of Prospective screening? *[AIIMS Nov 2001]*
    (a) Cervical Pap smear in a 40 years old female
    (b) Neonatal screening in a newborn for Hypothyroidism
    (c) Screening of immigrants in a country
    (d) Urine for sugar screening in a 40 years old male

17. In which of the following disease, screening procedure increases the overall survival maximum?
    [AIIMS May 2007, 08; NEET Pattern 2013; Bihar 2014]
    (a) Prostate cancer
    (b) Lung cancer
    (c) Colon cancer
    (d) Ovarian cancer

18. Most specific screening test for Vitamin D deficiency is:
    (a) 7-dehydrocholesterol *[NUPGET 2013]*
    (b) 1, 25 dihydroxy Vitamin D
    (c) 25 hydroxy Vitamin D
    (d) Serum calcium levels

19. Most reliable test for screening of diabetes mellitus:
    (a) GTT *[NEET Pattern 2012]*
    (b) Glycosylated hemoglobin
    (c) Fasting blood sugar
    (d) Urine for sugar

20. Blood screening is not done for: *[NEET Pattern 2012]*
    (a) HIV (b) HBV
    (c) EBV (d) HCV

21. Example of multiphasic screening is:
    [NEET Pattern 2016]
    (a) Chest X-ray for TB on large population
    (b) Annual health check up
    (c) Pap smear in old females
    (d) Mammography in all young females

CRITERIA FOR SCREENING

22. Correct statement among the following is
    [INICET July 2021]
    (a) Sensitivity depends on prevalence
    (b) Specificity depends on predictive value
    (c) In a population if the tests show more positive value in sensitivity, then there is lesser chance of people having the disease
    (d) Positive predictive value depends on prevalence

23. A total of 130 patients were screened for Disc prolapse by CT scan and confirmation of the disease was made by discectomy operation. Out of 56 patients who screened positive in CT scan, 46 were confirmed for disease in operation. Rest 74 patients who were screened negative in CT scan, only 40 patients were confirmed negative for the disease in operation. Calculate the Positive and Negative likelihood ratio. *[JIPMER May 2019]*
    (a) 2.875 and 0.531
    (b) 6.07 and 1.12
    (c) 1.12 and 6.07
    (d) 0.531 and 2.875

24. Screening test has the following features *except*:
    (a) Done on apparently healthy individuals
    (b) It is less accurate *[Karnataka 2009]*
    (c) Test results are arbitrary and final
    (d) It can be used as a basis for treatment

25. For the calculation of positive predictive value of a screening test, the denominator is comprised of:
    (a) True positives + False negatives *[AIPGME 99, 03]*
    (b) False positives + True negatives *[MH 2007]*
    (c) True positives + False positives
    (d) True positives + True negatives

26. Reliability of a test means: *[AIIMS Nov 2006]*
    (a) It measures what it is supposed to measure
    (b) It is able to correctly predict the presence of disease
    (c) It is able to correctly exclude the possibility of disease
    (d) It yields same reading/value when repeated under same conditions

27. Reliability of a screening test does not means:
    [AIIMS Nov 2006]
    (a) Reproducibility (b) Precision
    (c) Repeatability (d) Validity

28. True about the following is: *[AIPGME 1998]*

	MI present	MI absent
Positive ECG	300	100
Negative ECG	25	75

(a) Sensitivity is less than specificity
(b) Sensitivity is same as specificity
(c) PPV is more than NPV
(d) PPV is same as NPV

29. Positive predictive value is most affected by:
[AIPGME 1999]
   (a) Prevalence
   (b) Sensitivity
   (c) Specificity
   (d) Relative risk

30. A diagnostic test for a particular disease has a sensitivity of 0.90 and a specificity of 0.90. A single test is applied to each subject in the population in which the diseases population is 10%. What is the probability that a person positive to this test, has the disease? [AIIMS Nov 05]
   (a) 90%
   (b) 81%
   (c) 50%
   (d) 91%

31. In a group of patients presenting to a hospital emergency with abdominal pain, 30% of patients have acute appendicitis. 70% of patients with appendicitis have a temperature greater than 37.5 degree Celsius and 40% of patients without appendicitis have a temperature greater than 37.5 degree Celsius. Considering these findings, which of the following statements is correct? [AIIMS Nov 2004]
   (a) The sensitivity of temperature greater than 37.5 degree Celsius as a marker for appendicitis is 21/49
   (b) The specificity of temperature greater than 37.5 degree Celsius as a marker for appendicitis is 42/70
   (c) The positive predictive value of temperature greater than 37.5 degree Celsius as a marker for appendicitis is 21/30
   (d) The specificity of the test will depend upon the prevalence of appendicitis in the population to which it is applied

32. Specificity of a screening test is the ability of a test to detect:
[AIIMS Nov 2006; AIPGME 2000]
[UP 2000, DPG 2011, WB 2005]
[AIIMS May 2009, RJ 2002]
[NEET Pattern 2017]
   (a) True positives
   (b) False positives
   (c) False negatives
   (d) True negatives

33. Diagnostic power of the test is reflected by:
   (a) Sensitivity [AIPGME 2005]
   (b) Specificity [NEET Pattern 2015]
   (c) Predictive value
   (d) Population attributable risk

34. If the Hemoccult test is negative for screening of colonic cancer, no further test is done. If the hemoccult test is positive the individual will have a second stool sample tested with the Hemoccult II test. If this second for blood, the individual will be referred for more extensive evaluation. The effect of net sensitivity and net specificity of this method of screening is:
[AIIMS May 2005; JIPMER November 2017]
   (a) Net sensitivity and net specificity are both increased
   (b) Net sensitivity is decreased and net specificity is increased
   (c) Net sensitivity is increased and net specificity is decreased
   (d) Net sensitivity remains the same and net specificity is increased

35. A screening test is used in same way in two similar populations, but the proportion of false positive results among those who test positive in population A is lower than among those who test positive in population B. What is the likely explanation for this finding?
[AIIMS Nov 2008, AIIMS May 03; AIPGME 01]
   (a) The specificity of the test is lower in population A
   (b) The prevalence of disease is lower in population A
   (c) The prevalence of disease is higher in population A
   (d) The specificity of the test is higher in population A

36. A test for hepatitis C is performed for 200 patients with biopsy-proven disease and 200 patients known to be free of the disease. The test shows positive results on 180 of the patients with the disease, and negative results on 150 of the patients without the disease. Among those tested, this test therefore: [AIPGME 2002]
   (a) Has a positive predictive value of 90%
   (b) Has a negative predictive value of 75%
   (c) Has a sensitivity of 90%
   (d) Has a specificity of 82.5%

37. Due to an effective prevention program, the prevalence of an infectious disease in a community has been reduced by 90%. A physician continues to use the same diagnostic test for the disease that she has always used. How have the test's characteristics changed? [AIPGME 1992]
   (a) Its sensitivity has increased
   (b) Its positive predictive value has increased
   (c) Its negative predictive value has increased
   (d) The test's characteristics have not changed

38. Validity of a test is based upon all except: [AIIMS Nov 95]
[NEET Pattern 2013]
   (a) Sensitivity
   (b) Specificity
   (c) Precision
   (d) Accuracy

39. The probability of a test detecting a truly positive person from the population of diseased is the: [AIIMS Nov 98]
   (a) Sensitivity of the test
   (b) Specificity of the test
   (c) Positive predictive value of the test
   (d) Likelihood ratio

40. For the diagnosis of Deep Vein Thrombosis, 2 tests are done together, namely Impedance plethysmography and leg scanning after injecting 125I fibrinogen. This process will lead to: [AIIMS Nov 2006]
   (a) Increasing the positive predictive value
   (b) Increasing the negative predictive value
   (c) Increasing the pretest odds
   (d) Increasing the specificity

41. Blood pressure (BP) of Mr Ram is 120/80 mm Hg. Four different sphygmomanometries (I, II, III, IV) are used to measure his BP with three readings each. Based on their readings, match the sphygmomanometries with their respective accuracy and precision parameters:

Readings of sphygmomanometries		Parameters	
I	120/ 80, 120/ 80, 120/ 80	A	Precise but Inaccurate
II	140/ 96, 108/62, 96/82	B	Imprecise but Accurate
III	140/ 96, 140/ 96, 140/ 96	C	Precise and Accurate
IV	122/ 82, 120/ 80, 118/ 78	D	Imprecise and Inaccurate

(a) A – II, B – IV, C – I, D – III [DPG 2006]
(b) A – III, B – II, C – IV, D – I
(c) A – IV, B – III, C – II, D – I
(d) A – III, B – IV, C – I, D – II

42. Study this formula carefully:

$$\frac{\text{True positives}}{\text{True positive + False negatives}} \times 100$$

This denotes: [AIPGME 1996; 03]
(a) Sensitivity [DNB 2000, 2006, 2007]
(b) Specificity
(c) Positive Predictive value
(d) Negative Predictive value

43. Sensitivity indicates: [DPG 2008]
(a) Positivity in disease
(b) Detection of positivity cases not in disease
(c) It identify correctly those who have not in disease
(d) It depends upon positive cases having disease and negative cases having disease

44. In a population of 10000 people, the prevalence of a disease is 20%. The sensitivity of a screening test is 95% and specificity is 80%. The positive predictive value of the test will be: [AIIMS Nov 2009]
   [NEET Pattern 2015, 2017]
(a) 54.3% (b) 45.7%
(c) 15.3% (d) 98.5%

45. True about reliability of a test: [AIIMS Nov 2009]
(a) Gives same results on repeated tests
(b) Investigator's knowledge is important
(c) Consistency and reproducibility of the test are not a problem
(d) Extent of variation of measurement of contained behaviour

46. A test has high false positive rate in a community. True is:
   [AIIMS May 2010]
   [DNB 2011, WB 2008]
(a) High prevalence
(b) Low prevalence
(c) High sensitivity
(d) High specificity

47. A doctor order 6 tests for SLE. Which of the following is needed for inference? [AIIMS May 2010]
(a) Prior probability of SLE, sensitivity and specificity of test
(b) Incidence of SLE and predictivity of each test
(c) Incidence and prevalence of SLE
(d) Relative risk of SLE in the patient

48. A graph showing curves of Normal blood sugar level and Diabetic blood sugar level is shown below. Some area is found over-lapping in the two curves. Diagnostic cut-off point of 120 mg/dL is also marked. What does the shaded area (D) represent in the graph?
(a) True positive [AIPGMEE 2011]
(b) True negative
(c) False positive
(d) False negative

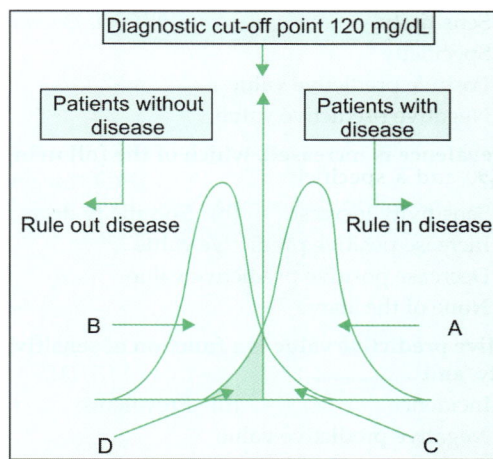

49. You have clinically diagnosed a patient as having SLE and ordered 6 tests, out of which 4 have come positive and 2 have come negative. To know the probability of SLE at this point, you need to know:
   [AIIMS November 2011] [AIPGME 2012]
(a) Incidence of SLE and Predictive value of each test
(b) Incidence and prevalence of SLE
(c) Relative risk of SLE in this patient
(d) Prior probability of each test, Sensitivity and specificity of each test

50. A new method of measuring Haemoglobin levels has been developed. Ten successive readings of a single sample are as follows: 9.4, 10.4, 9.6, 9.1, 10.8, 12.1, 10.1, 9.8, 9.2, 9.5. But the Haemoglobin measured by standard calorimetry was 10.2. Therefore the given method has:
   [AIIMS November 2011]
(a) Low validity, low reliability
(b) Low validity, high reliability
(c) High validity, low reliability
(d) High validity, high reliability

51. A city has a population of 10000 with 500 diabetic patients. A new diagnostic test gives true positive result in 350 patients and false positive result in 1900 patients. Which of the following is/are true regarding the test?
   [PGI May 2013]
(a) Prevalence is 5% (b) Sensitivity is 70%
(c) Specificity is 80% (d) Sensitivity is 80%
(e) Specificity is 70%

52. The formula A /A+B in the following table denotes?

Test result	Persons with disease	Persons without disease	Total
Positive	A	B	A + B
Negative	C	D	C + D

(a) Specificity [JIPMER May 2018, DPG 2008]
(b) Sensitivity
(c) PPV
(d) NPV

53. The ability of a test to correctly diagnose the percentage of sick people who are having the condition is called as:
    (a) Sensitivity [DNB December 2009]
    (b) Specificity
    (c) Positive predictive value
    (d) Negative predictive value

54. If prevalence is increased, which of the following will be seen? [PGI November 2013]
    (a) Sensitivity increase
    (b) Specificity decrease
    (c) Increase positive predictive value
    (d) Decrease positive predictive value
    (e) None of the above

55. Positive predictive value is a function of sensitivity, specificity and .... [AIIMS May 2014]
    (a) Incidence
    (b) Prevalence
    (c) Negative predictive value
    (d) Accuracy

56. True statement about PPV is: [NEET Pattern 2014]
    (a) It increases with prevalence
    (b) It decreases with prevalence
    (c) No relation with prevalence
    (d) Doubles with decrease in prevalence

57. 5000 persons underwent screening for a disease. Out of 500 diseased, 350 reported True positive and out of 4500 healthy, 3000 reported True negative. Which of the following is correct about this screening test?
     [NEET Pattern 2014]
    (a) Sensitivity 70%
    (b) Specificity 70%
    (c) Sensitivity 80%
    (d) Specificity 80%

58. A diagnostic test for a particular disease has a sensitivity of 0.90 and a specificity of 0.80. A single test is applied to each subject in the population in which the diseased population is 30%. What is the probability that a person, negative to this test, has no disease?
     [NEET Pattern 2014]
    (a) Less than 50%
    (b) 70
    (c) 95%
    (d) 72%

59. Recently a new Latex Agglutination Test was approved for Screening of a disease. Calculate Sensitivity and Specificity based on the findings given below:
     [AIIMS November 2015]

	Test positive	Test negative
Diseased	27	3
Non-diseased	5	95

    (a) Sensitivity 90%, Specificity 90%
    (b) Sensitivity 95%, Specificity 90%
    (c) Sensitivity 90%, Specificity 95%
    (d) Sensitivity 95%, Specificity 95%

60. A screening test was carried out among 114 population & 15 had the disease. 22 showed test positive among which 14 had the disease. What is the sensitivity of the test?
     [NEET Pattern 2015]
    (a) 37%
    (b) 63%
    (c) 93%
    (d) 100%

61. CA-125 is a marker for screening of Ovarian cancer. To characterize this test, histopathological confirmation of ovarian cancer was done in a cohort of patients. 60/100 women who tested positive for this test actually had ovarian cancer and 20/100 women who tested negative had ovarian cancer. What is the negative predictive value of this test? [AIIMS November 2016]
    (a) 20/100
    (b) 40/100
    (c) 60/100
    (d) 80/100

62. Sensitivity of a test is defined as:
     [NEET Pattern 2016, 2017]
    (a) Probability that a person with negative test do not have the disease in question
    (b) Probability that a person with positive test has indeed the disease in question
    (c) Ability of a test to identify correctly those who are having the disease
    (d) Ability of a test to identify correctly those who are not having the disease

63. A screening test is applied for screening of liver cancer in a population of 500. The test shows positive result in 80 individuals and negative in remaining 420. Out of 80 positive individuals 60 confirmed to be diagnosed liver cancer by diagnostic test and 20 were ruled out. Out of negative 420 individuals 40 had liver cancer. The sensitivity of the test is: [NEET Pattern 2017]
    (a) 60%
    (b) 80%
    (c) 90%
    (d) 95%

64. The Sensitivity of a given Screening test is quite high. It implies [AIIMS November 2017]
    (a) If test comes positive, patient has the disease
    (b) If test comes negative, patient does not have the disease
    (c) If disease is prevalent in the population and test comes positive, patient is likely to have the disease
    (d) If disease is rare in the population and test comes positive, patient is likely to have the disease

65. Out of 1000 population, a screening test found 90 to be diabetic correctly. Then a Gold standard test found 100 to be diabetic. What is the Sensitivity of the test?
     [NEET Pattern 2018]
    (a) 90/1000
    (b) 10/1000
    (c) 90/100
    (d) 110/1000

66. Which of the following statement is/are true?
     [PGI November 2017]
    (a) Sensitivity and specificity of test depend on prevalence of disease
    (b) Predictive value reflects the diagnostic power of the test

(c) Positive predictive value depend on prevalence of disease
(d) Sensitivity and specificity of test are characteristics of the test
(e) Sensitivity is Usefulness of a screening test

67. In a screening test for DM, Out of 1000 population 90 were positive. Then gold standard test was done in which 100 were positive calculate the sensitivity?
[NEET Pattern 2018]
(a) 90/100 (b) 100/110
(c) 80/100 (d) 100/100

68. If Two screening tests are used in Series, then there will be [AIIMS November 2018]
(a) Increased sensitivity and decreased specificity
(b) Increased specificity and decreased sensitivity
(c) Increased sensitivity and increased specificity
(d) Decreased sensitivity and decreased specificity

69. Probability that a person out of those tested positive on a screening test has in fact the disease is known as
[NEET Pattern 2019]
(a) Sensitivity (b) Specificity
(c) Positive predictive value
(d) Negative predictive value

Review Questions

70. False negative means: [Bihar 2006]
(a) Persons have disease but show negative test result
(b) Persons have not disease but show negative test result
(c) Persons have disease but show positive test result
(d) Persons have not disease but show positive test result

71. A screening test is more sensitive: [UP 2005, RJ 2007]
(a) Few false positive (b) Few false negative
(c) More false positive (d) More false negative

72. High false positive cases in a community signify that disease has: [AI 2001; UP 2008]
(a) High prevalence and Low incidence
(b) High incidence and Low prevalence
(c) Low prevalence and Low incidence
(d) High Incidence and High prevalence

73. Positive predictive value of a test does not depends upon:
[MP 2001]
(a) Sensitivity (b) Specificity
(c) Prevalence of disease (d) Incidence of disease

74. Sensitivity numerator is: [MP 2001]
(a) False positives [AIIMS May 2015]
(b) False negatives [AIIMS November 2015]
(c) True negatives
(d) True positives

75. A screening test was positive in 50% of diseased and 10% of healthy population. What is the specificity of the test?
[MP 2006]
(a) 0.5 (b) 0.9
(c) 0.83 (d) 0.064

76. True positive cases are detected by:
[MH 2000; RJ 2006; NEET Pattern 2015]
(a) Specificity
(b) Sensitivity
(c) Positive predictive value
(d) Negative predictive value

MISCELLANEOUS

77. Two researchers rated 50 images for needing further study. The researchers (A and B) either said Yes (for further study) or No (No further study needed). 20 images were rated Yes by both whereas 15 images were rated No by both. Overall, rater A said Yes to 25 images and No to 25. Overall, Rater B said Yes to 30 images and No to 20. Calculate Kappa statistic in the given question:
[INICET May 2023]
(a) 0.13 (b) 0.26
(c) 0.40 (d) 0.70

78. Bands used for Confidence intervals in Kaplan Meier Curve [INICET May 2023]
(a) Kolmogorov-Smirnov bands
(b) Berk and Jones bands
(c) Hall Wellner bands
(d) Hall and Wood bands

79. What is External validity of a study?
[INICET November 2021]
(a) Replicability
(b) Generalization
(c) Objectivity
(d) Causality

80. Which of the following option is true about ROC curve?
[JIPMER May 2019]
(a) It is a method of evaluating the quality/performance of tests
(b) It is plotted as test Sensitivity as x-coordinate versus its 1-Specificity (False positive rate FPR) as the y-coordinate
(c) A perfect test has an area under the ROC curve (AUROCC) of >1
(d) A decrease in sensitivity results in decrease in specificity

81. Screening in general population done in cancers of:
(a) Breast [PGI Dec 02]
(b) Colon
(c) Cervix
(d) Ovarian
(e) Pancreatic

82. Which of the following is not useful as a screening method? [AIIMS PGMEE November 2013]
(a) Pap smear for Cervical cancer
(b) CA-125 for Ovarian cancer
(c) Office endometrial washing for Endometrial cancer
(d) USG in Endometrial cancer

83. Screening test for Breast and Genital tract malignancy is: *[AIIMS November 2014]*
    (a) CA-125
    (b) Mammography
    (c) Office endometrial aspiration
    (d) Pap smear

84. Best time to screen in Breast self-examination (BSE) technique is *[NEET Pattern 2014]*
    (a) 1 week before the menstruation
    (b) 1 week after the menstruation
    (c) During ovulation
    (d) 2-3 days post-ovulation

85. Screening is not useful for: *[AIIMS PG May 2015]*
    (a) Carcinoma colon
    (b) Breast carcinoma
    (c) Prostate carcinoma
    (d) Testicular carcinoma

86. Which of these is the best for determining the threshold for diagnosis of a positive test? *[AIIMS November 2016]*
    (a) Pre-test probability
    (b) Receiver operator characteristic curve
    (c) Pearson coefficient
    (d) Analysis of Variance

Review Question

87. The method of choice of tuberculosis detection mass screening is: *[TN 2003]*
    (a) Tuberculin test
    (b) Mass Miniature Radiography (MMR)
    (c) Sputum smear examination by direct microscopy
    (d) Sputum culture

Explanations

CONCEPTS IN SCREENING

1. **Ans. (a) Screening tests define risk of passing genetic disorder; (d) Usually involve invasive procedures**
   [Ref. Park 26/e p924]
   Genetic screening/testing
   - Genetic testing is a type of medical test that identifies changes in genes, chromosomes, or proteins
   - It is a process to analyze blood or skin for the systematic search for persons with a particular genotype in a defined population (usually invasive procedures)
   - In order to locate this faulty gene, scientists search for variations in larger pieces of DNA called "markers", latter are found nearby the DNA and become the basis of genetic screening
   - The results of a genetic test can confirm or rule out a suspected genetic condition or help determine a person's chance of developing or passing on a genetic disorder

2. **Ans. (c) 1, 4** *[Ref. Park 26/e p152-153]*
   Screening for Cancers
   - For colorectal cancer, Colonoscopy is the ideal screening test
   - For breast cancer if mammography is done at 40 years age, females it's prevalence will increase (Below 40 years its not useful due to breast tissue density)
   - For Cervical cancer, Pap smear is used (VIA is better and more cost-effective though)
   - For Oral cancer, Bimanual oral palpation is used

3. **Ans. (a) Its screening test for Cervical cancer**
   [Ref. Park 26/e p432]
   - Trichomonads may be viewed on Pap smear, but this test yields low sensitivity and should not be relied on for diagnosis of T. vaginalis infection
   - Sensitivity of Pap smear for detecting trichomonads is 40-60% and Specificity approaches 95% in the hands of trained technicians
   - False-positive results are also common with this technique.

4. **Ans. (c) 21 years to 65 years age** *[Ref. Park 26/e p432]*
   Updated Cervical Cancer Screening Guidelines (ACOG)
   - *Age less than 21 years:* No Screening required
   - *Age 21-29 years:* Cytology alone once every 3 years
   - *Age 30-65 years:* Cytology alone once every 3 years OR Primary hrHPV testing alone once every 5 years OR Co-testing (hrHPV testing + Cytology) once every 5 years
   - *Age more than 65 years:* No Screening required (after prior negative results)
   - *Hysterectomy with removal of cervix:* No Screening required (if no history of high grade precancerous lesions or cervical cancer)

5. **Ans. (c) B and C** *[Ref. Park 27/e p152]*
   - Screening programmes are most useful if it can be applied before a final critical point in a disease (i.e. point after which attempted treatment of disease may not yield desirable beneficial effects); but they cannot detect a disease before B (Point of first possible detection)
   - Thus a screening test is most useful if applied between B (Point of first possible detection) and C (Final critical point)
   - It is of no use if applied after a final critical point.

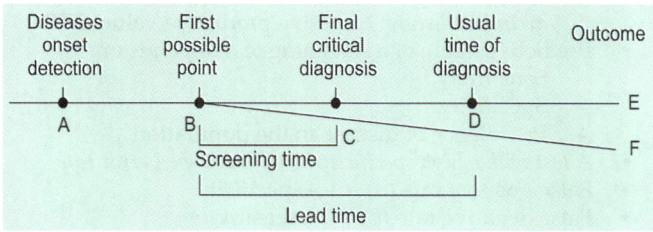

Model for early detection programmes

   - B – C: Screening time
   - B – D: Lead Time
     * Lead time is the advantage gained by screening (leading the time of diagnosis): Early detection of disease (B rather than D) will ensure earlier institution of treatment, thus better prognosis

6. **Ans. (b) Hidden portion of the iceberg**
   [Ref. Park 27/e p151]
   - *Differences in portions of iceberg phenomenon of disease:*

	Tip of iceberg	Submerged part of iceberg
Composition	Clinical cases	Latent, inapparent, presymptomatic, undiagnosed and undiagnosed cases and carriers
Visibility to clinician	Visible	Invisible
Prime importance for	Clinician	Epidemiologist
Detection	Diagnostic tests	Screening tests
Useful level of prevention	Secondary	Secondary

   - *Iceberg phenomenon of a disease is not shown by:*
     - Rabies
     - Tetanus
     - Measles
     - Rubella
   - *Iceberg phenomenon of a disease is also known as: Biological spectrum of a disease*

7. **Ans. (d) Negative predictivity** *[Ref. Park 27/e p156]*
   - *Negative predictive value [NPV]:* Ability of a screening test to identify correctly all those who do not have the

disease, out of all those who test negative on a screening test

$$NPV = \frac{d}{c + d} \times 100 = \frac{TN}{TN + FN} \times 100$$

ALSO REMEMBER
- *'Usefulness of a screening test'* is given by: Sensitivity
- *Statistical index of diagnostic accuracy:* Sensitivity
- *Diagnostic power of a screening test:* Predictive accuracy
  - *Diagnostic power of a screening test to correctly identify a disease:* Positive predictive value (PPV)
  - *Diagnostic power of a screening test to correctly exclude a disease:* Negative predictive value (NPV)
- Predictive value of a screening test depends on:
  - Sensitivity
  - Specificity
  - Prevalence of disease in the population
- *A test with a high specificity has a low Type I error rate*
- False positive rate (α) = 1 – specificity
- False negative rate (β) = 1 – sensitivity
- Power of a test (sensitivity) = 1 – β
- Receiver operating characteristic (ROC) curve, is a graphical plot between:
  - Sensitivity and (1 – specificity) OR
  - True positive rate and false positive rate
- *Efficiency of a Screening Test [E]:* the percentage of the times that the test give the correct answer compared to the total number of tests

$$E = \frac{TP + TN}{TP + TN + FP + FN} \times 100 = \frac{a + d}{a + b + c + d} \times 100$$

- *Youden's J statistic [Youden's index]:* Is a single statistic that captures the performance of a test
  Y = Sensitivity + Specificity - 1

8. **Ans. (d) First possible point of detection and usual time of diagnosis** [Ref. Park 27/e p151]
9. **Ans. (d) Early diagnosis can change disease course because of effective treatment** [Ref. Park 27/e p153]
10. **Ans. (d) Use of clinical or laboratory tests to detect disease in individual seeking health care for other reasons** [Ref. Park 27/e p151]
11. **Ans. (d) 1, 4, 5 and 7** [Ref. Park 27/e p151]
12. **Ans. (d) All of the above** [Ref. Park 27/e p151]

    Criteria for Ideal Screening Test
    - Acceptability, Repeatability (Reliability, Precision, Reproducibility), Validity
    - Safety, Rapidity, Yield, Simplicity, Ease of administration, Cheaper

13. **Ans. (b) Easy to perform; (d) More specific** [Ref. Park 27/e p151]

Review Question

14. **Ans. (a) Lead time** [Ref. Park 27/e p151]

TYPES OF SCREENING

15. **Ans. (b) Immigrant screening** [Ref. Encyclopedia of Immigrant Health by Loue 1/e (Volume 1) p1330]
    - *Prospective screening:* People screened for other's benefit with essential purpose of Disease control
    - *Examples:* Screening of immigrants, HIV screening among Sex workers.

16. **Ans. (c) Screening of immigrants in a country** [Ref. Park 27/e p153]
    - *Screening of disease:* Is used to search for an unrecognized diseases or defect, in apparently healthy individuals, by means of rapidly applied tests, examinations or other procedures
    - *Types of screening:*

	Prescriptive screening	Prospective screening
Definition	People screened for own's benefit	People screened for other's benefit
Essential purpose	Case detection	Disease control
Request for screening	No specific request	Specific request from authority
Example[s]	Neonatal screening Pap smear Urine for sugar	HIV screening among sex workers Screening of immigrants

ALSO REMEMBER
NEONATAL SCREENING (NNS):
- NNS is primarily a Secondary Level of Prevention
- *Neonatal hypothyroidism [NNH]:*
  - Most common neonatal disorder to be screened is Neonatal hypothyroidism [NNH]
  - *Blood sample of choice:* Umbilical cord blood
  - *Detection of:* TSH, T4
- *Phenylketonuria [PKU]:*
  - *PKU is an autosomal recessive trait* with a frequency of 1 in 10,000 births
  - *Enzyme deficient in PKU:* Phenylalanine hydroxylase
  - *Treatment of PKU:* restricting or eliminating foods high in phenylalanine, such as breast milk, meat, chicken, fish, nuts, cheese, legumes and other dairy products
  - *Guthrie Test:* Is done in neonates for mass screening of Phenylketonuria (PKU)
    1. *Guthrie test was the first screening test used in neonates*
    2. *Blood sample* is collected by heel prick of the baby 7 –10 days after birth
    3. *Guthrie Test is negative* in first 0 – 3 days of life
    4. *Guthrie test can detect* PKU, Galactosemia and Maple syrup urine disease
    5. *Chemicals detected*: Phenylalanine, Phenylpyruvate and Phenyllactate
    6. It is a semi-quantitative test
  - Currently, Guthrie test has been replaced by *Tandem mass Spectrometry* (TMS)

17. **Ans. (c) Colon cancer** *[Ref. CMDT 2014 p1571]*
    - *Colorectal cancer is ideal for screening:* as it is a common disease affecting 6% of men and women, which is fatal in half of the cases, yet it is curable if detected at an early stage

18. **Ans. (c) 25 hydroxy Vitamin D** *[Ref. Clinical Laboratory Medicine by McClatchey, 2/e p446]*

19. **Ans. (c) Fasting blood sugar** *[Ref. Park 27/e p449]*

20. **Ans. (c) EBV** *[Ref. Transfusion Guidelines for Clinicians by K Bhardwaj, 1/e p110]*

21. **Ans. (b) Annual health check up** *[Ref. Park 27/e p152]*

    TYPES OF SCREENING
    - Mass screening: Screening of whole population or a subgroup irrespective of individual's risk
      – Example: Chest X-ray for TB on large population
    - High risk (Selective) screening: Screening applied selectively to high risk groups based on epidemiological research
      – Examples: Cervical cancer screening in lower socioeconomic strata, Diabetes screening in members of a family with history, HIV screening in risk groups
    - Multiphasic screening: Application of two or more screening tests in combination to a large number of people at one time
      – Example: Annual health check ups
    - Multipurpose screening: Screening of a population by more than one test done simultaneously to detect more than one disease
      – Example: Screening of a pregnant women for VDRL, HIV, HBV by serological tests on a blood sample
    - Opportunistic and case finding screening: If there is no accurate or precise diagnostic test for the disease and where the frequency of its occurrence in the population is small; an objective is to detect disease and bring patients to treatment
      – Example: RHD in children

CRITERIA FOR SCREENING

22. **Ans. (d) Positive predictive value depends on prevalence** *[Ref. Park 26/e p155]*
    - *Baye's Theorem:* Gives relationship between PPV of a screening test and Sensitivity, Specificity & Prevalence of disease in a population
    - PPV is directly proportional to Prevalence
    - NPV is inversely proportional to Prevalence

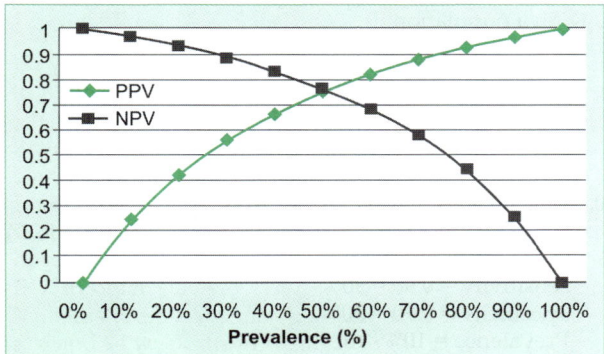

23. **Ans. (a) 2.875 and 0.531** *[Ref. Primary Care Medicine by Goroll 6/e p12]*

    In the given question, first we'll have to construct the 2×2 screening test table correctly (a=46, a+b =56, d=40, c+d=74 are given)

	Disease present	Disease absent	Total
ST positive	46 (a)	10 (b)	56
ST negative	34 (c)	40 (d)	74

    - **So,** Sensitivity = a/a+c × 100 = 46/(46+34) × 100 = 57.5% (0.575)
    - Specificity = d/b+d × 100 = 40/(10+40) × 100 = 80% (0.80)
    - **Now,** Positive likelihood ratio = Sensitivity/(1-Specificity) = 0.575/ (1-0.80) = 2.875
    - Negative likelihood ratio = (1-Sensitvity)/Specificity = (1-0.575)/0.80= 0.531.

24. **Ans. (d) It can be used as a basis for treatment** *[Ref. Park 27/e p151]*

25. **Ans. (c) True positives + False positives** *[Ref. Park 25/e p152]*
    - *Evaluation of screening test:*

Criteria	Numerator	Denominator
Sensitivity	True positives (a)	True positives + False negatives (a + c)
Specificity	True negatives (d)	True negatives + False positives (b + d)
PPV	True positives (a)	True positives + False positives (a + b)
NPV	True negatives (d)	True negatives + False negatives (c + d)
% False positives	False positives (b)	True negatives + False positives (b + d)
% False negatives	False negatives (c)	True positives + False negatives (a + c)

    - *Positive predictive value [PPV]:* Ability of a screening test to identify correctly all those who have the disease, out of all those who test positive on a screening test
      – PPV of a screening test depends on:
        1. Sensitivity
        2. Specificity
        3. Prevalence of disease in the population
      – PPV of a screening test is directly proportional to prevalence of disease in the population
        PPV α Prevalence of disease
    - As the prevalence of a disease increases in a population, PPV increases for the screening test

    > **ALSO REMEMBER**
    > - PPV is also known as *'post-test probability of a disease'* or *'precision rate'*
    > - *Baye's Theorem:* Gives relationship between PPV of a screening test and Sensitivity, Specificity and Prevalence of disease in a population
    > - NPV is inversely proportional to Prevalence of disease in a population
    >
    > $$PPV = \frac{[Sensitivity \times Prevalence]}{[Sensitivity \times Prevalence] + [(1 - Specificity)(1 - Prevalence)]} \times 100$$

26. **Ans. (d) It yields same reading/value when repeated under same conditions**   *[Ref. Park 27/e p154-156]*
    - *Reliability of a test:* Test gives consistent results when repeated more than once on the same individual or material, under the same conditions
    - *Reliability is also known as:* Repeatability, Precision or Reproducibility
    - *Reliability is measured by:*
        - Pearson product-moment correlation coefficient
        - Cronbach's alpha (internal consistency)
    - *Reliability of a test depends on:*
        - Observer variation:
            1. Intra-observer variation: Same observer taking 2 or more readings give varied results
            2. Inter-observer variation: Variation between different observers on same subject/material
        - Biological [subject] variation: occur due to
            1. Changes in parameters observed
            2. Variation in perceptions and answers of patients
            3. Regression to the mean
        - Errors relating to technical methods: occur due to
            1. Defective instruments
            2. Erroneous calibrations
            3. Faulty reagents
            4. Inappropriate/unreliable test

    > **ALSO REMEMBER**
    > - *Intra-observer variation can be minimized by:* taking average of readings
    > - *Inter-observer variation can be minimized by:*
    >   - Standardization of procedures/classifications
    >   - Intensive training of all observers
    >   - Making use of 2 or more observers for independent assessment
    > - *Accuracy:* degree of closeness of a measured or calculated quantity to its actual (true) value
    > $$\text{Accuracy} = \frac{TP + TN}{TP + FP + FN + TN}$$
    > - *Precision:* the degree to which further measurements or calculations show the same or similar results
    >   - *Reliability is precision, while validity is accuracy*
    > - Reliability is inversely related to random error

27. **Ans. (d) Validity**   *[Ref. Park 27/e p154]*
    - *Validity:* Refers to what extent the test measures which it purports to measure (adequacy of measurement)
    - *Validity has 2 components:*
        - Sensitivity
        - Specificity

28. **Ans. (d) PPV is same as NPV**   *[Ref. Park 27/e p156]*

Criteria	MI present	MI absent
Positive ECG	300 (TP a)	100 (FP b)
Negative ECG	25 (FN c)	75 (TN d)

    - Sensitivity = $\frac{a}{a+c} \times 100 = \frac{TP}{TP+FN} \times 100$

    - Sensitivity = $\frac{300}{300+25} \times 100 = 92\%$

    - Specificity = $\frac{d}{b+d} \times 100 = \frac{TN}{TN+FP} \times 10$

    - Specificity: $\frac{75}{75+100} \times 100 = 43\%$

    - Positive predictive value (PPV)

      $= \frac{a}{a+b} \times 100 = \frac{TP}{TP+FP} \times 100$

    - PPV = $\frac{300}{300+100} \times 100 = 75\%$

    - Negative predictive value (NPV)

      $= \frac{d}{c+d} \times 100 = \frac{TN}{FN+TN} \times 100$

    - NPV = $\frac{75}{25+75} \times 100 = 75\%$

    - Therefore,
        - Sensitivity > PPV OR NPV > Specificity
        - PPV = NPV

29. **Ans. (a) Prevalence**   *[Ref. Simple Biostatistics by Indrayan and Indrayan, 1/e p58]*
    - *Baye's Theorem:* Gives relationship between PPV of a screening test and Sensitivity, Specificity and Prevalence of disease in a population

    $$PPV = \frac{[\text{Sensitivity} \times \text{Prevalence}]}{[\text{Sensitivity} \times \text{Prevalence}] + [(1 - \text{Specificity})(1 - \text{Prevalence})]} \times 100$$

    - *Actual Baye's Theorem:* Gives relationship between Post-test probability of a disease in a population (PTP = PPV) and Sensitivity, Specificity and Post-test probability of a disease in a population (pTP = Prevalence)

    $$PTP = \frac{[\text{Sensitivity} \times pTP]}{[\text{Sensitivity} \times pTP] + [(1 - \text{Specificity})(1 - pTP)]} \times 100$$

    - Post-test probability of a disease in a population (PTP) IS SAME AS PPV
    - Pre-test probability of a disease in a population (pTP) IS SAME AS Prevalence

    > **ALSO REMEMBER**
    > - NPV is inversely proportional to Prevalence of disease in a population
    >
    > $$NPV = \frac{\text{Specificity} \times (1 - \text{Prevalence})}{[\text{Specificity} \times (1 - \text{Prevalence})] + [(1 - \text{Sensitivity}) \times \text{Prevalence}]} \times 100$$

30. **Ans. (c) 50%**   *[Ref. Simple Biostatistics by Indrayan and Indrayan, 1/e p58]*

    In the given question,
    Sensitivity = 0.90 = 90%
    Specificity = 0.90 = 90%
    Prevalence = 10%

Thus,

$$PPV = \frac{90 \times 10}{[90 \times 10] + [(100-90)(100-10)]} \times 100 = 50\% (0.50)$$

$$= 50\% (0.50)$$

- **Alternate way of solving such questions:** Construct a hypothetical table of screening test (FOLLOW RULES: Disease on top of table, screening test results on left side of table). Always take round values (e.g. 100, 1000, etc. as total population)

Results of a screening test for a disease		Disease	
		Present	Absent
Results	Positive	a (TP)	b (FP)
	Negative	c (FN)	d (TN)
	Total	a + b	b + d

Now taking hypothetically, a + b + c + d (total population) = 1000,
Prevalence = 10% (given in question); No. of cases (a + c) = 100
Thus, No. of healthy population (b + d) = Total population – cases = 1000 – 100 = 900
Since sensitivity $\left(\frac{a}{a+c} \times 100\right) = 0.90\% = 90\%$; a = 90 and c = 10
Similarly, specificity $\left(\frac{d}{b+d} \times 100\right) = 0.90\% = 90\%$; d = 810 and b = 90

Thus table will be as follows,

Results of a screening test for a disease		Disease	
		Present	Absent
Results	Positive	90	90
	Negative	10	810
	Total	100	900

Now, $PPV = \frac{a}{a+b} \times 100 = \frac{90}{90+90} \times 100 = 50\% (0.50)$

31. **Ans. (b) The specificity of temperature greater than 37.5 degree Celsius as a marker for appendicitis is 42/70**
    [Ref. Park 27/e p155]
    - In the given question, disease is Acute appendicitis and screening test is temperature (Positive if ≥ 37.5°C)
    - Taking a hypothetical total population (a + b + c + d) = 100, Prevalence of Acute appendicitis = 30%; cases (a + c) = 30
    Healthy population (without acute appendicitis; b + d) = 100 – 30 = 70
    a = TP = 70% of (a + c) = 21
    b = FP = 40% of (b + d) = 28
    c = FN = 30% of (a + c) = 9
    d = TN = 60% of (b + d) = 42
    Therefore,

- Sensitivity = $\frac{a}{a+c} \times 100 = \frac{21}{30} \times 100$

- Specificity = $\frac{d}{b+d} \times 100 = \frac{42}{70} \times 100$

- Positive predictive value (PPV)
  = $\frac{a}{a+b} \times 100 = \frac{21}{49} \times 100$

- Negative predictive value (NPV)
  = $\frac{d}{c+d} \times 100 = \frac{42}{51} \times 100$

32. **Ans. (d) True negatives** *[Ref. Park 27/e p155–156]*
    - Specificity of a screening test is the ability of a test to detect: True negatives
    - Sensitivity of a screening test is the ability of a test to detect: True positives
    - 'Usefulness of a screening test' is given by: Sensitivity
    - Statistical index of diagnostic accuracy: Sensitivity

> **ALSO REMEMBER**
> - Out of those disease in a population, few are correctly picked as positive by a screening test, this is: Sensitivity of a screening test
>   - Sensitivity = $\frac{a}{a+c} \times 100$
> - Out of those healthy in a population, few are correctly picked as not having the disease by a screening test, this is: Specificity of a screening test
>   - Specificity = $\frac{d}{b+d} \times 100$
> - Out of those shown positive by a screening test in a population, those who actually have the disease, this is: PPV of a screening test
>   - Positive predictive value (PPV) = $\frac{a}{a+b} \times 100$
> - Out of those shown negative by a screening test in a population, those who actually don't have the disease, this is: NPV of a screening test
> - Negative predictive value (NPV) = $\frac{d}{c+d} \times 100$

33. **Ans. (c) Predictive value** *[Ref. Park 27/e p156]*
    - Diagnostic power of a screening test: Predictive accuracy (it tells the actual no. of people having the disease or not having the disease out of those shown positive or negative by a screening test, respectively)
      – Diagnostic power of a screening test to correctly identify a disease: Positive predictive value (PPV)
      – Diagnostic power of a screening test to correctly exclude a disease: Negative predictive value (NPV)

34. **Ans. (b) Net sensitivity is decreased and net specificity is increased** *[Ref. Simple Biostatistics by Indrayan and Indrayan, 1/e p56]*
    SCREENING TESTS USED IN SERIES: A population is subjected to one screening test followed by a second screening test; 2nd screening test is applied on those individuals only who test positive on the 1st screening test
    - Combined sensitivity of 2 tests A and B in series: Sensitivity (A) × Sensitivity (B)

- Combined specificity of 2 tests A and B in series: Specificity (A) + Specificity (B) − [Specificity (A) × Specificity (B)]

SCREENING TESTS USED IN PARALLEL: A population is subjected to two (or more) screening tests at the same time; each of the individuals is subjected to both (or all) screening tests
- Combined sensitivity of 2 tests A and B in parallel: Sensitivity (A) + Sensitivity (B) − [Sensitivity (A) × Sensitivity (B)]
- Combined specificity of 2 tests A and B in parallel: Specificity (A) × Specificity (B)

	Tests in series	Tests in parallel
Combined sensitivity	Decreases	Increases
Combined specificity	Increases	Decreases
Combined PPV	Increases	Decreasee
Combined NPV	Decreases	Increases

35. **Ans. (c) The prevalence of disease is higher in population A** [Ref. Simple Biostatistics by Indrayan and Indrayan, 1/e p 58]

Results of a screening test for a disease		Disease	
		Present	Absent
Results	Positive	a (TP)	b (FP)
	Negative	c (FN)	d (TN)

- Total population having the disease [cases]: 'a + c' (TP + FN)
- Total population not having the disease [healthy]: 'b + d' (FP + TN)
- Total population: a + b + c + d = TP + FP + FN + TN
- PPV depends on sensitivity, specificity and prevalence of disease in the population

Now in this question, a screening test is used in same way in two similar populations; thereby the screening test will have similar sensitivity and specificity in both populations
PPV = a/(a + b) × 100, thus b (False Positive rate) is inversely proportional to PPV; and PPV is directly proportional to Prevalence of disease in a population,
So, False Positive rate (FP rate) is inversely proportional to the prevalence of disease in the population
Therefore, if the same screening test is having lower FP rate in population A (as compared to a similar population B), then this could be explained by higher prevalence of disease in population A
Also,
Prevalence of disease:

$$\frac{\text{Cases}}{\text{Total population}} \times 100 = \frac{a+c}{a+b+c+d} \times 100$$

Therefore, as b (FP rate) is lower in population A, prevalence of disease will be higher in this population

36. **Ans. (c) Has a sensitivity of 90%** [Ref. Park 27/e p155]
Now as given in the question, a + c (cases) = 200; b + d (healthy) = 200
Also, test shows positive results on 180 of the patients with the disease (200), so a (TP) = 180 and c (FN) = 20; and negative results on 150 of the patients without the disease, so d (TN) = 150 and b (FP) = 50

Results of a screening test for a disease	Hepatitis C	
	Present	Absent
Results Positive	180	50
Negative	20	150
Total	200	200

- Sensitivity $= \frac{a}{a+c} \times 100 = \frac{TP}{TP+FN} \times 100$
  - Sensitivity $= \frac{180}{180+20} \times 100 = 90\%$
- Specificity $= \frac{d}{b+d} \times 100 = \frac{TN}{TN+FP} \times 100$
  - Specificity: $\frac{150}{150+50} \times 100 = 75\%$
- Positive predictive value (PPV)
  $= \frac{a}{a+b} \times 100 = \frac{TP}{TP+FP} \times 100$
  - PPV $= \frac{180}{180+50} \times 100 = 78\%$
- Negative predictive value (NPV)
  $= \frac{d}{c+d} \times 100 = \frac{TN}{FN+TN} \times 100$
  - NPV $= \frac{150}{20+150} \times 100 = 88\%$

37. **Ans. (c) Its negative predictive value has increased** [Ref. Simple Biostatistics by Indrayan and Indrayan, 1/e p58]
- PPV and NPV of a screening test depends on:
  - Sensitivity
  - Specificity
  - Prevalence of disease in the population

In this question, since a physician continues to use the same diagnostic test for the disease that she has always used, sensitivity and specificity of the test will remain same
But predictive value of a test (PPV and NPV) depends on prevalence of a disease in a population
- PPV is directly proportional to prevalence of disease in the population
  - PPV á Prevalence of disease
  - As the prevalence of a disease increases in a population, PPV increases for the screening test
- NPV is inversely proportional to Prevalence of disease in a population
  - NPV α 1/Prevalence of disease
  - As the prevalence of a disease increases in a population, NPV decreases for the screening test

Therefore, since the prevalence of an infectious disease in a community has been reduced by 90%, its PPV will reduce and its NPV will increase

38. **Ans. (c) Precision** [Ref. Park 27/e p154]
- Validity: Refers to what extent the test measures which it purports to measure (adequacy/accuracy of measurement)

Screening of Disease

- *Validity has 2 components:*
  - Sensitivity
  - Specificity
- *Inherent properties of a screening test:*
  - Sensitivity
  - Specificity
  - Predictive accuracy

> **ALSO REMEMBER**
> - *Accuracy:* degree of closeness of a measured or calculated quantity to its actual (true) value
> - *Accuracy* = [(sensitivity) (prevalence)] + [(specificity) (1 – prevalence)]
> - *Efficiency/ Accuracy of a Screening Test [E]:* the percentage of the times that the test give the correct answer compared to the total number of tests
>
> $$E = \frac{TP + TN}{TP + TN + FP + FN} \times 100 = \frac{a + c}{a + b + c + d} \times 100$$
>
> - *Precision:* the degree to which further measurements or calculations show the same or similar results
>   - *Precision is also known as:* Reliability, Repeatability, Consistency or Reproducibility
> - *Precision versus Accuracy:*
>
> | | Precision | Accuracy |
> | --- | --- | --- |
> | Definition | Repeatability, reliability, consistency, reproducibility of a test | Degree of closeness of a measured or calculated quantity to its actual (true) value |
> | Test[s] | Range chart
R – chart | Mean chart
Levy Jennings (LJ) chart
Shewhart control chart |
>
> - *Reliability is precision, while validity is accuracy*
> - PPV is also known as 'post-test probability of a disease' or 'precision rate'
> - Levy Jennings (LJ) chart is a 'test of accuracy and test of loss of precision'

39. **Ans. (a) Sensitivity of the test** [Ref. Park 27/e p155]
    - *Sensitivity of a screening test detects:* true positives among all diseased
    - *Specificity of a screening test detects:* true negatives among all healthy
    - *PPV detects:* true positives among all those who are positive on a screening test
    - *NPV detects:* true negatives among all those who are negative on a screening test

> **ALSO REMEMBER**
> - *Likelihood ratio:* Incorporates both the sensitivity and specificity of the test and provides a direct estimate of how much a test result will change the odds of having a disease
>   - *Likelihood ratio for a positive result [LR+]* tells you how much the odds of the disease increase when a test is positive
>
> $$LR^+ = \frac{Sensitivity}{1 - Specificity}$$
>
>   - *Likelihood ratio for a negative result [LR-]* tells you how much the odds of the disease decrease when a test is negative
>
> $$LR^- = \frac{1 - Sensitivity}{Specificity}$$
>
> - *Post-test odds [the chances that patient has a disease]:* Once you have specified the pre-test odds (the likelihood that the patient would have a specific disease prior to testing), you multiply them by the likelihood ratio
> $Odds_{post} = Odds_{pre} \times$ Likelihood ratio

40. **Ans. (b) Increasing the negative predictive value**
    [Ref. Simple Biostatistics by Indrayan and Indrayan, 1/e p56]
    In the given question, 2 tests - Impedance Plethysmography and leg scanning after injecting 125I fibrinogen are done together, for the diagnosis of Deep Vein Thrombosis. Therefore these are two tests in done in parallel

41. **Ans. (d) A – III, B – IV, C – I, D – II** [Ref. A Dictionary of Public Health by J Kishore, p5, 410]
    - *Accuracy:* degree of closeness of a measured or calculated quantity to its actual (true) value
    - *Precision:* the degree to which further measurements or calculations show the same or similar results
      - Precision is also known as: Reliability, Repeatability, Consistency or Reproducibility
    - *Accuracy* = [(sensitivity) (prevalence)] + [(specificity) (1 – prevalence)]
    - $Accuracy = \frac{TP + TN}{TP + FP + FN + TN} \times 100$
    - *Reliability is precision, while validity is accuracy*

42. **Ans. (a) Sensitivity** [Ref. Park 27/e p155]

43. **Ans. (a) Positivity in disease; (d) It depends upon positive cases having disease and negative cases having disease**
    [Ref. Park 27/e p155]

44. **Ans. (a) 54.3%** [Ref. Park 27/e p155]
    In the given question,
    Sensitivity = 95%
    Specificity = 80%
    Prevalence = 20%
    Thus,
    $$PPV = \frac{[95 \times 20]}{[95 \times 20] + [(100 - 80)(100 - 20)]} \times 100 = 54.3\%$$

45. **Ans. All choices** [Ref. Park 27/e p154]
    RELIABILITY OF A TEST
    - Gives same results on repeated tests: Reliability
    - Investigator's knowledge is important
    - Consistency and reproducibility of the test are not a problem
    - Extent of variation of measurement of contained behaviour

46. **Ans. (c) High sensitivity** [Ref. Park 27/e p155]

Results of a screening test for a disease		Disease	
		Present	Absent
Results	Positive	a (TP)	b (FP)
	Negative	c (FN)	d (TN)

- Total population having the disease (cases): 'a + c' (TP + FN)
- Total population not having the disease (healthy): 'b + d' (FP + TN)
- Total population: a + b + c + d = TP + FP + FN + TN

Now, both cases (a + c) and healthy (b + d) are fixed in a population.

Thus if b (FP) increase, then d (TN) will reduce.

In the given question, higher FP (b) means a lower d (TN) or low specificity. Now both sensitivity and specificity are inversely related.

Thus Sensitivity will increase, will be higher

47. **Ans. (a) Prior probability of SLE, sensitivity and specificity of test** [Ref. Simple Biostatistics by Indrayan and Indrayan, 1/e p107-08; AIIMS 2011]
    - Post-test probability of a disease in a population (PTP) IS SAME AS PPV
    - Pre-test probability of a disease in a population (pTP) IS SAME AS Prevalence

    In the given question, a patient is clinically diagnosed as having SLE

    Thus, to determine the probability of SLE at this point (Post-test probability of SLE OR PPV), one would need to know Prior probability of SLE (Pre-test probability OR Prevalence of SLE); sensitivity and specificity of each test

48. **Ans. (d) False negative** [Ref. Park 27/e p156]

    In the given graph, Persons on the right side of diagnostic point (i.e., blood sugar level > 120 mg/dl) are declared as having the disease (= A + C). Similarly, those on the left side of diagnostic point (i.e., blood sugar level < 120 mg/dL) are declared as not having the disease (= B + D).

    Since A + C = Declared diseased; A = True positives and C = False positives

    AND since B + D = Declared non-diseased; B = True negative and D = False negative

49. **Ans. (d) Prior probability of each test, Sensitivity and specificity of each test** [Ref. Simple Biostatistics by Indrayan and Indrayan, 1/e p58]

50. **Ans. (c) High validity, low reliability** [Ref. Park 27/e p154]
    - Reliability is precision (repeatability) and Validity is accuracy (close to true/actual value)

    In the given question, 10 successive readings are all different and they have a mean value of 9.4+10.4+9.6+9.1+10.8+12.1+10.1+9.8+9.2+9.5/10 = 10.0

    Thus it has low reliability (non-consistent) and high validity (close to true/actual value of 10.2)s

51. **Ans. (a) Prevalence is 5%; (b) Sensitivity is 70%; (c) Specificity is 80%** [Ref. Park 27/e p155]

52. **Ans. (c) PPV** [Ref. K. Park 22/e p131-32, 24/e p152]

53. **Ans. (a) Sensitivity** [Ref. Park 27/e p155]

54. **Ans. (c) Increase positive predictive value** [Ref. Park 27/e p156]

55. **Ans. (b) Prevalence** [Ref. Park 27/e p156]

56. **Ans. (a) It increases with prevalence** [Ref. Park 27/e p156]

57. **Ans. (a) Sensitivity 70%** [Ref. Park 27/e p155]

58. **Ans. (c) 95%** [Ref. Park 27/e p155]

59. **Ans. (c) Sensitivity 90%, Specificity 95%** [Ref. Park 27/e p155]

    In the given question, first make the table in correct format as below,

	Diseased	Non-diseased
Test positive	27 (a)	5 (b)
Test negative	3 (c)	95 (d)

    Now, Sensitivity = a/(a + c) × 100 = 27/30 × 100 = 90%
    Specificity = d/(b + d) × 100 = 95/100 × 100 = 95%

60. **Ans. (c) 93%** [Ref. Park 27/e p155]
    In the given question, a + b + c + d = 114; a + c = 15; a + b = 22; a = 14

	Disease present	Disease absent	
ST positive	14 (a)	08 (b)	22
ST negative	01 (c)	91 (d)	92
	15	99	114

    Sensitivity = a/(a+c) × 100 = 14/15 × 100 = 93.3%

61. **Ans. (d) 80/100** [Ref. Park 27/e p155]
    In the given question,
    Total positive on test (a+b) = 100; Diseased out of positive (a) = 60
    So, c = 40
    Total negative on test (c+d) = 100; Diseased out of negative (c) = 20
    So, d = 80

	Disease present	Disease absent	
Test positive	60 (a)	40 (b)	100
Test negative	20 (c)	80 (d)	100

    NPV = d/(c+d) × 100 = 80/100 × 100 = 80% (80/100)

62. **Ans. (c) Ability of a test to identify correctly those who are having the disease** [Ref. Park 27/e p155]
    - *Sensitivity:* Ability of a test to identify correctly those who are having the disease
    - *Specificity:* Ability of a test to identify correctly those who are not having the disease
    - *Positive predictive value:* Probability that a person with positive test has indeed the disease in question
    - *Negative predictive value:* Probability that a person with negative test do not have the disease in question

63. **Ans. (a) 60%** [Ref. Park 27/e p155]
    In the given question,
    - Total population (a + b + c + d) = 500

- Total positive results (a + b) = 80
- Total negative results (c + d) = 420
- Out of total positives 80 (a + b), 60 (a) confirmed to be diagnosed Liver cancer
- Out of total positives 80 (a + b), 20 (b) ruled out for Liver cancer
- Out of total negatives 420 (c + d), 40 (c) had Liver cancer

So, out of total negatives 420 (c + d), 380 (d) ruled out for Liver cancer

Therefore, 2 × 2 table construction

	Liver cancer present	Liver cancer absent	Total
Screening test positive	60 (a)	20 (b)	80
Screening test negative	40 (c)	380 (d)	420

- Sensitivity = a/(a + c) × 100 = 60/(60 + 40) × 100 = 60%

64. **Ans. (c) If disease is prevalent in the population and test comes positive, patient is likely to have the disease** *[Ref. Park 27/e p155]*
    - A positive screening test is always followed by a confirmatory diagnostic test
    - Sensitivity is ability of a screening test to identify correctly all those who have the disease (cases)
    - A screening test with high sensitivity would suggest that those testing positive are extremely likely to have the condition(especially if prevalence of disease is high in population) and should progress to having a diagnostic test
    - If a disease is very rare in the population, then positive test is more likely to be a false positive (rather than being a true positive)

65. **Ans. (c) 90/100** *[Ref. Park 27/e p155]*
    In the given question,
    - Total population (a + b + c + d) = 1000
    - Total diabetic (a + c) = 100 (Diseased confirmed by Gold standard test)
    - Total positives on a Screening test (a) = 90
    Thus,
    - Sensitivity of screening test = a/(a + c) × 100 = 90/100 × 100 = 90% = 0.90 = 90/100

66. **Ans. (b) Predictive value reflects the diagnostic power of the test; (c) Positive predictive value depend on prevalence of disease; (d) Sensitivity and specificity of test are characteristics of the test; (e) Sensitivity is usefulness of a screening test** *[Ref. Park 27/e p156]*

67. **Ans. (a) 90/100** *[Ref. Park 25/e p149]*
    - Sensitivity = Total correctly diagnosed positive/Total diseased × 100 = 90/100 × 100 = 90%

    Note: Its' not mentioned in the question how many were True positives or False positives in 90 who tested positive; so we have to presume its near 90%.

68. **Ans. (b) Increased specificity and decreased sensitivity** *[Ref. Simple Biostatistics by Indrayan and Indrayan, 1/e p56]*

Two Screening Test Used in Series
- A population is subjected to one screening test followed by a second screening test; 2nd screening test is applied on those individuals only who test positive on the 1st screening test. So, automatically overall Sensitivity will decrease
- Specificity is Inverse of Sensitivity, so overall Specificity will decrease
- Combined sensitivity of 2 tests A and B in series: Sensitivity (A) × Sensitivity (B)
- Combined specificity of 2 tests A and B in series: Specificity (A) + Specificity (B) – [Specificity (A) × Specificity (B)]

69. **Ans. (c) Positive predictive value** *[Ref. Park 27/e p156]*

Screening test table

Results of a screening test for a disease		Disease	
		Present	Absent
Results	Positive	a (TP)	b (FP)
	Negative	c (FN)	d (TN)

Now, **in the given question**
- Persons those have been tested positive on a screening test: a + c (TP + FP)
- Person who in fact is having the disease: a (TP), c (FN)

So, a person who has tested positive on a screening test has in fact the disease = a/ (a+c) = Positive predictive value

Review Questions

70. **Ans. (a) Persons have disease but show negative test result** *[Ref. Park 27/e p155]*
71. **Ans. (b) Few false negative** *[Ref. Park 27/e p155]*
72. **Ans. (b) High incidence and Low prevalence** *[Ref. Park 27/e p155]*
73. **Ans. (d) Incidence of disease** *[Ref. Park 27/e p155]*
74. **Ans. (d) True positives** *[Ref. Park 27/e p155]*
75. **Ans. (b) 0.9** *[Ref. Park 27/e p155]*
76. **Ans. (b) Sensitivity** *[Ref. Park 27/e p155]*

MISCELLANEOUS

77. **Ans. (c) 0.40** *[Ref. Statistical Concepts by DLH Vaughn 1/e p649]*

Kappa coefficient (K)
- Indicates the extent of agreement between frequencies of two sets of data collected on two different occasions
- Formula: K = O-E/(1 – E)
- Interpretation:
  – 0 = agreement equivalent to chance.
  – 0 – 0.20 = slight agreement.
  – 0.21 – 0.40 = fair agreement.
  – 0.41 – 0.60 = moderate agreement.
  – 0.61 – 0.80 = substantial agreement.
  – 0.81 – 0.99 = near perfect agreement
  – 1 = perfect agreement.

In the given question,
- Step 1: Calculate O (the observed agreement):
  – 20 images were rated Yes by both.

- 15 images were rated No by both.
- So, O = Number in agreement/total = (20 + 15)/50 = 0.70
- Step 2: Find the probability that the raters would randomly both say Yes.
  - Rater A said Yes to 25/50 images, or 50% (0.5)
  - Rater B said Yes to 30/50 images, or 60% (0.6)
  - Total probability of the raters both saying Yes randomly is: $0.5 \times 0.6 = 0.30$
- Step 3: Calculate the probability that the raters would randomly both say No.
  - Rater A said No to 25/50 images, or 50% (0.5)
  - Rater B said No to 20/50 images, or 40% (0.4)
  - Total probability of the raters both saying No randomly is: $0.5 \times 0.4 = 0.20$
- Step 4: Calculate E. Add your answers from Step 2 and 3 to get the overall probability that the raters would randomly agree. E = 0.30 + 0.20 = 0.50
- Step 5: K = O−E/(1 − E) = (0.70 − 0.50)/(1 − 0.50) = 0.40

78. **Ans. (c) Hall Wellner bands**
    [Ref. Statistics for Bioengineering Sciences by Vidakovic 1/e p18]
    - Along with the Kaplan–Meier estimates, one usually gets an estimate of the standard error of the survival probability estimate at each time point, and possibly the upper and lower limits of a confidence interval
    - It is standard practice when plotting KM estimates of the survival curve to include curves that connect these pointwise confidence intervals into confidence bands
    - The confidence bands are interpreted as a visual display of the precision of the estimated curve (random function)
    - Two methods are available to construct the confidence bands for KM curves
      - The first has been proposed by Hall and Wellner (1980) (HW)
      - The second, proposed by Nair (1984), is called "Equal precision" (EP)

79. **Ans. (b) Generalization**   *[Ref. Park 26/e p153]*
    - Internal validity is the extent to which a research study establishes a trustworthy cause-and-effect relationship
    - External validity is the extent to which you can generalize the findings of a study to other situations, people, settings and measures

80. **Ans. (a) It is a method of evaluating the quality/performance of tests**
    [Ref. A Dictionary of Public Health by J Kishore, p446-47]
    - **Receiver Operator Characteristic (ROC) Curve** is a graphical representation between sensitivity and specificity of a diagnostic test, 'drawn between Sensitivity and (1 − Specificity)' (ROC curve is drawn between True positives and False positive error rate)
    - It is a method of evaluating the quality/performance of tests
    - In clinical tests, ROC curve is 'used to determine a cut-off point'

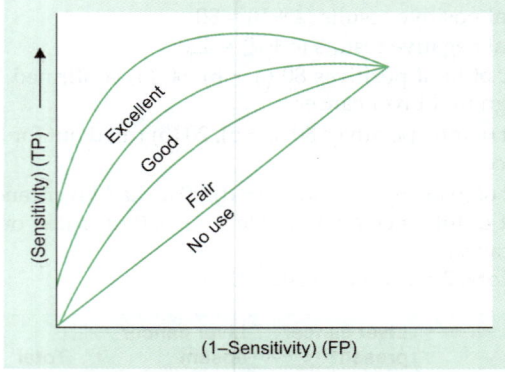

81. **Ans. All CHOICES**   *[Ref. Park 27/e p155-156]*
82. **Ans. (b) CA-125 for Ovarian cancer**   *[Ref. Holland Fries Cancer Medicine 8, Volume 8, p441]*
    EXPLANATION
    - *Endometrial cancer screening:*
      - Pap smear (Not much useful; only recommended for Cervical cancer)
      - Ultrasonography
      - Office endometrial washings
      - Colour flow imaging
    - *Ca-125 in not useful in screening ovarian cancers:*
      - CA125 increases only in late stages of cancer
      - CA125 gives a lot of False positive results
      - CA125 WITH USG is a good screening test

83. **Ans. (a) CA-125**   *[Ref. Primary Care Medicine by Goroll & Mulley, 6/e p824]*
    - CA 125 as marker of carcinomas
      - Ovarian cancer (Most common use)
      - Endometrial cancer
      - Fallopian tube cancer
      - Breast cancer
      - Lung cancer
      - GIT cancer
      - Pancreatic cancer

84. **Ans. (b) 1 Week after the menstruation**   *[Ref. Health Promotion in Nursing by Huerta, 3/e p240]*

85. **Ans. (d) Testicular carcinoma**   *[Ref. Internal Medicine by Stoller, p6]*
    - Screening is NOT routinely recommend for following carcinomas:
      - Testicular carcinoma
      - Lung carcinoma
      - Ovarian carcinoma

86. **Ans. (b) Receiver operator characteristic curve**
    [Ref. Henry's Clinical Diagnosis and Management by Laboratory Methods by McPherson 22/e p88]
    USES OF ROC CURVES
    - Determining the threshold for screening/diagnosis of a positive test
    - Comparison of two or more screening/diagnosis tests of a disease with each other

Review Question

87. **Ans. (c) Sputum smear examination by direct microscopy**
    [Ref. Park 20/e p164; Park 21/e p169, Park 22/e p195]

Chapter 5: Communicable and Non-communicable Diseases

COMMUNICANBLE DISEASES

GENERAL EPIDEMIOLOGY

Period of Communicability
- *Chickenpox:* 1–2 days before to 4–5 days after appearance of rash[Q]
- *Measles:* 4 days before to 5 days after appearance of rash[Q]
- *Rubella:* 7 days before symptoms to 7 days after appearance of rash
- *Mumps:* 4–6 days before symptoms to 7 days thereafter
- *Influenza:* 1–2 days before to 1–2 days after onset of symptoms
- *Diphtheria:* 14–28 days from disease onset[Q]
- *Pertussis:* 7 days after exposure to 3 weeks after paroxysmal stage
- *Meningocccus:* Until absent from nasal and throat discharges[Q]
- *Tuberculosis:* As long as not treated
- *Poliomyelitis:* 7–10 days before and after onset of symptoms[Q]
- *Hepatitis A:* 2 weeks before to 1 week after onset of jaundice
- *Hepatitis B:* Till disappearance of HBsAg & appearance of anti-HBs[Q]
- *Tetanus:* None[Q]

> **Key points**
> *Period of Infectivity:*
> - Chickenpox: 1–2 days before to 4–5 days after appearance of rash
> - Measles: 4 days before to 5 days after appearance of rash

Common Gestational Periods for Vertical Transmission of Diseases
- *Congenital Varicella:* First trimester[Q]
- **Congenital Rubella:** First trimester[Q]
- *Congenital Parvovirus:* Second Trimester[Q]
- *Congenital Syphilis:* Third trimester[Q]
- *Congenital Toxoplasmosis:* Third trimester
- **Congenital Hepatitis B:** Third trimester[Q]
- **Congenital CMV:** Third trimester[Q]
- **Congenital HIV:** During delivery[Q]
- **Congenital Hepatitis C:** During delivery[Q]
- **Congenital Herpes:** During delivery[Q]

> **Key points**
> MC time of Vertical transmission Congenital Rubella: First trimester

Incubation Periods of Common Diseases

Disease	Causative organism	IP
Smallpox	Variola virus	7–14 days
Chickenpox	Human (alpha) herpes virus 3[Q]	14–16 days
Measles (Rubeolla)	RNA paramyxovirus[Q]	10–14 days[Q]
Rubella (German Measles)	RNA Togavirus[Q]	14–21 days
Mumps	RNA Myxovirus	14–21 days
Influenza	Orthomyxovirus	18–72 hours[Q]
Diphtheria	Corynebacterium diphtheriae	2–6 days[Q]
Pertussis (Whooping cough)	Bordetella pertussis	7–14 days
Meningococcal meningitis	Neisseria meningitis	3–4 days

> **Key points**
> Measles (Rubeolla) RNA paramyxovirus[Q] IP 10–14 days[Q]

Contd...

Key points

Hepatitis A Enterovirus 72^Q (Picornavirus) IP 15–45 days IP

Key points

Hepatitis B Hepadna virus 45–180 days IP

Key points

Staphylococcal food poisoning Staphylococccus aureus 1–6 hours IP

Key points

Yellow fever Flavivirus fibricus IP 2–6 days

Key points

Ebola virus IP 2–21 days

Contd...

Disease	Causative organism	IP
SARS	Corona virus^Q	3–5 days
Tuberculosis	Mycobacterium tuberculosis	Weeks–years
Poliomyelitis	Poliovirus	7–14 days^Q
Hepatitis A	Enterovirus 72^Q (Picornavirus)	15–45 days^Q
Hepatitis B	Hepadna virus	45–180 days^Q
Hepatitis C	Hepacivirus	30–120 days
Hepatitis D	Deltavirus	30–90 days
Hepatitis E	Calcivirus	21–45 days
Cholera	Vibrio cholerae	1–2 days^Q
Typhoid fever	Salmonella typhi	10–14 days^Q
Staphylococcal food poisoning	Staphylococccus aureus	1–6 hours^Q
Ascariasis	Ascaris lumbricoides	2 months
Ancylostomiasis (Hookworm)	A. duodenale	5 weeks–9 months
Guinea worm (Dracunculiasis)	Dracunculus medinensis	1 year
Dengue	Arbovirus	3–10 days^Q
Malaria	Plasmodium vivax	8–17 days
	Plasmodium falciparum	9–14 days^Q
	Plasmodium malariae	18–40 days
	Plasmodium ovale	16–18 days
Lymphatic filariasis	Wuchereria bancrofti^Q	8–16 months^Q
Rabies	Lyssavirus type 1 (Rhabdovirus^Q)	3–8 weeks
Yellow fever	Flavivirus fibricus^Q	2–6 days^Q
Japanese encephalitis	Group B arbovirus (Flavivirus)	5–15 days
KFD	Arbovirus (Flavivirus)	3–8 days
Chikungunya fever	Chikungunyavirus (Arbovirus A)	4–7 days
Leptospirosis	Leptospira interrogans	4–20 days
Bubonic plague	Yersinia pestis	2–7 days
Pneumonic plague	Yersinia pestis	1–3 days
Septicemic plague	Yersinia pestis	2–7 days
Scrub typhus	Rickettsia tsutsugamushi^Q	10–12 days
Q fever	Coxiella burnetti^Q	2–3 weeks
Taeniasis (Tapeworms)	T. solium, T. saginata	8–14 weeks
Leishmaniasis (Kala azar)	L. donovani	1–4 months
Trachoma	Chlamydia trachomatis	5–12 days
Tetanus	Clostridium tetani	6–10 days^Q
Yaws	Treponema pertenue^Q	3–5 weeks
HIV/AIDS	HIV/HTLV–III/LAV	Months–10 years^Q
Swine flu	H1N1 Type A Influenza	1–4 days^Q
Crimean Congo Fever	Nairovirus^Q	1–3 days
NIPAH Virus	Hendra/Henapi virus^Q	14–16 days
Ebola Virus	Ebola virus	2–21 days
Anthrax	Bacillus anthracis	1–7 days
Brucellosis	Bacillus melitensis	5–60 days
COVID-19	SARS-CoV-2	1–14 days

Important Human Parasites

Parasite	Causative organism
Roundworm	Ascaris sp. Ascaris lumbricoides^Q
Balantidiasis	Balantidium coli
Tapeworm	Taenia solium/saginata
Coccidia	Cryptosporidium
Guinea worm	Dracunculus medinensis^Q
Amoebiasis	Entamoeba histolytica
Pinworm	Enterobius vermicularis^Q
Liver fluke	Fasciola hepatica^Q
Giardia	Giardia lamblia
Hookworm	Necator americanus^Q
Head louse	Pediculus humanus
Body louse	Pediculus humanus corporis
Crab louse	Phthirus pubis
Scabies	Sarcoptes scabiei^Q
Strongyloidiasis	Strongyloides stercoralis
Toxocariasis	Toxocara canis, Toxocara cati
Toxoplasmosis	Toxoplasma gondii
Trichinosis	Trichinella spiralis
Whipworm	Trichuris trichiura, Trichuris vulpis

Host of a Disease

- HOST: A person or other animal, including birds & arthropods, that affords subsistence or lodgement to an infectious agent under natural (as opposed to experimental) conditions
    - *Primary (definitive) host:* host in which parasite attains maturity or passes its sexual stage^Q
    - *Secondary (intermediate) host:* Host in which parasite is in larval or asexual stage^Q

Disease	Parasite	Host Primary	Host Secondary
Malaria^Q	Plasmodium	Anopheles	Man
Tapeworm	Taenia solium	Man	Pigs
Tapeworm	Taenia saginata	Man	Cattle
Guinea worm^Q	Dracunculus medinensis	Man	Cyclops
Filariasis	Wuchereria bancrofti	Man	Culex
Hydatid Disease^Q	Echinococcus	Dog	Sheep, Cattle, Man
Sleeping sickness	Trypanosomes	Man	Tse tse fly

- *Obligate host:* Only Host for a Parasite, e.g., Man in Measles, Man in Typhoid Fever^Q
- *Transport host:* A carrier in which the organism remains alive but does not undergo development
- *Paratenic host:* Is similar to an intermediate host, only that it is not needed for the parasite's development cycle to progress
    - *Difference between a paratenic and reservoir host:* Latter is a primary host, whereas paratenic hosts serve as "dumps" for non-mature stages of a parasite which they can accumulate in high numbers
- *Dead-end host:* Is an intermediate host that does generally not allow transmission to the definite host, thereby preventing the parasite from completing its development. For example, humans are dead-end hosts for Echinococcus canine tapeworms

Arboviral Infections in India^Q

Group A (Alpha viruses)	Others
Sindbis	Sandfly fever
Chikungunya	Umbre
Group B (Flaviviruses)	Chandipura
JE	Ganjam
KFD	Minnal
Dengue	Dhori
West Nile fever	African Horse sickness

COVID-19 DISEASE

COVID-19 Timeline

- *Global*
  - *December 2019:* Wuhan Municipal Health Commission, Hubei Province China, reported a cluster of cases of Pneumonia of unknown origin (PUO)
  - *07 January 2020:* Chinese authorities identifies "novel coronavirus, nCoV"
  - *13 January 2020:* A case of novel coronavirus reported in Thailand, the first recorded case outside of China
  - *30 January 2020:* WHO declares novel coronavirus outbreak as PHEIC (Public Health Emergency of International Concern)
  - *11 February 2020:* WHO declares the new coronavirus disease to be called COVID-19; New coronavirus was named SARS-CoV-2
  - *11 March 2020:* WHO declares COVID-19 as a Global Pandemic
  - *08 December 2020:* First dose of Covid vaccine administered globally (in United Kingdom)
- *Indian*
  - *30 January 2020:* India reports its First cases of COVID-19 from Thrissur, Kerala
  - *25 March 2020:* Nation-wide lockdown imposed
  - *16 January 2021:* First dose of Covid vaccine administered in India; India begins one of the world's biggest COVID-19 vaccination programmes
  - *December 2021:* DGCI approves Covaxin for use in 12-18 years old children
  - *December 2021:* Booster drive, 15-18 years old children vaccination drive announced

COVID-19 Situation Update

- *Global Situation Update [as on 01 June 2023]*
  - 689 million cases, 6.88 million deaths, 661 million recoveries, 0.99% Case fatality rate

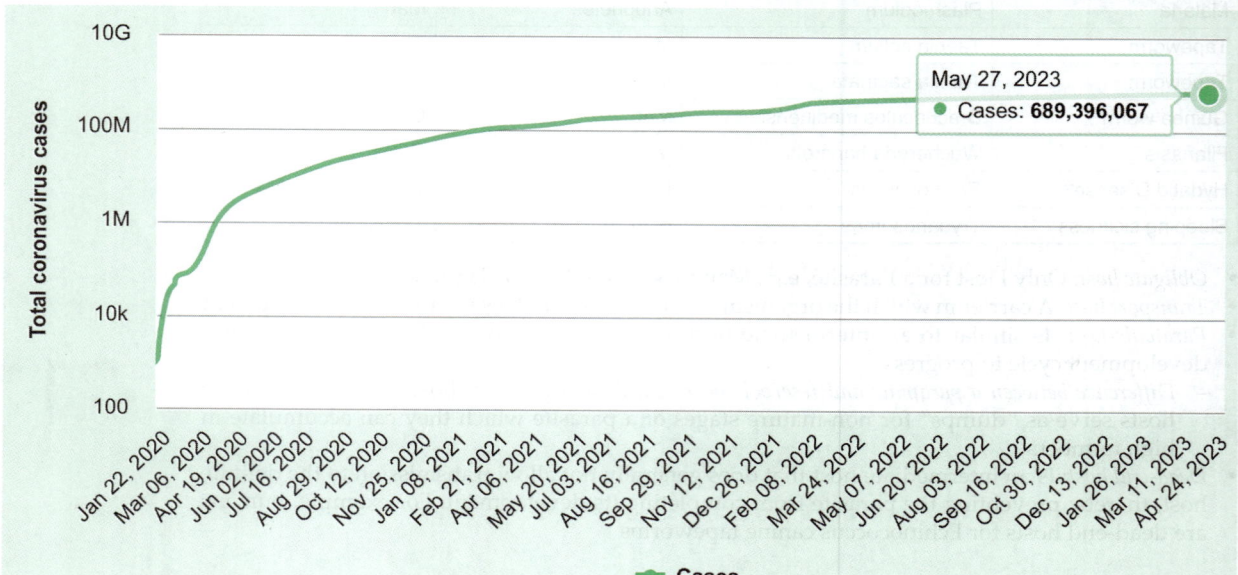

- *Indian Situation Update [as on 01 June 2023]*
  - 44.9 million cases, 0.53 million deaths, 44.4 million recoveries, 1.18% Case fatality rate

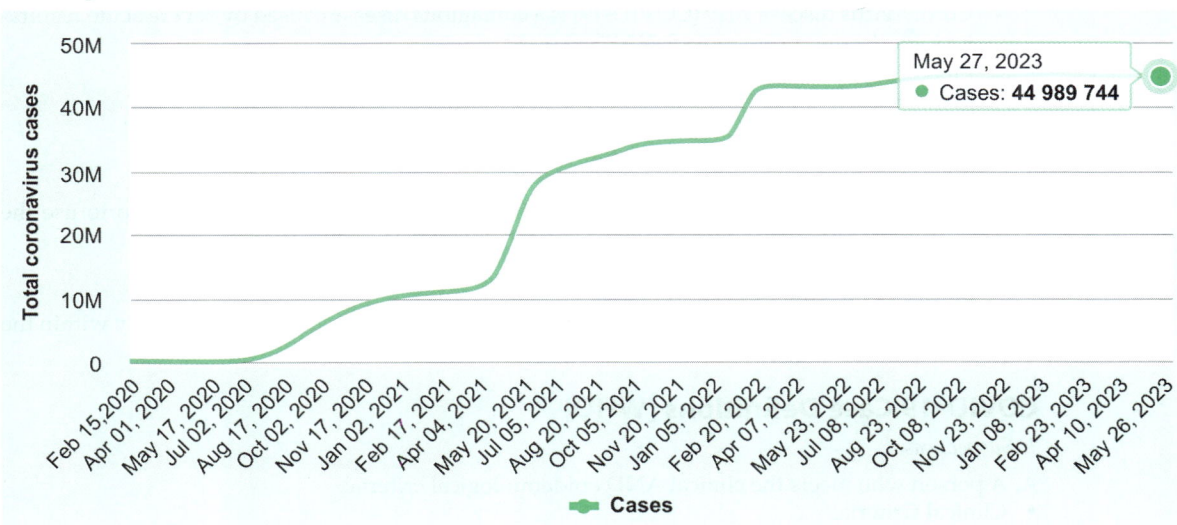

COVID-19 Major Variants (As on 01 June 2023)

- VOC: Variants of Concern

WHO label	Lineage	Date of designation
Omicron	B.1.1.529	26-Nov-2021

(© Table created by Dr Vivek Jain 2023-24)

- VBM: Variants Being Monitored

WHO label	Lineage	Date of designation
Alpha	B.1.1.7	21-Sept-2021
Beta	B.1.351	21-Sept-2021
Gamma	P.1	21-Sept-2021
Delta	B.1.617.2	14-Apr-2022
Epsilon	B.1.427 B.1.429	21-Sept-2021
Eta	B.1.525	21-Sept-2021
Iota	B.1.526	21-Sept-2021
Kappa	B.1.617.1	21-Sept-2021
N/A	B.1.617.3	21-Sept-2021
Zeta	P.2	21-Sept-2021
Mu	B.1.621 B.1.621.1	21-Sept-2021

(© Table created by Dr Vivek Jain 2023-24)

COVID-19 Epidemiology

- *Causative Agent : Coronavirus 'SARS-CoV-2'*
  - Subfamily Orthocoronavirinae, family Coronaviridae, genus Betacoronavirus, order Nidovirales, and realm Riboviria
  - Enveloped viruses with a positive-sense single-stranded RNA genome and a nucleocapsid of helical symmetry
  - Characterized by "Club-shaped spikes" projecting from their surface (Image looks like Solar corona on Electron micrographs)
  - Group of RNA viruses that cause diseases in mammals and birds

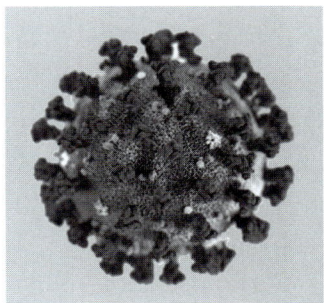

- In humans they can result in mild illnesses (e.g., common cold) or the more lethal illnesses (e.g., SARS, MERS and COVID-19
- COVID-19 Disease
  - Coronavirus disease 2019 (COVID-19) is a contagious disease caused by severe acute respiratory syndrome coronavirus 2 (SARS-CoV-2)
  - First known case was identified in Wuhan, China, in December 2019
  - The disease has since spread worldwide, leading to an ongoing pandemic
- Transmission Dynamics
  - Incubation period: 1-14 days (median 5.1 days)
  - Route(s) of transmission:
    - Respiratory route (Aerosolised droplet transmission); virus has been shown to use the angiotensin-converting enzyme 2 (ACE2) receptor for cell entry
    - Fomite borne transmission
  - Source of Infection: COVID-19 cases
  - Period of Infectivity: Starts 2 days prior to onset of symptoms and declines rapidly within the first week of symptom onset

COVID-19 Case Definitions [WHO]

1. Suspect case

A. A person who meets the clinical AND epidemiological criteria:
- Clinical Criteria:
  - Acute onset of fever AND cough; OR
  - Acute onset of ANY THREE OR MORE of the following signs or symptoms: Fever, cough, general weakness/fatigue, headache, myalgia, sore throat, coryza, dyspnoea, anorexia/nausea/vomiting, diarrhoea, altered mental status
  AND
- Epidemiological Criteria
  - Residing or working in an area with high risk of transmission of virus: closed residential settings, humanitarian settings such as camp and camp-like settings for displaced persons; any time within the 14 days prior to symptom onset; or
  - Residing or travel to an area with community transmission any time within the 14 days prior to symptom onset; or
  - Working in any healthcare setting, including with in health facilities or within the community; any time within the 14 days prior of symptom onset

B. A patient with severe acute respiratory illness:
- SARI: Acute respiratory infection with history of fever or measured fever of ≥38 C°; and cough; with onset within the last 10 days; and requires hospitalization

2. Probable Case
A. A patient who meets clinical criteria above AND is a contact of a probable or confirmed case, or linked to a COVID-19 cluster
B. A suspect case with chest imaging showing findings suggestive of COVID-19 disease
C. A person with recent onset of anosmia (loss of smell) or ageusia (loss of taste) in the absence of any other identified cause.
D. Death, not otherwise explained, in an adult with respiratory distress preceding death AND was a contact of a probable or confirmed case or linked to a COVID-19 cluster

3. Confirmed Case
A. A person with a positive Nucleic Acid Amplification Test (NAAT) including RT-PCR or any other similar test approved by ICMR
B. A person with a positive SARS-CoV-2 Antigen-RDT AND meeting either the probable case definition or suspect criteria OR
C. An asymptomatic person with a positive SARS-CoV-2 Antigen-RDT who is a contact of a probable or confirmed case

Clinical Features of COVID-19 Disease

- Fever, cough, general weakness/fatigue, headache, myalgia, sore throat, coryza, dyspnoea, anorexia/nausea/vomiting, diarrhoea, altered mental status
- Loss of smell (anosmia) or loss of taste (ageusia) preceding the onset of respiratory symptoms (Anosmia increase the pre-test probability of presence of SARS-COV-2)

- Older people and immune-suppressed patients in particular may present with atypical symptoms such as fatigue, reduced alertness, reduced mobility, diarrhoea, loss of appetite, delirium, and absence of fever
- Children might not have fever or cough as frequently as adults.

Risk Factors for Severe COVID-19 Disease

- Age more than 60 years
- Underlying comorbidity: Non-communicable diseases [Cardiovascular disease, hypertension, and CAD, DM (diabetes mellitus)] and other immunocompromised states, chronic lung/kidney/liver disease, cerebrovascular diseases and obesity.

Clinical Severity of COVID-19 Disease

Clinical Severity	Clinical presentation	Clinical parameters	Management Site
MILD	Uncomplicated upper respiratory tract infection, may have mild symptoms (fever, cough, sore throat, nasal congestion, malaise, headache)	Without shortness of breath or Hypoxia (normal saturation)	Covid Care Centre OR Home (as per home isolation guidelines)
MODERATE	Pneumonia with no signs of severe disease	Dyspnoea and/or hypoxia, fever, cough, including SpO_2 90 to ≤93% on room air, RR ≥ 24/minute	Dedicated Covid Health Centre (DCHC)
SEVERE	Severe Pneumonia	Pneumonia plus one of the following; RR >30 breaths/min, severe respiratory distress, SpO_2 <90% on room air	Dedicated Covid Hospital (DCH)
	Acute Respiratory Distress Syndrome (ARDS)	*Onset:* New or worsening respiratory symptoms within one week of known clinical insult *Chest imaging (Chest X-ray and portable bed side lung ultrasound):* Bilateral opacities, not fully explained by effusions, lobar or lung collapse, or nodules. *Origin of Pulmonary infiltrates:* Respiratory failure not fully explained by cardiac failure or fluid overload. Need objective assessment (e.g. echocardiography) to exclude hydrostatic cause of infiltrates/oedema if no risk factor present. *Oxygenation impairment in adults:* MILD ARDS: 200 mm Hg < PaO_2/FiO_2 ≤ 300 mm Hg (with PEEP or CPAP ≥5 cm H_2O) *MODERATE ARDS:* 100 mm Hg < PaO_2/FiO_2 ≤200 mm Hg with PEEP ≥5 cm H_2O) *SEVERE ARDS:* PaO_2/FiO_2 ≤ 100 mm Hg with PEEP ≥5 cm H_2O)	
	Sepsis	Acute life-threatening organ dysfunction caused by a dysregulated host response to suspected or proven infection (Altered mental status, difficult/fast breathing, low oxygen saturation, reduced urine output, fast heart rate, weak pulse, cold extremities or low blood pressure, skin mottling, or laboratory evidence of coagulopathy, thrombocytopenia, acidosis, high lactate or hyperbilirubinemia.	
	Septic Shock	Persisting hypotension despite volume resuscitation, requiring vasopressors to maintain MAP ≥65 mm Hg and serum lactate level >2 mmol/L	

(© Table created by Dr Vivek Jain 2022-23)

COVID-19 Laboratory Diagnosis

- *Samples Collected [Transported at 4°C, Vaccine carrier to Lab]*
  - Nasopharyngeal and oropharyngeal swab: Dacron or polyester flocked swabs*
  - Bronchoalveolar lavage: Sterile container
  - Tracheal aspirate, nasopharyngeal aspirate or nasal wash: Sterile container
  - Sputum: Sterile container
  - Tissue from biopsy or autopsy including from lung: Sterile container
  - Serum (2 samples – acute and convalescent): Serum separator tubes

[PREFERRED SAMPLE is Throat and nasal swab in viral transport media (VTM) and transported in cold chain; ALTERNATE SAMPLE is Nasopharyngeal swab/BAL/endotracheal aspirate mixed with VTM and transported in cold chain] [Use PPE for Sample Collection]

- *Recommended Test for Diagnosis: RT-PCR*
  - Real time or Conventional RT-PCR test (or any other test approved for diagnosis of COVID-19 by ICMR) is recommended for diagnosis
  - Rapid Antigen Tests are recommended in specific situation.

COVID-19 Clinical Management Guidelines in Adults (MoHFW, GOI)

1. Management of Mild Cases
- Physical distancing, indoor mask use and strict hand hygiene
- Symptomatic management for fever and cough
- Fluids intake to maintain hydration
- Warm water gargles, steam inhalation multiple times a day
- Monitor temperature and oxygen saturation 2-4 times per day (SpO_2 probe to fingers)
- Seek immediate medical attention if: Difficulty in breathing or High-grade fever/severe cough, particularly if lasting for >5 days or A low threshold to be kept for those with any of the high-risk or co-morbid features
- Drug Treatment for patients with mild cases:
  - Tab Paracetamol/Tab Naproxen
  - Tab Ivermectin/Tab Hydroxychloroquine
  - Inhalational Budesonide
  - Systemic oral steroids not indicated in mild disease

2. Management of Moderate Cases
- Symptomatic treatment: Paracetamol for fever/pain, anti-tussives for cough
- Adequate hydration to be ensured
- Oxygen Support: Target SpO_2: 92-96% (88-92% in patients with COPD)
- Anticoagulation: Un-Fractionated Heparin or Low Molecular Weight Heparin
- Anti-inflammatory or immunomodulatory therapy
- Consider IV methylprednisolone or IV Dexamethasone
- Antibiotics should not be prescribed routinely
- Awake proning manoeuvres
- Control of co-morbid condition
- Monitoring: Clinical Monitoring, Serial CXR/HRCT chest If there is worsening, Lab monitoring (CRP, D-dimer, CBC, KFT, LFT, IL-6 levels)

3. Management of Severe Cases
- Early supportive therapy and monitoring
  - Symptomatic treatment with paracetamol and antitussives to continue
  - Maintain euvolemia
  - Respiratory support: Supplemental oxygen therapy (Target $SpO_2 \geq 90\%$ in non-pregnant adults and $SpO_2 \geq 92–96\%$ in pregnant patients)
  - Anti-inflammatory or immunomodulatory therapy: Inj Methylprednisolone
  - Anticoagulation: Unfractionated heparin or Low Molecular Weight Heparin
  - Monitoring: Serial CXR. HRCT chest to be done ONLY if there is worsening; Lab monitoring (CRP, D-dimer 24-48 hourly; CBC, KFT, LFT daily; IL-6 to be done if deteriorating)
- Management of hypoxemic respiratory failure and ARDS
  - High-Flow Nasal Cannula oxygenation (HFNO) or Non-invasive mechanical ventilation
  - Endotracheal intubation
  - Mechanical ventilation using lower tidal volumes and lower inspiratory pressures
  - Prone ventilation to be considered when there is refractory hypoxemia
  - Extracorporeal life support (ECLS) for patients with refractory hypoxemia despite lung protective ventilation

- Management of Septic shock
  - Standard care: Antimicrobial therapy and fluid loading and vasopressors for Hypotension
- Other Therapeutic Measures
  - Obstetric, neonatal, and intensive care specialist care: For pregnant patients categorized as severe
  - Psychological counselling
  - Investigational therapies: Plasma therapy, Remdesivir, Tocilizumab

COVID-19 Infection Prevention and Control Practices

1. At Triage
- Give patient a 3-layer surgical mask
- Direct patient to an earmarked separate area/isolation room
- Keep at least 6 feet distance between suspected patients and other patients.
- Instruct all patients to cover nose/mouth during coughing/sneezing with tissue/flexed elbow
- Perform hand hygiene after contact with respiratory secretion

2. Apply Standard Precautions
- Hand hygiene
- Personal protective equipment (PPE)
- Appropriate patient placement; prevention of needle-stick or sharps injury; linen management, safe BMW waste management; cleaning and disinfection of equipment; and cleaning of the environment

3. Apply Droplet and Airborne Precautions
- N-95 mask
- Eye protection (face-shield or goggles)
- PPE (with gloves, long-sleeved gowns, eye protection, particulate respirators N95)
- Negative pressure rooms (Minimum of 12 air change/hour)

4. Apply Contact Precautions
- PPE (triple layer medical mask or N95 respirator, eye protection, gloves and gown) Disposable or dedicated equipment (stethoscopes, blood pressure cuffs and thermometers)
- If shared among patients, clean and disinfect instruments between each patient use
- Refrain from touching their eyes/nose/mouth with potentially contaminated gloved/un-gloved hands
- Avoid contaminating environmental surfaces
- Adequate room ventilation
- Avoid movement of patients or transport
- Perform hand hygiene

5. COVID-19 Vaccines
See Chapter 3.

COVID-19 Clinical Management Guidelines in Children (<18 Years Age)

1. Clinical Severity of COVID-19 in Children

Clinical severity	Clinical presentation	Management site
Asymptomatic	• Suspected contact [RAT or RTPCR negative or NA] • Incidentally detected [RAT or RTPCR positive]	Home isolation (tele consultation SOS)
Mild	• Sore throat, rhinorrhoea • Cough without breathing difficulty • SpO_2 ≥94% on room air • Other symptoms	Home isolation (tele consultation SOS) OR COVID Care Centre
Moderate	In addition to symptoms (Mild), Check for Pneumonia • Rapid respiration (age-based): <2 months RR ≥60/min; 2–12 months, RR ≥50/min; 1–5 years, RR ≥40/min; >5 years, RR ≥30/min; AND/OR SpO_2 90–93% on room air • Other symptoms	Admit in DCHC OR COVID-19 Hospital
Severe	• SpO_2 <90% on room air • Any of the following: Signs of severe pneumonia, ARDS, Septic shock, MODS, Pneumonia with cyanosis, Grunting, Severe retraction of chest, Lethargy, Somnolence, Seizure • Other symptoms	Admit in HDU/ICU of COVID-19 Hospital

(© Table created by Dr Vivek Jain 2022-23) (MODS: Multiorgan dysfunction syndrome)

2. COVID-19 Clinical Management Guidelines in Children (MoHFW, GOI)
- Management of Asymptomatic Cases
  - Infants and younger children to stay under immediate care of parents/guardians
  - No specific medication required
  - Continue medications for other conditions, if any
  - COVID appropriate behaviour (mask, strict hand hygiene, physical distancing)
  - Fluids and feeds: Maintain hydration, nutritious diet
  - Contact the doctor in case of appearance of symptoms
  - Investigations needed: NONE
- Management of Mild Cases
  - For fever, give Paracetamol
  - For cough, give throat soothing agents and warm saline gargles in older children and adolescents
  - Fluids and feeds: Maintain hydration, nutritious diet
  - No other COVID-19 specific medication needed
  - Antimicrobials are NOT indicated
  - Maintain monitoring chart (RR, chest indrawing, cold extremities, urine output, oxygen saturation, fluid intake, activity level, especially for young children)
  - COVID appropriate behaviour (mask, strict hand hygiene, physical distancing)
  - Contact the doctor in case of deterioration of symptoms
  - Investigations needed: NONE
- Management of Moderate Cases
  - Initiate oxygen if SpO_2 is <94% (Maintain 94-96%)
  - Maintain fluid and electrolyte balance
  - Encourage oral fluids (breast feeds in infants)
  - Initiate IV fluid therapy if oral intake is poor
  - Corticosteroids are NOT required
  - Paracetamol
  - Anti-microbials (if superadded bacterial infection)
  - Supportive care for comorbid conditions, if any
  - Investigations needed:
    - Baseline: CBC including ESR, Blood glucose
    - Chest X-ray
- Management of Severe Cases
  - Immediate oxygen therapy (Target SpO_2 94-96%)
  - Maintain fluid and electrolyte balance
  - Corticosteroids therapy to be initiated
  - Anticoagulants may also be indicated
  - In ARDS or shock, initiate necessary management
  - Antimicrobials to be (if superadded bacterial infection)
  - Organ support in case of organ dysfunction (e.g. renal replacement therapy)
  - Investigations needed:
    - Baseline: CBC including ESR, Blood glucose, CRP, LFT, KFT, Serum ferritin, D-Dimer
    - Chest X-ray
- Must Know
  - Steroids are not indicated and are harmful in asymptomatic and mild cases of COVID-19 (Indicated only in hospitalized severe and critically ill COVID-19 cases under strict supervision)
  - Anticoagulants are Not indicated routinely
  - Remdesivir (an emergency use authorization drug) is NOT recommended in children
  - CT chest is not indicated in diagnosis or management of COVID-19 infection in children

COVID-19 BMW Management (CPCB Guidelines)

Refer to Chapter 12

PERSONAL PROTECTIVE EQUIPMENT (PPE) MEDICAL

What is PPE?

- Personal protective equipment (PPE) - Medical is protective clothing, goggles, or other garments or equipment designed to protect the health personnel's body from injury or infection

Communicable and Non-communicable Diseases

- The hazards addressed by PPE include physical hazards, biohazards and airborne particulate matter
- PPE acts as a barrier between infectious materials such as viral and bacterial contaminants and skin/mouth/nose/or eyes (mucous membranes); and, the barrier has the potential to block transmission of contaminants from blood, body fluids, or respiratory secretions
- PPE is commonly used in health care settings such as hospitals, doctor's clinicsd and clinical laboratories
- Effective use of PPE includes properly removing and disposing of contaminated PPE to prevent exposing both the wearer and other people to infection

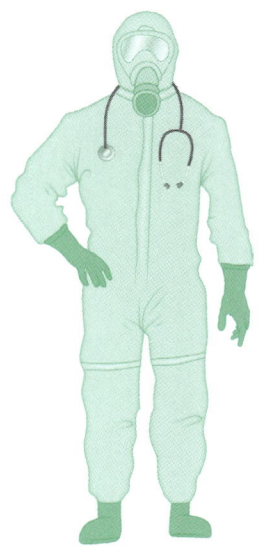

Components of PPE
- Gloves, gowns, shoe covers, head covers, masks (N95, Surgical mask), respirators, eye protection, face shields, hazmat suite, and goggles

Principles of PPE
Healthcare workers must follow the basic principles below to ensure that no infectious material reaches unprotected skin or mucous membranes while providing patient care
- Donning of PPE:
  - PPE must be donned correctly in proper order before entry into the patient care area
  - PPE should not be later modified while in the patient care area
- During Patient Care:
  - PPE must remain in place and be worn correctly for the duration of work in potentially contaminated areas
  - PPE should not be adjusted during patient care
  - Visibly contaminated outer gloves can be changed while in the patient room and patient care can continue
  - If during patient care any breach in PPE occurs (e.g., a tear develops in an outer glove, a needlestick occurs, a glove separates from the sleeve), the healthcare worker must move immediately to the doffing area to assess the exposure; the facility exposure management plan should be implemented
- Doffing of PPE:
  - PPE must be removed slowly and deliberately in the correct sequence to reduce the possibility of self-contamination or other exposure

PPE in Covid Pandemic (Exposure to SARS-CoV-2)
- Standard and transmission-based precautions to be followed
- PPE components:
  - Gloves (cover the wrists of the gown), goggles, gown (covering body at least from the neck to the mid-calf), a respirator with a rating of N95 or higher (or mask), and a face shield
  - Disposable N95 respirators must be certified by the National Institute for Occupational Safety and Health (NIOSH)

COVID-19 PPE BMW Management Guidelines: 4th Revision (CPCB 2020-21)
See Chapter 12

AAROGYA SETU

- Description: Aarogya Setu is an Indian COVID-19 "contact tracing, syndromic mapping and self-assessment" digital service, primarily a mobile app, developed by the National Informatics Centre under the Ministry of Electronics and Information Technology
- Primary function: "Mobile Application" to spread awareness for COVID-19 among citizens of India
- The main functions include:
  - Self-assessment of risk (User status)
  - COVID-19 Updates (gives updates on local and national COVID-19 cases): Tells about total no. of affected people in a given area
  - Covid vaccination status update for citizens

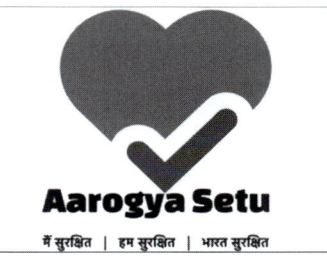

- Contact tracing
- Syndromic Mapping
- E-pass integration
- The app reached more than 100 million installs in 40 days
- This replaces the App "CORONA-KAVACH"

MUCORMYCOSIS: BLACK FUNGUS

Introduction
- Description: A "serious but rare" fungal infection that is frequently harmless for the immunocompetent, BUT can cause severe, frequently life-threatening infections
- Types of Mucormycosis: Rhinocerebral (sinus and brain), Pulmonary (lung), Cutaneous (skin), Gastrointestinal, Bones and Joints, Disseminated mucormycosis

Epidemiology of Mucormycosis
- Causative agent: Group of moulds - Mucormycetes
- Location: Environment, Soil
- Route of transmission: Aerosolised and dispersed by either inhalation (3-11 microns) or cutaneous/percutaneous route
- Predisposing factors of Mucormycosis in Covid Infection: Hyperglycemia in uncontrolled diabetes, Diabetic ketoacidosis, Organ/bone marrow transplantation, Neutropenia, Trauma/burns, Malignant hematologic disorders, Deferoxamine therapy (patients on hemodialysis), Rampant overuse and irrational use of steroids/broad-spectrum antibiotics, Pre-existing co-morbidities, Prolonged ICU stay, Breakthrough infections in Anti–fungal prophylaxis

Diagnosis of Mucormycosis
- Microscopic Pathologic appearance: Ribbon-like hyphae which branch at 90°, "Antlers of a moose appearance", Non-septate, Blood vessel/Angioinvasion, Haemorrhagic infarction, Coagulation necrosis, Infiltration by neutrophils, Perineural invasion
- Diagnosis:
  - Biopsy and Fungal culture (Direct detection of the fungus: Lung fluid, blood, serum, plasma, urine AND Matrix-assisted laser desorption/ionization: Identification of species)
  - Radiology: CT scan (Mucosal thickening, Bony erosions) AND MRI scan (Black turbinate sign)
  - Blood tests: CBC (Neutropenia)/Iron levels/blood glucose/bicarbonate/electrolytes
  - Endoscopic examination of nasal passages

Treatment and Prevention of Mucormycosis
- Treatment of Mucormycosis:
  - Aggressive therapy - Disfiguring surgical debridement + Adjunctive toxic antifungal therapy
  - Drugs used: Inj. Amphotericin B Deoxycholate, Liposomal Amphotericin B, Inj. Amphotericin B Lipid Complex, Posaconazole, Isavuconazole
- Prevention of Mucormycosis:
  - General measures "AVOID CONTACT WITH DECAYING ORGANIC MATTER" - Wearing a face mask in dusty areas, Washing hands,. Avoiding direct contact with water-damaged buildings, Protecting skin/feet/hands from exposure to soil or manure
  - Among COVID Positives: Prophylactic antifungals in high-risk groups, Strict Diabetes control & DKA management, Avoid unnecessary steroids/antibiotics, Early reporting of symptoms, Use clean distilled water for humidifiers during oxygen therapy.

SMALLPOX and CHICKENPOX

Smallpox

- *Epidemiological reasons/basis for Smallpox eradication^Q:*
  - No known animal reservoir
  - No long term carrier state
  - Infection provides lifelong immunity
  - Case detection simple due to characteristic rash
  - Subclinical cases did not transmit the disease
  - A highly effective vaccine was available
  - International cooperation

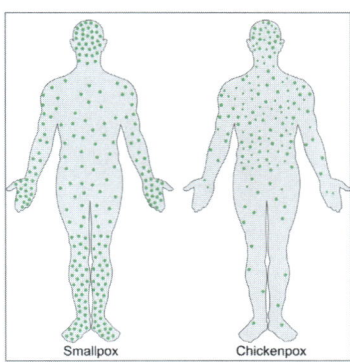

Small pox vs Chicken pox Rash

Chickenpox

- *Synonym:* 'Varicella'
- *Causative agent:* Varicella zoster virus [Human (alpha) Herpes Virus–3]^Q
- *Incubation period:* 14–16 days^Q
- *Source of infection:* Case (person-to-person contact)
- *Mode of transmission:* Air droplets (respiratory)
- *Period of communicability:* 1-2 days before to 4-5 days after appearance of rash
- *Secondary Attack rate^Q:* 90%
- *Rash:* Had to be differentiated from rash of Smallpox

Chickenpox rash	Smallpox rash
Dew drop on rose petal appearance^Q	—
Centripetal distribution^Q	Centrifugal distribution
Pleomorphic rash^Q	Non-pleomorphic
Superficial & Unilocular	Deep seated & Multilocular
Inflammation around vesicles present	No inflammation around vesicles
Affects flexor surfaces, involves axilla	Affects extensor surfaces, spares axilla
Spares palms and soles	Affects palms and soles
Rapid evolution	Slow evolution
Scabs form after 4–7 days	Scabs form after 10–14 days

> **Key points**
>
> **Chicken pox rash**
> - Dew drop on rose petal appearance
> - Centripetal distribution
> - Pleomorphic rash

- *MC late complication of chickenpox:* Shingles (caused by reactivation of the virus decades after the initial episode of chickenpox)
- *Most rapid and sensitive means of diagnosis^Q:* Examination of vesicle fluid under electron microscope (shows round particles)
- *Congenital Varicella:* Most threatening if transmitted in Ist trimester of pregnancy
- *Live attenuated Chickenpox Monovalent Vaccine:*
  - Strain: OKA strain
  - Seroconversion: >90%
  - Schedule for 12 months–12 years age: 6 weeks or 3 month interval
  - Schedule for >13 years age: 4-6 weeks interval
- *MMRV Combination Vaccine:*
  - Age group: 9 months–12 years
  - Minimum interval between 2 doses: 4 weeks
  - Preferable schedule: 2nd dose 6 weeks-3 months later or at 4-6 years age
- *Varicella Zoster immunoglobulin (VZIG):*
  - Given within 72 hours of exposure
  - Dose: 1.25–5.0 mL intramuscularly
  - Reserved for:
    - Immunosuppressed contacts of acute cases
    - Newborn contacts

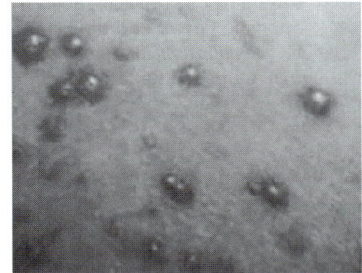

Chickenpox rash

MONKEYPOX

- *Causative agent:* Monkeypox virus, a double-stranded DNA virus in the genus Orthopoxvirus (family Poxviridae)

- Incubation period: 4–21 days
- Transmission:
  - Any close physical contact with monkeypox blisters or scabs (including during sexual contact, kissing, cuddling or holding hands)
  - Touching clothing, bedding or towels used by someone with monkeypox
  - Coughs or sneezes of a person with monkeypox when they're close to you
- Clinical presentation:
  - Invasion period (0–5 days): Fever, intense headache, lymphadenopathy, back pain, myalgia and intense asthenia
  - Skin eruption usually begins within 1–3 days of appearance of fever; the rash tends to be more concentrated on the face and extremities rather than on the trunk
  - 41% of cases of monkeypox were among HIV-positive patients between May and July 2022
  - Case fatality rate (Recently): 3–6%

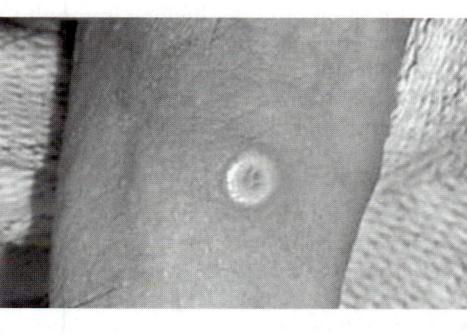

- Treatment:
  - First line antiviral treatment: Tecovirimat, or the smallpox treatment Brincidofovir
  - Supportive care (including antipyretic, fluid balance and oxygenation)
  - Empirical antibiotic therapy (secondary bacterial infection) or Aciclovir (Varicella zoster infection)
- Prevention: Vaccination against smallpox is assumed to protect against human monkeypox infection.

MEASLES

> **Key points**
>
> **MEASLES:**
> - Incubation Period: 10-14 days
> - No carriers
> - Secondary attack rate of Measles^Q: 80%
> - Koplik spots (buccal mucosa opposite Lower 2nd molar)
> - MC complication in young children: Otitis media

Measles (Rubeola)

- *Causative agent:* RNA paramyxovirus (so for only one serotype known)
- **Incubation Period: 10-14 days**^{Q}
- *Source of Infection:* cases (carriers are not known to occur^Q)
- *Mode of transmission:* Air droplets (respiratory)
- *Period of Communicability*^{Q}: 4 days before and 5 days after the appearance of rash (*Rash:* Retro-auricular origin^Q)
  - Measles is highly infectious during pro-dromal period and during eruption
- Measles has no second attacks (life long immunity seen)
- *Secondary attack rate of Measles*^{Q}: 80%
- *Measles shows a cyclical trend*^{Q}: Increase every 2-3 years
- *Pathogonomic clinical feature of Measles*^{Q}: Koplik spots (buccal mucosa opposite Lower 2nd molar)
- **MC complication of measles in young children**^{Q}: **Otitis media**
  - SSPE (Subacute Sclerosing Pan Encephalitis) is a rare complication of measles^Q: 1 per 10,000–100,000 cases (7-10 years after initial infection)
- *Measles is prevented by:*
  - *Active immunization by measles vaccine:*
  - Live, attenuated
  - *Strains:* Edmonston Zagreb (MC), Schwarez, Moraten
  - Passive immunization by measles immunoglobulin (WHO recommended dose: 0.25 mL/kg body weight^Q)
- *Treatment of Measles:*
  - No specific treatment
  - Supportive measures: Symptomatic treatment, Nutritional support, Breastfeeding (where appropriate), ORS
  - Vitamin A supplementation: All cases of severe Measles, All areas with high case fatality rates
    - To all cases: 2 doses, a dose each on Day 0 and Day 1 (50,000 IU <6 months age, 100,000 IU 6-11 months age, 200,000 IU ≥ 1 years age)
    - If Clinical signs of deficiency: 3rd dose 4–6 weeks later

WHO Measles Elimination Strategy^Q: 'Catch up, Keep up, Follow up'
- *Catch up:* Nationwide, vaccination campaign targeting all children 9 months to 14 years of age, irrespective of history of Measles disease or vaccination status
- *Keep up:* Routine services aimed at vaccinating more than 95% of each successive birth cohort
- *Follow up:* Subsequent nationwide vaccination campaigns conducted every 2–4 years targeting usually all children born after the catch-up campaign.

Accelerated Measles Mortality Reduction Strategy (WHO-UNICEF)
- Two doses of Measles containing vaccine (MCV) to all children through routine and supplementary immunization activities

Global Measles and Rubella Strategic Plan 2012–2020
- High population coverage with 2 doses of Measles and Rubella containing vaccines
- Effective surveillance
- Outbreak preparedness
- Generate Public confidence in vaccination
- Research and development

RUBELLA

Rubella (German Measles)
- *Causative agent:* RNA virus of Togavirus family^Q
- *Incubation period:* 14–21 days^Q (~18 days)
- *Source of infection:* Cases or subclinical cases
  - 'No known carrier state' for postnatally acquired rubella^Q
- *Mode of transmission:* Air droplets (respiratory)
- *Period of communicability:* One week prior to onset of symptoms to one week after rash appears
- *Immunity for Rubella:*
  - Single attack confers life long immunity (Second attacks rare)
  - 40% of reproductive age group females are susceptible in India^Q
  - Infants protected till 4-6m age
- *Most widely used test for diagnosis:* Heme-agglutination Inhibition test (HAI)

Key points
Rubella *Incubation period:* 14–21 days

Rubella Vaccine
- *Type of vaccine:* Live attenuated, 'strain RA 27/3'^Q [Vaccine virus non-communicable]
- *Dose and route:* 0.5 ml, subcutaneous
- Rubella vaccine is contraindicated in pregnancy and not given to infants
  - *If female vaccinated for rubella:* Advice against pregnancy for next 3 months^Q
- *Priority groups for rubella vaccination in India:*
  - *1st PRIORITY:* **15–49 years reproductive age group females**^Q
  - *2nd priority:* All children 1–14 years age
  - *3rd priority:* Routine universal immunization of all children aged 1

Key points
Rubella Vaccine
Live attenuated, 'strain RA 27/3'

Congenital Rubella Syndrome (CRS)
- *CRS is said to have occurred if*^Q:
  - Infant has IgM rubella antibodies shortly after birth, or
  - IgG antibodies persist for more than 6 months
- Major determinant of extent of fetal infection in CRS: Gestational age at which fetal transmission occurs
- *Infection in I trimester:* MOST DISASTROUS TIME^Q
  - Abortions
  - Still births
  - Skin lesions: blueberry muffin lesions^Q
  - **'Triad of Congenital Rubella Syndrome'** [*Congenital heart defects (MC is PDA*^Q*) + Cataracts + Sensorineural deafness*]
- *Infection in early part of II Trimester:* Deafness (only)

Key points
Rubella
Infection in I trimester: MOST DISASTROUS TIME

- *Infection after 16 weeks POG:* No major abnormalities
- *Risk of fetal damage in CRS:*

Stage of gestation	% fetuses infected	% fetuses damaged among infected	Overall risk of damage
< 11 weeks	90	100	90
11–16 weeks	55	37	20
17–26 weeks	33	0	0
27–36 weeks	53	0	0

> **Key points**
> MUMPS
> MC complication^Q: Aseptic meningitis

MUMPS

- *Causative agent:* Myxovirus parotiditis (RNA paramyxovirus)
- *Incubation Period:* 14-21 days^Q
- *Source of Infection:* Clinical & subclinical cases
- *Mode of transmission:* Air droplets (respiratory)
- *Period of Communicability:* 4-6 days before to 7 days after onset of symptoms
- Mumps show life long immunity
- *Secondary attack rate of Mumps^Q:* 86%
- *Clinical features:*
    - Salivary (esp. Parotid) glands involvement^Q
    - MC complication^Q: Aseptic meningitis
    - MC complication in adolescents^Q: Orchitis, Oopheritis
- *Mumps is prevented by:* Active immunization by Mumps vaccine:
    - *Type:* Live attenuated vaccine^Q
    - *Strain:* Jeryll Lynn strain^Q

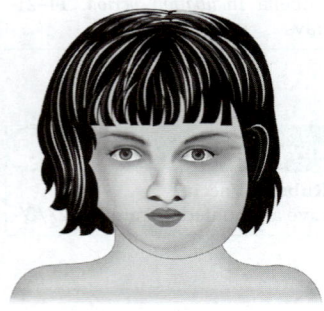

Mumps

INFLUENZA

Influenza

- *Causative agent:* Orthomyxovirus, 3 types: A, B, C
    - *Type A:* MC cause of outbreaks/epidemics^Q; Only cause of pandemics^Q
    - Type B
    - *Type C:* Not circulating currently
- *Currently circulating influenza viruses in world:*
    - **H_1N_1 (Type A)–Cause of Swine flu^Q**
    - H_2N_2 (Type A)
    - **H_5N_1 (Type A)–Cause of Avian influenza (Bird flu)^Q**
    - H_3N_2
    - H_7N_9
    - H_5N_6
    - Type B
- *Cyclical trends in Influenza^Q:*
    - Type A epidemics every 2–3 years
    - Type B epidemics every 4–7 years
    - Type A pandemics every 10–15 years
- *Antigenic variations in Influenza:* (MC in Type A^Q)

> **Key points**
> H_1N_1 (Type A)–Cause of Swine-flu

	Antigenic shift^Q	Antigenic drift^Q
Occurs due to	Genetic recombination/reassortment/rearrangement	Point mutation^Q
Nature	Sudden	Gradual/insidious
May lead to	Pandemics^Q	Epidemics

- *Incubation period:* 18–72 hours^Q
- *Period of infectivity:* 1–2 days before to 1–2 days after onset of symptoms^Q

Avian Influenza

- Also known as 'Bird flu' or 'Highly pathogenic avian influenza'

- *Causative agent*[Q]: H5N1 (Type A Influenza virus)
- *Avian Influenza is a Pandemic:* Origin from Hong Kong (1997)
- *Drug of choice*[Q]: Oseltamivir (Tamiflu) 75 mg BD × 5 days (contraindicated in infants)

Influenza: Pandemic (H1N1) Influenza 2009 [NEW NOMENCLATURE: Influenza A (H_1N_1) pdm 09]

- *WHO declaration of Influenza pandemic:* 11 June 2009
  - *World is now post-pandemic EXCEPT:* INDIA and NEW ZEALAND (locally intense transmission)
  - *Problem statement India:* 37000 cases, 1833 deaths [May 2009–August 2010]
- *Incubation period:* 1–4 days
- *Clinical features:*
  - *Uncomplicated influenza:* Influenza like illness (Fever, cough, sorethroat, rhinorrhoea, headache, muscle pain), GIT illness (diarrhoea WITHOUT dehydration)
  - *Complicated/severe influenza:* Pneumonia, CNS involvement, Severe diarrhoea, Secondary complications,
  - Exacerbation of chronic diseases
  - *Progressive disease:* Oxygen impairment/cardiopulmonary insufficiency, CNS complications, Invasive secondary bacterial infection, Severe dehydration
- *Risk factors of severe disease*[Q]:
  - Infants and children < 2 years
  - Pregnant females
  - COPD
  - Chronic cardiac disease
  - Metabolic disorders
  - Chronic renal/hepatic/neurological/hemoglobinopathies/immunosuppression (INCLUDING HIV) disorders
  - Children on aspirin therapy
  - Persons aged > 65 years
  - Morbid obesity
- *Laboratory diagnosis:*
  - **Most timely and sensitive detection: RT-PCR test**[Q]
  - **Samples: Nasopharyngeal + throat swabs** [Tracheal/bronchial aspirates in lower respiratory tract infection cases][Q]
  - *Point-of-care/Rapid diagnostic tests:* Not recommended
- *Duration of isolation:* for 7 days after onset of illness OR 24 hours after resolution of fever/respiratory symptoms whichever is longer
- *Antiviral therapy:*
  - *Severe/progressive clinical illness:* Oseltamivir[Q] (if not available or resistance, use Zanamivir)
  - *High risk of severe/complicated illness:* Oseltamivir OR Zanamivir
  - *Not high risk OR Uncomplicated confirmed/suspected illness:* No need of treatment
  - *Dosage:*
    - Oseltamivir 75 mg BD × 5 days
    - Zanamivir 2 inhalations (2 × 5 mg) BD × 5 days

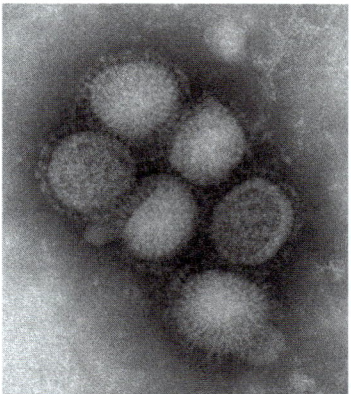

H1N1 virus

> **Key points**
> DOC for H_1N_1
> - Oseltamivir 75 mg BD × 5d

Oseltamivir Dosages[Q]

Treatment	Prophylaxis
By weight <15 kg: 30 mg BD × 5 days 15–23 kg: 45 mg BD × 5 days 24–39 kg: 60 mg BD × 5 days ≥ 40 kg: 75 mg BD × 5 days	By weight <15 kg: 30 mg OD × 10 days 15–23 kg: 45 mg OD × 10 days 24–39 kg: 60 mg OD × 10 days ≥ 40 kg: 75 mg OD × 10 days
For infants < 3 months: 12 mg BD × 5 days 3–5 months: 20 mg BD × 5 days 6–11 months: 25 mg BD × 5 days	For infants < 3 months: Not recommended unless critical 3-5 months: 20 mg OD × 10 days 6-11 months: 25 mg OD × 10 days

Avian Influenza H$_7$N$_9$

- Origin: China 2013
- Spread to: Hong Kong
- *Disease burden:*
  - *Cases:* 1567
  - *Deaths:* 615
  - *Case fatality rates:* 33%
- *MC age group affected:* Older males (>50 years age)
- *Mode of transmission:* Respiratory (Live bird markets)
  - Human to human transmission: Rare but possible
- *Treatment:* Neuraminidase inhibitors
  - Oseltamivir
  - Zanamivir

Vaccines for Influenza

- *Killed vaccines:*
  - 2 doses, 3–4 weeks apart, 0.5 ml (for age > 3 years), subcutaneous
  - 70–90% protective efficacy; duration 3–6 months
  - Is rarely associated with Guillain-Barré Syndrome^Q (GBS)
- *Live attenuated vaccines:*
  - Stimulate local + systemic immunity
  - Antigenic variations presents difficulties in manufacture
- *Newer vaccines^Q:*
  - *Split–virus vaccine:*
    - Also known as 'Sub-virion vaccine'
    - Highly purified
    - Lesser side effects
    - Less antigenic–multiple injections required
    - Useful for children
  - *Neuraminidase–specific vaccine:*
    - Sub-unit vaccine containing N-antigen
    - Permits subclinical infection–long lasting immunity
  - *Recombinant vaccine:*
    - Antigenic properties of virulent strain transferred to a less virulent strain
  - *Contraindications to Inactivated Influenza vaccines:*
    - Severe allergy to chicken eggs
    - History of hypersensitivity/anaphylactic reactions previously
    - Development of Guillain-Barré Syndrome (GBS) within 6 weeks of vaccine
    - Infants less than 6 months age
    - Moderate-to-severe illness with fever

H$_1$N$_1$ (Swine Flu) Vaccine

- *H$_1$N$_1$ Inactivated vaccine:* Single i/m injection
  - *Strain:* A/California/7/2009 (H1N1) V like strain^Q
  - *Storage temperature:* +2° to +8° C
  - *Contraindications:* History of anaphylaxis/severe reaction/Guillian Barre Syndrome, Infants < 6 months, Moderate-to severe illness with fever
  - *Protective immunity:* Develops after 14 days (NOT 100%)
- *H$_1$N$_1$ Live attenuated vaccine:* Nasal spray
  - *Side effects:* Rhinorrhoea, nasal congestion, cough, sore throat, fever, wheezing, vomiting
- *Priority groups (in order) for Influenza vaccines:*
  - Pregnant women^Q
  - Age > 6 months with chronic medical conditions
  - 15-49 years healthy young adults
  - Healthy young children
  - Healthy adults 49-65 years
  - Healthy adults >65 years

> **Key points**
>
> H$_1$N$_1$ Inactivated vaccine: Strain: A/California/7/2009

Revised/New Seasonal Influenza A (H_1N_1) Guidelines on Categorization of Seasonal Influenza A H_1N_1 Cases (MoHFW, GOI)[Q]

Category A	Category B1	Category B2	Category C
Mild fever *plus* Cough/Sore throat *with or without* • Bodyache • Headache • Diarrhea • Vomiting	Category-A *plus* • High grade fever • Severe sore throat	Category A *plus* • Children with mild illness with predisposing risk factors • Pregnant women • Persons >65 years • Patients with Lung disease/Heart disease/Liver disease/Kidney disease/Blood disorders/Diabetes/Neurological disorders/Cancer/HIV/AIDS/Long term cortisone therapy	Category A and B *plus* • Breathlessness • Chest pain • Drowsiness • Hypotension • Hemoptysis • Cyanosis • Children with somnolence • High persistent fever • Inability to feed well • Convulsions • Shortness of breath • Difficulty in breathing • Worsening of chronic disease
Treatment Guidelines			
• No testing • No Oseltamivir • Treat symptomatically • Home isolation • Reassess after 48 hrs.	• Home isolation • May need Oseltamivir • No testing required	• Home isolation • Give Oseltamivir • No testing required • BSA where required	• Immediate hospitalization • Start Oseltamivir • Send throat swab

(*BSA: Broad spectrum antibiotics)

DIPHTHERIA

Diphtheria

- *Causative agent:* Corynebacterium diphtheriae, a gram positive non-motile organism
- Diphtheria is an endemic disease in India
- *Source of infection:* Case or carrier
  - Carriers are more important as source of infection: 95% of total disease transmission[Q]
  - Nasal carriers are more dangerous than throat carriers[Q]
  - Incidence of carriers in a community: 0.5-1%
  - Immunization does not prevent carrier state[Q]
- *Incubation Period:* 2-6 days[Q]
- *Mode of transmission:* droplet infection (main mode), directly from cutaneous lesions and fomites
- *Period of Infectivity:* 14-28 days from onset of disease; longer for carriers[Q]
  - A case/carrier may be considered non-communicable when at least 2 cultures from nose and throat, 24 hrs apart, are negative[Q]
- **MC Subtype: Faucial (Tonsillar + Pharyngeal)**

> **Key points**
>
> *Carriers are more important as source of infection:* Diphtheria

DPT Vaccine

Refer to Chapter 3, Theory

Schick Test

- *Schick Test:* An intradermal test of immunity status and hypersensitivity to Diphtheria toxin
- *Dose:* 0.2 ml (1/50 MLD) of Schick test toxin in test arm and 0.2 ml of heat inactivated toxin in opposite 'control' arm
- *Interpretations of Schick Test:*

Observation		Reading	Interpretation[Q]
Test arm	**Control arm**		
No reaction	No reaction	NEGATIVE	Immune to diphtheria
Red flush	No reaction	POSITIVE	Susceptible to diphtheria

Contd...

Contd...

Observation	Reading		Interpretation[Q]
Red flush fading by 4th day	Red flush fading by 4th day	PSEUDOPOSITIVE	Hypersensitivity
Red flush	Pseudopositive	COMBINED	Susceptibility & Hypersensitivity

(Red flush = Positive reaction)

- Schick test negative if, >0.03 units antitoxin per ml in blood serum
- *Schick test has been replaced by:* Hemagglutination Test[Q]
- *Hemagglutination Test:* Measurement of serum antitoxin level

Treatment with Diphtheria Antitoxin

Type of Diphtheria	Antitoxin dose
Anterior nasal diphtheria	10,000–20,000 Units
Tonsillar diphtheria	15,000–25,000 Units
Pharyngeal/Laryngeal diphtheria (<48 hours duration)	20,000–40,000 Units
Nasopharyngeal disease	40,000–60,000 Units
Extensive disease (>3 days) Or with brawny swelling of neck	80,000–120,000 Units

WHOOPING COUGH

Pertussis/Whooping Cough

- *Causative agent:* Bordetella pertussis (5% cases by B. parapertussis)
- Also known as *'Whooping Cough'* or *'100 Day Cough'*[Q]
  - Paroxysms of cough are followed by an inspiratory whoop (high pitch)
- *Incubation period:* 7–14 days
- *Source of Infection:* Case
  - There is no subclinical or chronic carrier state[Q]
  - Neither vaccination nor infection confers long-term immunity
- *Secondary Attack rate:* > 90%[Q]
- *Incidence and fatality:* Females > Males
- Leukocytosis does not correlates with the severity of cough
- *Chief complications:* Brochitis, bronchopneumonia, bronchiectasis, subconjunctival hemorrhages, epistaxis, hemoptysis, punctuate cerebral hemorrhages, convulsions and coma.
- *Laboratory diagnosis:* Culturing of nasopharyngeal swabs on Bordet-Gengou medium, polymerase chain reaction (PCR), immunofluorescence (DFA), and serological methods
- *Drug of choice*[Q]: Erythromycin (40 mg/kg QID × 10 days)
- *Vaccines:* DPT [Refer to Chapter 3, Theory]

> **Key points**
> Drug of choice[Q] of Pertussis Erythromycin

MENINGOCOCCAL MENINGITIS

Meningococcal Meningitis/Cerebrospinal Fever

- *Causative agent:*
  - N. meningitidis, a gram negative diplococci
  - Serotypes A, B, C, D, 29E, W135, X, Y
- Meningococcal disease is endemic in India
- *Carriers are the more important source of infection than cases*[Q]
  - Mean duration of Temporary carriers: ~ 10 months
  - During epidemics, carrier rate may go up to 70-80%
- *Mode of Transmission:* Droplet infection
- *Incubation Period:* 2-10 days (average 3-4 days)
- *Case Fatality Rate (CFR) of Meningococcal meningitis*[Q]: 80%
  - With early diagnosis and treatment, CFR < 10%
- *Drugs of Choice:*

Management	Drug of choice
Treatment of cases	Penicillin
Treatment of carriers	Rifampicin[Q]
Chemoprophylaxis of contacts	Rifampicin[Q]/ceftriaxone

- Treatment with Penicillin does not eradicate carrier state[Q]

> **Key points**
> Chemoprophylaxis of contacts of Meningococcus: Rifampicin

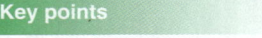

Meningococcal Vaccine

- *Type of Vaccine:* Killed vaccine, cellular fraction
- *Dose:* 0.5 mL
- *Route:* Subcutaneous
- *Site:* Antero-lateral thigh. Middle one-third
- Booster every 3 years
- Available for group A, C, W135 and Y meningococci
  - *Vaccine is not available for Group B meningococcus:* Group B polysaccharide is non-immunogenic^Q
- Contraindications^Q:
  - Pregnancy
  - Infants and children < 2 years of age (due to development of immunologic tolerance)

> **Key points**
> Vaccine is not available for Group B meningococcus

ACUTE RESPIRATORY TRACT INFECTIONS (ARIS)/PNEUMONIA (NEW GUIDELINES IMNCI 2017)

If 2 months–5 years age child with Wheezing with Fast breathing/Chest indrawing
- Rapidly acting inhaled bronchodilator trial up to 3 times 15-20 minutes apart
- Count the breaths and look for chest indrawing again
- Now classify.

Type of ARI	Signs/Symptoms	Management
No Pneumonia **GREEN**	No signs of severe or very severe pneumonia • Cough/cold	AT HOME • Inhaled bronchodilator × 5 days* • Soothe throat with safe remedy • If cough > 14 days, refer for TB assessment • If recurrent wheeze, refer for Asthma assessment • Follow-up in 5 days (if no improvement) • Advise mother when to return immediately
Pneumonia (Not severe) **YELLOW**	• Chest indrawing • Fast breathing present RR >50 (2-12 months) RR >40 (12 months-5 years)	AT PHC • Oral Amoxycillin × 5 days • Inhaled bronchodilator × 5 days* • Soothe throat with safe remedy • If cough > 14 days, refer for TB assessment • If recurrent wheeze, refer for Asthma assessment • Follow-up in 3 days • Advise mother when to return immediately • If Chest indrawing in HIV exposed/infected: Give 1st dose of Amoxycillin and Refer

Severe Pneumonia OR Very Severe Disease
 	
PINK
	• Stridor in calm child
	• Any general danger sign
	  – Inability to breastfeed/drink
	  – Vomit out everything
	  – Prior H/o convulsions
	  – Convulsing now
	  – Lethargy/unconscious
		REFER TO CHC/HOSPITAL
		• First dose of referral antibiotic*
		• Diazepam, if Convulsing now
		• Treat to prevent Low sugar
		• Keep the child warm

(* If wheezing disappeared after rapidly acting bronchodilator trial)

If 0-2 months old Young Infant
- Count the breaths (recount, if >60/min)
- Look for severe chest indrawing.

Very Severe Disease
 	
PINK
	• Any of the following signs
	  – Not feeding well
	  – Convulsions
	  – Fast breathing (>60/min)
	  – Severe chest indrawing
	  – Fever ≥ 37.5° C
	  – Body temperature < 35.5° C
	  – No movement or movement only on stimulation
		REFER TO CHC/HOSPITAL
		• First dose of referral antibiotic (i/m)
		• Treat to prevent low sugar
		• Advise mother how to keep child warm

Integrated Global Action Plan for Prevention and Control of Pneumonia & Diarrhoea (GAPPD)

- Specific Goals for 2025:
    - Reduce Pneumonia mortality in Under-five < 3 per 1000 LB
    - Reduce Diarrhoea mortality in Infants < 1 per 1000 LB
    - Reduce Incidence of Severe Diarrhoea in Under-fives by 75% (2010 baseline)
    - Reduce Incidence of Severe Pneumonia in Under-fives by 75% (2010 baseline)
    - Reduce Global no. of Stunted Under-fives by 40% (2010 baseline)

    Coverage targets:

By End-2025	By End-2030*
90% full dose coverage of each vaccine#	Drinking water
90% access to Diarrhoea, Pneumonia management#	Sanitation in HCF (2030) & H (2040)
>50% coverage of Exclusive breastfeeding (0-6 m)	Hand-washing facilities
Elimination of Pediatric HIV	Clean and safe energy technologies

(# 80% coverage in each district) (* Universal access in Health care facilities HCF & Homes H)

TUBERCULOSIS

Tuberculosis Situation in India

- *Incidence TB cases:* 2.7 million (27% of Global)
- *Mortality of TB:* 4,40,000 (31% of Global)
- *Incidence HIV-TB:* 92,000 (9% of Global)
- *Mortality of HIV-TB:* 9,700 (4% of Global)
- *MDR-TB:* 130,000 (24% of Global)
- *Children with TB:* 342,000 (31% of Global)

Epidemiological Facts: Tuberculosis

- Global population infected asymptomatically with TB: 33%
- Estimated case of TB previous year, globally: 10 million
- 1 case of Infectious Pulmonary TB can infect: 10-15 persons per year
- Majority of cases, global: >15 years adults (90%)
- Country with highest no. of cases: India
- Male: Female ratio: 1.7:1
- Country with highest number of MDR-TB cases: India (24%)
- Treatment success rates: 82% (TB), 77% (HIV-TB), 55% (MDR TB), 34% (XDR TB)

Epidemiological Indices for TB

- *Incidence of TB infection (Annual infection rate, Annual risk of infection- ARI):* Percentage of population under study who will be newly infected with TB among non-infected in 1 year
    - *Expresses attacking force of TB in community*
    - **In developing countries 1% ARI corresponds to: 50 SS +ve cases per 100,000 general population**[Q]
    - Tuberculin conversion index is the 'best indicator for evaluation of TB problem and its trend' in the community[Q]
- *Prevalence of TB infection:* Percentage of individuals who show a positive reaction to standard tuberculin test
    - Represent cumulative experience of population in 'recent as well as remote infection' with TB[Q]
    - Tuberculin test is the 'only way of estimating the prevalence of infection in a population'[Q]
- *Incidence of disease:* Percentage of new TB cases per 1000 population
    - Reveals trend of problem, including impact of control measures
    - Is of utility only in countries where high proportion of new cases are detected and notification is reliable
    - Sputum smear examination (AFB) is a reliable method for estimation[Q]

> **Key points**
> 1% ARI corresponds to: 50 SS +ve cases per 100,000 general population

- *Prevalence of disease or case rate:* Percentage of individuals whose sputum is positive for TB bacilli on microscopic examination^Q
  - 'Best available practical index to estimate case load' in community^Q
  - Age specific prevalence is most relevant index

Tuberculin/PPD

- *Tuberculin^Q:* Purified protein derivative (PPD) has replaced the antigen old tuberculin (OT)
  - *Tuberculins have also been prepared from atypical mycobacterium:* PPD-Y (M. Kansasii), PPD-B (Battey mycobacterium), Scrofula (M. scrofulaceum)
- Discovered by Von Pirquet (1907)
  - *Standard PPD (PPD-S) contains^Q:* 50,000 tuberculin units (TU) per mg [1TU= 0.00002 mg PPD]
  - **WHO advocates 'PPD-RT-23 with Tween-80'^Q**
- *Dosage:* First strength (1TU), Intermediate strength (5TU), Second strength (250TU)
- *Tuberculin test conversion* is defined as an increase of 10 mm or more within a 2-year period, regardless of age^Q
- *Tuberculin test in use:*
  - *Mantoux intradermal test:* More precise test of tuberculin sensitivity
  - *Heaf test:* Quick, easy, reliable and cheap, preferred for testing large groups
  - *Tine multiple puncture test* unreliable, not recommended
- Tuberculin test is the 'only way of estimating the prevalence of infection in a population'^Q
- Tuberculin test has lost its sensitivity as an indicator of the true prevalence of infection, in countries with high coverage of BCG^Q
  - True prevalence rates are exaggerated by infection with atypical mycobacteria and boosting effect of a second dose of tuberculin

Mantoux Test (Tool for detection of TB infection) (Pirquet Test)

- *Tuberculin test conversion*: Increase of > 10 mm within 2 years period
- **Dose^Q: 1 TU of PPD in 0.1ml injected intradermally on forearm**
- *WHO advocated preparation^Q:* PPD–RT-23 with Tween–80
- Is a test of prognostic significance
- Has limited validity due to lack of specificity
- *Readings^Q:* **Result read after 72 hrs (3d)**
- Only induration is measured:
  - *Induration >9 mm:* Positive (Past OR current infection with TB)^Q
  - *Induration 6-9 mm:* Doubtful (M. tuberculosis or Atypical mycobacteria)
  - *Induration <6 mm:* Negative^Q
- False Reactions:

False +ve Mantoux^Q	False –ve Mantoux^Q
Faulty technique of injection	Pre-allergic phase
Using degraded tuberculin	High fever
Too deep injection	Measles and chickenpox
Infection of other mycobacterium^Q	Whooping cough
Repeated tuberculin testing	Malnutrition
Prior BCG vaccine^Q	HIV/AIDS^Q
	Use of anti-allergic drugs
	Use of immunosuppressants

> **Key points**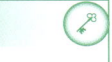
>
> **MANTOUX TEST:**
> - Dose^Q: 1 TU of PPD in 0.1ml
> - Readings^Q: Result read after 72 hrs (3d)

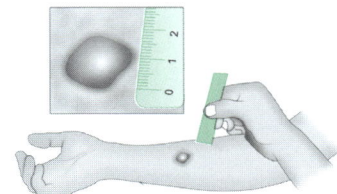

Mantoux Test

- *Results of tuberculin test must be interpreted carefully:* The person's medical risk factors determine at which increment (5 mm, 10 mm, or 15 mm) of induration the result is considered positive
  - *5 mm or more is positive in:*
    - HIV-positive person^Q
    - Recent contacts of TB case
    - Persons with nodular or fibrotic changes on chest X-ray consistent with old healed TB

- Patients with organ transplants
- Other immunosuppressed patients
- *10 mm or more is positive in:*
  - Recent arrivals (less than 5 years) from high-prevalence countries
  - Injection drug users
  - Residents and employees of high-risk congregate settings (e.g., prisons, nursing homes, hospitals, homeless shelters, etc.)
  - Mycobacteriology lab personnel
  - Persons with clinical conditions that place them at high risk (diabetes, prolonged corticosteroid therapy, leukemia, end-stage renal disease, chronic malabsorption syndromes, low body weight)
  - Children less than 4 years of age, or children and adolescents exposed to adults in high-risk categories
- *15 mm or more is positive in:*
  - Persons with no known risk factors for TB[Q]

Sputum Microscopy and Culture

- *Sputum smear examination (Z-N Staining) by direct microscopy:* is the 'method of choice as a case finding tool for tuberculosis'[Q]
- *Sputum culture examination:* is offered as a centralized service at district and regional chest clinic laboratories
  - Only meant for chest symptomatic who are smear negative
  - Useful for carrying out sensitivity tests and monitoring drug treatment

Mass Miniature Radiography (MMR[Q])

- Is not used now as a case finding tool
- Only useful:
  - As an additional criterion for diagnosis of Pulmonary TB, when none sputum smear is positive out of two
  - To exclude bronchiectasis/aspergilloma in frequent/severe is positive sputum smear cases
  - In suspected complication in a breathless patient needing specific treatment (e.g. pneumothorax, pericardial effusion, pleural effusion)

Guidelines for Chemoprophylaxis in Children (< 6 years)

(Who come in contact with a Sputum positive TB case)

IF	AND	THEN
Symptoms of TB	Clinician declares TB	Cat I DOTS given
No symptoms of TB	Tuberculin test NA	Isoniazid 5 mg/kg X 6 months[Q]
	Tuberculin test available	Isoniazid 5 mg/kg X 3 months, then do test If induration < 6 mm: Stop INH, Give BCG If induration > 6 mm: Continue INH for 3 months

(INH: Isoniazid; NA: Not available)

TB and Co-morbidities

- TB and HIV:
  - 10% activation of dormant TB over lifetime increases to 10% activation in one year
  - HIV-TB co-infection increases chances of TB disease 25-30 times more than in those infected with TB only
  - Diagnosis problems: Higher chances of Negative sputum smears (Use sputum culture), Chest x-ray less useful, Tuberculin test failure; Extrapulmonary TB more common
- TB and Diabetes:
  - Diabetes account for 20% of all TB
  - Diabetes account for 105 of Smear positive TB

- TB and Tobacco:
  - 38% TB deaths are associated with Tobacco use
  - 3-times higher prevalence of TB among smokers
  - 3-4 times higher mortality due to TB among smokers
  - **5R's to quit Tobacco**: **R**elevance of quitting, **R**isk of continuing, **R**eward of quitting, **R**oadblock to quitting, **R**epeat at each visit

The End TB Strategy 2016–2035^Q

- *Vision*: A world free of TB
  - Zero deaths, disease and suffering due to TB
- *Goal*: End the Global TB Epidemic

Indicators	Milestones^Q		Targets^Q	
	2020	2025	SDG 2030	End TB 2035
Reduction in number of TB deaths compared with 2015 (%)	35%	75%	90%	95%
Reduction in TB incidence rate compared with 2015 (%)	20% (< 85/100,000)	50% (< 55/100,000)	80% (< 20/100,000)	90% (< 10/100,000)
TB-affected families facing catastrophic costs due to TB (%)	Zero	Zero	Zero	Zero

Latent Tuberculosis (LATENT TB, LTBI)

- *Description:* Latent tuberculosis is where a patient is infected with Mycobacterium tuberculosis, but does not have active tuberculosis disease
  - Latent TB are NOT INFECTIOUS
- *Main risk:* 10% will go on to develop active TB at a later life
- *Tests used to identify patients with latent TB:*
  - Tuberculin skin tests (Montaux test, Heaf test, Tine test)
  - alpha-interferon tests

National Reference Laboratories for TB in India

- National Institute for Research in Tuberculosis (NIRT), Chennai^Q
- National Tuberculosis Institute (NTI), Bangalore^Q
- National Institute of TB and Respiratory Diseases (NITRD), Delhi
- Delhi and National Japanese Leprosy Mission for Asia (JALMA)—Institute of Leprosy and other Mycobacterial Diseases, Agra^Q
- Regional Medical Research Centre (RMRC), Bhubaneswar
- Bhopal Memorial Hospital and Research Centre (BMHRC), Bhopal

Revised National TB Control Program and NTEP 2020

Also Refer to Chapter 6, Theory

POLIOMYELITIS

Poliomyelitis Situation 2023 WORLD [as on 30 May 2023]

- Total cases: 20 WPV + 105 cVDPV
- 3 endemic countries:^Q Afghanistan, Pakistan, Mozambique

Poliomyelitis Situation 2023 INDIA [as on 30 May 2023]

- Total cases: NIL wild virus case [No case has been reported in India from 13 January 2011 onwards]
- India declared 'Polio-Free' on 27 March 2014
- Zero VDPV case (P2) reported from India

Poliomyelitis Disease

- *Causative agent:* Poliovirus (serotypes 1, 2 and 3)
    - P1 is MCC of epidemics[Q]
    - P2 is Most antigenic and Most easily eradicable (Eradicated on 20 Sep 2015))
    - **P3 is MCC of VAPP**[Q] (Vaccine associated paralytic poliomyelitis)–1 per 2.7 million chance[Q]
- *Reservoir:* Man[Q] (No chronic carriers[Q])
- MC clinical occurrence: Subclinical cases[Q]
    - For every 1 clinical case of polio: there are 1000 subclinical cases in children and 75 subclinical cases in adults[Q]
- *Infectious material:* Faeces and oro-pharyngeal secretions[Q]
- *Period of communicability:* 7-10 days before and after onset of symptoms
- *Risk factors for precipitation of an attack:*
    - Fatigue
    - Trauma
    - Intramuscular injections
    - Operative procedures (Tonsillectomy) esp. in epidemics of polio
    - Administration of Alum containing DPT vaccine
- *Incubation period:* 3–35 days (usually 7–14 days[Q])
- *Clinical presentation:*

Clinical spectrum	Infections	Remarks
Inapparent (Subclinical)	95%[Q]	No presenting symptoms; recognisable by isolation or rising antibody titres
Abortive polio (Minor illness)	4–8%	Mild or self-limiting illness; recognisable by isolation or rising antibody titres
Non-paralytic polio	1%	Synonymous with aseptic meningitis
Paralytic polio	< 1%	Descending asymmetric flaccid paralysis

Key points

- P1 is MCC of epidemics
- P3 is MCC of VAPP
- For every 1 clinical case of polio: there are 1000 subclinical cases

Available Diagnostic Tests for Poliomyelitis

- *Stool examination:*
    - Isolation of wild poliovirus from stool is 'the recommended method for laboratory confirmation of paralytic poliomyelitis'[Q]
    - Recommended in every case of AFP
    - Virus usually can be found in the feces from onset to up to < 8 weeks after paralysis, with 'the highest probability of detection during the first 2 weeks after paralysis onset'[Q]
- *Cerebrospinal Fluid (CSF) examination:*
    - Not recommended for purposes of surveillance[Q]
    - Not likely to yield virus, so collection is not recommended for culture
    - However, the CSF cell count, gram stain, protein, and glucose may be very useful in eliminating other conditions that cause AFP
- *Throat examination:*
    - Not recommended for purposes of surveillance[Q]
    - Not as likely as stool to yield virus and thus specimen collection from this site is not recommended
- *Blood examination:*
    - Not recommended for purposes of surveillance[Q]
    - Not likely to yield virus, and current serologic tests cannot differentiate between wild and vaccine virus strains
    - Interpretation of the serologic data can often be misleading
    - Collection of blood specimens for culture or serology not recommended

Key points

Polio diagnosis: Isolation of wild poliovirus from stool is the recommended method

Vaccines for Poliomyelitis

Refer to Chapter 3 Theory

HEPATITIS

Types of Viral Hepatitis

Type	Causative agent	Incubation period^Q	Common mode(s) of transmission
Hepatitis A	Enterovirus 72^Q (picornavirus)	15–45 days^Q	Faecal-oral^Q, sexual
Hepatitis B	Hepadnavirus^Q	45–180 days^Q	Sexual, perinatal, percutaneous
Hepatitis C	Hepacivirus (Flavivirus)	30–120 days	Percutaneous
Hepatitis D	Viriods like	30–90 days	Sexual, perinatal, percutaneous
Hepatitis E	Calcivirus (alphavirus like)	21–45 days	Faecal-oral^Q

Hepatitis A

- *Causative agent:* Enterovirus 72^Q (Picorna virus)
- *Incubation period:* 15-45 days^Q
- *Period of infectivity:* 2 weeks before to 1 week after onset of jaundice
- *Sex distribution:* Equal in both sexes
  - Children: More infected but mild or subclinical
- *Reservoir:* Human cases
- *Modes of transmission:*
  - **Faecal oral (Most common^Q)**
  - Parenteral
  - Sexual
- *Disinfectant:*
  - Formalin
  - UV rays
  - Boiling for 5 min
  - Autoclaving

Key points

Modes of transmission of Hepatitis A:
Faecal oral (Most common^Q)

Hepatitis B

- Also known as *'Serum hepatitis$^{Q'}$*
- *Causative agent:* Hepatitis B virus (HBV)–a Hapdnavirus
  - Is double shelled DNA virus–'Dane's particle$^{Q'}$
  - Discovered by Bloomberg
- *Reservoir of infection:* Man (case or carrier)
- *Incubation period:* 45–180 days^Q (6 weeks–6 months)
  - Median IP < 100 days^Q
- *Modes of transmission:* Blood borne, sexual, parenteral, perinatal^Q
- *Markers of Hepatitis B infection (in order of appearance in serum^Q):*
  - *HBsAg (Hepatitis B surface antigen):*
    - Also known as 'Australia antigen'^{Q}
    - First antigen to appear in serum–'first evidence of infection'^{Q}
    - **'Epidemiological marker of Hepatitis B infection'^{Q}**
  - *HBcAg (Hepatitis B core antigen):*
    - Alone does not appear in serum^Q
  - *HBeAg (Hepatitis B envelope antigen):*
    - Is a secretory form of HBcAg
    - 'Indicates active viral replication'^{Q}
    - **'Is a marker of infectivity for Hepatitis B'^{Q}**
    - *Persistence beyond 3 months:* Increased likelihood of chronic Hepatitis B
  - *Anti-HBc (Antibody to Hepatitis B core antigen):*
    - First antibody to appear in serum^Q
    - **IgM Anti-HBc indicates a diagnosis of acute Hepatitis B^Q**
    - IgG Anti-HBc persists indefinitely
  - *Anti-HBe (Antibody to Hepatitis B envelope antigen):*
    - Signals 'stoppage of active viral replication'^{Q}
  - Indicates 'end of period of infectivity'^{Q}

Key points

Hepatitis B
- Incubation period: 45–180 days
- HBsAg
  'Epidemiological marker
- HBeAg
  Is a marker of infectivity
- IgM Anti-HBc indicates a diagnosis of acute Hepatitis B

- Anti-HBs (Antibody to Hepatitis B surface antigen):
  - Last antibody to appear in serum
  - Signals 'recovery, end of period of communicability'[Q]
- Serologic patterns in Hepatitis B:

HBsAg	Anti HBs	Anti HBc	HBeAg	Anti HBe	Interpretation
+	–	IgM	+	–	Acute hepatitis B[Q]
+	–	IgG	+	–	Chronic hepatitis B with active viral replication[Q]
+	–	IgG	–	+	Chronic hepatitis B with low viral replication
+	+	IgG	+ or –	+ or –	Chronic hepatitis B with heterotypic Anti-HBs
–	–	IgM	+ or –	–	Acute hepatitis B[Q]
–	+	IgG	–	+ or –	Recovery from Hepatitis B (Immunity)[Q]
–	+	–	–	–	Vaccination (Immunity)[Q]
–	–	IgG	–	–	False positive

- Vaccines for Hepatitis B:
  - Plasma derived vaccine:
    - Is formalin inactivated sub-unit vaccine[Q]
    - Is based on HBsAg
    - Derived from carriers of Hepatitis B
  - rDNA yeast derived vaccine:
    - Recombinant DNA vaccine (genetically engineered)
- Hepatitis B Immunoglobulin:
  - Required for immediate protection:
    - Surgeons, nurse, laboratory workers
    - Newborn infants of carrier mothers
    - Sexual contacts of acute Hepatitis B patients
    - Ideally administered within 6 hours[Q] (not later than 48 hours)
  - Dose: 0.05–0.07 mL/kg, 2 doses 30 days apart

5Cs for Hepatitis Testing (WHO)

- Consent
- Confidentiality
- Correct test results
- Counselling
- Connection

Guidelines for the Prevention, Care and Treatment of Persons Living with Chronic Hepatitis B Infection

- Promote use of simple, non-invasive diagnostic tests to assess stage and eligibility for treatment
- Priorities treatment for those with most advance liver disease and highest risk of mortality
- Use of Nucleos(t)ide analogues with high barrier of drug resistance (Tenofovir and Entecavir, and Entecavir in age 2-11 years)
- *Other recommendations*: Regular monitoring for disease progression/drug-toxicity, Lifelong treatment in those with cirrhosis, Early detection of liver cancer

Global Health Sector Strategy on Viral Hepatitis 2016–2021

- *Vision*: Eliminate Viral Hepatitis as a Public Health Problem
- *Global Targets*:
  - Reduce new cases of Chronic HBV/HCV infections by 90%
  - Reduce deaths due to Viral hepatitis by 65%
- Key Interventions:

Preventive Interventions	• 3-dose Hepatitis B vaccine for infants • Prevention of MTCT of Hepatitis B through Birth dose of Hepatitis B vaccine • Blood safety, Injection safety • Harm reduction for persons using drugs
Treatment Interventions	• Diagnosis of HBV, HCV • Treatment of HBV, HCV

Hepatitis E

- *Synonym:* Enterically transmitted hepatitis non-A, non-B [HNANB^Q]
- *Description:* HEV is essentially a waterborne disease, transmitted through water or food supplies, contaminated by faeces
- *Incubation Period:* 2–9 weeks
- *HEV in pregnancy:* Fulminant form is common in Hepatitis E infection during Pregnancy (up to 20% cases) with a high case fatality rate^Q (up to 80%)

Key points

Hepatitis E: Enterically transmitted hepatitis non-A, non-B

DIARRHOEAL DISEASES (CHOLERA and TYPHOID)

Oral Rehydration Solution (ORS)

- ReSoMal (Rehydration Solution for Malnourished): Is recommended for severely malnourished children

Composition^Q (grams)	Osmolar concentration (mmol/litre)	
1 WHO ORS packet +	Sodium	45
2 litres water +	Potassium	40
50 grams sugar +	Chloride	70
40 grams electrolyte/mineral solution	Citrate	7
	Glucose	125
	Mg^{++} Zn^{++} Cu^{++}	4
	Total	300

- New WHO recommended reduced osmolarity oral rehydration solution (Low Na ORS):^{Q}

Composition^Q (grams)		Osmolar concentration^Q (mmol/litre)	
Sodium chloride	2.6	Sodium	75
Potassium chloride	1.5	Potassium	20
Sodium citrate	2.9	Chloride	65
Glucose	13.5	Citrate	10
		Glucose	75
Total	20.5	Total	245

Cholera

- Cholera is an acute diarrhoel disease caused by Vibrio cholerae
- Vibrio cholerae: 'Gram-negative bacterium' that produces cholera toxin (enterotoxin), which act on c-AMP system of mucosal cells of epithelium lining of the small intestine (to cause massive diarrhea)
  - Classical biotype
  - El Tor biotype [Serotypes: Ogawa (Earlier MC in India^Q), Inaba and Hikojima]
  - Recently El Tor Hybrid subtype has become MC in India
- *Incubation period^Q:* 1–2 days (Few hours–5 days)
- *Reservoir:* Human beings only
- Rice-watery diarrhoea^Q
- *Essentials for treatment of cholera:* Water and electrolyte replacement (ORS)

Key points

Stools in Cholera: Rice-watery diarrhoea

Guidelines for Cholera Control (WHO)

- *Verification of diagnosis:*
  - Identifying Vibrio cholerae 01 in stools OF FEW PATIENTS is sufficient
  - It is 'not necessary to culture stools of all cases or contacts'
- *Notification:*
  - Cholera is a notifiable disease locally, nationally and internationally^Q
  - Under International Health Regulations, Cholera is notifiable to WHO by national govt WITHIN 24 HOURS (no. of cases & deaths to be reported daily and weekly)
  - An area is declared free of Cholera when TWICE the IP has elapsed since last case^Q
- *Early case finding:* through aggressive case search

Key points

Cholera is a notifiable disease

- Establishment of treatment centres
- *Rehydration therapy:* through ORS
- *Adjuncts to therapy:* Only antibiotics may be used when vomiting stops

Group	Antibiotic of choice^Q
Treatment	
Adults	Doxycycline
Children	Azithromycin
Pregnancy	Azithromycin
Chemoprophylaxis	Tetracycline^Q

> **Key points**
> Mass chemoprophylaxis IS NOT ADVISED in cholera

- *Epidemiological investigations:* General sanitation measures, epidemiological studies
- *Sanitation measures:* Water control, excreta disposal, food sanitation, disinfection
- *Chemoprophylaxis:*
    - Mass chemoprophylaxis IS NOT ADVISED for total community; is only advisable for household contacts or a closed community^Q
    - Drug of choice for chemoprophylaxis: Tetracycline^Q
    - To prevent one case of cholera, 10,000 persons need to be given chemoprophylaxis
- Vaccination
- *Health education:* **MOST EFFECTIVE prophylactic measure**^{Q}

> **Key points**
> *Health education:* MOST EFFECTIVE prophylactic measure in cholera

Typhoid Fever

- *Causative agent:* Salmonella typhi
- *Reservoir of infection:* Man (cases and carriers)
    - Cases
    - Carriers
    - Incubatory carriers
    - *Convalescent carriers:* excrete bacilli for 6–8 weeks
    - *Chronic carrier:* excrete bacilli for > 1 year after clinical attack^Q
- *Source of infection:* faeces, urine of cases/carriers (primary source) and water, food fingers, flies (secondary source)
- *IP:* **10-14 days**^{Q}
- *Mode of transmission:* Faeco-oral route, urine-oral route
- *Clinical features*^{Q}:
    - 'Pea Soup diarrhoea'
    - Splenomegaly, relative bradycardia, dicrotic pulse, abdominal distension and tenderness
    - Rose spots^Q (2nd week)
    - Intestinal perforation (3rd week^Q) may be one of the complications
- *Laboratory Diagnosis:* **'BASU'** Mnemonic

Test of diagnosis	Time of diagnosis^Q	Remarks
Blood culture	1st week	Mainstay of diagnosis
Antibodies (Widal test)	2nd week	Moderate sensitivity & specificity
Stool culture	3rd week	
Urine test	4th week	
Newer tests		
IDL Tubex test		Detects IgM antibodies
TYPHI DOT		Detects IgM & IgG antibodies
TYPHI DOT-M		Detects IgM antibodies
DIPSTICK TEST		Detects IgM antibodies

- *Drug of choice:*
    - *Cases:* Cephalosporins (Ceftriaxone), Quinolones
    - *Carriers:* Ampicillin/Amoxycillin + Probenecid × 6 weeks
- *Immunisation for Typhoid:*
    - TYPHORAL (Live oral Ty21a^Q) vaccine:
    - Contains >10^9 viable organism of attenuated S. typhi^Q
    - *Schedule:* One capsule each on days 1, 3, 5 (booster of 3 doses, once every 3 years)

- *Protection duration:* 3 years
- *TYPHIM Vi Vaccine:*
  - Vi- Polysaccharide containing single dose i.m. or subcutaneous
  - Not given in age < 2 years
- *TAB vaccine:*
  - Contains S.typhi, S.paratyphi A and S.paratyphi B

Diarrhoea Control Measures

- Oral Rehydration Therapy (First 4 hours: 75 ml/kg):

Age	Weight (kg)	ORS solution
< 4 months	<5 kg	200–400 mL
4–11 months	5.0–7.9 kg	400–600 mL
1–2 years	8.0–10.9 kg	600–800 mL
2–4 years	11–15.9 kg	800–1200 mL
5–14 years	16–29.9 kg	1200–2200 mL
≥ 15 years	≥ 30 kg	2200–4000 mL

(Solution used: WHO Reduced Osmolarity ORS)

- Intravenous Rehydration (Total dose 100 mL/kg):

Age	First give 30 mL/kg	Then give 70 mL/kg
Infants	1 hour	5 hours
>1 year age	30 minutes	2.5 hours

(Solution used: Ringer lactate/Hartmann solution, Diarrhoea treatment solution (DTS))

- Maintenance Therapy:

Amount of Diarrhea	Amount of Oral Fluid
Mild diarrhoea (<1stool/2 hours)	100 ml/kg BW until diarrhoea stops
Severe diarrhoea (>1stool/2 hours)	10-15 ml/kg BW per hour

- Appropriate feeding
- Chemotherapy:
  - Vibrio cholerae: Doxycycline, Tetracycline, TMP-SMX, Erythromycin
  - Shigella: Ciprofloxacin
- Zinc supplementation:
  - Infants < 6 months age: 10 mg/day × 10–14 days
  - Children > 6 months age: 20 mg/day × 10–14 days

WORM INFESTATIONS

Guinea Worm (Dracunculiasis)

- *Causative agent:* Dracunculus medinensis (nematode)
- *Guineaworm disease in India:*
  - *Last case in India:* July 1996 (Jodhpur, Rajasthan)
  - *India certified for Elimination of Guineaworm (WHO):* Feb 2000[Q]
  - *India certified Guineaworm disease free:* Feb 2001[Q]
- *Reservoir of infection:* An infected person (no animal reservoir)
- *Type of biological transmission:* Cyclo-developmental transmission[Q]
- *Type of disease:* Water based disease[Q] (Cyclops play a role in transmission)
- *Mode of transmission:* Consumption of water containing Cyclops harbouring infective stage of parasite[Q]
- *Guineaworm is amenable to eradication:*
  - Provision of safe drinking water
  - Control of Cyclops
  - Health education
  - Active surveillance for cases
- *Treatment of cases:* Niridazole[Q], Mebendazole and Metronidazole

> **Key points**
> Guineaworm
> Type of biological transmission: Cyclo-developmental transmission

- No drug is effective for preventing disease transmission
- No drug is suitable for mass treatment

Roundworm (Ascariasis)

- *Importance:*
  - Is MC helminthic infection^Q
  - Is MC worm infestation in India^Q
- *Causative agent:* Ascaris lumbricoides
- *Reservoir of Infection:* Man^Q
- *Mode of transmission:* Faecal-oral route^Q
- *Incubation Period:* 2 months
- *Drugs of choice:*
  - Albendazole^Q
  - Mebendazole
  - Pyrantel

Hookworm (Ancylostomiasis)

- *Causative agent^Q:*
  - Ancylostoma duodenale
  - Necator americanus
- *Reservoir of Infection:* Man
- *Mode of transmission:* Direct penetration of skin of foot and by oral route^Q
- *Incubation Period:*
  - 5 weeks - 9 months (A. duodenale)
  - 7 weeks (Necator americanus)
- *Hookworm infection is also known as:* miners' anaemia, tunnel disease, brickmaker's anaemia, Egyptian chlorosis
  - Average blood loss in hookworm infection: 0.03-0.2 ml/worm/day^Q
- *Hookworm infection is associated with:*
  - Iron Deficiency Anemia^Q
  - Hypoalbuminemia
- *Cutaneous larva migrans:* a skin disease in humans, caused by the larvae of various nematode parasites, the most common of which is Ancylostoma braziliense^Q
- *Drugs of choice^Q:*
  - Albendazole (A. duodenale)
  - Mebendazole (N. americanus)
- *Endemic Index (Chandler's Index^Q):*
  - CI is average no of hookworm eggs per gram of faeces for the 'entire community'^{Q}
  - Interpretation of CI: Kato-katz Technique is employed

Average no of eggs/gm stools	Interpretation
<200	Not much significance
200–250	Potential danger
250–300	Minor public health problem
> 300^Q	Important public health problem

Tapeworm (Taeniasis)

- *Causative agent:*
  - Taenia solium
  - Taenia saginata
- *Hosts of Infection:*

	Definitive host	Intermediate host^Q
Taenia solium	Man	Pig
Taenia saginata	Man	Cattle

- *Mode of transmission:*
  - Ingestion of infective cysticerci in beef (T. saginata) or pork (T. solium)
  - Ingestion of food/water/vegetables contaminated with eggs

---

Key points

Roundworm: Is MC helminthic infection

Key points

Roundworm
Durg of choice: Albendazole

Key points

Hookworm infection is associated with: Iron Deficiency Anemia

Key points

Definitive host in Tapeworms: Man

- *Incubation Period:* 8-14 weeks
- *Drugs of choice*^{Q}:
  - Praziquantel
  - Niclosamide
  - Albendazole (Cysticercosis)

National Deworming Day (NDD)

- *National Deworming Day (NDD)*: 10th February^Q
- *Objective*^{Q}: Deworm all Pre-school and School aged children (both enrolled and unenrolled) through Schools and Anganwadi centers
- *Target beneficiaries*^{Q}: 1-19 years age (Both boys and girls)
- *Linkage with*: Vitamin A prophylaxis program^Q
- *Dosage*^{Q}:
  - *1–2 years age*: Half tablet 400 mg Albendazole stat
  - *2–19 years age*: Full tablet 400 mg Albendazole stat

DENGUE AND YELLOW FEVER

Dengue Fever and Related Syndromes

- *Dengue viruses are arboviruses (Flavivirus) which may result in:*
  - Asymptomatic infection
  - Dengue
  - Dengue hemorrhagic fever (DHF)
  - Dengue shock syndrome (DSS)
- Dengue viruses have 4 serotypes^Q (Den 1, 2, 3, 4)
- *Vector for dengue:* Aedes aegypti^Q
- *Reservoir:* Man, Mosquito^Q
- *Incubation period:* 3–10 days

> **Key points**
> Vector for dengue: Aedes aegypti

Clinical Diagnosis of Dengue

1. **Dengue Fever (Break-bone fever)**
- Probable diagnosis:
  - Acute febrile illness *plus*
  - ≥ 2 of the manifestations (Headache, Retro-orbital pain, Myalgia, Rash, Arthralgia/bone pain, Hemorrhagic manifestations, Leucopenia WBC <5000/cu.mm., Thrombocytopenia Platelets <1.5 Lac/cu.mm., Rising hematocrit 5-10%) *plus*
  - ≥ 1 of the events (Supportive serology on single serum sample/Comparable IgG titre with ELIA/IgM antibody test positive, Same location/time as of confirmed cases of Dengue)
- Confirmed Diagnosis: Probable case *plus* >1 of the following:
  - Dengue virus isolation (Serum/CSF/Autopsy samples)
  - >4-fold increase in Serum IgG (HAI test) or Increase in IgM antibody
  - Dengue virus detection in Tissue/CSF/Serum (Immunohistochemistry/IF/ELISA)
  - Detection of Dengue virus genomic sequences (RT-PCR)
2. **Dengue Hemorrhagic Fever**
- All of the following:
  - Acute onset of fever, 2-7 days duration
  - Hemorrhagic manifestations (Positive tourniquet test/Petechiae, echhymoses, purpura/Bleeding from mucosa, GIT, Injection sites, etc.)
  - Platelet count ≤ 100,000 cells/cu.mm.
  - Plasma leakage (Rising hematocrit, hemoconcentration >20%/Pleural effusion, ascites/Hypoprotenemia)
3. **Dengue Shock Syndrome**
- DHF criteria plus Signs of Shock
  - Tachycardia/Cool extremities/Weak pulse/Lethargy/Restlessness
  - Pulse pressure <20 mm Hg with increased Diastolic pressure (e.g. 100/80)
  - Hypotension (Systolic <80 mm Hg for age <5 years/80-90 mm Hg for older children and adults)

Laboratory Diagnosis of Dengue
- *Virus isolation*: Serum/Plasma/Plasma, washed buffy coat/Autopsy tissue/Mosquitoes
- *Viral nucleic acid detection*: RT-PCR assay
- Immunological response and Serological tests: Heme-agglutination inhibition assay (HIA)/Complement fixation (CF)/Neutralization test (NT)/IgM Capture (MAC-ELISA)/Indirect IgG-ELISA/IgM:IgG ratio
- *Viral antigen detection*: **Non-structural protein (NS-1)**
- *Rapid diagnostic test*: IgM, IgG
- Hematological assessment

Global Strategy for Dengue Prevention and Control 2021–2030
- *Goal:* Reduce the global burden of Dengue
- *Objectives (2010-2020 levels as base line):*
  - To build capacity in countries to detect, prevent and respond dengue outbreaks
  - To reduce preventable dengue deaths to zero
  - To reduce the burden of disease in countries and reduce incidence by 25%.

Dengue Vaccine - DENGVAXIA (CYD-TDV)
- *Importance*: WHO Endorsed World's First-ever Vaccine for Dengue Fever
  - Approved for use in 11 countries: Mexico, Philippines, Indonesia, Brazil, El Salvador, Costa Rica, Paraguay, Guatemala, Peru, Thailand, and Singapore
- *Type of vaccine*: Live recombinant tetravalent vaccine^Q
  - *Diluent*: Saline
  - No adjuvant
  - No preservatives
- *Strain*: **CYD-TDV**^{Q}
- *Age group*: 9-45 years age living in endemic areas
- *Schedule*: 3 injections spaced out over one year (0, 6 months, 12 months)^Q
- *Contraindications*: Allergy, Immunosuppression, HIV, Pregnancy, Breastfeeding
- *Production of vaccine*:
  - Live attenuated tetravalent chimeric vaccine made using recombinant DNA technology
  - Replacement of PrM (pre-membrane) and E (envelope) structural genes of the Yellow fever attenuated '*17D strain vaccine*'^{Q} with those from four dengue serotypes

Yellow Fever (Yellow Jack/Black Vomit/American Plague)
- *Causative agent*: Flavivirus fibricus (Togavirus Family, Gp B Arbovirus)
- *Reservoir of Infection*^{Q}:
  - *Forest (Sylvian) Cycle:* Monkeys and Forest mosquitoes
  - *Urban Cycle:* Man (Sub clinical and clinical cases) and Aedes aegypti
- *Period of Communicability:*
  - *Man:* first 3–4 days of illness
  - *Mosquitoes:* Lifelong (after extrinsic IP of 8-12 days^Q)
- *Immunity:* Single attack provides life long immunity
  - *Infants born of Immune mothers have antibodies upto:* 6 months of life
- *Incubation Period:* 3-6 days^Q
  - IP of 6 days recognized under International Health Regulations^Q
- *Case fatality rate*^{Q}: 80%
- *Yellow Fever Vaccine:*
  - Live attenuated, lyophilized (Freeze dried) vaccine^Q
  - **Strain: 17D strain (Chick Embryo grown)**^{Q}
  - *Cold chain Temperature:* –30° to + 5°C
  - *Reconstitution with Diluent:* Cold physiological saline^Q
  - *After reconstitution, use within:* ½ hour^Q
  - *Dose:* 0.5 mL (irrespective of age)
  - *Route:* Subcutaneous^Q
  - *Site:* At Insertion of Deltoid
  - *Immunity lasts:* From 7 days of Vaccination till 35 years^Q
  - **WHO recommended validity of Vaccination Certificate for International travel: from 10 days to LIFELONG**^{Q}

> **Key points**
> Incubation Period: 3-6 days in YF

> **Key points**
> Strain: 17D strain in YF vaccine

> **Key points**
> WHO recommended validity of Vaccination Certificate for International travel: from 10 days to Lifelong for YF

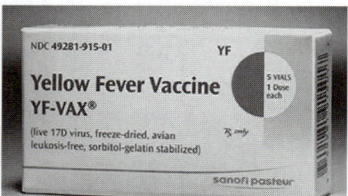

YF Vaccine

- YF vaccine is the only Live vaccine that can be administered in Pregnancy (if there is risk of exposure)^Q
- Yellow Fever Vaccine and Cholera Vaccine cannot be given together: Maintain a gap of 3 weeks or more between them^Q
- Indices of Surveillance of Aedes Mosquitoes^Q

$$\text{Container Index} = \frac{\text{No of containers showing breeding of Aedes larvae C+}}{\text{Total no of containers surveyed C}} \times 100$$

$$\text{House index} = \frac{\text{No of Houses showing breeding of Aedes Larvae H+}}{\text{Total no of Houses surveyed H}} \times 100$$

$$\text{Breteau Index} = \frac{\text{No of containers showing breeding of Aedes Larvae C+}}{\text{Total no of houses surveyed H}} \times 100$$

- YF Control measures:
  - Distance around airports to be kept free of aedes breeding: **400 m**^{Q}
  - Breteau Index (Aedes aegypti index) should be **< 1%** in towns and seaports^Q

> **Key points**
> YF Control measures:
> - Distance around airports to be kept free of aedes breeding: 400 m^Q
> - Breteau Index (Aedes aegypti index) should be <1% in towns and seaports

EYE (Elimination Yellow fever Epidemic) Strategy [WHO, UNICEF, GAVI]

3 Strategic Objectives	5 Competencies of Success
- Project at-risk population - Prevent international spread of YF - Contain outbreaks rapidly	- Affordable vaccines and sustained vaccine market - Strong political commitment at all levels - High level governance with long term partnerships - Synergies with other health programs and sectors - Research and development

MALARIA

Anopheles Mosquito

There are over 55 species of anopheline mosquitoes in India:
- *An. culicifacies:* Vector of rural malaria^Q
- *An stephensi:* Vector of urban malaria^Q; breed in overhead tanks^Q
- *An. fluviatilis:* Efficient vector; highly anthrophilic; breed in moving water
- *An. sundaicus:* Breed in brackish water
- An. dirus
- An. minimus
- An. philippinensis
- An. maculates

> **Key points**
> *An. culicifacies:* Vector of rural malaria
> *An stephensi:* Vector of urban malaria

Epidemiology of Malaria in India

- *Incubation period:*

Type	Incubation period
Plasmodium vivax	8–17 days (14 days)
Plasmodium falciparum^Q	9–14 days (12 days)
Plasmodium malariae	18–40 days (28 days)
Plasmodium ovale	16–18 days (17 days)

- *Season:* Most common in July–November
- *Definitive host:* Anopheles mosquito (Intermediate host: Man^Q)
  - Is seen in both rural as well as urban areas
- *Vector:* An. culicifacies (rural) and An. stephensi (urban)
- 22% population lives in high transmission area (>1 case/1,000 population)
- 0.84 million cases, 104 deaths [2017]
- 66% Plasmodium falciparum cases

Modes of Malaria Transmission

- *Bite of female anopheline mosquitoes:*
  - *Infective forms:* Sporozoites^Q

- *Injection of blood of a malaria patient containing asexual forms:* 'Trophozoite induced malaria'[Q]
  - Transfusion malaria[Q]
  - Congenital malaria
  - Malaria in drug addicts

Life Cycle of Mosquito

- *Hosts involved in transmission of malaria*[Q]:

Man	Female anopheles mosquito
Secondary host	Primary host
Intermediate host	Definitive host
Asexual cycle	Sexual cycle
Schizogony	Sporogony

- *Human cycle of Plasmodium:*
  - *Pre-erythrocytic schizogony:*
    - Development of sporozoites in liver parenchyma
    - Liberated merozoites are called as 'Cryptozoites'
    - No clinical manifestation; No pathological change
    - Blood is sterile
  - *Erythrocytic schizogony:*
    - Parasite resides inside RBCs; passes through stages of Trophozoite, Schizont, Merozoite
    - Parasitic multiplication brings clinical attack of malaria
  - *Gametogony:*
    - Some merozoites develop in RBCs of spleen and bone marrow to form 'Gametocytes'
  - *Exo-erythrocytic schizogony:*
    - Persistence of late tissue phase in liver[Q]
    - Seen in P.vivax and P. ovale
    - Cause relapses in Vivax and Ovale malaria
    - Liberated merozoites are known as 'Phanerozoites'
- *Mosquito cycle of Plasmodium:*
  - *Completion of gametogony:*
    - Exflagellation of microgamete and maturation of gametes
    - Fusion of gametes form 'Zygote'; zygote matures to 'Ookinite'
  - *Sporogony:*
    - Oookinite develops into 'Oocyst'
    - On 10th day of infection, oocyst ruptures, releasing sporozoites; sporozoites reach salivary glands
    - Mosquito at this stage is capable of transmitting infection

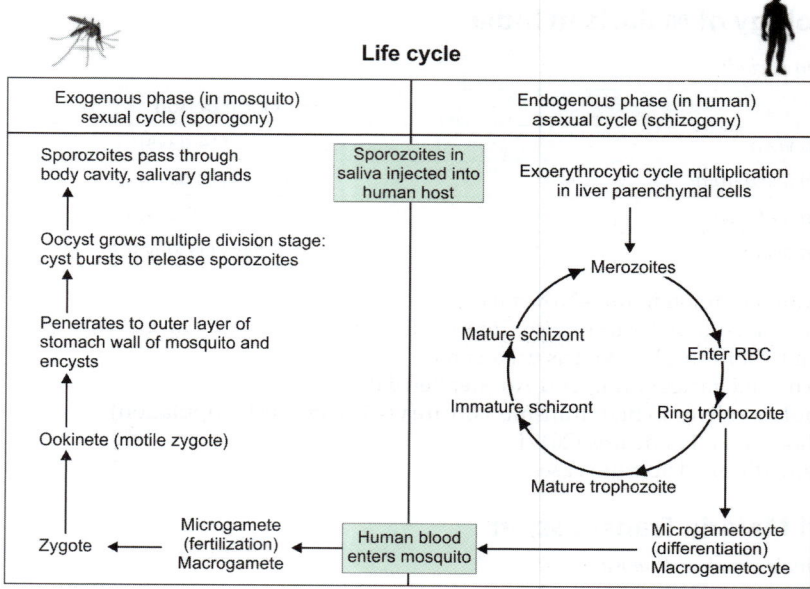

Malariometric Measures in Pre-eradication Era

- *Spleen rate:* Percentage children 2–10 years age showing enlargement of spleen
  - Index used for measuring endemicity of malaria in a community^Q
- Average enlarged spleen
- *Parasite rate:* Percentage children 2–10 years age showing parasites in blood films
- Parasite density index
- *Infant parasite rate:* Percentage infants showing parasites in blood films
  - Is 'most sensitive index of recent malaria transmission' in a locality^Q
  - If IFR is zero for 3 consecutive years, it is regarded as absence of malaria transmission (even though anopheline may remain)
- *Proportional case rate:* Is no. of clinical malaria cases diagnosed per 100 patients attending hospitals and dispensaries

> **Key points**
> *Infant parasite rate:* 'most sensitive index of recent malaria transmission'

Malariometric Measures in Eradication Era

- *Annual parasitic incidence (API):* Sophisticated measure of malaria incidence in a community^Q

$$\text{API} = \frac{\text{Confirmed cases during one year}}{\text{Population under surveillance}} \times 1{,}000$$

- *Annual blood examination rate (ABER):* (Index of operational efficiency^Q)

$$\text{ABER} = \frac{\text{Number of slides examined}}{\text{Population}} \times 100$$

- *Annual falciparum incidence (AFI)*
- *Slide positivity rate (SPR)*

$$\text{SPR} = \frac{\text{No. of blood semears + ve for parasite}}{\text{No. of blood smears examined}} \times 100$$

- *Slide falciparum rate (SFR)*

> **Key points**
> **API:** Sophisticated measure of malaria incidence

> **Key points**
> **ABER:** (Index of operational efficiency^Q)

New Malaria Treatment Guidelines in India (2013 onwards)^Q

See Annexure 12

Malaria Vaccine MOSQUIRIX (RTS, S)

- A recombinant protein-based malaria vaccine
  - World's first licensed malaria vaccine (July 2015) to be used in African babies
  - World's first vaccine licensed for use against a parasitic disease of any kind
- *Efficacy:* 26–50% in infants and young children
- *Components and mechanism:*
  - Engineered using genes from the repeat and T-cell epitope in the pre-erythrocytic circumsporozoite protein (CSP) of the Plasmodium falciparum malaria parasite and a viral envelope protein of the hepatitis B virus (HBsAg), to which was added a chemical adjuvant (AS01) to increase the immune system response
  - Infection is prevented by inducing humoral and cellular immunity, with high antibody titers, that block the parasite from infecting the liver

National Framework for Malaria Elimination in India 2016–2030

- *Vision:* Eliminate malaria nationally and contribute to improved health, quality of life and alleviation of poverty
- *Goals:*
  - Eliminate malaria (zero indigenous cases) throughout country by 2030^Q
  - Maintain malaria-free status in areas where malaria transmission has been interrupted and prevent re-introduction of malaria.
- *Objectives*^Q:
  - Eliminate malaria from 26 low (Category 1), moderate (Category 2) transmission areas by 2022

- Reduce incidence < 1 case per 1000 population per year by 2024
- Interrupt indigenous transmission of malaria throughout the entire country, including all high transmission states and UTs (Category 3) by 2027
- Prevent the re-establishment of local transmission of malaria in areas where it has been eliminated and maintain national malaria-free status by 2030 and beyond

Categories of States/UTs	Definition
Category 0 Prevention of re-establishment phase	States/UTs with zero indigenous cases of malaria
Category 1 Elimination phase	States/UTs (15) API < 1 case per 1000 population at risk
Category 2 Pre-elimination phase	States/UTs (11) with an API < 1 case per 1000 population at risk, but few districts are reporting an API > 1/1000
Category 3 Intensified control phase	States/UTs (10) with an API > 1 case per 1000 population at risk or above

Global Technical Strategy for Malaria (2016-2030)

Goals	Milestones		Targets
	2020	2025	2030
Reduce mortality	≥ 40%	≥ 75%	≥ 90%
Reduce Incidence	≥ 40%	≥ 75%	≥ 90%
Elimination	≥ 10 countries	≥ 20 countries	≥ 35 countries
Re-establishment	Prevention	Prevention	Prevention

LYMPHATIC FILARIASIS

Problem Statement of Lymphatic Filariasis

- *Global:* Affects 120 million people in 120 countries^Q; 1.1 billion people live in areas with risk of infection
- *SEAR:* 600 million live in endemic areas; 60 million infected
- *India:* Lymphatic filariasis is a major public health problem in India with 553 million people at risk in 233 districts; heavily endemic in UP, Bihar, Jharkhand, Andhra Pradesh, Orissa, Tamil Nadu, Kerala, Gujarat

Lymphatic Filariasis

- *Description:* Lymphatic Filariasis covers infection with 3 closely related nematode worms
- *Causative Agents:*^{Q}
  - Wuchereria bancrofti
  - Brugia malayi
  - Brugia timori
- *Definitive Host:* Man
- *Intermediate Host:* Mosquito
- *Vectors of Lymphatic filariasis:*
  - *Bancroftian filariasis:* Culex, Anopheles, Aedes
  - *Brugian filariasis:* Mansonia, Anopheles, Coquillettidia
- *Main Vectors of Lymphatic filariasis in India:*
  - *Bancroftian Filariasis:* Culex quinquefasciatus (C. fatigans^Q)
  - *Brugian Filariasis:* Mansonia annulifers, Mansonia uniformis^Q
- *Mode of Transmission:* Bite of Infected Vector mosquito
- *Stages of filariasis:*
  - *Pre-Patent Period:* Time interval between inoculation of Infective larvae and first appearance of detectable microfilariae (Mf)
  - *Clinical Incubation Period:* Time interval between invasion of infectve larvae to development of clinical manifestations(~ 8-16 months)
  - *Mosquito becomes infective:* When third stage larvae migrates to Proboscis of mosquito vector
  - *Asymptomatic amicrofilaraemia stage:* Absence of Mf or clinical manifestations

> **Key points**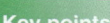
>
> **Bancroftian Filariasis:** Vector is Culex quinquefasciatus (C. fatigans)

- *Asymptomatic microfilaraemia:* Blood positive for Mf but no clinical manifestations; act as carriers and an important source of infection
- *Occult Filariasis (cryptic filariasis):* No clinical manifestations or Mf in blood
- Due to a hypersensitivity reaction to Filarial Antigens
- *Example:* Tropical pulmonary eosinophilia

Filaria Detection Tests

- *MC method used for epidemiological assessment of Lymphatic Filariasis (through mass blood survey):* Thick film using 20 cu. mm. of capillary blood (collected between 830 pm up to 12 midnight^Q)
- *Most sensitive method for detecting low density microfilaraemia:* Membrane Filter Concentration Method
- *DEC Provocation test (100 mg DEC oral):* Mf can be induced to appear in blood during daytime
  - Blood is examined 1 hour after DEC administration
- *Good method to detect low density microfilariaemia, when other methods fail:* Xenodiagnosis
  - Mosquitoes allowed to feed on patients, then dissected 2 weeks later

Treatment of Filariasis

- *Chemotherapy of Filariasis^Q:* **Diethylcarbamazine (DEC)**
  - *Bancroftian filariasis:* 6mg/kg/day × 12 days (Total 72 mg/kg^Q)
  - *Brugian filariasis:* 3-6 mg/kg/day × 6-12 days (Total 18-72 mg/kg)
  - DEC is effective in killing Mf
  - No effect on Infective (stage III) larvae
  - Uncertain effect on adult worm
- *Filariasis never causes explosive epidemics.* Favourable factors for success of control programme are:
  - Parasite does not multiply in Insect vector
  - Infective larvae do not multiply in Human Host
  - Life cycle of parasite is quite long (15 years or more)
- *DEC medicated salt:*
  - *Dose:* 1-4 gm DEC/kg of salt^Q
  - Is a type of Mass Treatment^Q (using very low dose of drug)
  - Treatment duration: 6-9 months
- National Filaria Control Programme (NFCP), 1955 is now a component of National Vector Borne Diseases Control Programme (NVBDCP), 2003-04
  - NVBDCP covers Malaria, Filariasis, Japanese Encephalitis, Kala Azar, Chikungunya fever and Dengue^Q

> **Key points**
>
> *Chemotherapy of Filariasis^Q:* Diethylcarbamazine (DEC)

Assessment of Filaria Control Programmes

Methods	Parameters	Inclusions
Clinical	Incidence of acute manifestations	Adenolymphangitis, epididymoorchitis, Lymphoedema, Hydrocoele, Chyluria
	Prevalence of Chronic Manifestations	
Parasitological	Mf rate (species specific)	% showing Mf in blood in population
	Filarial Endemicity Rate	Mf in blood and/or disease manifestations
	Microfilarial density (Intensity of infecn)	No Mf per unit volume (20 mm³) blood
	Average infestation rate (Prevalence of Mf)	Average no of Mf per positive slide.
Entomological	Vector density per 10 hour man catch % mosquito with Infective stage III Larvae Annual biting rate Types of larval breeding places	

Global Program to Eliminate Lymphatic Filariasis (GPELF) [WHO]

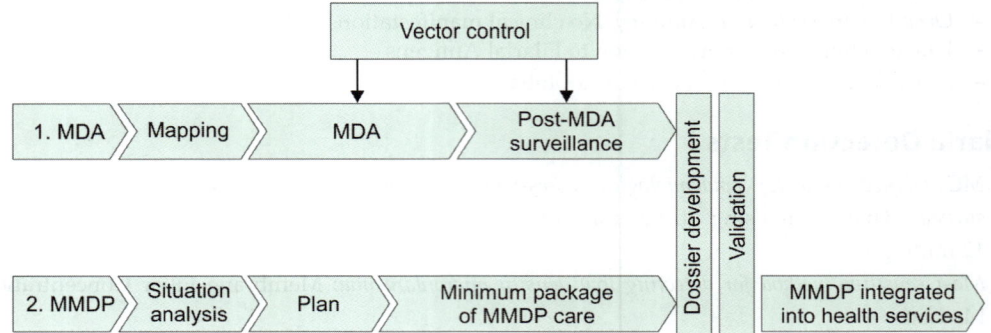

1. **Stop the spread of infection—Mass drug administration (MDA):** Annual MDA for > 5 years with a coverage of > 65% of the total at-risk population:
   - 6 mg/kg of body weight Diethylcarbamazine citrate (DEC) + 400 mg Albendazole; or
   - 150 µg/kg of body weight Ivermectin + 400 mg Albendazole (in areas that are also endemic for Onchocerciasis);
   - 400 mg Albendazole preferably twice per year (in areas that are also endemic for Loa loa).
   - Alternative and equally effective community-wide regimen in endemic regions: Common table salt or cooking salt fortified with DEC
2. **Alleviate suffering:** Morbidity management and disability prevention (MMDP)
   - Minimum recommended package of care to manage lymphedema and hydrocele
   - These services should be available within primary health care systems

Accelerated Plan for Elimination of Lymphatic Filariasis (APELF), India 2018

- Triple Drug Therapy or IDA (Ivermectin, Diethylcarbamazine DEC and Albendazole)
- Community engagement for successful MDA implementation
- DEC-medicated salt
- House-to-house visit advocacy

RABIES

Rabies (Hydrophobia^Q)

- Hydrophobia is pathognomic^Q (though few consider Aerophobia as pathognomic)
  - Causative agent: Lyssavirus Type 1 (Bullet shaped neurotropic RNA virus).
- Types of rabies virus: Street virus and Fixed virus

Characteristics	Street Virus (SV)	Fixed Virus (FV)
Source	Naturally occurring cases	Serial brain passage of SV
Incubation period	20–60 days	4–6 days
Pathogenicity	For all mammals	Sometimes pathogenic
Negri Bodies	Formed	Not formed
Importance	Cause rabies	Used for vaccine preparation^Q

- *Incubation period:* Variable [4 days to many years; ~ 3 to 8 weeks]
- Rabies is a dead-end infection in man^Q
- *Negri bodies (Pathognomic of Rabies^Q):* Intracytoplasmic eosinophilic inclusion bodies with basophilic granules in neurons
- *Mode of transmission:*
  - Animal bites (dogs, cats, monkeys, cow, goat, sheep, buffalo, horses EXCEPT RAT BITE and HUMAN BITE^Q)

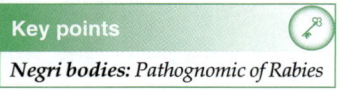

Key points

Negri bodies: Pathognomic of Rabies

- Licks (on abraded skin or abraded/unabraded mucosa)
- Aerosols (Rabies infected bats^Q)
- Person to person: Rare but possible
- Corneal and organ transplantation

Water: An Effective Natural Barrier against Rabies

- *Rabies-free area:* No case of Rabies in man or animals for past 2 years^Q
- *Rabies is not found in:*
  - Australia^Q
  - Cyprus
  - Ireland
  - Japan
  - Britain
  - Lakshadweep (India)^Q
  - China (Taiwan)
  - Iceland
  - Malta
  - New Zealand
  - Andaman and Nicobar Islands (India)^Q

Local Wound Treatment

- *Cleansing:* Flush and wash wound area with plenty of soap and running water for minimum 5-10 minutes^Q
- *Suturing:* not recommended; if necessary, do 24–48 hours later^Q
- *Anti-rabies serum:* Local application with prior sensitivity testing
- *Observe animal:* for 10 days^Q

Type of Contact, Exposure and Recommended Post-exposure Prophylaxis (PEP)

Category	Type of contact	Recommended PEP^Q
I	Touching or feeding of animals Licks on intact skin Contact of intact skin with secretions/excretions of rabid animal/human case	None, if reliable case history is available
II	Nibbling of uncovered skin Minor scratches or abrasions without bleeding	Wound management Anti-rabies vaccine
III	Single or multiple transdermal bites or scratches, licks on broken skin Contamination of mucous membrane with saliva (i.e. licks)	Wound management Rabies immunoglobulin Anti-rabies vaccine

Vaccines Approved for ID Use in the Country

- Purified Chick Embryo Cell Vaccine (PCECV) - Rabipur, Vaxirab N
- Purified Vero Cell Rabies Vaccine (PVRV) - Verorab, Abhayrab, Indira

Vaccines Approved for IM Use in the Country

- *Cell Culture Vaccines:* Human Diploid Cell Vaccine (HDCV), Purified Chick Embryo Cell Vaccine (PCECV), Purified Vero Cell Rabies Vaccine (PVRV)
- Purified Duck Embryo Vaccine (PDEV)

New Recommended Regimens/Schedules [NEW GUIDELINES]

Type of prophylaxis	Regimen
Post Exposure Intramuscular	
Essen Regimen (1-1-1-1-1)^Q	Day 0, 3, 7, 14, 28
Post Exposure Intradermal	
Updated Thai Red Cross Regimen (2-2-2-0-2)^Q	Day 0, 3, 7, 28
Post-exposure in vaccinated individuals^Q	Day 0, 3
Pre-exposure prophylaxis^Q	Day 0, 7, 21/28

- Minimum potency: 2.5 IU per i/m dose
- **Zagreb Regimen of Rabies vaccine** (intramuscular post-exposure):
  - 4-dose abbreviated multisite regimen
  - 2-0-1-0-1 (2 doses on Day 0, 1 dose on Day 7, 1 dose on Day 21)

For New WHO Rabies Vaccination Guidelines, Refer to Annexure 22

Other Management Guidelines

- *Anti Rabies serum*:
  - *Horse Antirabies Serum:* 40 IU/kg on Day 0 (50% in Wound, 50% i.m)
  - *Human Rabies Immunoglobulin*^{Q}: **20 IU/kg** (maximum in wound, rest i.m gluteal) (Concentration 150 IU/mL)
  - *Serum Sickness with Horse Serum:* 15–45%
- *Persons under Antirabic treatment should avoid:*
  - Alcohol (during and 1 month after treatment)
  - Undue physical and mental strain and late nights
  - Corticosteroids and other immunosuppressive agents
- *Intramuscular injections of Cell Culture and Purified Duck Embryo Vaccines:* Deltoid (not in Buttocks)
  - Volume of intradermal dose of Rabies Vaccine is 1/5th of intramuscular dose
  - Sites for intradermal rabies vaccines: Deltoid, Lateral thigh, Suprascapular region, Lower quadrant of abdomen
  - Booster injections in Pre-exposure prophylaxis: at intervals of 2 years
- *Immunisation of Dogs:* Primary Immunisation at 3-4 months and boosters at regular intervals
  - *BPL inactivated NTV:* Single dose 5 ml for dogs (3 ml for cats), revaccination after 6 months, subsequently every year
  - *Modified Live Virus Vaccine:* Single dose 3 ml, boosters every 3 years
- *Most logical and cost effective approach for control of Urban Rabies:* Elimination of stray dogs and swift mass immunisation
  - At least 80% of entire dog Population of the area must be immunized

> **Key points**
> *Dose of Human Rabies Immunoglobulin:* 20 IU/kg

Rabies to be a Notifiable Disease in India

- WHO's Rabies Elimination Plan "Zero by 30": The Global Strategic Plan to Prevent Human Deaths from Dog-Transmitted Rabies by 2030
- MoHFW to make 'Rabies Disease Notifiable in India': India to make Rabies Disease Notifiable, mandatory for ALL government and private health facilities
- Tests approved for Diagnosis:

Main tests	Other tests
• ELISA (Enzyme-linked immunosorbent assay) • FAT (fluorescent antibody test) • Direct-FAT (Direct fluorescent antibody test) • MI (Mouse inoculation test) • RTPCR (Reverse transcription PCR)	• DRIT (Direct rapid immunohistochemical test) • FAVN (Fluorescent antibody virus neutralization) • IFA (Indirect immunofluorescence) • IHC (Immunohistochemistry on formalin-fixed samples) • RTCIT (Rabies cell culture inoculation test) • RFFIT (Rapid Fluorescent Foci Inhibition Test)

(Table © Dr Vivek Jain 2022-23)

National Action Plan for Dog Mediated Rabies Elimination from India by 2030

- *Vision:* To achieve zero human deaths due to dog-mediated Rabies by 2030
- *Mission:* To progressively reduce and ultimately eliminate human Rabies in India through sustained, mass dog vaccination and appropriate post-exposure treatment
- Core Components of NAPRE:
  - *Human health component:* To prevent human deaths due to Rabies by ensuring timely access for post-exposure prophylaxis for all animal bite victims and creating well responsive Public Health System
  - *Animal health component:* To achieve at least 70% Anti Rabies vaccination coverage among dogs in a defined geographical area annually for 3 consecutive years

JAPANESE ENCEPHALITIS

Japanese Encephalitis (JE)

- *Causative agent:* Group B arbovirus (Flavivirus)
- *Host factors:*
  - **Pigs are 'Amplifier Hosts'**[Q]**:** Pigs themselves do not manifest overt symptoms but circulate the virus
  - *Cattle and buffaloes are 'Mosquito attractants':* Infected but not the natural hosts of JE virus
  - Horses are only domestic animals which show signs of encephalitis due to JE virus
  - *Birds are also involved in Natural History:* pond herons, cattle egrets, poultry and ducks
  - *Man is an 'Incidental Dead end Host'*[Q]**:** Man to Man transmission is not seen. 85% cases occur in Children < 15 years of age
- *Vectors of JE*[Q]: Culicine mosquitoes and some Anophelines
  - Culex tritaeniorhynchus (most important vector), Culex vishnuii and Culex gelidus
- *IP of JE in man:* 5–15 days (9–12 days in mosquitoes)
- *Case fatality rate:* 20–40% (may reach upto 58%)
- *Epidemiology in India:*
  - JE has been reported by 26 states and UT's in India
  - Gorakhpur District of UP contribute the largest no of cases[Q]
  - 85% of cases of JE are reported in age below 15 years BUT JE IS INFREQUENT IN INFANCY[Q]
  - Not all humans bitten by mosquitoes develop the disease: Ratio of JE overt disease to inapparent infection varies from 1:300 to 1:1000[Q]
  - **Endemicity of JE in India: 1-2 cases per village**[Q]

> **Key points**
> Pigs are 'Amplifier Hosts' in JE

> **Key points**
> Vectors of JE:
> Culex tritaeniorhynchus

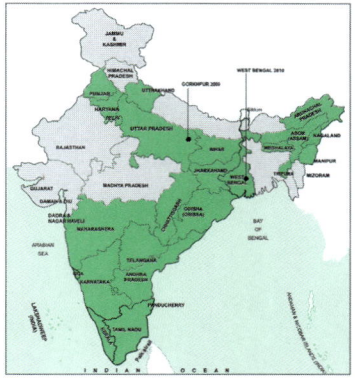
JE in India

JE Vaccines

Vaccine	Strain(s)[Q]
Mouse brain derived, purified & inactivated vaccine	Nakayama Strain Beijing Strain
Cell culture derived, inactivated vaccine	Beijing P3 Strain
Cell culture derived, live attenuated vaccine	SA 14-14-2 Strain (in India)

- *Mouse brain derived inactivated vaccine:*
  - 2 primary doses 4 weeks apart, booster after 1 year and subsequently at 3 yearly intervals until the age of 10-15 years
  - Dose: 0.5 ml for children aged < 3 years (1 ml for age > 3 years)
  - *Route:* Subcutaneous
  - Vaccine is most useful in interepidemic period
  - *Pre-exposure prophylaxis:* 3 Primary doses on day 0, 7, 28 (or 2 primary doses 4 weeks apart)
  - Booster after 1 year and then every 3 years

KFD

Kyasanur Forest Disease (KFD)

- KFD is also known as **'Monkey Disease'**[Q]
- *Causative agent:* Group B Togavirus (Flavivirus)
- *Reservoir:* Rats and squirrels
- *Amplifier hosts:* Monkeys[Q]
- Man is 'incidental dead-end host'
- *Vectors of KFD:*
  - **In India: Hemophysalis spinigera**[Q] **(Hard Tick)**
  - *Outside India:* Soft Tick[Q]
- *IP:* 3–8 days
- *Control measures*[Q]:
  - Control of ticks
  - Restriction of cattle movement
  - Vaccination: Killed KFD vaccine
  - Personal protection: through repellants

> **Key points**
> - KFD is also known as 'Monkey Disease'
> - Vectors of KFD:
>   In India: Hemophysalis spinigera[Q] (Hard Tick)

PLAGUE

Plague

> **Key points**
>
> *Vector of Plague:* Rat flea (Xenopsylla cheopsis)

- *Synonyms:* Black Death, Mahamari, The great death
- *Causative agent:* Yersinia pestis^Q (Gram negative, non-motile cocco-bacillus)
  - Bipolar staining with Wayson's stain^Q
- *Reservoir of Infection:* Wild rodents (Tatera indica in India^Q)
- *Source of Infection:* Infected rodents, fleas and cases of pneumonic plague
- *Commonest and most efficient vector of Plague:* **Rat flea (Xenopsylla cheopsis^Q)**
  - Both sexes of fleas bite and transmit the disease
- *Mode of transmission:* Bite of an infected flea, direct contact with tissues of infected animal or droplet infection (pneumonic plague)
- *Types of Plague:*

Type	IP	Remarks
Pneumonic Plague	1-3 days	Complication of Bubonic-Septicemic plague
Bubonic Plague	2-7 days	MC type of Plague^Q
Septicemic Plague	2-7 days	Occurs of Accidental laboratory infections

- *Drug of choice for treatment^Q:* **Streptomycin** 30 mg/kg i.m. × 7-10 days
- *Drug of choice for chemoprophylaxis^Q:* **Tetracycline** 500 mg QID × 5 days

Flea Indices in Plague

- *Total flea index:* Is average no. of fleas of all species per rat
- *Cheopsis index:* Is average no. of X. cheopsis per rat; Is an **'indicator of potential explosiveness'** if outbreak occurs^Q
- *Specific percentage of fleas:* Percentage of different fleas
- *Burrow index:* Average no. of fleas per species per rodent burrow

RICKETTSIAL DISEASES

Rickettsial Zoonoses

Description: Are a group of specific communicable diseases caused by Rickettsial organisms and transmitted to man by Arthropod vectors (Q fever excepted)

Disease	Agent	Vector	Reservoir
Typhus Group^Q			
Epidemic typhus	R. prowazekii^Q	Louse^Q	Humans^Q
Murine typhus	R. typhi	Flea	Rodents
Scrub typhus	R. tsutsugamushi^Q	Trombiculid mite	Rodents
Spotted Fever Gp			
Indian Tick typhus	R. conori	Tick	Rodents, dogs
RMSF	R. rickettsii	Tick	Rodents, dogs
Rickettsial pox	R. akari	Mite	Mice
Others			
Q Fever	Coxiella burnetii^Q	NIL^Q	Cattle, sheep, goat
Trench Fever	Bartonella quintana	Louse^Q	Humans^Q

Epidemic Typhus

- *Is a type of rickettsial disease of typhus group:*
  - *Recrudescent form of Epidemic typhus:* Brill Zinsser Disease^Q
  - Was the **'most formidable rickettsial disease in past'**
- *Causative agent:* R. prowazekii^Q
- *Vector^Q:* Louse (P. capitis, P. corporis)

> **Key points**
>
> *Vector:* Louse for epidemic Typhus

- *Mode of transmission*^{Q}: (IS NOT BY LOUSE-BITE)
  - Scratching and inoculation with infected louse faeces
  - Crushing infected louse on body
  - Inhalation of infected louse faeces or dust
- *Clinical picture:* Prolonged febrile illness, vasculitis
- *Drug of choice:* Tetracycline^Q
- Under International Health Regulations (IHRs), 'Louse borne typhus is a disease under surveillance'

Endemic Typhus

- Is also known as **'Flea borne typhus' or 'Murine typhus'**^{Q}
- *Causative agent:* Rikettsia typhi (R. mooseri)
- *Reservoir:* Rats
- *Mode of transmission:* Rat flea (Xenopsylla cheopsis^Q)–BUT NOT THROUGH BITE, rather through faeces inoculation on skin or inhalation of dried infective faeces
- *Incubation period:* 1–2 weeks
- *Weil-felix reaction:* Becomes positive with Proteus OX-19 in 2nd week
- *Drug of choice:* Tetracycline^Q

Scrub Typhus

- Most widespread Rickettsial Disease^Q
- *Causative agent:* **Rickettsia tsutsugamushi**^{Q}
- *Vector:* **Trombiculid Mite**^{Q} (Leptotrombidium delinese and L. akamushi)
- *IP:* 10-12 days
- *Typical clinical features:* Eschar (punched out ulcer covered with a blackened scar, indicates location of mite bite)
- Weil Felix Reaction is strongly positive with Proteus strain OXK

> **Key points**
>
> *Scrub Typhus:*
> - Causative agent: Rickettsia tsutsugamushi^Q
> - Vector: Trombiculid Mite^Q

Q Fever

- *Causative agent:* **Coxiella burnetii**^{Q}
  - Only Rickettsial disease without any vector^Q (soft tick in few animal cases)
  - Only Rickettsial disease without any skin lesion^Q
- *Mode of Transmission:* Inhalation of Infected dust, Aerosol transmission, direct contact, Contaminated food like meat, milk and milk products^Q
- IP: 2-3 weeks
- *Clinical features:*
  - Acute onset with fever, chills, general malaise and headache
  - 'Pneumonia like picture'^{Q}
  - Absence of rash/local lesion
  - Inapparent infections
- *Treatment:*
  - Tetracycline^Q
  - Pasteurization/Boiling of milk

> **Key points**
>
> **Q Fever**
> *Mode of Transmission:* Inhalation of Infected dust

LEISHMANIASIS

Leishmaniasis

Causative agent of Leishmaniasis:

Types of Leishmaniasis	Causative agent
Visceral Leishmaniasis (Kala Azar)	Leishmania donovani^Q
Cutaneous Leishmaniasis (Oriental Sore)	Leishmania tropica^Q
Mucocutaneous Leishmaniasis	Leishmania braziliensis

- *Reservoir of Infection:* Dogs, jackals, foxes, rodents and other mammals
  - Indian Kala Azar is a non-zoonotic infection: Man as reservoir

> **Key points**
>
> Vectors: Female phlebotamine sandflies for Kala Azar

- *Peak age of Kala Azar in India:* 5–9 years
- *Vectors:* **Female phlebotamine sandflies**

Types of Leishmaniasis	Vector^Q
Visceral Leishmaniasis (Kala Azar)	Phlebotamus argentipes
Cutaneous Leishmaniasis (Oriental Sore)	Phlebotamus papatasi
Mucocutaneous Leishmaniasis	Phlebotamus sergenti

- *Habitat of Sandfly:* Cracks and crevices of walls, tree holes caves^Q
- *Insecticide of choice for sandfly^Q:* DDT (sprayed only up to a height of 6 feet from floor) 1–2 gm/sq. metre
- *Mode of transmission:*
  - Bite of female phlebotamine sandflies
  - Contamination of bite wound
  - Contact (crushing of insects while feeding)
  - Blood transfusion
- *IP:* 10 days to 2 years (average 1–4 months)
- *Aldehyde Test of Napier:*
  - Becomes Positive after 2-3 months of disease onset and reverts to negative 6 months after cure
  - Useful Test for surveillance^Q (but not for diagnosis)
  - *Non-specific test:* Positive in many chronic infections where albumin: globulin ratio is reversed
- *Serological tests:*
  - *ELISA:* for diagnosis as well as epidemiological field survey^Q
  - **rk 39 dipstick test^Q**
  - Indirect Flourescent Antibody Test (IFAT)
  - Direct Agglutination Test (DAT)
- *Leishmanin (Montenegro) test^Q:*
  - *Procedure:* Intradermal injection of 0.1 mL leishmanin (a preparation of 10^6/mL washed promastigotes suspended in 0.5% phenol saline) on flexor surface of forearm
  - *Examine after 48-72 hrs:*
    - *Induration > 5 mm:* positive
    - *Induration < 5 mm:* negative
  - *Useful Test for:*
    - Immunity status^Q
    - Inferring endemicity or epidemicity of infection
    - Identifying groups at risk of infection
  - Test results in Leishmaniasis:

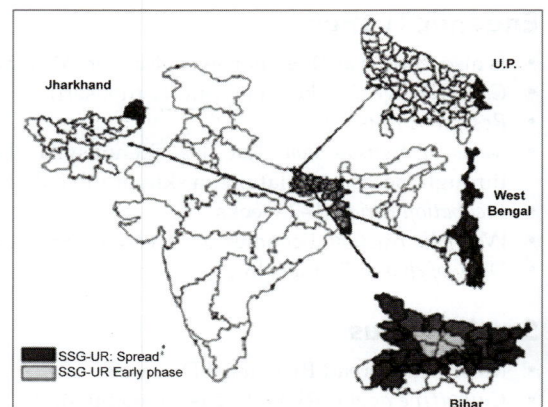

Kala Azar in India

Type of Leishmaniasis	Test Result
Visceral Leishmaniasis (Kala azar)	
Active Phase	Negative
Within 1 yr of recovery	Positive
Cutaneous Leishmaniasis	Positive
Mucocutaneous Leishmaniasis	
4-6 weeks after onset	Positive

Active Surveillance in Kala Azar

- Quarterly case searches
- '*Kala Azar fortnight*': Peripheral health workers and volunteers do door-to-door search, refer the cases of KA/PKDL to treatment centers for definitive diagnosis and treatment

Prophylaxis and Treatment

- There are no drugs available for personal prophylaxis of Kala azar^Q
- Drugs used in *Treatment of Leishmaniasis*^{Q}:
  - Sodium stibogluconate
  - Miltefosine
  - Pentamidine
  - Ketoconazole
  - Sitamaquine
  - Mepacrine
  - Paramomycin
  - Amphotericin B
  - Allopurinol
  - Urea stibamine

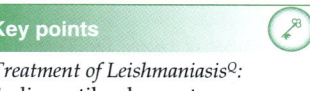

Key points

Treatment of Leishmaniasis^Q:
Sodium stibogluconate–

NEW Kala-azar Treatment Guidelines, NVBDCP 2017-2018

- **Treatment of choice for Kala-azar:**
  - **First line** ^{Q}: **Liposomal Amphotericin B (LAMB)** Single dose 10 mg/kg
  - Second line: Paromomycin + Inj. Miltefosine (Combination regimens)
  - Third line: Amphotericin B emulsion
  - Fourth line: Miltefosine capsules
  - Fifth line: Inj. Amphotericin B deoxycholate (Multiple doses)
- PKDL:
  - Miltefosine 100 mg BD X 12 weeks
  - Infusion Amphotericin B deoxycholate 1 mg/kg/day X 4 months
- Under-trial: Inj. Amphotericin B emulsion.
- Treatment is DOT (Direct observed Theory) for Miltefosine

Accelerated Plan for Kala-azar Elimination 2017

- **Goal:** To improve health status of vulnerable and at-risk populations living in Kala azar endemic areas by elimination of Kala-azar, so that it longer remains a public health problem by end of 2017
- **Target:** Incidence <1/10,000 population at sub-district level.

Kala Azar Elimination from India

- India is committed to eliminating Kala Azar from the country by 2023
- 632 (99.8%) endemic blocks have already achieved elimination status

TRACHOMA

Trachoma (Rough Eye)

- *Causative agent:* Chlamydia trachomatis (immune types A, B, C)
  - Sexually transmitted C. trachomatis (serotypes D, E, F, G, H, I, J, K) may cause a milder infection *'Inclusion Conjunctivitis'*
- IP: 5-12 days^Q
- *Mode of transmission:*
  - Direct or indirect contact with ocular discharges or fomites
  - Eye seeking flies
  - Venereal transmission
- *MC infected age group:* 2-5 yrs aged children
- *Communicability:* Trachoma is a disease of low infectivity
- *Reservoir of infection:* Children with active disease, chronically infected older children and adults
- *Predisposing factors:* Direct sunlight, dust, smoke and irritants (such as kajal or surma)
- *Field diagnosis of Trachoma:* At least 2 of following diagnostic criteria in children 0-10 years age^Q
  - Follicles on upper Tarsal conjunctiva
  - Limbal follicles or their sequelae (Herbert's Pits^Q)
  - Conjunctival scarring (Trichiasis, Entropion)
  - Vascular pannus
- *WHO classification of Trachoma:*
  - *TIF (Trachomatous Inflammation Follicular):* Presence of > 5 large follicles on upper tarsal conjunctiva^Q

> **Key points**
> Treatment of choice for Trachoma: Azithromycin 20 mg/kg oral stat

- TII (Trachomatous Inflammation Intense): Obscuration of > 50% of deep tarsal vessels of upper tarsal conjunctiva

Trachoma Treatment

- *Treatment of choice for Trachoma:* **Azithromycin** 20 mg/kg oral stat^Q
- *Current WHO recommendations for antibiotic treatment of trachoma:*
  - *District level prevalence is > 10% in 1-9 years old children:* Mass treatment with Azithromycin^Q
  - *District level prevalence is 5-10% in 1-9 years old children:* Targeted treatment with Azithromycin (the identification and treatment of all members of any family in whom one or more members have follicular trachoma)
  - *District level prevalence is < 5% in 1-9 years old children:* Azithromycin distribution may not be necessary
- *Mass treatment for Trachoma:* [NEW GUIDELINES–WHO]
  - *Indication of mass treatment in Trachoma:* > 10% prevalence of severe and moderate Trachoma in children < 10 yrs of age [NEW GUIDELINES–WHO]^Q
  - *Treatment:* 1% tetracycline ointment BD for 5 consecutive days each month or OD for 10 days each month for 6 consecutive months, or for 60 consecutive days^Q

> **Key points**
> Indication of mass treatment in Trachoma: > 10% prevalence

India Now Free from 'Infective Trachoma'!

- *Elimination criteria (WHO)^Q*: Prevalence of Active trachoma infection among children (< 10 years): < 5%
- National Trachoma Survey Report (2014–17) findings:
  - Prevalence of Active trachoma infection among children (< 10 years): 0.7%
  - Trachoma is no longer a public health problem in India
  - India has met the goal of Trachoma elimination (WHO GET 2020)
  - *Major contributor*: SAFE Strategy
- *Next aim*: To eliminate Trachomatous trichiasis (TT) from the country
- *National Trachoma Prevalence Surveys & Trachoma Rapid Assessment Surveys conducted by*: Dr. Rajendra Prasad Centre for Ophthalmic Sciences (AIIMS, New Delhi), NPCB and MOHFW

> **Key points**
> SAFE Strategy^Q (WHO)
> Surgery:
> Antibiotic use:
> Facial cleanliness
> Environmental improvement^Q

TETANUS

Tetanus

- *Causative agent:* Clostridium tetani (Gram +ve, anaerobic, drumstick appearance)
- *Reservoir:* Natural habitat is soil and dust
- IP: 6-10 days (1 day to several months)^Q
- *Period of communicability:* None^Q (no person to person transmission)
- *Mode of transmission:* Contamination of Wounds with spores
- *Tetanus toxin:* Second most lethal toxin (Most lethal toxin is Botulinum toxin^Q)
  - **Lethal dose for a 70 kg man: 0.1 mg**^{Q}
  - *Acts on 4 areas of nervous system:*
    - Motor End Plates in Skeletal System
    - Spinal Cord
    - Brain
    - Sympathetic System
  - *Principal action:* Blocks inhibition of Spinal reflexes
  - Sensitivity to toxin is more in males
- *Herd Immunity in Tetanus:* Does not protect the individual
- *Tetanus is best prevented by:* Active immunisation with Tetanus toxoid (TT)
- Aim of active Immunisation with TT:
  - Vaccinate the entire community
  - Ensure protective level of antitoxin ~ 0.01 IU/mL serum throughout life

> **Key points**
> Period of communicability: None for Tetanus

> **Key points**
> Herd Immunity in Tetanus: Does not protect

Tetanus Toxoid in Pregnancy

Refer to Chapter 3, Theory

Prevention of Tetanus in Wound

Immunity Category	Treatment by type of wound	
	Wounds < 6 hrs old, clean, non-penetrating, with negligible tissue damage	Other Wounds
A	Nothing more required	Nothing more required
B	Toxoid 1 dose	Toxoid 1 dose
C	Toxoid 1 dose	Toxoid 1 dose + Human Tetanus Immunoglobulin
D	Toxoid complete course	Toxoid complete course + Human Tetanus Immunoglobulin

Where,
A. Complete course of toxoid or booster dose in previous 5 years
B. Complete course of toxoid or booster dose in previous 5-10 years
C. Complete course of toxoid or booster dose in >10 years ago
D. Has not had a complete course of toxoid or status is unknown.

Neonatal Tetanus/8th Day Disease[Q]

- *NNT has a marked seasonal incidence in India:* > 50% of total annual cases occur in months of July, August and September
- *Cleans for safe delivery for prevention of NNT:*

3 Cleans	5 Cleans[Q]	7 Cleans
Clean Hands	Clean Hands	Clean Hands
Clean delivery surface	Clean delivery surface	Clean delivery surface
Clean Cord care	Clean Cord cut/blade	Clean Cord cut/blade
	Clean cord tie	Clean cord tie
	Clean cord stump	Clean cord stump
		Clean towel
		Clean water

> **Key points**
> **NNT Elimination level:** < 0.1/1000 LB

- 7 Cleans are proposed under RCH-III
- Clean cord stump implies 'No Applicant'
- Clean towel and clean water are for hands washing
- NNT Elimination (Classification of districts, India is based on 3 parameters: incidence rate, TT-2 or booster coverage and % attended deliveries)

Classification	Rate	TT-2 coverage	Attended deliveries
NNT High Risk	> 1/1000 LB	< 70%	< 50%
NNT Control	< 1/1000 LB	> 70%	>50%
NNT Elimination[Q]	< 1/1000 LB	> 90%	> 75%

- **India was Declared Maternal & Neonatal Tetanus eliminated in August 2015. (Certified 14 July 2016)**

LEPROSY/HANSEN'S DISEASE

Leprosy Situation in India [2022]

- *Prevalence:* 0.41 per 10000 population[Q]
- *Annual new case detection rate:* 4.5 per 100,000 population

Classification in Leprosy

Classifications of Leprosy:

Ridley Jopling classification[Q]	Indian classification	Madrid classification
TT (Tuberculoid)	Indeterminate	Indeterminate
BT (Borderline Tuberculoid)	Tuberculoid	Tuberculoid
BB (Borderline borderline)	Borderline	Borderline
BL (Borderline Lepromatous)	Lepromatous	Lepromatous
LL (Lepromatous Leprosy)	Pure Neuritic[Q]	

(Pure neuritic type Leprosy (Indian classification): No skin lesions)

- *Operational Classification of Leprosy (according to skin smear positivity) to serve as a basis for Chemotherapy:*

	Paucibacillary Leprosy (PBL)	**Multibacillary Leprosy (MBL)**
	BI < 2	BI ≥ 2
Included types	Indeterminate Polar tuberculoid (TT) Border tuberculoid (BT)	Polar lepromatous (LL) Borderline lepromatous (BL) Mid-borderline (BB)
Multidrug therapy^Q (MDT) in NLEP (Drugs)	Rifampicin 600 mg OAMS Dapsone 100 mg daily	Rifampicin 600 mg OAMS Dapsone 100 mg daily Clofazimine 300 mg OAMS, 50 mg daily
Treatment duration^Q	6 months	12 months
Follow up^Q (after treatment)	Annually for 2 yrs	Annually for 5 yrs

(BI: Bacteriological Index; OAMS: Once a month supervised)

Epidemiology of Leprosy

- *Description:* Chronic infectious disease caused by *Mycobacterium leprae* and affecting mainly peripheral nerves
  - Leprosy is a disease of 'high infectivity but low pathogenicity'
  - Attack rate of Leprosy among house-hold contacts: 4.4–12%
  - Youngest case of Leprosy in India: 2 ½ month infant^Q
  - Leprosy is often known as a 'Social disease'
  - Is probably the oldest disease known to mankind^Q
- *Mode of transmission of Leprosy:*^{Q}
  - Droplet infection (MC^Q)
  - Contact transmission (Direct skin to skin or indirect with soil/fomites)
  - Breast milk from lepromatous mothers
  - Transplacental
  - Insect vectors
  - Tattooing needles
- *Diagnosis of leprosy under NLEP* is currently based on clinical grounds^Q
  - *PBL:* 1–5 skin lesions
  - *MBL:* > 5 skin lesions

> **Key points**
> *Diagnosis of Leprosy*
> *PBL:* 1–5 skin lesions
> *MBL:* > 5 skin lesions

Important Points of Leprosy

- *Level of Leprosy for declaring it as a Public Health Problem:* >1/10,000^Q
- *Elimination Level of Leprosy:* <1/10,000^Q
  - India eliminated Leprosy in December 2005^Q
- *Goal for Leprosy under National Health Policy 2002:* Elimination by 2005
- Leprosy exhibits 'both cell mediated immunity (CMI) and humoral immunity'^{Q}

> **Key points**
> *Elimination Level of Leprosy:* <1/10,000

Tests for Detecting Immunity in Leprosy

Tests of Cell Mediated Immunity^Q	**Tests of Humoral Immunity**^{Q}
Lepromin test	FLA–ABS Test
Lymphocyte transformation test	Monoclonal antibodies test
Leucocyte migration inhibition test	ELISA tests
	Radioimmunassay

Lepromin Test

- Test of CMI in Leprosy^Q
- Test: 0.1 ml Lepromin intradermal on inner aspect of forearm
- *Antigens used in Lepromin test:*^{Q}
  - Dhamendra antigen (extensively used in India)
  - Mitsuda antigen

> **Key points**
> *Lepromin Test Readings:* After 48 hours and after 21 days

- WHO recommended concentration of Dhamendra Antigen: 1/16
- Readings: After 48 hours and after 21 days^Q
- Reactions in Lepromin test:
  - **Early Reaction (FERNANDEZ REACTION^Q):**
    - Read at 48 hours^Q
    - Redness > 10 mm indicates +ve test
    - Indicates prior exposure or infection
    - Delayed type of hypersensitivity^Q
    - Induced by soluble components of leprosy bacilli
    - Superior to late reaction
    - Corresponds to Mantoux Reaction (TB)^Q
  - **Late Reaction (LATE MITSUDA REACTION^Q):**
    - Read at 21 days^Q
    - Nodule > 5 mm diameter is +ve
    - Indicates cell mediated immunity^Q
    - Induced by bacillary component of antigen
    - BCG vaccine can convert it from −ve to +ve
- Value of Lepromin test:
  - Is not a diagnostic test^Q
  - Uses of Lepromin test^Q:
    - Evaluation of CMI status of patients
    - Aid to confirm the classification of Leprosy
    - Estimation of prognosis of cases
  - Drawbacks of Lepromin test as a diagnostic test:
    - Positive in non-cases
    - Negative in lepromatous and near-lepromatous cases
- Interpretation of Lepromin Test:

Reaction	Interpretation
++ to +++	Tuberculoid Leprosy (TT)^Q
+ to ++	Maculo-anaesthetic Leprosy (MA)
− or + or +	Intermediate Leprosy (I)
+ to ++	Borderline Tuberculoid Leprosy (BT)
+ or +	Borderline Borderline Leprosy (BB)
− or +	Borderline Lepromatous Leprosy (BL)
−	Lepromatous Leprosy (LL)

Key points

Uses of Lepromin test:
- Evaluation of CMI status
- Aid to confirm the classification
- Estimation of prognosis

Definitions under National Leprosy Elimination Program (NLEP)

- *Paucibacillary Leprosy (PBL):* 1–5 skin lesions and/or only one nerve involvement
- *Multibacillary Leprosy (MBL):* 6 or more skin lesions and/or more than one nerve involvement
- *Adequate treatment:* Patient has received 6 months of therapy in 9 months (for PBL) or 12 months of therapy within 18 months (for MBL)^Q
- *Regular treatment:* Received MDT for two-thirds of total duration of therapy, i.e. 4 months for PBL (out of 6 months of duration of therapy) and 8 months for MBL (out of 12 months of duration of therapy)^Q
- *Case:* Clinical signs of leprosy (with or without bacteriological confirmation of diagnosis) and who has not yet completed a full course of treatment with Multi-Drug Therapy (MDT)
- *Newly diagnosed case:* Diagnosed case who has not taken MDT in past
- *Defaulter:* A leprosy patient on MDT, who has not collected treatment for 12 consecutive months^Q
- *Relapsed case:* A patient whose therapy was terminated successfully, completed adequately, who subsequently develops new signs and symptoms of disease. either during surveillance period or thereafter

Key points

Defaulter: A leprosy patient on MDT, who has not collected treatment for 12 consecutive months

Leprosy is not Amenable to Eradication^Q

- Long and variable incubation period **(Most important reason)**^Q
- Disputed modes of transmission

- Presence of sub-clinical cases and our inability to detect them
- Complicated spectrum of disease manifestations
- Failure of cell mediated immunity in lepromatous cases
- Bacterial resistance and persistence in the human body
- Absence of a vaccine
- Social and cultural taboos leading to concealment of disease
- Discovery of extra-human reservoir

WHO's Global Leprosy Strategy 2021-2030

- Vision: Zero leprosy
    - Zero infection and disease
    - Zero disability
    - Zero stigma and discrimination
- Goal: Elimination of leprosy
    - Interruption of transmission
- Global targets for 2030:
    - Target 1 - 120 countries reporting zero new autochthonous cases
    - Target 2 - 70% reduction in annual number of new cases detected
    - Target 3 - 90% reduction in rate (per million population) of new cases with grade 2 disability (G2D)
    - Target 4 - 90% reduction in rate (per million children) of new child cases with leprosy.

HIV/AIDS

HIV Epidemiology

Route of transmission	% of total cases (India)	Efficiency of route
Sexual	87[Q]	0.01–1%[Q]
Blood and blood products	1[Q]	> 90%[Q]
Sharing needles/syringes	2	0.3%
Mother to child transmission	5	3%

- *Causative organism:* Human immunodeficiency virus (HIV) [Human T-Lymphotropic virus–III (HTLV–III); Lymphadenopathy virus (LAP)]
    - *Chances of HIV transmission in presence of STDs:* Increases 8–10 times[Q]
    - AIDS (Acquired Immunodeficiency Syndrome) is also known as 'Slim Disease'
- *Reservoir:* Cases and carriers
    - *Source:* Virus is in greatest concentration in blood, semen and CSF (lower concentrations in tear, saliva, breast milk, urine, cervical and vaginal secretions)
- *Basic modes of transmission[Q]:*
    - Sexual (MC)
    - Blood and blood products
    - Needles/syringes
    - Mother to Child transmission (MTCT)
- *IP:* Few months to 10 years
- **MC Opportunistic Infection (OI) in AIDS**
    - *World:* Pneumocystis carinii pneumonia (PCP)
    - *India:* Tuberculosis (> Candida > PCP)
- *Epidemiological pattern of HIV epidemic in India:* Type 4 pattern [Epidemic starts from highest risk group (commercial sex workers, homosexuals, drug users) to bridge population (clients of sex workers, STD patients, migrant population, partners of drug users), and then to general population]

> **Key points**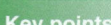
>
> **MC Opportunistic Infection (OI) in AIDS**
> - World: Pneumocystis carinii pneumonia
> - India: Tuberculosis

HIV Situation in India [2021]

- *Total no. of HIV cases:* Less than 2.4 million
- *Prevalence of HIV:* 0.21%
- *Classification of states:*

Groups with states/UTs	Criteria of prevalence in	
	High risk groups	Antenatal clinics
Group I (High Prevalence)^Q: Maharashtra, Tamil Nadu, Andhra Pradesh, Karnataka, Manipur, Nagaland, Mizoram, Telangana	>5%	>1%
Group II (Moderate Prevalence): Gujarat, Goa, Pondicherry	>5%	<1%
Group III (Low Prevalence): Remaining states & UTs	<5%	<1%

> **Key points**
> *Prevalence of HIV: 0.26% (India)*

- *Categorization of Districts*:

District	Criteria^Q
A	>1% ANC/PTCT prevalence anytime anywhere in last 3 years
B	<1% ANC/PTCT prevalence everywhere in last 3 years PLUS >5% prevalence in any HRG (CSW/MSM/IDU/STD)
C	<1% ANC/PTCT prevalence everywhere in last 3 years PLUS <5% in all STD clinic attendees/HRG with known hotspots (Migrants/Truckers/Factory workers/Tourists)
D	<1% ANC/PTCT prevalence everywhere in last 3 years PLUS <5% in all STD clinic attendees/HRG OR Poor HIV data with no known hotspots

(ANC Antenatal clinic; PTCT Parent to Child Transmission)

Age and Sex distribution of HIV/AIDS in India [2006]:

Distribution of HIV/AIDS cases	Cumulative cases
Age distribution	
0–14 years	5%
15–29 years	32%
30–44 years^Q	56%
> 45 years	7%
Sex distribution	
Male	71%
Female	29%

- *First case of HIV/AIDS: 1986 (Chennai, Tamil Nadu)^Q*
- **National AIDS Control Programme (NACP) launched: 1987^Q**
- *National AIDS Prevention and Control Policy (NAPCP): 2001*

Mother to Child Transmission (MTCT) of HIV

- *MTCT in developing countries (India): 30%^Q*
- *MTCT in developed countries: 20%*
- *Prevention of MTCT in India:*

Modality	Dose/type	Reduction in MTCT by	Post-modality MTCT in India
Zidovudine	Mother: 300 mg BD from 36 wks POG + 300 mg 3 h during delivery Child: 2 mg/kg 6 h × 6 wks	66%^Q	10%
Nevirapine	Single oral dose Mother: 200 mg at labor onset Child: 2 mg/kg^Q within 72 hrs of birth^Q	50%^Q	15%^Q
Caesarean section	Elective CS	50%	15%

Triple ARV Prophylaxis for PMTCT of HIV (3TC + TDF + EFV)^Q

- Description: New modality introduced under NACP for Prevention of Mother to Child Transmission of HIV in India
- Three drugs used in combination:

Clinical scenario	Regimen for prophylaxis
Those requiring ARV prophylaxis	TDF + 3TC + EFV (FDC Single pill)^Q Tenofovir 300 mg once daily plus Lamivudine 300 mg once daily plus Efavirenz 600 mg once daily
Those with prior exposure of NNRTI (NVP/EFV)	TDF + 3TC + LPV/r Tenofovir 300 mg once daily plus Lamivudine 300 mg once daily plus Lopinavir/Ritonavir 400/100 mg twice daily

- **Duration of prophylaxis:**
  - Start at 14 weeks POG
  - Continue through out pregnancy, delivery, lactation
  - End after 1 week of breastfeeding cessation
- **Breastfeeding in Triple ARV prophylaxis:**
  - Exclusive breastfeeding: Continue for 0-6 months age
  - Breastfeeding with complimentary feeding: Continue for 1 year or 2 years (those who had received Pediatric ART) age
- **Infant diagnosis:**
  - Repeat testing at 6 weeks age, 6 months, 12 months and 6 weeks after cessation of breastfeeding
  - Confirmation of HIV status of all at 18 months age
- **Postpartum Infant ARV prophylaxis: Nevirapine till 6 weeks age**

Revised PPTCT Guidelines (NACO 2012)

- ARV given to mother during pregnancy, intrapartum and through postpartum period and also to infant
- All Infants born to women who are receiving ART/maternal triple ARV prophylaxis/who present directly-in-labor and receive intra partum ARV prophylaxis: Daily NVP prophylaxis at birth, continue for minimum 6 weeks^Q (irrespective of exclusively breastfeeding or replacement feeding)
- If infant is born to woman who presented directly-in-labor and received intrapartum ARV prophylaxis: Daily NVP prophylaxis for the infant continue until mother initiated on ART/ ARV prophylaxis and complete minimum 6 weeks of therapy^Q

Birth weight	NVP daily dose (mg)	NVP daily dose (mL)	Duration
< 2000 gm	2 mg/kg OD	0.2 mL/kg OD	Upto 6 weeks** irrespective of exclusively breast fed or exclusive replacement fed
2000–2500 gm	10 mg OD	1 mL OD	
> 2500 gm	15 mg OD	1.5 mL OD	

(Strength: 10 mg NVP in 1 mL suspension)

New Revised ARV Regimen Guidelines for PEP HIV, NACP 2021

- Post-exposure Prophylaxis (PEP) for HIV/AIDS must be administered immediately (PREFERABLY within 2 hours, MAXIMUM within 72 hours of exposure)
- Duration of PEP is 28 days, irrespective of Regimen type

Exposed person	Preferred PEP Regimen	Alternate PEP Regimen
Adolescents and Adults (>10 years age, >30 kg weight)	• Tenofovir (300 mg)# + • Lamivudine (300 mg)# + • Dolutegravir (50 mg)#	• Tenofovir (300 mg)# + • Lamivudine (300 mg)# + • Lopinavir (200 mg)/Ritonavir (50 mg) 2 Tabs BD OR • Tenofovir (300 mg)# + • Lamivudine (300 mg)# + • Efavirenz (600 mg)#
Children (≥6 years age and ≥20 kg weight)	• Zidovudine (*) + • Lamivudine (*) + • Dolutegravir (50 mg) 1 Tab OD	**If Hb <9 gm/dL:** Abacavir (*) + • Lamivudine (*) + • Dolutegravir (50 mg) 1 Tab OD
Children (≤6 years age and ≤20 kg weight)	• Zidovudine (*) + • Lamivudine (*) + • Lopinavir/Ritonavir (*)	**If Hb <9 gm/dL:** Abacavir (*) + • Lamivudine (*) + • Lopinavir/Ritonavir (*)

(Table © Dr Vivek Jain 2022-23) (* Dosage as per weight band; #FDC 1 Tab OD)

HIV/AIDS Situation in World [2012]

- *Total no. of People Living with HIV/AIDS [PLHA]:* 34 million
- *HIV prevalence:* 0.8%
- *MC opportunistic Infection:* Pneumocystis carinii pneumonia^Q

National AIDS Control Programme, India

- *National AIDS Control Programme (NACP) launched:* 1987
- *Screening tests used:* ELISA/RAPID/SIMPLE (ERS)^Q
- *Confirmatory diagnostic test used:* Western Blot Assay (WBA)^Q

For further details Refer to Chapter 6, Theory

Key points

Antiretroviral (ARV) treatment started in AIDS if: CD4 count is ANY CD4 count

Key points

- Screening tests used: ELISA/RAPID/SIMPLE
- Confirmatory diagnostic test used: Western Blot Assay (WBA)

WHO Clinical Staging for HIV Infection (13 years or older)

- **Stage 1:** *(Performance scale 1:* Asymptomatic, normal activity)
  - Asymptomatic
  - Persistent generalized lymphadenopathy
- **Stage 2:** *(Performance scale 2:* Symptomatic, normal activity)
  - Weight loss <10% of body weight
  - Minor muco-cutaeous manifestations
  - Herpes zoster in last 5 years
  - Recurrent URTIs
- **Stage 3:** *(Performance scale 3:* Bed-ridden <50% days in last month)
  - Weight loss > 10% of body weight
  - Unexplained chronic diarrhea > 1 month
  - Unexplained prolonged fever > 1 month
  - Oral candidiasis (Thrush)
  - Oral hairy leucoplakia
  - Pulmonary TB
  - Severe bacterial infection
- **Stage 4:** *(Performance scale:* Bed-ridden > 50% days in last month)
  - HIV wasting syndrome (Weight loss > 10% + Chronic diarrhea + prolonged fever)
  - Pnemocystis carinii pneumonia
  - Toxoplasmosis of brain
  - Cryptosporiodosis with diarrhea, > 1 month
  - Cryptococcosis, extrapulmonary
  - CMV of organ (except liver, spleen, lymphnodes)
  - Herpes virus (mucocutaneous > 1 month or visceral)
  - Progressive multifocal leucoencephalopathy (PML)
  - Any disseminated endemic fungal infection
  - Candidiasis (Oesophagus, trachea, bronchi or lungs)
  - Atypical mycobacteria (disseminated)
  - Non- typhoid salmonella septicaemia
  - Extrapulmonary TB
  - Lymphoma
  - Kaposi's sarcoma
  - HIV encephalopathy

WHO Clinical Staging for HIV Infection (for Children)

- **Stage 1:**
  - Asymptomatic
  - Persistent generalized lymphadenopathy
- **Stage 2:**
  - Unexplained chronic diarrhea
  - Severe persistent or recurrent candidiasis (outside neonatal period)
  - Weight loss or failure to thrive
  - Persistent fever
  - Recurrent severe bacterial infections

- Stage 3:
  - AIDS–defining opportunistic infections
  - Severe failure to thrive
  - Progressive encephalopathy
  - Malignancy
  - Recurrent septicaemia or meningitis

Initiation of ART under NACP, India [New 2017 Guidelines]

- NACP, Govt of India has adopted WHO Guidelines on ART Initiation in 2017
- New Guideline: **Start ART irrespective of CD4 count**, Clinical staging, Age or Population.

> **Key points**
>
> *Start ART India CD4 any count*

National Strategic Plan for HIV/AIDS and STI, 2017-24

- Vision of the NACO: Paving the way for an AIDS free
- Goals: *Three Zeros*
  - Zero new infections
  - Zero AIDS-related deaths
  - Zero discrimination
- Objectives of NSP:
  - Reduce 80% new infections by 2024
  - 95% of estimated PLHIV know their status by 2024
  - 95% PLHIV have ART initiation and retention by 2024 (sustained viral suppression)
  - Eliminate MTCT of HIV & Syphilis by 2020
  - Eliminate HIV related stigma and discrimination by 2020
  - Facilitate sustainable HIV services delivery by 2024
- Targets by 2020:
  - 75% reduction in new HIV infections
  - **90-90-90**^{Q}: 90% of those who are HIV positive in the country know their status, 90% of those who know their status are on treatment and 90% of those who are on treatment experience effective viral load suppression
  - Elimination of mother-to-child transmission of HIV and Syphilis
  - Elimination of stigma and discrimination
- Targets by 2024:
  - 80% reduction in new HIV infections
  - **95-95-95**^{Q}: Ensuring that 95% of those who are HIV positive in the country know their status, 95% of those who know their status are on treatment and 95% of those who are on treatment experience effective viral load suppression
- Expected Outcome: Ending of AIDS by 2030
  - Enactment of the 'HIV/AIDS Bill' as a law
  - Implementation of the 'Test and Treat' policy

Global Alliance for Ending Aids in Children by 2030

- Initiative launched by: WHO, UNICEF and UNAID
- Based on four pillars:
  - Early testing and optimized comprehensive, high quality treatment and care for infants, children, and adolescents living with HIV to achieve universal coverage of ART and viral suppression
  - Closing the treatment gap for pregnant and breastfeeding women living with HIV and optimizing continuity of treatment towards the goal of elimination of vertical transmission
  - Preventing new HIV infections among pregnant and breastfeeding adolescents and women
  - Addressing rights, gender equality, social/structural barriers that hinder access.

STIs (OTHER THAN HIV)

Sexually Transmitted Infections (STIs)

Common sexually transmitted infections (STIs)^Q:

STI	Causative agent
5 Classical STD's Syphilis Gonorrhoea Chanchroid LGV Donovanosis	Treponema pallidum Neisseria gonorrhoeae Hemophilus ducreyi^Q Chlamydia trachomatis Calymmatobacterium granulomatis^Q
HIV/AIDS	**Human immunodeficiency virus**
Hepatitis A	Enterovirus 72 (Picornavirus)^Q
Hepatitis B	Hepadnavirus (Dane's particle)
Hepatitis C	Hepacivirus
Hepatitis D	HDV
Genital and anal warts	Human Papilloma Virus^Q
Scabies	Sarcoptes scabei^Q
Pubic louse	Phthirus pubis
Trichomoniasis	Trichomonas vaginalis (MC in World)

> **Key points**
>
> **5 Classical STDs —**
> *Syphilis*
> *Gonorrhoea*
> *Chanchroid*
> *LGV*
> *Donovanosis*

- *Other sexually transmitted agents include:*
  - Streptococcus group B^Q
  - Campylobacter
  - Ureaplasma urealyticum
  - Entamoeba histolytica
  - Shigella
  - Human (beta) herpes virus 5
  - Candida albicans^Q
  - Molluscum contagiosum
  - Mycoplasma hominis
  - Giardia lambia
  - Human (alpha) herpes virus 1, 2

- *Incubation periods of STIs:*

STI	Incubation period^Q
Syphilis^Q	9–90 days
LGV^Q	3–12 days
Donovanosis^Q	3–21 days
Chancroid^Q	3–5 days
Gonorrhoea^Q	1–5 days
Molluscum contagiosum	14–50 days
HIV/AIDS^Q	Months–10 years

Endemic Treponematoses

Disease	Causative agent	Mode of transmission	DOC
Pinta	Treponema carateum	Non venereal (direct contact)	Benzathine Penicillin G^Q
Yaws	**Treponema pertenue^Q**	**Non venereal^Q** (direct contact with secretions from infectious lesions, fomites, insect vectors)	**Benzathine Penicillin G^Q**
Endemic syphilis	Treponema pallidum	Non venereal	Benzathaine Penicillin G
Syphilis	Treponema pallidum	Venereal	Benzathaine Penicillin G

> **Key points**
>
> Yaws Caused by:
> Treponema pertenue

Yaws/Pian/Bubas/Framboesia

- *Causative agent:* Treponema pertenue^Q
- *IP:* 3-5 days

- Clinical features: h
  - *Early Yaws:* Mother Yaws^Q followed by generalized eruption
  - *Late Yaws:* by end of 5 yrs
    - *Crab Yaws^Q:* Lesions of soles and palms
    - *Gangosa^Q:* Destructive lesions of soft palate, hard palate and nose
    - *Goundu^Q:* osteo-periostitis of Superior maxillary bone^Q
- India has been declared Free: May 2016
- Man is the only known reservoir of Yaws^Q (but no natural immunity)
- Yaws provide partial immunity to venereal syphilis
- *WHO recommended treatment policies for Yaws:*

> **Key points**
> Yaws has been declared eliminated from India in May 2016 [Certified 14 July 2016]

Treatment policy	Recommended for type of area	Prevalence	Treatment given to
Total mass treatment	Hyperendemic	> 10%	Entire population with cases
Juvenile mass treatment	Mesoendemic	5-10%	All cases, all 0-15 yr children contacts
Selective mass treatment	Hypoendemic	< 5%	Cases, contacts of infectious cases

- With decline of Yaws, emphasis of control strategy has shifted to 'surveillance & containment'
- *Epidemiologically Yaws is not vulnerable to eradication^Q:*
  - Cases are contagious for months or years after onset of symptoms
  - Latent cases occur frequently (treponemes persist in CSF & lymph nodes even after cure)
  - Immunity acquired is only partial
  - Disease is not fatal
  - Accurate diagnosis by non- medical personnel is a problem
  - No vaccine available for Yaws

Syndromic Approach (Simplified STD Treatment)

- *Concept:* The traditional method of diagnosing STDs is by laboratory tests, which are very often unavailable or too expensive
  - Syndromic Management of STDs has been recommended by WHO since 1990 which is 'based on symptoms and clinical signs'^Q
- *Importance of Syndromic Approach:* Through this approach, a health worker at the most peripheral level without using laboratory support, can diagnose reproductive infections and accordingly prescribe treatment or advise referral of the patient.

> **Key points**
> Syndromic Management of STDs has been 'based on symptoms and clinical signs'

- *Main features of Syndromic Approach:*
  - Classification of the main causative pathogens by the clinical syndromes they produce
  - Use of flow charts to manage a particular syndrome
  - Treatment for all important causes of the syndrome
  - Notification and treatment of sex partners
  - No expensive laboratory procedures required
- *Advantages of Syndromic Approach:*
  - Permits STD treatment without costly laboratory tests
  - Offers accessibility, immediate, effective and efficient treatment
- *Disadvantage of Syndromic Approach:*
  - Over-treatment in some patients (esp. in vaginal discharge)
- *Syndromes in Syndromic Approach^Q:*
  - *Urethral discharge:* Is usually due to gonococcal or non-gonococcal (chlamydial) urethritis
  - *Vaginal discharge:* Is usually due to gonococcal or non-gonococcal cervicitis or vaginitis (trichomoniais, candidiasis or bacterial vaginosis). Speculum examination for establishing diagnosis
  - *Genital ulcer:* Due to syphilis, chanchroid, LGV, granuloma inguinale or herpes infection
  - *Inguinal swelling (Bubo):* Usually due to LGV
  - Lower abdominal pain/PID

STD Colour Coded Kits

Kit^Q	Colour^Q	Syndrome^Q	Contents
1	Grey	Urethral/Anorectal/Cervical discharge/SS#	Azithromycin, Cefixime
2	Green	Vaginal discharge	Secnidazole, Fluconazole
3	White	Genito-ulcerative disease (Non-herpetic)	Azithromycin, Benzathain penicillin
4	Blue	Genito-ulcerative disease (Non-herpetic)*	Azithromycin, Doxycycline
5	Red	Genito-ulcerative disease (Herpetic)	Acyclovir
6	Yellow	Lower abdominal pain	Cefixime, Metronidazole, Doxycycline
7	Black	Inguinal bubo	Azithromycin, Doxycycline

(*For patients allergic to penicillin, #SS Scrotal swelling)

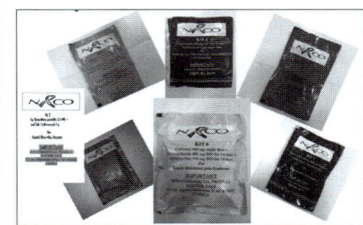
STD Color coded kits

Case Detection in a STD Control Programme

- Screening
- *Contact tracing:* Sexual partners of diagnosed patients are identified, located, investigated and treated
  - Is one of the best methods of controlling the spread of infection
  - Is relatively expensive (in low prevalence)
  - Key to success is patient himself (who must disclose all sexual contacts voluntarily)
- *Cluster testing:* Screening of all persons of either sex, who move in the same socio-sexual environment of the patient^Q
  - It almost doubles the number of cases found

> **Key points**
>
> **Case Detection in a STD Control Programme**
> - Screening
> - Contact tracing
> - Cluster testing

Suraksha Clinic

- *Description:* Chain of RTI/STI clinics to provide reproductive and sexual health services^Q
- *Established by:* National AIDS Control Program, NACO
- *Purpose:* Control of STI/RTIs viz., HIV, Syphilis, Gonorrhea, Herpes, Chlamydia, Genital warts
- *Facilities^Q:*
  - Blood sample testing
  - Counseling
  - Syndromic case management (RTI/STI/RPR kits)

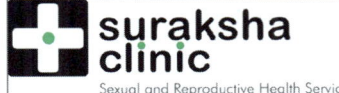
Suraksha Clinic

MISCELLANEOUS (COMMUNICABLE DISEASES)

Zoonoses

- *Zoonoses:* An infection or infectious disease transmissible under natural conditions from vertebrate animals to man
- Classification of Zoonoses based on direction of transmission:
  - *Anthropozoonoses^Q:* Infections transmitted from animals (zoo) to man (anthro):
    - Rabies^Q Plague^Q
    - Anthrax^Q Hydatid disease^Q
    - Trichinosis
  - *Zooanthroponoses^Q:* Infections transmitted from man (anthro) to animals (zoo):
    - Human TB in cattle^Q
  - *Amphixenosis:* Infections transmitted in either direction between animals and man:
    - Trypanosoma cruzi
    - Schistosoma japonicum

Food Poisoning

Incubation period of food poisoning:

Food poisoning	Incubation period
Salmonella^Q	12–24 hours
Staphylococcal^Q	1–6 hours

Contd...

Contd...

Food poisoning	Incubation period
Botulism	12–36 hours
Cl. perfirengens	6–24 hours
B. cereus (emetic form)	1–6 hours
B. cereus (diarrhoel form)	12–24 hours

- *Staphylococcal Food Poisoning:*
  - *Agent:* Enterotoxins of Staphylococcus aureus
  - Toxins formed at 35°–37° C
  - Toxins are relatively heat stable and resist boiling for 30 min or more
  - **Incubation period: 1–6 hours**
  - IP is short because of 'preformed toxin'
  - *Mechanism of food poisoning:* Intra-dietetic toxins (ingestion of toxins pre-formed in food, in which bacteria have grown)
- *Botulism food poisoning:*
  - *Agent:* Clostridium botulinum type A, B, E
  - *IP:* 12–36 hours
  - *Mechanism of food poisoning:* Intra-dietetic toxins
  - *Prominent symtoms:* GIT SYMPOTOMS ARE SLIGHT[Q]
    - Dysphagia[Q]
    - Diplopia[Q]
    - Dysarthria[Q]
  - *Prophylaxis:* 50,000–100,000 units anti-toxin
  - *Treatment:* Guanidine hydrochloride
- *Clostridium perfringens food poisoning:*
  - *Agent:* Clostridium perfringens (welchii)
  - *IP:* 6–24 hours
  - Rapid recovery with no deaths
- *Bacillus cereus food poisoning:*
  - *Agent:* Bacillus cereus
  - *IP:* 1–6 hours (emetic form), 12–24 hours (diarrhoeal form)

Brucellosis

- *Also known as:* Undulant fever[Q], Malta fever, Mediterranean fever
- *Causative agent:* Brucella species
  - **Brucella melitensis: Most virulent and invasive species**[Q]
  - *Brucella abortus:* Less virulent, primarily affect cattle
  - *Brucella suis:* Intermediate virulence, infects pigs
  - *Brucella canis:* Parasite of dogs
- *Reservoir:* Cattle, sheep, goats, swine, buffaloes, horses, dogs[Q]
- Modes of transmission[Q]:
  - *Contact infection:* Direct contact with infected tissues, blood, urine, vaginal discharge, aborted fetuses and **ESPECIALLY placenta**[Q]
  - *Food-borne infections:* Raw milk/dairy products, fresh raw vegetables, water
  - Air-borne infection: aerosol
- *Incubation period:* usually 1–3 weeks
- *Most striking feature:* Severity of illness and absence of clinical illness
- *Most rational approach for prevention:* Control and eradication of infection from animal reservoirs
- *Only satisfactory solution aimed at eradication:* Slaughter of infected animals, with full compensation paid to farmers
- *Antibiotic of choice:* Tetracycline 500 mg QID × 3 weeks[Q]

Crimean Congo Fever (CCF)

- *Type of disease:* Zoonosis of domestic/wild animals which may affect human beings
- *Causative agent:* Nairovirus[Q] (Bunyavirus)
- *Vector:* Hyalomma ticks[Q] (Hard ticks)

Key points

Incubation period: 1–6 hours for staphylococcal FP

Key points

Prominent symptoms in Botulism FP: GIT SYMPOTOMS ARE SLIGHT
- Dysphagia
- Diplopia
- Dysarthria

Key points

Antibiotic of choice: Tetracycline for Brucellosis

Key points

Congo fever:
- Vector: Hyalomma ticks[Q] (Hard ticks)
- Drug of choice: Ribavirin

- *Incubation period:* 1-13 days (Median 5-6 days)
- *Case fatality rate:* 30%^{Q}
- *Drug of choice:* Ribavirin^Q
- *Situation in India:* Exotic-Epidemic in India (Gujarat, Rajasthan, UP, Tamilnadu, Kerala)

Amoebiasis

- *Causative agent:* Entamoeba histolytica (7 pathogenic + 11 non-pathogenic zymodymes)
- Amoebiasis affects 15% of Indian population
- *Source of infection:* Cysts (NOT trophozoites)
- *Reservoir:* Man
- *Period of communicability:* Upto years (till cysts excreted)
- *Modes of transmission:*^{Q}
  - Faecal-oral
  - Sexual (Oro-rectal in homosexuals)
  - Vectors (Flies, Cockroaches, rodents)
- *Incubation period:* 2-4 weeks
- *Diagnosis:*
  - *Readily diagnostic test:* Trophozoites containing RBCs in freshly passed mucus per rectum
  - *Most sensitive serological test:* Indirect hemagglutination test
- *Treatment:*
  - *Symptomatic:* Metronidazole^Q
  - *Asymptomatic:* Diodohydroxyquin

> **Key points**
>
> Modes of transmission of Amoebiasis:
> - Faecal-oral
> - Sexual
> - Vectors

Hand Hygiene Guidelines (WHO)

- *Hand-Hygiene Modalities:*
  - *If hands are NOT visibly soiled:* Rub them with Alcohol base sanitizer (20–30 seconds)
  - *If hands are visibly soiled:* Wash hands with soap and water (40–60 seconds)
- 5 Check-points/Moments for Hand hygiene:
  - Before touching a patient
  - Before cleaning/aseptic procedure
  - After body fluid exposure risk
  - After touching a patient
  - After touching patient surroundings

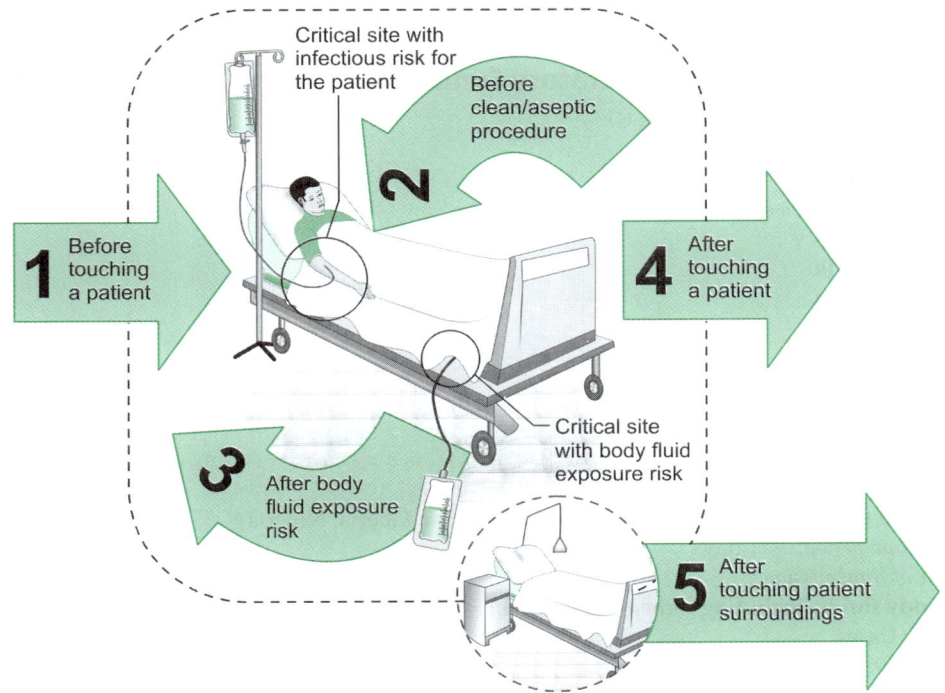

EMERGING AND RE-EMERGING DISEASES

NIPAH Virus

- *Genus*: Henapi virus
- Incubation period: 4-14 days
- *Transmission in India*:
  - *Occurrence*: West Bengal, Kerala
  - *Route*: **Consumption of fruits contaminated with bats (Pteropus: 'Flying foxes') secretions**
- *Clinical presentation*: Encephalitis
- *Case fatality rate*: 50%
- *Vaccine*: NONE for humans
- *Treatment*: Intensive supportive care

SARS Severe Acute Respiratory Syndrome

- *Causative agent:* Coronavirus[Q]
- *Origin:* China, 2002
  - Total cases: 8422
  - Total deaths: 916
- *Route of transmission:* Air droplets
- *Vaccine:* None
- *Treatment:*
  - Antipyretics
  - Supplemental Oxygen
  - Mechanical ventilation

H7N9 Avian Influenza

- *Occurrence:* First time among humans
- *Origin:* **March 2013, China**[Q]
- *Incubation period:* 1-10 days (~5 days)
- *Route of transmission:* Air droplets
- *Case fatality rate:* 33%[Q]
- *Vaccine:* NONE
- *Treatment:* Neuraminidase inhibitors
  - Oseltamivir
  - Zanamivir

MERS-CoV Middle East Respiratory Syndrome - Corona Virus

- *Cause:* Betacoronavirus (lineage C)[Q]
- *Origin:* Saudi Arabia, 2012[Q]
- *Incubation period:* 2-14 days[Q]
- *Route of transmission:*
  - Air droplets
  - **Camel milk**
  - Camel meat
- *Source:* Camels
- *Reservoir:* Bats
- *Case fatality rate:* 30%
- *Treatment:* None

Ebola Virus Disease[Q]

- *Current outbreak:* South Africa (Sierra Leone, Guinea, Liberia, Nigeria)[Q]
- *Incubation period:* 2-21 days
- *Route of transmission*[Q]:
  - **Body fluids** (including semen, breast milk)
- *Source:* Cases
- *Reservoir:* **Bats**[Q]
- *Case fatality rate*[Q]*:* 40%

- *Treatment:*
  - Rehydration
  - Symptomatic

H5N6 Avian Influenza
- First detected: 2015, China
- A subtype of the species Influenza A virus (sometimes called bird flu virus)
- Four known cases, three fatal, have occurred in humans

Zika Virus Disease
- Cause: Zika virus (Flavivirus), Positive sense RNA
- Transmission:
  - Mosquito bites: **Infected Aedes species mosquito** (A. aegypti^Q and A. albopictus)
  - Mother to child: At time of delivery (NOT via Breastfeeding)
  - Blood transfusion and sexual contact
- Specific associations:
  - Newborns (Vertical transmission): Microcephaly^Q, Chorioretinal scarring, Hydrops fetalis
  - Adults: Guillain–Barré syndrome^Q
- Diagnosis (WHO): RT-PCR testing on Serum (1-3 days of symptom onset) or Saliva (3-5 days)
- Lab diagnosis in India: NCDC, New Delhi and NIV, Pune
- Treatment: No specific treatment
- Public health emergency declaration by WHO: February 2016
- Zika virus in India: Few cases reported in India in Gujarat and Tamil Nadu (2017).

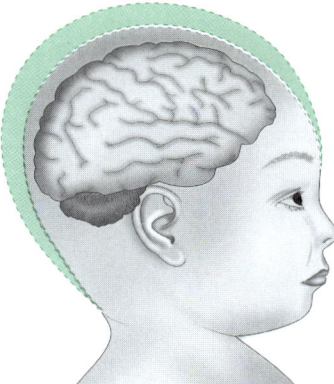

Microcephaly in Zika virus disease

List of Emerging Diseases likely to cause Major Epidemics (WHO)
• Crimean Congo hemorrhagic fever
• Ebola virus disease and Marburg
• Lassa fever
• MERS and SARS coronavirus diseases
• Nipah virus disease
• Rift Valley fever

H5N1 Avian Influenza
- Also known as 'Bird flu' or 'Highly pathogenic avian influenza'
- *Avian Influenza is a Pandemic:* Origin from Hong Kong (1997)
- First human case in India reported from Haryana in July 2021
- *Causative agent:* H5N1 (Type A Influenza virus)
- *Transmission:* Consumption of raw infected meat, contact with an infected bird's faeces, or secretions from its nose, mouth or eyes
- *Symptoms:*
  - Fever, cough, sore throat, muscle aches, conjunctivitis, and, in severe cases, breathing problems and pneumonia
  - Case fatality rate >50%
- *Treatment:*
  - Drug of choice: Oseltamivir (Tamiflu) 75 mg BD × 5 days (contraindicated in infants)
  - Zanamivir
- *Prevention:*
  - Conventional cooking (temperatures at or above 70°C) will inactivate the H5N1 Virus; properly cooked poultry meat is therefore safe to consume
  - Wash hands with warm water and soap, before and after handling foods
  - Avoid open-air markets or contact with live birds and poultry
  - Avoid eating raw eggs

Crimean Congo Fever (CCF)
- Reported in India since 2001
  - *Initial reports:* Ahmedabad – Gujarat (2010)
  - *Recent reports:* Gujarat, Rajasthan UP (2011-2015)

- *Type of disease:* Zoonosis of domestic/wild animals which may affect human beings
- *Causative agent:* Nairovirus, order Bunyavirus, genus Orthonairovirus, family Nairoviridae of RNA viruses
- *Transmission:* Vector is Hyalomma ticks (Hard ticks)
- *Incubation period:* 1–13 days (Median 5–6 days)
- *Symptoms:* Fever, muscle pains, headache, vomiting, diarrhoea, and petechial hemorrhages
- *Case fatality rate:* 30%
- *Drug of choice:* Ribavirin

West Nile Fever

- Re-occurrence in India reported from Mallapuram, Kerala in March 2021
- *Causative agent:* West Nile virus - single-stranded RNA virus, family Flaviviridae, genus Flavivirus
- *Transmission:*
    - Vector is Culex pipiens (and other Culicine species)
    - "Bird–mosquito–bird" transmission cycle
- *Incubation period:* 2–14 days
- *Symptoms:* 80% asymptomatic, fever, headache, vomiting, rash, encephalitis, meningitis
- *Prevention:*
    - No vaccine exists for prevention
    - Source reduction
    - Wear long sleeved shirts and long pants
    - Mosquito bed nets, Window and door screens, Insect repellents

Norovirus

- Occurrence in India reported from Wayanad, Kerala in November 2021
- *Synonym:* Winter Vomiting Bug
- *Causative agent:*
    - *Family Caliciviridae:* Single-stranded positive-sense RNA, non-enveloped viruses
    - *Genus Norovirus:* Has one species - Norwalk virus
- *Transmission:*
    - *Faecal-oral route:* Contaminated food or water or person-to-person contact
    - Contaminated surfaces or through air from the vomit of an infected person.
- *Symptoms:* Common cause of gastroenteritis
    - Symptoms usually develop 12–48 hours after being exposed, and recovery typically occurs within 1–3 days
    - Non-bloody diarrhoea, vomiting, and stomach pain
    - Fever, headaches may also occur
    - Complications are uncommon, but may include dehydration
- *Diagnosis:* PCR, Quantitative PCR assays
- *Prevention:*
    - Hand-washing with soap and water
    - Prevention of nosocomial infections
- *Treatment:*
    - There is no specific medicine
    - Management of dehydration caused by fluid loss in vomiting and diarrhoea
    - Mitigate symptoms using antiemetics and antidiarrheal

H10N3 Avian Influenza

- First human case in World reported from Zhenjiang, Jiangsu, China in May 2021
- Transmission (Possible route): Exposure to infected poultry or contaminated environments
- Human to human transmission not yet established
- Vaccine: NONE

NON-COMMUNICABLE DISEASES

CORONARY HEART DISEASE

Prudent Diet (Dietary Goals)

- *Description*: Dietary modification is the principal preventive strategy for prevention of CHD
- *WHO recommended changes*: [GOAL^Q : Cholesterol/HDL Ratio <3.5]
  - Reduction of fat intake to <20–30% of total energy intake^Q
  - Consumption of saturated fats <7% of total energy intake^Q
  - Reduction in dietary cholesterol to <200 mg per day
  - Increase in complex carbohydrate consumption
  - Reduction of salt intake to <5 gms per day^Q
  - Avoidance of alcohol consumption

> **Key points**
> **GOAL^Q of Prudent Diet:** Cholesterol/HDL Ratio < 3.5

Coronary Heart Disease

- *Coronary Heart Disease (CHD) or Ischemic Heart Disease (IHD):* Impairment of heart function due to inadequate flow to heart as compared to its needs, caused by obstructive changes in coronary circulation to heart
- *CHD manifests as:*
  - Angina pectoris
  - Myocardial infarction
  - Irregularities of the heart
  - Cardiac failure
  - Sudden death
- *Pattern of CHD in India^Q:*
  - Occurs a decade earlier then with age incidence in developed nations
  - Peak period is 51–60 years age
  - Males affected more than females
  - Hypertension and Diabetes mellitus account for > 40% cases
  - Heavy smoking is responsible for a large no. of cases
- *Risk factors of CHD:*

Non-modifiable risk factors^Q	Modifiable risk factors^Q
Age	Cigarette smoking
Sex	High blood pressure
Family history	Elevated serum cholesterol
Genetic factors	Diabetes
Personality (Type A) (?)	Obesity
	Sedentary habits
	Stress

Smoking as a Risk Factor for CHD

- Modifiable major risk factor
- 25% of CHD deaths under 65 years age
- Causes Sudden death from CHD, especially in men < 50 years age
- Degree of risk of developing CHD is directly related to no. of cigarettes smoked per day^Q
- Filter cigarettes are probably not protective^Q
- Synergistic with other risk factors like hypertension and hypercholesterolemia^Q
- Risk of death from CHD decreases on cessation of smoking
  - Risk declines substantially within 1 year of cessation
  - After 10–20 years, it is same as that of non-smokers^Q
  - Those with history of myocardial infarction–risk of fatal occurrence reduced by 50%

> **Key points**
> *Most direct association with CHD:* LDL cholesterol

Important Facts of CHD

- *Single most useful test for identifying individuals at high risk of CHD:* Blood pressure^Q
  - Systolic BP better predictor of CHD than Diastolic BP^Q

> **Key points**
> - Mean serum cholesterol level associated with high risk of CHD: >200 mg/dl
> - Protective for CHD: HDL cholesterol (>30 mg/dL)

- Most direct association with CHD: LDL cholesterol – Cholesterol/HDL ratio < 3.5
  - HDL cholesterol > 30 mg/dL
- Better predictors of CHD: Apolipoprotein A–I and Apolipoprotein B^Q
- Alcohol intake as an independent risk factor for CHD: > 75 grams per day
- Mean serum cholesterol level associated with high risk of CHD: >200 mg/dL^Q
  - Threshold level: 220 mg/dl is protective
- Protective for CHD: HDL cholesterol (>30 mg/dl)^Q
- Clinical goal of CHD prevention: Cholesterol/HDL ratio <3.5^Q

HYPERTENSION

- Hypertension (HT) is the MC cardiovascular disorder^Q
- Single most useful test to identify high risk of CHD: Blood Pressure^Q
- Systolic BP is a better predictor of CHD than diastolic BP
- Prevalence of HT in India (1977-78):

> **Key points**
> Systolic BP is a better predictor of CHD than diastolic BP

	Males	Females
Urban	59.9 per 1000	69.9 per 1000
Rural	35.5 per 1000	35.9 per 1000

- Population strategy for prevention of Hypertension: Is primary level of prevention
  - Nutrition (Reduction of salt intake to < 5 grams a day, moderate fat intake, avoidance of alcohol intake, restriction of energy intake as per body needs)
  - Weight reduction (BMI <25)
  - Exercise promotion
  - Behavioural changes (reduction of stress and smoking, doing yoga and meditation)
  - Health education
  - Self care
- **Rule of Halves^Q:** Hypertension is an 'Iceberg disease'. Only about half of hypertensive subjects in general population of most of the developed countries are aware of condition, only half of those aware of the problem were being treated and only half of those treated were considered adequately treated

> **Key points**
> Hypertension is an 'Iceberg disease'

A Total population
B Hypertensive
C Symptomatic hypertensive
D Diagnosed hypertensive
E Treated
F Adequately treated

Rule of Halves

- **Tracking of Blood Pressure^Q:** If BP of individuals were followed up over a period of years from early childhood into adult life, then those having high BP would continue into same 'track' as adults
  - Low BP tends to remain low and high BP tends to become higher as individuals grow older

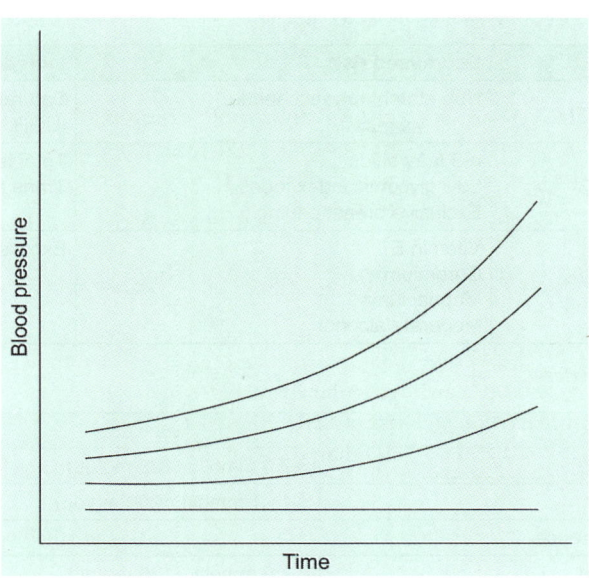

Tracking of blood pressure

- *Goal of population strategy (Primary prevention) for HT control:* To shift the community distribution of BP towards lower levels or 'biological normality'

NEW BP Classification (ACC/AHA Guidelines) 2017

SBP		DBP	JNC-VII	ACC/AHA 2017
< 120	And	< 80	Normal BP	Normal BP
120-129	And	< 80	Pre-hypertension	Elevated BP
130-139	And	80-89	Pre-hypertension	Stage 1 hypertension
140-159	Or	90-99	Stage 1 hypertension	Stage 2 hypertension
≥ 160	Or	≥ 100	Stage 2 hypertension	Stage 2 hypertension

(ACC/AHA: American College of Cardiology and American Heart Association).

Lifestyle Modifications to Manage Hypertension

Modification	Recommendation	Approx. SBP
Weight reduction	Maintain BW, Normal BMI 18.5–24.99	5–20 mm Hg/10 kg BW loss
Adopt DASH diet plan	Diet rich in fruits/vegetables, Low fat dairy products (Reduced Saturated fat, Total fat)	8–14 mm Hg
Dietary sodium reduction	<100 mEq/day (2.4 gm Sodium/6 g Sodium chloride)	2–8 mm Hg
Physical activity	Regular aerobic physical activity (>30 min/day, most days of week)	4–9 mm Hg
Moderation of alcohol consumption	Limit alcohol consumption < 2 drinks/day	2–4 mm hg

DIABETES MELLITUS

- *Evidence of Life style factors and risk of Diabetes:*

Evidence	Decreased risk	Increased risk
Convincing	Voluntary weight loss Physical activity	Overweight, obesity Abdominal obesity Physical inactivity Maternal diabetes

Contd...

Contd...

Evidence	Decreased risk	Increased risk
Probable	Non-starch polysaccharide	Saturated fats IUGR
Possible	n-3 fatty acids Low glycemic index foods Exclusive breastfeeding	Total fat intake Trans fatty acids
Insufficient	Vitamin E Chromium Magnesium Moderate alcohol	Excess alcohol

- *WHO Diagnostic Criteria:*

Diabetes	
Fasting plasma glucose	> 7.0 mmol/L (126 mg/dL)
2-hour plasma glucose	> 11.1 mmol/L (200 mg/dL)
Impaired Glucose Tolerance	
Fasting plasma glucose	< 7.0 mmol/L (126 mg/dL)
2-hour plasma glucose	7.8-11.1 mmol/L (140-200 mg/dL)
Impaired fasting glucose	
Fasting plasma glucose	6.1-6.9 mmol/L (110-125 mg/dL)
2-hour plasma glucose	< 7.8 mmol/L (140 mg/dL)

Glycaemic Index

- *Definition*: Area under the 2-hour glucose response curve (AUC)
- *Low glycaemic index foods*: Less readily digestible and lower absorption of sugar
- *Classification of Glycaemic Index (GI)*:

Classification	GI range	Examples
Low GI	≤ 55	Most fruits and vegetables (EXCEPT potato/water-melon/sweet potato), Whole grains, Beans, Pasta, Lentils
Medium GI	56–69	Sucrose, Basmati rice, Brown rice
High GI	≥ 70	Corn flakes, Baked potato, White bread, Candy bar, Syrupy food, Jasmine rice

Diabetic Foot

- Diabetic foot is a common devastating and debilitating complication of diabetes that can lead to amputation
- *DF Triopathy:* Infection, ischemia and neuropathy

Types of Diabetic foot complications	Lesions
Type 1 Diabetic foot complications (Infective)	Wet gangrene, cellulitis, necrotizing fasciitis, abscess
Type 2 Diabetic foot complications (non-Infective)	Trophic ulcer, claw toe, Charcot foot, ischemic ulcer, hammer toe, dry gangrene
Type 3 Diabetic foot complications (Mixed) [When type 2 diabetic foot complications get infected]	Non healing ulcer with osteomyelitis

- LFT Screening tool - Triple assessment for foot (Amit Jain) is an original new, simple, practical screening tool developed from India for diabetic foot
    - *Look component:* Inspect the dorsum, plantar and inter- digital region for ulcer/pre-ulcerative lesions or infection
    - *Feel component:* Assess the blood supply to foot by palpating posterior tibial/anterior tibial/dorsalis pedis arteries
    - *Test component:* Check for sensation

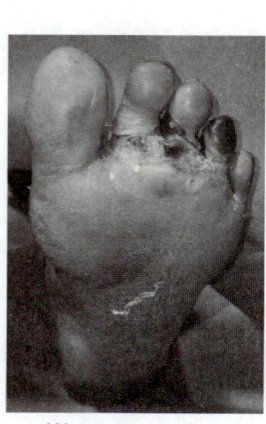

Wet gangrene foot

RHEUMATIC FEVER (RF)

- *Causative agent:* Group A beta hemolytic streptococci^Q
  - Serotype M type 5 has highest 'rheumatogenic potential'^{Q}
  - Recently Coxsackie virus B4 has been suggested as a 'causative factor' & Streptococcus acting as a 'conditioning agent'
- RF is a disease of childhood & adolescence (5–15 yrs) affecting both sexes equally
- *RF is not a communicable disease:* but it results from a communicable disease (streptococcal pharyngitis)
- *MC cause of Heart disease in 5–30 yrs age group (globally)^Q:* RF
- *Prevalence of RHD in India:* 5–7 per 1000 in 5–15 yrs age group^Q
  - RF occurs in 1–3% of Streptococcal infection
- *Eradication of Grp A Streptococcus is not possible:* Due to high carrier rate
- *MC cardiac lesion seen in RF:*
  - *In children:* Mitral regurgitation^Q
  - *In adults:* Mitral stenosis^Q
- *MC ECG finding in RF:* First degree AV block^Q
- *Diagnosis of RF is by employing NEW Revised Jones criteria^Q:*

> **Key points**
> *Prevalence of RHD in India:* 5-7 per 1000 in 5–15 yrs age group
> *MC cardiac lesion seen in RF:*
> - *In children:* Mitral regurgitation^Q
> - *In adults:* Mitral stenosis
> *Diagnosis of RF is by employing Revised Jones criteria*

NEW Revised Jones Criteria

A. For all patient populations with evidence of preceding GAS infection	
Diagnosis: Initial ARF	2 Major manifestations OR 1 major plus 2 minor manifestations
Diagnosis: Recurrent ARF	2 Major OR 1 major and 2 minor OR 3 minor manifestations
B. Major criteria	
Low-risk populations	Moderate- and high-risk populations
Carditis - Clinical and/or subclinical Arthritis - Polyarthritis only Chorea Erythema marginatum Subcutaneous nodules	Carditis - Clinical and/or subclinical Arthritis–Monoarthritis/polyarthritis, Polyarthralgia Chorea Erythema marginatum Subcutaneous nodules
C. Minor criteria	
Low-risk populations	Moderate- and high-risk populations
Polyarthralgia Fever (≥38.5°C) ESR ≥60 mm (1st hour)/CRP ≥3.0 mg/dL Prolonged PR interval*	Monoarthralgia Fever (≥38°C) ESR ≥30 mm/h and/or CRP ≥3.0 mg/dL Prolonged PR interval*

(*after accounting for age variability, unless Carditis is a major criterion)
(ARF: Acute rheumatic fever; CRP, C-reactive protein; ESR, erythrocyte sedimentation rate; and GAS, group A streptococcal infection) (Low-risk populations are those with ARF incidence ≤2 per 100,000 school-aged children or all-age rheumatic heart disease prevalence of ≤1 per 1000 population per year)

- *Prevention of RF with Benzathine benzyl penicillin^Q:*

Type of prevention	Adults	Children	Remarks
Primary	1.2 million units	600,000 units	Single dose intramuscular
Secondary	1.2 million units	600,000 units	3 weekly intervals for 5 yrs or till 18 yrs age (whichever is later)

- Oral penicillin (Penicillin V or G) X 10 days is the 'least expensive method' of giving penicillin to eradicate Streptococci from throat
- Secondary prevention for patients with carditis: Continue for 10 yrs after the last attack or at least until 25 yrs age (whichever is longer)

CANCERS

NEW WHO Cancer Data—Globocan 2020 (Top 5 causes)

- Incidence of Cancer WORLD

Total Population	Males	Females
1. Breast 2. Lung 3. Colorectum 4. Prostate 5. Stomach	1. Lung 2. Prostate 3. Colorectum 4. Stomach 5. Liver	1. Breast 2. Colorectum 3. Lung 4. Cervix-uteri 5. Thyroid

- Prevalence and Mortality of Cancer WORLD

Prevalence	Mortality
1. Breast 2. Colorectum 3. Prostate 4. Lung 5. Thyroid	1. Lung 2. Colorectum 3. Liver 4. Stomach 5. Breast

- Incidence of Cancer INDIA

Total Population	Males	Females
1. Breast 2. Lip/Oral cavity 3. Cervix-uteri 4. Lung 5. Colorectum	1. Lip/Oral cavity 2. Lung 3. Stomach 4. Colorectum 5. Oesophagus	1. Breast 2. Cervix-uteri 3. Ovary 4. Lip/Oral cavity 5. Colorectum

- Prevalence and Mortality of Cancer INDIA

Prevalence	Mortality
1. Breast 2. Cervix-uteri 3. Lip/Oral cavity 4. Ovary 5. Prostate	1. Breast 2. Cervix-uteri 3. Lip/Oral cavity 4. Lung 5. Esophagus

OBESITY

Criteria for Assessment of Obesity

- Body Mass Index (Quetelet's Index^Q):

Key points

$$BMI = \frac{Weight\ (Kg)}{Height^2\ (m)^2}$$

$$BMI = \frac{Weight\ (Kg)}{Height^2\ (m)^2}$$

Classification of adults according to BMI:

Classification	BMI		
	Global population^Q	Asian population	Indian population^Q
Underweight	< 18.5	< 18.5	< 18.5
Normal BMI	18.5-24.99	18.5-22.99	18.5-22.99
Overweight	25-29.99	23-26.99	23-24.99
Obesity	≥ 30.0	≥ 27.0	≥ 25.0

Classification of obesity based on BMI^Q:

Classification	BMI
Pre-obese (overweight)	25.0-29.99
Obesity Grade I	30.0- 34.99
Obesity Grade II	35.0-39.99
Obesity Grade III (Morbid obesity)	≥ 40.0

Classification of underweight based on BMI:

Classification	BMI
Grade I Underweight	17.0-18.49
Grade II Underweight	16.0-16.99
Grade III Underweight	< 16.0

- *Ponderal index^Q:*

$$PI = \frac{\text{height (cm)}}{3\sqrt{\text{body weight (kg)}}}$$

- *Broca index^Q:*
  Ideal weight = Height (cms)–100
- *Lorentz formula:*

$$LF = Ht (cm)-100 - \frac{Ht(cm)-150}{2(women) \text{ or } 4(men)}$$

- *Corpulence index (normal ≤ 1.2)^Q:*

$$CI = \frac{\text{Actual weight}}{\text{Desirable weight}}$$

- *Skin fold thickness (SFT):*
  - Rapid & non-invasive method of fat assessment
  - 'Herpenden skin callipers' are good for estimation of SFT^Q
  - *Main drawback:* Poor repeatability (Poor precision)
  - *Measurement at 4 sites:* Mid-triceps, biceps, sub-scapular, supra-iliac regions
    - Sum ≥ 50 mm in girls indicate obesity
    - Sum ≥ 40 mm in boys indicate obesity
  - *Single best measurement site of skin fold thickness:* **Mid triceps**^{Q}
    - 18 mm in boys indicate obesity
    - 32 mm in girls indicate obesity
- *Waist circumference (WC) & waist: hip ratio (WHR):*
  - Good predictor of risk of cardiovascular diseases
  - High WHR indicates abdominal fat accumulation
    - WHR > 1.0 in men indicate obesity^Q
    - WHR > 0.85 in women indicate obesity^Q
  - Cut-offs for waist circumference in India:

Populations	Cut-off for WC^Q
Indian	
Males	90 cm
Females	80 cm
Global	
Males	102 cm
Females	88 cm

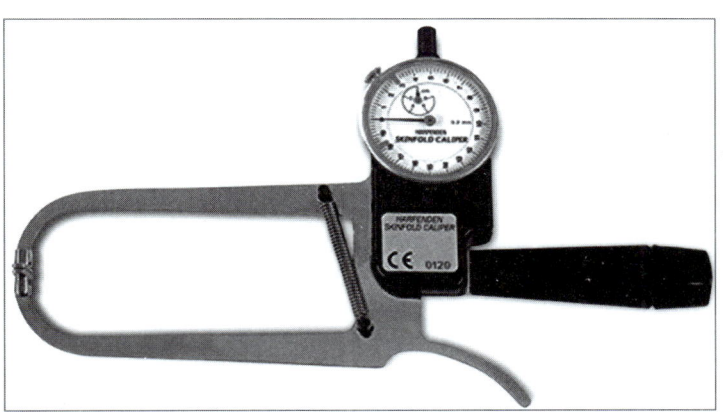

Herpenden Calipers

> **Key points**
> *Single best measurement site of skin fold thickness:* Mid triceps

- *Waist: Height Ratio (WHtR)^Q:*
  - WHO has declared **WHtR as 'best indicator of cardiovascular risk'**
  - WHtR is 'age and sex independent'
  - Cut-off for WHtR: 0.5
- *Other indicators:*
  - Total body water
  - Total body potassium
  - Body density

> **Key points**
> WHO has declared WHtR as 'best indicator of cardiovascular risk'

Weight Control Measures

- *Dietary changes:*
  - Reduce proportions of carbohydrates and fats (energy dense foods)
  - Increase fibre consumption
  - Ensure adequate levels of essential nutrients
- Increased physical activity
- *Others:*
  - Drugs
  - Surgical treatment
  - Health education

BLINDNESS

Blindness Situation

National Blindness and Visual Impairment Survey Report 2015-2019

Category	Presenting Visual Acuity*
Blindness	< 3/60
Visual impairment (VI)	< 6/18
Early visual impairment (EVI)	< 6/12 – 6/18
Moderate visual impairment (MVI)	< 6/18 – 6/60
Moderate severe visual impairment (MSVI)	<6/18 – 3/60
Severe visual impairment (SVI)	< 6/60 – 3/60
Functional low vision: A person with impairment of visual functioning even after treatment and/or standard refractive correction, and a visual acuity of less than 6/18 to light perception, or a visual field of less than 10 degree from the point of fixation, but who uses, or is potentially able to use, vision for planning and/or execution of a task	

(Table © Dr Vivek Jain 2022-23) (* in better eye with available correction)

Prevalence and Causes of Blindness & VI in India

- **Prevalence of blindness in all age groups: 0.36%**
- Prevalence of visual impairment (VI-Blindness+MSVI) in all age groups: 2.55%
- **Major Causes of Blindness in population aged ≥ 50 years: Cataract 66.2%,** Corneal opacity including trachomatous 8.2%, Cataract surgical complications including PCO 7.2%, Posterior segment disease excluding DR & ARMD 5.9%, Glaucoma 5.5%
- Major Causes of Blindness in population aged 0-49 years: Corneal opacity 37.5%, All globe/CNS abnormality Amblyopia, Phthisis, Other/undetermined
- Major Causes of Visual Impairment in population aged ≥ 50 years: Cataract 71.2%, Refractive error 13.4%, Cataract surgical complications including PCO 5.9%
- Major Causes of Visual Impairment in population aged 0-49 years: Refractive error 29.6%, Cataract, All globe/CNS abnormality Amblyopia, Corneal opacity

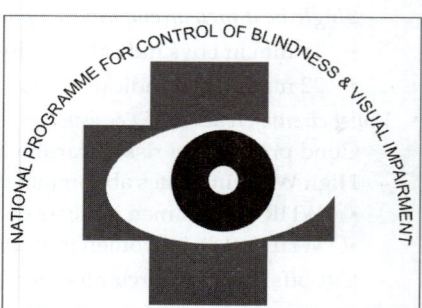

	World	India (NPCB, India)
Blindness	'visual acuity of <3/60 in better eye with best possible correction'	'visual acuity of <3/60 in better eye with best possible correction' [New Guideline 2017-2018]
Prevalence	0.6% [2002]	0.36% [2015–19]
Causes	**Cataract (48%)—MCC^Q** Glaucoma (12%) Uveitis (10%) ARMD Trachoma Corneal opacity Corneal opacity Others	**Cataract–MCC^Q** Refractive Error Glaucoma Posterior segment pathology Corneal opacity Other causes

Definitions of Blindness

- WHO defines Blindness as 'visual acuity of **<3/60** in better eye with best possible correction'^Q
- National Programme for Control of Blindness (NPCB), India defines Blindness as 'visual acuity of **<3/60** in better eye with best possible correction'^Q [New Guideline 2017-2018]
- American Medical Association definition of blindness: 'Central visual acuity of 20/200 or less in the better eye with corrective glasses'^Q (or central visual acuity of more than 20/200 if there is a visual field defect in which the peripheral field is contracted to such an extent that the widest diameter of the visual field subtends an angular distance less than 20 degrees in the better eye)

> **Key points**
> - WHO defines Blindness as 'visual acuity of <3/60
> - National Programme for Control of Blindness (NPCB), India defines Blindness as 'visual acuity of <3/60

WHO and NPCB Definitions

WHO–ICD	Visual Acuity	NPCB, India
Low Vision		
Category 1	<6/18–6/60	Low Vision^Q
Category 2	<6/60–3/60	Economic Blindness^Q
Blindness		
Category 3	<3/60–1/60	Social Blindness^Q
Category 4	<1/60–PL+	Manifest Blindness
Category 5	PL–	Absolute Blindness

(PL+: Perception of Light; PL–: No perception of light)

- *Revised Categories of Visual Impairment:*

Category	VA less than	VA equal or better than
0: Mild/No visual impairment		6/18
1: Moderate visual impairment	6/18	6/60
2: Severe visual impairment	6/60	3/60
3: Blindness	3/60	1/60
4: Blindness	1/60	Light perception
5: Blindness	No light perception	No light perception
9	Undetermined/Unspecified	Undetermined/Unspecified

Vision Impairment [ICD-11, WHO]

- Distance Vision impairment:

Category of VI	Definition
Mild VI	Presenting visual acuity <6/12
Moderate VI	Presenting visual acuity <6/18
Severe VI	Presenting visual acuity <6/60
Blindness	Presenting visual acuity <3/60

- Near Vision impairment: Presenting near vision acuity <N6 or N8 at 40 cms with existing correction
- Major causes of VI & Blindness:

Moderate-Severe VI	Blindness
Uncorrected refractive errors (53%)	Un-operated cataract (35%)
Un-operated cataract (25%)	Uncorrected refractive errors (21%)
ARMD, Glaucoma, Diabetic retinopathy	Glaucoma (8%)

Low Vision

- *Low Vision (Visual Acuity < 6/18–6/60):* Is an important cause of sub-optimal visual functioning.
- *Major causes of Low Vision in India:* (are similar to causes of blindness)
  - Cataract (77%)–MCC of Low Vision in India^Q
  - Refractive Error (19%)

> **Key points**
> Cataract (77%)–MCC of Low Vision in India

- Central corneal opacity
- Pterygium
- Peripheral corneal opacity
- Other causes

> **Key points**
>
> *Vision 2020– The Right To Sight:* to reduce avoidable (preventable and curable) blindness by 2020

Vision 2020

- *Vision 2020– The Right To Sight:* A global initiative by WHO and International NGOs to reduce avoidable (preventable and curable) blindness by 2020[Q]
- *Aim of Vision 2020:* To reduce the current projection of 75 million blind people by the year 2020 to a target of 25 million
- Vision 2020 will be implemented as '4 five-year plans', starting in 2000, 2005, 2010 and 2015 respectively

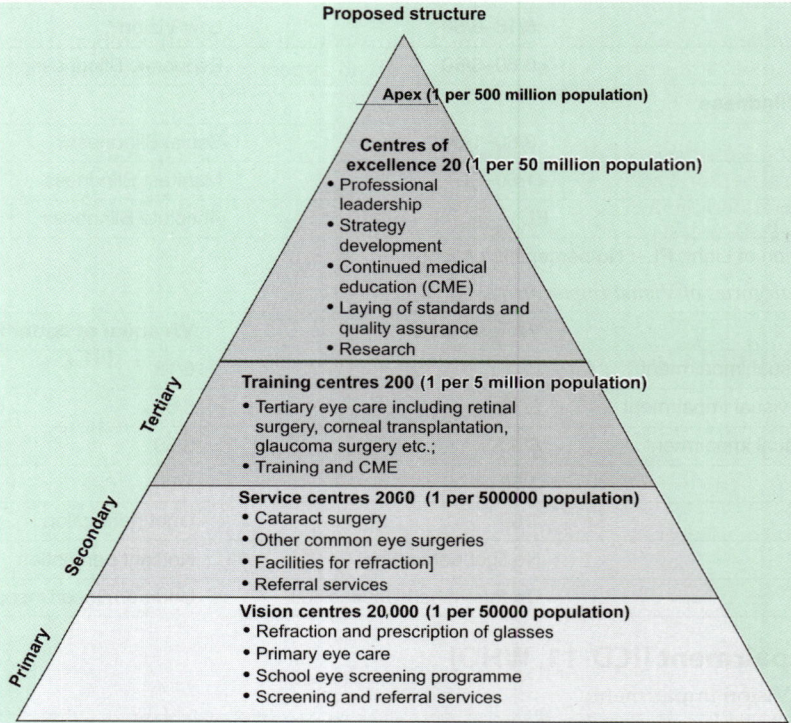

Proposed structure for vision 2020: The right to sight

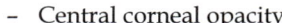

Vision 2020

Global Vision 2020 (5 diseases[Q])	Indian Vision 2020 (7 diseases[Q])
Cataract	Cataract
Refractive errors and low vision	Refractive errors and low vision
Childhood blindness	Childhood blindness
Trachoma	Trachoma (Focal)
Onchocerciasis	Glaucoma
	Diabetic retinopathy
	Corneal blindness

- *Basic Strategies Under Vision 2020:*
  - Disease prevention and control
  - Training of personnel
  - Strengthening the existing eye care infrastructure
  - Use of appropriate and affordable technology
  - Mobilization of resources
- *Recommended human resources and service facilities for Indian Vision 2020:*

Global Eye Health Action Plan 2014-2019

- Main Aim: To reduce avoidable Visual Impairment (VI) as a Global Public Health problem, and to secure access to rehabilitation services for the VI

- 5 Principles and Approaches:
  - Universal access and equity
  - Human rights
  - Evidence based practice
  - Life course approach
  - Empowerment of people with VI
- Global Target: Reduction in prevalence of Avoidable VI by 25% by 2019 (from baseline 2010)
- 3 Indicators:
  - Prevalence and causes of VI
  - Number of eye care personnel
  - Cataract surgery

STROKE (APOPLEXY)

- *WHO definition:* Rapidly developing clinical signs of local (or global) cerebral dysfunction, lasting more than 24 hours or leading to death, with no apparent cause other than vascular origin
  - 24 hour threshold EXCLUDES transient ischemic attacks (TIA)
- *Causes of stroke:*
  - **Cerebral thrombosis (MCC of stroke or apoplexy^Q)**
  - Cerebral hemorrhage
  - Subarachnoid hemorrhage
  - Cerebral embolism

MISCELLANEOUS (NON-COMMUNICABLE DISEASES)

Prevention and Control of Non-Communicable Diseases (NCDs)

- *Population strategy:*
  - Focus on control of underlying causes (riak factors) in whole populations, 'not merely by individuals'
  - *Principle:* Small changes in risk factor levels in total populations can achieve the biggest reduction in mortality, thus aim should be 'to shift the whole curve or risk factors towards biological normality'
  - *Specific interventions/Dietary changes:* (PRUDENT DIET- DIETARY GOALS^Q)
  - Primordial prevention
- *High risk strategy:*
  - *Identifying risk:* By using simple tests for blood pressure, serum cholesterol measurement
  - *Specific advice:* To those identified at high risk
- *Secondary prevention:*
  - *Aim:* to prevent reoccurrence and progression of NCDs

WHO STEP wise Approach^Q

- *STEP wise approach to Surveillance (STEPS):* Is a simple, standardized method by WHO for surveillance
- *Is of two types:*
  - STEP wise approach to chronic disease risk factor surveillance
  - STEP wise approach to Stroke surveillance
- *Comprises of 3 steps:*

STEPS	Core	Expanded
STEP 1^Q Behavioural measurements	Tobacco use Alcohol consumption Diet Physical activity History of raised BP History of diabetes	Tobacco use Alcohol consumption Diet Physical activity History of raised BP History of diabetes
STEP 2^Q Physical measurements	Height & weight Waist BP	Hip circumference Heart rate
STEP 3^Q Biochemical measurements	Blood glucose Blood lipids	Triglycerides HDL cholesterol

> **Key points**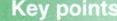
>
> **STEP wise approach** to chronic disease risk factor surveillance

Accidents and Injuries in India (in Order of Decreasing Numbers)
- Road traffic accidents^Q
- Work related injuries
- Burns
- Violence, Suicide
- Poisoning
- Drowning

Accidents and Injuries: Burns
- *Description:* Injury to skin and other organic tissue due to heat/radiation/radioactivity/electricity/friction/chemicals
- *Problem statement:*
    - Global: 11 million severe burns, 195,000 deaths per year
    - India: 1 million moderate/severe burn cases per year
- *Risk factors:*
    - Children, Young women more commonly affected in houses
    - Low, middle income countries
    - Hazardous occupations
    - Poverty, overcrowding, lack of proper safety measures
    - Young girls placement in household works
    - Underlying medical conditions (Epilepsy, peripheral neuropathy, disabilities)
    - Alcohol abuse, smoking
    - Easy access to chemicals used for assault
    - Kerosene use as a fuel source
    - Inadequate safety measures for LPG, electricity
- *Prevention strategy - First aid:*
    - DO's:
        - Remove clothing, irrigate burns
        - Use cool running water
        - Extinguish flames (roll on ground, blanket/water/extinguisher use)
        - Dilute chemicals (in chemical burns)
        - Wrap patient in clean cloth, transfer to health facility
    - DON'Ts :
        - Don't start first-aid before ensuring your won safety
        - Don't apply paste/oil/turmeric/raw cotton
        - Don't apply ice
        - Avoid prolonged cooling with water (to prevent hypothermia)
        - Don't open blisters without availability of topical antibiotics
        - Don't apply any material directly to wound
        - Avoid topical medication until patient is in appropriate medical care

Accidents and Injuries: Snake Bite
- *Problem statement:*
    - 5 million snake bites per year
    - 2.5 million snake bite poisonings per year
    - 0.1 million deaths per year
    - 0.3 million amputations and permanent disabilities
- *Clues of severe envenoming:*
    - Snake identified as dangerous
    - Rapid early extension of local swelling from site of bite
    - Early tender enlargement of local lymph nodes
    - Early systemic symptoms: Hypotension, shock, nausea, vomiting, diarrhoea, severe headache, heaviness of eyelids, excessive drowsiness, ptosis/ophthalmoplegia
- *National Snake-bite First-Aid Protocol (Government of India, 2007):*
    - Reassure the patient: 70% bites are non-poisonous; 50% bites from poisonous snakes actually envenomate patient
    - Immobilise like a fractured limb: Don't apply tight ligatures
    - Don't give alcoholic beverages, stimulants
    - Remove constricting items/clothings

- Don't incise or manipulate bite site (No ice application)
- Transport patient to a medical facility
- *Anti-venom:*
  - First developed by: Albert Calmette
  - Description: Polyvalent nature, intravenous route

Oral Diseases

- Oral Diseases (WHO): A state of being free from chronic mouth and facial pain, oral and throat cancer, oral infection and sores, periodontal (gum) diseases, tooth decay, tooth loss, and other diseases and disorders that limit an individual's capacity in biting, chewing, smiling, speaking and psychological well being
- Oral disease burden in India:
  - Common disorders: Periodontal diseases (>90%), Dental caries (40-45%), Malocclusion (30% of children)
  - Other disorders: Oral cancers, Oral manifestations of HIV (72% of HIV patients), Oro-dental trauma, Cleft lip and palate, and noma (Oro-facial gangrene)
- Risk factors: Modifiable risk factors (Tobacco use, Alcohol consumption, Unhealthy diets high in free sugars) common to major NCDs (CVDs, Diabetes, Cancer, Chronic respiratory diseases)
- Prevention of Oral Diseases
  - Promoting a well-balanced diet: Low in free sugars, With adequate fruit and vegetable intake
  - Reducing smoking, use of smokeless tobacco, alcohol consumption
  - Reduce risk of facial injuries: Encouraging use of protective equipment in sports and when travelling in motor vehicles

PYQs: Quick Review for NEET

Respiratory Diseases	
Small Pox was declared Eradicated on	8 May, 1980
Rash type in Chickenpox is	Pleomorphic and Dew-drop like
TB Research Centre is located at	Chennai
Chicken pox vaccine is type of	Live attenuate vaccine
Koplik Spots are diagnostic of	Measles (Lower 2nd molar)
Incubation Period for Measles is	10-14 days
Highly Pathogenic Avian Influenza (Bird Flu) is by	Type A (H5N1 strain) virus
Hundred Day Cough is	Pertussis (Whooping Cough)
DOC for Chemoprophylaxis of Meningococcal Meningitis	Rifampicin
Positive Schick Test indicates	Susceptibility to Diphtheria
Inability to drink in Pneumonia is a sign of	Very Severe Disease
Sputum +ve TB patients on chemotherapy should be isolated for	3 weeks
SARS is caused by	Corona Virus
WHO has recommended 'DANISH 1331' strain for	BCG Vaccine
Overall Prevalence of TB infection	30-40%
Avian Influenza DOC	Oseltamivir 150 mg BD × 5 days
Incubation period for Measles	10 days
Koplik spots are seen in disease	Measles
MDR TB is Resistance to	INH and Rifampicin
SSPE is seen in	Measles
Isolation in Tuberculosis is	Not beneficial
IP of Influenza is	18–72 hours
Number of sputum positive cases of tuberculosis per lakh in India	75

Contd...

Contd...

Congenital rubella syndrome triad is	Cataract, Deafness, PDA
Drug resistance in retreatment of TB	13–17%
White death is	Tuberculosis
White plague is	Tuberculosis
Pleomorphism is seen in	Chickenpox
Three-day disease is	Rubella
DOC for carriers of Typhoid	Ampicillin
TB bacilli in 1 mL expectoration of an active case of TB	10,000
Measles vaccine is generally not given before age	9 months
Diphtheria carrier are diagnosed by	Throat culture
Neurological complications of DPT are due to	Pertussis component
Anti-tubercular drug which causes Optic neuritis	Ethambutol
One TB infected person can infect how many people in one year	10 people per year
Mycobacterium tuberculosis infection in humans is MC due to	Inhalation
Incubation period of Chicken pox is	14-16 days
Measles turn infectious _____ days before onset of rash	4 days
95% carrier and 5% cases are seen in disease	Diphtheria
Herd immunity threshold for diphtheria is	83-86%
Most common influenza virus causing disease	Type A Influenza
H1N1 strain of influenza is responsible for	Swine flu
Incubation period of chickenpox is	14-16 days
Secondary attack rate of Mumps is	> 85%
Isolation period of TB is	3 weeks after treatment
MC complication of Chicken pox is	Bacterial infection of skin
Herd immunity threshold for Measles	85-90%
Infective period for Diphtheria	14-28 days from disease onset
Intestinal Diseases	
For every 1 clinical case of Poliomyelitis, there are	1000 subclinical Cases
HBeAg in Hepatitis B is Marker of	Infectivity/Viral Replication
Concentration of Sodium in mmol/L in Low osmolarity ORS	75 mmol/L
Dose of ORS for a child with weight 12 kg	900 ml
ORS Solution should be used within	24 Hours
Typhoid oral vaccine regimen	1, 3, 5 days
Enteric Fever includes	Typhoid and Para-typhoid Fevers
Dysphagia, dysarthria and diplopia seen in	Clostridium botulinum food poisoning
Isolation period of Hepatitis A	3 weeks
1955 Hepatitis outbreak is Delhi was	Hepatitis E
Incubation period in Staphylococcal food poisoning	1-6 hours
Chances of Viral Hepatitis Type C becoming a chronic infection	50% or more
Chandler's Index for Hookworms is	Average no. of Eggs/gm of stool
Reservoir of Polio	Man (only)
HEV transmission route	Faecal-oral route
Typhoid diagnosed in 1st week by	Blood Culture
DOC Cholera (Pregnancy)	Azithromycin (Earlier Furazolidone)
Persistent Diarrhoea in infants of more than	14 days

Contd...

Contd...

ORS should be discarded after	24 hours of preparation
Total osmolarity of WHO Reduced Osmolarity ORS	245 mmol/L
First outbreak of Hepatitis E in Delhi	1955
Chandler's index is used for	Ankylostoma duodenale
MC food poisoning	Staphylococcus
Sodium ion content in ORS	75 mmol/L
In ORS, Na+ absorption is due to	Glucose
Chandler's index is based on	Hookworm eggs/gram faeces of community
MC type of Vibrio cholerae in India	Hybrid form
Epidemiological marker of Hepatitis B is	HBs Ag
Ratio of Sodium : Glucose in WHO Reduced Osmolarity ORS	1 : 1
Wild poliomyelitis is still endemic in	Pakistan, Afghanistan, Nigeria
Guinea worm infestation used to be common in workers of	Step wells
In Polio sensory loss is	Absent
Intestinal perforation in typhoid occurs in	Early III week
Cause of Fulminant hepatitis in pregnancy	Hepatitis E
Food poisoning in less than 6 hours	Staphylococcal FP
Chandler's index is	Hookworm eggs/gm stool
Best treatment for diarrhoea	ORS
Chandler's Index major public health problem if	More than 300
Dracunculiasis was more common in state of	Rajasthan
Infectious hepatitis/Epidemic jaundice is	Hepatitis A
Virus causes Fulminant hepatitis during pregnancy	Hepatitis E
Incubation period of Poliomyelitis is	7-14 days
Arthropod Borne Diseases	
MC arboviral disease is	Dengue
Presumptive Treatment in Malaria	Chloroquine
Malaria exhibits _____ biological transmission	Cyclo-propogative transmission
Vector of urban malaria	Anopheles stephensi
Tourniquet test (dengue) is positive if	>20 petechial spots/sq. inch in cubital fossa
Classical dengue fever is transmitted by	Aedes mosquito
Infective stage of Plasmodium to man	Sporozoite
Elimination of Lymphatic Filariasis as a global public health problem by	2020
Malaria is transmitted by	Female anopheles mosquito
Drug preferred for Chloroquine-resistant malaria in pregnancy	Quinine
Most virulent Plasmodium species	Plasmodium falciparum
Stage of Plasmodium responsible for relapses	Merozoites
Cycle that is seen in RBCs in malaria	Endogenous
Best dengue diagnosis in first week	NS1 antigen
Best indicator for malaria prevalence in a community	Spleen rate
Babesiosis is transmitted via	Ticks
Relapse in Malaria is due to	Hypnozoites
Maximum spread of malaria occurs in ____ month	September-October
Zoonoses	
Only communicable disease of man that is always fatal	Rabies
Main Vector for Yellow Fever is	Aedes aegypti

Contd...

Contd...

Pigs in Japanese Encephalitis are	Amplifier Hosts
Injected in and around the wound in class III rabies bite	Anti rabies serum
KFD is transmitted in India by	Haemaphysalis (Hard tick)
Main reservoir of Plague in India	Tatera indica (Wild Rodent)
Scrub typhus is caused by	Rickettsia tsustsugamushi
Strain of Yellow fever vaccine	17 D
Kala Azar is caused by	L. donavani
Schedule of intradermal rabies vaccine	2-2-2-0-2 (Thai updated Red cross regimen)
Leishmaniasis (Kala Azar) is transmitted by	Sand Fly (Phlebotamus)
Vector of KFD in India	Hemophysalis (Hard Tick)
Japanese encephalitis is transmitted by	Culex tritaeniorhynchus
Reservoir in Chikungunya fever	Primates (monkeys)
MC location of Hydatid cysts in body	Postero-superior lobe of liver
In the case of dog bite the biting animal should be observed for at least	10 days
Yersinia pseudotuberculosis disease resembles	Typhoid/Appendicitis (in humans)
IP of Yellow fever	2–6 days
R. prowazekii is transmitted by	Louse
Validity of YF vaccination Certificate	10 days - Lifelong
Epidemic typhus main mammalian reservoir	Human beings
Cheopis index is	Average number of cheopis per rat
Intermediate host for Hydatid disease is	Sheep (& pigs, cattle, horses, camels, man)
Soft Tick is vector of	Q fever, Relapsing Fever, KFD (outside India)
Q-fever is caused by	Coxiella burnetti
Q-fever is transmitted by	Inhalation of infected dust
Last outbreak of Plague	Dangud, Uttrakashi (2004)
Amplifier host of Japanese encephalitis	Pigs
Vector of Yellow fever	Aedes aegypti
1994 epidemic in India	Plague
Dose of equine anti-rabies immunoglobulin (ERIG)	40 IU per kg of body weight
Hydatid cyst is seen MC in	Liver
Disease with highest case fatality rate	Rabies
Quarantine period for Yellow fever	6 days
Q-fever is caused by	Coxiella burnetti
Vector of Scrub typhus	Trombiculid mite
Leptospirosis is transmitted by	Infected rat's urine
White leprosy is	Leishmaniasis
Flea-borne typhus is	Murine/Endemic typhus
"Rabies free" area has no case of indigenously acquired rabies for	> 2 years
Plague is transmitted by	Rat flea (Xenopsylla cheopsis)
Mammalian reservoir for R. prowazekii	Humans
Scrub typhus is caused by	R. tsutsugamushi
Quintan fever is caused by	B. quintana
Major reservoir of KFD	Squirrels (& Rats)
Quarantine period for Plague	6-7 days
MC variety of Plague	Bubonic

Contd...

Contd...

Reservoir for Scrub typhus	Rodents
Rickettsial disease not producing rash	Q-fever
Surface Infections	
Elimination Level for leprosy	<1 case per 10,000 population
MDT for PBL is given for	6 months
Leprosy is Public health problem if prevalence is more than	1 per 10,000 population
Yaws is caused by	Treponema pertenue
Slims' Disease is	AIDS
Lyme disease is transmitted by	Ticks (Ixodes ticks)
DOC for Lymphogranuloma venerum in India	Doxycycline
8th Day Disease is	Tetanus neonatorum
NNT is prevented by	Tetanus toxoid
Lymphogranuloma venereum is caused by	Chlamydia trachomatis
Dome shaped centrally umbilicated papules seen in	Molluscum contagiosum
Elimination Level of Neonatal tetanus is	<0.1 case per 1,000 Live births
HIV MTCT rate in India	30 %
Erythema nodosum is seen in treatment of _____ type of Leprosy	Lepromatous leprosy
HIV MTCT rate due to breastfeeding	12-16 %
As per WHO, Leprosy is a public health problem if prevalence is	> 0.01%
HIV MTCT Prevention efficacy of Nevirapine	50%
Cluster testing is useful in detecting cases of	STDs
Zidovudine is C/I with antiretroviral drug	Stavudine
Best marker of HIV progression in human body (NACP)	CD4 : CD8 ratio
MC Opportunistic Infection in HIV in World	Pneumocystis carinii Pneumonia (TB–India)
Blood screening before transfusion in India is done for	HIV, HBV, HCV, Malaria, Syphilis
Average incubation period for HIV	10 years
Mistuda reaction is read at	21st day
Scabies is caused by	Sarcoptes scabei
Incubation period of Chancroid is	4-7 days
HIV mainly affects cell type	Helper T-cells (CD4)
Prophylaxis for anthrax	Doxycycline
MC nerve involved in leprosy	Ulnar N
World AIDS day is on	01 December
"3 by 5" initiative implemented by WHO in 2003 for AIDS means	Provide ART to 3 million HIV by 2005
Indian states reporting maximum number of AIDS cases till now	Tamil Nadu
Advice to couple with both HIV+	Use condoms
Minimum duration of PEP for HIV	4 weeks
Lepromin test is strongly positive in	Tuberculoid leprosy
Duration of Multidrug Therapy to resolve Paucibacillary leprosy	6 months
Single drug treatment of trachoma	Azithromycin
First case of AIDS was reported in	1981 (USA)
World population affected with trachoma	500 million
Not a bridging population in HIV transmission	Male homosexuals
Man is dead end for	Rabies, Tetanus, Japanese encephalitis
Neonatal tetanus incidence < 1/1000 LB, TT2 coverage > 70% is	NNT control

Contd...

Contd...

Lymphogranuloma venerum is caused by	Chlamydia trachomatis (L1, L2, L2a or L3)
Granuloma inguinale caused by	Klebsiella granulomatis (Calymmatobacterium)
Minimum oil immersion fields examined for Leprosy	Minimum 100 OIFs
First test to be conducted for HIV	ELISA
'Sparsh' is an awareness campaign for	Leprosy in India
Most efficient rout of transmission of HIV	Blood & blood product
Colored kit for STD treatment is _____ approach	Syndromic
Emerging & Reemerging Infections	
DOC for Crimean Congo Fever	Ribavirin
Ocular disease not seen in India	Onchocerciasis
Mode of spread of Ebola virus	Body luids
Zika virus is transmitted by mosquito	Aedes mosquito
Non-communicable diseases	
Prevalence of Blindness in India	1.05%
WHO Blindness is	<3/60 in better eye
MCC of Blindness	Cataract
Rule of Halves is seen in	Hypertension
MC cause of heart disease in 5-30 years old is	Rheumatic fever
WHO Criteria for diagnosis of RF/RHD are based on	Revised Jones Criteria
MC Cancer in India is	Lung Cancer (M); Breast cancer (F)
Prevalence of blindness in India is	1.05%
Ideal cholesterol level should be below	200 mg/dL
Pap Smear should be done	Beginning of sexual activity, then every 3 years
BMI formula is	Weight (Kgs)/Height^2 (m^2)
Waist Hip Ratio indicates Obesity in Women when it is	> 0.85
India was certified free of Dracunculiasis on	February 2001
Corpulence index measures	Obesity
Prophylactic treatment of Rheumatic heart disease	Benzathaine penicillin
BMI of Normal Asian Men	18.5-22.99
Base population for population based cancer registry is	2–7 million
MC cancer of females in India	Breast cancer
MCC cancer death among males in India	Lung cancer
Low vision is	<6/18 in better eye
Ischemic heart disease is associated with mostly	LDL cholesterol
Cholesterol with high-risk of CHD	LDL cholesterol
Tracking of BP (Hypertension) means	Hypotensive remain hypotensive
MC carcinoma in World	Breast cancer
Chimney Sweep's Cancer is also known as	Carcinoma scrotum
Quetelet index is represented by	BMI (Weight/[Height]2)
Age-distribution showed by Breast carcinoma	Bimodal
Prevalence of RHD in India in 5-15 years age group	5-7 per 1000
Corpulence index is	Actual weight/Desired weight
Waist to hip ratio which indicates obesity in men	> 1.0
Obesity index defined as Height (cms)–100	Broca's index
A person is underweight if BMI is	< 18.5

Multiple Choice Questions

GENERAL EPIDEMIOLOGY

1. Match the following Diseases with their Longest Incubation periods [INICET May 2023]

Diseases	Incubation period
A- SARS	1- 21 days
B- Chicken pox	2- 90 days
C- Syphilis	3- 50 days
D- Hepatitis A	4- 10 days

   (a) A-2, B-4, C-3, D-1
   (b) A-4, B-1, C-2, D-3
   (c) A-2, B-1, C-4, D-3
   (d) A-4, B-1, C-3, D-2

2. Endogenous transmission of which organism is found in India? [INICET May 2022]
   (a) Ebola
   (b) Crimean congo hemorrhagic fever
   (c) Yellow fever
   (d) Hendra virus

3. Following disease has highest mortality after clinical manifestations develop [INICET November 2020]
   (a) H1N1 Influenza
   (b) NIPAH
   (c) Ebola
   (d) Rabies

4. Maternal antibodies do not provide protective immunity to neonate in [NEET PG Pattern January 2020]
   (a) Diphtheria
   (b) Pertussis
   (c) Tetanus
   (d) Polio

COVID-19 DISEASE

5. Drugs used in the treatment of severe COVID-19 infection in children include [INICET July 2021]
   (a) Steroids
   (b) Remdesivir
   (c) Ivermectin
   (d) All of the above

6. You will sanitize your hands under the following conditions (MULTIPLE RESPONSE) [INICET November 2020]
   (a) Before examining the patient
   (b) After examining the patient
   (c) After touching patients' surroundings
   (d) When you see your hands are visibly soiled

7. All are helpful in COVID 19 prevention/disinfection except: [AIIMS June 2020]
   (a) 70% ethanol
   (b) 1% Gluteraldehyde
   (c) Hand washing
   (d) Use of mask

8. Handling of Viral specimens of SARS CoV 2 requires Biosafety level: [AIIMS June 2020]
   (a) BSL-1
   (b) BSL-2
   (c) BSL-3
   (d) BSL-4

SMALLPOX and CHICKENPOX

9. A 25 years old male has been diagnosed with Varicella (Chicken pox). Advice for the contacts of the case would be [NEET PG Pattern 2023]
   (a) Isolation for 6 days
   (b) Isolation for 6 days + VZIG within 72 hours + Acyclovir
   (c) Isolation for 14 days + VZIG within 48 hours
   (d) VZIG alone is sufficient

10. A school going cousin of a 23 years old woman, living in the same house, contracts Varicella. The woman was advised Varicella antibody test that was found to be negative. What is your best statement? [NEET PG Pattern September 2021]
    (a) Woman is susceptible to Zoster
    (b) Woman is susceptible to Chicken pox
    (c) Woman is immune to Chicken pox
    (d) Woman is immune to Zoster

11. The infectivity of chickenpox lasts for: [AIPGME 2002] [UP 2002]
    (a) Till the last scab falls off
    (b) 6 days after onset of rash
    (c) 3 days after onset of rash
    (d) Till the fever subsides

12. Chickenpox is characterised by all except: [AIIMS May 1995]
    (a) Scabs are infective
    (b) Pleomorphic stages
    (c) Rashes symmetrical centripetal dew-drop like
    (d) Palms and soles not affected by rash

13. Smallpox eradication was successful due to all of the following reasons except: [AIPGME 2011] [AIIMS Nov 2010]
    (a) Subclinical cases did not transmit the disease
    (b) A highly effective vaccine was available

(c) Infection provided lifelong immunity
(d) Cross-resistance existed with animal pox

14. All of the following are true about Varicella virus *except*: [AIIMS Nov 2010]
    (a) 10-30% chances of occurrence
    (b) All stages of rash are seen at the same time
    (c) Secondary attack rate is 90%
    (d) Rash commonly seen in flexor area

15. Secondary attack rate of chickenpox is: [NEET Pattern 2013]
    (a) 60
    (b) 50
    (c) 90
    (d) 40

16. Chickenpox is infective: [NEET Pattern 2014]
    (a) 2 days before and 2 days after rash appearance
    (b) 2 days before and 5 days after rash appearance
    (c) 4 days before and 4 days after rash appearance
    (d) 4 days before and 5 days after rash appearance

17. True about chickenpox are all *except*:
    (a) Caused by Herpes simplex type-3
    (b) SAR is 90% [NEET Pattern 2016]
    (c) Superficial rash
    (d) Single stage of rash is seen

18. Varicella zoster virus infection is more likely to occur in which of the following months? [NEET Pattern 2017]
    (a) March
    (b) August
    (c) October
    (d) November

19. Shingles is caused by: [NEET Pattern 2018]
    (a) Variola major
    (b) Varicella zoster virus
    (c) CMV
    (d) Toxoplasma

20. True about Chickenpox infection: [NEET Pattern 2017]
    (a) Centrifugal distribution
    (b) Centripetal distribution
    (c) Severe prodromal symptoms
    (d) Involves mainly extensor surface

MEASLES

21. A 5 years old child presented to OPD at a PHC with a history of fever and rash. On examination, the child has Koplik spots in the buccal mucosa. Diagnosis is: [NEET PG Pattern 2020, 2023]
    (a) Chicken pox
    (b) Measles
    (c) Mumps
    (d) Rubella

22. A women had two children named Ram and Shyam. One day, Shyam had Measles with fever and rash. After few days, Ram developed the same symptoms. He was reported to the sub-centre. Which of the following is/are correct? [INICET May 2022]
    (a) Ram is the index case
    (b) Shyam is primary case
    (c) Ram got infected from Shyam
    (d) If mother had reported when Shyam got infection, Ram could have been vaccinated

23. Which of the following is not true of Measles?
    (a) High secondary attack rate [AIPGME 2008]
    (b) Only one strain causes infection
    (c) Not infectious in pro-dromal stage
    (d) Infection confers lifelong immunity

24. Which of the following is the 'Least common' complication of measles? [AIIMS May 2006, May 2007; NEET Pattern 2014]
    (a) Diarrhea   (b) Pneumonia
    (c) Otitis media (d) SSPE

25. Which of the following statements is true about the epidemiological determinants of measles? [AIIMS Nov 2005]
    (a) Measles virus survives outside the human body for 5 days
    (b) Carriers are important sources of infection
    (c) Secondary attack rate is less than that of rubella
    (d) Incidence of measles is more in males than females

26. True about measles is all *except*: [AIPGME 1996]
    (a) Kopliks spots appear as rash disappears
    (b) It is prevented by both active and passive immunization
    (c) Otitis media and meningitis are the most common complications
    (d) TB is aggravated in post measles

27. All are true regarding measles vaccine *except*: [AIPGME 1996]
    (a) Freeze dried live attenuated vaccine
    (b) Single intramascular dose of 0.5 mL
    (c) Is occasionally associated with TSS
    (d) Contraindicated in pregnancy

28. True about measles: [PGI June 04]
    (a) Koplik spot appears in Prodromal stage
    (b) Fever stops after onset of Rash
    (c) Vaccine given at 9 months
    (d) It is not diagnosed when coryza and rhinitis is absent
    (e) Incubation period is 6 days

29. Koplik spots are seen in: [DNB December 2011; Bihar 2006]
    (a) Prodromal stage   (b) Incubation
    (c) Eruptive   (d) Convalescent stage

30. Most common cause of death due to measles is:
    (a) Pneumonia [AP 2014]
    (b) Secondary bacterial infection [Bihar 2006]
    (c) Measles encephalitis
    (d) Otitis media

31. Post-exposure Measles vaccine must be given within ... day(s) of exposure: [NEET Pattern 2015]
    (a) 1 day   (b) 3 days
    (c) 7 days   (d) 10 days

32. Supplementary immunization service for measles immunization: [NEET Pattern 2015]
    (a) Keep up with >95% immunized
    (b) Catch up
    (c) Follow up   (d) All of the above

33. True about Measles: [NEET Pattern 2016]
    (a) More in summer   (b) Two types of vaccine
    (c) Infectivity decreases after appearance of rash
    (d) Incubation period is 10-14 days

34. True about Measles rash appearance
    (a) Along with Koplik spots [NEET Pattern 2016]
    (b) 1-2 days before Koplik spots
    (c) 1-2 days after Koplik spots
    (d) Post-measles stage

35. Period of isolation for Measles is from: [AIIMS November 2018]
    (a) Onset of catarrhal symptoms to 3 days after
    (b) Onset of catarrhal symptoms to 7 days after
    (c) Onset of catarrhal symptoms to 6 days after
    (d) Onset of catarrhal symptoms to 8 days after

Review Questions

36. To eradicate measles the percentage of infant population to be vaccinated is at least ____%:
    [DNB 2001, 05; NEET Pattern 2012]
    (a) 70   (b) 80
    (c) 85   (d) 95

37. In Measles, infective period is:
    [UP 2008; NEET Pattern 2017]
    (a) 3 days before and 4 days after the appearance of rash
    (b) 4 days before and 3 days after the appearance of rash
    (c) 4 days before and 5 days after the appearance of rash
    (d) 5 days before and 4 days after the appearance of rash

38. All are true about measles except: [MP 2000]
    (a) Both active and passive immunization are given simultaneously
    (b) Flaring up of TB
    (c) Most infectious during rashes
    (d) Causes pneumonia and otitis media

39. A baby was given a dose measles vaccine at 6 months of age due to epidemic of measles/malnutrition. Correct regarding giving subsequent dose will be: [MH 2007]
    (a) Give one more dose as soon as possible
    (b) Give after 14-16 months with booster dose
    (c) Give after 9 months age
    (d) No dose required

RUBELLA

40. A premature baby having Low birth weight is delivered today. On examination, the baby is having cataract (bilateral), PDA and possibly hearing impairment. Underlying cause could be [NEET PG Pattern 2023]
    (a) CMV
    (b) Toxoplasmosis
    (c) HSV
    (d) Rubella

41. Recommended vaccination strategy for rubella is to vaccinate first and foremost: [AIPGME 2007; RJ 2008]
    (a) Women 15-49 yrs
    (b) Infants
    (c) Adolescent girls
    (d) Children 1-14 yrs

42. Risk of the damage of fetus by maternal rubella is maximum if mother gets infected in: [AIIMS Nov 2005]
    (a) 6-12 weeks of pregnancy [AIIMS 1997]
    (b) 20-24 weeks of pregnancy
    (c) 24-28 weeks of pregnancy
    (d) 32-36 weeks of pregnancy

43. All of the following statements are true about Congenital Rubella except: [AIIMS 2011, AIPGME 2005]
    (a) It is diagnosed when the infant has IgM antibodies at birth
    (b) It is diagnosed when IgG antibodies persist for more than 6 months
    (c) Most common congenital defects are deafness, cardiac malformations and cataract
    (d) Infection after 16 weeks of gestation results in major congenital defects

44. MMR vaccine is recommended at the age of:
    [NEET Pattern 2013]
    (a) 9-12 months   (b) 15-18 months
    (c) 2-3 years   (d) 10-19 years

45. Rubella is caused by: [NEET Pattern 2019]
    (a) Orthomyxovirus   (b) Paramyxovirus
    (c) Toga virus   (d) Arbovirus group B

46. Congenital Rubella Syndrome include all except:
    (a) Cataract [NEET Pattern 2019]
    (b) VSD
    (c) Intracerebral hemorrhage
    (d) SN deafness

MUMPS

47. M.C. complication of mumps in children is: [RJ 2004]
    (a) Pneumonia   (b) Pancreatitis
    (c) Aseptic meningitis (d) Encephalitis

48. Incubation period of Mumps is: [NEET Pattern 2013]
    (a) 7 days (b) 10 days
    (c) 14 days (d) 18 days

INFLUENZA

49. Recent Influenza Pandemic was due to which strain?
    [NEET PG Pattern January 2020]
    (a) H1N1 (b) H5N1
    (c) H7N7 (d) H3N2

50. Regarding Influenza, not true statement is:
    [AIIMS November 2019]
    (a) Secondary attack rate 5-15%
    (b) Virus shedding present before the patient presents with symptoms
    (c) 1-5 years age is not a high risk age group
    (d) Aquatic birds are reservoir

51. Which of the following is not true about influenza virus?
    [AIIMS June 1999]
    (a) Influenza virus A is subject to frequent antigenic variations
    (b) Antigenic drift is a gradual antigenic change over a period of time
    (c) Antigenic shift is due to genetic recombination of virus
    (d) Major epidemics are due to antigenic drift

52. Newer Influenza vaccine includes: [PGI June 08]
    (a) Split – virus vaccine
    (b) Neuraminidase
    (c) Live attenuated vaccine
    (d) Killed vaccine
    (e) Recombinant vaccine

53. True about epidemiology of influenza:
    (a) Asymptomatic seen rarely [PGI June 05]
    (b) Incubation period 10-12 hrs
    (c) Pandemic rare
    (d) Extra human reservoir not seen
    (e) All ages and sex equally affected

54. Which of the following is true about influenza:
    (a) Affects all ages and sexes [PGI June 06]
    (b) I. P 18 – 72 hrs
    (c) Pandemics rare
    (d) Asymptomatics rare
    (e) No animal reservoir

55. Which of the following lead to an outbreak of Influenza in China in 2013? [PGI May 2013]
    (a) H1N1 (b) H3N2
    (c) H2N2 (d) H7N9
    (e) H5N1

56. Pig in H1N1 influenza acts as: [DNB December 2010]
    (a) Carrier (b) Amplifying host
    (c) Reservoir (d) Vector

57. Major reason for H5N1 not to become a global pandemic is: [AIIMS November 2014]
    (a) Route of transmission is not respiratory
    (b) Man to man transmission is rare
    (c) Does not cause serious disease among humans
    (d) Restricted to few countries only

58. All are used in treatment of Influenza B except:
    [NEET Pattern 2015]
    (a) Oseltamivir (b) Zanamivir
    (c) Premavir (d) Ribavirin

59. True about Influenza infectivity: [NEET Pattern 2016]
    (a) Communicable period is 5 days before to 5 days after the onset of symptoms
    (b) Source of infection is clinical case
    (c) There are no subclinical cases
    (d) All are correct

60. What is common to H5N1 and H7N7 strains of Influenza?
    [NEET Pattern 2016]
    (a) Frequently endemic infection in man
    (b) Have same frequency of antigenic variation
    (c) Strains of Avian influenza
    (d) All are correct

61. Not used for treatment and/or prophylaxis of Seasonal influenza: [NEET Pattern 2015]
    (a) Amantadine
    (b) Rimantadine
    (c) Oseltamivir
    (d) Acyclovir

62. According to WHO, a conformed case of swine flu (HINI) was defined as a person with acute febrile respiratory illness with laboratory conferment WHO laboratories by all of the following tests *except*:
    [NEET Pattern 2016]
    (a) Real time PCR
    (b) Viral culture
    (c) 4 fold rise in virus specific neutralizing antibodies
    (d) ELISA

63. High risk group for Influenza is: [PGI November 2017]
    (a) Morbid obese
    (b) Young adult
    (c) Children <18 months
    (d) Pregnant women
    (e) Elderly person

DIPHTHERIA

64. A 3 years old child diagnosed provisionally with Diphtheria and on examination he has a grayish white pseudomembrane around his tonsils (image shown). The child has a 6 years old sibling at home, who is fully immunized as per the Immunization schedule. What is the best measure to prevent Disease in the sibling of the child?
    [NEET PG Pattern January 2020]

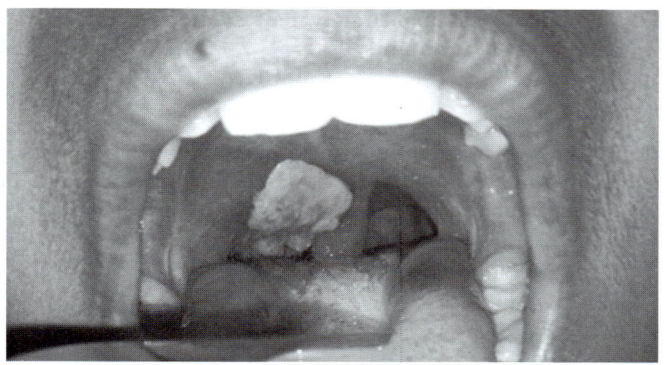

(a) Full course of DPT vaccine given
(b) Booster dose of DPT
(c) Nothing is required to be done
(d) Prophylactic erythromycin to be given

65. True about Diphtheria are all *except*:
   (a) Carriers are more common sources of infection than cases *[AIPGME 1996] [AIIMS Nov 1996]*
   (b) Incubation period is 2-6 days
   (c) 25 Lf of diphtheria toxoid are present per ml in DPT vaccine
   (d) Diphtheria is an endemic disease in India

66. A herd immunity of over .... % is considered necessary to prevent epidemic spread of diphtheria: *[NEET Pattern 2012; DNB 2000]*
   (a) 50%   (b) 55%
   (c) 60%   (d) 70%

67. Management of non-immunized diphtheria contacts include all except: *[PGI November 2014]*
   (a) Prophylactic penicillin
   (b) Single dose of toxoid
   (c) Daily throat examination
   (d) Daily throat swab culture
   (e) Weekly throat swabs examination

68. Incubation period of Diphtheria and Salmonella is: *[NEET Pattern 2015]*
   (a) 1-2 days & 20-40 days
   (b) 2-6 days & 7-21 days
   (c) 2-6 days & 10-14 days
   (d) 1-2 days & 10-14 days

69. In recent surveillance reports cases of diphtheria are reducing. This is due to: *[NEET Pattern 2016]*
   (a) Chemoprophylaxis
   (b) Improved standard of living
   (c) Vaccination
   (d) Health education

70. Dose of Diphtheria antitoxin is: *[NEET Pattern 2019]*
   (a) 5000-10000 Units
   (b) 10000-15000 Units
   (c) 50000-100000 Units
   (d) 1000-5000 Units

71. Drug of choice for Prophylaxis against Diphtheria is: *[NEET Pattern 2019]*
   (a) Ciprofloxacin   (b) Amoxycillin
   (c) Erythromycin   (d) Cotrimoxazole

Review Question

72. Treatment of choice for diphtheria carriers is: *[DNB 2003]*
   (a) Erythromycin   (b) Tetracycline
   (c) Penicillin   (d) DPT

WHOOPING COUGH

73. Which of the following statements is true regarding pertussis? *[AIPGME 2002]*
   (a) Neurological complication rate of DPT is 1 in 50000
   (b) Vaccine efficacy is more than 95%
   (c) Erythromycin prevents spread of disease between children
   (d) Leukocytosis correlates with the severity of cough

74. True regarding pertussis is all *except*: *[AIIMS Nov 1997, AIIMS May 1995]*
   (a) It is associated with an inspiratory whoop
   (b) It is a droplet infection
   (c) Parapertussis causes more severe disease than pertussis
   (d) Pneumonia is most common complication

75. True about Pertussis is/are: *[PGI May 2012]*
   (a) Incubation period is 7-14 days
   (b) Main source of infection is chronic carriers
   (c) Can affect any age
   (d) Secondary attack rate in unimmunised persons is 90%
   (e) More common in Summers

76. True about Pertussis is: *[NEET Pattern 2015]*
   (a) Most of the infections are subclinical
   (b) Most infective stage is Paroxysmal stage
   (c) Drug of choice is Erythromycin
   (d) Cerebellar ataxia may be a chronic common complication

Review Questions

77. Treatment for pertussis contacts children for: *[UP 2000]*
   (a) Prophylactic antibiotic for 10 days
   (b) Prophylactic antibiotic for 14 days
   (c) Prophylactic antibiotic for 12 days
   (d) Prophylactic antibiotic for 11 days

78. About pertussis true is: *[MP 2000]*
   (a) Secondary attack rate 90%
   (b) No cross immunity with parapertussis
   (c) Most infectious during paroxysmal stage
   (d) Affects only humans

MENINGOCOCCAL MENINGITIS

79. True about meningococcal meningitis is:
    [AIIMS May 1994]
    (a) Causative agent is a Gram –ve diplococci
    (b) Cases are the most important source of infection
    (c) Treatment with penicillin eradicates carrier state
    (d) Vaccine can be given in pregnancy

80. Xavier and Yogender stay in the same hostel of the same university. Xavier develops infection with Group B meningococcus. After a few days, Yogender develops infection due to Group C meningococcus. All the following are true statements *except*: [AIPGME 2002]
    (a) Educate students about meningococcal transmission and take preventive measures
    (b) Chemoprophylaxis against both Group B and Group C
    (c) Vaccine prophylaxis of contacts of Xavier
    (d) Vaccine prophylaxis of contacts of Yogender

81. Vaccine for meningococcal meningitis should be routinely given to: [AIIMS PGMEE May 2013]
    (a) Laboratory workers
    (b) Young adolescents
    (c) 4-8 years old children
    (d) Elderly population

82. Prophylaxis of meningococcal meningitis is:
    [WB 2008, DNB December 2009]
    (a) Ciprofloxacin (b) Rifampicin
    (c) Penicillin (d) Gentamicin

83. WHO criteria for High endemicity for Meningococcal disease include: [AIIMS PGMEE May 2013]
    (a) 0.1% (b) 0.01%
    (c) 0.001% (d) 1.0%

84. Meningococcal vaccine available is:
    [NEET Pattern 2013]
    (a) ACW135Y
    (b) ABCW135
    (c) CYW135B
    (d) ABCY

85. With reference to meningococcal meningitis, which one of the following statements is not correct?
    [UPSC CMS 2015]
    (a) Fatality in untreated cases is 60%
    (b) Disease spreads mainly by droplet infection
    (c) Treatment of cases has no significant effect in epidemiological pattern of disease
    (d) Mass chemoprophylaxis causes immediate drop in incidence rate of cases

86. Meningococcal vaccine contains:
    [NEET Pattern 2017]
    (a) 50 mcg of polysaccharide of each strain
    (b) 100 mcg of polysaccharide of each strain
    (c) 1000 mcg of polysaccharide of each strain
    (d) 5000 mcg of polysaccharide of each strain

87. How many doses of monovalent meningococcal 'C' vaccine is given in Infants? [NEET Pattern 2017]
    (a) One (b) Two
    (c) Three (d) Four

88. In a case of meningitis, Neisseria meningitides was grown in culture after 48 hours. Which measure is to be taken immediately? [NEET Pattern 2017]
    (a) Isolation of contacts
    (b) Antibiotic treatment of contacts
    (c) Vaccination of contact
    (d) All of the above

ARI

89. A 2-year-old female child was brought to a PHC with a history of cough and fever for 4 days with inability to drink for last 12 hours. On examination, the child was having weight of 5 kg and respiratory rate of 45/minute with fever. The child will be classified as suffering from:
    [AIPGME 2004, 2005, AIIMS June 2000]
    (a) Very severe disease (b) TB
    (c) Pneumonia (d) No Pneumonia

90. A child aged 24 months was brought to the Primary Health Centre with complaints of cough and fever for the past 2 days. On examination, the child weighed 11 Kg respiratory rate was 38 per minute, chest indrawing was present. The most appropriate line of management for this patient is? [AIPGME 2002, IPGME 2003]
    (a) Classify as pneumonia and refer urgently to secondary level hospital
    (b) Classify as pneumonia, start antibiotic and advise to report after 2 days
    (c) Classify as severe pneumonia, start antibiotics and refer urgently
    (d) Classify as severe pneumonia and refer urgently

91. A 10-month-old child is brought to a PHC with history of cough and cold. On examination, he has respiratory rate of 48 breaths per minute and there is absence of chest indrawing. His weight is 5 kg. He is probably suffering from: [AIIMS November 2014]
    (a) No pneumonia
    (b) Pneumonia
    (c) Severe pneumonia
    (d) Very severe pneumonia

92. Not evaluated in Clinical evaluation pneumonia at PHC:
    [NEET Pattern 2014]
    (a) Respiratory rate (b) Inability to feed
    (c) Oxygen saturation (d) Chest in drawing

93. Fast breathing in a 6-month old infant is taken as:
    [NEET Pattern 2019]
    (a) >60 breaths/min
    (b) >50 breaths/min
    (c) >40 breaths/min
    (d) >30 breaths/min

Review Question

94. Respiratory rate can be diagnosed as fast breathing in a less than 2-month-old infant, if respiratory rate/minute is more than: [Kolkata 2004]
    (a) 29
    (b) 39
    (c) 49
    (d) 59

TUBERCULOSIS

95. MDR TB is resistance to [NEET PG Pattern 2022]
    (a) Rifampicin, Isoniazid and Fluoroquinolone
    (b) Rifampicin, Isoniazid and Kanamycin
    (c) Rifampicin and Kanamycin
    (d) Isoniazid and Rifampicin

96. All are targeted in End TB strategy *except*: [NEET Pattern 2017]
    (a) 95% reduction in deaths due to TB
    (b) 90% reduction in Incidence of TB
    (c) 0% TB-affected families facing catastrophic costs
    (d) 0% HIV-TB coinfection rate

97. If the objective of the investigator is to assess the incidence of tuberculosis infection in a community, the most appropriate methodology would be to: [AIIMS Nov 2005, 2006, AIPGME 2007]
    (a) Identify all individuals with positive tuberculin test
    (b) Perform sputum examination of chest symptomatics
    (c) Identify new converters to Tuberculin test
    (d) Screen all under-five children with Tuberculin test

98. Point of control in tuberculosis the infection is:
    (a) < 1% in 0-14 group of children [AIPGME 1991]
    (b) > 1% is all children 0-5 yrs age group
    (c) < 1% in 15-49 of age group
    (d) < 2% in 0-14 group

99. The most appropriate test to assess the prevalence of tuberculosis infection in a community is:
    [AIIMS May 1992; AIPGME 2004; NEET Pattern 2014]
    (a) Mass Miniature Radiography
    (b) Sputum examination
    (c) Tuberculin test
    (d) Clinical examination

100. National Tuberculosis Institute is located at:
     [AIIMS Nov 2003; DNB 2003]
     (a) New Delhi
     (b) Chingelput
     (c) Bangalore
     (d) Chennai

101. Decrease in which of the following parameters indicate the decrease in tuberculosis problem in India?
     (a) Incidence of infection [DPG 2004]
     (b) Prevalence of infection
     (c) Incidence of disease
     (d) Prevalence of disease

102. The overall prevalence of tuberculosis infection in India as per 4th round of longitudinal survey was:
     [Karnataka 2004]
     (a) 20%
     (b) 30%
     (c) 40%
     (d) 50%

103. The percentage of positive Mantoux test in Indian if 20-40 yrs age group is: [PGI Dec 03]
     (a) < 5%
     (b) 5 – 10%
     (c) 20 – 30%
     (d) > 50%
     (e) > 80%

104. Population of a village on 1st June 2007 is 16,500. Since 1st January 2007, 22 new cases of TB were detected. Total registered cases were 220. What is the incidence of TB? [AIPGME 2010]
     (a) 133 per 100,000
     (b) 121 per 100,000
     (c) 111 per 100,000
     (d) 100 per 100,000

105. McKneown's Theory states that reduced prevalence of Tuberculosis occurs due to: [AIPGME 2011]
     (a) Enhanced knowledge and awareness
     (b) Medical advancements
     (c) Behavioural modification
     (d) Social and environmental factors

106. A lactating woman has sputum positive Tuberculosis and her neonate child is 3 months old. What is the recommended chemoprophylaxis? [AIIMS May 2011]
     (a) INH 3 mg/kg for 3 months
     (b) INH 5 mg/kg for 3 months
     (c) INH 3 mg/kg for 6 months
     (d) INH 5 mg/kg for 6 months

107. Incidence of TB in a community measured by:
     [DNB December 2011; NEET Patterns 2014, 2018]
     (a) Sputum smear +
     (b) Tuberculin test +
     (c) Sputum culture
     (d) Mantoux test +

108. One of the following is known as Tuberculin Conversion Index: [NUPGET 2013]
     (a) Incidence of infection
     (b) Prevalence of infection
     (c) Incidence of disease
     (d) Prevalence of disease

109. Xpert MTB/RIF test is used to detect: [PGI May 2013]
     (a) For assessing resistance to isoniazid
     (b) For assessing multi drug resistant TB
     (c) For assessing rifampicin resistance
     (d) Monitoring drug response in MDR TB
     (e) Diagnosis of TB

110. TB multidrug regimen is given to: [NEET Pattern 2013]
     (a) Prevent resistance
     (b) Broad spectrum
     (c) Prevent side effects
     (d) None

111. Contacts of Sputum positive tuberculosis patient who should be given preventive chemotherapy:
     (a) Pregnant women [NEET Pattern 2014]
     (b) Old people
     (c) Children above 6 years
     (d) Children below 6 years

112. Tuberculin test is a cheap and easily available test. In which of the following situations there is high failure in interpretation of result? [AIIMS PG May 2015]
    (a) Environmental mycobacterium infections are less
    (b) High prevalence of immunized people
    (c) High prevalence of disease
    (d) Lesser number of HIV positive cases

113. What is true about TB in a diabetic?
    (a) Severity of TB increases [NEET Pattern 2015]
    (b) Incidence of TB increases
    (c) Course of TB disease changes
    (d) All of the above

114. WHO defines Multi-drug resistant (MDR) Tuberculosis strain as one that is: [UPSC CMS 2015]
    (a) At least resistant to INH
    (b) At least resistant to Rifampicin
    (c) Resistant to INH and Rifampicin with or without resistant to other anti TB drugs
    (d) Resistant to Streptomycin only

115. According to WHO Guidelines, Latent TB investigation is not done in: [AIIMS November 2015]
    (a) Patient on TNF inhibitors
    (b) Silicosis
    (c) Chronic alcoholism
    (d) Dialysis

Review Questions

116. Tuberculin unit is: [DNB 2003]
    (a) 0.0001 mg
    (b) 1 unit of PPD RT3
    (c) 0.1 mg BCG
    (d) None of the above

117. True about tuberculosis: [MP 2000]
    (a) >10^4 bacilli are required in sputum for detection
    (b) Mantoux test can differentiate between BCG and infection
    (c) Can be grown on ordinary culture media
    (d) Drug sensitivity is tested by Schick test

118. In India, a tubercular mother is advised for all except:
    (a) Give baby BCG [RJ 2003]
    (b) ATT to mother
    (c) With hold Breastfeeding
    (d) None of these

POLIOMYELITIS

119. Which type of sample can be used to isolate poliovirus earliest? [AIIMS Nov 2004]
    (a) Stool
    (b) Blood
    (c) Throat
    (d) CSF

120. True about oral polio vaccine: [PGI June 03]
    (a) Poliomyelitis in recipients
    (b) Poliomyelitis in contact of recipient
    (c) Guillain-barre syndrome
    (d) Vomiting and fever

121. True about complete eradication of poliomyelitis from India is: [AIIMS PGMEE November 2013]
    (a) From 2012 onwards, no vaccine associated polio case has been detected
    (b) Last polio case in India was reported in 13 January 2011
    (c) Mostly IPV is used currently
    (d) India is the only country which is not able to eliminate it completely

122. Regarding poliovirus responsible for poliomyelitis all are true except: [DNB June 2010]
    (a) Type 3 is most common is India
    (b) Type 1 is most common in India
    (c) Type 1 is responsible for most epidemics
    (d) Type 2 is eradicated worldwide

123. Which of the following is not a type of Vaccine derived polio virus? [AIIMS November 2014]
    (a) cVDPV
    (b) iVDPV
    (c) aVDPV
    (d) mVDPV

124. Which of the following serotypes of Polio virus is most commonly associated with vaccine associated paralytic poliomyelitis? [PGMCET 2015]
    (a) Serotype 1
    (b) Serotype 2
    (c) Serotype 3
    (d) Serotype 1 and 2

125. Which of the following is least suggestive of poliovirus infection? [UPSC CMS 2015]
    (a) Low grade fever and malaise with complete resolution in 2 to 3 days
    (b) Biphasic illness with several days of fever, then meningeal symptoms and asymmetric flaccid paralysis 5 to 10 days later
    (c) Descending motor paralysis with preservation of tendon reflexes and absent sensation
    (d) Failure to isolate a virus from the CSF in the presence of marked meningismus

126. Paralysis in Polio is characterized by:
    (a) Exaggerated tendon reflexes [NEET Pattern 2017]
    (b) Symmetrical paralysis
    (c) Tonic paralysis
    (d) Lower motor neuron type

Review Questions

127. Mg++ is used in OPV vaccine as: [Kolkata 2008]
    (a) Stabilizer
    (b) Adjuvant
    (c) Preservative
    (d) Vehicle

128. Wrong about polio patient who had paralysis: [RJ 2006]
    (a) Most predominant polio virus during epidemic is type I
    (b) Sub clinical infection common
    (c) Can transmit It by nasal discharge
    (d) Can be given vaccine

129. All are true about SALK vaccine *except*: [RJ 2009]
    (a) It prevents paralysis
    (b) Oral polio can be given as booster
    (c) It is contraindicated in immunocompromised patients
    (d) Easily transported

HEPATITIS

130. A person reported with Chronic Hepatitis B, which of the following Serum markers are likely to be seen in profile? [INICET May 2022]
    (a) HbsAg +
    (b) Anti HBs +
    (c) Anti HBc +
    (d) HBV DNA +

131. A 35 years old patient reported suffering with malaise and fatigue since last 2 months. On laboratory examination, his serum parameters depicted HBsAg + with IgM core antibody +. Diagnosis is [NEET PG Pattern 2022]
    (a) Chronic hepatitis B
    (b) Chronic hepatitis C
    (c) Acute hepatitis B
    (d) Acute hepatitis C

132. Hepatitis-B subunit vaccine is derived from which antigen? [INICET November 2021]
    (a) HBeAg
    (b) HBsAg
    (c) HBcAg
    (d) HB DNA

133. A man presents with the following Serum markers profile for Hepatitis B. PROFILE: HBsAg–, HBeAg –, Anti HBc IgG + [INICET November 2021]
    Stage of infection is:
    (a) Precore mutant infection
    (b) Chronic Hepatitis B
    (c) Window period
    (d) Remote recovered

134. Intern had a prick from positive Hepatitis B patient. Anti HBs values were 91 mIU/L of the intern while patient was HBsAg positive. Next line of management will be: [AIIMS June 2020]
    (a) 1 dose of HBIG and be revaccinated as soon as possible
    (b) 1 dose of Hepatitis B vaccine
    (c) 1 dose of HBIG and 1 dose of Hepatitis B vaccine
    (d) No post-exposure HBV management is necessary

135. Which of the following is not transmitted through sexual route? [AIPGME 2003]
    (a) Hepatitis A
    (b) Hepatitis E
    (c) Both Hepatitis A and Hepatitis E
    (d) Hepatitis D

136. Which of the Hepatitis B Virus serological marker indicates the first evidence of Hepatitis B infection? [Karnataka 2009]
    (a) Anti-HBs
    (b) Anti-HBc
    (c) HBeAg
    (d) HBsAg

137. Which of the following is true about HCV screening? [PGI Dec 04]
    (a) Medical students are screened before their joining
    (b) IV drug abuser are prone to infection
    (c) Blood products taken before 1997 should be screened
    (d) Long term hemodialysis
    (e) Interferon is treatment

138. Hepatitis A true is: [PGI June 06]
    (a) Causes mild illness in children
    (b) 3% incidence of carrier state
    (c) Sexual route common
    (d) 10% transform into HCC
    (e) Vertical Transmission never seen

139. Which of the following is/are seen in Acute Hepatitis-B? [PGI May 2011]
    (a) HBsAg
    (b) Anti-HBs
    (c) Anti-HBc
    (d) HBeAg
    (e) Anti-HBe

140. Both HBsAg and HBeAg are positive in: [AIIMS PGMEE May 2013]
    (a) Acute infectious Hepatitis B [AIIMS Nov 2014]
    (b) Chronic Hepatitis B
    (c) Recovery phase of Hepatitis B
    (d) Individuals vaccinated with Hepatitis B

141. Acute Hepatitis B marker(s) is/are: [PGI May 2012]
    (a) HBsAg
    (b) Anti HBs
    (c) Anti HBc
    (d) HBeAg
    (e) Anti HBe

142. A mother is HBsAg positive at 32 weeks of pregnancy. What should be given to the newborn to prevent neonatal infection? [NEET Pattern 2013]
    (a) Hepatitis B vaccine + Immunoglobulin
    (b) Immunoglobulin only
    (c) Hepatitis B vaccine only
    (d) Immunoglobulin followed by vaccine 1 month later

143. A nurse was diagnosed to have HBeAg and HBsAg in serum. Most likely she is having:
    (a) Chronic hepatitis B [AIIMS November 2014]
    (b) HBV + HBE coinfection
    (c) Active and infectious Hepatitis B disease
    (d) Recovery from Hepatitis B

144. Seen in Superinfection of HDV is: [NEET Pattern 2015]
    (a) IgM Anti-HBc, IgM Anti-HDV
    (b) IgM Anti-HBs, HDVAg, IgM Anti-HDV, HDV RNA
    (c) IgM Anti-HBc, HDVAg, IgM Anti-HDV, HDV RNA
    (d) HDVAg, IgM Anti-HDV, HDV RNA

145. Which of the following viral markers signifies the ongoing viral replication in the case of Hepatitis-B infection? [UPSC CMS 2015]
    (a) Anti-HBs
    (b) Anti-HBc
    (c) HBe Ag
    (d) HBs Ag

146. A person shows HBsAg +, AntiHBc IgG +, HBeAg+, AntiHBe Ab -. Diagnosis: [NEET Pattern 2015]
    (a) Acute Hepatitis B
    (b) Vaccination
    (c) Recovery from Hepatitis B
    (d) Chronic Hepatitis B with high infectivity

Review Question

147. Hepatitis A virus shedding in faeces is: [UP 2004]
    (a) One week before the symptoms appear
    (b) Two weeks after the symptoms appear
    (c) Two weeks before the symptoms and two week thereafter
    (d) One week before the symptoms and one week thereafter

DIARRHEAL DISEASES (CHOLERA AND TYPHOID)

148. Which of the following statements is/are true regarding Typhoid disease? (Multiple response) [INICET May 2022]
    (a) For prevention of typhoid most important step is immunization
    (b) Proper disposal of feces, safe water supply, personal hygiene is more important than immunization
    (c) Resistance to drugs in typhoid is less severe than that of TB
    (d) Person to person transmission is present in 10% cases

149. A 32 years old patient develops vomiting 3-4 hours after eating a meal. What is the most likely cause? [NEET PG Pattern January 2020]
    (a) Staphylococcus aureus
    (b) Salmonella enteritidis
    (c) Clostridium botulinum
    (d) Clostridium perfirengens

150. The freshly prepared ORS (Oral Rehydration Solution) should not be used after: [AIPGME 1993]
    (a) 6 hours
    (b) 12 hours
    (c) 18 hours
    (d) 24 hours

151. A 5-year-old boy passed 18 loose stools in last 24 hours and vomited twice in last 4 hours. He is irritable but drinking fluids. The optimal therapy for this child is:
    (a) Intravenous fluids [AIPGME 2003]
    (b) Oral rehydration therapy
    (c) Intravenous fluid initially for 4 hours followed by oral fluids
    (d) Plain water add libitum

152. Which of the following is the drug of choice for chemoprophylaxis of cholera? [AIIMS May 2005; UP 2004; NEET Pattern 2013]
    (a) Tetracycline
    (b) Doxycycline
    (c) Furazolidon
    (d) Cotrimoxazole

153. The usual incubation period for typhoid fever is: [AIIMS May 1994; NEET Patterns 2012, 13]
    (a) 10-14 days
    (b) 3-5 days
    (c) 21-25 days
    (d) Less then 3 days

154. The drug of choice for treating cholera in children is: [AIIMS Nov 2005; UP 2004]
    (a) Tetracycline
    (b) Doxycycline
    (c) Furazolidone
    (d) Cotrimoxazole

155. True about citrate in ORS: [AIIMS June 1997]
    (a) Increases shelf life
    (b) Nutritious
    (c) Cheaper
    (d) Tastier

156. The sodium content of ReSoMal (rehydration solution for malnourished children) is: [AIPGME 2006]
    (a) 90 mmol/L
    (b) 60 mmol/L
    (c) 45 mmol/L
    (d) 30 mmol/L

157. Which one of the following gives strong evidence of Typhoid Fever carrier status: [AIIMS Nov 2008]
    (a) Isolation of Core antigen
    (b) Isolation of Vi antigen
    (c) Persistence of Vi antibodies
    (d) Demonstration of Typhoid bacilli in stools

158. For controlling an outbreak of cholera, all of the following measures are recommended *except*:
    (a) Mass chemoprophylaxis [AIPGME-1992 and 2003]
    (b) Proper disposal of excreta [AIIMS 1991, 1997]
    (c) Chlorination of water
    (d) Early detection and management of cases

159. A convalescent case of cholera remains infective for: [DPG 2005; NEET Pattern 2017]
    (a) < 7 days
    (b) 7-14 days
    (c) 14-21 days
    (d) 21-28 days

160. Ringer lactate true is: [PGI Dec 07]
    (a) Cl^- - 111
    (b) Na^+ - 45
    (c) K^+ - 5
    (d) Lactate – 29
    (e) Ca^{+2} - 5

161. A 12 kg child with diarrhoea, fluid to be replaced in first 4 hours: [NEET Pattern 2013]
    (a) 0-400 ml
    (b) 400-800 ml
    (c) 800-1200 ml
    (d) 1200-1600 ml

162. Which is true of typhoid? [DNB 2008]
    (a) Female carriers are less common
    (b) Male carriers though less are more dangerous
    (c) Gall bladder usually not involved in carrier state
    (d) Tetracycline is the DOC for carriers

163. ORS contains 75 mmol/litre of: [NEET Pattern 2013; DNB December 2011]
    (a) Sodium
    (b) Potassium
    (c) Glucose
    (d) Chloride

164. Dehydration in a child with diarrhoea, thirst present, tears absent is: [NEET Pattern 2013]
    (a) Mild
    (b) Moderate
    (c) Severe
    (d) None

Communicable and Non-communicable Diseases

165. New WHO ORS osmolarity is:
 [NEET Patterns 2012, 2017; PGMCET 2015]
 (a) 270 (b) 245
 (c) 290 (d) 310

166. Which of the following about the composition of new ORS is wrong: [DNB June 2009]
 (a) NaCl- 2.6 grams/litre
 (b) KC1- 1.5 grams/litre
 (c) Glucose - 13.5 grams/litre
 (d) Total osmolarity - 300 mmol/litre

167. True of 8th Pandemic of Cholera: [PGI May 2014]
 (a) Started in Bangladesh
 (b) Originated in 2012
 (c) Due to O139 El Tor (d) Low attack rate
 (e) Low proportion of adults in endemic regions

168. A village affected with epidemic of cholera, what is the 1st step which should to be taken in village to decrease the death from cholera? [NEET Pattern 2014]
 (a) Safe water supply and sanitation
 (b) Cholera vaccination to all individuals
 (c) Primary Chemoprophylaxis
 (d) Treat everyone in the village' with tetracycline

169. Mechanism of action of Cholera toxin is through:
 [NEET Pattern 2015]
 (a) Gangliosides (b) Adenyl cyclase
 (c) Gangliosides + Adenyl cyclase
 (d) Exotoxin

170. Chemoprophylaxis is indicated in the following conditions except: [UPSC CMS 2015]
 (a) Cholera (b) Meningococcal meningitis
 (c) Plague (d) Typhoid

171. Main function of Sodium citrate in ORS:
 [NEET Pattern 2016]
 (a) To increase absorption of glucose by cotransport
 (b) To correct electrolyte imbalance
 (c) To correct acidosis
 (d) To correct dehydration

172. Ideal treatment of stools to prevent contamination in Cholera epidemic is: [NEET Pattern 2016]
 (a) Cresol
 (b) Bleaching powder
 (c) Sodium hypochlorite
 (d) Phenol

173. Vi polysaccharide dose can be given first at the age of:
 [NEET Pattern 2016]
 (a) 6 months (b) 12 months
 (c) 18 months (d) 24 months

174. Schedule of Typhoid oral vaccine is:
 [NEET Pattern 2017]
 (a) Day 1, 2, 3 (b) Day 2, 3, 5
 (c) Day 1, 3, 5 (d) Day 2, 4, 6

175. According to WHO, all are true about Reduced Osmolarity ORS (in mmol/L) except: [NEET Pattern 2017]
 (a) Glucose - 90
 (b) Na - 75
 (c) Potassium - 20
 (d) Citrate - 10

Review Questions

176. Which is true of typhoid? [DNB 2008]
 (a) Female carriers are less common
 (b) Male carriers though less are more dangerous
 (c) Gallbladder usually not involved in carrier state
 (d) Tetracycline is the DOC for carriers

177. Isolation in patient with Salmonellosis is done:
 (a) Till fever subsides [AP 2006]
 (b) Till Widal becomes negative [UP 2002]
 (c) Till 3 stool test are negative
 (d) For 48 hrs of Chloramphenicol treatment

178. Best disinfectant for cholera stools is: [MP 2000]
 (a) Bleaching powder (b) Cresol
 (c) Coal-tar (d) Formalin

WORM INFESTATIONS

179. All of the following statements regarding dracunculiasis are true except: [AIIMS Nov 2004]
 (a) India has eliminated this disease
 (b) Niridazole prevents transmission of the disease
 (c) The disease is limited to tropical and subtropical regions
 (d) No animal reservoir has been proved

180. Chandlers Index is used in epidemiological studies of
 [AIIMS Dec 1998, Nov 1993; NEET Pattern 2013; UPSC CMS 2015]
 (a) Round worms
 (b) Hookworms
 (c) Guinea worms
 (d) Sand fly

181. Chandlers index for Hookworm. When it is health problem? [NEET Patterns 2013, 14]
 (a) >300 (b) >200
 (c) >100 (d) >50

182. Uses of Chandler's index for hookworm include all except: [AIIMS PGMEE 2014]
 (a) Assessment of endemicity
 (b) Monitoring individual treatment
 (c) Monitoring mass treatment of community
 (d) Comparison of worm load in different populations

183. WHO considerations regarding Dracunculosis eradication, all are true except: [NEET Pattern 2014]
 (a) Drinking piped water and installation of hand pumps
 (b) DDT
 (c) Health education and awareness of public
 (d) Control of Cyclops

Review Question

184. Chandler's index is:
[NEET Pattern 2014; MP 2001 AP 2006; DPG 2004]
(a) No. of eggs of hook work in 100 gram soil
(b) No. of eggs of hookworm in per gram soil
(c) No. of eggs of hookworm in per gram stool
(d) Percentage of stool specimens positive for hookworms

DENGUE

185. Dengue discharge protocol includes
[AIIMS November 2019]
(a) 24 hours after Recovery from shock
(b) Urine volume > 200 ml
(c) 24 hours after absence of fever with use of Paracetamol
(d) Return of normal appetite

186. Dengue virus appears to have a direct man-mosquito-man cycle in India. The mechanism of dengue virus survival in the inter-epidemic period is: [DPG 2011]
(a) Non-human reservoir
(b) Dormant or latent phase in man
(c) Transovarian transmission of the virus
(d) Poor housekeeping by the public

187. True about Dengue fever is/are: [PGI May 2011]
(a) Is the most common arboviral infection
(b) Can be both epidemic as well as endemic
(c) Can survive in ambient temperature
(d) Incidence decreasing in India in last 2-3 decades
(e) Vector is Aedes aegypti

188. Which is not true of Dengue fever? [NUPGET 2013]
(a) Aedes aegypti is the principal vector
(b) Break bone fever is characteristic
(c) Serotype 4 is more dangerous than other serotypes
(d) Torniquet test is positive

189. All are true about Dengue hemorrhagic fever *except*:
[AIIMS November 2014]
(a) Lamivudine is drug of choice
(b) Malnutrition is protective
(c) Transmitted by Aedes
(d) Causative agent belongs to Flaviviradae group

190. A 20-year-old male is diagnosed as a case of dengue fever at a Primary Health Centre. What are the suitable measures to be taken for the prevention and control of dengue in that area? [UPSC CMS 2015]
(a) Case management for DF and DHF and vaccination
(b) Case management for DF and DHF, isolation and individual protection from mosquitoes
(c) Case management for DF and DHF, isolation and individual protection from mosquitoes and vaccination
(d) Case management for DF and DHF, isolation and individual protection from mosquitoes and environmental measures for elimination of breeding places

191. Which of the following statement is/are true about Dengue? [PGI November 2017]
(a) According to WHO dengue is classified only in 2 category DF and DHF
(b) Subsequent infection with different strain produces severe form of dengue
(c) Most infection with dengue virus is asymptomatic
(d) Vector is Aedes mosquito
(e) Provides life long immunity

Review Questions

192. Which is not true about dengue hemorrhagic fever?
[Bihar 2006]
(a) Thrombocytopenia   (b) Hepatomegaly
(c) Shock   (d) Plasma leaking

193. Infective period of Aedes mosquito for Classical Dengue fever (break-bone fever) is: [AIIMS 1988; Karnataka 1987; MH 1997; Manipal 1997; SGPGI 1996; TN 1993, 1991; UP 1996; UPSC 1986; TN 2000]
(a) 10-20 days   (b) 20-30 days
(c) 30-40 days   (d) Lifelong

194. Which of the following statement regarding dengue is correct: [Kolkata 2004]
(a) Caused by 3 serotypes of dengue virus
(b) It is endemic in India
(c) Aspirin is used for treatment
(d) Clinical course of dengue is more fulminant in children than adults

MALARIA

195. Which of the following are included in Malaria Vector Indices?
1. Human blood index
2. Biting density
3. Slide positivity rate
4. Inoculation rate

Use the following key to mark correct answer
[AIIMS May 2019]
(a) 1, 3
(b) 2, 4
(c) 1, 2, 3, 4
(d) 1, 2, 4

196. Malaria control means [AIIMS November 2019]
(a) To reduce Malaria mortality to Zero
(b) To prevent local transmission for 3 years
(c) To reduce Malaria disease so that it's no longer a Public health problem
(d) To reduce Incidence to Zero

197. API is: [AIIMS May 1993]
(a) Annual parasitic index
(b) Average parasitic index

(c) Animal parasite interval
(d) Annual parasitic incidence

198. The infective form of malarial parasite through a blood transfusion is: [AIIMS June 1997]
    (a) Trophozoite (b) Merozoite
    (c) Sporozoite (d) Schizont

199. In a Chloroquine resistant zone the presumptive treatment of malaria to be given is: [AIIMS May 02, Nov 1999]
    (a) Chloroquine + primaquine 45 mg
    (b) Chloroquine + pyrimethamine
    (c) Sulphalene 1000 mg
    (d) Sulphadoxine + pyrimethamine

200. In high-risk areas the radical treatment for Plasmodium vivax infection after microscopic confirmation is administration of tablets primaquine in the daily dosage of: [AIIMS May 1993]
    (a) 0.25 mg/kg body weight
    (b) 0.50 mg/kg body weight
    (c) 0.75 mg/kg body weight
    (d) 1.00 mg/kg body weight

201. The most sensitive index of recent transmission of malaria in a community is: [AIIMS Nov 1993, 2003, Feb 1997, AIPGME 1996]
    (a) Spleen rate [DPG 2005, MP 2005]
    (b) Infant parasite rate [MH 2006, JIPMER 1999]
    (c) Annual parasite incidence
    (d) Slide positivity rate

202. Species of Anopheles transmitting malaria is urban areas is: [DPG 2007, NEET Pattern 2017]
    (a) Stephensi (b) Culcifacies
    (c) Minimus (d) Fluviatilis

203. The peaks of fever in malaria coincide with the release of successive broods of ....into the blood stream: [Karnataka 2008]
    (a) Sporozoites (b) Trophozoites
    (c) Merozoites (d) Hypnozoites

204. True about epidemiology of malaria: [PGI Dec 06]
    (a) Extrinsic incubation period 0-14 days
    (b) In India common during January to June
    (c) Man acts as definitive host
    (d) Rare in urban areas
    (e) Mosquito acts as definitive host

205. Malaria is transmitted by: [PGI Dec 07]
    (a) Anopheles stephensi
    (b) Anopheles dirus
    (c) Culex
    (d) Phlebotamus

206. All of the following factors are responsible for resurgence of Malaria except: [AIPGME 2011]
    (a) Drug resistance (b) Use of bed-nets
    (c) Vector resistance (d) Mutation in parasite

207. Plasmodium ovale in India has been reported from: [PGI May 2011]
    (a) Maharashtra (b) Madhya Pradesh
    (c) Manipur (d) Gujarat
    (e) Odisha

208. True about Malaria in India is/are: [PGI November 2012]
    (a) 1.5 million cases annually
    (b) Quinine drug of choice in severe malaria in pregnancy
    (c) Anopheles culicifacies is vector in Urban malaria
    (d) Plasmodium ovale is not seen in India
    (e) Falciparum malaria is most common type

209. Prophylaxis for malaria not used: [NEET Pattern 2013]
    (a) Doxycycline (b) Artesunate
    (c) Chloroquine (d) Mefloquine

210. Chemoprophylaxis of Malaria can be done by all except: [NEET Pattern 2012] [NEET Pattern 2013]
    (a) Chloroquine (b) Mefloquine
    (c) Proguanil (d) Primaquine

211. Throughout the country every year anti-malaria month is observed during the month of: [PGMCET 2015; UP 2005]
    (a) July (b) January
    (c) June (d) December

212. Consider the following statements regarding falciparum malaria:
    1. Mortality rises steeply when proportion of infected erythrocytes increases >3%
    2. Patient may develop hypoglycemia even when not treated with Quinine
    Which of the statements given above is/are correct? [UPSC CMS 2015]
    (a) 1 only (b) 2 only
    (c) Both 1 and 2 (d) Neither 1 nor 2

213. Extrinsic incubation period of Plasmodium is: [NEET Pattern 2016]
    (a) 7-10 days (b) 10-20 days
    (c) 20-25 days (d) 21-30 days

214. Species of Anopheles causing malaria in Andaman & Nicobar Island? [NEET Pattern 2015]
    (a) Anopheles stephensi
    (b) Anopheles dirus
    (c) Anopheles culicifacies
    (d) Anopheles epiroticus

215. Specific content in malaria vaccine is: [NEET Pattern 2017]
    (a) Gametocytic protein (b) Polysaccharide sheath
    (c) Sporozoite protein (d) Lipoprotein envelop

216. Plasmodium species known for Relapses in Malaria is: [AIIMS November 2017]
    (a) Vivax, Falciparum (b) Falciparum, Malariae
    (c) Vivax, Malariae (d) Vivax, Ovale

217. Which of the following is NOT an indicator for Malaria surveillance in a population? [NEET Pattern 2019]
    (a) Annual parasite index
    (b) Annual parasite incidence
    (c) Annual falciparum incidence
    (d) Slide falciparum rate

Review Questions

218. If API >2, the vector is resistant to DDT, the malathion spray should be done every: [UP 2006]
    (a) One round of malathion every month
    (b) 2 round or malathion every month
    (c) 1-2 round of malathion every 3 months
    (d) 3 round of malathion every 3 months

219. A malarial survey is conducted in 50 villages having a population of 1 lakh. Out of 20000 slides examined, 500 turned out to be malaria positive. The annual parasite incidence is: [Kolkata 2008]
    (a) 20   (b) 5
    (c) 0.5   (d) 0.4

220. Among various species of mosquitoes belonging to anopheles genus, one that is highly anthrophilic and transmits even at low density is: [MH 2003]
    (a) Anopheles sundicans
    (b) Anopheles fluvitalis
    (c) Anopheles stephensi
    (d) Anopheles culicifacies

LYMPHATIC FILARIASIS

221. A 32 years old male patient comes to OPD with fever and swelling of lower limbs. He tests positive for Filarial antigen. Next step for diagnosis is [NEET PG Pattern 2023]
    (a) DEC provocation test
    (b) PBS
    (c) Bone marrow aspiration
    (d) Lymph node biopsy

222. DEC is used extensively in the chemotherapy of Filariasis. It is most effective against: [AIIMS May 1993]
    (a) Microfilariae
    (b) Adult worm
    (c) Infective stage larvae
    (d) All of the above

223. The organism most commonly causing genital filariasis in most parts of Bihar and Eastern U.P. is:
    (a) *Wuchereria bancrofti*
    (b) *Brugia malayi*
    (c) *Onchocerca volvulus*
    (d) *Dirofilaria*

224. The currently given regimen for Bancroftian filariasis is: [AIPGME 1991]
    (a) DEC – 6 mg/Kg /day × 21 days
    (b) DEC – 6 mg/Kg /day × 12 days
    (c) DEC – 100 mg/day × 21 days
    (d) DEC – 100 mg/day × 12 days

225. The DEC-medicated salt for mass treatment in lymphatic filariasis was shown to be safe, cheap and effective in: [Karnataka 2008]
    (a) Goa
    (b) Daman and Diu
    (c) Andaman and Nicobar islands
    (d) Lakshadweep islands

226. All of the following are helpful for elimination of filariasis, *except*: [AIIMS PGMEE May 2012]
    (a) Microfilariae do not multiply in vectors
    (b) They multiply in humans
    (c) Larvae are deposited on skin surface where they can't survive
    (d) Mass drug administration

227. All of the following are true about filariasis *except*: [DNB December 2011]
    (a) It is sheathed
    (b) Tail end is free from nuclei and unsheathed
    (c) Has nocturnal activity
    (d) Day time resides inside the lymphatics

228. Diagnosis of Filariasis is confirmed most commonly done by: [NEET Pattern 2017, 2018]
    (a) Clinical features
    (b) Detection of microfilariae
    (c) PCR
    (d) Serological test

Review Questions

229. Life cycle of filarial in the mosquito is described as: [AP 2005; NEET Patterns 2017, 2018]
    (a) Cyclopropagative   (b) Cyclodevelopmental
    (c) Propagative   (d) None

230. The Clinical incubation period of Filariasis is: [TN 2003]
    (a) 10 to 20 days
    (b) 3 to 6 months
    (c) 6 to 12 months
    (d) 8 to 16 months

RABIES

231. A splenectomised person (done 5 years ago) as well the dog who bite him, both have been vaccinated previously. Antibiotic used in a case of dog bite is: [INICET May 2023]
    (a) Metronidazole
    (b) Ciprofloxacin
    (c) Amoxycillin + Clavulanic acid
    (d) Only observation of dog is sufficient

232. A child presents with a dog bite from a street dog. On examination, an abrasion of 1.5 cm is present, with slight oozing. Which of the following statements are correct?
 [INICET November 2022]
 1. Category 3 wound
 2. Wash the wound with normal tap water for 15-20 minutes
 3. Clean the wound with spirit
 4. Loose suturing of the wound with a proper dressing
 5. Equine immunoglobulin is given at a dose of 40 IU/kg of body weight, twice
 6. Intradermal vaccine is administered on days 0, 3, 7, 28
 (a) 2, 3, 5, 6
 (b) 1, 2, 5, 6
 (c) 1, 2, 3, 5
 (d) 1, 2, 3, 6

233. Rabies Immunoglobulin, true is/are: (Multiple response) [INICET May 2022]
 (a) Not useful after 72 hours
 (b) Maximum dose in deltoid muscle
 (c) Dose 20 IU per kg
 (d) If human IG is not present, then give equine IG

234. Most logical and cost-effective approach of controlling Rabies in Urban population [NEET PG Pattern 2022]
 (a) Test all the dogs for Rabies
 (b) Remove stray dogs and vaccinate the dog population
 (c) Administer Rabies vaccine to the entire human populations
 (d) Health education of people

235. A child has received full Rabies vaccination in December 2018 and now presented with oozing wound on Great toe and the pet had vaccination also. Next line of management is [AIIMS November 2019]
 (a) No vaccine required
 (b) RIG + 5 doses of vaccine
 (c) 5 doses of vaccines only
 (d) 2 doses of Rabies vaccine

236. Pre-exposure prophylaxis for Rabies is given on:
 [AIPGME 96, AIPGME 98; NEET Pattern 2014]
 (a) Days 0, 3, 7, 14, 28, 90
 (b) Days 0, 3, 7, 28, 90
 (c) Days 0, 3
 (d) Days 0, 7, 28

237. For the treatment of case of class III dog bite, all of the following are correct except: [NEET Pattern 2013]
 (a) Give Immunoglobulins for passive immunity
 (b) Give ARV [AIPGME 2005]
 (c) Immediately stitch wound under antibiotic coverage
 (d) Immediately wash wound with soap and water

238. Which of the following statements about rabies is FALSE?
 [DPG 2004]
 (a) Convulsions are generally not seen in a patient with rabies
 (b) Presence of meningitis suggests against the diagnosis of rabies
 (c) Intracytoplasmic basophilic inclusion bodies are seen in brain cells
 (d) Incubation period is approximately 20 to 80 days

239. Rabies in not found in: [DPG 2006]
 (a) Lakshadweep Islands
 (b) Rajasthan
 (c) Meghalaya
 (d) Odisha

240. Bite of which of the following animals do not result in human rabies? [DPG 2007]
 (a) Dog (b) Mouse
 (c) Horse (d) Cat

241. Characteristic features of Rabies include all except:
 [NUPGET 2013]
 (a) Can manifest as ascending paralysis
 (b) Hematogenous spread to brain
 (c) Can be transmitted by bites other than dogs also
 (d) In invariably fatal

242. Number of doses of Rabies HDCV vaccine required for pre-exposure prophylaxis: [NEET Pattern 2013]
 (a) 5 (b) 2
 (c) 3 (d) 1

243. A 10-year-old child with unprovoked Dog bite comes to you. Appropriate action is: [AIIMS PG May 2015]
 (a) Withhold vaccine and observe dog for 10 days
 (b) Give cell culture derived vaccine
 (c) No further action is necessary
 (d) Kill the dog and send brain for biopsy

244. For the prevention of human rabies, immediate flushing and washing the wound(s) in animal bite cases, with plenty of soap and water, under running tap should be carried out for how much time? [PGMCET 2015]
 (a) 2 minutes (b) 1 minute
 (c) 15 minutes (d) 5 minutes

245. Intramuscular dose of Rabies vaccine for pre-exposure prophylaxis: [NEET Pattern 2017]
 (a) 0.1 mL (b) 1 mL
 (c) 2 mL (d) 5 mL

246. Which of the following is/are true about post-exposure prophylaxis in Rabies? [PGI 2017]
 (a) Category I: Both vaccine and immunoglobulin are given
 (b) Immunoglobulin not required if prior full vaccination is received
 (c) Local wound cleaning is done in all cases of dog wound
 (d) Category I: Requires vaccination only
 (e) Vaccine is stopped if within 3 days of bite, dog dies

Review Questions

247. Rabies free country is: [DNB 2000, 04, 05]
    (a) China (b) Russia
    (c) Australia, UK (d) France

248. All these Rabies vaccines are commercially available except: [UP 2000]
    (a) Killed sheep brain
    (b) Human diploid vaccine
    (c) Vero-continuous cell vaccine
    (d) Recombinant glycoprotein vaccine

249. A patient presents with dogs bite in the palm fingers and oozing of blood on the neck regions, belongs to which class of the exposures: [UP 2008]
    (a) Class I (b) Class II
    (c) Class III (d) None

250. Nervous tissue Rabies vaccines are usually manufactured from: [MP 2007]
    (a) Sheep (b) Human diploid cell
    (c) Duck embryos (d) Chick embryos

251. Rabies does not occur in which of the following parts of India? [MH 2003]
    (a) Daman and Diu
    (b) Andaman and Nicobar Islands
    (c) Dadra and Nagar Havelli
    (d) Puducherry

YELLOW FEVER

252. A patient with history of travel to Africa developed jaundice with hemorrhagic fever and conjunctival effusion. He was given treatment but died. Which of the following vaccines could have prevented his death? [NEET PG Pattern 2022]
    (a) 17D vaccine
    (b) Nakayama strain
    (c) Ra 27/3 strain
    (d) Jeryll lynn strain

253. The incubation period of yellow fever is: [AIIMS May 04]
    (a) 3 to 6 days (b) 3-4 weeks
    (c) 1 to 2 weeks (d) 8-10 weeks

254. All are features of yellow fever except: [AIIMS June 1997]
    (a) Subclinical cases present
    (b) Fatality rate > 90%
    (c) One attack gives life long immunity
    (d) Hepatic and renal involvement in severe cases

255. According to International Health Regulations, there is no risk of spread of yellow Fever if the Aedes aegypti index remains below: [AIPGME 2004]
    (a) 1% (b) 5% [NEET Pattern 2013]
    (c) 8% (d) 10%

256. All are true for Yellow Fever except: [AIPGME 2003]
    (a) Causative agent is Flavivirus fibricus
    (b) Case fatality is up to 80 %
    (c) Validation of Vaccination Certificate begins after 10 days and lasts till 10 years
    (d) Incubation period is 16-46 days

257. True about yellow fever: [PGI June 04]
    (a) I.P. is 10-14 days (b) Transmitted by Aedes
    (c) It is found in Asia
    (d) Incidence is increased by humidity
    (e) It is a flavivirus

258. Yellow fever certificate of vaccination is valid for: [NEET Pattern 2012; UP 2001; DNB December 2010]
    (a) 1 year (b) 10 years
    (c) 35 years (d) Lifelong

259. To prevent yellow fever Aedes aegypti index should be less than……..: [DNB December 2010, 11]
    (a) 0.5% (b) 1%
    (c) 2% (d) 5%

260. All are true about Yellow Fever except: [AIIMS Nov 1999]
    (a) Incubation period is 3-6 days
    (b) Validity of International certificate of Vaccination lasts up to 10 years
    (c) Urban form is controlled by 17 D vaccine
    (d) Aedes aegypti index should not be more than 10% to ensure freedom from yellow Fever

261. Which of the following statements about yellow fever is not correct? [NEET Pattern 2016]
    (a) Yellow fever is caused by Flavivirus fibricus
    (b) One attack of yellow fever gives life-long immunity
    (c) India is yellow fever "receptive area"
    (d) The validity of yellow fever vaccination certificate begins 10 days after the date of vaccination and extends up to 5 years

Review Question

262. Which if the following is the 'YELLOW FEVER' reference centre? [MH 2008]
    (a) Haffkin's institute, Mumbai
    (b) Central Institute, Kasauli
    (c) NIN, Hyderabad
    (d) AIIMS, Delhi

JAPANESE ENCEPHALITIS

263. Match the following for Japanese encephalitis [INICET November 2021]
    A. Culex   1. Accidental host
    B. Man   2. Reservoir host
    C. Pig   3. Amplifier host
    D. Ardeid birds   4. Vector
                      5. Paratenic host

(a) A-4, B-1, C-2, D-3
(b) A-4, B-1, C-3, D-2
(c) A-4, B-2, C-3, D-1
(d) A-2, B-4, C-3, D-1

264. Acute encephalitis syndrome cases are being reported from Gorakhpur, Uttar Pradesh. The Heath team decides for mass vaccination which comes under Universal immunization program. Identify the vaccine type and route.
 [NEET PG Pattern September 2021]
 (a) Live attenuated intramuscular
 (b) Killed subcutaneous
 (c) Killed intramuscular
 (d) Live attenuated subcutaneous

265. All are true regarding Japanese encephalitis disease, except: [NEET PG Pattern January 2020]
 (a) Man act as Reservoir
 (b) Vector is Culex vishnuii
 (c) Pig vaccination control transmission
 (d) None is true

266. Vector for Zika virus disease is
 [NEET PG Pattern January 2020]
 (a) Anopheles stephensi
 (b) Phelebotomus
 (c) Aedes Aegypti
 (d) Culex

267. All are true about Japanese Encephalitis except:
 [AIPGME 1996, Dec 98, AIIMS May 97]
 (a) Man is incidental dead-end host
 (b) Culicines and anophelines are vectors involved
 (c) Case fatality rate is over 90%
 (d) 85% of cases occur in children <15 years age

268. True statement regarding Japanese Encephalitis is:
 [AIPGME 2011]
 (a) 70% of cases are reported from infants
 (b) Ratio of clinical apparent to non-apparent infections is 1:100
 (c) Mosquito bite is always associated with the disease
 (d) Epidemic is declared if there are 2-3 cases in a village

269. Which of the following is not true regarding Japanese encephalitis vaccine? [AIIMS PG May 2015]
 (a) Booster doses are given after 1 year and repeated every 3 years
 (b) Not given for infants less than 6 months age
 (c) Two primary doses given to children aged 1-3 years age
 (d) In endemic areas, vaccination is given to cover children 1-9 years age

270. Amplifier host in Japanese encephalitis:
 [NEET Pattern 2017]
 (a) Horse   (b) Pigs
 (c) Dogs   (d) Monkey

271. Bird-Arthropod-Man transmission is seen in:
 (a) Plague
 (b) Japanese encephalitis
 (c) *Paragonimus westermani* [NEET Pattern 2019]
 (d) *Plasmodium falciparum*

Review Questions

272. Not true about Japanese's encephalitis is:
 (a) Man to man transmission [Bihar 2006]
 (b) Vector is culex. tritaeniorhynchus
 (c) Rice field
 (d) Horse shows symptom

273. Major determinant to eradication of Japanese encephalitis is: [RJ 2007]
 (a) No effective vaccine
 (b) Breeding place of vector
 (c) Large no. of in apparent infections
 (d) Numerous animal hosts

KFD

274. Which of these is NOT useful in the prevention of KFD?
 [AIIMS May 2001]
 (a) Vaccination
 (b) Deforestation
 (c) Prevention of roaming cattle
 (d) Personal protection

275. The vector for KFD is: [AIIMS May 1993]
 (a) Aedes aegypti   (b) Haemaphysalis
 (c) Culex   (d) Xenopsylla

PLAGUE

276. A patient is a known case of Inguinal buboes. He now presents with Multiple buboes in axilla and groin. Identify the vector [NEET PG Pattern September 2021]
 (a) Sandfly
 (b) Phlebotomus bug
 (c) Triatominae bug
 (d) Xenopsylla cheopsis

277. All are true about Plague except:
 (a) Domestic rat "Rattus rattus" has been incriminated as main reservoir [AIPGME 1997]
 (b) Both sexes of rat flea bite to transmit the disease
 (c) IP for bubonic plague is 1-3 days
 (d) Infants under 6 months are not given the killed vaccine

278. The most effective method to break transmission chain in plague is: [AIIMS May 2002]
 (a) Early diagnosis and treatment
 (b) Control of fleas
 (c) Control of rodents
 (d) Vaccination

279. All of the following statements about plague is wrong, except: [AIIMS May 2004]
    (a) Domestic rat is the main reservoir
    (b) Bubonic is the most common variety
    (c) The causative bacillus can survive up to 10 years in the soil of rodent burrows
    (d) The incubation period for pneumonic plague is one to two weeks

280. Plague epidemic in Surat in 1995 has occurred after a silence period of: [DPG 2005]
    (a) 18 years   (b) 20 years
    (c) 28 years   (d) 30 years

281. Maximum Explosiveness of Plague (Severity of spreading) is determined by: [DPG 2006, 11; NEET Pattern 2013; DNB 2011]
    (a) Total flea index   (b) Cheopsis index
    (c) Borrow index   (d) Specific percentage of fleas

Review Question

282. The highly infections clinical form of plague is: [TN 2003]
    (a) Bubonic plague   (b) Pneumonic plague
    (c) Septicaemic plague   (d) All of the above

RICKETTSIAL DISEASES

283. A military soldier presents with fever rash and myalgia. There is an absence of rash in palms and soles. History of louse infestation present in the same battalion. Causative organism is [NEET PG Pattern 2022]
    (a) R. prowazekii
    (b) R. conori
    (c) R. typhi
    (d) R. akari

284. Which of the following pairs of 'Rickettsial Diseases– Insect vectors' is wrongly matched? [AIPGME 96]
    (a) Epidemic typhus – Louse
    (b) Scrub typhus - Flea
    (c) Rocky Mountain spotted fever - Tick
    (d) Rickettsial pox - Mite

285. A patient complained of chills and fever following a louse bite 2 weeks before. He had rashes all over the body and was delirious at the time of presentation to the hospital and subsequently went into coma. A provisional diagnosis of vasculitis due to Rickettsial infection was made. Which one of the following can be the causative agent? [AIPGME 2006]
    (a) Rickettsia typhi
    (b) Rickettsia rickettsiae
    (c) Rickettsia prowazekii
    (d) Rickettsia akari

286. It is true regarding endemic typhus that: [AIPGME 07]
    (a) Man is the only reservoir of infection
    (b) Flea is a vector of the disease
    (c) The rash developing into eschar is a characteristic presentation
    (d) Culture of the etiological agent in tissue culture is diagnostic modality

287. Mode of transmission of Q fever is: [AIIMS May 04]
    (a) Bite of infected louse   [DNB 2008]
    (b) Bite of infected tick
    (c) Inhalation of aerosol
    (d) Bite of infected mite

288. A man presents with fever and chills 2 weeks after a louse bite. There was a maculo-papular rash on the trunk which spread peripherally. The cause of this infection can be: [AIIMS May 2003; NEET Pattern 2017]
    (a) Scrub typhus   (b) Endemic typhus
    (c) Rickettsial pox   (d) Epidemic typhus

289. All of following statements are true regarding Q fever, except: [AIIMS May 2003, AIPGME 1996]
    (a) It is a zoonotic infection
    (b) Human disease is characterized by an interstitial pneumonia
    (c) No rash is seen
    (d) Weil-Felix reaction is very useful for diagnosis

290. All are true about Scrub typhus except: [AIPGME 2010]
    (a) Mite is a vector
    (b) Adult mite feeds on vertebral host
    (c) Caused by R. tsutsugamushi
    (d) Tetracycline is treatment

291. Rickettsiae are transmitted by: [PGI May 2011]
    (a) Flea   (b) Louse
    (c) Mosquito   (d) Mite
    (e) Fly

292. Epidemic typhus causes & vector: [NEET Patterns 2013, 2015; DNB 2010; UP 2005]
    (a) Rickettessia prowazki & louse
    (b) R. typhi & mite
    (c) R. conori & tick
    (d) R. akari & mite

293. Vagabond disease transmitted by: [NEET Pattern 2013]
    (a) Louse   (b) Mite
    (c) Tick   (d) Black fly

294. Rickettsial pox is caused by: [DNB December 2009]
    (a) Rickettsia ricketsiae   (b) Rickettsia akari
    (c) R. typhi   (d) Rickettsia conori

295. Endemic typhus is transmitted by: [DNB December 2009; NEET Pattern 2012; UP 2006]
    (a) Flea   (b) Tick
    (c) Mite   (d) Mosquito

296. Rickettsial disease: [NEET Pattern 2015]
    (a) Weil disease
    (b) Rocky mountain spotted fever
    (c) Leptospirosis
    (d) Trichomoniasis

297. How transmission of Epidemic typhus does takes place by louse? [NEET Pattern 2016]
    (a) Bite of louse
    (b) Eating infected material
    (c) Crushing louse on body
    (d) All of the above

298. Drug of choice for Scrub typhus is: [AIIMS November 2017]
    (a) Azithromycin (b) Chloramphenicol
    (c) Doxycycline (d) Ciprofloxacin

299. Quintan fever is caused by: [NEET Pattern 2017]
    (a) *Rickettsia typhi* (b) *Bartonella*
    (c) *Coxiella burnetti* (d) *Rickettsia conorii*

Review Questions

300. Organism that does not need vector for transmission:
    (a) Rickettsia prowazekii [Kolkata 2005]
    (b) Rickettsia rickettsii
    (c) Coxiella burnetii
    (d) Borrelia recurrentis

301. Trombiculid mite can transmit:
    [MP 2004, RJ 2000, DNB 2006; NEET Pattern 2013]
    (a) Indian tick typhus (b) Scrub typhus
    (c) Relapsing fever (d) Q. fever

302. Arthropods are vector for all *except*:
    [MH 2007; NEET Pattern 2015]
    (a) Scrub typhus
    (b) Epidemic typhus
    (c) Q-fever
    (d) Rocky mountain sportted fever
    (d) Flea

303. Rash starting peripherally is a feature of: [RJ 2007]
    (a) Epidemic types
    (b) Endemic Typhus
    (c) Scrub typhus
    (d) Indian tick typhus

304. Rash is absent in: [RJ 2008] [NEET Pattern 2017]
    (a) Epidemic types (b) Endemic typhus
    (c) Scrub typhus (d) Q-fever

LEISHMANIASIS

305. Reservoir of Indian Kala-azar is: [AIIMS May 03]
    (a) Man (b) Rodent
    (c) Canine (d) Equine

306. All are used in treatment of Visceral Leishmaniasis *except*:
    (a) Sitamaquine [AIIMS Nov 2009]
    (b) Paramomycin
    (c) Hydroxychloroquine
    (d) Miltefosine

307. Woman traveling from Bihar to Delhi is suspecting to have Kala-azar. Suitable investigation is:
    [NEET Pattern 2016]
    (a) P24 antigen (b) rk-39 test
    (c) Combo RDT (d) HRP-2 antigen

308. Kala-azar is endemic in all *except*: [NEET Pattern 2018]
    (a) Bihar (b) UP
    (c) Assam (d) Jharkhand

309. Each of the following statements concerning Kala-azar is correct *except*: [NEET Pattern 2018]
    (a) Kala-azar is caused by Leishmania donovani
    (b) Kala-azar is transmitted by the bite of sandflies
    (c) Kala-azar occurs primarily in rural Latin America
    (d) Kala-azar can be diagnosed by finding amastigotes in bone marrow

Review Questions

310. Kala-azar is transmitted by: [TN 2005]
    (a) Phlebotomus sergenti
    (b) Phlebotomus papatasii
    (c) Phlebotomus argentipes
    (d) All of the above

311. All the following statements are true for Indian Kala-azar *except*: [MP 2009]
    (a) It is transmitted by the bite of an infected sandfly
    (b) Dog is the reservoir of infection
    (c) The causative parasite is cultivated in the NNN medium
    (d) The disease is endemic in Bihar

TRACHOMA

312. For a Case presenting with Trachoma in a PHC OPD, SAFE-strategy was applied. Which one of the following is not correct? [INICET July 2021]
    (a) Surgery for trichiasis
    (b) Antibiotics
    (c) Face cleaning
    (d) Evaluation of control program

313. SAFE strategy include all the following *except*:
    (a) Screening [AIIMS Nov 2006]
    (b) Antibiotics
    (c) Face washing
    (d) Environmental improvement

314. True about trachoma is: [AIPGME 1996]
    (a) Is a disease of high infectivity
    (b) Prevalence of severe and moderate trachoma in > 1 % in children less than 10 years is indication for mass treatment
    (c) Irritants like kajal or surma also predispose
    (d) Is a non-avoidable cause of blindness in India

315. For the field diagnosis of trachoma, the WHO recommends that follicular and intense trachoma inflammation should be assessed in: [AIIMS May 2003]
    (a) Women aged 15-45 years
    (b) Population of 10 to 28 year range
    (c) Children aged 0-10 years
    (d) Population above 25 years of age irrespective of sex

316. In the grading of Trachoma, Trachomatous Inflammation-follicular is defined as the presence of: [AIPGME 2004]
    (a) Five or more follicles in the lower tarsal conjunctiva
    (b) Three or more follicles in the lower tarsal conjunctiva
    (c) Five or more follicles in the upper tarsal conjunctiva
    (d) Three or more follicles in the upper tarsal conjunctiva

317. Mass treatment of trachoma is undertaken, when the prevalence is more than: [DPG 2005]
    (a) 3%
    (b) 5%
    (c) 6%
    (d) 10%

318. Azithromycin mass treatment is given in community when prevalence of Trachoma is more than: [AIIMS November 2011]
    (a) 4%
    (b) 6%
    (c) 8%
    (d) 10%

TETANUS

319. A 40 years old male presented to emergency with TT course received 10 years ago. On examination the wound is clean cut and <6 hours old. Management will include: [NEET PG Pattern 2023]
    (a) Single dose TT
    (b) Complete course TT
    (c) Complete course TT with TIG
    (d) No treatment is required

320. What should be the minimum dose of tetanus antitoxin in body to provide optimal protection?: [AIIMS June 2020]
    (a) > 0.1 IU/ml
    (b) > 0.01 IU/ml
    (c) > 0.001 IU/ml
    (d) > 5 IU/ml

321. Patient reports 4 hours after a having a clean wound without laceration. He had taken TT 10 years before. The next step in management is: [NEET PG Pattern January 2020]
    (a) Full course TT is given
    (b) Single dose of TT
    (c) Tetanus immunoglobulin +First dose TT
    (d) Tetanus immunoglobulin + TT Full course

322. A person has received complete immunization against tetanus 10 years ago, now he presents with a clean wound without any lacerations from an injury sustained 3 hours ago. He should now be given:
    (a) Full course of tetanus toxoid [AIPGME 01]
    (b) Single dose of tetanus toxoid [NEET Pattern 2013]
    (c) Human tetanus globulin
    (d) Human tetanus globulin and single dose of toxoid

323. Neonatal tetanus is said to be eliminated when the rate is: [AIIMS Feb 1997; NEET Pattern 2013; DNB 2008]
    (a) > 10 per 1000 LB
    (b) > 1 per 1000 LB
    (c) < 1 per 1000 LB
    (d) < 0.1 per 1000 LB

324. All the following are done to prevent tetanus neonatorum except: [AIPGME 2007]
    (a) Two TT doses to all pregnant women
    (b) TT to all females in reproductive age group
    (c) TT to all newborns
    (d) Injection penicillin to all neonates

325. All of the following statements are true about Clostridium tetani infection except: [AIIMS Nov 2010]
    (a) Main reservoir is soil, animal intestine and human intestine
    (b) Main mode of transmission is through trauma and contaminated wound
    (c) Herd immunity does not have much value
    (d) Seen commonly in winter and dry climate

326. All are true regarding Clostridium tetani infection except: [AIPGME 2011]
    (a) Incubation period 6-10 days
    (b) 3 primary doses of vaccine required for full protection
    (c) Man-to-man transmission
    (d) Produces heat-resistant spores

327. An adult, previously unimmunized against Tetanus presents with a clean non-penetrating wound sustained 2 hours previously. What tetanus prophylaxis is advised? [Karnataka 2011]
    (a) Only through cleaning of wound
    (b) Tetanus toxoid 1 dose
    (c) Tetanus toxoid complete course
    (d) Tetanus toxoid complete course + human tetanus immunoglobulin

328. True about Tetanus is all except: [AIIMS PGMEE November 2012]
    (a) Tetanus protection 5 years if previously immunized
    (b) Herd immunity present
    (c) Can't be eradicated
    (d) Elimination is less than 1 case per 1000 live births

Review Questions

329. The period of communicability of Tetanus is: [UP 2007, RJ 2001]
    (a) 7 days
    (b) 14 days
    (c) 21 days
    (d) None

330. A person had clean non-penetrating wound four hours back. He had a complete course of toxoid eleven years ago. What treatment is recommended? [MP 2009]
    (a) No toxoid is required
    (b) Toxoid one dose
    (c) Toxoid complete course
    (d) Toxoid complete course+Human tetanus Ig

331. Indicators of the Elimination of NEONATAL TETNUS includes the following *except*? [MH 2008]
    (a) Incidence rate <0.1/1000 live births
    (b) > 90% coverage of 3 antenatal visits
    (c) TT2 injection coverage in pregnant mothers >90%
    (d) None

LEPROSY

332. False about Leprosy is: [AIPGME 1991]
    (a) It has been eliminated from India
    (b) It can be transmitted through breast milk
    (c) Lepromin test is not a diagnostic test
    (d) MDT is contraindicated during pregnancy

333. Leprosy can be transmitted through all *except*:
    [AIIMS 1991; AIPGME 2004]
    (a) Mother to child   (b) Breast milk
    (c) Insect vectors   (d) Tattooing needles

334. Leprosy is considered a public health problem if the prevalence of leprosy is more than:
    [DNB 2008 AIPGME 03, AIIMS Dec 1998]
    (a) 1 per 10,000   (b) 2 per 10,000
    (c) 5 per 10,000   (d) 10 per 10,000

335. In the management of leprosy, Lepromin test is most useful for: [AIPGME 2003]
    (a) Herd immunity   (b) Prognosis
    (c) Treatment
    (d) Epidemiological investigations

336. A patient with leprosy had slightly erythematous, anesthetic plaques on the trunk and upper limbs. He was treated with paucibacillary multidrug therapy (PB-MDT) for 6 moths. At the end of 6 months, he had persistent erythema and induration in the plaque. The next step of action recommended by the World Health Organization (WHO) in such a patient is: [AIIMS May 2001]
    (a) Stop antileprosy treatment
    (b) Continue PB-MDT till erythema subsides
    (c) Biopsy the lesion to document activity
    (d) Continue Dapsone alone for another 6 months

337. In the management of leprosy, Lepromin test is not useful for: [AIIMS Nov 2008, AIPGME 1991]
    (a) Diagnosis
    (b) Prognosis
    (c) Confirmation of classification
    (d) Evaluation of cell mediated immunity

338. All of the following statements about leprosy are true *except*: [AIPGME 2004]
    (a) Multibacillary leprosy is diagnosed when there are more than 5 skin patches
    (b) New case detection rate is an indicator for incidence of leprosy
    (c) A defaulter is defined as a patient who has not taken treatment for 6 months or more
    (d) The target for elimination of leprosy is to reduce the prevalence to less than 1 per 10,000 population

339. All of the following are tests used to detect Cell mediated immunity in Leprosy *except*: [AIIMS Feb 1997]
    (a) Lepromin Test
    (b) Lymphocyte Transformation Test
    (c) Leucocyte Migration Inhibition Test
    (d) FLA-ABS Test

340. Erythema Nodosum Leprosum (ENL) occurs:
    [Karnataka 2007; DNB December 2011]
    (a) Due to Lepromin test reaction
    (b) In those with tuberculoid leprosy
    (c) As a reaction to multidrug therapy
    (d) In those with lepromatous leprosy

341. True about epidemiology of leprosy: [PGI Dec 08]
    (a) If high prevalence of cases seen in childhood, it means disease is under control
    (b) Lepra bacilli cannot survive outside human body
    (c) Bacterial load is high in tuberculoid variety
    (d) Insect can transmit the disease
    (e) Relapse rate is indictor of efficacy of the drug

342. Which of the following about lepromin test is not true?
    (a) It is negative in most children in first six months
    (b) It is a diagnostic test   [AIIMS May 2010]
    (c) It is an important aid to classify type of leprosy disease
    (d) BCG vaccination may convert lepra reaction from negative to positive

343. Leprosy is not yet eradicated because:
    [AIIMS PGMEE May 2012]
    (a) No effective vaccine
    (b) Highly infectious but low pathogenicity
    (c) Only humans are reservoir
    (d) Long incubation period

344. Prevalence of leprosy in India per 10,000 is?
    (a) >1   (b) 0.88   [DNB June 2011]
    (c) 0.71   (d) 0.69

345. Ridley Jopling Leprosy classification is a type of:
    [AIIMS PGMEE May 2013]
    (a) Clinical, bacteriological, Immunological, epidemiological classification
    (b) Clinical, bacteriological, Immunological, therapeutic classification
    (c) Clinical, bacteriological, Immunological, histological classification
    (d) Operational classification

346. Lepromin test is used for all of the following *except*:
    [MP 2009] [NUPGET 2013]
    (a) Classify the lesions of leprosy patients
    (b) Determine the prognosis of disease
    (c) Assess the resistance of individuals to leprsoy
    (d) Diagnosis of leprosy

347. **True regarding Leprosy:** *[PGI November 2014]*
    (a) Clofazimine included in treatment regimen
    (b) Any positive smear 1+ is MBL
    (c) Grenz zone in Lepromatous spectrum
    (d) All deformity cases are MBL
    (e) MBL recommended treatment for 12 months duration

348. **4 Split skin smears of a single patient Two samples with 10 bacilli out of 100 hpf and 2 samples with >1000 bacilli out of average fields Bacteriological index?**
    (a) 3.5
    (b) 4.5 *[NEET Pattern 2015]*
    (c) 5.5
    (d) 6.5

349. **Annual new case detection rate of Leprosy in India is:** *[AIIMS November 2017]*
    (a) 0.64/10000
    (b) 9.71/10000
    (c) 0.64/100000
    (d) 9.71/100000

350. **Leprosy prevalence case rate in India as per March 2016:** *[AIIMS November 2017]*
    (a) 0.66/10000
    (b) 0.66/100000
    (c) 9.7/10000
    (d) 9.7/100000

351. **Which of the following may be used as Candidate vaccine(s) in Leprosy?** *[PGI November 2017]*
    (a) BCG vaccine
    (b) Killer M. Leprae + BCG vaccine
    (c) M. Indicus Pranii
    (d) BCG vaccine + M. vaccae
    (e) None

Review Questions

352. **Treatment of leprosy a/c to WHO is done by all drugs, except:** *[Bihar 2005]*
    (a) Dapsone
    (b) Clofazimine
    (c) Ciprofloxacin
    (d) Rifampicin

353. **Which of the following is true statement about leprosy:** *[PGI 1998] [UP 2004]*
    (a) Two plus (2+) indicates 2 different site
    (b) 7 sites are needed
    (c) Paucibacillary leprosy bacterial index is less than 2
    (d) Various sites needed

354. **In paucibacillary leprosy the single drug dapsone is continue for:** *[UP 2008]*
    (a) 9 days
    (b) 90 days
    (c) 180 days
    (d) 10 days

355. **In multi-bacillary leprosy, bacterial index is more than:** *[RJ 2005]*
    (a) 1
    (b) 2
    (c) 5
    (d) 10

356. **Which of the following measurements indicates whether leprosy cases are being detected early or not?** *[RJ 2007]*
    (a) New case detection rate
    (b) Proportion of children among new cases
    (c) Proportion of new cases with disability
    (d) Prevalence rate of disease

HIV

357. **A nurse got a NSI (Needle stick injury) from a HIV infected needle. Which of the following statements are True/False regarding the management?** *[AIIMS November 2019]*
    (a) Zidovudine used a monotherapy in PEP
    (b) Washing hands advised with soap and water
    (c) HIV status of nurse must be known before PEP
    (d) Repeat HIV testing at 6 weeks
    (e) Lamivudine + Tenofovir + Efavirenz for 4 weeks

358. **The commonest mode of transmission of AIDS in India (in descending order) is:** *[AIPGME 2002]*
    (a) Transplacental, homosexual, heterosexual
    (b) Homosexual, heterosexual, transplacental
    (c) Heterosexual, transplacental, homosexual
    (d) Heterosexual, homosexual, transplacental

359. **The first country in the South East Asian Region (SEAR) to report AIDS was:** *[Karnataka 2007]*
    (a) Sri Lanka
    (b) India
    (c) Thailand
    (d) Bangladesh

360. **The highest number of AIDS cases in India have occurred in the age group of:** *[Karnataka 2005]*
    (a) 0-14 years
    (b) 15-29 years
    (c) 30-44 years
    (d) Above 45 years

361. **WHO Stage IV HIV includes all except:** *[AIIMS May 2009]*
    (a) Toxoplasmosis
    (b) Pneumocystis carinii
    (c) HIV wasting syndrome
    (d) Oral thrush

362. **Major signs for AIDS case definition according to WHO are:** *[PGI June 03]*
    (a) Generalised lymphadenopathy
    (b) Prolong fever more than 1 month
    (c) Prolong cough for > 1 month
    (d) Chronic diarhoea > 1 month
    (e) Weight loss > 10%

363. **Regarding Epidemiology of HIV True is:**
    (a) Mother to Child Transmission is 25%
    (b) Seminal secretion are highly Infectious than vaginal Secretion
    (c) Infectious in window period
    (d) Southern Africa have 72% of total global burden
    (e) Children rarely affected

364. Which of the following is used to prevent transmission of HIV from an infected pregnant mother to newborn child?
 [AIIMS November 2011]
 (a) Lamivudine (b) Nevirapine
 (c) Stavudine (d) Didanosine

365. Risk of mother to child HIV transmission in pregnant woman at the time of delivery, and after delivery in non-breastfeeding woman is:
 [AIIMS PGMEE November 2013]
 (a) 5-10% (b) 10-15%
 (c) 15-30% (d) More than 50%

366. HIV post exposure prophylaxis should be started within:
 [NEET Pattern 2012]
 (a) 24 hours (b) 48 hours
 (c) 72 hours (d) 6 hours

367. HIV transmission Mother to child can be stopped by all *except*: *[AIIMS PGMEE May 2013]*
 (a) Caesarean section
 (b) Vitamin A supplementation
 (c) Stopping Breastfeeding
 (d) Zidovudine to mother antenatal and newborn after delivery

368. MC subtype of HIV in India is: *[NEET Pattern 2013]*
 (a) HIV-A (b) HIV-B
 (c) HIV-C (d) None of the above

369. HIV sentinel surveillance is used to identify/calculate:
 [AIIMS PGMEE November 2012]
 (a) High risk population
 (b) Prevalence of HIV
 (c) Trend finding among populations
 (d) All of the above

370. Antiretroviral prophylaxis decrease the chance of transmission of HIV to fetus during pregnancy of HIV to fetus during pregnancy by: *[Bihar 2014]*
 (a) 35% (b) 45%
 (c) 50% (d) 65%

371. HIV virus was discovered in the year:
 (a) 1981 (b) 1983 *[AIIMS May 2014]*
 (c) 1986 (d) 1996

372. Most effective to prevent HIV Vertical transmission:
 [NEET Pattern 2015]
 (a) HAART (b) Nevirapine
 (c) Zidovudine (d) Elective CS

373. Post-exposure prophylaxis against HIV infection should not be delayed beyond: *[UPSC CMS 2015]*
 (a) 4 hours (b) 8 hours
 (c) 24 hours (d) 48 hours

374. Which states are qualified as high prevalence states in the context of HIV/AIDS? *[UPSC CMS 2015]*
 (a) When prevalence in high risk groups is more than 5%, and less than 1% in antenatal women
 (b) When prevalence in high risk groups is more than 5%, and 1% or more in antenatal women
 (c) When prevalence in high risk groups is less than 5%, and more than 1% in antenatal women
 (d) None of these

375. Which one of the following tests has the highest chance of detecting HIV infection in a blood donor during the window period? *[UPSC CMS 2015]*
 (a) Demonstration of antibody to HIV by ELISA
 (b) CD4 count
 (c) P24 antigen detection
 (d) Western blot test

376. False regarding HIV 1 & 2 is: *[NEET Pattern 2015]*
 (a) HIV 2 discovered in West Africa 1986
 (b) Resembles Simian virus
 (c) Blood screened for both HIV 1 & 2
 (d) HIV 2 is more dangerous

377. True about post-exposure prophylaxis in HIV:
 [NEET Pattern 2016]
 (a) Should be given in 5 days of exposure
 (b) Single dose Nevirapine prevents mother to child transmission
 (c) Given for 2 weeks
 (d) Standard protocol is to use any two NRTs with no other drugs

378. Which of the following is defined as Generalized HIV epidemic? *[NEET Pattern 2017]*
 (a) Prevalence in pregnant women > 0.5%
 (b) Prevalence in a population > 0.5%
 (c) Prevalence in pregnant women > 1%
 (d) Prevalence in a population > 1%

379. If in a state prevalence of HIV is >5% in high risk group but in antenatal women it is <1%. The state belongs to:
 [NEET Pattern 2017]
 (a) High prevalence state
 (b) Moderate prevalence state
 (c) Low prevalence state
 (d) Very low prevalence state

380. Average Incubation period of HIV to AIDS transformation is: *[NEET Pattern 2018]*
 (a) 1 year (b) 2 years
 (c) 5 years (d) 10 years

381. Maximum chances of HIV transmission are associated with? *[PGI May 2018]*
 (a) Receptive anal sex
 (b) Insertive anal sex
 (c) Receptive oral sex
 (d) Insertive oral sex
 (e) Vaginal sex

382. Slogan of World AIDS Day 2017 is *[JIPMER May 2018]*
 (a) Unite for HIV (b) HIV wellness
 (c) Right to health (d) Everyone counts

383. A resident got Needle stick injury (NSI) while taking sutures of a HIV positive patient. Which of the following statements is incorrect regarding HIV transmission? [NEET Pattern 2019]
    (a) Three drug combination to be preferred for Post exposure prophylaxis (PEP)
    (b) 28 day prescription for PEP to be done
    (c) PEP to be offered within maximum 72 hours
    (d) High chances of HIV transmission

384. True regarding mother to child transmission of HIV is: [NEET Pattern 2019]
    (a) Rate of transmission is 80-90%
    (b) Very low chance of transmission of mother is newly infected
    (c) Transmission is direct relationship with the maternal viral Load
    (d) Elective caesarean section has no role in prevention

Review Questions

385. About epidemiology of AIDS all are true except:
    (a) In India it is mainly caused by HIV-1 [MP 2002]
    (b) Maternofetal transmission is the most common mode of transmission
    (c) I.V. drug abuse increases the risk
    (d) Medical personnel are at higher risk of getting infection with HIV

386. All the following statements are true for the viral genome in HIV, except: [MP 2009]
    (a) They are diploid
    (b) They consist of DNA dependent DNA polymerase activity
    (c) They consist of three major genes-gag, pol and env-characteristic of all retroviruses
    (d) They are most complex of human retroviruses

387. From epidemiological point of view of AIDS, which of the following states in India is put in Group I (i.e. general epidemiological cases of HIV > 5% high risk and HIV > 1% ANC)? [MH 2003]
    (a) Assam   (b) Mizoram
    (c) Nagaland   (d) Tripura

388. Window period for HIV infection is: [RJ 2005]
    (a) 3-12 weeks   (b) 8-20 weeks
    (c) 6-24 weeks   (d) None

389. Most common mode of HIV transmission from mother to child: [RJ 2005]
    (a) 1st trimester (b) 2nd transmission
    (c) Perinatal   (d) Breastfeeding

STI'S (OTHER THAN HIV)

390. In India, Pre-transfusion routine blood screening is recommended for all, except: [INICET May 2022]
    (a) HIV   (b) HBV
    (c) Malaria   (d) Dengue

391. Which of the following is the causative agent of STD disease Donovanosis? [NEET PG Pattern January 2020]
    (a) Hemophilus ducreyi
    (b) Klebsiella granulomatis
    (c) Leishmania donovani
    (d) Treponema pallidum

392. Match the STD Color Coded Kits with their Numbers [INICET July 2021]

STD Kit Color	Syndrome
A. White	1. Urethral/cervical discharge
B. Grey	2. Genital ulcer disease
C. Green	3. Lower abdominal pain
D. Yellow	4. Vaginal discharge

   (a) A-1, B-2, C-3, D-4
   (b) A-4, B-2, C-1, D-3
   (c) A-3, B-1, C-2, D-4
   (d) A-2, B-1, C-4, D-3

393. All the following are causative agents of sexually transmitted infections except: [AIPGME 1991]
    (a) Candida   (b) Group B streptococcus
    (c) Hepatitis B   (d) Echinococcus

394. The syndromic management of urethral discharge includes treatment of: [AIIMS Dec 1992]
    (a) Neisseria gonorrhoeae and herpes genitalis
    (b) Chalamydia trachomatis and herpes genitalis
    (c) Neisseria gonorrhoeae and Chlamydia trachomatis
    (d) Syphilis and chancroid

395. In India, syndromic approach is used for management of: [AIIMS November 2011]
    (a) Chancroid and Chancre
    (b) Chancroid and Herpes genitalis
    (c) Chancroid, Chancre and Herpes genitalis
    (d) Chancre and Herpes genitalis

396. True about incubation periods of STDs:
    (a) Syphilis 10-90 days [PGI May 2011]
    (b) LGV 3-10 days
    (c) Donovanosis 3-20 days
    (d) Chancroid 21-28 days
    (e) Gonorrhea 2-14 days

397. A sexually active, long distance truck driver's wife comes with vaginal discharge. Under Syndromic approach, which drug should be given? [AIIMS PGMEE May 2012]
    (a) Metronidazole, Azithromycin, Fluconazole
    (b) Metronidazole
    (c) Azithromycin
    (d) Metronidazole and fluconazole

398. Case detection in STDs is done by all except: [NUPGET 2013]
    (a) Screening   (b) Contact tracing
    (c) Cluster testing (d) Notification

399. Drug of choice for Scabies in pregnancy is:
 [NEET Pattern 2014]
 (a) Ivermectin (b) Crotaminton
 (c) Benzyl benzoate (d) Permethrin

Review Question

400. Method of case detection in control of sexually transmitted diseases in which person names the persons moving in same socio-sexual environment? [MH 2007]
 (a) Contact tracing
 (b) High risk screening
 (c) Selective screening
 (d) Cluster testing

OTHER COMMUNICABLE DISEASES

401. Mass Drug Administration is not helpful for:
 [AIIMS November 2019]
 (a) Lymphatic filariasis
 (b) Vitamin A deficiency
 (c) Worm infestation
 (d) Scabies

402. Which of the following statements about Yaws is not true? [AIPGME 2008]
 (a) Spread by sexual transmission
 (b) Caused by Treponema pertenue
 (c) Has cross immunity with Syphilis
 (d) Cannot be differentiated serologically from Treponema pallidum

403. Dhamendra's Index and Jopling's classification deals with: [AIPGME 2008]
 (a) TB (b) Leprosy
 (c) Syphilis (d) Polio

404. The following are characteristic features of staphylococcal food poisoning, except: [AIIMS May 2004]
 (a) Optimum temperature for toxin formation is 37°C
 (b) Intra-dietetic toxins are responsible for intestinal symptoms
 (c) Toxins can be destroyed by boiling for 30 minutes
 (d) Incubation period is 1-6 hours

405. Iceberg phenomenon is not seen in:
 [NEET Pattern 2017; AIIMS Nov 1993]
 (a) AIDS (b) TB
 (c) Poliomyelitis (d) Measles

406. All of the following diseases can be transmitted during the incubation period except: [AIIMS June 1997]
 (a) Measles (b) Tuberculosis
 (c) Hepatitis A (d) Pertussis

407. In all of the following diseases chronic carriers are found except: [AIIMS Sep 96, May 2006; June 1998]
 (a) Measles (b) Typhoid
 (c) Hepatitis B (d) Gonorrhea

408. Brucellosis can be transmitted by all of the following modes, except: [AIIMS May 2006-2007, Nov 2006]
 (a) Contact with infected placenta
 (b) Ingestion of raw vegetables from infected farms
 (c) Person to person transmission
 (d) Inhalation of infected dust or aerosol

409. In which of these conditions is post exposure prophylaxis NOT useful? [AIIMS May 2001, Nov 2004]
 (a) Measles (b) Rabies
 (c) Pertussis (d) Hepatitis B

410. "Hundred day cough" is the name of: [AIIMS Feb 1997]
 (a) Cough due to Bordetella pertussis
 (b) Cough due to haemophylus influenzae
 (c) Cough due to adenovirus
 (d) Cough due to respiratory syncytial virus

411. Which one of the following diseases CANNOT be eradicated: [AIPGME 1992, 2003]
 (a) Leprosy (b) Tuberculosis
 (c) Measles (d) Pertussis

412. '3 by 5 Initiative' was launched in developing countries to combat: [AIIMS May 2005]
 (a) Tuberculosis (b) Malaria
 (c) SARS (d) HIV/AIDS

413. Intermediate host for Taenia saginata is:
 (a) Man (b) Cattle [AIIMS May 1994]
 (c) Pig (d) Fish

414. A synthetic "cocktail" vaccine SPf66 has shown potential for the protection against: [AIIMS June 1997]
 (a) Dengue/DHF (b) Japanese encephalitis
 (c) Falciparum malaria (d) Lymphatic filariasis

415. All of the following are blood-borne infections except:
 [AIIMS Nov 2003]
 (a) Hepatitis B (b) Hepatitis C
 (c) Hepatitis E (d) Hepatitis G

416. Carriers are important in all the following except:
 [AIPGME 2002, 2011, AIPGME 2007; DNB 2003]
 (a) Polio (b) Typhoid [AIIMS Dec 98]
 (c) Measles (d) Diphtheria

417. Man in the only host for: [DPG 2006]
 (a) Trichuris trichura
 (b) Dracunculus medinensis
 (c) Onchocerca volvolus
 (d) Wuchereria bancrofti

418. Which of the following is not administered by intradermal route? [DPG 2007, 2008]
 (a) BCG (b) Insulin
 (c) Mantoux (d) Drug sensitivity injection

419. Disease caused by arboviruses include: [PGI June 02]
 (a) Yellow fever (b) Japanese encephalitis
 (c) Trench fever (d) Epidemic typhus
 (e) Dengue

420. Cluster testing is the term used during: [RJ 2007]
    (a) UIP Survey for polio [Karnataka 2007]
    (b) Screening for STDs [DNB 2000, 2005, 2006]
    (c) Exposing the body for hypopigmented patches
    (d) Testing contacts of typhoid cases [AIPGME 2002]

421. Incubation period less than few hours: [PGI Dec 2K]
    (a) Hepatitis – A   (b) Food poisoning
    (c) Influenza   (d) Rabies

422. Post exposure prophylaxis in healthcare professional is indicated in infections with: [PGI Dec 08]
    (a) HBV   (b) Rabies
    (c) Diphtheria   (d) Measles
    (e) Tetanus

423. Epidemic caused by type A arbovirus in India is: [DPG 2008]
    (a) Chikungunya   (b) KFD
    (c) Yellow fever (d) Dengue

424. Karatomalacia is seen in which of the following diseases: [PGI June 02; PGI 2001]
    (a) Measles   (b) Diarrhea
    (c) Mumps   (d) Rubella
    (e) Chickenpox

425. Pandemics are caused by: [PGI June 05]
    (a) Hepatitis-B   (b) Influenza-A
    (c) Influenza-B   (d) Influenza-C

426. Animal to man transmission seen in: [PGI Dec 08]
    (a) Rabies   (b) Japanese encephalitis
    (c) HIV   (d) Mumps
    (e) Tetanus

427. Vector-borne diseases are: [PGI Dec 08]
    (a) Epidemic typhus   (b) Japanese encephalitis
    (c) Tetanus   (d) Hanta virus disease
    (e) KFD

428. Viruses documented to cause fetal damage: [PGI June 05]
    (a) Hepatitis B   (b) Varicella
    (c) Measles   (d) Parvovirus

429. Which of the following is not transmitted by lice? [AIIMS May 2009; NEET Pattern 2017]
    (a) Trench fever   (b) Relapsing fever
    (c) Q fever   (d) Epidemic typhus

430. Mass prophylaxis is given for all except: [AIIMS Nov 2010]
    (a) Lymphatic filariasis   (b) Vitamin A deficiency
    (c) Scabies   (d) Worm infestation

431. Modes of transmission of amoebiasis are all except: [AIIMS Nov 2010]
    (a) Faecal-oral   (b) Oro-rectal
    (c) Vertical transmission
    (d) Through cockroaches

432. Arthropod-borne disease not seen in India is: [AIPGME 2011]
    (a) West Nile fever
    (b) Dengue infection
    (c) Kyasanur Forest disease
    (d) Yellow fever

433. All are true about Yaws except: [AIPGME 2011]
    (a) Caused by Treponema pertenue
    (b) Transmitted non-venerally
    (c) Secondary Yaws can involve bones
    (d) Later stages involve heart and nerves

434. Tetracycline is used in the prophylaxis of: [AIPGME 2011]
    (a) Cholera   (b) Brucellosis
    (c) Leptospirosis (d) Meningitis

435. Maternal antibodies do not occur for: [DPG 2011]
    (a) Polio   (b) Diphtheria
    (c) Whooping cough   (d) Tetanus

436. Brucellosis is transmitted by: [PGI May 2011]
    (a) Cattle   (b) Camel
    (c) Sheep   (d) Goat
    (e) Dogs

437. Which is not transmitted by Aedes aegypti? [DNB June 2011]
    (a) Yellow fever
    (b) Dengue
    (c) Japanese encephalitis
    (d) Filariasis

438. Maternal antibodies are present in the newborn against all of the following disease except: [DNB 2008]
    (a) Diphtheria   (b) Tetanus
    (c) Pertussis   (d) Measles

439. Mass prophylaxis not done in: [AIIMS PGMEE November 2012]
    (a) Scabies
    (b) Lymphatic filariasis
    (c) Vitamin A deficiency
    (d) Worm infestation

440. Rat is associated with: [DNB June 2010; NEET Patterns 2014]
    (a) Leptospirosis   (b) Measles
    (c) Tetanus   (d) Influenza

441. Incubation period of which disease is less than 7 days: [NEET Pattern 2012]
    (a) Cholera   (b) Measles
    (c) Leishmaniasis   (d) Mumps

442. Which of the following is a zoonotic disease? [NEET Pattern 2012] [NEET Pattern 2013]
    (a) Hydatid cyst   (b) Malaria
    (c) Filariasis   (d) Dengue fever

443. **Subclinical infection is seen in all** *except*:
 [NEET Pattern 2012]
 (a) Mumps (b) Poliomyelitis
 (c) Measles (d) Rubella

444. **Second attack rate is minimum in:** *[NEET Pattern 2013]*
 (a) TB (b) Diphtheria
 (c) Measles (d) Whooping cough

445. **Post-exposure prophylaxis exist for all** *except*:
 [NUPGET 2013]
 (a) Measles (b) Hepatitis C
 (c) Varicella zoster (d) HIV

446. **Scabies treatment(s) include:** *[PGI May 2012]*
 (a) Gammexene (b) Crotamiton
 (c) 5% Permethrin (d) Isoniazid
 (e) Sulphur ointment

447. **Zoonotic disease of viral etiology include:**
 [NUPGET 2013]
 (a) Q fever (b) Rickettsiae disease
 (c) Rabies (d) Rubella

448. **Isolation period, false is:** *[AIIMS May 2013]*
 (a) Chickenpox – 6 days after onset of rash
 (b) Herpes zoster – 6 days after onset of rash
 (c) Measles – up to 3 days after onset of rash
 (d) German measles – 7 days after onset of rash

449. **True about Leptospirosis is/are:** *[PGI November 2012]*
 (a) It is a Zoonosis
 (b) Incubation period is 2–3 months
 (c) Transmission occurs through direct skin contact
 (d) Drug of choice is Penicillin
 (e) Is a Spirochaetal disease

450. **Following are examples of human "dead end" disease** *except*:
 [NEET Pattern 2013]
 (a) Bubonic plague
 (b) Japanese encephalitis
 (c) Hydatid disease
 (d) Leishmaniasis

451. **Which disease does not occur as seasonal variation?**
 [NEET Pattern 2012]
 (a) Measles (b) Rubella
 (c) Gastroenteritis (d) Cerebra meningitis

452. **The following fall under the category of enzootic** *except*:
 [DNB 2007]
 (a) Influenza
 (b) Anthrax
 (c) Brucellosis
 (d) Endemic typhus

453. **Tick-borne relapsing fever is caused by:**
 (a) Borrelia recurrentis *[DNB December 2010]*
 (b) Borrelia burgdorferi
 (c) Rickettsia prowazeki
 (d) Borellia hermsii

454. **Viral hemorrhagic fever(s) seen in India is/are:**
 [PGI November 2013]
 (a) KFD
 (b) Dengue fever
 (c) Crimean Congo fever
 (d) Yellow fever
 (e) Hanta fever

455. **Saddleback fever is known as:** *[NIMHANS 2014]*
 (a) Brucellosis (b) Dengue fever
 (c) Malaria fever (d) Typhoid fever

456. **Chemoprophylaxis is not required in:** *[AIIMS May 2014]*
 (a) Conjunctivitis (b) Meningitis
 (c) Measles (d) Plague

457. **Following is NOT caused by virus:**
 (a) Rocky mountain spotted fever
 (b) KFD *[NEET Pattern 2014]*
 (c) Dengue
 (d) Yellow fever

458. **Regarding Non-industrial anthrax, true is/are:**
 [PGI November 2014]
 (a) Common in veterinarians
 (b) Seasonal pattern
 (c) Common in butchers
 (d) Cutaneous form most common
 (e) More commonly inhalational than industrial form

459. **Not true about Ebola virus is:** *[PGI November 2014]*
 (a) Caused by ss Negative strand RNA virus
 (b) Bats most likely reservoir
 (c) Incubation period is less than 48 hours
 (d) Sexual transmission possible
 (e) Oseltamivir is quite effective in treatment

460. **Zoonoses include:** *[PGI November 2014]*
 (a) Plague (b) Rabies
 (c) Anthrax (d) Tetanus
 (e) Brucellosis

461. **Incubation period less than 5 days is:**
 [PGI November 2014]
 (a) Influenza
 (b) Salmonella typhi
 (c) Vibrio parahemolyticus
 (d) Yersinia
 (e) Swine flu

462. **Metazoonoses include:** *[JIPMER 2014]*
 (a) Plague (b) Rabies
 (c) Schistosomiasis (d) Brucellosis
 (e) Yellow fever

463. **MC Shigella subtype in India is:** *[NEET Pattern 2015]*
 (a) Shigella dysenteriae
 (b) Shigella flexneri
 (c) Shigella boydii
 (d) Shigella sonnei

464. Consider the following diseases:
    1. Measles
    2. Polio
    3. Staphylococcal food poisoning
    4. Typhoid

    Which of the above are the correct examples for incubation period of 10-14 days? [UPSC CMS 2015]
    (a) 1 and 3
    (b) 2 and 4
    (c) 1 and 4
    (d) 3 and 4

465. Post exposure prophylaxis is given in:
    (a) Hepatitis A infection [PGI November 2017]
    (b) Hepatitis B infection
    (c) Hepatitis C infection
    (d) Rabies
    (e) Varicella zoster virus infection

466. Cattle and sheep livestock is natural host for: [NEET Pattern 2017]
    (a) Crimean Congo fever
    (b) Dengue
    (c) KFD
    (d) Yellow fever

467. Viral hemorrhagic fever includes? [PGI May 2018]
    (a) Yellow fever
    (b) West Nile fever
    (c) Lassa fever
    (d) Ross fever
    (e) Crimean Congo fever

468. Vector-borne diseases are? [PGI May 2018]
    (a) Dengue
    (b) KFD
    (c) Japanese encephalitis
    (d) Plague
    (e) Yellow fever

Review Questions

469. Inclusion body in neuron is seen in: [DNB 2001]
    (a) Rabies
    (b) Diphtheria
    (c) Yellow fever
    (d) Japanese encephalitis

470. Agent can be used in bioterrorism: [Bihar 2005]
    (a) Plague
    (b) Typhoid
    (c) *Streptococcus*
    (d) *Staph. aureus*

471. Incubation period is less than 1 week in: [UP 2003]
    (a) Cholera
    (b) Enteric fever
    (c) Hepatitis B
    (d) Chickenpox

472. Subacute Sclerosing panencephalitis (SSPE) is caused by: [UP 2005]
    (a) Measles
    (b) Mumps
    (c) Rubella
    (d) Smallpox

473. Clinical features of Botulism are all except: [UP 2006]
    (a) Diarrhea
    (b) Dysarthria
    (c) Ocular nerve paralysis
    (d) Blurring of vision

474. Amphixenosis is: [UP 2007]
    (a) Ascaris lumbricoidis
    (b) Entrobius - vermicularis
    (c) Anthrax
    (d) T. cruzi

475. Following are examples of human "dead end" disease *except*: [UP 2007]
    (a) Bubonic plague
    (b) Japanese encephalitis
    (c) Hydatid disease
    (d) Leishmaniasis

476. Shortest Incubation period is associated with: [AP 2002]
    (a) Influenza
    (b) Cholera
    (c) Syphilis
    (d) AIDS

477. Disease transmitted by water is: [AP 2003]
    (a) Hepatitis B
    (b) Polio
    (c) Japanese encephalitis
    (d) Dengue fever

478. Which of the following flavi virus is closely related to Russian spring summer encephalitis causing virus: [AP 2004]
    (a) Dengue
    (b) Chikungunya
    (c) KFD
    (d) Yellow fever

479. Which statement is not true in arboviral disease?
    (a) Japanese encephalitis is transmitted by culex
    (b) KFD is transmitted by Ticks [AP 2005]
    (c) Filariasis is transmitted by Aedes mosquito
    (d) Dengue is transmitted by Aedes mosquito

480. All of the following are Anthropozoonotic diseases except: [AP 2008]
    (a) Plague
    (b) Rabies
    (c) Hydatid cyst
    (d) Dracunculosis

481. Leptospira icterohaemorrhagiae infection is transmitted by the following animals:
    [AP 1987; NIMHANS 2001; TN 1995; TN 2000]
    (a) Rats
    (b) Dogs
    (c) Birds
    (d) Bats

482. Patients are to be isolated in all of the following diseases except: [TN 2003]
    (a) AIDS
    (b) Smallpox
    (c) Anthrax
    (d) Plague

483. Tick-borne disease is: [Kolkata 2004]
    (a) Tularemia
    (b) Q fever
    (c) Relapsing fever
    (d) Rocky mountain spotted fever

484. Aedes transmit which of the following disease in India: [Kolkata 2004]
    (a) Dengue
    (b) Chikungunya fever
    (c) Malaria/Filaria
    (d) Japanese encephalitis

485. Cyclopropogative cycle is seen is:
    [Kolkata 2009; NEET Patterns 2012, 2016]
    (a) Malaria
    (b) Filaria
    (c) Yellow fever
    (d) Plague

486. Food poisoning is caused by all *except*: [MP 2000]
    (a) *Staphylococcus aureus*
    (b) *Clostridium difficile*
    (c) *Vibrio parahaemolyticus*
    (d) *Bacillus cereus*

487. Isolation is not useful in: [MP 2002]
    (a) Polio   (b) Cholera
    (c) Measles   (d) Diphtheria

488. Which of the following is most prevalent presently in India: [MP 2002]
    (a) Polio   (b) Dracunculiasis
    (c) Plague   (d) Kala-azar

489. Iceberg phenomena is seen in all *except*: [MP 2003]
    (a) Leprosy   (b) Rabies
    (c) Hypertension   (d) Tuberculosis

490. Due to epidemiological reasons chemoprophylaxis is most impractical in the control of: [MH 2003]
    (a) Measles   (b) Cholera
    (c) Diphtheria   (d) Tuberculosis

491. Plague is what type of zoonosis? [MH 2005; JIPMER 2014]
    (a) Cyclozoonosis   (b) Direct zoonosis
    (c) Sapro-zoonosis   (d) Meta zoonosis

492. Which is not a zoonotic disease? [RJ 2002]
    (a) Brucellosis   (b) Malaria
    (c) Rabies   (d) Trichinoses

493. Which is not a zoonotic disease? [RJ 2003]
    (a) Tetanus   (b) Rabies
    (c) Brucellosis   (d) Hydatid disease

494. Shortest incubation period is of: [RJ 2004]
    (a) Diphtheria   (b) Rubella
    (c) Smallpox   (d) Chickenpox

495. Which one of the following is an Index of communicability of an infection? [RJ 2009]
    (a) Carrier rate
    (b) Prevalence rate
    (c) Secondary attack rate
    (d) Primary attack rate

EMERGING AND RE-EMERGING INFECTIONS

496. Not true for Ebola virus disease: [AIIMS June 2020]
    (a) Commonly transmitted through Nosocomial route
    (b) Spread by mosquito
    (c) Filovirus
    (d) Man is an accidental dead end host

497. Confirmed clinical cases have been reported from India for which of the following viral hemorrhagic fevers recently? [AIIMS November 2017]
    (a) Yellow fever   (b) Marburg fever
    (c) Crimean Congo fever   (d) Hanta virus

498. Vector of Crimean Congo hemorrhagic fever: [NEET Pattern 2018]
    (a) Brucella suis   (b) Hyalomma tick
    (c) Brucella abortus   (d) Brucella canis

CORONARY HEART DISEASE

499. Mrs. X, plasma glucose level 160 mg/dl. What will you advise regarding the non-pharmacological management of the disease? [INICET May 2022]
    (a) Not more than 30% calories should come from the fat
    (b) <5000 mg/day Sodium
    (c) Diet with Total cholesterol less than 100 mg per day
    (d) Diet including 80g dietary fibre daily

500. "MONICA Project" is associated with [NEET PG Pattern January 2020]
    (a) Risk factor intervention trials for CVD
    (b) Oslow diet/smoking intervention study
    (c) Monitoring of trends and determinants in Cardiovascular disease
    (d) Lipid Research Clinics study

501. Following dietary changes are advised to reduce prevalence of coronary heart disease *except*: [AIPGME 1997, 04]
    (a) Increased complex carbohydrate intake
    (b) Saturated fat intake less than 10% of total energy intake
    (c) Salt intake less than 20 g/day
    (d) Reduce fat intake to 20-30% of total energy intake

502. Which one of the following statements about influence of smoking on risk of coronary heart disease (CHD) is not true? [AIPGME 2005] [AIPGME 1999]
    (a) Risk of death from CHD decreases from cessation of smoking [AIPGME 1999]
    (b) Filters provide a protective effect for CHD
    (c) Influence of smoking is synergistic to other risk factors for CHD
    (d) Influence of smoking is directly related to number of cigarettes smoked per day

503. Which of the following is maximally associated with Coronary heart disease? [AIIMS Nov 2010]
    (a) HDL   (b) VLDL
    (c) LDL   (d) Chylomicrons

504. Which of the following is not a dietary modification recommended in high risk cardiovascular group? [AIPGME 2011]
    (a) LDL cholesterol less than 100 mg/dL
    (b) Avoid alcohol
    (c) Saturated fat intake 7% of total calories
    (d) Salt intake less than 5 grams

505. Inability to perform any work without discomfort is: [AIIMS November 2014]
    (a) NYHA 1   (b) NYHA 2
    (c) NYHA 3   (d) NYHA 4

506. Which of the primordial prevention strategies is not for coronary heart disease (CHD)? [NEET Pattern 2016]
    (a) Take healthy diet containing adequate amounts of macro and micro nutrients
    (b) Regular physical activity
    (c) Management of hypertension and diabetes
    (d) Prevention of tobacco use

507. Primary prevention in Myocardial infarction are all except: [NEET Pattern 2018]
    (a) Maintenance of normal body weight
    (b) Change in life style
    (c) Change in nutritional habits
    (d) Screening for hypertension

Review Questions

508. False about coronary heart disease: [AP 2007]
    (a) Indian CHD occurs 1 decade later than Western CHD
    (b) Heavy cigarette smoking is a risk factor
    (c) Males are affected more than females
    (d) None

509. All of the following are true about coronary heart diseases in India except: [MP 2000]
    (a) Smoking predisposition seen
    (b) Mean age of patient is 10-20 years more than that of western
    (c) Seen more in males
    (d) DM predisposition to MI is seen

510. Best-know large sample study programme for coronary heart disease is: [MH 2003; NEET Pattern 2013]
    (a) Framingham study   (b) North kerelia study
    (c) Standford study   (d) Oxford study

511. Modifiable risk factors in coronary artery disease are all except: [MH 2005]
    (a) Personality   (b) Smoking
    (c) Obesity   (d) Hypertension

HYPERTENSION

512. A person who has lower blood pressure during childhood tends to have low blood pressure during adulthood too. This is known as: [NEET PG Pattern 2023]
    (a) STEPS approach
    (b) Rule of halves
    (c) Tracking phenomenon
    (d) None of the above

513. True about hypertension, the primary prevention includes: [PGI June 06]
    (a) Weight reduction
    (b) Exercise promotion
    (c) Reduction of salt intake
    (d) Early diagnosis of hypertension
    (e) Self care

514. Tracking of BP implies: [NEET Pattern 2014]
    (a) BP increase with age
    (b) BP decreases with age
    (c) BP of hyoptensive become hypertensive
    (d) BP of hyoptensive remain hypotensive

515. What is DASH? [NEET Pattern 2017; PGMCET 2015]
    (a) Dietary approaches to stop hypertension
    (b) Domestic approach to safeguard hepatitis
    (c) Dietary approaches to stop hyperlipidemia
    (d) Domestic approaches to stop hypertension

516. Diet to be prescribed in hypertension: [NEET Pattern 2015]
    (a) Fruits, vegetables and low salt diet
    (b) Proteins, fibres and low salt diet
    (c) Carbohydrate, fibres and low salt diet
    (d) Fruits, vegetables, Low fat dairy foods

RHEUMATIC FEVER

517. A child presented with manifestations of Streptococcal infection but no carditis. What will you suggest for secondary prevention? [NEET PG Pattern 2022]
    (a) Single dose of Inj. Benzathine penicillin
    (b) Lifelong benzathine penicillin 3 weekly once
    (c) 3 weekly benzathine penicillin injection for 5 years or till 18 years whichever is later
    (d) 3 weekly benzathine penicillin injection for 5 years or till 25 years whichever is later

518. All of the following statements about rheumatic fever/heart disease epidemiology in India are true except: [AIIMS Nov 2002]
    (a) Its prevalence varies between 2 and 11 per 1000 children aged 5-16 years
    (b) Mitral regurgitation is the commonest cardiac lesion seen
    (c) It occurs equally in females and males
    (d) Rheumatic fever occurs in about 2% of streptococcal sore throats

519. All are true about rheumatic fever in India except: [AIIMS Dec 1994]
    (a) RF is reported in 1-3% of streptococcal infections
    (b) More commonly seen in 5-15 years age group
    (c) Except carditis, other manifestations do not cause permanent damage
    (d) In Revised Jones' Criteria, evidence of preceding streptococcal infection is taken for last 21 days

520. All of the following are Major criteria of Jones in Rheumatic fever except: [AIIMS Nov 2010]
    (a) Pancarditis
    (b) Arthritis
    (c) Chorea
    (d) Elevated ESR

521. Not included among major criteria in acute rheumatic fever is: [AIIMS PGMEE May 2013]
    (a) Erythema marginatum
    (b) Polyarthralgia
    (c) Chorea
    (d) Pancarditis

522. Erythema marginatum accompany the following in Acute rheumatic fever: [NEET Pattern 2015]
    (a) Carditis
    (b) Arthritis
    (c) Subcutaneous nodules
    (d) Chorea

523. Jai Vigyan National Mission is for: [NEET Pattern 2017]
    (a) Adolescent girls health
    (b) Mother & child health [MCH]
    (c) Science & technology
    (d) Child labour prevention

CANCERS

524. HPV infection may lead to (Multiple response) [INICET May 2022]
    (a) Cervical cancer
    (b) Anal cancer
    (c) Oropharyngeal cancer
    (d) Laryngeal papillomatosis

525. The most common cancer affecting Indian urban women in Delhi, Mumbai and Chennai is: [DNB 2007, AIPGME 2005]
    (a) Cervical cancer
    (b) Ovarian cancer
    (c) Breast cancer
    (d) Uterine cancer

526. The most common cancer, affecting both males and females of the world, is: [AIIMS May 2005, Dec 1994]
    (a) Cancer of the pancreas NEET Pattern 2013
    (b) Buccal mucosa cancer
    (c) Lung cancer
    (d) Colorectal cancer

527. The most common malignant tumor of adult males in India is: [AIPGME 2004]
    (a) Oropharyngeal carcinoma
    (b) Gastric carcinoma
    (c) Colorectal carcinoma
    (d) Lung cancer

528. The most common type of cancer among females in India is: [Karnataka 2005]
    (a) Cervical cancer
    (b) Breast cancer
    (c) Ovarian cancer
    (d) Colonic cancer

529. Habits and customs are conducive to cancer as evident below except: [Karnataka 2006]
    (a) Kangri cancer in Kashmir due to hot pot in winter
    (b) Oral cancer due to pan chewing in India
    (c) Penile cancer and cervical cancer following circumcision
    (d) Lung cancer due to smoking

530. Which of the following can be prevented by screening: [PGI June 08]
    (a) Ca cervix
    (b) Ca Breast
    (c) Ca Prostate
    (d) Ca Lung
    (e) Ca Colon

531. Highest increase in survival rate is seen after screening of: [AIIMS May 2011]
    (a) Carcinoma cervix
    (b) Carcinoma lungs
    (c) Carcinoma colon
    (d) Carcinoma breast

532. Current cancer patients in India reported annually: [AIIMS PGMEE November 2012]
    (a) 0.5 million
    (b) 1 million
    (c) 5 millions
    (d) 10 millions

533. Globally most common cancer is: [NUPGET 2013]
    (a) Colorectal cancer
    (b) Bladder cancer
    (c) Lung cancer
    (d) Oropharyngeal cancer

534. Tobacco responsible for oral cancer is: [NEET Pattern 2014]
    (a) 100%
    (b) 40%
    (c) 90%
    (d) 60%

535. Maximum mortality in India among women is due to which carcinoma? [NEET Pattern 2015]
    (a) Lungs
    (b) Cervix-uteri
    (c) Ovary
    (d) Breast

536. Which of the following is the MC malignant tumor in Adult males in India? [UPSC CMS 2015]
    (a) Lung cancer
    (b) Oropharyngeal carcinoma
    (c) Gastric carcinoma
    (d) Colorectal carcinoma

537. MCC of Cervical cancer in India is: [NEET Pattern 2015]
    (a) HPV 31, 33
    (b) HPV 6, 11
    (c) HPV 16, 18
    (d) HPV 31, 45

538. Population-based registries are better than hospital based registries due to the following reasons except: [NEET Pattern 2017]
    (a) May be used for etiological studies
    (b) Help in assessing the effectiveness of control program
    (c) Measure the burden of disease in a defined population
    (d) Provide readily accessible information about patients and treatment outcome

539. Which of the following is not a goal of Population based cancer registry? [NEET Pattern 2018]
    (a) Administrative information
    (b) Determination of cancer rates and trends
    (c) Patterns of care and outcomes
    (d) Cancer prevention

Review Questions

540. Best method of screening for early detection of carcinoma breast in young woman is: [Bihar 2004]
    (a) Regular X-rays
    (b) Self examination
    (c) Mammography
    (d) Regular biopsies

541. "Field carcinogenesis" is seen in: [UP 2000]
    (a) Head and neck carcinoma
    (b) Colon carcinoma
    (c) Brain tumor
    (d) Breast carcinoma

542. Risk factors for Cancer cervix are increased by the following: [MP 2007]
    (a) Less than 20 years of age
    (b) Late marriage
    (c) Upper socio-economic class
    (d) Early marriage

543. Which is not a predisposing factor for carcinoma cervix? [RJ 2001]
    (a) Early marriage
    (b) Early coitus
    (c) Early child bearing
    (d) Single child birth

OBESITY

544. What will be the BMI of a male whose weight is 89 kg and height is 172 cm?
    [NEET Pattern 2018; AIPGME 2005; DNB 2007]
    (a) 27 (b) 30
    (c) 33 (d) 36

545. All of the following sites are used for measuring skin fold thickness to assess obesity except: [AIPGME 2004]
    (a) Mid-triceps
    (b) Biceps
    (c) Subscapular
    (d) Anterior abdominal wall

546. A patient is called obese if BMI is: [AIPGME 2007; NEET Pattern 2013]
    (a) 20-30 (b) > 25
    (c) > 30   (d) > 40

547. Internationally accepted method of measuring obesity is: [DPG 2006]
    (a) BMI (b) Ponderal index
    (c) Lorentz index (d) Corpulence index

548. Which of the following should be done to reduce obesity? [DPG 2006]
    (a) Regular exercise with same amount of food
    (b) Decrease fat intake but have stomach full
    (c) Reduce the amount of fat in diet only
    (d) Reduce intake of fats, carbohydrates and protein

549. An adult is considered to be overweight if he/she has the BMI: [Karnataka 2009]
    (a) >18.5 (b) > 20
    (c) > 25   (d) None of the above

550. Obesity indices are: [PGI June 02]
    (a) Broca's index (b) Ponderal index
    (c) Quetelet index (d) Corpulence index

551. Calculate BMI if weight in kilograms is 98 and height in centimeters is 175: [DNB December 2009, 11]
    (a) 28 (b) 32
    (c) 36 (d) 40

552. What will be the BMI of a male whose weight is 89 kg and height is 172 cm? [DNB 2007]
    (a) 27 (b) 30
    (c) 33 (d) 36

553. Which index of obesity does not include height?
    [NEET Patterns 2018, 13; DNB June 2010; AIPGME 1991]
    (a) BMI (b) Ponderal's index
    (c) Broca's index (d) Corpulence index

554. Normal range of BMI Asian individual is: [DNB December 2010]
    (a) 18.5 to 24.99 (b) 22.5 to 24.99
    (c) 18.5 to 22.5   (d) 18.5 to 22.99

555. Height in centimetres by cube root of body weight is also known as: [DNB December 2011; NEET Pattern 2017]
    (a) Quetelet index
    (b) Broca index
    (c) Ponderal's index
    (d) Corpulence index

556. Corpulence index means: [DNB 2008]
    (a) Measurement of obesity
    (b) Measurement of copper level in serum
    (c) Measurement of iron losses in faeces
    (d) Pressure difference b/w chambers of heart

557. Which is the cutoff level of Waist-Hip Ratio in Women indicating abdominal fat accumulation? [PGMCET 2015]
    (a) 0.75 (b) 0.85
    (c) 0.95 (d) 1.05

558. Corpulence Index is given by: [NEET Pattern 2017]
    (a) Actual weight – Desirable weight
    (b) Actual weight/Desirable weight
    (c) Desirable weight/Actual weight
    (d) Height (cms) – 100

559. Lethal BMI among males is: [NEET Pattern 2018]
    (a) < 11 (b) < 13
    (c) < 16 (d) < 18.5

560. What should be the value of BMI to be considered as "Lethal" in men? [NEET Pattern 2018]
    (a) 12
    (b) 18
    (c) 13
    (d) 14

Review Questions

561. Abdominal fat accumulation is assessed by: [MP 2005]
    (a) Corpulence index
    (b) Broca's index
    (c) Ponderal index
    (d) Waist to hip ratio

562. BMI (body mass index) is defined as:
    [JIPMER 2000; All India 2005, MH 2005, DPG 2006]
    (a) $\dfrac{Weight\ (kg)}{(Height)^2\ (meters)}$
    (b) $\dfrac{Weight\ (Kg)}{(Height)^{16}\ (cm)}$
    (c) $\dfrac{Midarm\ circumference\ (cm)}{Head\ circumstance\ (cm)}$
    (d) Midarm circumference (cm) between ages of 1-5 years

BLINDNESS

563. Taking the definition of blindness as visual acuity less than 3/60 in the better eye, the number of blind persons per 100,000 population in India is estimated to be:
    (a) 500
    (b) 700 [AIIMS Nov 2003]
    (c) 1000
    (d) 1500

564. Under NPCB in India, cutoff for blindness is defined as having a vision of: [AIPGME 2000; PGMCET 2015]
    (a) < 3/60 in worse eye
    (b) < 6/60 in better eye
    (c) < 3/60 in better eye
    (d) < 6/60 in worse eye

565. Disease not included in Vision 2020, India is:
    [AIPGME 2005; NEET Pattern 2012]
    (a) Cataract
    (b) Glaucoma
    (c) Diabetic retinopathy
    (d) Onchocerciasis

566. The commonest cause of low vision in India is:
    (a) Uncorrected refractive errors [AIPGME 2004, 03]
    (b) Cataract
    (c) Glaucoma
    (d) Squint

567. According to the National Programme for Control of Blindness (NPCB) survey (1986-89), the highest prevalence of blindness in India is in: [AIIMS Dec 1991]
    (a) Jammu and Kashmir
    (b) Odisha
    (c) Bihar
    (d) Uttar Pradesh

568. Blindness can be seen in: [PGI Dec 2K]
    (a) Measles
    (b) Mumps
    (c) Rubella
    (d) Coxsackie

569. If Blindness is surveyed using Schools as compared to Population Surveys, then estimation of prevalence of blindness will have: [AIIMS PGMEE May 2013]
    (a) Overestimation
    (b) Underestimation
    (c) Remains same
    (d) None of them is used for evaluation

570. Disability certificate is given for poor vision if visual acuity is 4/60, in tune of visual impairment as a percentage: [AIIMS PGMEE November 2012]
    (a) 1
    (b) 0.4
    (c) 0.3
    (d) 0.75

571. Arrange the causes of Blindness as per National Survey 2006-07 in India (increasing order of percentage):
    [NEET Pattern 2015]
    (a) Refractive error, Glaucoma, Corneal opacity, Cataract
    (b) Corneal opacity, Glaucoma, Refractive error, Cataract
    (c) Cataract, Refractive error, Glaucoma, Corneal opacity
    (d) Glaucoma, Refractive error, Corneal opacity, Cataract

572. Which of the following is not an Avoidable cause of blindness? [NEET Pattern 2017]
    (a) Cataract
    (b) Vitamin A deficiency
    (c) Refractive errors
    (d) Retinal dystrophies

Review Questions

573. WHO defines blindness if the visual acuity is less than:
    [UP, 2006, Bihar 2004; NEET Pattern 2013]
    (a) 3/60
    (b) 18/38
    (c) 9/60
    (d) 6/6

574. Most common cause of ocular morbidity in India is:
    [UP 2000]
    (a) Cataract
    (b) Xerophthalmia
    (c) Trachoma
    (d) Refraction error

575. Most common cause of blindness due to easily preventable cause in children:
    [RJ 2001; NEET Pattern 2017]
    (a) Diabetes
    (b) Trachoma
    (c) Vit. A deficiency
    (d) Cataract

MISCELLANEOUS (Non-communicable diseases)

576. WHO STEPwise approach include all, except:
    [NEET PG Pattern 2022]
    (a) Physical
    (b) Psychological
    (c) Behavioural
    (d) Therapeutic

577. Stanford-three-community study, The North Kerelia project and Lipid Research Clinics study are types of:
    (a) Cohort studies [AIPGME 2004]
    (b) Nested case control studies
    (c) Case series report studies
    (d) Risk factor intervention trials

578. Most common cause of stroke in India is: [AIIMS Dec 1994]
    (a) Cerebral thrombosis
    (b) Cerebral embolism
    (c) Cerebral hemorrhage
    (d) Subarachnoid hemorrhage

579. Which one of the following is NOT a characteristic of non-communicable disease: [AIPGME 1993]
    (a) Well-defined etiological agent
    (b) Multifactorial causation
    (c) Long latent period
    (d) Variable onset

580. The preferred public health approach to control non-communicable diseases is: [AIIMS Nov 02]
    (a) Shift the population curve of risk factors by a population based approach
    (b) Focus on high risk individuals for reduction of risk
    (c) Early diagnosis and treatment of indentified cases
    (d) Individual disease based vertical Programmes

581. WHO STEPS is used for: [AIIMS May 2009]
    (a) Communicable diseases [NEET Pattern 2013]
    (b) Non-communicable diseases
    (c) Immunodeficient diseases
    (d) Autoimmune diseases.

582. Rural and urban population differ in incidence in all diseases except: [AIPGME 2010]
    (a) Bronchitis   (b) TB
    (c) Lung cancer   (d) Mental illness

583. Diabetes mellitus is best diagnosed by: [AIIMS November 2011]
    (a) Fasting blood sugar (FBS) > 100 mg/dL and Postprandial blood sugar (PPBS) > 140
    (b) FBS >125 mg/dL and PPBS >199 mg/dL
    (c) HbA1c = 5.5%
    (d) FBS > 70 md/dL

584. True about Road traffic accidents: [PGI May 2011]
    (a) Most common cause of accidental deaths in India
    (b) More in USA in motor-car users than pedestrians
    (c) More in number than self-inflicted injuries in India
    (d) More in number than railway accidents in India
    (e) Contribute 50% of all injury related deaths in India

585. In India causing maximum death among the following is: [NEET Pattern 2013]
    (a) Drowning
    (b) Road traffic accident
    (c) Burns
    (d) Poisoning

586. Most reliable test for screening of diabetes mellitus [NEET Pattern 2012]
    (a) Random blood sugar   (b) Fasting blood sugar
    (c) Glucose tolerance test (d) Urine sugar

587. According to NCRB Report 2014, Suicide rate in India is: [NEET Pattern 2015]
    (a) 1.1 per 100,000 population
    (b) 10.6 per 100,000 population
    (c) 25.8 per 100,000 population
    (d) 30.9 per 100,000 population

588. According to NCRB 2014, Most common means of Suicide in India is: [NEET Pattern 2015]
    (a) Self-poisoning
    (b) Self-immolation
    (c) Drowning
    (d) Hanging

589. Haddon matrix is related to: [AIIMS PG May 2015]
    (a) Hypertensive disorders
    (b) Communicable diseases
    (c) Maternal and child mortality
    (d) Injury prevention

590. Smoking is preventive for: [NEET Pattern 2015]
    (a) Lung cancer   (b) Chronic bronchitis
    (c) Ulcerative colitis (d) CHD

591. Prevalence of Diabetes in India in adult population: [NEET Pattern 2017]
    (a) 1-2%   (b) 3-5%
    (c) 5-6%   (d) 7-8.5%

592. A person is said to killed by road traffic accident if he dies within how many days of accident? [NEET Pattern 2017]
    (a) 12 days   (b) 30 days
    (c) 40 days   (d) 47 days

593. WHO criteria for diagnosis of diabetes is: [NEET Pattern 2017]
    (a) Venous blood fasting sugar 140 to 200 mg/100 mL
    (b) Venous blood fasting sugar 120 to 180 mg/100 mL
    (c) Venous blood fasting sugar 120 to 200 mg/100 mL
    (d) Venous blood fasting sugar 140 to 180 mg/100 mL

594. According to WHO Global Action Plan for Prevention and Control of Non-communicable Diseases 2013-2020, targeted reduction in prevalence of raised blood pressure is: [NEET Pattern 2018]
    (a) 10%   (b) 25%
    (c) 33%   (d) 50%

595. The Glycemic index for Glucose is [NEET Pattern 2018]
    (a) 0.5   (b) 1
    (c) 1.5   (d) 2

Review Questions

596. Which is the least common cause of heart disease in India? [Bihar 2004]
    (a) Rheumatic   (b) Hypertensive
    (c) Ischemic   (d) Congenital

597. **Primordial prevention in myocardial infarction are all except:** [Bihar 2004]
    (a) Maintenance of normal body weight
    (b) Change in life style
    (c) Change in nutritional habits
    (d) Screening for hypertension

598. **Following is not a risk factor for development of diabetes mellitus:** [MP 2001]
    (a) Sedentary life style
    (b) Protein energy malnutrition in infancy
    (c) Excessive intake of alcohol
    (d) High intake of vitamin-A

599. **The North Kerelia project evaluate risk factors of:** [MP 2005]
    (a) Diabetes
    (b) Coronary heart disease
    (c) Cancers
    (d) Obesity

600. **Glycosylated haemoglobin reflects the mean blood glucose level of previous:** [AP 2003]
    (a) 15 days
    (b) 1 month
    (c) 3 months
    (d) 6 months

Explanations

GENERAL EPIDEMIOLOGY

1. **Ans. (b) A-4, B-1, C-2, D-3**
   [Ref. Park 27/e p161, 191, 248, 379]

2. **Ans. (b) Crimean congo hemorrhagic fever**
   [Ref. Mourya, D.T., Yadav, P.D., Gurav, Y.K. et al. Crimean Congo hemorrhagic fever serosurvey in humans for identifying high-risk populations and high-risk areas in the endemic state of Gujarat, India. BMC Infect Dis 19, 104 (2019)]
   - India reported its first CCHF case in the Ahmedabad, Gujarat (2011)
   - Since then, several sporadic cases and outbreaks of CCHF have been reported from the states of Gujarat, Rajasthan and Uttar Pradesh
   - Majority of CCHF cases have been published from various districts of Gujarat thus making Gujarat an endemic state for CCHF disease in India

3. **Ans. (d) Rabies** *[Ref. Park 26/e p318]*
   - Rabies disease has case fatality rate close to 100%
   - Till date only 3 rabies cases on record have survived

4. **Ans. (b) Pertussis** *[Ref. Park 25/e p177]*
   - Infants are susceptible form Birth in Pertussis as maternal antibodies do not appear to provide protection

COVID-19 DISEASE

5. **Ans. (a) Steroids** *[Ref. Guidelines for Management of COVID-19 in Children (below 18 years) MOHFW, GOI June 2021 p1]*

   Severe Covid in Children, MoHFW Guidelines 2021
   - *Clinical diagnosis:* SpO_2 <90% on room air AND any of the following (Signs of severe pneumonia, ARDS, Septic shock, Multi-organ dysfunction syndrome, or Pneumonia with cyanosis/grunting/severe retraction of chest/lethargy/somnolence/seizure)
   - *Investigations baseline:* CBC including ESR, blood glucose, CRP, LFT, KFT, serum ferritin, D-Dimer, Chest X-Ray
     – CT chest is NOT indicated in diagnosis or management of COVID-19 infection in children
   - *Management:*
     – Immediate Oxygen therapy (Target SpO_2 94–96%)
     – Maintain fluid and electrolyte balance
     – Corticosteroids therapy to be initiated
     – Anticoagulants may also be indicated
     – In case ARDS or shock develops, initiate necessary management
     – Antimicrobials if there is evidence/suspicion of superadded bacterial infection
     – Organ support in case of organ dysfunction e.g. renal replacement therapy
     – Remdesivir (an emergency use authorization drug) is NOT recommended in children

6. **Ans. (a), (b), (c)** *[Ref. Hand Hygiene Brochure WHO p5]*

   HAND HYGIENE GUIDELINES (WHO)
   - *If hands are NOT visibly soiled:* Rub them with Alcohol base sanitizer (20–30 seconds)
   - *If hands are visibly soiled:* Wash hands with Soap and water (40–60 seconds)

   5 Check-points/Moments for Hand hygiene:
   - Before touching a patient
   - Before cleaning/aseptic procedure
   - After body fluid exposure risk
   - After touching a patient
   - After touching patient surroundings

   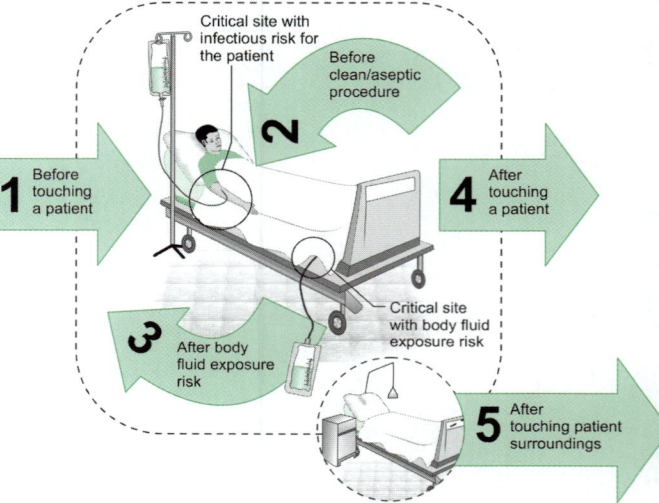

7. **Ans. (b) 1% Gluteraldehyde**
   [Ref. COVID19 – All you need to know! CDC Document]
   For COVID prevention/disinfection, CDC recommendations include:
   - 70% ethanol based sanitizers
   - Hand washing with Soap and water for minimum 20 seconds
   - Use of Mask (Especially N95)

8. **Ans. (b) BSL-2**
   [Ref. Interim Laboratory Biosafety Guidelines for Handling and Processing Specimens Associated with Coronavirus Disease 2019 (COVID-19). CDC 2019]

   Biosafety Levels for COVID-19
   - *BSL-2 Laboratory:* For handling Routine Diagnostic Testing Procedures using Standard Precautions (Processing, Staining and microscopic analysis, Examination of bacterial cultures, Pathologic examination and processing of tissues, Molecular analysis, Final packaging, Electron microscopic studies, Routine antibody or antigen detection tests)

- *BSL-3 Laboratory:* Virus isolation in cell culture and initial characterization of viral agents recovered in cultures of SARS-CoV-2

SMALLPOX and CHICKENPOX

9. **Ans. (a) Isolation for 6 days** [Ref. Park 27/e p163]

   Management of Contacts of a Varicella case
   - Isolation for 6 days after onset of rash
   - Varicella vaccination is useful if given to susceptible contacts within 5 days (preferably 72 hours) of first exposure
   - High-risk susceptible contacts where vaccination is not indicated, such as neonates, pregnancy and immunosuppressed persons, should be offered VZIG within 72 hours of exposure

10. **Ans. (b) Woman is susceptible to Chicken pox** [Ref. Park 26/e p158-159]

    Anti-Varicella/Varicella Zoster Virus (VZV)/Chickenpox IgG; Varicella immunity test
    - *Negative:* Indicates no detectable Varicella IgG antibodies. A negative results indicate no current or previous infection with Varicella virus. Such individuals are presumed to be susceptible to primary infection.
    - *Equivocal:* Equivocal results are indeterminate. Patient may or may not have immunity to Varicella Virus. It is not acceptable proof of immunity.
    - *Positive:* Indicates evidence of Varicella IgG antibodies and suggests past or current infection with Varicella virus. Antibodies obtained via acquired immunity or immunization and probable protection from clinical infection. (Immunity).

11. **Ans. (b) 6 days after onset of rash** [Ref. Park 27/e p159]
    - Period of communicability:
      - *Chickenpox:* 1–2 days before to 4–5 days after appearance of rash
      - *Measles:* 4 days before to 5 days after appearance of rash
      - *Diphtheria:* 14–28 days from disease onset
      - *Poliomyelitis:* 7–10 days before and after onset of symptoms

> **ALSO REMEMBER**
>
> **CHICKENPOX:**
> - Also known as 'Varicella'
> - *Causative agent:* Varicella zoster virus [Human (alpha) Herpes Virus – 3]
> - *Secondary attack rate:* 90%
> - *Incubation period:* 14–16 days
> - *Rash:*
>
> | Chickenpox rash | Smallpox rash |
> |---|---|
> | Dew drop on rose petal appearance | No dew drop |
> | Centripetal distribution | Centrifugal distribution |
> | Pleomorphic rash | Non-pleomorphic |
>
> - *MC late complication of Chickenpox:* Shingles (caused by reactivation of the virus decades after the initial episode of chickenpox)
> - *Aspirin must not be given to children with chickenpox:* Risk of Reye's Syndrome

- *Strain of Live attenuated Chickenpox Vaccine:* OKA strain
- *Congenital Varicella:* Most threatening if transmitted in Ist trimester of pregnancy

12. **Ans. (a) Scabs are infective** [Ref. Park 27/e p161]

13. **Ans. (d) Cross-resistance existed with animal pox** [Ref. Park 27/e p159]
    - *Epidemiological Reasons/Basis For Smallpox Eradication:*
    - No known animal reservoir
    - No long term carrier state
    - Infection provides lifelong immunity
    - Case detection simple due to characteristic rash
    - Subclinical cases did not transmit the disease
    - A highly effective vaccine was available
    - International cooperation

14. **Ans. (a) 10–30% chances of occurrence** [Ref. Park 27/e p161]
    - Single attack of Varicella gives durable (lifelong) immunity

15. **Ans. (c) 90** [Ref. Park 27/e p161]

16. **Ans. (b) 2 days before and 5 days after rash appearance** [Ref. Park 27/e p161]

17. **Ans. (d) Single stage of rash is seen** [Ref. Park 27/e p161]
    - Chicken pox rash shows Pleomorphism (All stages of rash at same time in same area)

18. **Ans. (a) March** [Ref. Clinical Maternal-Fetal Medicine by Winn, 1/e p263]
    - Infection with varicella occurs year-round, although incidence is found to peak in March, April and May in temperate climates

19. **Ans. (b) Varicella zoster virus** [Ref. Park 27/e p161]
    - Herpes zoster, also known as zoster and shingles, is caused by the reactivation of the varicella-zoster virus (VZV), the same virus that causes varicella (chickenpox)
    - VZ Virus is Human (Alpha) Herpes Virus 3

20. **Ans. (b) Centripetal distribution** [Ref. Park 27/e p159]
    Smallpox rash is Centrifugal (lesions concentrated on the face and distal extremities; fewer lesions on the trunk); Chickenpox rash is Centripetal (lesions concentrated on the trunk)

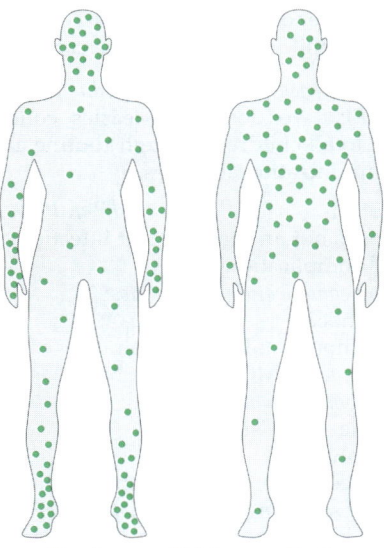

Smallpox vs Chickenpox Rash

MEASLES

21. Ans. (b) Measles [Ref. Park 27/e p165]
- Pathognomonic clinical feature of Measles: Koplik spots (buccal mucosa opposite Lower 2nd molar)

22. Ans. (b) Shyam is primary case; (c) Ram got infected from Shyam; (d) If mother had reported when Shyam got infection, Ram could have been vaccinated [Ref. Park 26/e p164]

In the given question,
- First Shyam got Measles, so Shyam is the Primary case for the family
- After few days, Ram developed the same symptoms, So Ram is the Secondary case
- To be effective, Measles vaccine must be given to contacts within 3 days of exposure. So, if mother had reported when Shyam got infection, Ram could have been vaccinated

23. Ans. (c) Not infectious in pro-dromal stage [Ref. Park 27/e p165]
- **MEASLES (RUBEOLA):**
- *Period of Communicability:* 4 days before and 5 days after the appearance of rash (*Rash:* Retro-auricular origin)
  - Measles is highly infectious during pro-dromal period and during eruption
  - Period of communicability declines rapidly after appearance of rash
- Measles has no second attacks (life long immunity seen)

> **ALSO REMEMBER**
> - WHO Measles elimination strategy comprises a 3-Part Vaccination strategy, 'Catch up, Keep up, Follow up'
>   - *Catch up:* One time nationwide, vaccination campaign targeting all children 9 months to 14 years of age, irrespective of history of Measles disease or vaccination status
>   - *Keep up:* Routine services aimed at vaccinating more than 95% of each successive birth cohort
>   - *Follow up:* Subsequent nationwide vaccination campaigns conducted every 2 – 4 years targeting usually all children born after the catch-up campaign

- *Accelerated Measles Mortality Reduction Strategy (WHO-UNICEF):* Two doses of Measles containing vaccine (MCV) to all children through routine and supplementary immunization activities.

24. Ans. (d) SSPE [Ref. Park 27/e p165-166]
- Measles is not an unimportant infection: It does lead to several complications
- *Common complications of Measles:*
  - Diarrhoea
  - Pneumonia and other respiratory complications
  - Otitis media: MC complication of Measles in children
- *Serious complications of Measles:*
  - Febrile convulsions
  - Encephalitis
  - Sub-acute sclerosing pan-encephalitis (SSPE)
- *Sub-acute sclerosing pan-encephalitis (SSPE):*
  - Also known as 'Dawson's disease', 'Dawson's encephalitis'
  - Rare complication of Measles developing 7 – 10 years after Measles infection (Fatality 10–20%)
  - Characterised by progressive mental deterioration leading to paralysis (persisting virus in brain)
  - Frequency: 1 per 10,000–100,000 cases of natural Measles

> **ALSO REMEMBER**
> - MC complication of Mumps: Aseptic meningitis

25. Ans. (c) Secondary attack rate is less than that of rubella [Ref. Park 27/e p165]

SAR of measles = 80% and Rubella = 90%

26. Ans. (a) Kopliks spots appear as rash disappears [Ref. Park 27/e p165]

MEASLES (RUBEOLA):
- *Incubation Period:* 10-14 days
- *Causative agent:* RNA paramyxovirus (so for only one serotype known)
- *Source of Infection:* cases (carriers are not known to occur)
- *Period of Communicability:* 4 days before and 5 days after the appearance of rash (Rash: Retro-auricular origin)
- Measles has no second attacks (life long immunity seen)
- *Secondary attack rate of Measles:* 80%
- *Measles shows a cyclical trend:* Increase every 2-3 years
- *Blood cell type predominantly infected in Measles:* Monocyte
- *Pathognomic clinical feature of Measles:* Koplik spots (on buccal mucosa opposite Lower 2nd molar)
- *Pathognomic microscopic feature of Measles:* Warthin Finkledy cells (multinucleated giant cells)
- *MC complication of measles in young children:* Otitis media
- *SSPE (Subacute Sclerosing Pan Encephalitis) is a rare complication of measles:* 1 per 10,000–100,000 cases of Measles (7-10 years after initial infection)
- *Epidemic of measles occur:* If proportion of susceptible children is >40%
- *If Measles is introduced in a virgin community:* it infects >90% children
- *Eradication of Measles:* Requires a vaccination coverage >96%
- *Baby measles (Exanthem subitum-roseola infantum):* Sixth disease (three day fever)
- *German Measles:* Rubella

> **ALSO REMEMBER**
> - Measles is prevented by:
>   - *Active immunization by measles vaccine:*
>   - *Passive immunization by measles immunoglobulin*

27. Ans. (b) Single intramuscular dose of 0.5 mL [Ref. Park 27/e p166]

28. Ans. (a) Koplik spots appear in Prodromal stage; (b) Fever stops after onset of Rash; (c) Vaccine given at 9 months [Ref. Park 27/e p165]

29. Ans. (a) Prodromal stage [Ref. Park 27/e p165]

30. Ans. (b) Secondary bacterial infection [Ref. Infections of Central Nervous System by Scheld, 4/e p126]

31. **Ans. (b) 3 days** [Ref. Park 27/e p165]
    - Post-exposure Measles vaccine must be given within: 3 days of exposure
        - IP for Naturally acquired Measles: 10 days
        - IP for Vaccine induced Measles: 7 days

> **ALSO REMEMBER**
> - *Measles Outbreak Control Measures:*
>   - Isolation for 7 days after Onset of rash
>   - Immunization of contacts within 2 days of exposure
>   - Immunoglobulin administration within 3-4 days of exposure (if vaccine contraindicated)
>   - Prompt immunization at beginning of Epidemic

32. **Ans. (d) All of the above**
    [Ref. WHO Measles Field Guide, p34]
    - Supplemental Immunization Activities (SIAs)/Mass immunisation campaigns: Necessary to reach never-vaccinated children who have never had measles disease and to provide an opportunity for a second dose for cases of primary vaccine failure
    - All children in the target age group and geographic area will be eligible to receive a dose of measles vaccine irrespective of past immunisation or history of clinical measles

33. **Ans. (d) Incubation period is 10-14 days**
    [Ref. Park 27/e p165]
    - **MEASLES TRANSMISSION**
    - Measles case is infective 4 days before to 5 days after appearance of rash
    - More commonly seen in winters and early spring in India
    - Incubation period: 10-14 days
    - Only one type of vaccine (Live attenuated)

34. **Ans. (c) 1-2 days after Koplik spots** [Ref. Medical Microbiology by Murray 7/e p516, Park 25/e p161–162]
    - **RASH IN MEASLES**
    - Starts 12-24 hours after appearance of Koplik spots
    - Retro-auricular origin spreads to other parts of body (fades in opposite direction)
    - Takes 1-2 days to cover body
    - Fever highest and patient sickest on day of rash

35. **Ans. (a) Onset of catarrhal symptoms to 3 days after**
    [Ref. Park 27/e p168]
    - Period of infectivity of Measles: 4 days before to 5 days after rash appearance
    - Period of Isolation for Measles: Onset of Catarrhal stage through 3rd day of rash

Review Questions

36. **Ans. (d) 95** [Ref. Park 27/e p168]
37. **Ans. (c) 4 days before and 5 days after the appearance of rash** [Ref. Park 27/e p165]
38. **Ans. (a) Both active and passive immunization are given simultaneously** [Ref. Park 27/e p166-167]
39. **Ans. (c) Give after 9 months age**
    [Ref. Park 27/e p166]

RUBELLA

40. **Ans. (d) Rubella** [Ref. Park 27/e p169]
    - Classical Triad of Congenital Rubella Syndrome includes Sensorineural deafness, Congenital heart defects (MC is PDA) and Cataract

41. **Ans. (a) Women 15-49 yrs** [Ref. Park 27/e p170]
    - *Priority groups for rubella vaccination in India:*
        - *1st PRIORITY:* 15 – 49 years reproductive age group females
        - *2nd priority:* All children 1 – 14 years age
        - *3rd priority:* Routine universal immunization of all children aged 1

> **ALSO REMEMBER**
> - 'Forchheimer's sign' occurs in 20% of cases, and is characterized by small, red papules on the area of the soft palate

42. **Ans. (a) 6-12 weeks of pregnancy** [Ref. Park 27/e p169]
    - **Congenital Rubella Syndrome (Crs):**
    - CRS is said to have occurred if:
        - Infant has IgM rubella antibodies shortly after birth, or
        - IgG antibodies persist for more than 6 months
    - *Major determinant of extent of fetal infection in CRS:* Gestational age at which fetal transmission occurs,
        - *Infection in I trimester:* MOST DISASTROUS TIME
            1. Abortions
            2. Still births
            3. *Skin lesions:* blueberry muffin lesions
            4. 'Triad of Congenital Rubella Syndrome'
                i. Sensorineural deafness
                ii. Congenital heart defects (MC is PDA)
                iii. Cataracts
        - *Infection in early part of II Trimester:* Deafness (only)
        - *Infection after 16 weeks POG:* No major abnormalities
    - *Risk of fetal damage in CRS:*

Stage of gestation	% fetuses infected	% fetuses damaged among infected	Overall risk of damage
< 11 weeks	90	100	90
11 – 16 weeks	55	37	20
17 – 26 weeks	33	0	0
27 – 36 weeks	53	0	0

- *Other manifestations of CRS may include:* spleen, liver or bone marrow problems, mental retardation, microcephaly, low birth weight, thrombocytopenic purpura (characteristic 'blueberry muffin' rash), hepatomegaly, micrognathia

43. **Ans. (d) Infection after 16 weeks of gestation results in major congenital defects** [Ref. Park 27/e p169]
44. **Ans. (b) 15-18 months** [Ref. Park 27/e p170]
45. **Ans. (c) Toga virus** [Ref. Park 27/e p169]
    - **Toga Viruses and Diseases**
    - *Alpha viruses*: Eastern Equine encephalitis, Western Equine encephalitis, Venezuelan Equine encephalitis, Chikungunya fever
    - *Rubiviruses*: Rubella (enveloped single-stranded positive-sense RNA virus)

46. **Ans. (c) Intracerebral hemorrhage** [Ref. Park 27/e p169]

Congenital Rubella Syndrome (CRS) Manifestations
- *Classic triad (Greg's Triad)*: Sensorineural deafness, Eye abnormalities (microphthalmia, cataract and retinopathy), Congenital Heart Diseases (PDA, VSD, ASD, Coarctation of aorta)
- *Other manifestations*: Spleen, liver and bone marrow involvement, mental retardation, microcephaly, Low Birth Weight, hepatomegaly, micrognathia, thrombocytopenic purpura (leading to the characteristic Blueberry Muffin Rash)
- *Predisposition to*: Developmental delay, growth retardation, autism, schizophrenia, learning disabilities, diabetes, glaucoma

MUMPS

47. **Ans. (c) Aseptic meningitis** [Ref. Park 27/e p171]
48. **Ans. (d) 18 days** [Ref. Park 27/e p171]

INFLUENZA

49. **Ans. (a) H1N1** [Ref. Park 25/e p169]
    - Most recent influenza pandemic occurred in 2009, caused by an influenza A (H1N1) virus
    - It is estimated to have caused between 100,000–400,000 deaths globally in the first year alone

50. **Ans. (c) 1–5 years age is not a high risk age group** [Ref. Park 25/e p167]
    - High risk groups for influenza include <5 years age, >65 years age, DM/CHD/Kidney aliments/Respiratory ailments

51. **Ans. (d) Major epidemics are due to antigenic drift** [Ref. Park 27/e p172-178]

INFLUENZA
- *Antigenic variations in Influenza:* (MC in Type A)

	Antigenic shift	Antigenic drift
Occurs due to	Genetic recombination/reassortment/rearrangement	Point mutation
Nature	Sudden	Gradual/insidious
May lead to	Epidemics/Pandemics	Sporadic cases

- *Incubation period:* 18–72 hours
- *Vaccines for Influenza:*
    - Killed vaccines:
        - 2 doses, 3-4 weeks apart, 0.5 ml (for age >3 years), subcutaneous
        - 70–90% protective efficacy; duration 3–6 months
        - Is rarely associated with Guillain-Barré Syndrome (GBS)
    - Live attenuated vaccines:
        - Stimulate local + systemic immunity
        - Antigenic variations presents difficulties in manufacture
    - Newer vaccines:
        - Split virus vaccine: 'Sub-virion vaccine', lower antigenicity, fewer side effects
        - Neuraminidase specific vaccine: 'Subunit vaccine'
        - Recombinant vaccine

52. **Ans. (a) Split – virus vaccine; (b) Neuraminidase; (e) Recombinant vaccine** [Ref. Park 23/e p168–169]
    - *Newer Influenza Vaccines:*
        - *Split – virus vaccine:*
            - Also known as 'Sub-virion vaccine'
            - Highly purified
            - Lesser side effects
            - Less antigenic – multiple injections required
            - Useful for children
        - *Neuraminidase – specific vaccine:*
            - Sub-unit vaccine containing N-antigen
            - Permits subclinical infection – long lasting immunity
        - *Recombinant vaccine:*
            - Antigenic properties of virulent strain transferred to a less virulent strain

> **ALSO REMEMBER**
> - H1N1 (Swine flu) Vaccine:
> - H1N1 Inactivated vaccine: Single i/m injection
>   - Strain: A/California/7/2009 (H1N1) V like strain
>   - Storage temperature: +2° to +8° C
>   - Contraindications: History of anaphylaxis/severe reaction/Guillian-Barré Syndrome, Infants <6months, Moderate-to-severe illness with fever
>   - Protective immunity: Develops after 14 days (NOT 100%)
> - H1N1 Live attenuated vaccine: Nasal spray
>   - Side effects: Rhinorrhoea, nasal congestion, cough, sore throat, fever, wheezing, vomiting
> - Priority groups (in order) for Influenza vaccines:
>   - Pregnant women
>   - Age > 6 months with chronic medical conditions
>   - 15-49 years healthy young adults
>   - Healthy young children
>   - Healthy adults 49-65 years
>   - Healthy adults >65 years

53. **Ans. (e) All ages and sex equally affected** [Ref. Park 27/e p172-173]

54. **Ans. (a) Affects all ages and sexes; (b) I.P. 18 – 72 hours** [Ref. Park 27/e p173]

55. **Ans. (d) H7N9** [Ref. WHO H7N9 Avian Influenza 2013 document]

56. **Ans. (c) Reservoir** [Ref. Park 27/e p174]

57. **Ans. (b) Man to man transmission is rare** [Ref. Park 27/e p173]

Reasons for H5N1 not becoming Global Pandemic
- Absence of efficient human to human mode of transmission (Major reason)
- Absence of replication in humans
- Absence of serious disease in humans

58. **Ans. (d) Ribavirin** [Ref. Manson's Tropical Diseases, 24/e p168–169]
    - Neuraminidase inhibitors such as Oseltamivir, Zanamivir, and Peramivir, which inhibit the viral enzyme neuraminidase in both influenza virus A and B, are effective for treatment and prophylaxis of influenza

- Amantadine and Rimantadine are active only against Influenza A

59. Ans. (b) Source of infection is clinical case
[Ref. Park 27/e p173]

INFLUENZA TRANSMISSION
- Period of infectivity: 1–2 days before and 1–2 days after onset of symptoms
- *Source*: Case or Subclinical case
- Incubation period: 18–72 hours

60. Ans. (c) Strains of Avian influenza
[Ref. Animal Influenza by Swayne Fig 5.1]

H7N7 INFLUENZA
- H7N7 virus infection in humans is uncommon, but has been documented in persons who have direct contact with infected birds, especially during outbreaks among poultry
- More common in Horses
- In humans, H7N7 virus infections cause mild to moderate illness
- Unusual zoonotic potential represents a pandemic threat

61. Ans. (d) Acyclovir
[Ref. Pediatric Critical Care by Fuhrman 5/e p691]
- Amantadine, Rimantadine, Oseltamivir and Zanamivir are approved for prophylaxis of Seasonal influenza

62. Ans. (d) ELISA *[Ref. Park 23/e p169]*
- WHO case definition for Pandemic (H1N1) 2009 virus infections in humans: An individual with laboratory confirmed pandemic (H1N1) 2009 virus infection by one or more of the following tests:
  - Polymerase chain reaction (PCR)
  - Viral culture
  - 4-fold rise in pandemic (H1N1) 2009 virus virus-specific neutralizing antibodies.

63. Ans. (a) Morbid obese; (c) Children <18 months; (e) Elderly person *[Ref. Park 27/e p173, 175]*

High Risk Groups (HRG) in Influenza

HRG for Influenza Mortality	HRG for H1N1 Influenza Severe Disease
Old persons >65 years Children <18 months Diabetes CHD Kidney ailments Respiratory ailments Obesity Morbid obesity	Infants, Young children <2 years Pregnant women Old persons >65 years Asthma, COPD Metabolic disorders (DM) Chronic cardiac/renal/hepatic disease Neuro-conditions Hemoglobinopathies Immunosuppression (HIV) Children on Chronic Aspirin

DIPHTHERIA

64. Ans. (c) Nothing is required to be done
[Ref. Park 27/e p180]

Management of Contacts of Diphtheria
- If primary immunization or booster dose received within last 2 years: Nothing to be done
- If primary immunization or booster dose received more than 2 years before: 1 booster dose of Diphtheria toxoid
- Non-immunized close contact: Prophylactic Penicillin/Erythromycin, 1000–2000 units Diphtheria antitoxin, Active immunization against Diphtheria
- Medical surveillance of contacts: Daily for at least once a week post-exposure
- Bacteriological surveillance: Swabbing at weekly intervals

65. Ans. (c) 25 Lf of diphtheria toxoid are present per ml in DPT vaccine *[Ref. Park 27/e p180]*
- DPT VACCINE:
  Refer to Chapter 3, Theory

> **ALSO REMEMBER**
> - *Tests of immunity status:*
>
> | Disease | Tests of immunity status | Antigen used |
> |---|---|---|
> | Diphtheria | Schick test | Schick toxin |
> | Tuberculosis | Montaux test | PPD |
> | Leprosy | Lepromin test | Dhamendra Antigen |
> | Kala azar | Montenegro (Leishmanin) test | Leishmanin Antigen |

66. Ans. (d) 70% *[Ref. Park 27/e p180]*

67. Ans. (b) Single dose of toxoid; (d) Daily throat swab culture *[Ref. Park 27/e p180]*

Management of diphtheria contacts
- Immunisation:
  - If primary immunization or booster was received in previous 2 years: No further action
  - If primary immunization or booster was received more than 2 years ago: 1 booster dose
  - If unimmunized contact: Active immunization + 1000-2000 units Antitoxin + Prophylactic penicillin/erythromycin
- Examination:
  - *Physical examination*: Daily for 1 week after exposure
  - *Throat swabbing*: Weekly for several weeks

68. Ans. (c) 2-6 days & 10-14 days *[Ref. Park 25/e p174, 258]*

69. Ans. (c) Vaccination *[Ref. Park 27/e p180]*
- Available retrospective data in India indicate declining trend in Diphtheria cases
- It is due to increased coverage of child population by immunization

70. Ans. (c) 50000-100000 Units *[Ref. Park 27/e p180]*

Diphtheria Antitoxin

Diphtheria type	Antitoxin dose
Anterior nasal diphtheria	10,000–20,000 Units
Tonsillar (Faucial) diphtheria	15,000–25,000 Units
Pharyngeal/Laryngeal <48 hours duration diphtheria	20,000–40,000 Units
Nasopharyngeal diphtheria	40,000–60,000 Units
Extensive disease >3 days duration/Brawny neck swelling	80,000–120,000 Units

71. Ans. (c) Erythromycin [Ref. Park 27/e p180]

Drug of Choice in Diphtheria

Diphtheria	Drug(s) of choice
Prophylaxis of Diphtheria	Erythromycin
Prophylaxis of Household contacts	Erythromycin
DOC for Unimmunized contacts	Erythromycin + Antitoxin + Toxoid
DOC for Carriers	Erythromycin
DOC for Cases	Penicillin/Erythromycin

Review Question

72. Ans. (a) Erythromycin [Ref. Park 27/e p180]

WHOOPING COUGH

73. Ans. (c) Erythromycin prevents spread of disease between children [Ref. Park 27/e p182]
    - Pertussis (Whooping Cough):
    - Leukocytosis does not correlates with the severity of cough
    - *Drug of choice:* Erythromycin (40 mg/kg QID X 10 days)
    - *Vaccines:*
        – DPT:
            ▪ Killed acellular bacilli 20,000 million per dose (0.5 ml)
            ▪ Pertussis component leads to neurological complications after 2 years of age (@ 1 per 1,70,000 vaccinees)
            ▪ Vaccine efficacy is 50 – 60 % (2 doses) and 70% (3 doses)
        – Pertussis killed whole cell vaccine
    - DOC for cases and contacts: Erythromycin (for 10 days)

74. Ans. (c) Parapertussis causes more severe disease then pertussis [Ref. Park 27/e p182]

75. Ans. (a) Incubation period is 7-14 days; (c) Can affect any age; (d) Secondary attack rate in unimmunised persons is 90% [Ref. Park 27/e p182]

76. Ans. (c) Drug of choice is Erythromycin [Ref. Park 27/e p182]

    PERTUSSIS
    - Source of Infection: Cases
    - Subclinical cases DO NOT exist
    - Infective period: Catarrhal stage (1 week after exposure to 3 weeks after onset of paroxysmal stage)
    - Drug of choice: Erythromycin (40 mg/kg in 4 divided doses X 10 days)
    - Complications: Bronchitis, bronchopneumonia, bronchiectasis, convulsions, coma

Review Questions

77. Ans. (a) Prophylactic antibiotic for 10 days [Ref. Park 27/e p182]

78. Ans. (a) Secondary attack rate 90%; (b); (d) [Ref. Park 27/e p182]

MENINGOCOCCAL MENINGITIS

79. Ans. (a) Causative agent is a Gram –ve diplococci [Ref. Park 27/e p184]

> **ALSO REMEMBER**
> - Case Fatality Rate (CFR) of Meningococcal meningitis: 80%
>   – With early diagnosis and treatment, CFR declines to < 10%
> - Meningococcal disease is endemic in India
> - Treatment with Penicillin doesn't eradicate the carrier state in meningococcal meningitis
> - Isolation of cases is not useful in epidemics of meningococcal meningitis as carriers outnumber case

80. Ans. (c) Vaccine prophylaxis of contacts of Xavier [Ref. Park 27/e p185]
    - No vaccine prophylaxis can be given to contacts of Xavier as there is no effective vaccine available for Group B Meningococcus.

> **ALSO REMEMBER**
>
> **MENINGOCOCCAL MENINGITIS:**
> - *Causative agent:* Neisseria meningitidis
>   – *Most lethal form:* B
>   – *Epidemics:* A, C > B > W-135, Y
> - *Reservoir:* Human beings (only)
> - *Waterhouse-Friderichsen syndrome:* A massive, usually bilateral, hemorrhage into the adrenal glands caused by fulminant meningococcemia
> - *Case fatality rate:* 80% (10% in early diagnosis and treatment)
> - *Diagnosis:* Culturing the organism on a chocolate agar plate (*Specimen:* CSF)

81. Ans. (b) Young adolescents [Ref. CDC Meningococcal Vaccine Guidelines 2014]
    Meningococcal Vaccine Recommendations:
    - *Routinely*:
        – All adolescents 11-12 years age (1st dose at 11-12 years age, followed by Booster dose at 16 years age)
    - *Other groups*:
        – Adolescents 13-18 years
        – Young people 19-21 years
        – 2 years and above (Splenectomized/Chronic diseases/Lab workers/Travelers to endemic areas)

82. Ans. (b) Rifampicin [Ref. Park 27/e p184]

83. Ans. (b) 0.01% [Ref. Park 27/e p184]
    WHO Classification of Meningococcal areas:
    - Low endemicity: < 2 cases per 100,000 population per year
    - Moderate endemicity: 2-10 cases per 100,000 population per year

- High endemicity: > 10 cases per 100,000 population per year (0.01%)
- Epidemic: > 100 cases per 100,000 population per year (0.1%)

84. Ans. (a) ACW135Y [Ref. Park 27/e p185]

85. Ans. (a) Fatality in untreated cases is 60% [Ref. Park 27/e p184]

86. Ans. (a) 50 mcg of polysaccharide of each strain [Ref. Park 27/e p185]

    Meningococcal Polysaccharide Vaccines
    - Types: Bivalent (a, C), Trivalent (A, C, W135), Quadrivalent (A, C, W135, Y)
    - Vaccines contain 50 mcg of each individual polysaccharides
    - Single dose > 2 years age, Subcutaneous
    - MC adverse effects: Pain, Redness at site

87. Ans. (b) Two [Ref. Park 27/e p185]

    Monovalent Men A Conjugate Vaccine
    - 2 months -11 months age: 2 doses (Interval 2 months) and 1 booster dose after 12 months
    - 1 year - 29 years age: 1 dose

88. Ans. (b) Antibiotic treatment of contacts [Ref. Park 27/e p185]

    Meningococcal Meningitis Prevention & Control
    - Treatment of cases:
      - Antibiotics started < 48 hours of illness save 95% lives
      - Drug of choice: Penicillin (Ceftriaxone if allergic to Penicillin)
      - Epidemics: Single dose Long-acting Chloramphenicol or Ceftriaxone
    - Treatment of carriers: Rifampicin
    - Treatment of contacts:
      - Start treatment < 24 hours of identification of index case
      - Drugs used: Rifampicin, Ciprofloxacin, Ceftriaxone, Azithromycin

ARI

89. Ans. (a) Very severe disease [Ref. Park 27/e p187]
    - Inability to feed and severe malnutrition (weight 5 kg at 2 years age) makes the child as having Very Severe Pneumonia.

90. Ans. (b) Classify as pneumonia, start antibiotics and advice to report after 3 days [Ref. Park 27/e p188]
    - **In the given question,** a child aged 24 months weighed 11 Kg, respiratory rate was 38 per minute, chest indrawing was present,
    - Chest indrawing makes the child pneumonia, start antibiotics and repeat after 3 days

> **ALSO REMEMBER**
> - *Acute Respiratory Tract Infections (ARI) Control Programme:*
>   - Started as a pilot project in 1990
>   - Currently is a part of RCH Programme – II (2004 – 09)

91. Ans. (d) Very severe pneumonia [Ref. Park 27/e p188-189]

    In the question, child 10 month has respiratory rate 48/minute (normal), and absence of chest indrawing (a feature of Severe pneumonia).
    But, child has weight 5 kg (Expected weight at 10 months age is 9-9.5 kg). So this child is Severe malnutrition according to Gomez classification
    Hence, it is a case of Very severe pneumonia

92. Ans. (c) Oxygen saturation [Ref. Park 27/e p188-189]

93. Ans. (b) >50 breaths/min [Ref. Park 27/e p187]

Fast Breathing in Children (New IMNCI Guidelines)

Age group	Respiratory rate	Classification
12 months–5 years	>40/minute	Pneumonia
2–12 months	>50/minute	Pneumonia
<2 months	>60/minute	Very severe disease

Review Question

94. Ans. (d) 59 [Ref. Park 27/e p187-189]

TUBERCULOSIS

95. Ans. (d) Isoniazid and Rifampicin [Ref. Park 26/e p208]
    - Multidrug Resistant TB (MDR–TB): Resistance to Isoniazid and Rifampicin 'with or without resistance to other drugs

96. Ans. (d) 0% HIV-TB co-infection rate [Ref. Park 27/e p237-238]

The End TB Strategy 2016-2035^Q
- *Vision*: A world free of TB
  - Zero deaths, disease and suffering due to TB
- *Goal*: End the Global TB Epidemic

Indicators	Milestones^Q		Targets^Q	
	2020	2025	SDG 2030	End TB 2035
Reduction in number of TB deaths compared with 2015 (%)	35%	75%	90%	95%
Reduction in TB incidence rate compared with 2015 (%)	20% (<85/100,000)	50% (<55/100,000)	80% (<20/100,000)	90% (<10/100,000)
TB-affected families facing catastrophic costs due to TB (%)	Zero	Zero	Zero	Zero

ALSO REMEMBER

- *3 by 5 Initiative:* Launched by WHO and UNAIDS on 1st Dec 2003
  - *Target:* To provide antiretroviral treatment (ART) to 3 million people living with HIV/AIDS (PLHA) in developing countries by end of 2005
  - *Ultimate goal:* To provide universal access to treatment for HIV/AIDS to all those who need it
- *Catch up – Keep up – Follow up strategy:* WHO Measles elimination strategy comprises a 3-Part Vaccination strategy:
  - *Catch up:* One time nationwide, vaccination campaign targeting all children 9 months to 14 years of age, irrespective of history of Measles disease or vaccination status
  - *Keep up:* Routine services aimed at vaccinating more than 95% of each successive birth cohort
  - *Follow up:* Subsequent nationwide vaccination campaigns conducted every 2 – 4 years targeting usually all children born after the catch-up campaign.
- *WHO Intensive PULSE strategy:* Is for prevention and control of Poliomyelitis
- *Roll Back Malaria Initiative:* Launched by WHO, UNICEF, UNDP and World Bank in 1998
  - Strengthen health system
  - Ensure proper and expanded use of insecticide treated bed nets (ITBN)
  - Ensure adequate access to basic healthcare and training of healthcare workers
  - Encourage simpler and effective means of administering medicines
  - Encourage development of more effective drugs and vaccines
- *SAFE Strategy:* Recommended by WHO for global elimination of blinding trachoma
  - Surgery
  - Antibiotic use
  - Facial cleanliness
  - Environmental improvement
- *Accelerated Measles Mortality Reduction Strategy (WHO-UNICEF):* Two doses of Measles containing vaccine (MCV) to all children through routine and supplementary immunization activities
- *Right to Sight Initiative (VISION 2020):* To eliminate all causes of avoidable blindness by 2020
- *GET Initiative:* Alliance for Global Elimination of Trachoma by 2020

ALSO REMEMBER

- *Tuberculin:* Purified protein derivative (PPD) has replaced the antigen old tuberculin (OT)
  - WHO advocates 'PPD-RT-23 with Tween-80'
  - *Dosage:* First strength (1TU), Intermediate strength (5TU), Second strength (250TU)
  - *Tuberculin test in use:*
    - *Mantoux intradermal test:* More precise test of tuberculin sensitivity
    - *Heaf test:* Quick, easy, reliable and cheap, preferred for testing large groups
    - *Tine multiple puncture test:* Unreliable, not recommended
  - *Tuberculin test conversion:* It is defined as an increase of 10 mm or more within a 2-year period, regardless of age
- *Mantoux test:*
  - *Dose:* 1 TU of PPD in 0.1ml injected intradermally on forearm
  - Result read after 72 hrs (3d)
  - Only induration is measured:
    - *Induration > 9 mm:* Positive
    - *Induration 6 – 9 mm:* Doubtful (M. tuberculosis or Atypical mycobacteria)
    - *Induration < 6 mm:* Negative
  - Is a test of prognostic significance
- *Sputum smear examination (Z-N Staining) by direct microscopy:* It is the 'method of choice as a case finding tool for tuberculosis'
- *Sputum culture examination:* Is offered as a centralized service at district and regional chest clinic laboratories
  - only meant for chest symptomatic who are smear negative
  - useful for carrying out sensitivity tests and monitoring drug treatment

97. Ans. (c) Identify new converters to Tuberculin test
    [Ref. Park 27/e p216]

98. Ans. (a) <1% in 0-14 group of children
    [Ref. Park 21/e p169, Park 22/e p170]
    - Control of a disease includes:
      - Reducing incidence of disease
      - Reducing duration of disease (and risk of transmission)
      - Reducing the effects of infection (including physical and psychological complications)
      - Reducing financial burden to the community
    - WHO definition of TB control: Prevalence of natural infection in the age group 0 – 14 years is of the order of 1%

99. Ans. (c) Tuberculin test [Ref. Park 27/e p216]

    TUBERCULIN TEST:
    - Discovered by Von Pirquet (1907)

- Tuberculin test is the 'only way of estimating the prevalence of infection in a population'
- Positive reaction to the test: evidence of past or present infection by M. tuberculosis
- Tuberculin test has lost its sensitivity as an indicator of the true prevalence of infection, in countries with high coverage of BCG; True prevalence rates are exaggerated by:
  - Infection with atypical mycobacteria
  - Boosting effect of a second dose of tuberculin

ALSO REMEMBER
- **Mantoux Test:**
  - 1 Tuberculin Unit (TU) in 0.1 mL
  - *False Reactions:*

False +ve Mantoux	False –ve Mantoux
Faulty technique of injection	Pre-allergic phase
Using degraded tuberculin	High fever
Too deep injection	High fever
Infection of other mycobacterium	Measles and Chickenpox
	Whooping cough
Repeated tuberculin testing	Malnutrition
Prior BCG vaccine	HIV/AIDS
	Use of anti-allergic drugs
	Use of immunosuppressants

100. Ans. (c) Bangalore   *[Ref. Park 19/e p151, 20/e p161]*

ALSO REMEMBER
- NEERI is credited with 'Nalgonda Technique' for defluoridation of water
- CDRI is credited with development of 'Centchroman', a non-hormonal non-steroidal oral contraceptive pill
- Location of headquarters of International health agencies.

International Health Agency	Location of Headquarters
WHO	Geneva, Switzerland
UNICEF	New York, USA
FAO	Rome, Italy
ILO	Geneva, Switzerland

101. Ans. (a) Incidence of infection   *[Ref. Park 27/e p210]*

102. Ans. (c) 40%   *[Ref. Park 27/e p210]*
- Prevalence of TB infection in India: 40%

103. Ans. (c) 20 – 30%   *[Ref. Park 27/e p208-210]*
- **Tuberculosis Situation In India:**
- *Country with highest TB burden in world*: India
- *Infected with TB (Mantoux positive):* Two out of five Indians (40%)
- *Annual risk of becoming infected with TB:* 1.5%
- *Lifetime risk of disease among infected:* 10%
- *Indians developing TB everyday:* 5000
- *Sputum positive every year:* 0.8 million
- *TB deaths per year:* 0.37 million

104. Ans. (a) 133 per 100,000   *[Ref. Park 27/e p208-210]*
- *Incidence of TB:* Is percentage of new cases (confirmed by bacteriological examination) per 1000 population
  Incidence of TB = New cases/Total population × 1000
- **In the given question:** New cases of TB are 22, and total population is 16, 500.
- Thus, Incidence of TB = 22/16500 × 1000 = 1.33 per 1000 population
- Or Incidence of TB = 133 per 100,000 population

105. Ans. (d) Social and environmental factors
- Thomas McKeown attributed the modern rise in the world population, AND DECLINE OF TB from the 1700s to the present to broad economic and social changes (especially diet and nutrition – "Nutritional Determinism") rather than to targeted public health or medical interventions

106. Ans. (d) INH 5 mg/kg for 6 months   *[Ref. Park 23/e p215]*
- *Guidelines for Chemoprophylaxis in children (< 6 years) who come in contact with a Sputum positive TB case:*

IF	AND	THEN
Symptoms of TB	Clinician declares TB	Cat I DOTS given
No symptoms of TB	Tuberculin test NA	Isoniazid 5 mg/kg × 6 months
	Tuberculin test	Isoniazid 5 mg/kg × 3 months, then do test
		If induration < 6 mm: Stop INH, Give BCG
		If induration > 6 mm: Continue INH for 3 months

(INH: Isoniazid; NA: Not available)

107. Ans. (a) Sputum smear +   *[Ref. Park 27/e p214]*

108. Ans. (a) Incidence of infection   *[Ref. Park 27/e p210]*

109. Ans. (c) For assessing rifampicin resistance; (e) Diagnosis of TB   *[Ref. Tuberculosis: Diagnosis and Treatment by Timothy, 23/e p197]*

110. Ans. (a) Prevent resistance   *[Ref. Park 27/e p222]*

111. Ans. (d) Children below 6 years   *[Ref. Park 27/e p214]*

112. Ans. (b) High prevalence of immunized people   *[Ref. Park 27/e p231]*
- In countries with high coverage of BCG vaccine (India has 89% BCG coverage), which produces tuberculin hypersensitivity, Tuberculin test has lost its sensitivity as an indicator of true prevalence of infection

113. Ans. (d) All of the above   *[Ref. Park 27/e p236]*
TUBERCULOSIS AND DIABETES
- Diabetes is an independent risk factor for Tuberculosis
- Diabetes account for 15% of all Tuberculosis (21% of Smear +ve TB)
- Higher 2-3 times risk of progression from Latent to Active TB
- More severe clinical course
- Late diagnosis
- High risk of death in TB treatment
- High risk of relapse after TB treatment
- Higher risk of other infections

114. Ans. (c) Resistant to INH and Rifampicin with or without resistant to other anti TB drugs

[Ref. Park 27/e p222]

115. **Ans. (c) Chronic alcoholism** *[Ref. Guidelines on the management of latent tuberculosis infection, WHO p13]*

   LATENT TUBERCULOSIS INFECTION (LTBI)
   - *Latent TB*: Latent tuberculosis infection (LTBI) is defined as a state of persistent immune response to stimulation by Mycobacterium tuberculosis antigens without evidence of clinically manifested active TB

SYSTEMATIC TESTING & TREATMENT **Strong recommendation** • People living with HIV • Contacts of pulmonary TB case • Anti-TNF treatment • Dialysis • Organ or hematologic transplantation • Silicosis **Conditional recommendation** • Prisoners • Health workers • Immigrants from high burden countries • Homeless persons • Illicit drug users	**LTBI testing procedures** • Interferon-gamma release assays (IGRA) • Mantoux tuberculin skin test (TST) **Systematic testing NOT recommended** • Diabetes • Harmful alcohol use • Tobacco smokers • Underweight people [*Mnemonic*: **D**rugs **H**arm **U**nderage **T**eens]

Review Questions

116. **Ans. (b) 1 unit of PPD RT3** *[Ref. Park 27/e p216]*

117. **Ans. (a) >10⁴ bacilli are required in sputum for detection** *[Ref. Park 27/e p214-215]*

118. **Ans. (c) With hold breastfeeding** *[Ref. Park 27/e p230]*

POLIOMYELITIS

119. **Ans. (a) Stool** *[Ref. Park 27/e p241-242]*
   - *Stool examination*:
     - Isolation of wild poliovirus from stool is *'the recommended method for laboratory confirmation of paralytic poliomyelitis'*
     - Recommended in every case of AFP
     - Virus usually can be found in the feces from onset to up to < 8 weeks after paralysis, with 'the highest probability of detection during the first 2 weeks after paralysis onset'

120. **Ans. (a) Poliomyelitis in recipients; (b) Poliomyelitis in contacts of recipients** *[Ref. Park 27/e p244-245]*
   - OPV has a rare complication of Vaccine associated paralytic Poliomyelitis (VAPP)
     - *In vaccines:* 1 in 2.7 million
     - *In Close contacts of vaccines:* 1 in 5 million
   - Poliomyelitis Situation 2016 WORLD [as on 01 January 2017]
     - Total cases: 35 WPV + 3 cVDPV
     - 3 endemic countries: Afghanistan, Pakistan, Nigeria
   - Poliomyelitis Situation 2016 INDIA [as on 01 January 2017]
     - Total cases: NIL wild virus case [No case has been reported in India from 13 January 2011 onwards]
     - India declared 'Polio-Free' on 27 March 2014
     - 1 VDPV case (P2) reported from India

121. **Ans. (b) Last polio case in India was reported in 13 January 2011** *[Ref. NPSP GOI Website]*

   CURRENT POLIO SITUATION 2018
   - Current situation in India:
     - No wild case of Polio in India currently (2011 onwards)
     - Last case was reported on 13 January 2011 (FREE on 27 March 2016)
     - VDPV in India: 1 cases P2
     - OPV_b is mostly used in India (Routine immunizations, as well as Pulse Polio Immunization)

122. **Ans. (a) Type 3 is most common is India** *[Ref. Park 27/e p241]*

123. **Ans. (d) mVDPV** *[Ref. Park 27/e p242]*

   Vaccine derived polio virus (VDPV)
   - Properties of VDPV:
     - Occurs due to Sabin (OPV) vaccine: cVDPV Poliovirus type 2 (MC)
     - Clinical presentation indistinguishable from Wild poliovirus (WPV)
     - cVDPV present similar public health threat like WPV
     - iVDPV prolonged infection may transmit virus to others
   - Incidence of VDPV: 4 cases per million birth cohort per year
   - Types of VDPV:
     - cVDPV: Person-to-person transmission in community
     - iVDPV: Isolates from immunodeficient persons
     - aVDPV: Ambiguous from healthy person or sewage isolates
   - Key risk factors for cVDPV emergence:
     - Development of immunity gaps (due to low OPV coverage)
     - Prior elimination of WPV types
     - Low routine immunization coverage with trivalent OPV
     - Insensitive AFP surveillance
   - Diagnosis:
     - Real time Reverse transcription
     - PCR nucleic acid amplification

124. **Ans. (c) Serotype 3** *[Ref. Park 27/e p242]*
   - VAPP is MC associated with P3 (60%) > P2 > P1 of Sabin (OPV)

125. **Ans. (c) Descending motor paralysis with preservation of tendon reflexes and absent sensation** *[Ref. Park 27/e p243]*

126. **Ans. (d) Lower motor neuron type** *[Ref. Hutchison's Atlas of Pediatric Physical Diagnosis 1/e p271]*

   Types of Paralytic Poliomyelitis
   - Spinal poliomyelitis (MC type): Lower motor neuron lesion of the anterior horn cells of Spinal cord which affects the muscles of the legs, arms and/or trunk asymmetrically
   - Bulbar poliomyelitis: Involvement of Lower cranial nerves

- Bulbospinal poliomyelitis: Involvement of both Bulbar cranial nerves and Spinal cord

Review Questions

127. Ans. (a) Stabilizer [Ref. Park 27/e p244-245]

128. Ans. (c) Can transmit it by nasal discharge [Ref. Park 27/e p244-245]

129. Ans. (c) It is contraindicated in immunocompromised patients [Ref. Park 27/e p244]

HEPATITIS

130. Ans. (a) HbsAg+; (c) Anti HBc+; (d) HBV DNA+ [Ref. Park 26/e p249]
     - Chronic hepatitis B with active viral replication: HBsAg+, IgG Anti HBc+, HBeAg+, HBV DNA+
     - Chronic hepatitis B with low viral replication: HBsAg+, IgG Anti HBc+, Anti HBe+, HBV DNA+

131. Ans. (c) Acute hepatitis B [Ref. Park 26/e p249]
     - Acute Hepatitis B cases have HBsAg+, IgM Anti HBc+, HBeAg+ (Infectivity)

132. Ans. (b) HBsAg [Ref. Park 26/e p249]
     - Active component in Hepatitis B Subunit Recombinant vaccine is HBsAg

133. Ans. (b) Chronic hepatitis B [Ref. Park 26/e p249]
     - Chronic hepatitis B with active viral replication: HBsAg+, IgG Anti HBc+, HBeAg+, HBV DNA+
     - Chronic hepatitis B with low viral replication: HBsAg+, IgG Anti HBc+, Anti HBe+, HBV DNA+

134. Ans. (d) No post-exposure HBV management is necessary [Ref. Hepatitis B and Healthcare Personnel, IAC]

     PEP Guidelines for Hepatitis-B Exposure

HBsAg status of patient	Anti HBs levels of exposed persons	Management
+	<10 mIU/ml	HBIG + Hepatitis B Vaccine
–	<10 mIU/ml	Hepatitis B Vaccine
+/–	≥10 mIU/ml	No further action

135. Ans. (b) Hepatitis E [Ref. Park 27/e p261]
     - Types of Viral Hepatitis:

Type	Causative agent	Incubation period	Common mode(s) of transmission
Hepatitis A	Enterovirus 72 (picornavirus)	15–45 days	Faecal-oral, sexual
Hepatitis B	Hepadnavirus	45–180 days	Sexual, perinatal, percutaneous
Hepatitis C	Hepacivirus (Flavivirus)	30–120 days	Percutaneous
Hepatitis D	Viriods like	30–90 days	Sexual, perinatal, percutaneous
Hepatitis E	Calcivirus (alphavirus like)	21–45 days	Faecal-oral

> **ALSO REMEMBER**
> - MC cause of fulminancy in viral hepatitis: Hepatitis D
> - MC cause of chronicity in viral hepatitis: Hepatitis C
> - MC cause of carriers in viral hepatitis: Hepatitis B
> - MC cause of cancers in viral hepatitis: Hepatitis C
> - Prognosis in viral hepatitis: Hepatitis A > Hepatitis E > Hepatitis D (acute) > Hepatitis C > Hepatitis D (chronic) > Hepatitis B
> - Hepatitis caused by a DNA virus: Hepatitis B
> - World Hepatitis Day: May 19 (2008); July 28 (2011-14)

136. Ans. (d) HBsAg [Ref. Park 27/e p252]

137. Ans. (a) Medical students screened before their joining; (b) IV drug abuser are prone to infection; (d) Long term hemodialysis; (e) Interferon is treatment [Ref. Park 27/e p258-259]
     - **HEPATITIS C:**
     - Is major cause of parenterally transmitted non-A, non-B hepatitis (PT-NANB)
     - Infection in world: 3% (Infection in blood donors in India: 2%)
     - Is a leading reason for liver transplantation
     - Risk of maternal-neonatal transmission is small
     - IP: 6 – 7 weeks
     - Chronicity: 50%

138. Ans. (a) Cause mild illness in children [Ref. Park 27/e p249]
     - Key facts about Epidemiology of hepatitis A infection:
       – Causative agent: Enterovirus 72 (Picorna virus)
       – Disinfectant:
         - Formalin
         - UV rays
         - Boiling for 5 min
         - Autoclaving
       – Reservoir: Human cases
       – Period of infectivity: 2 weeks before to 1 week after onset of jaundice
       – Children: More infected but mild or subclinical
       – Sex distribution: Equal in both sexes
       – Modes of transmission:
         - Faecal oral (Most common)
         - Parenteral
         - Sexual
       – Carrier stage and carcinoma (HCC): Generally not seen in Hepatitis A

139. Ans. (a) HbsAg; (c) Anti-HBc; (d) HBeAg [Ref. Park 27/e p252]
     - Serologic patterns in Hepatitis B:

HBsAg	Anti-HBs	Anti-HBc	HBeAg	Anti-HBe	Interpretation
+	–	IgM	+	–	Acute Hepatitis B
+	–	IgG	+	–	Chronic Hepatitis B + replication
–	+	IgG	–	+	Recovery from Hepatitis B
–	+	–	–	–	Vaccinated individuals

140. Ans. (a) Acute infectious Hepatitis B
[Ref. Park 27/e p252]

SEROLOGIC PATTERNS IN HEPATITIS B

HBsAg	Anti-HBs	Anti-HBc	HBeAg	Anti-HBe	Interpretation
+	–	IgM	+	–	Acute Hepatitis B
+	–	IgG	+	–	Chronic Hepatitis B + replication
–	+	IgG	–	+	Recovery from Hepatitis B
–	+	–	–	–	Vaccinated individuals

141. Ans. (a) HBsAg; (c) Anti HBc; (d) HBeAg
[Ref. Park 27/e p252]

142. Ans. (a) Hepatitis B vaccine + Immunoglobulin
[Ref. Park 27/e p254]

143. Ans. (c) Active and infectious Hepatitis B disease
[Ref. Park 27/e p254]

HBsAg plus HBEAg in serum
- Acute hepatitis B
- Active and Infectious hepatitis B
- Chronic hepatitis B with Active viral replication (high infectivity)

144. Ans. (d) HDVAg, IgM Anti-HDV, HDV RNA
[Ref. Liver Disease in Children by Frederick, 3/e p428, 24/e p235]

SEROLOGIC DIFFERENTIATION OF HEPATITIS B AND D

	IgM AntiHBc	HDVAg	IgM AntiHDV	HDV RNA
Acute HBV	+	–	–	–
Acute HDV coinfection	+	+	±	+
Acute HDV superinfection	–	+	+	+
Chronic HDV	–	–	+	+

145. Ans. (c) HBe Ag [Ref. Park 27/e p252]
146. Ans. (d) Chronic Hepatitis B with high infectivity
[Ref. Park 27/e p252-253]
- AntiHBc IgG+ indicate Chronic disease
- HBeAg indicate Active viral replication (High infectivity)

Review Question

147. Ans. (c) Two weeks before the symptoms and two week thereafter [Ref. Park 27/e p251]

DIARRHEAL DISEASES (CHOLERA AND TYPHOID)

148. Ans. (b) Proper disposal of feces, safe water supply, personal hygiene is more important than immunization
[Ref. Park 26/e p275]
- The control of typhoid fever must be through improved sanitation and domestic/personal hygiene
- Complementary approaches to prevention include immunization which is the only specific preventive measure likely to provide highest benefit for the money spent

149. Ans. (a) Staphylococcus aureus [Ref. Park 25/e p261]
- Incubation period of food poisoning: Salmonella 12–24 hours, Staphylococcal 1–6 hours, Botulism 12–36 hours, Cl. perfirengens 6–24 hours, B. cereus (emetic form) 1–6 hours, B. cereus (diarrhoel form) 12–24 hours

150. Ans. (d) 24 hours [Ref. Park 27/e p266]
- Oral Rehydration Solution ORS:
- *Reduced Osmolarity Oral Rehydration Solution (Low Na ORS):* WHO NEW ORS

Composition (grams)		Osmolar concentration (mmol/litre)	
Sodium chloride	2.6	Sodium	75
Potassium chloride	1.5	Potassium	20
Sodium citrate	2.9	Chloride	65
Glucose	13.5	Citrate	10
		Glucose	75
Total	20.5	Total	245

ALSO REMEMBER
- ORS is the 'most important discovery of 20th century'
- As many as 90-95% of all cases of cholera and acute diarrhoea can be treated by oral fluids alone
- *Inclusion of trisodium citrate instead of sodium bicarbonate in WHO ORS:* Makes the product more stable and results in less stool output
- *Low Osmolarity ORS:* Reduces stool output by 20%, vomiting by 30% and need for unscheduled intravenous therapy
- *WHO/UNICEF recommended oral rehydration formulation:* Reduced Osmolarity Oral Rehydration Solution (Low Na ORS)
- *Initial amount of ORS required for dehydration:* 75 ml per kg
- Intravenous rehydration:
  - *Ringer's lactate solution (Hartmann's solution):* Best commercially available solution
  - *Diarrhoea treatment solution (DTS):* WHO recommended ideal polyelectrolyte solution for intravenous solution
  - *Normal saline:* Poorest solution

151. Ans. (b) Oral rehydration therapy [Ref. Park 27/e p266]
- Intravenous rehydration infusion is usually required ONLY FOR initial rehydration of severely dehydrated patients who are in shock or unable to drink
  - **In the given question**, a 5 year old boy passed 18 loose stools in last 24 hours and vomited twice in last 4 hours, He is irritable BUT DRINKING FLUIDS,
  - Thus intravenous therapy is not indicated

- Also plain water will not replace the salts lost in stools and vomiting
- So, ideal treatment is Oral rehydration therapy

152. Ans. (a) Tetracycline [Ref. Park 27/e p268]

Group	Antibiotic of choice
Treatment	
Adults	Doxycycline
Children	Azithromycin
Pregnancy	Azithromycin
Chemoprophylaxis	Tetracycline

153. Ans. (a) 10-14 days [Ref. Park 27/e p277]

154. Ans. NONE (NOW Azithromycin, earilier Furazotidone) [Ref. Park 27/e p274-275]

- Cholera is an acute diarrhoel disease caused by Vibrio cholerae
  - Classical biotype
  - El Tor biotype [Serotypes: Ogawa (MC in India), Inaba and Hikojima]
- *Vibrio cholerae:* 'Gram-negative bacterium' that produces cholera toxin (enterotoxin), which act on c-AMP system of mucosal cells of epithelium lining of the small intestine (to cause massive diarrhea)
- *Incubation period:* 1 – 2 days (Few hours – 5 days)
- *Reservoir:* Human beings only
- *Essentials for treatment of cholera:* Water and electrolyte replacement (ORS)

> **ALSO REMEMBER**
> - *Cholera stools appearance:* 'RICE WATERY diarrhoea'
> - *Father of Public Health:* Cholera (although some regard John Snow as the same)
> - *Most susceptible blood group to cholera:* Blood group O (> B > A > AB)
> - *Recent most cholera outbreak:* Iraq (UN 2007)
> - *History of cholera:*
>   - *John Snow (1813-1858):* Found the link between cholera and contaminated drinking water (1854 using Spot maps)
>   - Robert Koch identified V. cholerae with a microscope as the bacillus causing the disease (1885)
>   - *Cholera morbus:* Used in 19th and early 20th centuries for both non-epidemic cholera and other gastrointestinal diseases (sometimes epidemic) that resembled cholera

155. Ans. (a) Increases shelf life [Ref. Park 27/e p266]

- In WHO ORS, sodium bicarbonate has been replaced by trisodium citrate:
- Makes the product more stable
- Results in less stool output (especially in high-output diarrhoea like cholera) as it increases intestinalabsorption of sodium and water

156. Ans. (c) 45 mmol/L [Ref. OP Ghai 7/e p71-72, Park 23/e p232-247]

157. Ans. (b) Isolation of Vi antigen [Ref. Park 27/e p277]

- *Laboratory Diagnosis:* **'BASU' Mnemonic**

Test of diagnosis	Time of diagnosis	Remarks
Blood culture	1st week	Mainstay of diagnosis
Antibodies (Widal test)	2nd week	Moderate, Sens, Spec
Stool culture	3rd week	
Urine test	4th week	
Newer tests		
IDL Tubex test		Detects IgM antibodies
TYPHI DOT		Detects IgM and IgG Ab
TYPHI DOT-M		Detects IgM antibodies
DIPSTICK TEST		Detects IgM antibodies
Isolation of Vi Ag		Detects carriers

> **ALSO REMEMBER**
> - *In chronic cases of Typhoid, organisms persist in:* Gall Bladder and Biliary tract
>   - Typhoid Mary, who gave rise to 1300 cases, was a chronic carrier
>   - Vi antibodies are in 80%
>   - *Most Successful approach to treatment:* Cholecystectomy + Ampicillin therapy
> - Immunization doesn't give 100% protection

158. Ans. (a) Mass chemoprophylaxis [Ref. Park 27/e p275]

> **ALSO REMEMBER**
> - Drugs for chemoprophylaxis:

Disease	Chemoprophylaxis
Cholera	Tetracycline/Furazolidone
Bacterial conjunctivitis	Erythromycin ointment
Diphtheria	Erythromycin and 1st dose of vaccine
Influenza	Amantadine
Malaria	
< 6 Wk	Doxycycline
≥ 6 Wk	Mefloquine
Meningococcal meningitis	Rifampicin
Plague	Tetracycline
Typhoid	NONE

- *Chemoprophylaxis is Primary level of prevention (Mode of Intervention: Specific protection)* as risk factors are present but disease has not yet taken place

159. Ans. (c) 14-21 days [Ref. Park 27/e p272]

- *Types of carriers in Cholera:*

Type of carrier	Duration	Remarks
Preclinical (incubatory)	1 – 5 days	Are potential patients
Convalescent	2 – 3 weeks	Not received effective antibiotic treatment
Contact (Healthy)	< 10 days	Due to subclinical infection; cause spread
Chronic	Up to 10 years	Gallbladder infected

160. **Ans. (a) Cl⁻ –111; (d) Lactate-29**
 [Ref. Internet, Park 23/e p226]
 - *Composition of Ringer Lactate:*
   – Sodium ion: 130 mmol/L
   – Potassium ion: 4 mmol/L
   – Chloride ion: 109 mmol/L
   – Calcium ion: 1.5 mmol/L
   – Lactate ion: 28 mmol/L

161. **Ans. (c) 800-1200 mL** *[Ref. Park 27/e p267]*

162. **Ans. (b) Male carriers though less are more dangerous** *[Ref. Park 27/e p277]*

163. **Ans. (a) Sodium; (c) Glucose** *[Ref. Park 27/e p266]*

164. **Ans. (b) Moderate** *[Ref. Recent Advances in Paediatrics by Suraj Gupte, 1/e p181]*

165. **Ans. (b) 245** *[Ref. Park 27/e p266]*

166. **Ans. (d) Total osmolarity – 300 mmol/l** *[Ref. Park 27/e p266]*

167. **Ans. (a) Started in Bangladesh; (c) Due to O139 El Tor; (e) Low proportion of adults in endemic regions** *[Ref. Medical Microbiology, Samuel Baron, 4/e chapter24]*

168. **Ans. (a) Safe water supply and sanitation** *[Ref. Park 27/e p274-275]*

169. **Ans. (c) Gangliosides + Adenyl cyclase** *[Ref. Park 27/e p271-272]*

CHOLERA ENTEROTOXIN
- *Light (L) toxin*: Binds with Ganglioside in Epithelial cell membrane
- *Heavy (H) toxin*: Activates Adenyl cyclase in Epithelial cell wall which increase cAMP, leading to outpouring of isotonic fluid in lumen of intestine

170. **Ans. (d) Typhoid** *[Ref. Park 27/e p278-279]*

COMMON DISEASES CHEMOPROPHYLAXIS
- *Bacterial Conjunctivitis, Pertussis, Diphtheria*: Erythromycin
- *Plague, cholera*: Tetracycline
- *Meningococcal meningitis*: Rifampicin > Sulfazine
- *Influenza*: Amantadine
- *Tetanus*: Penicillin
- *Malaria*: Doxycycline, Mefloquine

171. **Ans. (c) To correct acidosis** *[Ref. Textbook of Pharmacology by Seth 3/e pIX.22]*

CITRATE IN ORS
- Base is added in the form of bicarbonate, citrate or lactate for correction of acidosis resulting due to loss of alkali in stools
- Trisodium citrate is more stable than Sodium bicarbonate
- Increase intestinal absorption of sodium and water
- Results in les stool output in High output diarrhoea (Cholera)

172. **Ans. (a) Cresol** *[Ref. Park 27/e p275]*

CHOLERA STOOL DISINFECTION IN EPIDEMIC
- Most effective disinfectant is a Coal-tar disinfectant with RW coefficient >10 like Cresol
- Disinfectant with RWC <5 should not be used

173. **Ans. (d) 24 months** *[Ref. Park 27/e p279-280]*

Vi POLYSACCHARIDE TYPHOID VACCINE
- Purified Vi capsular polysaccharide from Ty2 S
- Does not elicit immune response <2 years age
- Licensed for use >2 years age
- 1 dose is required, produces protection after 7 days
- Revaccination recommended every 3 years

174. **Ans. (c) Day 1, 3, 5** *[Ref. Park 27/e p279]*

COMMONLY ASKED VACCINE SCHEDULES
- Hepatitis-B (Infants): 6, 10, 14 weeks OR 0, 6, 14 weeks
- Hepatitis-B (Adults): 0, 1, 6 months
- Typhoral (Ty21a): 1, 3, 5 days
- Rabies (Post-exposure Intramuscular): 1-1-1-1-1 (0, 3, 7, 14, 28 days)
- Rabies (Post-exposure Intradermal): 2-2-2-0-2 (0, 3, 7, 28 days)
- Rabies (Pre-exposure Intramuscular): 0, 7, 21/28 days

175. **Ans. (a) Glucose – 90** *[Ref. Park 27/e p266]*
- WHO Reduced Osmolarity ORS contains (in mmol/L) Sodium 75, Potassium 20, Chloride 65, Citrate 10, Glucose 75; Total Osmolar concentration is 245 mmol/L.

Review Questions

176. **Ans. (b) Male carriers though less are more dangerous** *[Ref. Park 27/e p277]*

177. **Ans. (c) Till 3 stool test are negative** *[Ref. Park 27/e p278]*

178. **Ans. (b) Cresol** *[Ref. Park 27/e p275]*

WORM INFESTATIONS

179. **Ans. (b) Niridazole prevents transmission of the disease** *[Ref. Park 27/e p288]*

> **ALSO REMEMBER**
> - Guineaworm is also known as 'medina worm'
> - *Most effective larvicide for Guineaworm control:* Abate (Temephos)
> - India was the first country to establish the National Guineaworm Eradication Programme (1983-84), as a centrally sponsored scheme (50 : 50 cost-sharing basis centre: state)

180. **Ans. (b) Hookworms** *[Ref. Park 27/e p288]*
- *Endemic Index (Chandler's Index):*
  – CI is average no of hookworm eggs per gram of faeces for the 'entire community'
  – Interpretation of CI:

Average no of eggs/gm stools	Interpretation
< 200	Not much significance
200-250	Potential danger
250-300	Minor public health problem
> 300	Important public health problem

  – Technique employed: Kato-katz Technique

ALSO REMEMBER
- Average blood loss in hookworm infection: 0.03 – 0.2 mL per worm per day
- Important human parasites:

Parasite	Causative organism	Parasite	Causative organism
Roundworm	Ascaris sp. Ascaris lumbricoides	Head louse	Pediculus humanus
Balantidiasis	Balantidium coli	Body louse	Pediculus humanus corporis
Tapeworm	Cestoda	Crab louse	Phthirus pubis
Coccidia	Cryptosporidium	Scabies	Sarcoptes scabiei
Guinea worm	Dracunculus medinensis	Strongyloidiasis	Strongyloides stercoralis
Amoebiasis	Entamoeba histolytica	Toxocariasis	Toxocara canis, Toxocara cati
Pinworm	Enterobius vermicularis	Toxoplasmosis	Toxoplasma gondii
Liver fluke	Fasciola hepatica	Trichinosis	Trichinella spiralis
Giardia	Giardia lamblia	Whipworm	Trichuris trichiura, Trichuris vulpis
Hookworm	Necator americanus, Ancylostoma duodenale		

181. Ans. (a) >300   *[Ref. Park 22/e p221]*
182. Ans. (b) Monitoring individual treatment
    [Ref. Park 22/e p221]
183. Ans. (b) DDT   *[Ref. Park 27/e p288]*

Review Question

184. Ans. (c) No. of eggs of hookworm in per gram stool
    [Ref. Park 21/e p221, Park 22/e p221]

DENGUE

185. Ans. (d) Return of normal appetite   *[Ref. Park 25/e p277]*

    Dengue Discharge Protocol
    - Absence of fever >24 hours, without use of anti-pyretics
    - Return of appetite
    - Visible clinical improvement
    - Good urine output
    - >2-3 days after recovery from shock
    - No respiratory distress from pleural effusion or ascites
    - Platelet count > 50,000/cu.mm.

186. Ans. (c) Transovarian transmission of virus
    [Ref. Park 27/e p290]
    - Aedes mosquito become infective by feeding on a patient from the day before onset to the 5th day (viraemia stage) of illness: After an extrinsic incubation period of 8-10 days, the mosquitoes become infective, it remains so for life
      - Transovarial transmission of dengue virus has been demonstrated in the laboratory

187. Ans. (a) Is the most common arboviral infection; (b) Can be both epidemic as well as endemic; (c) Can survive in ambient temperature; (e) Vector is Aedes aegypti
    [Ref. Park 27/e p288-299]

    Refer to Theory

188. Ans. (c) Serotype 4 is more dangerous than other serotypes   *[Ref. Park 27/e p290]*

189. Ans. (a) Lamivudine is drug of choice
    [Ref. K. Park 22/e p225; Infectious Diseases and Arthropods by J. Goddard, 2/e, p62]
    - Moderate to severe protein energy malnutrition reduces risk of DHF/DSS in dengue-infected children
    - *Treatment of DHF*: None specific
      - Paracetamol
      - ORS, Oral fluids
      - I/V fluids, IV colloids
      - Blood transfusion

190. Ans. (d) Case management for DF and DHF, isolation and individual protection from mosquitoes and environmental measures for elimination of breeding places
    [Ref. Park 27/e p295-298]

191. Ans. (b) Subsequent infection with different strain produces severe form of dengue; (c) Most infection with dengue virus is asymptomatic; (d) Vector is Aedes mosquito
    [Ref. Park 27/e p288-291]

Review Questions

192. Ans. (c) Shock   *[Ref. Park 27/e p293]*
193. Ans. (d) Lifelong   *[Ref. Park 27/e p290]*
194. Ans. (b) It is endemic in India   *[Ref. Park 27/e p289-298]*

MALARIA

195. Ans. (d) 1, 2, 4   *[Ref. Park 25/e p287]*

    Malaria Vector Indices
    - *Human blood index:* Proportion of freshly fed female Anopheline mosquitoes whose stomach contain human blood – "Indicate Degree of Anthrophilism"
    - *Sporozoite rate:* % female Anopheline mosquitoes with sporozoites in salivary glands
    - *Mosquito density:* Number of mosquitoes per man-hour-catch
    - *Man-biting rate ("Biting density"):* Average incidence of Anopheline bites per day per person (Determined by Standardized vector catches on human bait)
    - *Inoculation rate:* Man-biting rate X Infective sporozoite rate

196. Ans. (c) To reduce Malaria disease so that it's no longer a Public health problem   *[Ref. Park 25/e p282]*
    - *Malaria control:* To reduce Malaria disease so that it's no longer a Public health problem

- *Malaria elimination:* Reduction to Zero of incidence of infection (Complete interruption of transmission)
- *Certification of Malaria Elimination (WHO):* Chain of local malaria transmission by Anopheline mosquitoes has been fully interrupted in an entire country for at least 3 consecutive years

197. Ans. (d) Annual parasitic incidence [Ref. Park 27/e p306]
- *Annual parasitic incidence (API):* Sophisticated measure of malaria incidence in a community

$$\text{API} = \frac{\text{Confirmed cases during one year}}{\text{Population under surveillance}} \times 1000$$

198. Ans. (a) Trophozoite [Ref. Parasitology by KD Chatterjee, 12/e p86, Park 22/e p282–83]
- **Modes of Malaria Transmission:**
- Bite of female anopheline mosquitoes:
  – Infective forms: Sporozoites
- Injection of blood of a malaria patient containing asexual forms:'Trophozoite induced malaria'
  – Transfusion malaria
  – Congenital malaria
  – Malaria in drug addicts

199. Ans. (d) Sulphadoxine + pyrimethamine [Ref. Park 23/e p288]

200. Ans. (a) 0.25 mg/kg body weight [Ref. Anti malaria drug policy 2007, Park 23/e p288]
- *Please Refer to New Guildelines (Annexure 12)*

> **ALSO REMEMBER**
> - Mefloquine should be used ONLY in Plasmodium falciparum cases having proven resistance to chloroquine
> - *Primaquine is contraindicated in:* pregnant women, infants, G6PD patients *Mass treatment of Malaria (WHO recommendation):* In highly endemic areas (API > 5 per 1000 population)
>   – Mass prophylaxis in age < 5 years is not recommended

201. Ans. (b) Infant parasite site [Ref. Park 27/e p306]
202. Ans. (a) Stephensi [Ref. Park 27/e p304]
203. Ans. (c) Merozoites [Ref. Park 27/e p303]
Peaks of fever in malaria coincide with release of successive broods of Merozoites into the blood stream

204. Ans. (e) Mosquito acts as definitive host [Ref. Park 27/e p301-305]
- Epidemiology of Malaria in India:
  – Incubation period:

Malaria	Incubation period
Plasmodium vivax	14 days
Plasmodium falciparum	12 days
Plasmodium malariae	28 days
Plasmodium ovale	17 days

  – *Season:* Most common in July – November
  – *Definitive host:* Anopheles mosquito (*Intermediate host:* Man)
  – Is seen in both rural as well as urban areas
  – *Vector:* An. culicifacies (rural) and An. stephensi (urban)

205. Ans. (a) Anopheles stephensi; (b) Anopheles dirus [Ref. Park 27/e p304]

206. Ans. (b) Use of bed-nets [Ref. Park 21/e p712-14, Park 22/e p716-18]
- Resurgence of Malaria in India has occurred due to:
  – Drug resistance
  – Vector resistance
  – Mutation in parasite
- Use of bed-nets (primary level of prevention) is infact likely to reduce incidence of malaria

207. Ans. (d) Gujarat; (e) Odisha [Ref. Malaria Research Centre, India]
- Plasmodium ovale has been reported from Baroda, Gujarat and Koraput, Odisha in India

208. Ans. (a) 1.5 million cases annually; (b) Quinine drug of choice in severe malaria in pregnancy; (e) Falciparum malaria is most common type [Ref. Park 27/e p299-314]

209. Ans. (b) Artesunate [Ref. Park 27/e p313]
210. Ans. (d) Primaquine [Ref. Park 27/e p312]
211. Ans. (c) June [Ref. Park 22/e p387]
- Anti-malaria month is observed every year in month of June prior to onset of monsoon and transmission season to enhance awareness and encourage community participation

212. Ans. (c) Both 1 and 2 [Ref. Encyclopedia of Epidemiology, Volume 1 by Boslaugh 1/e p623]
- In Falciparum Malaria, once vital organ dysfunction occur or proportion of infected erythrocytes increases >3%, the mortality rises steeply
- Hypoglycemia is very common in Pregnant women with Falciparum malaria
  – It occurs in 50% of Quinine-treated patients

213. Ans. (b) 10-20 days [Ref. Park 27/e p303]
EXTRINSIC INCUBATION PERIOD OF PLASMODIUM
- Period for development of parasite from Gametocyte to Sporozoite stage in body of mosquito
- EIP is around 10-20 days

214. Ans. (d) Anopheles epiroticus [Ref. Park 27/e p301]
MAJOR ANOPHELES VECTORS IN INDIA
- An. culicifacies: Rural and Peri-urban areas (Peninsular India)
- An. stephensi: Urban and Industrial areas
- An. fluviatilis: Hilly areas, Forests, Forest fringes (East India)
- An. minimus: Foot-hills (North-eastern states)
- An. dirus: Forests (North-eastern states)
- An. epiroticus: Andaman & Nicobar Islands

215. Ans. (c) Sporozoite protein [Ref. Vaccines E-Book by Stanley A. Plotkin, 7/e p563]
Malaria Vaccine MOSQUIRIX (RTS, S)
- A recombinant protein-based malaria vaccine
- World's first licensed malaria vaccine (July 2015)

- *Development:* Engineered using genes from the repeat and T-cell epitope in the pre-erythrocytic circumsporozoite protein (CSP) of the Plasmodium falciparum malaria parasite and a viral envelope protein of the hepatitis B virus (HBsAg)
- Chemical adjuvant added: AS01

216. Ans. (d) Vivax, Ovale [Ref. Park 27/e p303]
Relapses in Malaria
- Vivax and Ovale malaria relapse generally after 3 years after first attack
- Recurrences of Falciparum disappear within 1-2 years
- Malariae has tendency to cause prolonged, low-level, asymptomatic parasitaemia

217. Ans. (a) Annual parasite index [Ref. Park 27/e p306]

Malariometric Measures

Pre-eradication Era	Eradication Era
• Spleen rate • Average enlarged spleen • Parasite rate • Parasite density index • Infant parasite rate • Proportional case rate	• Annual parasitic incidence (API) • Annual blood examination rate (ABER) • Annual falciparum incidence (AFI) • Slide positivity rate (SPR) • Slide falciparum rate (SFR)

Review Questions

218. Ans. (d) 3 round of malathione every 3 months
[Ref. Park 20/e p360]

219. Ans. (b) 5 [Ref. Park 27/e p306]

220. Ans. (b) Anopheles fluvitalis [Ref. Park 27/e p300-304]

LYMPHATIC FILARIASIS

221. Ans. (b) PBS [Ref. Park 27/e p318]
- MC method used for epidemiological assessment of lymphatic filariasis (through mass blood survey): Thick film using 20 cu. mm. of capillary blood (collected between 830 pm up to 12 midnight)

222. Ans. (a) Microfilariae [Ref. Park 27/e p319]
- *Chemotherapy of Filariasis:* Diethylcarbamazine (DEC)
    - Bancroftian filariasis: 6 mg/kg/day × 12 days (Total 72 mg/kg)
    - Brugian filariasis: 3-6 mg/kg/day × 6–12 days (Total 18–72 mg/kg)
- *DEC is effective in killing Mf:*
    - No effect on Infective (st age III) larvae
    - Uncertain effect on adult worm
- *DEC medicated salt:*
    - *Dose:* 1–4 gm DEC/kg of salt
    - Is a type of Mass Treatment (using very low dose of drug)
    - *Treatment duration:* 6–9 months
- National Filaria Control Programme (NFCP), 1955 is now a component of National Vector Borne Diseases Control Programme (NVBDCP), 2003–04
    - NVBDCP covers Malaria, Filariasis, Japanese Encephalitis, Kala Azar and Dengue

223. Ans. (a) Wuchereria bancrofti [Ref. Park 27/e p315]
- *Problem statement of Lymphatic filariasis:*
    - *Global:* Affects 120 million people in 120 countries; 1.1 billion people live in areas with risk of infection
    - *SEAR:* 600 million live in endemic areas; 60 million infected
    - *India:* Lymphatic filariasis is a major public health problem in India with 553 million people at risk in 233 districts; heavily endemic in UP, Bihar, Jharkhand, Andhra Pradesh, Orissa, Tamil Nadu, Kerala, Gujarat

> **ALSO REMEMBER**
> - *Subcutaneous Filariasis:* It is caused by
>   - Loa loa (the African eye worm)
>   - Mansonella streptocerca
>   - Onchocerca volvulus
>   - Dracunculus medinensis (the guinea worm)

224. Ans. (b) DEC – 6 mg/kg/day x 12 days
[Ref. Park 27/e p319]

225. Ans. (d) Lakshadweep islands [Ref. Park 27/e p320]
- DEC-medicated salt for mass treatment in lymphatic filariasis was shown to be safe, cheap and effective in: Lakshadweep islands

226. Ans. (c) Larvae are deposited on skin surface where they can't survive [Ref. Park 27/e p316]

227. Ans. (b) Tail end is free from nuclei and unsheathed
[Ref. Park 27/e p315-316]

228. Ans. (b) Detection of microfilariae
[Ref. Park 27/e p318]
- Standard/definitive method for diagnosing active Filariasis infection is the identification of microfilariae in a blood smear by microscopic examination
    - Microfilariae that cause Lymphatic filariasis circulate in the blood at night (Nocturnal periodicity)
    - Blood collection (20 cu. mm) should be done at night to coincide with the appearance of the microfilariae, and a thick smear should be made and stained with Giemsa or hematoxylin and eosin
    - For increased sensitivity, concentration techniques can be used
- Serologic techniques provide an alternative to microscopic detection of microfilariae for the diagnosis of lymphatic filariasis
    - Patients with active filarial infection typically have elevated levels of antifilarial IgG4 in the blood and these can be detected using routine assays

Review Questions

229. Ans. (b) Cyclodevelopmental [Ref. Park 27/e p316]

230. Ans. (d) 8 to 16 months [Ref. Park 27/e p317]

RABIES

231. Ans. (c) Amoxicillin + Clavulanic acid
[Ref. Wilderness Medicine E-Book by Auerbach 6/e p661]
- Prophylactic antibiotics (usually amoxicillin-clavulanate) should be given to asplenic individuals who have been bitten by a dog, even in the absence of infectious symptoms
- Amoxicillin and clavulanate is first-line therapy for the prophylactic treatment of dog, human, and cat bites
- Appropriate tetanus and rabies prophylaxis
- Local debridement and thorough cleaning of the wound

232. Ans. (d) 1, 2, 3, 6 [Ref. Park 27/e p325]
- A dog bite from a street dog leading to an abrasion of 1.5 cm is present, with slight oozing is category 3 bite
- Wash the wound with normal tap water for 15–20 minutes
- Clean the wound with spirit
- Vaccine schedule: 2-2-2-2-2 Intradermal (Day 0, 3, 7, 28) should be given with HRIG or ERIG single dose

233. Ans. (c) Dose 20 IU per kg; (d) If human IG is not present, then give equine IG [Ref. Park 26/e p321]

Rabies Immunoglobulin
- Dose of Human Rabies Immunoglobulin (HRIg): 20 IU/kg body weight
- Dose of Equine Rabies Immunoglobulin (ERIg): 40 IU/kg body weight
- RIg must be given as soon as possible
- RIg is NOT recommended beyond the 7th day of starting first dose of vaccine
- RIg must never be given intravenously
- Entire dose of RIg (or as much as possible) must be infiltrated around the wound(s) site(s). Remaining dose, if any, must be given intramuscularly in deltoid

234. Ans. (b) Remove stray dogs and vaccinate the dog population [Ref. Park 26/e p322]
- Since dogs are the primary source of infection, the most cost-effective (and logical) strategy is Elimination of stray dogs and ownerless dogs PLUS Swift mass immunization, in shortest possible time, of at least 80% of entire dog population of the area

235. Ans. (d) 2 doses of Rabies vaccine [Ref. Park 25/e p305]
- Rabies exposed patients who document previous complete pre-exposure vaccination or complete post-exposure prophylaxis with CCEEV: Give 1 dose IM or 2 doses CVV ID (day 0, 3)

236. Ans. (d) Days 0, 7, 28 [Ref. Park 27/e p326]

ALSO REMEMBER
- *World Rabies day:* September 28
- *First successful human antirabies vaccination performed by:* Louis Pasteur (1883)
- Serum antibodies take 7 days to appear after vaccination (Maximum level of Immunity achieved in days)
- *Best prophylaxis of Rabies in exposed persons:* Combined Vaccine and Immunoglobulin/Serum treatment
- *Best prophylaxis of Rabies in exposed persons:* Combined Vaccine and Immunoglobulin/Serum treatment

- *Anti Rabies serum:*
  - *Horse Antirabies Serum:* 40 IU/kg on Day 0 (50% in Wound, 50% i.m)
  - *Human Rabies Immunoglobulin:* 20 IU/kg (partly in wound, rest i.m gluteal)
- *Intramuscular injections of Cell Culture and Purified Duck Embryo Vaccines:* Deltoid (not in Buttocks)
- Volume of intradermal dose of Rabies Vaccine is 1/5th of intramuscular dose
- *Booster injections in Pre-exposure prophylaxis:* at intervals of 2 years

237. Ans. (c) Immediately stitch wound under antibiotic coverage [Ref. Park 27/e p324]
- Bite wounds should not be immediately sutured to prevent additional trauma, which may help spread of the rabies virus deeper into the tissues.
  - If suturing is necessary, it should be done 24–48 hours later, with minimal possible stitches, under cover of anti-rabies serum locally.
- *Rabies vaccine was first developed by:* Louis Pasteur (and Emile Roux)
- *Strain of Human Diploid Cell Vaccine:* Attenuated Pitman-Moore L503 strain
- *Induced Coma Treatment:* In 2005, the case of Jeanna Giese, a girl of 15 who survived acute, unvaccinated rabies was reported, indicating the successful treatment of rabies through induction of a coma

238. Ans. (c) Intracytoplasmic basophilic inclusion bodies are seen in brain cells [Ref. Internet www.cdc.gov, Park 21/e p250-57, Park 22/e p251-56]
- Incubation period of Rabies is 3 – 8 weeks (20–60 dasys)
- Patients of rabies could present atypically with aseptic meningitis
- Rabies may sometimes present as 'Convulsive Rabies'
- Negri bodies (Pathognomic of Rabies): Intracytoplasmic eosinophilic inclusion bodies in neurons. (Inside it contains basophilic formation)

239. Ans. (a) Lakshadweep Islands [Ref. Park 27/e p322]

240. Ans. (b) Mouse [Ref. Park 27/e p323]

241. Ans. (b) Hematogenous spread to brain [Ref. Park 27/e p323]

242. Ans. (c) 3 [Ref. Park 27/e p326]

243. Ans. (b) Give cell culture derived vaccine [Ref. Park 27/e p324]

244. Ans. (c) 15 minutes [Ref. Park 27/e p324]
LOCAL WOUND TREATMENT IN RABIES
- Purpose of local treatment is to remove as much virus as possible, from site of inoculation, before it is absorbed on local nerve endings
- Local wound treatment can reduce chances of Rabies by upto 80%
- Immediate flushing and washing wound area with plenty of soap and running water for minimum 15 minutes is of paramount importance
- *Suturing:* not recommended; if necessary, do 24–48 hours later under cover of Anti-rabies serum (Local application with prior sensitivity testing)

- Chemical treatment with virucidal agents (Alcohol, tincture, 0.01% aqueous iodine)

245. **Ans. (b) 1 mL** *[Ref. Park 27/e p325-326]*
    Rabies Vaccine Dosages
    - Intramuscular dose of Rabies vaccine for post-exposure prophylaxis: 1 mL
    - Intradermal dose of Rabies vaccine for post-exposure prophylaxis: 0.1 mL
    - Intramuscular dose of Rabies vaccine for pre-exposure prophylaxis: 1 mL
    - Intradermal dose of Rabies vaccine for pre-exposure prophylaxis: 0.1 mL

    ALSO REMEMBER
    Rabies Immunoglobulin Dosages
    - Dose of Human Rabies Immunoglobulin (HRIg): 20 IU/kg body wt
    - Dose of Equine Rabies Immunoglobulin (ERIg): 40 IU/kg body wt

246. **Ans. (b) Immunoglobulin not required if prior full vaccination is received; (c) Local wound cleaning is done in all cases of dog wound** *[Ref. Park 27/e p325-326]*
    Post Exposure Prophylaxis of Rabies Guidelines
    - Category-wise PEP measures:
      - Category I wound: None
      - Category II wound: Local treatment of wound + Immediate vaccination
      - Category III wound: Local treatment of wound + Immediate vaccination + Immediate immunoglobulin
    - PEP is discontinued if:
      - Suspected animal proved free of rabies by an appropriate laboratory
      - In case of domestic animal, latter remains healthy throughout 10 day observation period from day of bite
    - Rabies Immunoglobulin is NOT indicated in previously vaccinated individuals

Review Questions

247. **Ans. (c) Australia, UK** *[Ref. Park 27/e p322]*
248. **Ans. (d) Recombinant glycoprotein vaccine** *[Ref. Gupta and Mahajan 3/e p299]*
249. **Ans. (c) Class III** *[Ref. Park 23/e p279]*
250. **Ans. (a) Sheep** *[Ref. Park 23/e p279]*
251. **Ans. (b) Andaman and Nicobar Islands** *[Ref. Park 27/e p322]*

YELLOW FEVER

252. **Ans. (a) 17D vaccine** *[Ref. Park 26/e p323-324]*
    - Yellow fever is a disease common in Africa transmitted through Aedes mosquito
    - Symptoms include fever, muscle pain with prominent backache, headache, loss of appetite, and nausea or vomiting
    - There may be a second, more toxic phase within 24 hours of recovering from initial symptoms. It includes high fever, jaundice (yellowing of the skin and eyes, hence the name 'yellow fever'), dark urine and abdominal pain with vomiting

253. **Ans. (a) 3 to 6 days** *[Ref. Park 27/e p328]*
    - Incubation Period: 3 – 6 days
      - IP of 6 days recognized under International Health Regulations

254. **Ans. (b) Fatality rate > 90%** *[Ref. Park 27/e p328]*

255. **Ans. (a) 1%** *[Ref. Park 27/e p329]*
    - *International Health Regulations (IHRs) of WHO covers 7 diseases:*
      - Cholera
      - Plague
      - Yellow Fever
      - Smallpox
      - Wild Polio Virus
      - Human Influenza
      - SARS
    - *International measures to restrict the spread of Yellow Fever (IHRs):*
      - *Travellers:*
        - Must possess a valid International certificate of vaccination (validity 10 days – Lifelong) against YF before they enter 'YF receptive areas'
        - *If no such certificate available:* Quarantine for 6 days (Max I.P of YF) from date of leaving an infected area
        - *If traveller arrives before certificate becomes valid (10 days after vaccination):* Isolate till it becomes valid
      - *Mosquitoes:*
        - *Aircrafts/ships arriving from endemic areas:* Aerosol spray to kill insect vectors
        - *Airports/seaports kept free from vector breeding:* at least 400 meters around boundary
        - *Aedes aegypti index:* kept below 1%

    ALSO REMEMBER
    - *Reference centres for YF in India:*
      - National Institute of Virology (NIV), Pune
      - Central Research Institute (CRI), Kasauli
    - *Indices of Surveillance of Aedes mosquitoes:* Refer to Ans. 146, Theory
      - Breteau Index (Aedes aegypti index) should be < 1% in towns and seaports in endemic areas to ensure freedom from Yellow Fever

256. **Ans. (c) Validation of Vaccination Certificate begins after 10 days and lasts till 10 years; (d) Incubation period is 16–46 days** *[Ref. Park 27/e p329]*

257. **Ans. (b) Transmitted by Aedes; (d) Incidence is increased by humidity; (e) It is a flavivirus** *[Ref. Park 27/e p327-328]*

258. **Ans. (d) Lifelong**

259. **Ans. (b) 1%** *[Ref. Park 27/e p329]*

260. **Ans. (b) Validity of International certificate of Vaccination lasts up to 10 years; (d) Aedes aegypti index should not be more than 10% to ensure freedom from yellow Fever** *[Ref. Park 27/e p329]*

- *Indices of Surveillance of Aedes Mosquitoes:*

  $$\text{Container Index} = \frac{\text{Not of containers showing breeding of Aedes larvae}}{\text{Total no of containers surveyed}} \times 100 = \frac{C^+}{C} \times 100$$

  $$\text{House index} = \frac{\text{No of house showing breeeding of Aedes Larvae}}{\text{Total no of Houses surveyed}} \times 100 = \frac{H^+}{H} \times 100$$

  $$\text{Breteau Index} = \frac{\text{No of containers showing breeding of Aedes Larvae}}{\text{Total no of houses surveyed}} \times 100 = \frac{C^+}{H} \times 100$$

- Breteau Index (Aedes aegypti index) should be < 1% in towns and seaports in endemic areas to ensure freedom from Yellow Fever

> **ALSO REMEMBER**
> - *India is a 'Yellow Fever receptive' area:* Population is unvaccinated and susceptible to Yellow Fever. Vector Aedes aegypti is also found in abundance. Common monkey of India (Macacus spp) is also susceptible
> - International Health Regulations(IHR) covers 7 diseases:
>   - Cholera
>   - Plague
>   - Yellow Fever
>   - Smallpox
>   - Wild Polio Virus
>   - Human Influenza
>   - SARS
> - *Thermolability of vaccines:* sensitivity to heat
> - Reconstituted BCG > YF > OPV > Measles and Reconstituted Measles > Hep B > DPT > DT > BCG > TT
>   - *Most Thermolabile vaccine:* Reconstituted BCG
>   - *Most Thermostable vaccine:* TT
> - *Vaccines contraindicated in pregnancy:* All Live Vaccines (except Yellow fever) and Meningococcal Vaccine.

261. **Ans. (d) The validity of yellow fever vaccination certificate begins 10 days after the date of vaccination and extends upto 5 years** *[Ref. Park 27/e p327-329]*
   - Yellow fever vaccination certificate validity: 10 days TILL Lifelong (New Guideline by WHO)

Review Question

262. **Ans. (b) Central Institute, Kasauli** *[Ref. Park 27/e p329]*

JAPANESE ENCEPHALITIS

263. **Ans. (b) A-4, B-1, C-3, D-2** *[Ref. Park 26/e p326]*
   JE Epidemiology
   - Vector: Culex triteniorhynchus
   - Amplifier host: Pigs
   - Accidental host: Man
   - Reservoir host: Ardied birds (Herons, ducks, fowls)

264. **Ans. (d) Live attenuated subcutaneous** *[Ref. Park 26/e p328]*
   - All Japanese encephalitis (JE) cases are reported under Acute Encephalitis syndrome (AES)
   - Good protection is obtained through Live attenuated JE vaccine under NIS with strain SA-14-14-2
   - SA-14-14-2 is given 0.5 ml Subcutaneous
   - During 2011-2018, four districts of Gorakhpur division (Gorakhpur, Maharajganj, Deoria and Kushinagar) and three districts of Basti division (Basti, Sant Kabir Nagar and Sidharth Nagar) contributed to 86% of total AES cases of Uttar Pradesh

265. **Ans. (a) Man act as Reservoir** *[Ref. Park 25/e p312]*
   - Man is an Incidental 'Dead-end host' in Japanese encephalitis

266. **Ans. (c) Aedes Aegypti** *[Ref. Park 25/e p301]*
   - Zika virus disease is transmitted by bite of infected Aedes mosquito, mainly species Aedes aegypti

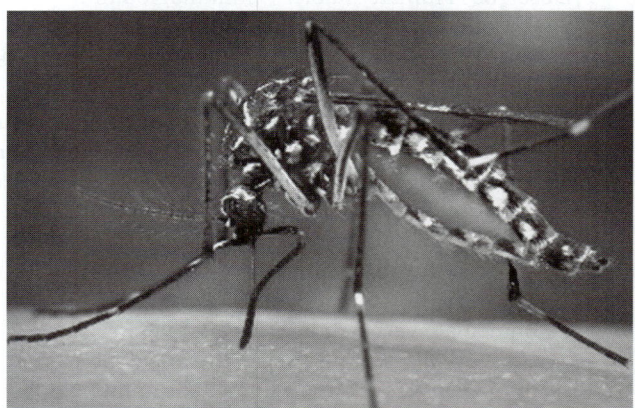

267. **Ans. (c) Case fatality rate is over 90%** *[Ref. Park 27/e p331]*
   - *Vectors of JE:* Culicine mosquitoes and some Anophelines
     - Culex tritaeniorhynchus (most important vector), Culex vishnuii and Culex gelidus
   - *Case fatality rate:* 20 – 40% (may reach up to 58%)

> **ALSO REMEMBER**
> - JE has been reported by 26 states and UT's in India
>   - Gorakhpur District of UP contribute the largest no of cases

268. **Ans. (d) Epidemic is declared if there are 2-3 cases in a village** *[Ref. Park 27/e p331-334]*
   - 85% of cases of JE are reported in age below 15 years BUT JE IS INFREQUENT IN INFANCY: Vaccination not recommended below 6 months age infants (as also interference from maternal antibodies)
   - *Not all humans bitten by mosquitoes develop the disease:* Ratio of JE overt disease to inapparent infection varies from 1:300 to 1:1000
   - *Endemicity of JE in India:* 1-2 cases per village

269. **Ans. (d) In endemic areas, vaccination is given to cover children 1-9 years age** *[Ref. Park 27/e p332-333]*
   JAPANESE ENCEPHALITIS VACCINES
   - *Mouse brain derived inactivated vaccine*:
     - 2 primary doses 4 weeks apart, booster after 1 year and subsequently at 3 yearly intervals until the age of 10–15 years

Communicable and Non-communicable Diseases | 385

- Dose: 0.5 ml for children aged < 3 years (1 ml for age > 3 years)
- Route: Subcutaneous
- *Pre-exposure prophylaxis*: 3 Primary doses on day 0, 7, 28 (OR 2 primary doses 4 weeks apart); then Booster after 1 year and then every 3 years
- *Cell culture based Live attenuated vaccine (SA-14-14-2 strain)*:
  - Single dose, followed by Single booster dose after 1 year

> **ALSO REMEMBER**
> - In endemic areas, JE vaccine is given to all children aged 1-15 years age
> - JE vaccine is not used below the age of 6 months:

270. **Ans. (b) Pigs** *[Ref. Park 27/e p332]*
    HOSTS IN JAPANESE ENCEPHALITIS
    - Primary maintenance host: Ardied birds (ducks, fowls, herons)
    - Major vertebrate host: Pigs
    - Amplifier host: Pigs
    - Mosquito attractants: Cattle, buffaloes
    - Incidental dead-end host: Man

271. **Ans. (b) Japanese encephalitis** *[Ref. Park 27/e p331]*
    Japanese encephalitis Transmission
    - JE virus infects several extra-human hosts (Birds, animals)
    - Basic cycles of JE transmission:
      - Pig – Mosquito – Pig
      - Ardied bird – Mosquito Ardied bird
    - Mosquito vectors: Culex tritaeniorhynchus (and C. vishnuii, C. gelidus)
    - Man is incidental dead-end host

Review Questions

272. **Ans. (a) Man to man transmission** *[Ref. Park 27/e p332]*
273. **Ans. (c) Large no. of in apparent infections** *[Ref. Park 27/e p331-333]*

KFD

274. **Ans. (b) Deforestation** *[Ref. Park 27/e p335]*
    - Control measures:
      - Control of ticks
      - Restriction of cattle movement
      - Vaccination: Killed KFD vaccine
      - Personal protection: through repellants

> **ALSO REMEMBER**
> - KFD belongs to 'Biosafety Level 4', highest risk category of pathogens

275. **Ans. (b) Haemaphysalis** *[Ref. Park 27/e p335]*
    - Vectors of KFD:
      - *In India*: Hemophysalis spinigera (Hard Tick)
      - *Outside India*: Soft Tick
    - Tick as vectors:

Hard tick as vector	Soft tick as vector
KFD (in India)	Q fever (in few animal cases)
Tularaemia	Relapsing fever
Babesiosis	KFD (outside India)
Tick paralysis	
Viral encephalitis	
Tick hemorrhagic fevers	

PLAGUE

276. **Ans. (d) Xenopsylla cheopsis** *[Ref. Park 26/e p337]*
    - Typical symptoms of bubonic plague infection are BUBOES (large, swollen, tender lymph nodes) usually occurring in the neck, armpit, and groin
    - Other symptoms include fever, malaise, headache, blister at the site of a flea bite, and red or purple rash on top of the enlarged lymph nodes
    - Vector of Bubonic plague is rat flea (Xenopsylla cheopsis)

277. **Ans. (a) Domestic rat "Rattus rattus" has been incriminated as main reservoir** *[Ref. Park 27/e p340–342]*

> **ALSO REMEMBER**
> - Pneumonic plague is the most virulent and least common form of plague
> - *Recent most outbreak of Plague:* Village Dangud, Uttrakashi district, Uttrakhand (2004)
> - Man has no natural immunity against Plague
> - A Rat flea may ingest upto 0.5 cu.mm of blood (containing as many as 5000 bacilli)
> - A partially blocked flea is more efficient transmitter of Plague than a totally blocked flea as it can live longer
> - 'Liasion rodents' between man and field rodents: Commensal rodents especially the peri-domestic species (eg. R.norvegicus)
> - *Most effective method to break chain of transmission of Plague:* Destruction of Rat fleas (by proper application of an effective insecticide)
> - *For effective control of Plague by insecticidal sprays:* Flea Index should drop down to zero within 48hrs of application
> - WHO recommendation on Plague vaccination: should be only for prevention and NOT FOR CONTROL of human plague

278. **Ans. (b) Control of fleas** *[Ref. Park 27/e p343]*
279. **Ans. (b) Bubonic is the most common variety** *[Ref. Park 27/e p342]*
280. **Ans. (c) 28 years** *[Ref. Park 20/e p256]*
    - Since the last reported cases in Karnataka in 1966, there have been no laboratory confirmed cases in India, till its reappearance in 1994 (Gap of 28 years)
    - In 1994, Bubonic Plague (Beed, Maharashtra) was followed by an outbreak of Pneumonic Plague (Surat, Gujarat)

- Overall 4780 suspected cases, 167 confirmed cases and 53 deaths
- In February 2002, outbreak of Pneumonic Plague (Gap of 8 years) in Hat Koti village, Shimla district, Himachal Pradesh
  - Overall 16 cases and 4 deaths
- In October 2004, Outbreak of Bubonic Plague in Dangud village, Uttarkashi, Uttrakhand.
  - Over all 8 cases and 3 deaths.

281. Ans. (b) Cheopsis index [Ref. Park 23/e p294]

Review Question

282. Ans. (b) Pneumonic plague [Ref. Park 27/e p341]

RICKETTSIAL DISEASES

283. Ans. (a) R. prowazekii [Ref. Park 26/e p343]
   - Epidemic Typhus is a type of rickettsial disease of typhus group:
   - *Causative agent:* R. prowazekii
   - *Vector:* Louse (P. capitis, P. corporis)
   - *Mode of transmission:* (IS NOT BY LOUSE-BITE) Scratching and inoculation with infected louse faeces, Crushing infected louse on body, Inhalation of infected louse faeces or dust

284. Ans. (b) Scrub typhus – Flea [Ref. Park 27/e p346]

> **ALSO REMEMBER**
> - 'Brill Zinnser Disease' is the recrudescent form of Epidemic Typhus (Louse borne typhus)
> - *Drug of choice for Rickettsial diseases:* Tetracycline

285. Ans. (c) Rickettsia prowazekii [Ref. Park 27/e p346]
286. Ans. (b) Flea is a vector of the disease [Ref. Park 27/e p347-348]
287. Ans. (c) Inhalation of aerosol [Ref. Park 27/e p348]
   - *Modes of Transmission of few important diseases:*

Disease	Mode(s) of transmission
Leptospirosis	Direct contact with urine/tissue of infected animal, contaminated food or water, droplet infection
Leprosy	Droplet infection, contact transmission, breast milk, insect vectors, tattoo needles, vertical transmission
Hepatitis A	Faecooral route, Parenteral, Sexual
Legionnaire's disease	Contaminated air conditioning supply
Plague	Bite of Flea (Xenopsylla)
Yaws	Non-venereal direct contact, fomites, vectors
Ancylostomiasis (Hookworm)	Direct penetration through skin, oral
Q fever	Inhalation of infected dust, Meat and milk products
Hydatid Disease (Echinococcus)	Food, water contaminated with eggs

288. Ans. (d) Epidemic typhus [Ref. Park 27/e p348-349]
289. Ans. (d) Weil Felix reaction is very useful for diagnosis [Ref. Park 27/e p346]
290. Ans. (b) Adult mite feeds on vertebral host [Ref. Park 27/e p347]
   - In Scrub typhus the nymphal and adult stages of the mite are free living in nature, they do not feed on vertebrate hostst
   - Larvae (chigger) feed on vertebrate hosts' and pick up rickettsiae
   - Larval stage 'act as a both reservoir and a vector'

291. Ans. (a) Flea; (b) Louse; (d) Mite [Ref. Park 27/e p346]
292. Ans. (a) Rickettessia prowazki & louse [Ref. Park 27/e p346]
293. Ans. (a) Louse [Ref. Medicine at a Glance by Davies, 3/e p446, 24/e p316]
294. Ans. (b) Rickettsia akari [Ref. Park 27/e p346]
295. Ans. (a) Flea [Ref. Park 27/e p346]
296. Ans. (b) Rocky mountain spotted fever [Ref. Park 27/e p346]
   - Weil disease and Leptospirosis are Spirochaetal diseases
   - Trichomoniasis is a protozoan parasitic STD
   - RMSF is caused by Rickettsia ricket sii

297. Ans. (c) Crushing louse on body [Ref. Park 27/e p348-349]
   EPIDEMIC TYPHUS TRANSMISSION BY LOUSE
   - Scratching and inoculating himself with louse faeces
   - Crushing an infected louse on person
   - Inhalation of infected louse faeces or dust

298. Ans. (c) Doxycycline [Ref. CRC Desk Reference of Clinical Pharmacology 1/e p61]
299. Ans. (b) Bartonella [Ref. Park 27/e p346]
   - Bartonella quintana infection (historically called 'trench fever') is a vector-borne disease primarily transmitted by the human body louse Pediculus humanus.

Review Questions

300. Ans. (c) Coxiella burnetii [Ref. Park 27/e p348]
301. Ans. (b) Scrub typhus [Ref. Park 27/e p347]
302. Ans. (c) Q-fever [Ref. Park 27/e p348]
303. Ans. (d) Indian tick typhus [Ref. Park 27/e p348]
304. Ans. (d) Q-fever [Ref. Park 27/e p348]

LEISHMANIASIS

305. Ans. (a) Man [Ref. Park 27/e p352]
   LEISHMANIASIS:
   - Leishmaniasis is also known as Leichmaniosis, Leishmaniose, *Orient Boils, Baghdad Boils, kala azar, black fever, sandfly disease, Dum-Dum fever, Espundia, White Leprosy*
   - *Leishmaniasis* is diagnosed in the haematology laboratory by direct visualization of the amastigotes (Leishman-Donovan bodies)
   - *Reservoir(s) of important diseases:*

Disease	Microorganism	Reservoir(s)
Epidemic Tyhus	Rickettsia prowazekii	Humans
Endemic Typhus	Rickettsia typhi	Rats
Scrub Typhus	Rickettsia tsutsugamushi	Trombiculid Mite
Indian Tick Typhus	Rickettsia conori	Rodents
RMSF	Rickettsia rickettsii	Rodents
Rickettsial Pox	Rickettsia akari	Mice
Trench fever	Bartonella quintana	Humans
Q fever	Coxiella burnetti	Cattle, sheep, goat
Dracunculiasis	Dracunculus medinensis	Humans
Ascariasis	Ascaris lumbricoides	Humans
Ancylostomiasis	Ancylostoma duodenale	Humans

306. **Ans. (c) Hydroxychloroquine** [Ref. Internet]
 - Sitamaquine is a new once-a day oral drug for treatment of Kala azar
 - Miltefosine and paramomycin have been recently included in Kala Azar Control component of NVBDCP

307. **Ans. (b) rk-39 test** [Ref. Park 27/e p353]
 RECOMBINANT K39 (rk39) TEST
 - Disease: Visceral leishmaniasis (Kala azar)
 - Antigen: Recombinant (r) K39 antigen derived mainly from L. chagasi
 - Solution: Colloidal gold
 - Time taken: <10 minutes

308. **Ans. (c) Assam** [Ref. Park 27/e p352]
 - Kala Azar is endemic in Bihar, UP, West Bengal, Jharkhand

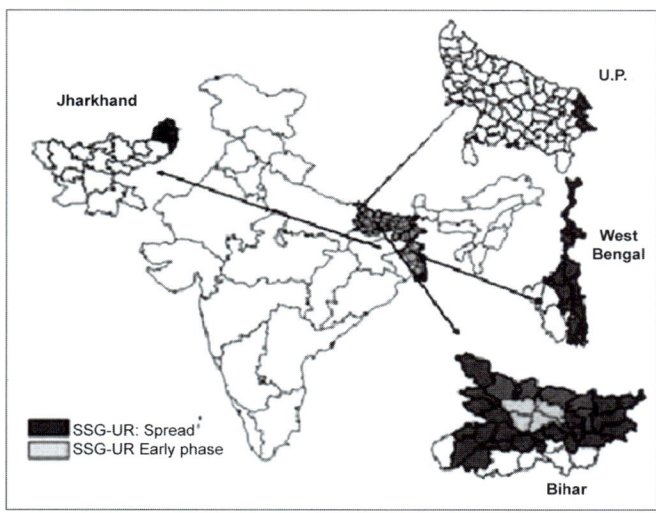

309. **Ans. (c) Kala-azar occurs primarily in rural Latin America** [Ref. Park 27/e p352]
 - India, Bangladesh, Brazil, Nepal, Ethiopia and Sudan contribute for 90% of Global cases of Kala azar.

Review Questions

310. **Ans. (c) Phlebotomus argentipes** [Ref. Park 27/e p353]

311. **Ans. (b) Dog is the reservoir of infection** [Ref. Park 27/e p352]

TRACHOMA

312. **Ans. (d) Evaluation of control program variables**
 [Ref. Trachoma control: the SAFE strategy by Lei Tian. Int J Ophthalmol. 2018; 11(12): 1887–1888]
 - The WHO developed SAFE strategy for the prevention and treatment of trachoma based on community intervention: Surgery for trachomatous trichiasis, aiming at reducing trachomatous trichiasis caused by eyelid entropion (**Surgery, S**); Application of antibiotics, especially the highly effective azithromycin, so as to eliminate infection of chlamydia trachomatis in trachoma patients (**Antibiotic, A**); Facial cleanliness for better personal hygiene (**Facial cleanliness, F**); Environmental improvement, in order to reduce the risk of infection and reinfection of Chlamydia trachomatis (**Environmental improvement, E**)

313. **Ans. (a) Screening** [Ref. National Health Programs of India by Dr. J. Kishore, 7/e p368, 8/e p428]
 - WHO has recommended 'SAFE Strategy' for global elimination of blinding trachoma:
   – *Surgery:* for Trichiasis and Entropion
   – *Antibiotic use:* Azithromycin is Drug of choice
   – Facial cleanliness
   – Environmental improvement

> **ALSO REMEMBER**
> - *WHO recommended strategy for measles elimination:* 'Catch up – Keep up – Follow up strategy', AMMRS
> - *WHO recommended strategy for polio eradication:* 'Pulse strategy'
> - *GET 2020:* The Alliance for the 'Global Elimination of Blinding Trachoma' by the year 2020 (GET 2020)

314. **Ans. (c) Irritants like kajal or surma also predispose** [Ref. Park 27/e p356-357]

 TRACHOMA (ROUGH EYE):
 - *Communicability:* Trachoma is a disease of low infectivity
 - *Predisposing factors:* Direct sunlight, dust, smoke and irritants (such as kajal or surma)
 - *Mode of transmission:*
   – Direct or indirect contact with ocular discharges or fomites
   – Eye seeking flies
   – Venereal transmission
 - *Treatment of choice for Trachoma:* Azithromycin 20 mg/kg oral stat
 - *Mass treatment for Trachoma:* [NEW GUIDELINES–WHO]
   – Indication of mass treatment:[3] 10 % prevalence of severe and moderate Trachoma in children < 10yrs of age
 - *Treatment:* 1% tetracycline ointment BD for 5 consecutive days each month or OD for 10 days each month for 6 consecutive months, or for 60 consecutive days.

> **ALSO REMEMBER**
> - *MC infected age group:* 2-5 yrs aged children

315. **Ans. (c) Children aged 0-10 years** [Ref. National Health Programs of India by Dr. J. Kishore, 7/e p365]

316. Ans. (c) Five or more follicles in the upper tarsal conjunctiva [Ref. National Health Programs of India by Dr. J. Kishore, 7/e p368, 8/e p429]

317. Ans. (d) 10% [Ref. Park 27/e p357]
- *Indication of mass treatment in Trachoma:* > 10 % prevalence of severe and moderate Trachoma in children < 10 yrs of age [NEW GUIDELINES–WHO]

318. Ans. (d) 10% [Ref. WHO Trachoma Control: A guide for programme managers, 2006; p21-22]
- Current WHO recommendations for antibiotic treatment of trachoma:
  – *District level prevalence is > 10% in 1-9 years old children:* Mass treatment with Azithromycin
  – *District level prevalence is 5-10% in 1-9 years old children:* Targeted treatment with Azithromycin (the identification and treatment of all members of any family in whom one or more members have follicular trachoma)
  – *District level prevalence is < 5% in 1-9 years old children:* Azithromycin distribution may not be necessary

TETANUS

319. Ans. (a) Single dose TT [Ref. Park 27/e p361]
- TT course received 10 years ago so category B, and he has a clean-cut wound so only 1 Booster TT dose is sufficient

320. Ans. (b) > 0.01 IU/ml [Ref. Park 26/e p355]
- Antitoxin activity is expressed in international units (IU) and a tetanus antitoxin level of 0.01 IU/ml serum, is considered the minimum protective level
- This "protective" level is based on animal studies that correlate antitoxin levels with symptoms or death

321. Ans. (b) Single dose of TT [Ref. Park 25/e p341]
- Patient belongs to Immunity Category C, so he will get Single dose TT (If it was >6 hours old, unclean, penetrating, with tissue damage then Single dose TT + TIG)

322. Ans. (b) Single dose of tetanus toxoid [Ref. Park 27/e p362]
- **In the given question,** a person has received complete immunization against tetanus 10 years ago
- Thus he is in immunity category B
- Now, he presents with a clean wound without any lacerations from an injury sustained 3 hours ago,
- Thus he should now be given single dose of tetanus toxoid

323. Ans. (d) < 0.1 per 1000 LB [Ref. Park 27/e p361]
- NNT Elimination (Classification of districts, India is based on 3 parameters: incidence rate, TT-2 or booster coverage and % attended deliveries)

Classification	Rate	TT-2 coverage	Attended deliveries
NNT High Risk	> 1/1000 LB	< 70%	< 50%
NNT Control	< 1/1000 LB	> 70%	>50%
NNT Elimination	< 0.1/1000 LB	> 90%	> 75%

- *Herd Immunity in Tetanus:* Does not protect the individual

324. Ans. (d) Injection penicillin to all neonates [Ref. Park 27/e p361]

325. Ans. (d) Seen commonly in winter and dry climate [Ref. Park 27/e p360-361]
Tetanus (especially NNT) hjas a marked seasonal incidence in India: > 50% cases in July-September

326. Ans. (c) Man-to-man transmission [Ref. Park 27/e p359]
- *Primary course of tetanus immunisation:* 3 doses of DPT at interval of 4-8 weeks starting at 6 weeks age (to be followed by boosters at 18 months, 5-6 years, 10 years and 16 years age)
- *Period of communicability:* NONE (not transmitted from person-to-person)
- *Incubation period:* 06-10 days
- *Reservoir:* Soil and dust (spores survive for years in soil)

327. Ans. (c) Tetanus toxoid complete course [Ref. Park 27/e p362]

328. Ans. (b) Herd immunity present [Ref. Park 27/e p359]

Review Questions

329. Ans. (d) None [Ref. Park 27/e p359]
330. Ans. (b) Toxoid one dose [Ref. Park 27/e p362]
331. Ans. (b) > 90% coverage of 3 antenatal visits [Ref. Park 27/e p361]

LEPROSY

332. Ans. (d) MDT is contraindicated during pregnancy [Ref. Park 27/e p362-378]
- Operational Classification of Leprosy (according to skin smear positivity) to serve as a basis for Chemotherapy:

	Paucibacillary Leprosy (PBL) BI < 2	Multibacillary Leprosy (MBL) BI > 2
Included types	Indeterminate Polar tuberculoid (TT) Border tuberculoid (BT)	Polar lepromatous (LL) Borderline lepromatous (BL) Mid-borderline (BB)
Multidrug therapy (MDT) in NLEP (Drugs)	Rifampicin 600 mg OAMS Dapsone 100 mg daily	Rifampicin 600 mg OAMS Dapsone 100 mg daily Clofazimine 300 mg OAMS and 50 mg daily
Treatment duration	6 months	12 months
Follow up (after treatment)	Annually for 2 yrs	Annually for 5 yrs

(*BI*: Bacteriological Index; *OAMS*: Once a month supervised)
* MBL cases are most important source of infection
* MDT is safe in pregnancy

> **ALSO REMEMBER**
> - *An infectious case of Leprosy can be rendered non-infectious by treatment with:*
>   - Dapsone for 90 days, or
>   - Rifampicin for 3 weeks
> - *Attack rate of Leprosy among house-hold contacts: 4.4 - 12%*
> - *Youngest case of Leprosy in India: 2 ½ month infant*
> - *Leprosy is often known as a 'Social disease'*
>   - Is probably the oldest disease known to mankind
> - *Mode of transmission of Leprosy:*
>   - Droplet infection
>   - Contact transmission (Direct skin to skin or indirect with soil/fomites)
>   - Other routes:
>   - Breast milk from lepromatous mothers
>   - Insect vectors
>   - Tattooing needles
> - *Diagnosis of leprosy under NLEP*: It is currently based on clinical grounds
>   - PBL: 1 – 5 skin lesions
>   - MBL: > 5 skin lesions

333. **Ans. None of the above**   *[Ref. Park 27/e p364]*
   - *Mode of transmission of Leprosy:*
     - Droplet Infection (Aerosols)
     - Contact Transmission (infectious patient and healthy susceptible)
     - Direct contact (skin to skin)
     - Indirect contact (soil, fomites, clothes and linen)
     - Breast milk from lepromatous mothers, transplacental
     - Insect vectors
     - Tattoo needles

334. **Ans. (a) 1 per 10,000**   *[Ref. National Health Programs of India by Dr. J. Kishore, 7/e p215]*
   - *Level of Leprosy for declaring it as a Public Health Problem:* >1/10,000
   - *Elimination Level of Leprosy:* <1/10,000 (adopted as a resolution by WHO in 1991, to eliminate leprosy as a public health problem by year 2000)
   - *Goal for Leprosy under National Health Policy (NHP) 2002:* Elimination of Leprosy by 2005
   - India eliminated Leprosy in December 2005 [India has so far eliminated 4 diseases, namely, Guineaworm– 2000, Leprosy – 2005, Yaws – 2016 – and NNT 2016]
   - *As on 2018, in India:*
     - Prevalence: 0.67 per 10,000
   - *Elimination level for Neonatal tetanus:*
     - Rate < 0.1 per 1000 live births
     - TT2 coverage > 90%
     - Attended deliveries > 75%
   - *Elimination level for Tuberculosis (WHO and STOP TB Strategy):* <1 case per million population (to eliminate TB as a public health problem)
   - *Criteria for tracking progress towards IDD elimination:*

Indicator	Goal
Proportion with enlarged thyroid (age 6 – 12 years)	< 5 %
Urinary Iodine Excretion below 100 mcg/litre	< 50 %
Urinary Iodine Excretion below 50 mcg/litre	< 20 %
Proportion of houses consuming adequately iodised salt	> 90 %

335. **Ans. (b) Prognosis**   *[Ref. Park 27/e p368]*
   - *Uses of Lepromin test:*
     - Evaluation of CMI status of patients
     - Aid to confirm the classification of Leprosy
     - Estimation of prognosis of cases
   Also Refer to Theory

> **ALSO REMEMBER**
> - Tests of immunity/susceptibility:
>   - *Schick Test:* Diphtheria
>   - *Mantoux Test:* Tuberculosis
>   - *Leishmanin (Montenegro) Test:* Leishmaniasis (Kala Azar)

336. **Ans. (a) Stop antileprosy treatment**   *[Ref. Internet; WHO Website, Park 21/e p299, Park 22/e p298]*
   - *According to WHO treatment guidelines for Leprosy:*
     - All MB (multibacillary) patients who have completed 12 or more doses of WHO MDT for multibacillary leprosy 'should be regarded as cured' and removed from the registers
     - However, as usual, all patients should be educated about the signs/symptoms of reactions and relapse and asked to report immediately to the nearest health centre when such problems arise
   - *It is not necessary to give MDT to PB patients until clinical inactivity:*
     - Clinical activity in PB leprosy does not necessarily imply direct correlation with bacterial multiplication
     - *In a large proportion of patients it is not possible to achieve clinical inactivity in six months even though all the organisms are killed:* Lesions become inactive gradually over a period of one to two years after the treatment has been discontinued

337. **Ans. (a) Diagnosis**   *[Ref. Park 27/e p368]*
338. **Ans. (c) A defaulter is defined as a patient who has not taken treatment for 6 months or more**
       [Ref. National Health Programs of India by Dr. J. Kishore, 8/e p362, Park 25/e p332–347]

> **ALSO REMEMBER**
> - *'Leprosy is not amenable to eradication' as it has:*
>   - Long and variable incubation period
>   - Disputed modes of transmission
>   - Presence of sub-clinical cases and our inability to detect them
>   - Complicated spectrum of disease manifestations
>   - Failure of cell mediated immunity in lepromatous cases

- Absence of a vaccine
- Social and cultural taboos leading to concealment of disease
- Discovery of extra-human reservoir
- *Definitions in Revised National Tuberculosis Control Programme (RNTCP):*
  - *New case:* Never taken treatment or took treatment less than 4 weeks
  - *Cured:* Follow up smears negative on 2 separate occasions including those at the end of treatment
  - *Relapse:* Returns sputum smear positive (ss+ve) after being declared cured
  - *Failure:* Remains or becomes ss+ve at or after 5 months of treatment
  - *Defaulter:* Who misses treatment for a continuous period of 2 months or more

339. **Ans. (d) FLA-ABS Test** *[Ref. Park 27/e p368]*

ALSO REMEMBER
- **LEPROMIN TEST:**
  - Is not a diagnostic test: It can yield false positive or false negative (esp. in lepromatous and near lepromatous cases)
  - Is a useful tool for evaluation of CMI status
  - Is widely used to aid classification of the disease
  - Is of great value in estimating the prognosis in Leprosy: Test is strongly positive in typical tuberculoid (TT) cases.
  - Typical lepromatous (LL) cases are lepromin negative indicating a failure of CMI
    1. Lepromin negative individuals are at a higher risk of developing Progressive Multibacillary Leprosy (MBL)
    2. Lepromin positive individuals either escape the clinical disease (the majority) or develop Paucibacillary Leprosy (PBL-the minority)
- **LTT and LMIT CMI Tests:**
  - Useful to detect sub-clinical infection
  - *Disadvantage:* cannot be applied on a mass scale in field conditions

340. **Ans. (d) In those with lepromatous leprosy** *[Ref. Park 27/e p372-373]*

341. **Ans. (d) Insect can transmit the disease** *[Ref. Park 27/e p364]*

342. **Ans. (b) It is a diagnostic test** *[Ref. Park 27/e p368]*

343. **Ans. (d) Long incubation period [SINGLE BEST ANSWER]** *[Ref. Park 22/e p291]*

344. **Ans. (d) 0.69 [Now 0.67]** *[Ref. Park 27/e p363]*

345. **Ans. (c) Clinical, bacteriological, Immunological, histological classification** *[Ref. Park 27/e p365]*

Classifications of Leprosy

Ridley Jopling classification	Indian classification	Madrid classification
TT (Tuberculoid)	Indeterminate	Indeterminate
BT (Borderline Tuberculoid)	Tuberculoid	Tuberculoid
BB (Borderline Borderline)	Borderline	Borderline
BL (Borderline Lepromatous)	Lepromatous	Lepromatous
LL (Lepromatous Leprosy)	Pure Neuritic	

- Ridley Jopling classification is based on Immuno-histological scale

346. **Ans. (d) Diagnosis of leprosy** *[Ref. Park 27/e p368]*

347. **Ans. (a) Clofazimine included in treatment regimen; (c) Grenz zone in Lepromatous spectrum; (e) MBL recommended treatment for 12 months duration** *[Ref. Park 27/e p371]*

348. **Ans. (a) 3.5** *[Ref. Park 27/e p367]*

RIDLEY'S LOGARITHMIC SCALE FOR BACTERIAL INDEX
- *Bacterial/Bacteriological) index (BI):* Density of bacilli in smears, including both living and dead bacilli
- *Ridley's logarithmic scale:* Based on the number of bacilli seen in an average High Power microscopic field, using an oil-immersion objective (1/12 in or 2 mm)
- *When several smears are taken:* Mean index is calculated

Score	Description
6+	Many clumps of bacilli in an average field (over 1000)
5+	100-1000 bacilli in an average field
4+	10-100 bacilli in an average field
3+	1-10 bacilli in 10 fields
2+	1-10 bacilli in 10 fields
1+	1-10 bacilli in 100 fields

In the given question, Two samples have 10 bacilli in 100 hpf (each 1+ score), and Two samples with >1000 bacilli in average filed (each 6+ score)

$$BI = \frac{1+1+6+6}{4} = 3.5$$

349. **Ans. (d) 9.71/100000** *[Ref. Park 27/e p362-363]*
- Annual New Case Detection Rate (ANCDR):
  - An important Indicator being used under the National Leprosy Eradication Program
  - Indicator is calculated at the end of March every year, wherein New Cases detected during the period April (Previous Calendar year) and March (current year) is used
  - ANCDR 2015-16: 9.71 per 100,000 population
- Prevalence Rate (PR):
  - Utilized in the program to measure achievements under NLEP
  - Monthly availability of PR also helped in keeping active track on the disease epidemiologically
  - PR 2015-16: 0.66/10,000 population

350. **Ans. (a) 0.66/10000** *[Ref. Park 27/e p363]*

Leprosy Situation in India [2017-18]
- New cases detected: 135, 485
- Annual new case detection rate, ANCDR: 9.27 per 100,000 population
- Prevalence rate, PR: 0.67 per 10,000 population
- Proportion of Cases: MB (49.57%), Female (39.17%), Child (8.7%), Grade II Deformity (3.87%), ST cases (18.80%), SC cases (18.78%)
- Gr. II Disability Rate: 3.94 per million population

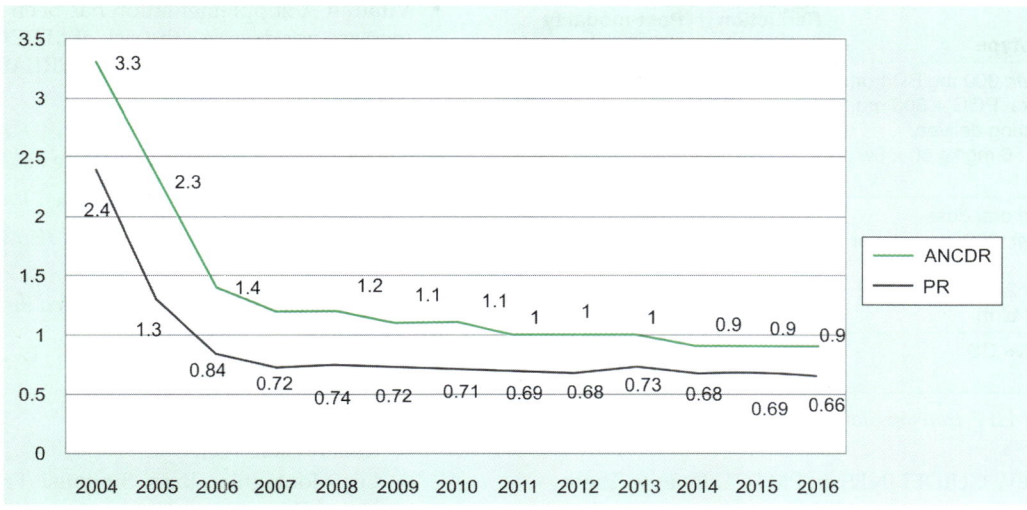

351. Ans. (a) BCG vaccine; (b) Killer M. Leprae + BCG vaccine; (c) M. Indicus Pranii
     [Ref. Essentials of Microbiology by Kumar 1/e p245]

Leprosy Vaccine Trials
- BCG Mycobacterium bovis (India)
- BCG plus Killed Mycobacterium leprae (India)
- Mycobacterium w MIP Mycobacterium Indicus Pranii (India)
- ICRC/Indian Cancer Research Center bacilli (India)
- Mycobacterium habana (India)
- Mycobacterium vaccae (Vietnam)

ALSO REMEMBER
- Addition of a preparation of killed M. vaccae to BCG did not enhance the protection afforded over that observed by either vaccine alone.

Review Questions

352. Ans. (c) Ciprofloxacin [Ref. Park 27/e p370-371]
353. Ans. (c) Paucibacillary leprosy bacterial index is less than 2 [Ref. Park 27/e p370]
354. Ans. (c) 180 days [Ref. Park 25/e p341]
355. Ans. (b) 2 [Ref. Park 27/e p370]
356. Ans. (d) Prevalence rate of disease [Ref. Park 27/e p363]

HIV

357. Ans. TRUE (b) Washing hands advised with soap and water; TRUE (e) Lamivudine + Tenofovir + Efavirenz for 4 weeks [Ref. Park 25/e p382]

    PEP for HIV (WHO 2016)
    - Initiated ideally within 72 hours
    - Wound/skin site should be washed immediately with soap and water, and exposed mucous membranes should be flushed with water (Use of caustic agents or antiseptics or disinfectants at the wound site is not recommended)
    - 3-drug regimen is preferably used (Lamivudine + Tenofovir + Efavirenz) for 4 weeks
    - HIV status assessment of exposed person should not be a barrier for initiating PEP

358. Ans. (c) Heterosexual, transplacental, homosexual [Ref. Park 27/e p396]

    - HIV transmission in India: [2010]

Route of transmission	Percentage of total cases	Efficiency of route
Sexual	87	0.01–1%
Blood and blood products	01	>90%
Sharing needles/syringes	02	0.3%
Mother to child transmission	05	30%

- Tamil Nadu in India has the largest number of HIV/AIDS cases; HIV prevalence has crossed 2% mark in Mumbai
- Age and Sex distribution of HIV/AIDS in India [2006]:

Distribution of HIV/AIDS cases	Cumulative cases
Age distribution	
0–14 years	5%
15–29 years	32%
30–44 years	56%
> 45 years	7 %
Sex distribution	
Male	71%
Female	29%

- Mother to Child Transmission (MTCT) of HIV:
  - MTCT in developing countries (India): 30%
  - MTCT in developed countries: 20%
  - Prevention of MTCT in India:

Modality	Dose/type	Reduction in MTCT by	Post-modality MTCT in India
Zidovudine	Mother: 300 mg BD from 36 wks POG + 300 mg 3h during delivery Child : 6 mg/kg 6h × 6w	66%	10%
Nevirapine	Single oral dose Mother: 200 mg at labor onset Child: 2mg/kg within 72 hrs of birth	50%	15%
Caesarean section	Elective CS	50%	15%

- Risk of HIV transmission with prolonged breast feeding: 12 – 15%
- For NEW GUIDELINES on PMTCT, Refer to Theory

359. Ans. (c) Thailand [Ref. Internet]
- First case of HIV reported:
  - USA: 1981
  - Thailand: 1984
  - India: 1986
  - Sri Lanka: 1987
  - Bangladesh: 1989

360. Ans. (c) 30-44 years [Ref. Park 27/e p396]
- HIV afflicted age groups in India: 30-44 years > 15-29 years > 45+ years > under 15 years

361. Ans. (d) Oral thrush [Ref. Park 27/e p398]

362. Ans. (a); (b); (d); (e) [Ref. Park 27/e p399]

363. Ans. (b) Seminal secretions are highly infectious than vaginal secretions; (c) Infectious in window period; (d) Southern Africa have 72% of global burden; (e) Children rarely affected [Ref. Park 27/e p392-393]
- Key facts about Epidemiology of HIV infection:
  - Reservoir: Cases and carriers
  - Source: Virus is in greatest concentration in blood, semen and CSF (lower concentrations in tear, saliva, breast milk, urine, cervical and vaginal secretions)
  - Children under 15 years make only 3% of cases
  - Basic modes of transmission:
    - Sexual
    - Blood and blood products
    - Needles/syringes
    - Mother to Child transmission (MTCT)
  - IP: Few months to 10 years

364. Ans. (b) Nevirapine; (a) Lamivudine [Ref. Park 27/e p402]

365. Ans. (c) 15-30% [Ref. Park 23/e p346]
HIV transmission in absence of intervention:
- MTCT of HIV in developed countries: 20% (15-25%)
- MTCT transmission of HIV in developing countries: 30% (25-35%)

366. Ans. (c) 72 hours [Ref. Park 27/e p405]

367. Ans. (b) Vitamin A supplementation [Ref. Park 27/e p498]

- Vitamin A supplementation has been shown to neither increase nor decrease the risk of MTCT of HIV
- Vitamin A supplementation INCREASE HIV transmission through breastfeeding

368. Ans. (c) HIV-C [Ref. HIV/AIDS Care and Counselling by ACV Dyk, 4/e p21]

369. Ans. (d) All of the above [Ref. Park 22/e p318, 322]

370. Ans. (d) 65% [Ref. HIV by HJ Makadon 3/e p299]

371. Ans. (b) 1983 [Ref. Black Death: AIDS in Africa by S Hunter 1/e p39]
HIV Discovery
- HIV-1 discovered in 1983
- HIV-2 discovered in 1986
- HIV discovered by:
  - Robert Gallo (USA)
  - Luc Montagnier, Barre Sinnousi (France) – Awarded Nobel Prize

372. Ans. (a) HAART [Ref. Perinatal and Pediatric HIV/AIDS by Mamatha, 1/e p344]
- Women enrolled on HAART (Triple ARV prophylaxis) had a much lower (1%) rate of HIV vertical transmission as compared to Zidovudine lone
- HAART showed similar rates of transmission when Zidovudine monotherapy was combined with single dose of Maternal or neonatal Nevirapine

373. Ans. NONE [Ref. Antiretroviral Therapy Guidelines for HIV-Infected Adults and Adolescents Including Post-exposure Prophylaxis, MOHFW, GOI. p78]
PEP INITIATION IN NACP
- PEP needs to be started as soon as possible after the exposure and within 72 hours
- In animal studies, initiating PEP within 12, 24 or 36 hours of exposure was more effective than initiating PEP 48 hours or 72 hours following exposure
- PEP is not effective when given more than 72 hours after exposure
- A baseline rapid HIV testing should be done before starting PEP

	HIV+ Asymptomatic	HIV+ Symptomatic	HIV status unknown
Mild exposure	Consider 2-drug PEP	Start 2-drug PEP	Usually no PEP/ Consider 2-drug PEP
Moderate exposure	Start 2-drug PEP	Start 3-drug PEP	Usually no PEP/ Consider 2-drug PEP
Severe exposure	Start 3-drug PEP	Start 3-drug PEP	Usually no PEP/ Consider 2-drug PEP

374. Ans. (b) When prevalence in high risk groups is more than 5%, and 1% or more in antenatal women [Ref. High risk pregnancy by Deshpande, 1/e p79]

375. Ans. (c) P24 antigen detection [Ref. Blood Banking and Transfusion Medicine by Hillyer 1/e p605]
HIV TESTS DURING WINDOW PERIOD
- HIV RNA genomic sequence detection by NAT (Nucleic acid amplification testing) - MOST SENSITIVE TEST
- p24 antigen capture ELISA

376. **Ans. (d) HIV 2 is more dangerous**
 [*Ref. New Scientist 18 Feb 1988 p27*]
 HIV-1 & HIV-2
 - HIV-1 was discovered in 1983 (USA)
 - HIV-2 was discovered in 1986 (West Africa)
 - HIV-1 and HIV-2 both have similar genetic structures EXCEPT that HIV-2 has vpx gene (instead of vpu gene)
 - SIV (Simian immunodeficiency virus) is a Lentivirus of primates that resembles HIV-1 and HIV-2 in morphology and attraction to CD4 cells

377. **Ans. (b) Single dose Nevirapine prevents mother to child transmission** [*Ref. Park 27/e p405*]
 POST-EXPOSURE PROPHYLAXIS IN HIV
 - Should be given in 3 days of exposure
 - Regimen with 2 drugs is effective BUT 3-drug regimen is preferred
 - A complete course of PEP comprises 28 days of medicine

378. **Ans. (c) Prevalence in pregnant women > 1%**
 [*Ref. ANAC's Core Curriculum for HIV/AIDS Nursing 3/e p10*]
 TYPES OF HIV EPIDEMICS (WHO/UNAIDS)
 - Low level epidemic: Prevalence consistently < 5% in all subgroups
 - Concentrated epidemic: Prevalence ≥ 5% in at least one Sub-groups but < 1% in Pregnant women
 - Generalized epidemic: Prevalence consistently > 1% in Pregnant women
 - Hyper-endemic (Proposed type): Prevalence > 15% in General population

379. **Ans. (b) Moderate prevalence state**
 [*Ref. Park 27/e p394*]

Groups with states/UTs	Criteria of prevalence in	
	High risk groups	Antenatal clinics
Group I (High Prevalence): Maharashtra, Tamil Nadu, Andhra Pradesh, Karnataka, Manipur, Nagaland, Mizoram, Telangana	>5%	>1%
Group II (Moderate Prevalence): Gujarat, Goa, Pondicherry	>5%	<1%
Group III (Low Prevalence): Remaining states & UTs	<5%	<1%

380. **Ans. (d) 10 years** [*Ref. AIDS Epidemiology and HIV Pathogenesis by Tan 1/e p271*]
 - Average incubation period for HIV (the time between infection with HIV and the development of AIDS) for adults not receiving treatment is about 10 years

381. **Ans. (a) Receptive anal sex** [*Ref. Park 27/e p396-397*]

HIV TRANSMISSION
- Any vaginal, anal or oral sex can transmit HIV
- Chances of transmission from Male-to-Female is twice as likely as from Female-to-Male
- Anal intercourse has higher risk than Vaginal route
- HIV transmission chances increase further in presence of mucosal/skin abrasions
- Risk increases in vaginal intercourse if woman is menstruating
- Adolescent girls (underdeveloped cervix as barrier) and Menopausal women (thinning of mucosa) increase the risk.

382. **Ans. (c) Right to health**
 [*Ref. UNAIDS Organization Website*]
 - Slogan for WAD 2017: Right to Health
 - Slogan for WAD 2018: Know your Status

383. **Ans. (d) High chances of HIV transmission**
 [*Ref. Park 27/e p396, 405*]
 Needle stick injury (NSI) and Post exposure prophylaxis (PEP) for HIV
 - NSI carry low risk of transmission 0.1-0.3% (It becomes significant among Injecting drug users due to repeated exposure)
 - PEP, to be effective, must be offered as early as possible: it must be offered ideally within 72 hours
 - 28 day prescription for PEP to be done
 - 3-drug combination is preferred for PEP: Lamivudine + Tenofovir + Lopinavir/ritonavir

384. **Ans. (c) Transmission is direct relationship with the maternal viral Load** [*Ref. Park 27/e p396*]
 Mother to Child Transmission (MTCT) of HIV
 - Rate of transmission is 20-30% (Developed-Developing nations)
 - MC time of transmission: During delivery
 - Higher risk of transmission: Newly infected mother, Mother with AIDS
 - Transmission is direct relationship with the maternal viral load:
   - Direct relationship between MTCT and maternal viral load with the disease transmission occurring at all levels of maternal viral load
   - Risk of MTCT is directly proportional to the viral load of HIV (More so with HIV-1)
 - Almost entire MTCT prevention is possible: ARV prophylaxis, Elective caesarean section (Before onset of labor and rupture of membranes), and avoidance of breastfeeding

Review Questions

385. **Ans. (b) Maternofetal transmission is the most common mode of transmission** [*Ref. Park 27/e p396-397*]
386. **Ans. (b) They consist of DNA dependent DNA polymerase activity** [*Ref. Harrison's 17/e p1140*]
387. **Ans. (c) Nagaland; (b) Mizoram**
 [*Ref. Park 23/e p344-345*]
388. **Ans. (a) 3-12 weeks** [*Ref. Park 27/e p397*]
389. **Ans. (c) Perinatal** [*Ref. Park 27/e p396-397*]

STI'S (OTHER THAN HIV)

390. **Ans. (d) Dengue** [*Ref. Park 26/e p491*]
 - In India, it is mandatory to test every unit of blood collected for hepatitis B, hepatitis C, HIV/AIDS, syphilis and malaria

- If donors test positive to any of the five infections, their blood is discarded. Although the blood policy advocates disclosure of TTI status, donors are not, in practice, informed about their results

391. **Ans. (b) Klebsiella granulomatis** [*Ref. Park 25/e p359*]
   - 5 Classical STD's include Syphilis (Treponema pallidum), Gonorrhoea (Neisseria gonorrhoeae), Chancroid (Hemophilus ducreyi), LGV (Chlamydia trachomatis), Donovanosis (Calymmatobacterium/Klebsiella granulomatis)

392. **Ans. (d) A-2, B-1, C-4, D-3** [*Ref. Park 26/e p491*]

   STD Colour Coded Kits
   - *Kit 1 (Grey) Urethral/Anorectal/Cervical discharge/Scrotal swelling:* Azithromycin, Cefixime
   - *Kit 2 (Green) Vaginal discharge:* Secnidazole, Fluconazole
   - *Kit 3 (White) Genito-ulcerative disease (Non-herpetic):* Azithromycin, Benzathine penicillin
   - *Kit 4 (Blue) Genito-ulcerative disease (Non-herpetic allergic to Penicillin):* Azithromycin, Doxycycline
   - *Kit 5 (Red) Genito-ulcerative disease (Herpetic):* Acyclovir
   - *Kit 6 (Yellow) Lower abdominal pain:* Cefixime, Metronidazole, Doxycycline
   - *Kit 7 (Black) Inguinal bubo:* Azithromycin, Doxycycline

393. **Ans. (d) Echinococcus** [*Ref. Park 27/e p380-381*]
   - Echinococcus is transmitted to humans by ingestion of eggs in dog's faeces.

> **ALSO REMEMBER**
> - *The 1st effective treatment for a STD:* Salvarsan (a treatment for syphilis)
> - *Sexually transmitted oral infections:*
>   - Common colds
>   - Influenza
>   - Staphylococcus aureus
>   - E. coli
>   - Candida albicans
> - *Echinococcus granulosus:*
>   - Also known as 'Dog Tape Worm'
>   - Dog – sheep cycle with man as intermediate dead end host
>   - *Definitive host:* Dog
>   - *Intermediate host:* Sheep
>   - *Infective stage:* Metacystode larva
>   - *Drug of choice:* Mebendazole
>   - *Casoni's test:* Immediate hypersensitivity skin test

394. **Ans. (c) Neisseria gonorrhoeae and Chlamydia trachomatis** [*Ref. National Health Programs of India by Dr. J. Kishore, 8/e p249, Park 27/e p390-391*]

395. **Ans. (c) Chancroid, Chancre and Herpes genitalis** [*Ref. National Health Programs of India by Dr. J. Kishore, 9/e p261-262*]

396. **Ans. (a) Syphilis 10-90 days; (b) LGV 3-10 days; (c) Donovanosis 3–20 days** [*Ref. Park 27/e p380-381*]

397. **Ans. (a) Metronidazole, Azithromycin, Fluconazole** [*Ref. Park 27/e p383*]

398. **Ans. (d) Notification** [*Ref. Park 25/e p357*]
399. **Ans. (d) Permethrin** [*Ref. Drugs in Pregnancy and Lactation by Briggs & Freeman, 8/e p1447*]

Review Question

400. **Ans. (d) Cluster testing** [*Ref. Park 27/e p388*]

Other communicable diseases

401. **Ans. (d) Scabies** [*Ref. Evidence-Based Dermatology by Williams 2/e p469*]
   - Mass Drug Administration is not helpful for Scabies
   - Scabies is best treated by Drug administration (DOC 5% Permethrin) on individual basis with treatment of all family members

402. **Ans. (a) Spread by sexual transmission** [*Ref. Park 27/e p390*]

403. **Ans. (b) Leprosy** [*Ref. Park 27/e p365*]

404. **Ans. (c) Toxins can be destroyed by boiling for 30 minutes** [*Ref. Park 27/e p281*]

405. **Ans. (d) Measles** [*Ref. Park 27/e p46, 165*]

406. **Ans. (b) Tuberculosis** [*Ref. Park 27/e p104*]
   - CARRIER: An infected person or animal that harbours a specific infectious agent 'in the absence of discernible clinical disease' and serves as a potential source of infection to others
   - *Characteristics of a carrier:*
     - Disease agent present in body
     - Absence of recognizable signs and symptoms of disease
     - Shedding disease agent (thus a source of infection)
   - *Incubatory carriers:* Shed infectious agent during the incubation period of the disease (esp. during last few days of IP). *For example:* Measles, Mumps, Polio, Pertussis, Influenza, Diphtheria, Hepatitis B, HIV

> **ALSO REMEMBER**
>
> **LATENT TUBERCULOSIS (LATENT TB, LTBI):**
> - Latent tuberculosis is where a patient is infected with Mycobacterium tuberculosis, but does not have active tuberculosis disease.
>   - Latent TB are NOT INFECTIOUS
>   - Main risk: 10% will go on to develop active TB at a later life
> - *Tests used to identify patients with latent TB:*
>   - Tuberculin skin tests (Montaux test, Heaf test, Tine test)
>   - a-interferon tests
> - *To give treatment for latent TB to someone with active TB is a serious error:* TB will not be adequately treated and there is a serious risk of developing drug-resistant strains of TB
> - *Several treatment regimens in use:*
>   - 9 months Isoniazid
>   - 6 months Isoniazid
>   - 4 months Rifampicin
>   - 3 months Isoniazid + Rifampicin
>   - 2 months Rifampicin + Pyrizinamide.

407. Ans. (a) Measles　　　　　　　[Ref. Park 27/e p104]
- *Chronic carriers:* A carrier who excretes bacilli for indefinite periods of time
  - Typhoid　　　　　　Dysentery
  - Hepatitis B　　　　　Cerebrospinal meningitis
  - Malaria　　　　　　Gonorrhoea
- There are no carriers in Measles

408. Ans. (c) Person to person transmission
　　　　　　　　　　　　　　　　　　[Ref. Park 27/e p337]
- *Modes of transmission of Brucellosis:*
  - *Contact infection:* direct contact with infected tissues, blood, urine, vaginal discharge, aborted fetuses and ESPECIALLY placenta
  - *Food-borne infections:* raw milk/dairy products, fresh raw vegetables, water
  - *Air-borne infection:* aerosol

409. Ans. (c) Pertussis　　　　　　[Ref. Park 27/e p183]
- The merit of hyperimmune globulin in pertussis prophylaxis has yet to be established. So far there is no evidence of its efficacy in well-controlled trials
- Post exposure prophylaxis of:
  - *H. influenza B:* Rifampicin × 4 days
  - *Hepatitis A:* Human normal Immunoglobulin
  - *Hepatitis B:* Human specific Immunoglobulin
  - *Meningococcal meningitis:* Rifampicin 600 mg BD × 2 days OR Meningococcal vaccine
  - *Rabies:* Human normal Immunoglobulin + Vaccine
  - *Tetanus:* Human normal Immunoglobulin + Vaccine
  - *Measles:* Vaccine within 3 days

> **ALSO REMEMBER**
> - *Types of immunoglobulins:*
>   - *IgG:* comprises 85% of total serum immunoglobulins, largely extravascular, 'only class of immunoglobulins to cross placenta'
>   - *IgM:* comprises 10% of total serum immunoglobulins, 'indicative of recent infection', has high agglutinating and complement-fixating ability
>   - *IgA:* comprises 15% of total serum immunoglobulins, predominantly found in secretions, 'primary defence mechanism at mucous membranes'
>   - *IgD:* exact function not known
>   - *IgE:* concentrated in submucous tissues, 'responsible for immediate allergic anaphylaxis reaction'
> - *Preparations of immunoglobulins:*
>
> | | Human normal Ig's | Human specific Ig's |
> |---|---|---|
> | Source | Antibody-rich fraction obtained from a pool of > 1000 donors | Plasma of recovered patients or immunized individuals |
> | Composition | > 90% IgG; less IgA | 5 times antibody potential of standard preparation |
> | Examples | Hepatitis A
Measles
Mumps
Rabies
Tetanus | Hepatitis B
Varicella
Diphtheria |

410. Ans. (a) Cough due to *Bordetella pertussis*
　　　　　　　　　　　　　　　　　　[Ref. Park 27/e p182]

> **ALSO REMEMBER**
> - *Hundred day cough:* Pertussis (Whooping cough)
> - *5 day fever:* Trench fever
> - *8th day disease:* Tetanus
> - *Black sickness:* Kala azar
> - *Black death:* Plague
> - *Cerebrospinal fever:* Meningococcal meningitis
> - *Breakbone fever:* Dengue
> - *Koch's phenomenon:* Tuberculosis
> - *Hansen's disease:* Leprosy
> - *Break-bone fever:* Dengue
> - *Slim disease:* AIDS
> - *First disease/Rubeolla:* Measles
> - *Second disease:* Scarlet fever
> - *Third disease/German Measles:* Rubella
> - *Fourth disease:* Duke's disease
> - *Fifth disease:* Erythema infectiosum (Parvovirus)
> - *Sixth disease/Baby Measles/3-day fever:* Exanthem subitum/Roseola infantum
> - *Barometer of Social Welfare (India):* Tuberculosis
> - *Father of Public Health:* Cholera
> - *River Blindness:* Onchocerciasis

411. Ans. (a) Leprosy　　　　　　　[Ref. Park 23/e p314]

412. Ans. (d) HIV/AIDS　[Ref. Park 20/e p299, Park 22/e p298]
- 3 BY 5 INITIATIVE: Launched by WHO and UNAIDS on 1st Dec 2003
  - *Target:* To provide antiretroviral treatment (ART) to 3 million people living with HIV/AIDS (PLHA) in developing countries by end of 2005

> **ALSO REMEMBER**
> - *WHO Intensive PULSE strategy:* Is for prevention and control of Poliomyelitis

413. Ans. (b) Cattle　[Ref. Textbook of Community Medicine by Sunder Lal, 2/e p511, Park 27/e p349]
- HOST: A person or other animal, including birds and arthropods, that affords subsistence or lodgement to an infectious agent under natural (as opposed to experimental) conditions
  - *Primary (definitive) host:* Host in which parasite attains maturity or passes its sexual stage
  - *Secondary (intermediate) host:* Host in which parasite is in larval or asexual stage

Disease	Parasite	Host Primary	Host Secondary
Malaria	Plasmodium	Anopheles	Man
Tapeworm	Taenia solium	Man	Pigs
Tapeworm	Taenia saginata	Man	Cattle
Guinea worm	Dracunculus medinensis	Man	Cyclops
Filariasis	Wuchereria bancrofti	Man	Culex
Hydatid disease	Echinococcus	Dog	Sheep, Cattle, Man
Sleeping sickness	Trypanosomes	Man	Tse tse fly

- *Obligate host:* Only Host for a Parasite. For example, Man in Measles, Man in Typhoid Fever
- *Transport host:* A carrier in which the organism remains alive but does not undergo development
- *Paratenic host:* It is similar to an intermediate host, only that it is not needed for the parasite's development cycle to progress. The difference between a paratenic and reservoir host is that the latter is a primary host, whereas paratenic hosts serve as "dumps" for non-mature stages of a parasite which they can accumulate in high numbers
- *Dead-end host:* Is an intermediate host that does generally not allow transmission to the definite host, thereby preventing the parasite from completing its development. For example, humans are dead-end hosts for Echinococcus canine tapeworms

Tapeworms:

Tapeworm	Causative organism
Pork tapeworm	Taenia solium
Beef tapeworm	Taenia saginata
Fish tapeworm	Diphyllobothrium latum
Dwarf tapeworm (Rat tapeworm)	Hymenolepsis nana

TAENIASIS:
- *Taeniasis are called as 'Cyclozoonoses':* Require more than one vertebrate host species (but no invertebrate host) to complete their developmental cycles
- T.solium and T.saginata may persist for several years in infected humans (small intestines)
- *Mode of transmission:*
  - Ingestion of infective cysticerci in undercooked beef (T.saginata) or pork (T.solium)
  - Ingestion of food, water or vegetables contaminated with eggs
  - Reinfection by reperistalsis of eggs (bowel to stomach)
- IP: 8-14 weeks
- *Most serious risk of T.solium infection:* Cysticercosis
- *Treatment:* Praziquantel and niclosamide
- *DOC Cysticercosis:* Albendazole
- *Most effective method to prevent food borne infections:* cooking of beef and pork

414. Ans. (c) Falciparum malaria   [Ref. Park 19/e p219]
- SPf 66: A synthetic 'Lytic Cocktail vaccine' developed for P. Falciparum has been extensively tested
  - Formulated as peptide-alum combination
  - Safe, effective and reduces risk of developing clinics malaria by 30%

415. Ans. (c) Hepatitis E   [Ref. Park 27/e p261]

HEPATITIS E:
- Enterically transmitted hepatitis non-A, non-B [HNANB]
- HEV is essentially a waterborne disease, transmitted through water or food supplies, contaminated by faeces
- Incubation Period: 2 – 9 weeks
- HEV in pregnancy: Fulminant form is common in Hepatitis E infection during Pregnancy (up to 20% cases) with a high case fatality rate (up to 80%)

416. Ans. (c) Measles   [Ref. Park 27/e p164]

417. Ans. (a) Trichuris trichura
   [Ref. Park 21/e p94, Park 22/e p95]
- *Obligate Host:* Means the only host
  - Man in Measles
  - Man in Typhoid

418. Ans. (b) Insulin
   [Ref. Park 21/e p168, 176, Park 22/e p172, 178]
- Insulin is given through sub-cutaneous route

419. Ans. (a) Yellow fever; (b) Japanese encephalitis; (e) Dengue
   [Ref. Park 27/e p288]
- *Arboviral infections (arthropod-borne viral infections) in India:*

Group A (Alphaviruses)	Others
Sindbis Chikungunya	Umbre Sathuperi Chandipura Chittor
Group B (Flaviviruses)	Ganjam Minnal Venkatapuram Dhori Kaisodi Sandfly fever African Horse Sickness Vellore
Dengue KFD JE West Nile	

420. Ans. (b) Screening for STD's   [Ref. Park 27/e p388-389]

421. Ans. (b) Food poisoning   [Ref. Park 27/e p280-281]
- *Incubation period of food poisonings:*

Food poisoning	Incubation period
Salmonella	12 – 24 hours
Staphylococcal	1 – 6 hours
Botulism	12 – 36 hours
Cl. perfirengens	6 – 24 hours
B. cereus (emetic form)	1 – 6 hours
B. cereus (diarrhoel form)	12 – 24 hours

422. Ans. (a) HBV; (b) Rabies; (d) Measles; (e) Tetanus
   [Ref. Park 21/e p139, 196, 255, 286, Park 22/e p141, 197, 285]
- *Diseases transmitted by needle stick injury:*

– HIV – HBV – HCV – Malaria – Syphilis – Leptospirosis – Blastomycosis – Brucellosis – Cryptococcosi	– Diphtheria – Ebola virus – Herpes simplex – Mycobacterium caviae – RMSF – Tuberculosis – Varicella zoster

423. Ans. (a) Chikungunya   [Ref. Park 27/e p335-336]

424. Ans. (a) Measles; (b) Diarrhea   [Ref. Park 27/e p164]
- *All cases of Measles should be treated with Vitamin A:* as many children develop acute deficiency of Vitamin A (Xerophthalmia) which may lead to Keratomalacia and blindness from corneal scarring
- *Diarrhoea is associated with Vitamin A deficiency too*

425. Ans. (b) Influenza-A [Ref. Park 27/e p174-175]
426. Ans. (a) Rabies; (b) Japanese encephalitis
 [Ref. Park 27/e p323, 332]
427. Ans. (a) Epidemic typhus; (b) Japanese encephalitis; (e) KFD [Ref. Park 27/e p105-106]
428. Ans. (b) Varicella; (d) Parvovirus [Ref. Park 27/e p104-105]
- *Vertical transmission of diseases:*

Disease	Most common time of transmission
Varicella	I trimester
Rubella	I trimester
Parvovirus	II trimester
Hepatitis B	III trimester
Toxoplasmosis	III trimester
Syphilis	III trimester
CMV	Any trimester
HIV	During delivery
Hepatitis C	During delivery

429. Ans. (c) Q fever [Ref. Park 27/e p348]
 Refer to Theory
430. Ans. (c) Scabies [Ref. Park 27/e p908]
- *Lymphatic filariasis:* DEC OR 'DEC + Albendazole/Ivermectin'
- *Vitamin A deficiency:* Single massive dose of Vitamin A (200,000 IU) to preschool children (aged 1-6 years) every 6 months
- *Worm infestation:* Periodic de-worming of Ascariasis (Roundworm) may be undertaken every 2-3 months
  - Undertaken where parasites & PEM highly prevalent
  - ONLY reduces worm load (DOESNOT interrupt transmission)
- *Scabies:* All family members (NOT community) must be treated simultaneously
431. Ans. (c) Vertical transmission [Ref. Park 27/e p283]
- *Modes of transmission of Amoebiasis:*
  - Faecal-oral
  - Sexual (Oro-rectal in homosexuals)
  - Vectors (Flies, Cockroaches, rodents)
432. Ans. (d) Yellow Fever [Ref. Park 27/e p328]
- Although Yellow fever has never been reported from Asia, the region is at risk because conditions required for transmission are present.
433. Ans. (d) Later stages involve heart and nerves
 [Ref. Park 27/e p390]
434. Ans. (a) Cholera [Ref. Park 27/e p274]
435. Ans. (c) Whooping cough [Ref. Park 27/e p181-182]
- Infants are susceptible to Pertussis infection from birth because maternal antibody does not appear to give them protection.
436. Ans. ALL CHOICES [Ref. Park 27/e p337]
437. Ans. (c) Japanese encephalitis [Ref. Park 27/e p331-332]
438. Ans. (c) Pertussis [Ref. Park 27/e p181-182]
439. Ans. (a) Scabies [Ref. Park 27/e p908]
440. Ans. (a) Leptospirosis [Ref. Park 27/e p338-339]
441. Ans. (a) Cholera [Ref. Park 27/e p273]
442. Ans. (a) Hydatid cyst [Ref. Park 27/e p350-351]
443. Ans. (c) Measles [Ref. Park 27/e p164-168]
444. Ans. (a) TB [Ref. Multiple sources]
445. Ans. (b) Hepatitis C [Ref. Park 27/e p259-260]
446. Ans. (a) Gammexene; (b) Crotamiton; (c) 5% Permethrin; (e) Sulphur ointment [Ref. Park 27/e p908]
447. Ans. (c) Rabies [Ref. Park 27/e p322]
448. Ans. (d) German measles – 7 days after onset of rash
 [Ref. Park 27/e p165-166]
449. Ans. (a) It is a Zoonosis; (c) Transmission occurs through direct skin contact; (d) Drug of choice is Penicillin; (e) Is a Spirochaetal disease [Ref. Park 27/e p338-339]
450. Ans. (d) Leishmaniasis [Ref. Park 27/e p352-353]
451. Ans. (c) Gastroenteritis [Ref. Park 27/e p264-265]
452. Ans. (a) Influenza [Ref. Park 27/e p102]
453. Ans. (d) Borellia hermsii [Ref. Principles and Practices of Paediatric Infectious Diseases, 4/e p959]
454. Ans. (a) KFD; (b) Dengue fever; (c) Crimean Congo fever; (e) Hanta fever
455. Ans. (b) Dengue fever [Ref. Emerging Biological Threats: A Reference Guide by JR Callahan, 1/e p63]
- Saddleback fever: Two peaks of fever separated by an afebrile period in-between
- Seen in: Dengue, Trench fever, Bartonellosis, Chikungunya, Colaradotick fever
456. Ans. (c) Measles [Ref. Park 27/e p164-165]
457. Ans. (a) Rocky mountain spotted fever
 [Ref. Park 27/e p345]
458. Ans. (a) Common in veterinarians; (b) Seasonal pattern; (c) Common in butchers; (d) Cutaneous form most common [Ref. Anthrax by Koehler, 1/e p9]
459. Ans. (c) Incubation period is less than 48 hours; (e) Oseltamivir is quite effective in treatment
 [Ref. Ebola Virus InfoPage, WHO International Website]
460. Ans. (a) Plague; (b) Rabies; (c) Anthrax; (e) Brucellosis
 [Ref. Park 27/e p322]
461. Ans. (a) Influenza; (d) Yersinia; (e) Swine flu
 [Ref. Park 27/e p321]
462. Ans. (a) Plague; (c) Schistosomiasis; (e) Yellow fever
 [Ref. Park 27/e p322]
463. Ans. (b) Shigella flexneri [Ref. Foodborne and Waterborne Bacterial Pathogens by Faruque, 1/e p91]
464. Ans. (c) 1 and 4 [Ref. Park 27/e p164, 277]
465. Ans. (a) Hepatitis A infection; (b) Hepatitis B infection; (d) Rabies; (e) Varicella zoster virus infection
 [Ref. Park 27/e p139]
466. Ans. (a) Crimean Congo fever [Ref. Desk Encyclopedia of Human and Medical Virology 1/e p29]

- Crimean-Congo hemorrhagic fever virus natural hosts include cattle, sheep, and goats

467. Ans. (a) Yellow fever; (c) Lassa fever; (e) Crimean Congo fever *[Ref. The Travel and Tropical Medicine Manual by Sanford 5/e p285]*

Syndromes of Arboviral Diseases
- Undifferentiated fever syndrome: Oropouche, Mayaro, Sandfly fever
- Dengue fever syndrome: Dengue, Chikungunya, O'nyong-nyong, Sindbis, West Nile, Ross River
- Syndrome of Hemorrhagic fevers: Lassa fever, Ebola, Marburg, Crimean-Congo, Argentine, Bolivian, Dengue, Yellow fever viruses
- Encephalitis

468. Ans. ALL OF THE CHOICES *[Ref. Park 27/e p288, 334, 332, 339, 327]*
- Dengue (Aedes aegypti), KFD (Hemophysalis – Hard tick), Japanese encephalitis (Culex tritaeniorhynchus), Plague (Xenpsylla – Rat flea), Yellow fever (Aedes aegypti) are common vector borne diseases.

Review Questions

469. Ans. (a) Rabies *[Ref. Park 27/e p323]*
470. Ans. (a) Plague *[Ref. Internet, Wikipedia]*
471. Ans. (a) Cholera *[Ref. Park 27/e p273]*
472. Ans. (a) Measles *[Ref. Park 27/e p164]*
473. Ans. (a) Diarrhea *[Ref. Park 27/e p281]*
474. Ans. (d) T. cruzi *[Ref. Park 25/e p98]*
475. Ans. (d) Leishmaniasis *[Ref. Park 21/e p94, Park 22/e p95]*
476. Ans. (b) Cholera *[Ref. Park 27/e p273]*
477. Ans. (b) Polio *[Ref. Park 27/e p243]*
478. Ans. (c) KFD *[Ref. Park 27/e p334]*
479. Ans. (c) Filariasis is transmitted by Aedes mosquito *[Ref. Park 27/e p315]*
480. Ans. (d) Dracunculosis *[Ref. Park 27/e p288]*
481. Ans. (a) Rats *[Ref. Park 27/e p338]*
482. Ans. (a) AIDS *[Ref. Park 27/e p133]*
483. Ans. (a) Tularemia; (d) Rocky Mountain spotted fever *[Ref. Park 25/e p316]*
484. Ans. (a) Dengue; (b) Chikungunya fever *[Ref. Park 27/e p897]*
485. Ans. (a) Malaria *[Ref. Park 27/e p106]*
486. Ans. (b) *Clostridium difficile* *[Ref. Park 27/e p280-281]*
487. Ans. (a) Polio *[Ref. Park 27/e p133]*
488. Ans. (d) Kala-azar *[Ref. Park 27/e p352]*
489. Ans. (b) Rabies *[Ref. Park 27/e p46]*
490. Ans. (d) Tuberculosis *[Ref. Park 27/e p139]*
491. Ans. (d) Meta zoonosis *[Ref. Park 27/e p323]*
492. Ans. (b) Malaria *[Ref. Park 27/e p322]*
493. Ans. (a) Tetanus *[Ref. Park 27/e p322]*
494. Ans. (a) Diphtheria *[Ref. Park 27/e p179]*
495. Ans. (c) Secondary attack rate *[Ref. Park 27/e p108]*

EMERGING AND RE-EMERGING INFECTIONS

496. Ans. (b) Spread by mosquito *[Ref. Park 26/e p401]*

Ebola Virus Disease
- *Cause:* Ebola virus (Filoviradeae)
- *Incubation period:* 2–21 days
- *Route of transmission:* Body fluids (including semen, breast milk)
- *Source:* Cases, Reservoir: Bats (Mammals are dead end host)
- *Case fatality rate:* 40%
- *Treatment:* Rehydration, Symptomatic

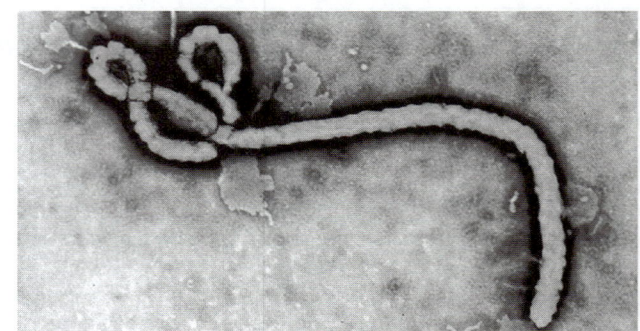

497. Ans. (c) Crimean Congo fever *[Ref. National Health Portal, GOI]*
- In India the first confirmed case of CCHF was reported during a nosocomial (Infections caught in hospitals) outbreak in Ahmadabad, Gujarat, in January 2011
- Subsequently outbreaks were reported from different districts of Gujarat every year
- During 2012–2015, several outbreaks and cases of CCHF transmitted by ticks via livestock and several nosocomial infections were reported in the states of Gujarat and Rajasthan
- Cases were documented from 6 districts of Gujarat (Ahmadabad, Amreli, Patan, Surendranagar, Kutch, and Aravalli) and 3 districts of Rajasthan (Sirohi, Jodhpur, and Jaisalmer)
- A CCHF case was also reported from Uttar Pradesh state

498. Ans. (b) Hyalomma tick *[Ref. Crimean-Congo Hemorrhagic Fever by Berger 1/e p12]*

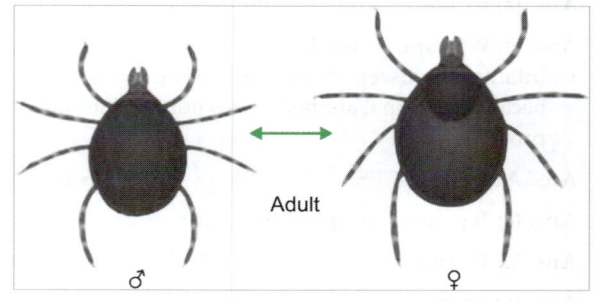

Hyalomma ticks

Vectors of Crimean Congo hemorrhagic fever
- MC tick species: Hyalomma, Dermacenter, Rhipicephalus, Ixodes
- Other tick species: Ambylomma

CORONARY HEART DISEASE

499. Ans. (a) Not more than 30% calories should come from the fat; (b) <5000 mg/day Sodium *[Ref. Park 26/e p728]*

Prudent Diet (Dietary Goals)
- A prudent diet may be associated with enhanced insulin sensitivity and a lower risk of type 2 diabetes—It is a dietary modification is the principal preventive strategy for prevention of CHD and other chronic diseases
- GOAL of Prudent Diet: Cholesterol/HDL Ratio <3.5
- WHO recommended changes:
  - Reduction of fat intake to <30% of total energy intake
  - Consumption of saturated fats <7% of total energy intake
  - Reduction in dietary cholesterol to <200 mg per day
  - Increase in complex carbohydrate consumption
  - Reduction of salt intake to <5 gms per day
  - Avoidance of alcohol consumption

500. Ans. (c) Monitoring of trends and determinants in Cardiovascular disease *[Ref. Park 25/e p397]*
- Multinational Monitoring of Trends and Determinants in Cardiovascular Disease (MONICA)
- WHO MONICA Project is designed to measure the trends in mortality and morbidity from Coronary heart disease (CHD) and stroke, and to assess the extent to which they are related to changes in known risk factors in different populations in 27 countries (10 years period)

501. Ans. (b); (c) Salt intake less than 20 g/day *[Ref. Park 27/e p422]*
- PRUDENT DIET (DIETARY GOALS): Dietary modification is the principal preventive strategy in the prevention of CHD. WHO recommended changes: [GOAL: Cholesterol/HDL Ratio <3.5]
  - Reduction of fat intake to <20–30% of total energy intake
  - Consumption of saturated fats <7% of total energy intake
  - Reduction in dietary cholesterol to <100 mg/1000 kcal/day
  - Increase in complex carbohydrate consumption
  - Reduction of salt intake to <5 gms per day
  - Avoidance of alcohol consumption

ALSO REMEMBER
CORONARY HEART DISEASE:
- *CHD is our modern epidemic (WHO):* CHD causes 25 – 30% of deaths in most industrialized countries
- *Simplest measure of burden of CHD:* Proportional mortality ratio
- *Case fatality rate of CHD:* Proportion of attacks fatal within 28 days of onset
- According to Ross, Incubation period of CHD may be > 10 years

- *Pattern of CHD in India:*
  - Occurs a decade earlier compared with age incidence in developed nations
  - Peak period is 51 – 60 years age
  - Males affected more than females
  - Hypertension and Diabetes mellitus account for > 40% cases
  - Heavy smoking is responsible for a large no. of cases
- *Single most useful test for identifying individuals at high risk of CHD:* Blood pressure
  - Systolic BP better predictor of CHD than Diastolic BP
- *CHD risk preventation:*
  - Cholesterol/HDL ratio < 3.5
  - HDL cholesterol > 30 mg/dL
- *Alcohol intake as an independent risk factor for CHD:* >75 grams per day.

502. Ans. (b) Filters provide a protective effect for CHD *[Ref. Park 27/e p420]*
- *Smoking as a risk factor for CHD:*
  - Modifiable major risk factor
  - 25% of CHD deaths under 165 years age
  - Causes Sudden death from CHD, especially in men < 50 years age
  - Degree of risk of developing CHD is directly related to no. of cigarettes smoked per day
  - Filter cigarettes are probably not protective
  - Synergistic with other risk factors like hypertension and elevated serum cholesterol
  - *Risk of death from CHD decreases on cessation of smoking:*
    1. Risk declines substantially within 1 year of cessation
    2. After 10–20 years, it is same as that of non-smokers
  - Those with history of myocardial infarction – risk of fatal occurrence reduced by 50%

ALSO REMEMBER
- *Mean serum cholesterol level associated with high risk of CHD:* >200 mg/dl
  - *Threshold level:* 220 mg/dl
  - *Most direct association with CHD:* LDL cholesterol
  - *Protective for CHD:* HDL cholesterol (>30 mg/dl)
  - *Clinical goal of CHD prevention:* Cholesterol/HDL ratio <3.5
  - *Better predictors of CHD:* Apolipoprotein A–I and Apolipoprotein B

503. Ans. (c) LDL *[Ref. Park 27/e p421]*
- Most direct association with CHD: LDL cholesterol

504. Ans. (a) LDL cholesterol less than 100 mg/dL *[Ref. Park 27/e p421]*

505. Ans. (d) NYHA 4 *[Ref. Comprehensive Coronary Care by Jowett & Thompson, 4/e p280]*

New York Heart Association (NYHA) Classification
- *Importance*: Scale used for quantification of degree of functional limitation imposed by Congestive health failure (CHF)

Class	Severity	Physical activity	Description
NYHA I	Mild asymptomatic	No limitation	Comfortable at rest and ordinary exertion
NYHA II	Mild symptomatic	Slight limitation	Comfortable at rest; ordinary exertion cause symptoms
NYHA III*	Moderate	Marked limitation	Comfortable at rest; less than ordinary activity cause symptoms
NYHA IV	Severe	Unable to carryout	Symptoms at rest

(*Class IIIa No dyspnoea at rest; Class IIIb Dyspnoea at rest)

506. Ans. (c) Management of hypertension and diabetes
 [Ref. Park 27/e p422]
- Management of hypertension and diabetes is High risk strategy – Primary level of prevention for CHD

507. Ans. (d) Screening for hypertension
 [Ref. Park 27/e p423]
- Screening for hypertension is Secondary level of prevention (Early detection)

Review Questions

508. Ans. (a) Indian CHD occurs 1 decade later than Western CHD [Ref. Park 27/e p420]

509. Ans. (b) Mean age of patient is 10-20 years more than that of western [Ref. Park 27/e p420]

510. Ans. (a) Framingham study [Ref. Park 27/e p423]

511. Ans. (a) Personality [Ref. Park 27/e p420]

HYPERTENSION

512. Ans. (c) Tracking phenomenon [Ref. Park 27/e p427]
 TRACKING OF BLOOD PRESSURE
- If BP of individuals were followed up over a period of years from early childhood into adult life, then those having high BP would continue into same 'track' as adults
- Low BP tends to remain low and high BP tends to become higher as individuals grow older

513. Ans. (a) Weight reduction; (b) Exercise promotion; (c) Reduction of salt intake; (e) Self care [Ref. Park 27/e p428]
- Population strategy for prevention of Hypertension:
  – Is primary level of prevention
  – Includes:
    - Nutrition (Reduction of salt intake to < 5 grams a day, moderate fat intake, avoidance of alcohol intake, resytriction of energy intake as per body needs)
    - Weight reduction (BMI <25)
    - Exercise promotion
    - Behavioural changes (reduction of stress and smoking, doing yoga and meditation)
    - Health education
    - Self care

514. Ans. (d) BP of hyoptensive remain hypotensive [Ref. Park 27/e p427]

515. Ans. (a) Dietary approaches to stop hypertension [Ref. DASH Guide by Chavez, 1/e p1]
 DASH DIET (DIETARY APPROACHES TO STOP HYPERTENSION)
- *Description*: Dietary pattern promoted to prevent and control hypertension
- DASH diet is rich in fruits, vegetables, and low-fat dairy foods with whole grains; includes meat, fish, poultry, nuts, and beans; and is limited in sugar-sweetened foods and beverages, red meat, and added fats
- DASH reduces SBP by 6 mm Hg, DBP by 3 mm Hg in high normal BP
- DASH leads to No changes in body weight
- DASH is adjusted based on daily intake of 1,600-3,100 calories

516. Ans. (d) Fruits, vegetables, Low fat dairy foods [Ref. DASH Guide by Chavez, 1/e p1]

RHEUMATIC FEVER

517. Ans. (c) 3 weekly benzathine penicillin injection for 5 years or till 18 years whichever is later [Ref. Park 26/e p426-427]
 Prevention of RF with Benzathine benzyl penicillin
- *Primary prevention*: 1.2 million units (600,000 units in children) Single dose intramuscular
- *Secondary prevention*: 1.2 million units (600,000 units in children) 3 weekly intervals for 5 years or till 18 years age (whichever is later

518. Ans. (b) Mitral regurgitation is the commonest cardiac lesion seen [Ref. Park 27/e p432]

> **ALSO REMEMBER**
> - *RF is not a communicable disease*: but it results from a communicable disease (streptococcal pharyngitis)
> - *MC cause of Heart disease in 5–30 yrs age group (globally)*: RF
> - *Prevalence of RHD in India*: 5–7 per 1000 in 5–15 yrs age group
>   – RF occurs in 1–3% of Streptococcal infection
> - *Eradication of Grp A Streptococcus is not possible*: In view of its high carrier rate
> - *MC ECG finding in RF*: First degree AV block
> - *Best indicator for evaluation of RF control programme*: Prevalence of RHD in 6–14 yrs school children
>   – Recommended periodicity of surveys: every 5 yrs
>   – Recommended sample size: 20,000–30,000
> - Except carditis, other major manifestations in RF do not cause permanent residual damage

519. **Ans. (d) In Revised Jones' Criteria, evidence of preceding streptococcal infection is taken for last 21 days**
 [Ref. Park 27/e p433]

520. **Ans. (d) Elevated ESR** *[Ref. Park 27/e p433]*

521. **Ans. (b) Polyarthralgia** *[Ref. Park 27/e p433]*

522. **Ans. (a) Carditis**
 [Ref. Dermatology by Bolognia 1/e p307]

 ERYTHEMA MARGINATUM
 - Migratory annular polycyclic eruption
 - Cutaneous manifestation of Acute Rheumatic fever (Seen in <10% patients)
 - Seen in conjunction with Carditis
 - Precedes joint manifestations

523. **Ans. (c) Science & technology** *[Ref. Information India 1997-98 And 1998-99 by Agrawal, p276]*
 - Indian Council of Medical Research initiated a Jai Vigyan Mission Mode Project on Control of RF/RHD in year 2000 with following components:
   - Study the epidemiology of Streptococcal sore throats
   - Establish registries for RF and RHD
   - Vaccine development for Streptococcal infection
   - Conducting advanced studies on pathological aspects of RF and RHD

ALSO REMEMBER
- Jai Vigyan Mission Mode Science and Technology Projects have been launched by Government of India, in various disciplines, as another step towards implementation of time bound technology development programmes

CANCERS

524. **Ans. (a) Cervical cancer; (b) Anal cancer; (c) Oropharyngeal cancer; (d) Laryngeal papillomatosis**
 [Ref. HPV and Cancer by Radosevich, 1/e p2-5]

 HPV-related Cancers
 - Cervical cancer (HPV 16,18)
 - Oropharyngeal cancers (HPV 16)
 - Genital warts (HPV 6,11)
 - Laryngeal papillomatosis (HPV 6,11)
 - Anal cancer
 - Penile cancer
 - Vaginal cancer
 - Vulvar cancer

525. **Ans. (c) Breast cancer** *[Ref. Cancer Registration in India – 50 Years of Cancer Control Programme in India, MoHFW]*
 - Most common cancer among females in India is Breast Cancer in both urban and rural areas *[NEW DATA RELEASED]*

526. **Ans. (c) Lung cancer** *[Ref. Park 27/e p434-437]*
 - The total cancer burden (in decreasing order) globally:
   - Lung cancer
   - Breast cancer
   - Colorectal cancer

ALSO REMEMBER
- Among Indian women, cancers of breast and cervix account for nearly 60% of all cancers
- *Beer consumption is associated with:* rectal cancer
- Alcohol contributes to: 3% of all cancer deaths
- *Environmental factors are responsible for:* 80-90% of all human cancers
- Occupational exposures (MC – Skin cancer) account for 1 – 5% of all cancers
- *MC cancer among females in India:* Breast cancer
- Gall bladder cancer has the highest age-adjusted incidence rate among females in Delhi

527. **Ans. NONE (Now Lip, Oral cavity cancer)**
 [Ref. Textbook of Community Medicine by Sunder Lal, 2/e p613, Park 27/e p436-437]
 Refer to theory for new data.

528. **Ans. (b) Breast cancer** *[Ref. Park 27/e p436]*

529. **Ans. (c) Penile cancer and cervical cancer following circumcision** *[Ref. Park 27/e p436-437]*
 - *Associations of few cancers:*

Association	Cancer associated
Smoking	Lung cancer
Tobacco chewing	Oral cancer
Using hot pot in winter	Kangri cancer
Beer consumption	Rectal cancer
Smoked fish consumption	Stomach cancer
High fat intake	Breast canvcer
Reduced fibre intake	Colo-rectal cancer
Aniline dyes exposure	Bladder cancer

530. **Ans. (a) Ca cervix; (b) Ca Breast; (c) Ca Prostate; (e) Ca Colon** *[Ref. Park 27/e p439]*
 - Lung cancer does not satisfy the criteria for suitability of a disease for Lung cancer

531. **Ans. (c) Carcinoma colon** *[Ref. CMDT 2014, p1571]*
 [Ref. Chapter 4]

532. **Ans. (b) 1 million** *[Ref. Park 27/e p436]*

533. **Ans. (c) Lung cancer** *[Ref. Park 27/e p436]*

534. **Ans. (c) 90%** *[Ref. Park 22/e p354]*

535. **Ans. (d) Breast** *[Ref. Park 27/e p436-437]*
 - Mortality due to cancers among women in India (2012): Breast (21.5%) > Cervix uteri (20.7%) > Colorectum > Ovary

536. **Ans. (b) Oropharyngeal carcinoma**
 [Ref. Park 27/e p436-437]
 CANCERS AMONG MALES IN INDIA
 - *Highest Incidence*: = Lip/Oral cavity > Lung Ca

537. **Ans. (c) HPV 16, 18**
 [Ref. Operative OBG by Malhotra 1/e p725]

CERVICAL CANCER
- MC in World: HPV 16, 18, 45, 31
- MC in India: HPV 16, 18 (76% of all cases)
- Single MCC in India: HPV 16 (59% of total cases)

538. **Ans. (d) Provide readily accessible information about patients and treatment outcome** [Ref. Park 27/e p438]
    - Hospital-based registries in Cancer:
        - Include all in-patients and out-patients treated in a hospital/institution
        - Uniformly collected data
        - Useful in evaluation of diagnostic and treatment programs if there is a long term follow-up of patients
    - Population-based registries in cancer:
        - Cover complete cancer situation in a given geographic area
        - Optimum base size of population 2-7 million
        - Provide incidence rate of cancer
        - Evaluate causes of cancer, surveillance of trends, planning and evaluation of operational activities

539. **Ans. (a) Administrative information** [Ref. Park 27/e p438]

Aims of Population Based Cancer Registry
- Provide incidence rates of cancers
- Epidemiological insight into etiology of cancer
- Surveillance of time trends
- Planning and evaluation of cancer control activities

Review Questions

540. **Ans. (b) Self examination** [Ref. Internet]
541. **Ans. (a) Head and neck carcinoma** [Ref. Internet]
542. **Ans. (d) Early marriage** [Ref. Park 27/e p439]
543. **Ans. (d) Single child birth** [Ref. Park 27/e p439]

OBESITY

544. **Ans. (b) 30** [Ref. Park 27/e p454]
    - Body Mass Index (Quetelet's Index):
      In the given question, Weight = 89 Kg and Height = 1.72 m
      Thus, $Wt/Ht^2 = 89/(1.72)^2 = 30$

545. **Ans. (d) Anterior abdominal wall** [Ref. Park 27/e p455]
546. **Ans. (c) > 30** [Ref. Park 27/e p454]
547. **Ans. (a) BMI** [Ref. Park 27/e p453-454]
    - BMI (Body Mass Index) or Quetelet's Index: although not an accurate measurement of fat accumulation, but is a widely used index of obesity (also is Broca's Index)

548. **Ans. (a) Regular exercise with same amount of food** [Ref. Park 27/e p455]
    WEIGHT CONTROL MEASURES:
    - *Dietary changes:*
        - Reduce proportions of carbohydrates and fats (energy dense foods)
        - Increase fibre consumption
        - Ensure adequate levels of essential nutrients
    - Increased physical activity
    - *Others:*
        - Drugs
        - Surgical treatment
        - Health education

549. **Ans. (c) > 25** [Ref. Park 27/e p454]
550. **Ans. (a) Broca's index; (b) Ponderal index; (c) Quetelet index; (d) Corpulence index** [Ref. Park 27/e p454]
551. **Ans. (b) 32** [Ref. Park 27/e p454]
552. **Ans. (b) 30** [Ref. Park 27/e p454]
553. **Ans. (d) Corpulence index** [Ref. Park 27/e p454]
554. **Ans. (d) 18.5 to 22.99** [Ref. Park 27/e p454]
555. **Ans. (c) Ponderal's index** [Ref. Park 27/e p454]
556. **Ans. (a) Measurement of obesity** [Ref. Park 27/e p454]
557. **Ans. (b) 0.85** [Ref. Park 23/e p400; WC & WHR, WHO Consultation 2008]

WHO CUT-OFF POINTS OF WHR

Indicator	Cut-off points	Risk of metabolic complications
Waist circumference	>94 cm (M); >80 cm (W)	Increased
Waist circumference	>102 cm (M); >88 cm (W)	Substantially increased
Waist–hip ratio	≥ 0.90 cm (M); ≥ 0.85 cm (W)	Substantially increased

(M: Men; W: Women)

558. **Ans. (b) Actual weight/Desirable weight** [Ref. Park 27/e p454]
    - Corpulence Index is an indicator of Obesity
    - CI = Actual weight/Desirable weight
    - Normal CI is up to 1.2

559. **Ans. (b) < 13** [Ref. Irwin and Rippe's Intensive Care Medicine 6/e p2187]
    - Lethal BMI among males: < 13
    - Lethal BMI among Females: < 11

560. **Ans. (c) 13** [Ref. Irwin and Rippe's Intensive Care Medicine 6/e p2187]
    - Lethal BMI among males: < 13
    - Lethal BMI among Females: < 11

Review Questions

561. **Ans. (d) Waist to hip ratio** [Ref. Park 27/e p454]
562. **Ans. (a)** $\dfrac{\text{Weight (Kg)}}{(\text{Height})^2 \text{ (meters)}}$ [Ref. Park 27/e p454]

BLINDNESS

563. **Ans. (b) 700** [Ref. The Principles and Practice of Community Ophthalmology, NPCB, Govt. of India, 2002; p29]

564. **Ans. (c) < 3/60 in better eye** [Ref. New Guidelines, NPCB, GOI 2017-18]

- *Legal blindness:* Is defined as visual acuity (vision) of 3/60 or less in the better eye with best correction possible
  - In many areas, people with average acuity who nonetheless have a visual field of less than 10 degrees (the norm being 180 degrees) are also classified as being legally blind.

565. Ans. (d) Onchocerciasis *[Ref. National Health Programs of India by Dr. J. Kishore, 7/e p368 and The Principles and Practice of Community Ophthalmology, NPCB, Govt. of India, 2002; p234-45]*

- *Vision 2020 – The Right To Sight:* A global initiative by WHO and International NGOs to reduce avoidable (preventable and curable) blindness by 2020

Global Vision 2020 (5 diseases)	Indian Vision 2020 (7 diseases)
Cataract	Cataract
Refractive errors and low vision	Refractive errors and low vision
Childhood blindness	Childhood blindness
Trachoma	Trachoma (Focal)
Onchocerciasis	Glaucoma
	Diabetic retinopathy
	Corneal blindness

ALSO REMEMBER
- India was the 'first country in the world to launch the National Programme for Control of Blindness' in 1976 with the goal of reducing the prevalence of blindness.

566. Ans. (b) Cataract *[Ref. The Principles and Practice of Community Ophthalmology, NPCB, Govt. of India, 2002; p36]*

ALSO REMEMBER
- WHO defines Blindness as 'visual acuity of <3/60 in better eye with best possible correction'
- National Programme for Control of Blindness (NPCB), India defines Blindness as 'visual acuity of <3/60 in better eye with best possible correction' [NEW GUIDELINES 2017-2018]
- *American Medical Association definition of blindness:* 'Central visual acuity of 20/200 or less in the better eye with corrective glasses' (or central visual acuity of more than 20/200 if there is a visual field defect in which the peripheral field is contracted to such an extent that the widest diameter of the visual field subtends an angular distance less than 20 degrees in the better eye)
- *Goal for Blindness in National Health Policy (NHP) 2002:* Reduce prevalence of Blindness to 0.5% by 2010
- *International symbol of blindness:* Long white cane.

567. Ans. (a) Jammu and Kashmir *[Ref. The Principles and Practice of Community Ophthalmology, NPCB, Govt. of India, 02; p34]*

- WHO – NPCB SURVEY OF BLINDNESS IN INDIA (1986–89):
- Prevalence of blindness: 1.49%
- Prevalence of one-eyed blindness: 0.8%
- *Economically blind (Visual acuity <6/60 in better eye) in India:* 11.92 million
- *One eye economically blind (Visual acuity <6/60 in worse eye):* 7.12 million
- *Low vision (<6/18 – 6/60 in better eye):* 28.56 million (MCC: Cataract)
- *Highest prevalence of blindness:* Jammu and Kashmir (2800/100,000 population)
- *Lowest prevalence of blindness:* Meghalaya (220/100,000 population)
- *Classification of states based on blindness prevalence:*

Category	% prevalence	States
Low	< 1	Delhi, Himachal Pradesh, Punjab, West Bengal, North East States
Moderate	1 – 1.49	Andhra Pradesh, Assam, Bihar, Gujarat, Haryana, Kerala, Karnataka
High	1.5 – 1.99	Maharashtra, Orissa, Tamil Nadu, Uttar Pradesh
Very high	> 2	Jammu and Kashmir, Madhya Pradesh, Rajasthan

ALSO REMEMBER
- About 80% of blindness is avoidable
- *Legal Blindness:* Visual acuity <3/60 OR Visual field <10° in better eye with best possible correction
- *Work Vision:* <6/60 (Economic Blindness)
- *Walk Vision:* <3/60 (Social Blindness)

568. Ans. (a) Measles; (c) Rubella *[Ref. Park 27/e p164-165]*

- *Severe Measles:* can lead to acute deficiency of Vitamin A, which may lead to:
  - Keratomalacia
  - Blindness from corneal scarring
- *Congenital Rubella:* may lead to
  - Cataract
  - Glaucoma
  - Retinopathy

569. Ans. (b) Underestimation *[Ref. Park 22/e p371, 27/e p457]*

Blindness situation in India:
- Estimated prevalence of Blindness in India (Total): 11.2 per 1000 population
- Estimated prevalence of Blindness in India (0-14 years): 0.1 per 1000 population
- Estimated prevalence of Blindness in India (15-49 years): 0.6 per 1000 population
- Estimated prevalence of Blindness in India (50+ years): 77.3 per 1000 population

  So if Schools are used where only refractive errors generally constitute blindness (that too very few are actually blind i.e. <3/60) AS COMPARED TO POPULATION (where age-related cataract constitute as major cause of blindness), it would lead to underestimation of prevalence of blindness in the country

570. Ans. (d) 0.75 *[Ref. Disability Guidelines, Office of the Commissioner for Persons with Disabilities p13]*

571. **Ans. (c) Cataract, Refractive error, Glaucoma, Corneal opacity** [Ref. Park 27/e p457]

CAUSES OF BLINDNESS IN INDIA
- Cataract (62.6%)
- Refractive error (19.7%)
- Other causes: Glaucoma > Posterior segment pathology > Corneal opacity > Surgical complications > Posterior capsular opacification

572. **Ans. (d) Retinal dystrophies** [Ref. Lecture Notes Ophthalmology by James 1/e p185]

Avoidable Causes of Blindness
- Preventable causes: Vitamin A deficiency, Trachoma, Onchocerciasis
- Treatable causes: Cataract, Refractive errors, Glaucoma

Review Questions

573. **Ans. (a) 3/60** [Ref. Park 27/e p456]
574. **Ans. (d) Refraction error** [Ref. Park 27/e p457]
575. **Ans. (c) Vit. A deficiency** [Ref. Park 27/e p457]

MISCELLANEOUS (NON COMMUNICABLE DISEASES)

576. **Ans. (b) Psychological; (d) Therapeutic** [Ref. WHO STEPwise Approach]
- STEPwise approach to surveillance (STEPS) is a simple, standardized method by WHO for surveillance. It is of two types:
  - STEPwise approach to chronic disease risk factor surveillance
  - STEPwise approach to Stroke surveillance
- Comprises of 3 steps:
  - STEP 1: Behavioural measurements
  - STEP 2: Physical measurements
  - STEP 3: Biochemical measurements

577. **Ans. (d) Risk factor intervention trials** [Ref. Park 27/e p423-424]

- **WIDELY REPORTED RISK FACTOR INTERVENTION TRIALS:**
- Stanford-three-community study:
  - *Aim:* To determine if community health education can reduce the risk of cardiovascular diseases
  - *Results:* Reduction seen 23 – 28%
- The North Kerelia project:
  - *Aims:* To reduce cardiovascular risk factor levels and to promote early diagnosis, treatment and rehabilitation of patients
  - *Results:* Reduction seen in CHD deaths in 10 years
- Multiple risk factor intervention trial (MRFIT):
  - *Aims:* To reduce cardiovascular risk factor levels (smoking, high BP, hypercholesterolemia)
  - *Results:* Non-significant reduction in reduction seen in CHD deaths in 10 years
  - *Interpretation:* Control group was not properly chosen (changed habits and lifestyle to an extent not anticipated by designers of trial)
- Oslow diet/smoking intervention study:
  - *Aim:* To determine if serum lipids lowering and smoking-cessation would reduce incidence of first attack of CHD in 40-50 yrs males
  - *Results:* Reduction of MI by 47%
  - *Importance:* With this study, primary prevention of CHD entered practical field of preventive medicine in an impressive manner.
- Lipid Research Clinics study:
  - *Aim:* To determine if reducing serum cholesterol (using cholestyramine) would prevent CHD events
  - *Results:* 8.5% reduction in total cholesterol, 12.6% reduction in LDL-cholesterol; 24% reduction in CHD and 19% reduction in non-fatal MI

578. **Ans. (a) Cerebral thrombosis** [Ref. Park 27/e p431]
- **STROKE (APOPLEXY):**
- *WHO definition:* Rapidly developing clinical signs of local (or global) cerebral dysfunction, lasting more than 24 hours or leading to death, with no apparent cause other than vascular origin
  - 24 hour threshold EXCLUDES transient ischemic attacks (TIA)
- *WHO definition:* Rapidly developing clinical signs of local (or global) cerebral dysfunction, lasting more than 24 hours or leading to death, with no apparent cause other than vascular origin
- *Causes of stroke:*
  - Cerebral thrombosis (MCC of stroke or apoplexy)
  - Cerebral hemorrhage
  - Subarachnoid hemorrhage
  - Cerebral embolism

579. **Ans. (a) Well-defined etiological agent** [Ref. Park 27/e p415]
- *Gaps in natural history of non-communicable diseases:*
  - Absence of a known agent
  - Multifactorial causation
  - Long latent period
  - Indefinite onset

> **ALSO REMEMBER**
> - *6 key sets of risk factors for non communicable diseases:*
>   - Cigarette use and other forms of smoking
>   - Alcohol abuse
>   - Failure/inability to obtain preventive health services
>   - Lifestyle changes (dietary patterns, physical activity)
>   - Environmental risk factors
>   - Stress factors
> - *Chronic diseases:* Comprises of all impairments or deviations from normal, which have one or more of the following characteristics:
>   - Are permanent
>   - Leave residual disability
>   - Are caused by non-reversible pathological alteration
>   - Require special training of patient for rehabilitation
>   - May be expected to require a long period of supervision, observation or care

580. **Ans. (a) Shift the population curve of risk factors by a population based approach** [Ref. Park 27/e p416]

581. **Ans. (b) Non-communicable diseases** [Ref. World Health Organisation]
    - *STEP wise approach to surveillance (STEPS):* Is a simple, standardized method by WHO for surveillance
    - Is of two types
    - STEP wise approach to chronic disease risk factor surveillance
    - STEP wise approach to Stroke surveillance
    - *Comprises of 3 steps:*

STEPS	CORE	EXPANDED
STEP 1	Tobacco use	Tobacco use
Behavioural measurements	Alcohol consumption	Alcohol consumption
	Diet	Diet
	Physical activity	Physical activity
	History of raisesd BP	History of raised BP
	History of dibetes	History of diabetes
STEP 2	Height and weight	Hip circumference and Heart rate
Physical measurements	Waist BP	
STEP 3	Blood glucose	Triglycerides and HDL choleterol
Biochemical measurement	Blood lipids	

582. **Ans. (b) TB** [Ref. Textbook of Community Medicine by Sunder Lal, 2/e p419, 591, 612]
    - TB in India (National TB Survey, ICMR 1955-58):
    - Rural population suffered as equally as urban population
    - Elderly suffered more than young ones
    - Mental illness in India
    - Prevalence rates are significantly higher in urban areas (Except for epilepsy and hysteria)
    - *Bronchitis and Lung Cancer in India:* Is more common in Urban areas.

583. **Ans. (b) FBS >125 mg/dL and PPBS >199 mg/dL** [WHO Guidelines]

    WHO GUIDELINES FOR DIAGNOSIS OF DIABETES MELLITUS
    - *Fasting plasma glucose level:* >126 mg/dL (>7 mmol/L)
    - *2-hour venous plasma glucose in Glucose tolerance test:* > 200 mg/dL (>11.1 mmol/L)
    - *Casual plasma glucose:* >200 mg/dL (>11.1 mmol/L)
    - *Glycated haemoglobin:* >6.5%

584. **Ans. ALL CHOICES** [Ref. Park 27/e p462-463]
    - *Accidents and injuries in India (in order of decreasing numbers):*
      – Road traffic accidents
      – Work related injuries
      – Burns
      – Violence, suicide
      – Poisoning
      – Drowning

585. **Ans. (b) Road traffic accident** [Ref. Park 27/e p463]

586. **Ans. (b) Fasting blood sugar** [Ref. Oxford Desk Reference OBG by Arulkumaran, 1/e, p201]

587. **Ans. (b) 10.6 per 100,000 population** [Ref. Accidental Deaths and Suicides in India 2014, National Crime Records Bureau, Ministry of Home Affairs, GOI p192]

    SUICIDES IN INDIA
    - *Suicide rate in India:* 10.6 per Lac population
    - *Highest number of Suicides:* Maharashtra
    - *Highest Suicide rate:* Puducherry > Sikkim
    - *Lowest Suicide rate:* Nagaland
    - *MC cause of Suicides:* Other family problems > Illness
    - *MC age group in Suicides:* 18-30 years (Males: Females = 2:1)
    - *MC mode of Suicides:* Hanging (> Self-poisoning > Self-immolation > Drowning)

588. **Ans. (d) Hanging** [Ref. Accidental Deaths and Suicides in India 2014, National Crime Records Bureau, Ministry of Home Affairs, GOI p207]

589. **Ans. (d) Injury prevention** [Ref. Textbook of Public Health and Community Medicine by Bhalwar, 1/e p1243]

    THE HADDON MATRIX
    - *Description:* One of the most successful theoretical approaches to injury prevention, developed by Dr William Haddon in the 1970s
    - *Principles of injury prevention based on the Haddon's Matrix:*
      – To reduce exposure to risk
      – To prevent road traffic crashes from occurring
      – To reduce the severity of injury in the event of crash
      – To reduce the consequences of injury through improved post-collision care
    - Haddon Matrix divides the timing of the injury event into three phases
      – Pre-injury phase: Goal is to eliminate any energy transfer to the host (Primary prevention)
      – Injury phase: Goal is to eliminate/reduce the amount of energy absorbed by the host once an energy transfer has occurred (Secondary prevention)
      – Post-injury phase: Introduces value criteria to consider when choosing an intervention strategy

Phase	Human Factors	Vector (Vehicles)	Physical environment	Socioeconomic environment
Pre-injury	Alcohol Intoxication	Instability in utility vehicles	Poor visibility of road hazards	Lack of knowledge regarding injury risks
Injury	Low resistance to energy	Sharp or pointed edges/ surfaces	Flammable building materials	Lack of enforcement of safety belt legislation
Post-injury	Conditions affecting energy tolerance	Rapidity of energy reduction	Emergency medical response	Lack of funding for emergency medical Services and rehabilitation services

590. Ans. (c) Ulcerative colitis [Ref. The Health Benefits of Tobacco by Douglass 1/e p24]

SMOKING IS PREVENTIVE FOR
- Ulcerative colitis
- Alzheimer's disease
- Parkinson's disease

591. Ans. (d) 7–8.5% [Ref. Diabetes - Clinician's Desk Reference by Leslie, 1/e p12]

Diabetes in India
- In 2008, an estimated 347 million people in the world had diabetes and the prevalence is growing, particularly in low- and middle-income countries
- India had 69.2 million people living with diabetes (8.7%) as per the 2015 data
- Of these, it remained undiagnosed in more than 36 million people

592. Ans. (b) 30 days [Ref. Road Safety Annual Report 2017 p12]

Road Fatality
- After 2005, person who died within 30 days of a road crash
- Before 2005, fatalities were counted within six days
- For international comparisons, a correction factor of 1.069 is applied for the years before 2005

593. Ans. (c) Venous blood fasting sugar 120 to 200 mg/100 mL [Ref. Park 27/e p450]

WHO Diagnostic Criteria for Diabetes Mellitus

	Cut-off (mmol/L)	Cut-off (mg/dL)
Diabetes		
Fasting plasma glucose	≥7 mmol/L	≥126 mg/dL
2-hour plasma glucose	>11.1 mmol/L	>200 mg/dL
Impaired glucose tolerance		
Fasting plasma glucose	<7 mmol/L	<126 mg/dL
2-hour plasma glucose	7.8–11.1 mmol/L	140–200 mg/dL
Impaired fasting glucose		
Fasting plasma glucose	6.1–6.9 mmol/L	110–125 mg/dL
2-hour plasma glucose	<7.8 mmol/L	<140 mg/dL

(Venous plasma glucose after 75 grams oral glucose load)

594. Ans. (b) 25% [Ref. Park 27/e p416]
WHO Global Action Plan for Prevention and Control of Non-communicable Diseases 2013-2020

GLOBAL ACTION PLAN FOR THE PREVENTION AND CONTROL OF NONCOMMUNICABLE DISEASES 2013–2020
- Vision: A world free of the avoidable burden of non-communicable diseases.
- Goal: To reduce the preventable and avoidable burden of morbidity, mortality and disability due to NCDs
- Voluntary global targets:
  - 25% relative reduction in the overall mortality from cardiovascular diseases, cancer, diabetes, or chronic respiratory diseases
  - ≥ 10% relative reduction in the harmful use of alcohol, as appropriate, within the national context
  - 10% relative reduction in prevalence of insufficient physical activity
  - 30% relative reduction in mean population intake of salt/sodium
  - 30% relative reduction in prevalence of current tobacco use in persons aged 15+ years
  - 25% relative reduction in the prevalence of raised blood pressure or contain the prevalence of raised blood pressure, according to national circumstances
  - Halt the rise in diabetes and obesity
  - ≥ 50% of eligible people receive drug therapy and counselling (including glycaemic control) to prevent heart attacks and strokes
  - 80% availability of the affordable basic technologies and essential medicines, including generics, required to treat major NCDs diseases in both public and private facilities

595. Ans. (b) 1 [Ref. Advanced Human Nutrition by Medeiros 4/e p74]
- Glycemic response (GR) of a food is a measure of that food's ability to raise blood sugar
- Glycemic index scale is 0 to 100 when using glucose as the standard.

Review Questions

596. Ans. (d) Congenital [Ref. Park 27/e p417-418]
597. Ans. (d) Screening for hypertension [Ref. Park 27/e p422]
598. Ans. (d) High intake of vitamin-A [Ref. Park 27/e p448-449]
599. Ans. (b) Coronary heart disease [Ref. Park 27/e p424]
600. Ans. (c) 3 months [Ref. Park 27/e p450]

CHAPTER 6: National Health Programmes, Policies and Legislations in India

SOME IMPORTANT HEALTH PROGRAMMES OF INDIA

Refer to Annexure 6

NATIONAL TB ELIMINATION PROGRAM (NTEP) 2020

Timeline of TB Programs in India
- *1962:* National TB Control Program (NTP) launched [Strategy: BCG vaccination, TB treatment]
- *1992–93:* Revised National TB Control Program (RNTCP) launched [Strategy: DOTS]
- *01 January 2020:* National TB Elimination Program (NTEP) launched

Estimates of TB Burden in India (2018)
- *Incidence TB cases:* 2.7 million (27% of Global)
- *Mortality of TB:* 4,40,000 (31% of Global)
- *Incidence HIV-TB:* 92,000 (9% of Global)
- *Mortality of HIV-TB:* 9,700 (4% of Global)
- *MDR-TB:* 130,000 (24% of Global)
- *Children with TB:* 342,000 (31% of Global)

National Strategic Plan (NSP) - TB 2017–25
- *VISION:* TB-Free India with zero deaths, disease and poverty due to TB
- *GOAL:* To achieve a rapid decline in burden of TB, morbidity and mortality while working towards elimination of TB in India by 2025
- NSP sets out the strategic direction and key initiatives that the MoHFW will undertake from 2017–25 for working towards achieving the goals of eliminating TB by 2025 (Achieve SDG and End TB targets for India)
- *Approach:* 'DETECT-TREAT-PREVENT-BUILD' approach
- *Strategic Focus Areas:*
  - Early diagnosis of all the TB patients
  - Prompt treatment with the right drugs and regimens
  - Patient financial and nutritional support
  - Active case finding
  - Contact tracing
  - LTBI management in high risk population
  - Airborne infection control

Vision and Goal of NTEP
- *Vision:* TB-Free India with zero deaths, disease and poverty due to TB
- Goal: To achieve a rapid decline in burden of TB, morbidity and mortality while working towards *"Elimination of TB in India by 2025"*
- Four Pillars: Build (strengthen sustain policies), Prevent, Detect, Treat

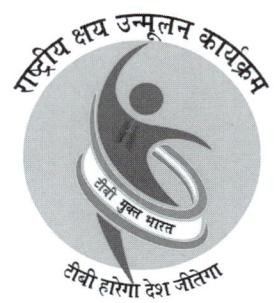

Definitions under NTEP

1. Presumptive TB Case Definitions
- *Presumptive Pulmonary TB:* A person with any of the symptoms and signs suggestive of TB, including: cough for 2 weeks or more, fever for 2 weeks or more, significant weight loss, haemoptysis, any abnormality in chest radiograph
- *Presumptive Paediatric TB:* A child with persistent fever and/or cough for 2 weeks or more, loss of weight/no weight gain and/or history of contact with infectious TB cases
    - *Weight criteria:* History of unexplained weight loss or no weight gain in past 3 months; loss of weight is defined as loss of >5% body weight as compared to highest weight recorded in last 3 months
    - In a symptomatic child, contact with a person with any form of active TB within last 2 years may be significant
- *Presumptive DR TB:* Patient who is eligible for Rifampicin resistant screening at the time of diagnosis or/and during the course of treatment for DS TB or H mono/poly. This includes following patients:
    - All Notified TB patients (Public and private)
    - Follow-up positive on microscopy including treatment failures on standard first line treatment and all oral H mono/poly regimen
    - Any clinical non-responder including paediatric (if specimen available)

2. Identification of Presumptive TB Patient
- *Active Case Finding:* When the Community health workers seeks for TB symptoms among the vulnerable key population
- *Passive Case Finding:* When the Patient Voluntarily reports symptoms to the Medical Officer
- *Intensified Case Findings:* When the Medical Officer searches for TB symptoms among the individual seeking care in the health facility e.g., ART Centre, Diabetic Clinics, NCD Clinics

3. Case Definitions
- *Microbiologically confirmed TB:* Microbiologically confirmed TB refers to a presumptive TB case from whom a biological specimen is positive for acid fast bacilli, or positive for Mycobacterium tuberculosis on culture, or positive for TB through Rapid Diagnostic molecular test
- *Clinically Diagnosed TB:* A clinically diagnosed TB refers to a presumptive TB case who is not microbiologically confirmed, but has been diagnosed with active TB by a clinician on the basis of X-ray abnormalities, histopathology or clinical signs with a decision to treat the patient with a full course of Anti-TB treatment

Diagnosis of TB under NTEP

- Diagnostic Tools for Microbiological confirmation of TB
    - *Sputum Smear Microscopy (for AFB):* Ziehl-Neelsen Staining, Fluorescence staining
    - *Culture:* Solid (Lowenstein Jensen) media, Automated Liquid culture systems (BACTEC MGIT 960, BacT Alert or Versatrek)
    - *Drug Sensitivity Testing:* Modified Proportionate Sensitivity Testing (PST) for MGIT 960 system, Economic variant of Proportion sensitivity testing (1%) using LJ medium
    - *Rapid molecular diagnostic tests:* Line Probe Assay (LPA) (MTB complex and detection of RIF & INH resistance and FQ and SLI resistance), Nucleic Acid Amplification Test (NAAT) (CBNAAT/TrueNat)
    - *Other tests:* Radiography, LF-LAM (Lateral Flow Urine Lipo Arabino Mannan for TB in HIV diagnosis), c-TB (Antigen used ESTA6, CFP10 for Skin testing in Latent TB diagnosis)
    - Serology is banned in India for TB diagnosis

- Diagnostic Algorithm for Adult Pulmonary TB (PTB)

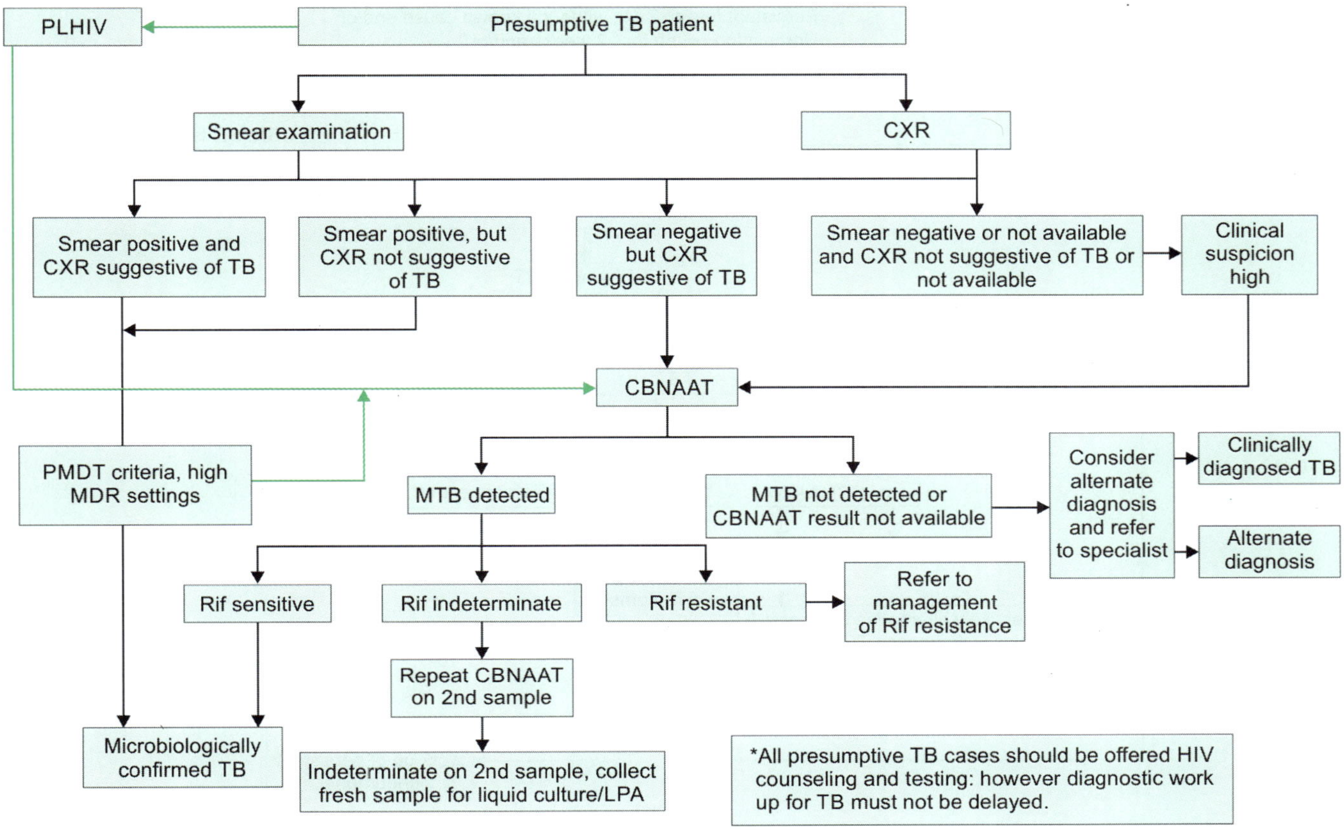

- Diagnostic Algorithm for Adult Extra Pulmonary TB (EPTB)

Diagnostic algorithm for extra pulmonary TB

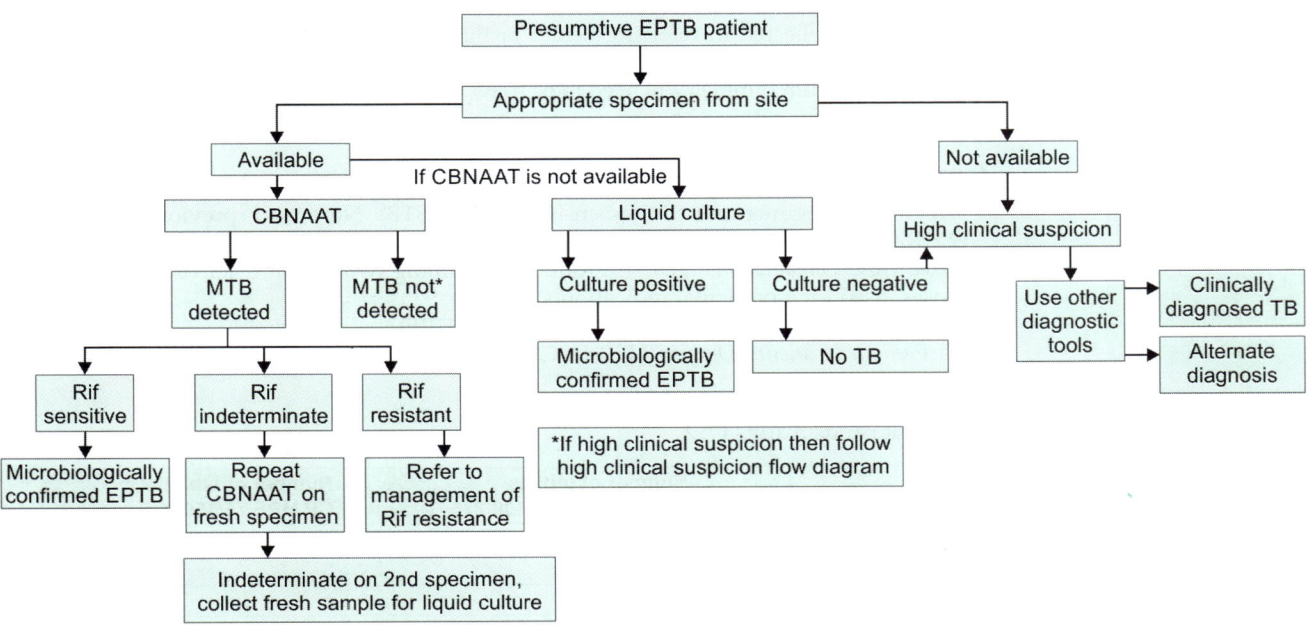

- Diagnostic Algorithm for Paediatric Pulmonary TB (PTB)

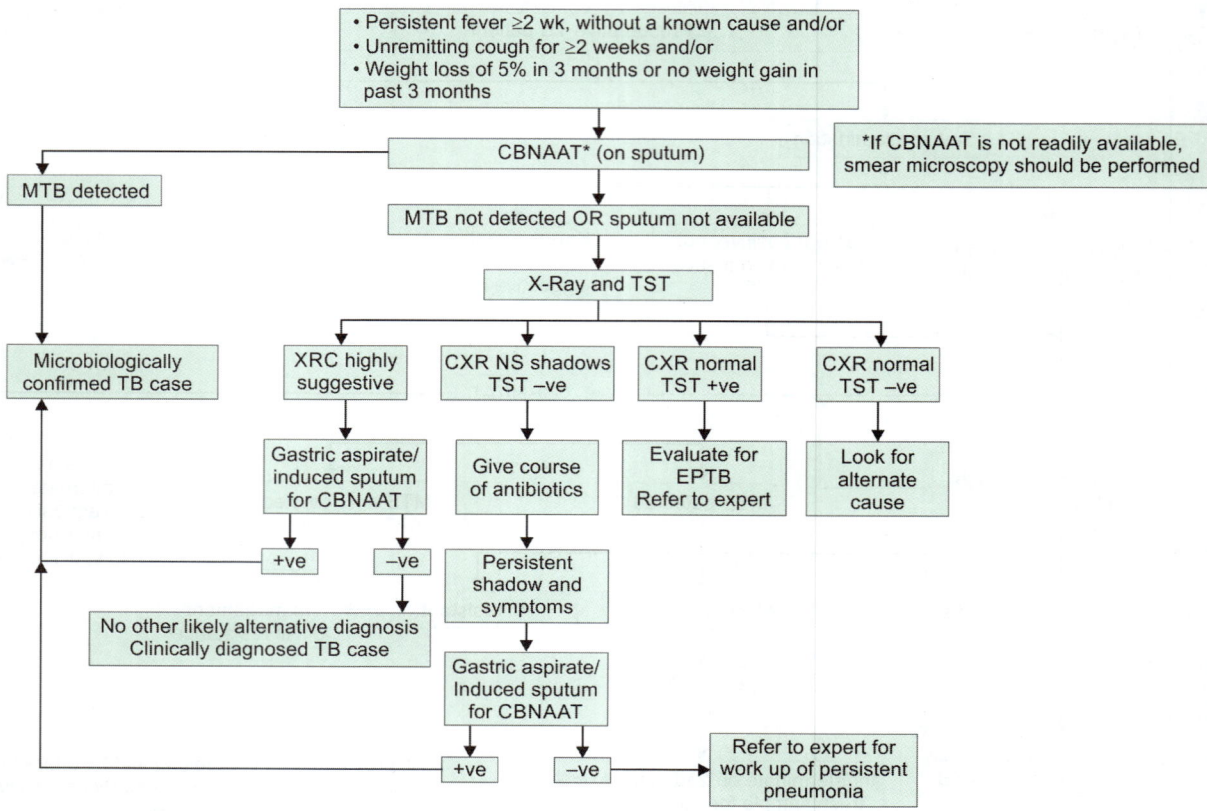

- Sputum Smear Collection under NTEP
    - For the diagnosis of tuberculosis, the two specimens of a patient i.e., "SPOT" and the other an early "MORNING" sample are collected
    - Sputum samples are collected in
    - Sputum collected in referring health facilities should be transported to the nearest DMC within 2 days
    - Fresh sputum samples will need to be transported from the DMC to the CBNAAT laboratory in cool chain within 72 hours

Treatment of TB under NTEP

- Treatment Regimen for Drug-Sensitive TB (DSTB) New and previously treated cases: 2 HRZE (IP 56 doses) + 4HRE (CP 112 doses)
- *Fixed Dose Combinations (FDCs):* Products containing two or more active ingredients in fixed doses, used for a particular indication(s)
    - *Adults:* 4-FDC (IP – HRZE) and 3-FDC (CP – HRE)
    - *Paediatric patients:* Dispersible 3-FDC (HRZ) and Dispersible 2-FDC (HR)

1. Weight Bands Based Treatment
- Weight bands Adults FIVE:

Weight category	Number of tablets IP HRZE 75/150/400/275	Number of tablets CP HRE 75/150/275
25–34 kg	2	2
35–49 kg	3	3
50–64 kg	4	4
65–75 kg	5	5
>75 kg	6	6

(IP: Intensive phase; CP: Continuation phase)

- Weight bands Paediatrics SIX:

Weight category	Number of tablets IP HRZ 50/75/150	Number of tablets IP E 100	Number of tablets CP HR 50/75	Number of tablets CP E 100
4–7 kg	1	1	1	1
8–11 kg	2	2	2	2
12–15 kg	3	3	3	3
16–24 kg	4	4	4	4
25–29 kg	3 + 1A*	3	3 + 1A*	3
30–39 kg	2 + 2A*	2	2 + 2A*	2

(IP: Intensive phase; CP: Continuation phase)

2. Long term Follow-up
- After completion of treatment, the patients should be followed up clinically at the end of 6, 12, 18 & 24 months.

3. Treatment under HIV-TB
- First Line ART for HIV-TB: TENOFOVIR 300 mg + LAMIVUDINE 300 mg + EFAVIRENZ 600 mg (FDC)
- Second Line ART for HIV-TB: Regimens available under NACP
    - Tenofovir + Lamivudine + PI (Atazanavir/ritonavir or Lopinavir/Ritonavir)
    - Zidovudine + Lamivudine+ PI (Atazanavir/ritonavir or Lopinavir/Ritonavir)
    - Stavudine+ Lamivudine + PI (Atazanavir/ritonavir or Lopinavir/Ritonavir)
    - Abacavir+ Lamivudine+ PI (Atazanavir/ritonavir or Lopinavir/Ritonavir)

INH Preventive Therapy

1. INH Preventive Therapy in Children
- Children <6 years of age in close contact (But TB excluded)
- HIV infected children who either had a known exposure to an infectious TB case or are Tuberculin skin test (TST) positive (>=5mm induration) but have no active TB disease
- All TST positive children who are receiving immunosuppressive therapy (e.g., Childrenwith nephrotic syndrome, acute leukaemia, etc.)
- A child born to mother who was diagnosed to have TB in pregnancy provided congenital TB has been ruled out

2. INH Preventive Therapy in Adults
- Adults and adolescents living with HIV unlikely to have active TB
- Children living with HIV who do not have poor weight gain, fever or current cough unlikely to have active TB
- Children living with HIV if evaluation shows no TB

3. Dose of IPT Used under NTEP
- *Adult and Adolescent:* Isoniazid 300 mg + Pyridoxine 50 mg per day × 6 months
- *Children above 12 months:* Isoniazid 10 mg/kg + Pyridoxine 25 mg per day × 6 months

NIKSHAY FLOW

- *Nikshay Entry:* Once the treatment regimen is finalized, all patients will be initiated on treatment after opening of the treatment card and entries are done in Nikshay
- *Patient flow in Nikshay:*
    - *Nikshay 1:* Initiating the patient on appropriate treatment regimen
    - *Nikshay 2:* Transfer/referral flow after initiation of treatment
    - *Nikshay 3:* Nikshay Aushadhi

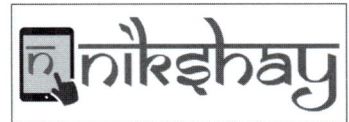

NIKSHAY MITRA INITIATIVE

- NMI is a part of Pradhan Mantri TB Mukt Bharat Abhiyaan launched by The President of India on September 9, 2022

- Nikshay Mitra is a government project that enables people to adopt tuberculosis patients and take care of their nutritional and medical requirement, with an aim to combat stigma associated with the disease
- Nikshay Mitra has a number of choices for help, including dietary, diagnostic, occupational, and supplementary nutritional supplements. In addition, they can select a support period of one to three years. They can select the state, district, building, and medical facilities. The district TB officer will make it easier to become Nikshay Mitra.
- *Objectives of the Initiative:*
  - Provide additional patient support to improve treatment outcomes of TB patients
  - Augment community involvement in meeting India's commitment to end TB by 2025
  - Leverage Corporate Social Responsibility (CSR) activities
- Additional assistance that may be provided by the Nikshay Mitra to on-treatment TB patients: Nutritional support, Additional investigations for the diagnosed TB patients, Vocational support, Additional nutritional supplements

Organisational Structure for NTEP

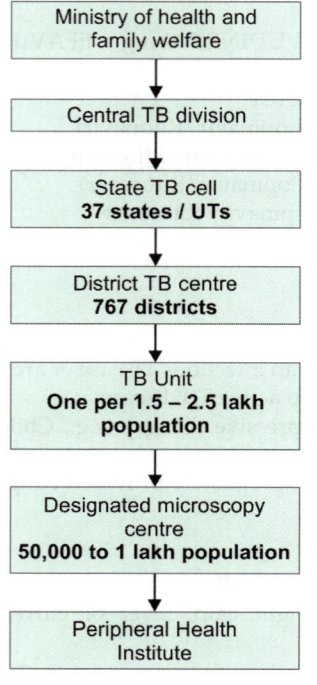

Supporting facilities
- National Institutes (3)
- National Reference Laboratories (6)
- Intermediate Reference Laboratories (29)
- State TB Training and Demonstration Centre (26)
- Culture and DST Laboratories (42)
- Nodal DR-TB Centre (154)
- CBNAAT Laboratories (1180)

Must Know Facts About NTEP

- Nikshay Poshan Yojana:
  - Financial incentive of Rs 500/- per month for each notified TB patient for duration for which the patient is on anti-TB treatment
  - All TB patients notified on or after 1st April 2018 including all existing TB patients under treatment are eligible to receive incentive
- All TB patients who have been diagnosed and registered under NTEP will be referred for screening for Diabetes
- Two new drugs named Bedaquiline and Delamanid with anti-TB effect were approved for treatment of multidrug resistant TB by The Central Drugs Standard Control Organization (CDSCO)

REVISED NATIONAL TB CONTROL PROGRAMME

Epidemiology of Tuberculosis in India

- *ARI (India):* 1–2% (average ARI = 1.7%)
- For every 1% rise of ARI, there are 50 SS +ve cases/lac population[Q]

Key points

For every 1% rise of ARI, there are 50 SS +ve cases/lac population[Q].

Index	Situation in India	Remark
Incidence of Infection	1–2% (~1.7%)	ARI – Tuberculin Conversion Index^Q
Prevalence of Infection^Q	40%	Standard Tuberculin Test^Q
Incidence of Disease	1.7 per 1000	New cases^Q
Prevalence of Disease	0.2%	All cases

> **Key points**
> ARI – Tuberculin Conversion Index^Q.

Key Notable Points regarding Tuberculosis

- Every TB sputum positive patient can infect up to 10–15 individuals in a year^Q
  - *Without treatment, 50% of TB patients will die, 25% will remain healthy and 25% will develop chronic infectious TB.*
- TB is 'Barometer of Social Welfare in India'^{Q}
- TB (AFB) Bacillus discovered by: Robert Koch^Q
  - *TB Bacilli are alcohol and acid fast^Q*
  - *Generation time of TB bacilli:* 20 hours^Q
  - *TB bacteria remain alive:* in sputum for 1 day and in droplet nuclei for 10 days^Q
- *Diagnosis in RNTCP:* Ziehl-Neelsen Staining^Q
- *World TB Day:* 24th March^Q
- TB was declared as *'Global emergency in 1983'* by WHO^Q
- TB is the MC Opportunistic Infection (OI) in HIV in India^Q
- *Elimination level for Tuberculosis (WHO and STOP TB Strategy)*^{Q}: <1 case per million population (to eliminate TB as a public health problem)
- *TB Institutes of importance in India*:
  - National Tuberculosis Institute (NTI) – Bengaluru^Q
  - Tuberculosis Research Centre – Chennai
  - LRS Institute of TB and Respiratory Diseases – New Delhi

> **Key points**
> **World TB Day:** 24th March.

> **Key points**
> **National Tuberculosis Institute (NTI)** – Bengaluru.

Annual Risk of Infection (ARI)

- *Definition*: Is the proportion of population which will be primarily infected with tuberculosis in course of 1 year
- *Public health importance*:
  - Is incidence of infection of TB
  - Is known as 'Tuberculin Conversion Index'^{Q}
  - Best indicator of trend of TB unaffected by current control measures^Q
  - Most informative index of magnitude of problem of TB^Q.

Zeihl Neelsen (ZN) Staining

- *Importance:* Sputum smear of a suspected TB patient is used for the diagnosis
- *Decolourizer:* 25% sulphuric acid^Q
- *Acid Fast Bacilli (AFB) of TB^Q:* 'Rod shaped' with 'beaded appearance' (Beads: Mycolic Acid^Q)
  - Minimum bacillary load for a positive result: >10,000 bacilli per mL sputum^Q
  - Results of ZN staining: Minimum 100 fields examined^Q

Grading of smears	Criterion
0	No bacilli per 100 oil immersion fields
Scanty	1–9 bacilli per 100 oil immersion fields
1+ grading	10–99 bacilli per 100 oil immersion fields
2+ grading	1–10 bacilli per oil immersion field
3+ grading	>10 bacilli per oil immersion field

Directly Observed Treatment Short Course (DOTS)

- *Description:* Is a community based Tuberculosis treatment and care strategy which combines the benefit of supervised treatment with community based care and support.

- Success of DOTS depend upon 5 componentsQ: [**Mnemonic: A G**ood **P**olitician **U**nderstands **D**evelopment]
    - **A**ccountability
    - **G**ood quality sputum microscopy
    - **P**olitical commitment
    - **U**ninterrupted supply of good quality drugs
    - **D**irectly observed treatment
- *Ensures high cure rates through 3 components:*
    - Appropriate medical treatment
    - Supervision and motivation by a health/non-health personnel
    - Monitoring of disease by health services
- DOTS is given by peripheral health staff – 'DOTS Agents' (MPWs, Voluntary workers like teachers, Anganwadi workers, Dais)
    - Incentive/honorarium paid: 1000/- (Cat I), 1000/- (Cat-II), 5000/-(Resistant patients) per patient completing treatment
- Drugs are supplied in 'patient-wise boxes containing full course of treatment'
    - Intensive phase: Each blister pack has one day's medication
    - Continuation phase: Each blister pack has one week's medication
- *Principles of DOTS administration:*
    - DOTS is directly observed treatment short course chemotherapy^Q
    - In DOTS during the intensive phase of treatment a health worker are other trained person watches as the patients swallows the drugs in his presence
    - During continuation phase the patient is issued medicine for one week in multiblister combipack of which the first dose is swallowed by the patient in the presence of health worker or trained person
    - Consumption of medicine in the continuation phase is also checked by return of empty multiblister combipack when patient come to collect medicine for the next week
    - In this programme alternate day treatment is used
    - Streptomycin is given in category II only
    - In category-1 new sputum smear, positive cases sputum examination is done in 2, 4 and 6 months.

Revised National Tuberculosis Control Programme (RNTCP)

- *Differences in National Tuberculosis Programme (NTP) and RNTCP:*

	NTP, 1962	RNTCP, 1992^Q
Objective	Early diagnosis & treatment	Breaking chain of transmission
Operational targets	Not defined	1. Cure rate >90% 2. Case finding >90%
Strategy	1. SCC supervised 2. Conventional	1. DOTS 2. Uninterrupted drug supply
Diagnosis	More emphasis on X-rays	Mainly sputum microscopy

- *Objectives of RNTCP **(90/90 Objectives)**:*
    - Detection of >90% of all incident TB cases including DR-TB & HIV-TB^Q
    - Successfully treat >90% of new smear positive cases & >85% of all previously treated TB patients^Q
- *History of RNTCP:*
    - RNTCP (based on DOTS strategy), began as a pilot in 1993 and was launched as a national programme in 1997
    - By 24th March 2006, the entire country was covered under DOTS
- *Infrastructure:*
    - The RNTCP designated 'Microscopy Centre' is established for approx. 100,000 population^Q (50,000 in hilly and mountainous areas)
    - Senior TB Laboratory Supervisor (STLS) is one for every 5 microscopy centres
        - 1 STLS per 5 lac population^Q
        - STLS rechecks all +ve slides and 10% of all –ve slides

Key points

Objectives of RNTCP^Q:
- To achieve a cure rate of atleast 90%.
- To achieve a case detection rate of 90%.

- *Diagnosis in RNTCP:*
  - In RNTCP, mainstay of diagnosis is Sputum microscopy; the sputum smears are stained for acid fast Bacilli (AFB) with 'Ziehl-Neelsen (ZN) Stain'
  - *Decolorizer:* 25% sulphuric acid
  - *Counter-stainQ:* 0.1% Loeffler's methylene blue (or 1% picric acid or 0.2% malachite green).

AFB Sputum Smears (SS) for Diagnosis of a Case of TB [New Guidelines]

- *Tuberculosis suspect:* A person with productive cough >2 weeks with or without hemoptysis, fever for >2 weeks, chest pain, weight loss, night sweats, and loss of appetite is subjected to 2 SS examinations
- Number of specimen(s) required for diagnosis of smear positive pulmonary Tuberculosis: TWO^Q
  - '2 sputum smears' over 2 days period:
    - *Spot Sample* (Day 1)
    - *Morning Sample* (Day 2)
- Chances of detecting smear positive cases:
  - With 1 Sample: 80%
  - With 2 Sample: 93%

  New Treatment Guidelines, See Annexure 8.

> **Key points**
> 1 STLS per 5 lac population.

Daily Self-administered Non-DOTS Regimes^Q [New Guidelines]

- *Indication:* ONLY if there are adverse reactions to drugs or patients compliance is not possible

Non-DOTS regime 1 (ND1) Pulmonary (SS+ve) seriously ill Extra-pulmonary seriously ill	2 (SHE) + 10 (HE)
Non-DOTS regime 2 (ND2) Pulmonary (SS–ve) not seriously ill Extra-pulmonary not seriously ill	12 (HE)

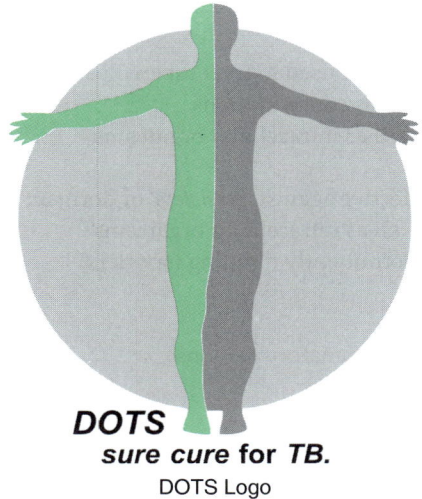

DOTS sure cure for TB.
DOTS Logo

Drug Resistance in TB

- *Primary (Initial) Resistance:* When a person contract infection from a person with resistant bacilli of TB
- *Secondary (Acquired) Resistance:* Resistance developing during the course of treatment for TB
- *Multidrug Resistant TB (MDR–TB)^Q:* Resistance to Isoniazid and Rifampicin 'with or without resistance to other drugs'
  - *Treatment of MDR-TB^Q:*
    - DOTS PLUS (Category IV)
    - Must be done on basis of sensitivity testing

> **Key points**
> **Treatment of MDR-TB^Q:**
> DOTS PLUS (Category IV)

- Directly observed therapy certainly helps to improve outcomes and is considered an integral part of MDR-TB treatment
- *Extensive Drug Resistant TB (XDR–TB)^Q:* Resistance to rifampicin and isoniazid AND to any member of the quinolone family AND to one of the injectable second-line drugs (kanamycin, capreomycin, or amikacin)
    - XDR–TB is MDR TB with further resistance to 3–6 classes of second line drugs (Older definition^Q)
    - Principles of treatment for MDR-TB and for XDR-TB are same
    - XDR-TB does not transmit easily in healthy populations, yet is capable of causing *'epidemics in populations which are already stricken by HIV'*
- *Drug Resistance (TB) in India:*

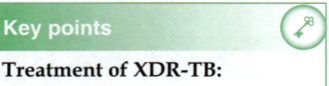

Key points

Treatment of XDR-TB: Category V

Primary drug resistance	3–13%
INH	11–22%
Rifampicin	0–12%
Acquired drug resistance	
INH	34–67%
Rifampicin	0–53%
MDR – TB^Q	3–42%

Antitubercular Drugs

Bactericidal drugs^Q	Bacteriostatic drugs^Q
Isoniazid Rifampicin Streptomycin Pyrazinamide	Ethambutol
Ciprofloxacin Ofloxacin Kanamycin	Thiacetazone Cycloserine PAS Ethionamide

- *Isoniazid:*
    - First effective bactericidal drug used to treat tuberculosis
    - May be bacteriostatic at lower concentrations
    - Acts on extracellular as well as intracellular organisms
- *Rifampicin:*
    - Only bactericidal drug effective against *'persisters'* or dormant bacilli in solid caseous lesions^Q
    - Acts on extracellular as well as intracellular organisms^Q
    - Acts best on slowly or intermittently dividing (spurters)^Q
- *Pyrazinamide:*
    - Acts on intracellular bacilli
    - Acts on bacilli at sites of inflammatory response

Dosages of Antitubercular Drugs

Drugs	Daily therapy^Q	Thrice weekly therapy^Q
Isoniazid	5 mg/kg	10–15 mg/kg
Rifampicin	10 mg/kg	10 mg/kg
Pyrazinamide	25 mg/kg	35 mg/kg
Streptomycin	15 mg/kg	15 mg/kg
Ethambutol	15 mg/kg	30 mg/kg

Important Facts of Antitubercular Drugs

- *Most effective anti-tubercular drug:* Rifampicin^Q
- *Most bactericidal antitubercular drug:* Rifampicin^Q

- *Most toxic antitubercular drug:* Isoniazid
- *Antitubercular drug causing rapid sputum conversion:* Rifampicin
- *Antitubercular drug causing orange discoloration of urine:* Rifampicin^Q
- *Antitubercular drug first to develop resistance:* Isoniazid^Q
- *Antitubercular drug contraindicated AIDS patients on Protease Inhibitors:* Rifampicin^Q
- *Antitubercular drug contraindicated in HIV:* Thiacetazone^Q (Exfoliative dermatitis)
- *Antitubercular drugs contained in all phases of all categories of DOTS:* Rifampicin and Isoniazid^Q
- *Injectable Antitubercular drug:* Streptomycin^Q
- *Antitubercular drug contraindicated in pregnancy:* Streptomycin^Q
- *Antitubercular drug contraindicated in children <6 years age:* Ethambutol^Q
- *Antitubercular drug causing Optic neuritis (Red-Green color blindness):* Ethambutol^Q
- *Antitubercular drug causing vestibular damage:* Streptomycin^Q

> **Key points**
>
> Antitubercular drug causing Optic neuritis (Red-Green color blindness): Ethambutol.

Groups of TB Drugs (WHO 2016)

	Group	Drug(s)
A	Fluoroquinolones	Levofloxacin, Moxifloxacin, Gatifloxacin
B	Second line injectables (SLI)	Amikacin, Capreomycin, Kanamycin (Streptomycin)
C	Other core Second line agents	Ethionamide/Prothionamide, Cycloserine/Terizidone, Linezolid, Clofazimine
D	Add-on agents*	**D1** Pyrazinamide, Ethambutol, High dose Isoniazid **D2** Bedaquiline, Delmanid **D3** PAS, Cilastatin4/Meropenem4, Amoxycillin-Clavulanate, (Thiacetazone)

(*Not part of Core MDR-TB regimens)

New Anti-tubercular Drugs

Bedaquiline

- Introduction: Diarylquinoline drug which targets Mycobacterial ATP synthase
- Extended half-life: Present even 5.5 months after stoppage
- Significant use in culture-conversion time for MDR-TB
- Patient selection criteria: Age 18 years or more with MDR-TB
- Contraindications: Pregnancy, Cardiac arrhythmia

Week 0–2	BDQ 400 mg daily + OBR (Optimized background regimen)
Week 3–24	BDQ 200 mg thrice a week + OBR (Optimized background regimen)
Week 25–End	Continue other 2nd line drugs as per RNTCP

Delamanid

- DCG India allow 50 mg usage as Combination regimen for Pulmonary MDT-TB.

NATIONAL POLIO ELIMINATION PROGRAMME (NPEP)

Pulse Polio Immunization (PPI) Programme in India

- *Launched in India:* 1995–96^Q (1st round on 9th Dec 1995 and 20th Jan 1996)
    - First PPI targeted children <3 years age
    - Later on WHO recommended age group be 0–5 years (1996–97)
- *Meaning of 'Pulse'^{Q}:* Sudden, simultaneous mass administration of Oral Polio Vaccine (OPV) on a single day to *'all children 0–5 years age'*, irrespective of their previous immunization status
    - PPI replaces wild virus with vaccine virus from the community
    - PPI is over and above routine immunization
- *Intensive Pulse Polio Immunization (IPPI)^Q:* Intensification of PPI has been done by adding additional rounds at fixed booths followed by *'house-to-house search-and-vaccinate'* component
- *Success of PPI (India):* 35000 cases annually in 1995–96 to NIL case in 2012

Basic Strategies to Eradicate Poliomyelitis from India[Q]
- Routine immunization
- PPI/National Immunization Day (NID)/Sub-NID (SNID)
- Surveillance of acute flaccid paralysis (AFP)
- Conduct extensive house-to-house immunization mopping-up campaigns

Vaccine Vial Monitor (VVM)
- *Description:* A simple tool (sticker on OPV vial) which enables vaccinator to know *'whether vaccine is potent'* at the time of administration[Q]
- Mandatory since 1998 for quality assurance
- WHO Grading of VVM (OPV):

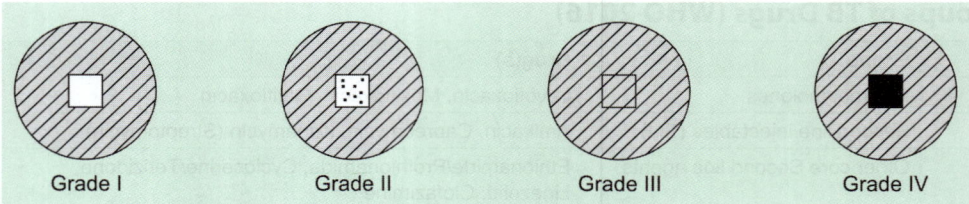

Vaccine Vial Monitor (VVM)

Acute Flaccid Paralysis (AFP) Case Investigation[Q]
- *Acute Flaccid Paralysis (AFP):* Acute onset (<4 weeks) in a child aged <15 years, or any case of paralytic illness in a person of any age when polio is suspected
    - *Acute:* rapid progression of from onset to maximum paralysis
    - *Flaccid:* loss of muscle tone, 'floppy' as opposed to spastic or rigid
    - *Paralysis:* weakness, loss of voluntary movement
- *Differential diagnosis of AFP[Q]:* Descending asymmetric flaccid LMN paralysis
    - Guillain Barre Syndrome (Cytologico-albuminic dissociation[Q])
    - Transverse myelitis (Normal CSF, sensory loss +, bladder dysfunction +)
    - Traumatic neuritis (any age, only one leg involved)
    - Other Non-polio enteric viruses: Coxsackie-B, ECHO, Enterovirus type 70 and 71, Mumps
- *Active case search in the community:* In the community where an AFP case resides or where an AFP case has visited during the incubation period for polio (4–25 days before paralysis onset[Q]), a house-to-house active case search is conducted to find additional AFP cases that may have occurred
    - This activity is carried out immediately along with ORI
    - A search is conducted for any children <15 years who have had the onset of AFP within the preceding 60 days[Q]
    - All cases that are found are investigated immediately, with collection from the case of two stool specimens before administration of OPV
- *Adequate stool sample collection[Q]:* From every case of AFP, stool samples are collected for diagnosis of cases of poliomyelitis
    - 2 stool samples
    - 24–48 hours apart
    - Within 14 days of onset of paralysis[Q] (or maximum 8 weeks)
    - Each 8 grams (adult thumb size) weight[Q]
    - Collect in clean, dry screw-capped container (need not be sterile, no preservative/transport media required)
    - Transport to laboratory in *'Reverse cold chain'*[Q] (+2° to +8°C)
    - Standard Lab Request Form (LRF) filled accompany the specimens
- *Outbreak response immunization (ORI):* Following the AFP case investigation and stool specimen collection, ORI is organized in community
    - Children aged 0–59 months are given one dose of OPV regardless of previous immunization[Q] (in the village/locality of the AFP case)

> **Key points**
> Transport to laboratory in 'Reverse cold chain'[Q] (+2° to +8°C).

- Travel history of the child with AFP may suggest additional places of stay where ORI should also be conducted
- Atleast 500 children are vaccinated[Q]
- **60-day follow-up in a case of Acute Flaccid Paralysis (AFP)[Q]:** The District Immunization Officer (DIO) must visit every case of AFP 60 days after onset of paralysis *'to confirm the presence or absence of residual weakness[Q]'*
  - Activity completed before 70th day
  - *Minimal levels of residual weakness can usually be detected by:*
    - Mid-arm or mid-thigh circumference: Reveal wasting on one side
    - Asymmetry in the skin folds on medial aspects of thigh

> **Key points**
> Visit every case of AFP 60 days after onset of paralysis 'to confirm the presence or absence of residual weakness[Q]'.

NEW WHO Indicators of AFP Surveillance & Laboratory Surveillance

Indicators of Surveillance Performance	
• Completeness of reporting • Sensitivity of surveillance • Completeness of case investigation • Completeness of follow-up • Laboratory performance	• ≥80% AFP surveillance reports received on time (Including zero reports) • Non-polio AFP rate >1/100,000 population* • ≥80% AFP cases should have "adequate" stool specimens# • ≥80% AFP cases for residual paralysis (>60 days of onset of paralysis) • 100% AFP case specimens be processed in a WHO-accredited laboratory^

(* ≥2/100,000 population in Endemic areas; ≥3/100,000 population in countries with recent outbreaks; annually in age <15 years)
(#2-specimens of sufficient quantity, collected >24 hours apart, <14 days onset of paralysis, arriving at laboratory by Reverse cold chain, with proper documentation)
(^Global Polio Laboratory Network)

Two indicators - Gold standard for AFP surveillance quality	
Non-polio AFP case rate	≥2 cases/100,000 children*
AFP cases with 2 adequate stool samples	≥80%

(* ≥3 cases/100,000 children in areas with new outbreaks; aged <15 years)

Timeliness in AFP Surveillance	
AFP cases investigated <48 hours	≥80%
AFP cases with 2 adequate stool specimens	≥80%
Specimens arriving at the laboratory in good condition	≥80%
Specimens arriving at a WHO-accredited laboratory <3 days of being sent	≥80%
Specimens for which laboratory results are sent <28 days of their receipt	≥80%

(© Tables Dr Vivek Jain 2019–20)

RCH PROGRAMME

RMNCH+A (Reproductive, Maternal, Newborn, Child and Adolescent Health) Strategy

- **PLUS indicates:**
  - Inclusion of adolescence as a distinct 'life stage'
  - Linking of maternal and child health to reproductive health and other components
  - Linking of community and facility-based care as well as referrals
- **Goals for RMNCH+A strategy (As per 12th Five year plan)[Q]:**
  - Reduction of IMR to 25 per 1,000 live births by 2017
  - Reduction in MMR to 100 per 100,000 live births by 2017
  - Reduction in TFR to 2.1 by 2017

Adolescents Priority interventions:	Reproductive health Priority interventions:
Nutrition; IFA supplementation Adolescent health clinics Information and counselling Menstrual hygiene Preventive health checkups	Community-based promotion and delivery of contraceptives Promotion of spacing methods (interval IUCD) Sterilization services (vasectomies and tubectomies) Comprehensive abortion care (includes MTP Act) Prevention and management of STI/RTI
New born and Child care Priority interventions:	**Pregnancy and Child birth Priority interventions:**
Home-based newborn care, prompt referral Child nutrition, Micronutrients supplementation Immunization IMNCI Facility-based care of the sick newborn Early detection and management of 4Ds	AN care & tracking of high-risk pregnancies Skilled obstetric care Immediate essential newborn care & resuscitation Emergency obstetric and new born care Postpartum care, IUCD and sterilization Implementation of PC & PNDT Act

(4Ds: Defects, Deficiencies, Diseases and Disability in children (0–18 years)

- **5 × 5 Matrix of RMNCH+A:** Minimum Essential commodities^Q

Reproductive health	Maternal health	Newborn health	Child health	Adolescent health
FP commodities: Tubal rings, CuT 380A, IUCD 375	Injection Oxytocin	Injection Vitamin K	ORS	Tablet Albendazole
OCPs, Mala N, Condoms	Tablet Misoprostol	Mucus extractor	Zinc dispersible tablets	Tablet Dicyclomine
Emergency contraceptive pills (LNG 1.5 mg)	Inj. Magnesium sulphate	Vaccines: BCG, OPV, HepB	Salbutamol syrup/ nebulising solution	
Pregnancy testing kits - Nischay			Vaccines: DPT, OPV, Measles, Hep-B, JE, Pentavalent vaccine	
Tablet Mifepristone			Syrup Vitamin A	

– All facilities must have IFA tablets, IFA syrup, PCM, Chloroquine, Dexamethasone, Trimethoprim-Sulphamethoxazole, Amoxycillin, Ampicillin, Gentamicin, Ceftriaxone, Thermometer, Weighing scale, BP apparatus, Stop watch, Cold box, Vaccine carrier, Oxygen Bag & mask, Testing equipments of Sugar/Hemoglobin/Urine

Components of Reproductive and Child Health Programme

- Community Needs Assessment Approach (CNAA)
- Integrated packages of services for mother and child
- MTP services at PHC and safe abortion
- Control and prevention of RTI/STI
- Adolescent health
- Services in urban slums
- Improving quality of services
- Unmet needs and sub-centre action plans
- Communication strategy
- Gender sensitiveness
- Greater involvement of Panchayati Raj Institutions (PRIs), NGOs and community

BEmONC and CEmONC Components[Q]

BEmONC	CEmONC
Basic Emergency Obstetric & Newborn Care	Comprehensive Emergency Obstetric & Newborn Care
24 hour delivery & neonatal services [Q]	Additional services
Level II facilities	Level III facilities
24 × 7 PHC, CHC [Q]	District hospital, 1 FRU per 500,000 population[Q]
Manual removal of placenta Antibiotics Anticonvulsants Uterotonics Vacuum assisted delivery MVA off retained products of conception Newborn resuscitation	All components of BEmONC Surgical capability Blood transfusion

(Level I facilities include other PHCs/Subcentres/delivery points; MVA: Manual vacuum aspiration)

Couple Protection Rate (CPR)

- *Definition[Q]:* Is defined as the percent of eligible couples protected against childbirth by one of the approved methods of family planning, i.e. condoms, oral pills, IUDs or sterilization
  - CPR is an indicator of 'contraceptive prevalence in a community'[Q]
  - Demographers believe that 'NRR = 1 can be achieved only with CPR >60%'[Q]: Thus goal under the earlier National Population Policy was CPR 60% by 2000
- *Effective Couple Protection Rate (ECPR):* Is defined as the percent of eligible couples 'effectively' protected against childbirth by one of the approved methods of family planning, i.e. condoms, oral pills, IUDs or sterilization.

IFA Tablets & Iron Deficiency Anemia

- *Iron and Folic Acid content per IFA tablet:* (See also Annexure 21)
  - Adult tablet: 100 mg elemental iron and 500 mcg folic acid[Q]
  - Pediatric tablet: 20 mg elemental iron and 100 mcg folic acid[Q]
  - For preterm infants, IFA tablet: 10–15 mg elemental iron and 100 mcg folic acid
- 'National Nutritional Anemia Prophylaxis Programme' was launched in 1970 to prevent nutritional anaemia in mothers and children
  - This programme is being taken up by MCH Division of Ministry of Health and Family Welfare; now it is part of RCH programme.
- *Prevalence of Iron Deficiency Anemia (IDA) in India:* [NFHS – 3, 2005–06]

Key points

IFA Adult tablet: 100 mg elemental iron and 500 mcg folic acid[Q].

Group	Anemia cut off level	Anemia type	Prevalence
Children (6–59 months)	<11.0 g/dL[Q] 10.0–10.9 g/dL 7.0–9.9 g/dL <7.0 g/dL	Any Mild Moderate Severe	70% 27% 40% 03%
Women (15–49 years)	<12.0 g/dL[Q] 10.0–11.9 g/dL 7.0–9.9 g/dL <7.0 g/dL	Any Mild Moderate Severe	55% 38% 15% 02%
Men (15–49 years)	<13.0 g/dL[Q] 12.0–12.9 g/dL 9.0–11.9 g/dL <9.0 g/dL	Any Mild Moderate Severe	24% 13% 10% 01%

Integrated Management of Neonatal and Childness Illness (IMNCI)

- *IMNCI is a* 'strategy for reducing morbidity and mortality associated with major causes of childhood illness'
- **Curative component includes management of** [Q]:
  - **Diarrhoea**
  - **Measles**
  - **Pneumonia**

Key points

IMNCI Curative component includes:
- Diarrhoea
- Measles
- Pneumonia
- Malaria
- Severe malnutrition and nutritional counseling

- Malaria
- Severe malnutrition and nutritional counseling
- *Health promotive and preventive component:*
  - Breast feeding
  - Nutritional counseling
  - Vitamin A and iron supplementation
  - Immunization
  - Treatment of helminthic infestation
- *Target:* Children <5 years age^Q
  - Children <2 months age
  - Children aged 2 months – 5 years
- *Components of IMNCI strategy:*
  - Improving case management skills of health care staff
  - Improving overall health systems
  - Improving family and community health practices
- *Case management process^Q:* Is presented in a series of charts (**Mnemonic: A C**ase **I**s **T**reated & **C**are **G**iven)
  - **A**ssess the young infant or child
  - **C**lassify the illness
  - **I**dentify the treatment
  - **T**reat the infant or child
  - **C**ounsel the mother
  - **G**ive follow-up care
- IMNCI is the Indian adaptation of IMCI (Integrated Management of Childhood Illness); major highlights of Indian adaptation are^Q,
  - Inclusion of early neonatal age (0–7 days age) in programme
  - Incorporating national guidelines on malaria, anemia, Vitamin-A supplementation and immunization schedule
  - Training of health workers begin with sick young infants up to 2 months
  - Proportion of training time devoted to sick young infant and sick child is almost equal
  - Is skill based
- For New IMNCI Pneumonia/ARI Guidelines, Refer to Chapter 5.

> **Key points**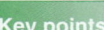
>
> **Colour Coding: IMNCI**
> - PINK: Pre-referral treatment + Refer urgently to hospital
> - YELLOW: Specific treatment at PHC
> - GREEN: Home based management

Quality Indicators to Monitor and Evaluate RCH Programme^Q

- No. of RTI/STI cases detected, treated, referred
- No. of ANC cases registered – Total and less than 12 weeks
- No. of pregnant females with 3 antenatal checkups
- No. of high risk pregnant females referred
- No. of pregnant females who had received 2 doses of TT
- No. of pregnant females under anaemia prophylaxis and treatment
- No. of ANC cases with complication referred to PHC/FRU
- No. of deliveries by trained and untrained birth attendant
- No. of women given 3 post natal checkups
- No. of newborns with birth weight recorded
- No. of children fully immunised
- No. of adverse effects following immunization (AEFI)
- No. of cases of ARI and diarrhoea under 5 years treated, referred, deaths
- No. of cases motivated, followed up for contraception.

Global Strategy for Women's, Children's and Adolescent's Health 2016–2030

- Vision: Every woman, child and adolescent realize their rights to physical and mental health and wellbeing, has economic and social opportunities, and is able to participate fully in shaping prosperous and sustainable society by 2030
- Global Strategy Goals: *'Survive, Thrive and Transform'*
- Survive (End preventable deaths):
  - MMR <70 per 100,000 LB
  - NNMR <12 per 1000 LB

- U5MR <25 per 1000 LB
- End epidemics of HIV, TB, Malaria, Neglected tropical diseases, and Other communicable diseases
- Reduce premature mortality from NCDs by 1/3, promote mental health and wellbeing
- Thrive (Ensure Health and Wellbeing):
  - End all malnutrition and address nutritional needs, Ensure universal access to sexual and reproductive health services, Ensure access to good quality early childhood development, Substantially reduce pollution related deaths/illnesses, Achieve universal health coverage
- Perform (Expand enabling environments):
  - Eradicate extreme poverty, Ensure completion of free equitable good quality primary/secondary education, Eliminate harmful practices/discrimination/violence against girls and women, Achieve universal and equitable access to safe and affordable drinking water and to adequate sanitation and hygiene, Enhance scientific research upgrade technological capabilities and encourage innovation, Provide legal identity for all (including birth registration), Enhance global partnership for sustainable development

NATIONAL PROGRAMME FOR CONTROL OF BLINDNESS AND VISUAL IMPAIRMENT (NPCBVI) NPCB UPDATES 2017–2018

- *Definition of Blindness (NPCB) in line with WHO definition*:
  - Presenting distance visually acuity <3/60 (20/400) in the better eye^Q
  - Limitation of field of vision to be <10 degrees from center of fixation
  - Expected outcome: Population of blind people in India reduce from 12 million to 8 million
  - Ultimate Goal (WHO Goal): Reduce Blindness prevalence (India) to 0.3% by 2020^Q
- Nomenclature of the scheme is also changed from 'National Program for Control of Blindness (NPCB)' to 'National Program for Control of Blindness and Visual Impairment' (NPCBVI)

Blindness in India

- *India is single largest contributor to global blind pool*
  - *Measured according to:* NPCB criterion (<3/60 in BEBPC^Q) [New Guidelines 2017–18]
  - *Total estimated no. of blind persons: 15 million*
- *Current prevalence:* 1.05% (Acc. of older guideline)
  - *State with highest prevalence of blindness:* Jammu & Kashmir^Q
  - *State with lowest prevalence of blindness:* Meghalaya
  - *Prevalence after correction:* 0.56% [2001–02]
  - *Prevalence of blindness in age >50 years:* 8.5%
  - *Prevalence of one-eyed blindness:* 0.8% (MCC: Cataract – 73%)
- India is 'overestimating the no. of blinds as per WHO definition$^{Q'}$
  - Since now WHO cutoff (<3/60 in BEBPC) is employed in India, estimated prevalence of blindness would be: 0.7%^{Q} (Estimate only)
- *Blindness in India includes:* Economic Blindness, Social Blindness, Manifest Blindness and Absolute Blindness (WHO blindness includes Social Blindness, Manifest Blindness and Absolute Blindness)
  - *MCC of Blindness (India):* Cataract^Q.

> **Key points**
> MCC of Blindness (India): Cataract^Q.

Strategies of National Programme for Control of Blindness (NPCB, 1976)

- Strengthening service delivery
- Developing human resources for eye care
- Promoting outreach activities and public awareness
- Developing institutional capacity
- To establish eye care facilities for every 5 lac persons

> **Key points**
> NPCB Blind <3/60

> **Key points**
> WHO Blind <3/60

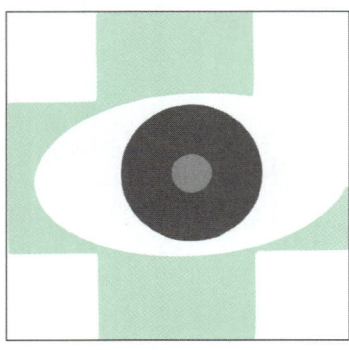

NPCB Logo

Revised Strategies of NPCB[Q]

- *To make NPCB more comprehensive by:*
  - Strengthening services for other causes of blindness like corneal blindness and refractive errors in school children
  - Improving follow-up services of cataract operated persons
  - Treating other causes of blindness like glaucoma
- To strengthen participation of voluntary organizations
- To shift from eye camp approach to fixed facility surgical approach[Q]
- To enhance coverage of eye services in tribal & underserved areas
- To expand World Bank project activities:
  - Construction of dedicated eye OTs and eye wards
  - Training of eye surgeons
  - Modern cataract surgery
  - Supply of ophthalmic equipment.

Organizational Structure for NPCB

Organizational level	Infrastructure developed/upgraded
Tertiary level	Regional institutes of Ophthalmology Upgraded medical colleges Medical colleges designated as training centers for PMOAs Eye banks
Secondary level	District hospitals upgraded NGO eye hospitals
Primary level	Sub-district level hospitals/CHCs Mobile Ophthalmic Units Upgraded PHCs Link workers/Panchayats

- NPCB was launched in 1976 as a '100% Centrally sponsored programme'
  - India was the 'first country to launch a national level programme for blindness'[Q]
- *Apex institute:* National Institute of Ophthalmology (Dr. Rajendra Prasad Centre for Ophthalmic Sciences [2007] AIIMS, New Delhi)[Q]
- *NPCB cut-off for blindness:* <3/60 in better eye
  - Prevalence of blindness in general population: *1.05% (MCC: Cataract 77%) [2007]*[Q]
  - Cataract surgery rate required to clear the backlog of blindness: *340 operations per lac population [2007]*[Q]
  - IOL implantations in cataract surgeries: *34% [2007]*[Q]

Definition and Causes of Blindness in NPCB

	World	India (NPCB, India)
Blindness[Q]	'Visual acuity of **<3/60** in better eye with best possible correction'	'Visual acuity of **<3/60** in better eye with best possible correction' [New Guideline 2017–18]
Prevalence	0.6% [2002]	0.36% (2019)
Causes[Q]	Cataract (48%) – MCC Glaucoma (12%) Uveitis (10%) ARMD Trachoma Corneal opacity Diabetic Retinopathy Others	Cataract (62%) – MCC Refractive Error (19.7%) Glaucoma Posterior segment pathology Corneal opacity Other causes

Important Points of Blindness

- *About 80% of blindness is avoidable*
- *Legal Blindness^Q:* Visual acuity <3/60 OR Visual field <10° in better eye with best possible correction
- *Work Vision^Q:* <6/60 (Economic Blindness)
- *Walk Vision^Q:* <3/60 (Social Blindness).

School Eye Screening (SES) Programme

- Focus on middle school (V – VIII class) covering 10–14 years age^Q
  - 150,000 children to be screened per block
- One trained teacher to handle 150 students^Q
  - 1 – day training for teacher at nearest PHC^Q
  - Teacher Kit: Vision screening cards, referral cards, tape/rope to measure 20 feet
- *Visual cut-off for referral to nearest PHC:* <6/9 in either eye^Q
- *Prerequisites for undertaking SES:*
  - Para-medical Ophthalmic Assistant (PMOA) available^Q
  - Relevant equipments procured
  - Optician contracted for providing spectacles

Vision 2020 – Right to Sight Initiative

Refer to Chapter 5, Theory

- *International organisations involved in Vision 2020:*^{Q}
  - WHO
  - Orbis
  - International Agency for Prevention of Blindness
  - International Eye Foundation
  - International Federation for Ophthalmological Societies
  - International Organisation against Trachoma
  - Rotary International
  - World Blind Union
  - World Council of Optometry
  - International Association of Lions Club
  - Sight Savers International
  - Helen Keller International.

Cataract Blindness Control Project (CPCB)

- The Government of India obtained a soft loan from the *'World Bank'*^{Q} to control cataract blindness in 7 states of country for the period 1994–2002
- *Activities undertaken in the project:*
  - Establishment and functioning of 'District Blindness Control Societies (DBCS)'
  - Construction of eye theatre/eye wards in District hospitals
  - Supply of Ophthalmic equipment
  - Intra-Ocular Lens (IOL) implantation in District Hospitals
  - Training of surgeons in IOL surgery, and
  - Assistance to NGOs for setting up of eye care facilities

NATIONAL HIV/AIDS CONTROL PROGRAMME (NACP)

NACP - IV (2012–17)

- Goal: Accelerate Reversal and Integrate Response
- Objectives^Q:
  - Reduce new infections by 50% (2007 Baseline of NACP III)
  - Provide comprehensive care and support to all persons living with HIV/AIDS and treatment services for all those who require it

HIV Screening in NACP

- *Tests for Screening of HIV^Q:* E/R/S Battery
  - ELISA (E) Test

> **Key points**
> **Tests for Screening of HIV:**
> – ELISA
> – RAPID
> – SIMPLE

- RAPID (R) Test
- SIMPLE (S) Test
- *Confirmatory diagnosis of HIV:* Western Blot Assay^Q
- *Screening strategies of HIV^Q:*
  - *Strategy I:* One out of three screening tests (E/R/S) are used
    - Done for screening every blood unit before transfusion
    - Does not recommend its use for diagnosis of HIV in a person
  - *Strategy II:* Two out of three screening tests (E/R/S) are used
    - Done for screening person who is symptomatic with any one of AIDS defining illness (NACO guidelines)
  - *Strategy III:* All three screening tests (E/R/S) are used
    - Done for screening person who is asymptomatic
- *ELISA Test:* first screening test commonly employed for HIV
  - It has a high sensitivity.

HIV Diagnosis Tests

- *Western Blot Assay (Immunoblot):* Is a method to detect a specific protein^Q in a given sample of tissue homogenate or extract.
  - Used as a confirmatory test for HIV (NACP, India).
  - *Based on detecting^Q:* Viral core protein (p24) and envelope glycoprotein (gp 41)
- p24 Antigen Test
- Nucleic-acid-based tests
- RT-PCR test
- Quantiplex bDNA or branched DNA test

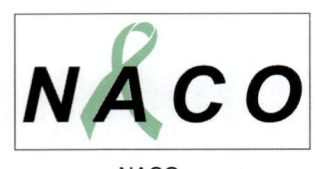

NACO

Targeted Interventions in NACP^Q

- *Basic purpose:* To reduce transmission of HIV amongst most vulnerable populations.
- *Approach:* Combines a comprehensive and integrated approach to vulnerable segments of population.
- *Main activities:*
  - Behaviour change
  - Communication
  - Treatment of STD
  - Create enabling environment to facilitate behaviour change
- *Segments of population covered^Q:*
  - Sex workers
  - Injecting Drug Users
  - Truckers
  - Homosexual men (MSM-Men having sex with men)
  - Migrant labourers
  - Transgender & Hijrås

Opt-in/Opt-out Testing

- *Opt-in testing^Q:* Testing is offered and the patient is required to actively give permission before it can occur
- *Opt-out testing^Q:* Means performing an HIV test after notifying the patient that the test is normally performed, but that the patient may elect to decline or defer testing; assent is then assumed unless the patient declines testing
  - WHO and CDC recommends opt-out testing policies in health care settings
  - Opt- out testing has a higher (85–98%) testing rate than opt- in testing (25–83%)
  - It does NOT eliminate the need for informed consent.

> **Key points**
> WHO and CDC recommends opt-out testing policies in health care settings.

LAC (Link ART Centre)

- Providing ARV drugs to patients on ART
- Monitoring of patients on ART
- Treatment of minor Opportunistic Infections (OIs)
- Identification and management of side-effects
- Reinforcement of drug adherence on every visit

LAC PLUS (LAC services PLUS Pre-ART Management)
- Help in integrating HIV care into general health system
- Reduce loss of patients between ICTC and Care Support and Treatment (CST) services

ART Plus[Q]
- Second line ART drugs in NACP

'ALL IN' Initiative (Global Initiative to End Adolescent AIDS)
- *Description:* A partnership between UNAIDS and UNICEF to reach adolescents with HIV services and to end the AIDS epidemic by 2030
- *Four key action areas:*
    - Adolescents as leaders and actors of social change
    - Improving data collection
    - Encouraging innovative approaches to reach adolescents
    - Placing adolescent HIV firmly on political agendas
- *Fast-Track Targets to be achieved by 2020:*
    - Reducing new HIV infections by at least 75%
    - Reducing AIDS-related deaths by 65%
    - Achieving zero discrimination
- *Main Goals:*
    - Ending adolescent AIDS by 2030
    - Ending the global AIDS epidemic as a public health threat

NATIONAL VECTOR BORNE DISEASES CONTROL PROGRAMME (NVBDCP)

Introduction to NVBDCP
- NVBDCP covers 6 vector borne diseases[Q] of public health importance in India:

Disease	Main vector
Malaria	Female Anopheles
Filariasis	Culex quinquefasciatus (C. fatigans)
Dengue	Aedes aegypti
Kala Azar	Sandfly (Phlebotamus)
Japanese Encephalitis	Culex tritaeniorhynchus
Chikungunya fever	Aedes aegypti

NVBDCP: MALARIA

Modified Plan of Operation (MPO)[Q]
- *Modified Plan of Operation (MPO):* In 1977, attempts at malaria eradication were given up and under review policy MPO was launched
- *Under MPO, areas were divided on the basis of API[Q]:*
- *Areas with API >2:*
    - Regular insecticide spray (interval 6 weeks)[Q]

Condition	Insecticide	Dose and frequency
Non-refractory to DDT	DDT	1.0 gm per square metre; 2 rounds
Refractory to DDT	Malathion	2.0 gm per square metre; 3 rounds
Refractory to Malathion	Pyrethroids	0.25 gm per square metre; 2 rounds

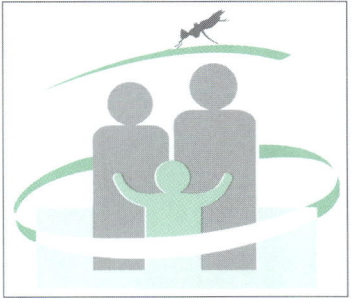

NVBDCP

- Entomological studies
- Malaria surveillance
- Treatment of cases
- Intensify efforts in rural areas (providing input under Plasmodium falciparum Containment Programme with SIDA)
- Decentralization of lab services to PHC level
- Establishment of Drug Distribution Centers (DDCs) and Fever Treatment Depots (FTDs)
- Areas with API <2:
    - Focal spray of DDT (or BHC or Malathion) if a case of Pf occurs in the area^Q
    - Active and passive surveillance
    - Presumptive treatment to all suspected fever cases
    - Ensuring radical treatment to those found positive on blood smear
    - Epidemiological investigation of case to determine causative factors

Fever Treatment Depots (FTDs) and Drug Distribution Centres (DDCs)

Fever Treatment Depots^Q	Drug Distribution Centres
FTD holder given training at PHC 1. Collection of blood smears 2. Giving presumptive treatment 3. Impregnation of bed nets 4. Promotion of larvivorous fishes	DDC established (if no FTD) 1. Giving presumptive treatment 2. Impregnation of bed nets 3. Promotion of larvivorous fishes

Malaria Diagnosis

- *Diagnosis of malaria in NVBDCP (malaria component):* Peripheral blood smear^Q
    - *Two types of smear,*
        - *Thick smear (Sensitivity):* Presence of malaria^Q
        - *Thin smear (Specificity):* Species identification^Q
    - *Stain used:* JSB (Jaswant Singh Bhattacharaya) Stain^Q
    - 1 microscope per 25,000 population at PHCs
    - Dipstick test in selected areas
    - 'Link Worker' per 2000 population^Q in high Pf areas (collects smears, provides presumptive treatment and forwards slides to PHCs)
    - 1 Fever Treatment Depot (FTD) in every village.
- *Rapid tests for diagnosis of Pf*:
    - Dipstick test (Pf Histidine rich protein II – HRP II)
    - Leishman stain
    - Field's stain
    - Acridine orange
- 'Dipstick Test' is used for the rapid diagnosis of Plasmodium falciparum (Pf)
    - Is a 'rapid whole blood immuno-chromatographic test'
    - Uses 2 antibodies specific for 'Pf Histidine Rich Protein II Antigen'^{Q}
    - Is a 'antigen capture assay'
    - Colloidal gold is used in the test card
    - Gives results in 3–5 minutes
    - Specificity and negative predictive value is 99%
    - Not as effective when parasite levels <100 parasites/mL of blood
- Optimal Test [Parasite-specific lactic dehydrogenase (LDH dipstick test)]: Positive in P.falciparum and P.vivax parasitaemia; It is a simple and rapid, and superior to HRP II^Q.

Enhanced Malaria Control Project (EMCP)

- World Bank supported project for six crore tribal population in 8 states
- *Selection criteria for PHCs in EMCP^Q*:
    - Annual parasitic incidence (API) >2 in last 3 yrs
    - Pf cases >30% of all malaria cases
    - 25% of population is tribal
    - Area has been reporting deaths due to malaria (and has flexibility to direct resources to needy areas in case of outbreak)

> **Key points**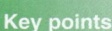
> *Malaria*: 1 microscope per 30,000 population.

Insecticide Treated Bed Nets (ITBN)

- Insecticide treated Bed nets (ITBN) Programme (esp. deltamethrin) has resulted in significant decline in malaria incidence and API
  - Average decline in anopheline mosquito density – 68%
  - Average decline in culicine mosquito density – 50%
- *Chemicals used in ITBN Programme:* Synthetic pyretheroids^Q
  - Deltamethrin: 2.5% in dosage of 25 mg/m²
  - Cyfluthrin: 5% in dosage of 50 mg/m²
  - Other insecticides used: Permethrin, Lambdacyhalothrin, Etofenprox, Cypermethrin
- *Effectiveness of pyrethroids^Q:* for 6–12 months (Retreatment every 6 months)
  - *Long-lasting insecticidal mosquito nets (LLINs):* Also use pyrethroid insecticides, and a chemical binder that allows the nets to be washed >20 times, allowing use for >3 years
- *Household bed nets used for mosquito control:*
  - No. of holes per square inch >150^Q
  - Diameter of each hole <0.0475 inch^Q
- *Common insect repellents:*
  - DEET (N, N-diethyl-m-toluamide) (Most commonly used)
  - Allethrin
  - Essential oil of the lemon eucalyptus [p-menthane-3, 8-diol (PMD)]
  - Icaridin (picaridin)
  - Nepetalactone (catnip oil)
  - Citronella oil
  - Permethrin
  - Soyabean oil
  - Neem oil.

Types of Drug Resistance in Malaria^Q

- *R1 resistance:* Recrudescence of infection between 7–28 days of treatment completion following initial resolution of symptoms and parasite clearance.
- *R2 resistance:* Patients with marked reduction of parasitemia (parasite count reduced by more than 75%) at 48 h but failed to clear parasites by day 7.
- *R3 resistance:* Patients whose parasitemia did not fall by more than 75% within 48 h or occasionally increased by day 7.

NVBDCP: LEISHMANIASIS

Introduction to Leishmaniasis

- *Leishmaniasis (Kala azar):* Is a group of protozoal diseases caused by Leishmania

Type of Leishmaniasis	Causative agent^Q
Visceral Leishmaniasis	Leishmania donovani^Q
Cutaneous/dermal Leishmaniasis	Leishmania tropica^Q
Muco-cutaneous Leishmaniasis	Leishmania braziliensis

- *Kala azar is transmitted by^Q:* Female Phlebotamus argentipes (Sandfly)
  - Sandfly cannot fly; it hops
  - Sandfly rests in cracks and crevices of walls^Q
  - *Insecticide of choice:* DDT^Q
    - 2 rounds of spray per year
    - Spray up to 6 feet height on walls
    - If DDT–resistant, use BHC
- Kala azar is known as 'Black Sickness'^Q

> **Key points**
>
> *Kala azar is transmitted by^Q:* Female Phlebotamus argentipes (Sandfly).

Sandfly

- *Sandfly is the vector of:^Q*
  - Visceral Leishmaniasis (Kala azar)

- Cutaneous Leishmaniasis (Oriental Sore)
- Sandfly Fever
- Oroya Fever
- Sandflies inject the infective stage, *metacyclic promastigotes*, during blood meals.

DDT

- DDT is Dichloro-Diphenyl-Trichloroethane
- Synthesized by: Othmar Zeidler^Q (1874)
- Insecticidal properties discovered by: Swiss scientist Paul H. Müller^Q (1939) [awarded the 1948 Nobel Prize in Physiology and Medicine^Q]
- Positive association found with: Liver, biliary tract and breast cancers.

Tests for Leishmaniasis

- *Parasitological diagnosis:* LD bodies in aspirates of spleen, liver, bone marrow, lymph nodes, skin
- *Hematological diagnosis:* Progressive leucopenia, anemia, reversed albumin: globulin ratio (raised IgG)
- *Aldehyde Test of Napier:* Used earlier for diagnosis but is a better test for surveillance^Q
  - Non-specific test
  - Demands use of venous blood
  - Detects raised globulins
  - False +ve in many chronic conditions where albumin: globulin ratio is reversed
- *Serological Tests:*
  - rK-39 Dipstick test^Q: Is for Visceral Leishmaniasis (Kala Azar)
  - ELISA
  - IFAT
  - Direct Agglutination Test
- *Leishmanin (Montenegro) Test:* Test of immunity status^Q
  - 0.1 mL (intradermal) washed promastigotes on forearm
  - Read after 48–72 hours^Q
    - Induration >5 mm is +ve.

> **Key points**
> rK-39 Dipstick test^Q: Is for Visceral Leishmaniasis (Kala Azar).

Treatment of Kala Azar^Q

- *1st Line^Q: Sodium stibogluconate* (i/v or i/m) 20 mg/kg × 20 days (antimonial compounds)
- 2nd Line: *Pentamidine* (i/v) 3 mg/kg × 10 days
- 3rd Line: *Amphotericin-B* (i/v) 1 mg/kg × 20 days (now considered as treatment of choice in many countries^Q)
- *Other drugs:*
  - Ketoconazole
  - Allopurinol
  - Paramomycin
  - Mepacrine (for dermal leishmaniasis)
  - New Wonder Drug: Miltefosine (oral) 2.5 mg OD × 4 weeks [Is now second line treatment].

Active Surveillance in Kala Azar

- Quarterly case searches
- 'Kala Azar fortnight': Peripheral health workers and volunteers do door-to-door search, refer the cases of KA/PKDL to treatment centers for definitive diagnosis and treatment

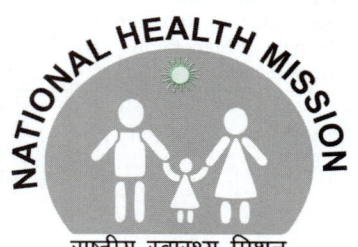

NHM Logo

NATIONAL HEALTH MISSION

- *Launched*: 2013
- *Composition*: NRHM + NUHM
- *Goals of NHM*: (According to XII FYP 2012–17)
  - Reduce MMR to 1/1000 live births
  - Reduce IMR to 25/1000 live births

- Reduce TFR to 2.1
- Prevention and reduction of anaemia in women aged 15–49 years
- Prevent and reduce mortality & morbidity from communicable, non-communicable; injuries and emerging diseases
- Reduce household out-of-pocket expenditure on total health care expenditure
- Reduce annual incidence and mortality from Tuberculosis by half
- Reduce prevalence of Leprosy to <1/10000 population and incidence to zero in all districts
- Annual Malaria Incidence to be <1/1000
- Less than 1 per cent microfilaria prevalence in all districts
- Kala-azar Elimination by 2015, <1 case per 10000 population in all blocks

NATIONAL RURAL HEALTH MISSION (NRHM)

Core Strategies of National Rural Health Mission (NRHM)

- Train and enhance capacity of Panchayati Raj Institutions (PRIs)
- Promote access to improved healthcare at household level (ASHA recruitment and training^Q)
- Health Plan for each village through Village Health Committee
- Strengthening sub-centre through an untied fund
- Strengthening existing PHCs and CHCs, and provision of 30–50 bedded CHC per lakh population (Indian public Health standards: IPHS^Q)
- Preparation and Implementation of an inter-sectoral District Health Missions
- Strengthening capacities for data collection, assessment and review for evidence based planning , monitoring and supervision.
- Formulation of transparent policies for development of human resources
- Developing capacities for preventive health care at all levels.
- Janani Suraksha Yojana (JSY) is a safe motherhood intervention under NRHM being implemented with by promoting institutional delivery amount the poor pregnant women^Q
- Promoting non- profit sector particularly in under served areas.

Key Strategies of NRHM

- *National Rural Health Mission 2005–12:* Provide every village in the country with a trained female community health activist – ASHA (Accredited Social Health Activist)^Q
- Develop 'Health Plan (VHP) for each village' through Village Health Samiti of Panchayat (PHS).
  - *ASHA will make VHPQ:* ASHA along with ANM, Aanganwadi Workers and community workers under the leadership of PHS
- 'Intersectoral District Health Plan (DHP)', prepared by District Health Mission (DHM) including drinking water, sanitation, hygiene and nutrition
  - Core unit of planning, budgeting and implementation: District^Q

Accredited Social Health Activist (ASHA)

- *Proposed population norm:* 2 ASHA worker per 1000 population^Q
- *ASHA is expected to act as,*
  - *Interface between:* Community and Health care system^Q
  - *Bridge between:* ANM and village^Q
  - *Accountable to:* Panchayat^Q
- *Selection criteria of ASHA:*
  - Woman resident of local community
  - Preferably 25–45 years age
  - Literate with formal education up to 10th class^Q (Relaxable for Tribal areas)
- *Responsibilities of ASHA^Q:*
  - Create awareness on health and its social determinants and mobilize the community towards local health planning and increased utilization and accountability of the existing health services
  - Promote good health practices and provide a minimum package of curative care as appropriate and feasible and make timely referrals
  - Provide information on determinants of health, on existing health services and the need for timely utilization of services

Key points

Norm: 2 ASHA worker per 1000 population.

Key points

ASHA education: Literate with formal education up to 10th class.

- Counsel women on aspects of reproductive and child health
- Mobilise the community and facilitate them in accessing health and health related services provided by the government
- Act as a depot holder for essential provisions like ORS, IFA tablets, chloroquine, disposable delivery kits, oral pills & condoms[Q]
- Provide primary medical care and act as DOTS provider[Q]
- Help develop a comprehensive village health plan[Q]
- Arrange escort/accompany pregnant women and children requiring treatment/admission to nearest health facility[Q]
- Be a part of JSY (Janani Suraksha Yojana) and help reduce MMR[Q]
- *Resource person for training of ASHA:* ANM and Anganwadi worker[Q]
- *Other roles of Anganwadi worker integrated with ASHA:*
  - Organisation of Health-day
  - IEC activities
  - Depot holder and issuing to ASHA
  - Update list of eligible couples and children
  - Mobilisation for food supplementation
- *Other roles of ANM worker integrated with ASHA:*
  - Organise meetings with ASHA
  - Participate and guide for organising Health-day
  - Updating eligible couple register
  - Motivating pregnant females for antenatal care
  - Educating ASHA for danger signals of pregnancy
  - Orient ASHA on OCPs.

> **Key points**
>
> *Resource person for training of ASHA:* ANM and Anganwadi worker[Q].

Indicators for Monitoring and Evaluation of ASHA's Work

- *Process indicators:*
  - No. of ASHAs selected
  - No. of ASHAs trained
  - % ASHAs attending review meeting after 1 year
- *Outcome indicators:*
  - % newborns weighed and families counseled
  - % deliveries with skilled assistance
  - % institutional deliveries
  - % JSY claims made to ASHA
  - Completed immunized 12–23 months age group
  - % unmet need in BPL
  - % fever cases received chloroquine within 1 weeks in endemic area
- *Impact indicators[Q]:*
  - Infant mortality rate (IMR)
  - Child malnutrition rates
  - No. of cases of TB/Leprosy detected as compared to last year.

ASHA Kits-composition

Drug Kit	Equipment Kit
• DDK for Clean deliveries at home • Tab. Paracetamol • Paracetamol syrup • Tab. Iron Folic Acid (L) • Tab. Punarvadu Mandur (ISM Preparation of Iron) • Tab. Dicyclomine • Tetracycline ointment • Zinc Tablets • Povidone Ointment Tube • G.V. Paint • Cotrimoxazole syrup • Pediatric Cotrimoxazole tablets	• Digital Wrist Watch • Thermometer • Weighing Scale (for newborn) • Baby Blanket • Baby Feeding spoon • Kit Bag • Communication Kit • Mucous Extractor

Contd...

Contd...

Drug Kit	Equipment Kit
• ORS Packets • Condoms • Oral pills (In cycles) • Spirit • Soap • Sterilized Cotton • Bandages, 4 cm × 4 meters • Nischay Kit • Rapid Diagnostic Kit • Slides for Malaria & Lancets • Emergency Contraceptive Pill • Sanitary napkins*	

(*Menstrual Hygiene amongst adolescent girls)

Janani Suraksha Yojana (JSY)

- Launched on 12th April 2005^Q
- Is modification of National Maternity Benefit Scheme^Q
- *Objectives of JSY:* Reduction of maternal mortality and infant mortality^Q (through institutional deliveries and care especially for poor women)
- *Salient features of JSY:*
  - Is 100% centrally sponsored^Q
  - Combines 'benefit of cash assistance with institutional care'^{Q}
  - Eligibility of cash assistance.
    - In low performing states (LPS): All women undergoing institutional deliveries
    - In high performing states (HPS): Below poverty linewomen aged 19 years and above and SC/ST pregnant women
  - Limitation of cash assistance:
    - In low performing states (LPS): All births in institutions
    - In high performing states (HPS): Up to 2 live births
- *JSY package:* [New guidelines 2017]^Q

> **Key points**
>
> **Janani Suraksha Yojana (JSY)**
> - Launched on 12th April 2005^Q
> - Is modification of National Maternity Benefit Scheme^Q.

Category	Rural areas			Urban areas		
	Mother's package	ASHA's package	Total package	Mother's package	ASHA's package	Total package
LPS	1400	600	2000	1000	400	1400
HPS	700	600	1300	600	400	1000

(LPS: Low performing states; HPS: High performing states)

NATIONAL RURAL HEALTH MISSION

New Initiatives

- Home delivery of contraceptives by ASHA
- District level household survey (DLHS-4) in 26 states/UTs
- Promotion of Menstrual hygiene in 152 districts
- Differential financial approach
- ASHA involvement in Home based newborn care (HBNC)
- Performance based funds allocation to states
- Village Health, Sanitation and Nutrition Committee (VHSNC)
- Mainstreaming of AYUSH

Janani-Shishu Suraksha Karyakram (JSSK)

- *Pregnant women components:*
  - Free deliveries (including caesarean section) in public health institutions
  - Free drugs and consumables

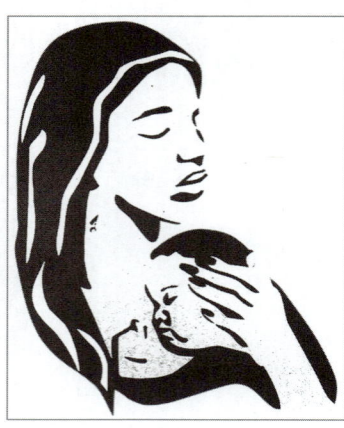

JSSK

- Free diet (Normal delivery: 3 days; Caesarean section: 7 days)
- Free diagnostics
- Free blood transfusion (whenever required)
- Free transport from home to institution
- Child health components:
  - *Nutritional rehabilitation centres (NRCs)*: Inpatient treatment of severely malnourished children and counselling of mothers on proper feeding
  - *Integrated management of neonatal and childhood illnesses (IMNCI)*: Management of common childhood illnesses
  - *Pre-service IMNCI*: Included in medical curriculum to generate trained IMNCI manpower
  - *Facility based IMNCI (F-IMNCI)*: Focus on inpatient management of major causes of neonatal and childhood mortality, viz. asphyxia, sepsis, low birth weight, pneumonia, diarrhoea, malaria, meningitis and severe malnutrition
  - *Facility based newborn care*:

Health facility	All newborns at birth	Sick newborns
MCH level I: PHC, Subcentre	Newborn care corner (NBCC) in labour room	Prompt referral
MCH level II: CHC, First referral unit (FRU)	NBCC in labour room and operation theatre	Newborn stabilization unit (NBSU)
MCH level III: District hospital	NBCC in labour room and operation theatre	Special newborn care unit (SNCU)

  - *Newborn care corner (NBCC)*: Space within delivery room for immediate care to newborns mandatory for all health facilities
  - *Newborn stabilization unit (NBSU)*: Facility within or near maternity ward where sick and low birth weight newborns can be cared for short periods
    - Location: CHCs, FRUs
    - Space required: 4 bedded unit and 2 beds for post-natal ward for rooming-in
  - *Special newborn care unit (SNCU)*: Neonatal unit near labour room to provide special care for sick newborns (EXCEPT assisted ventilation, major surgery)
    - Location: District hospitals, Sub-district hospitals having >3000 deliveries per year
    - Space required: 12 bedded unit and 4 additional beds for adult step-down
  - *Triage of sick newborns*:

Emergency signs	Priority signs	Non-urgent signs
Hypothermia (<36°C) Apnoea, gasping Severe respiratory distress Central cyanosis Shock Coma, convulsions Encephalopathy	Cold stress Respiratory distress Irritable/restless/jittery Abdominal distension Severe jaundice Severe pallor Bleeding from other sites Major congenital malformation Wt <1.8 or >4.0 kg	Transitional stools Possetting Minor birth trauma Superficial infections Minor malformations Jaundice All other cases
Initiate emergency treatment	*Assess and act rapidly*	*Assess and counsel*

  - *Home-based newborn care (HBNC)*:
    - Main person involved: ASHA
    - Other health personnel involved: ANM, Anganwadi worker, Medical officer
    - ASHA 6 visits in Institutional deliveries: Day 3, 7, 14, 21, 28, 42
    - ASHA 7 visits in Home based deliveries: Day 1, 3, 7, 14, 21, 28, 42
    - Other functions of ASHA (Paid ₹ 250/-):
      - Record birth weight
      - BCG, OPV, DPT to newborn
      - Birth registration
      - Mother/newborn safety till 42nd day

Nutrition Rehabilitation Centres (NRCs)

- *Description*:
  - Facility based units: To provide medical and nutritional care to Severe acute malnutrition (SAM) children under 5 years of age who have medical complications
  - Special focus: Skill improvement of mothers on child care and feeding practices
- *Services provided at NRCs*:
  - 24-hours care and monitoring of the child
  - Treatment of medical complications
  - Therapeutic feeding
  - Sensory stimulation and emotional care
  - Counselling on appropriate feed, care and hygiene
  - Demonstration and practice by doing of energy dense foods
  - Identification of contributory factors (Social assessment of family)
  - Follow-up of discharged children
- *SAM Management*:
  - **Stabilization phase (1–2 days)**: 'Starter diet' for nutritional and electrolyte balance
  - **Transition phase (2–3 days)**: Transition to 'Catch up diet' when there is beginning of loss of edema, return of appetite, no nasogastric tube/infusion/severe medical problems and child is alert and active; purpose to ensure that child tolerates increased energy/protein intake
  - **Rehabilitation phase**: Initiated when reasonable appetite (finishes >90% feed given), major loss of edema, and no other medical problem; purpose is promotion of rapid weight gain, stimulation of emotional/physical development and preparation for feeding at home
- *Micronutrient supplementation*:
  - Vitamin A to all children on Day 0, 1, 14 (50,000 IU <6 months age/100,000 IU 6–12 months age or weight <8 kg/200,000 IU >12 months age)
  - Daily basis supplementation for 2 weeks: Multivitamin (A, C, D, E, B12), Folic acid, Zinc, Copper, Iron)
- *Follow up of children discharged*: Home visits (by AWWs, ASHAs) and NRC visits

Navjat-Shishu Suraksha Karyakram (NSSK)

- Main objective: To train health personnel in basic newborn care and resuscitation

Rashtriya Bal Swasthya Karyakram (RBSK) 2013[Q]

- *Importance*: Child Health Screening and Early Intervention Services Programme under National Rural Health Mission[Q]
- *Target group*[Q]:
  - 0–6 years old children (Rural areas + Urban slums)
  - 6–18 years old children (Enrolled in government schools)
- *Targeted diseases (4D's)* [Q]:
  - Defects at birth
  - Diseases in children
  - Deficiency conditions
  - Developmental delays including disabilities
- Selected 34 diseases under RBSK:

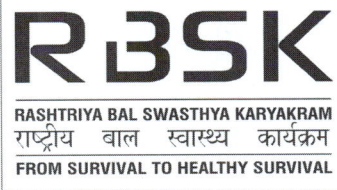

RBSK

Defects at birth	Deficiency conditions
Neural tube defects	Anemia (especially severe)
Down's syndrome	Vitamin A deficiency (Bitot spots)
Cleft lip/palate	Vitamin D deficiency (Rickets)
Talipes	Severe acute malnutrition
Dysplasia of hip	Goitre
Congenital cataract	
Congenital deafness	
Congenital heart disease	
Retinopathy of prematurity	

Contd...

Contd...

Diseases in children	Developmental delays including disabilities
Skin conditions (Eczema, Fungal, Scabies)	Vision impairment
Otitis media	Hearing impairment
Rheumatic heart disease	Neuro-motor impairment
Reactive airway disease	Motor delay
Dental conditions	Cognitive delay
Convulsive disorders	Language delay
	Behaviour disorder (Autism)
	Learning disorder
	Attention deficit hyperactivity disorder
	Congenital hypothyroidism, Sickle cell anemia, Beta thalassemia

- *Suggested composition of Mobile health team*:
    - 2 AYUSH Medical officers (1 male, 1 female)
    - 1 ANM/Staff nurse
    - Pharmacist

Rashtriya Kishor Swasthya Karyakram (RKSK) 2014

- Importance: India's First comprehensive adolescent health programme
- Target Group: Adolescents 10–19 years age (243 million; 21% of Indian population) in Urban and rural areas
    - Girls and Boys
    - Married and Unmarried
    - Poor and Affluent
    - School and Out of school
- **Strategy**[Q]: **RMNCH+A** (Reproductive, Maternal, New born, Child Health + Adolescent)

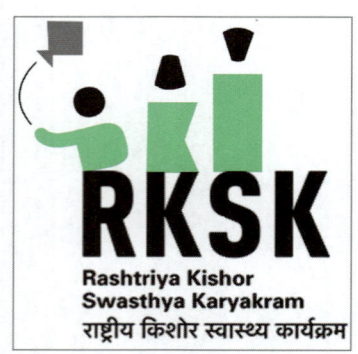
RKSK

7 Critical Components (7C's)[Q]	6 Strategic Priorities
Coverage	Nutrition
Content	Sexual and reproductive health (SRH)
Communities	Non-communicable diseases (NCDs)
Clinics	Substance misuse
Counselling	Injuries & violence (+ gender-based violence)
Communication	Mental health
Convergence	

National Urban Health Mission 2013

- *Description*: Subcomponent of National Health Mission (NHM), other component being NRHM
- *Coverage*[Q]: All state capitals, district headquarters and other cities/towns with a population of 50,000 and above (Cities and towns <50,000 population covered by NRHM)
- *Main aim*: To improve the health status of urban population particularly slum dwellers and other vulnerable sections by facilitating their access to quality health care
- *Expected outcomes of the programme*[Q]:
    - Reducing IMR in urban areas by 40% to 20 per 1000
    - Reduce MMR in urban areas by 50% to 1 per 1000
    - Achieve universal access to reproductive health including 100% institutional delivery
    - Achieve Total Fertility Rate of 2.1
    - Achieve all targets of Disease Control Programmes
- *Key components of NUHM*[Q]:
    - **U-PHC** (Urban - Primary Health Centre):
        1. 1 per 50,000 population (near or within a slum)[Q]
        2. OPD (consultation), basic lab diagnosis, drug/contraceptive dispensing and delivery of RCH services, as well as preventive and promotive aspects of all diseases

- **U-CHC** (Urban - Community Health Centre):
  1. 30–50 bedded U-CHC providing inpatient care in cities (>1 per 500,000 population)^Q
  2. 75–100 bedded U-CHC facilities in metros
- Subcentres: NOT ESTABLISHED in NUHM^Q
  1. Outreach services will be provided through Female Health Workers (FHWs)/Auxiliary Nursing Midwives (ANMs) headquartered at the UPHCs
- USHA (Urban Social Health Activist): 1 per 1000–2500 population^Q
- Mahila Aarogya Samiti (MAS): 1 per 250–500 population

NATIONAL LEPROSY ELIMINATION PROGRAMME (NLEP)

Multidrug Therapy (MDT) (See also Annexure 23)

Refer to Chapter 5, Theory
- *Drugs used in treatment of leprosy (Multi-Drug Therapy – MDT)*^{Q}:
  - *Rifampicin:* Bactericidal drug kills 99.9% organisms (600 mg dose)
  - *Clofazimine:* Bacteriostatic drug most active on daily administration
  - *Dapsone:* Safe drug in dose up to 100 mg
- *Other drugs effective in treatment of leprosy:*
  - Thioamides: Ethionamide & Prothionamide
  - Fluoroquinolones
  - Minocycline
  - Macrolides
- *Treatment of Single Skin Lesion (SSL) of Leprosy:*
  - *Previously:* ROM therapy
    - Rifampicin 600 mg
    - Ofloxacin 400 mg
    - Minocycline 100 mg
  - *Currently:* 6 month treatment as for Paucibacillary (PBL) Leprosy (Rifampicin and dapsone for 6 months)^Q.

NLEP Logo

Lepra Reactions

- *Lepra Reactions:* Is an inflammation that can affect skin patches, nerves, eyes and in few case, internal organs

- They can occur anytime in a leprosy patient:
  - Before diagnosis
  - At time of diagnosis
  - During treatment
  - After treatment has finished
- *Types of Lepra Reactions^Q:*

Type I Lepra reactions Reversal reactions	Type II Lepra reactions Erythema Nodosum Leprosum (ENL)
More common in Borderline leprosy^Q	More common in LL and BL leprosy^Q
Reddish & swollen skin lesions Painful, tender, swollen nerves Signs of nerve damage Fever & malaise Swollen hands & feet New skin lesions (rare)	Tender, reddish & transient skin nodules Occasionally painful & swollen nerves Fever, joint pains & malaise Eye involvement

- *Treatment of Lepra Reactions:*
  - *Type I (Reversal) Reactions:* Prednisolone (steroid^Q)
  - *Type II (ENL) Reactions:*
    - *Mild cases:* Analgesics or anti-pyretics like aspirin
    - *Severe cases:* Prednisolone (steroid^Q)
    - *During steroid withdrawal:* Clofazimine
- *Reversal Reaction Versus Relapse:*

	Reversal Reaction	Relapse
Time interval	During treatment or within 6 months of stopping treatment	Generally after 6 months of stopping treatment
Onset	Abrupt & sudden	Slow & insidious
Old lesions	Edematous, erythematous, tender	Erythematous & infiltration
New Lesions	Several appear	Few appear
Ulcerations	May take place	Does not occur
Nerve involvement	Multiple nerves involved, painful & tender	Single nerve involved, non-painful & non-tender
General condition	Fever, joint pains, malaise	Not usually affected
Response to steroids	Rapid	Nil

Infrastructure Norms under NLEP
- *SET Centre:* one per 20,000–25,000 population^Q
- *Urban Leprosy Centre (ULC):* one per 50,000 population^Q
- *Leprosy Control Unit (LCU):* one per 4–5 Lac population^Q.

Survey Education and Treatment (SET) Centre
- *A SET Centre is attached with:* PHC in rural area
- *Administrative control:* Medical Officer (PHC)
- *Population catered:* 20,000–25,000
- *Staff:* One paramedical worker
- *Functions:*
  - Detection of cases early by house-to-house survey
  - Health education about leprosy
  - Free treatment of all cases and follow-up
  - Contact tracing and their chemoprophylaxis with Dapsone

> **Key points**
> **SET Centre:** 1 per 20,000–25,000 population.

Simplified Information System (SIS)
- *Description^Q:* Is the Management and Information System (MIS) essential for the monitoring and evaluation of National Leprosy Eradication Programme (NLEP); It was started in 2002

- *Indicators of SIS (NLEP):*
  - Prevalence rate of leprosy
  - New case detection rate
  - Child proportion among new cases
  - Visible deformed case proportion among new cases
  - MBL (Multibacillary Leprosy) proportion among new cases
  - Female proportion among new cases
  - New case detection rate in Scheduled castes
  - New case detection rate in Scheduled tribes
  - Patient month blister calendar packs stock
  - Proportion of health subcentres providing MDT (Multidrug Therapy)
  - Absolute no. of patients made RFT (Released from treatment)

Newer Initiatives Under NLEP

- *Focussed Leprosy Elimination Plan (FLEP) 2005:*
  - Priority areas: Prevalence >3 per 10,000
  - Increased efforts on IEC, training and integrated service delivery
  - Week long 'Block Leprosy Awareness Campaign'
- *SAPEL and LEC^Q:*
  - Special Action Projects for Elimination of Leprosy (SAPEL) in Rural areas and Leprosy Elimination Campaigns (LEC) for Urban areas: To cover populations residing in difficult/inaccessible areas, which were not generally covered by regular programme activities.
- *Accompanied MDT^Q:* If patient is unable to come to collect his/her MDT from clinic, any responsible person from family or village can collect it.
  - Designed to help patients who have to interrupt their treatment due to any avoidable reason
  - Especially useful for irregular patients
  - Gives patients a choice: Patients can collect entire MDT course when diagnosed after proper counselling.

New Set of Indicators in Leprosy Control^Q

- *Operational Indicators:* Monitor functioning of control activities
  - No. of new cases detected
  - New cases with grade 2 disability per 100,000 population
  - Treatment completion/cure rate
- *Case detection indicators*
  - % of children (0–14 yrs) among new detected cases: A high prevalence of infection among children indicate that Leprosy is a active and spreading
  - % of females among new detected cases
  - % of Multi-bacillary cases on regular treatment
  - % of new cases with grade 2 disability
- *Quality of service indicators*
  - New cases % correctly diagnosed
  - No. of relapses
  - % treatment defaulters
  - % patients who develop new disability during MDT
- *Epidemiological indicators:* Evaluate effectiveness of programme^Q
  - Incidence
    - Most sensitive index of transmission^Q
    - Only index for measuring effectiveness of measures taken^Q
  - Prevalence
    - 'Is Measure of case load'^Q
    - Is useful in planning treatment services^Q

> **Key points**
> Incidence of Leprosy
> - Most sensitive index of transmission

Post-exposure Prophylaxis (PEP) for Leprosy: Directly Observed Rifampicin Supervised (DORSQ)

- Inclusion criteria for PEP:
  - A person who has been living/working/having social activities for >3 months and 20 hours/week with a newly detected case of leprosy in last 1 year
  - Age ≥ 2 years

- Exclusion criteria for PEP:
  - Pregnant women (PEP can be given after delivery)
  - Rifampicin therapy for any reason in last 2 years (e.g. for TB or Leprosy treatment)
  - History of liver disorders or renal disorders
  - Possible signs and/or symptoms of Leprosy
  - Possible signs and/or symptoms of TB
  - Acute febrile illness
- Post exposure prophylaxis with rifampicin
  - Contacts not meeting exclusion criteria will be given Rifampicin chemoprophylaxis
  - Suspect cases if confirmed will be given MDT
  - Administration of PEP has to be directly observed
- Single-dose Rifampicin post-exposure prophylaxis:
  - >35 kg: 600 mg
  - 20–35 kg: 450 mg
  - <20 kg: 10–15 mg/kg
- Contact categories:
  - Family contacts: All family members (Except those away during the last 1 year)
  - Household contacts: People living in the same house as the Index case
  - Neighbour contacts: All people living in 3 houses on either side and 3 houses across the street from Index case
  - Social contacts: People with whom the Index case is in contact for >20 hours/week for a cumulative of 3 months or more.

NATIONAL PROGRAMME FOR PREVENTION AND CONTROL OF DEAFNESS (NPPCD)

NPPCD

- *Long term objective:* To reduce disease burden by 25% by end of XI Five Year Plan^Q
- *Immediate objectives:*
  - To prevent avoidable hearing loss due to disease or injury
  - Early identification, diagnosis and treatment of ear problems responsible for hearing loss and deafness
  - To medically rehabilitate deaf persons of all age groups
  - To strengthen the existing inter-sectoral linkages for continuity of the rehabilitation programme, for deaf
  - To develop institutional capacity for ear care services by providing equipment, material and training personnel
- *Pilot project:* In first phase of implementation in 25 districts.

NATIONAL IODINE DEFICIENCY DISORDERS CONTROL PROGRAMME (NIDDCP)

NIDDCP

- National Goitre Control Programme (NGCP) launched in 1962 (100% centrally sponsored)
- National Iodine Deficiency Disorders Control Programme (NIDDCP) was launched in 1992.

Indicators to Monitor Success of NIDDCP

- *Process Indicators:* Indicators to monitor and evaluate the salt iodization process
  - Salt iodine content at the production site
  - Salt iodine content at point of packaging
  - Salt iodine content at wholesale and retail levels
  - Salt iodine content in households
- *Impact Indicators:* Indicators to assess baseline (Iodine Deficiency Disorders) IDD status and to monitor and evaluate the impact of salt iodization on the target population

- *Urinary Iodine Levels:* The *'principal impact indicator'*^{Q} recommended once a salt iodization programme has been initiated (changes in goitre prevalence lag behind changes in iodine status and therefore cannot be relied upon to reflect accurately current iodine intake, although they may be useful in following trends)
- *Goitre assessment:* (by palpation or by ultrasound) should remain a component of surveys to establish the baseline severity of IDD
- *Neonatal thyroid stimulating hormone (TSH) levels:* may also play a role here if a country already has in place a screening programme for hypothyroidism
- *Sustainability Indicators:* Indicators to assess whether iodine deficiency has been successfully eliminated and to judge whether achievements can be sustained and maintained for the decades to come
  - Median urinary iodine levels in the target population
  - Availability of adequately iodized salt at the household level
  - Set of programmatic indicators (as evidence of sustainability).

> **Key points**
> Urinary Iodine Levels: The **'principal impact indicator'**.

Important Points Regarding NIDDCP

- *Indicators for epidemiological assessment of iodine deficiency:*
  - Prevalence of goitre
  - Prevalence of cretinism
  - Urinary iodine excretion
  - Measurement of thyroid function (T4, TSH)
  - Prevalence of neonatal hypothyroidism
  - One-third of world population is exposed to the risk of IDD
- *Iodine deficiency as a major public health problem*^{Q}: Goitre prevalence >10%
- *Daily requirement of Iodine*^{Q}: 150 mcg (<1 teaspoon over lifetime^Q) supplied normally by well balanced diets and drinking water
- *WHO/UNICEF/ICCIDD recommended daily iodine intake:*

Group	Recommended daily intake
Preschool children (0–59 months)	90 mcg
School children (6–12 years)	120 mcg
Adults (>12 years)	150 mcg^Q
Pregnancy and lactation	250 mcg

> **Key points**
> *Daily requirement of Iodine*^{Q}: 150 mcg.

- *Iodised Oil:*
  - *Intramuscular Iodised Oil (poppy-seed oil):* Average dose 1 mL injection provided protection for 4 years^Q.
  - *Oral Iodised Oil:* 2 mL dose is effective for 2 years.
- *Most widely used prophylactic public health measure against endemic goiter:* Iodised salt^Q
  - Iodised salt is most convenient, effective and economical method of mass prophylaxis in endemic areas.
- *Standards of Iodised salt (Level of Iodization in salt):*^{Q}
  - At production level: 30 ppm
  - At consumer level: 15 ppm
- *Two-in-one salt:* National Institute of Nutrition (Hyderabad) developed *'Twin Fortified Salt'* also known as *'Double Fortified Salt' (DFS)*^{Q}
  - *DFS contains* salt, potassium iodate, ferrous sulphate and sodium hexa meta phosphate (It contains Iron and Iodine)
  - *DFS provides* 40 mcg Iodine and 1 mg Iron per gram of salt^Q.
- *DEC Medicated Salt:* is used for mass treatment of Filariasis; Treatment should be continued for 6–9 months
  - 1–4 gm DEC (diethylcarbamazine) per kg salt^Q

> **Key points**
> *Standards of Iodised salt (Level of Iodization in salt):*^{Q}
> - At production level: 30 ppm
> - At consumer level: 15 ppm.

- *In areas with mild-moderate iodine deficiency:* IQ of school children is lower by 13 points average
- *Global Iodine Deficiency Disorders (IDD) Day:* 21st October^Q
- *Criteria for tracking progress towards IDD elimination^Q:*

Indicator	Goal
Proportion with enlarged thyroid (age 6–12 years)	<5%
Urinary Iodine Excretion below 100 mcg/litre	<50%
Urinary Iodine Excretion below 50 mcg/litre	<20%
Proportion of houses consuming adequately iodised salt	>90%

NATIONAL PROGRAM FOR PREVENTION AND CONTROL OF FLUOROSIS (NPPCF) 2014

Goal
To prevent and control Fluorosis disease in the country.

Objectives
- To collect, assess and use the baseline survey data of fluorosis of Ministry of Drinking Water Supply
- Comprehensive management of fluorosis in the selected areas
- Capacity building for prevention, diagnosis and management of fluorosis cases

Case Definitions in NPPCF

1. Suspect case
- Dental Fluorosis (in children): Any case with a history of residing in an endemic area along with one or both of the followings:
  - Chalky white teeth/white spots on the white enamel surface
  - Transverse yellow, brown/black bands or spots on the enamel surface
- Skeletal Fluorosis: Any case with a history of residing in an area with Fluoride above 1.0 mg/l along with one or more of the followings health complaints
  - Severe pain and stiffness in neck, back bone (lumbar region), shoulder, knee and hip region. Pain may commence either in 1 or 2 or more joints. Patient has restricted mobility of cervical and/or lumbar spine and has to turn the whole body towards that side to see
  - Knock knee/Bow leg (In children, adolescents)
  - Inability to squat (advanced stage of Skeletal Fluorosis)
  - Ugly gait and posture (advanced stage of Skeletal Fluorosis)
- Non-Skeletal Fluorosis: Any case with a history of residing in an endemic area along with one or more of the following health complaints.
  - Gastro-intestinal problems: Consistent abdominal pain, intermittent diarrhea/Constipation, bloated feeling, nausea, loss of appetite
  - Neurological manifestations: Nervousness & depression, tingling sensation in fingers and toes, excessive thirst and tendency to urinate frequently (Polydipsia and polyuria)
  - Muscular manifestations: Muscle weakness & stiffness, pain in the muscle and loss of muscle power, unable to walk or work

2. Confirmation of a case: Any suspected case can be confirmed after retrieval of a clinical history, by the following tests:
- Any suspected case with high level of fluoride in urine (>1 mg/L)
- Any suspected case with interosseous membrane calcification in the forearm confirmed by X-ray Radiograph
- Any suspected case, if kidney ailment is prevailing, serum fluoride need to be tested, besides urine fluoride

NATIONAL PROGRAMME FOR PREVENTION AND CONTROL OF CANCER, DIABETES, CARDIOVASCULAR DISEASES AND STROKE (NPCDCS)

- Introduction:
  - Single centre for Cancer, Diabetes, Cardiovascular disease, Stroke[Q]
  - 100 districts in 21 states being covered in 11th Five year plan[Q]
  - 20,000 Subcentres and 700 Community health centres (CHCs) covered
- Activities at Sub-centres[Q]:
  - Health promotion for behaviour and lifestyle change
  - Opportunistic screening of BP, Blood glucose (Strip method) in age >30 years
  - Referral to CHC of cases of DM, HT
- Activities at CHCs:
  - Diagnosis and management at NCD clinic
  - Home visits by nurse for bedridden cases
  - Referral to District hospital for complicated cases
- Activities at District hospital[Q]:
  - Health promotion
  - Screening of population >30 years
  - Diagnosis and management of cardiovascular diseases
  - Home-based palliative care for chronic, debilitating, progressive patients
- Urban health check-up scheme for Diabetes and High BP:
  - Screen urban slum population
  - Screen population >30 years and pregnant females
- Cancer control in NPCDCS:
  - Regional cancer control scheme: Regional cancer centres to act as Referrral centres for complicated cases
  - Oncology wing development scheme
  - Decentralized NGO scheme: IEC activities and early cancer detection
  - IEC at Central level
  - Research and training

NATIONAL PROGRAM ON AMR CONTAINMENT

- *Background:* Antimicrobial resistance is a growing public health problem. GOI launched a "National Program on AMR Containment" during the 12th five-year plan (2012–2017) which is being coordinated by NCDC. The network of labs is being expanded in a phased manner and currently includes 35 state medical college labs in 26 States/UTs.
- *Main objectives:*
  - Establish a laboratory-based AMR surveillance system in the country to generate quality data on antimicrobial resistance
  - Carry out surveillance of antimicrobial usage in different health care settings
  - Strengthen infection control practices and promote rational use of antimicrobials through Antimicrobial stewardship activities
  - Generate awareness amongst health care providers and community on antimicrobial resistance and rational use of antimicrobials.
- *Activities carried out under the programme:*
  - AMR Surveillance carried out for "7 priority bacterial pathogens" - Klebsiella spp., Escherichia coli, Staphylococcus aureus, and Enterococcus spp., Pseudomonas spp, Acinetobacter spp., Salmonella enterica serotypes Typhi and Paratyphi
  - National Treatment Guidelines for antimicrobial use in infectious diseases
  - National Guidelines for Infection Prevention and Control in Healthcare facilities
  - IEC Activities
  - Strengthening Laboratory capacity for AMR detection

NATIONAL DIGITAL HEALTH MISSION 2020 (NDHM)

- *Aim:* To provide necessary support for 'integration of Digital Health Infrastructure' in India
- *Basis:* National Health Policy-2017, NHA- National Health Authority, "Universal Health Coverage"
- *Health ID:* Unique for every citizen of India having all the Health related information of the individual
- *Personal heal record:* Electronic record managed/shared by the individual itself
- *Digi-Doctor:* A comprehensive repository of all doctor's who are practicing modern allopathic system
- *Health Facility Registry:* A complete repository of all the facilities across the country including both Government Public & Private Hospitals, Pharmacies, Laboratories, Clinics & Imaging Centres
- Electronic Medical Records

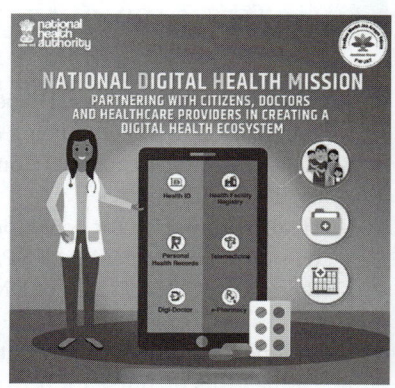

SUMAN SCHEME 2019

- *SUMAN:* Surakshit Matritva Aashwasan
- *Launched:* 10 October 2019
- *Goal:* To end all Maternal & new born deaths
- *Vision:* Achieve 'zero' maternal & new born deaths through quality care with dignity & respect
- *Beneficiaries:*
  – All Pregnant Mothers
  – All mothers upto 6 months post delivery
  – All sick newborns
- *Suman Service Guarantee:*
  – Basic Package
  – BEmONC package
  – CEmONC package

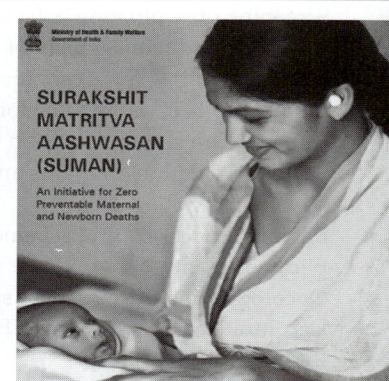

PMSMA

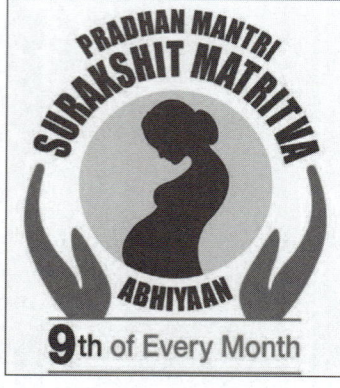

- *PMSMA:* Pradhan Mantri Surakshit Matritva Abhiyan
- *Aim:* To provide quality Antenatal care services for 2nd or 3rd trimester on 9th Date of Every Month
- *Description:* A minimum package of antenatal care services is to be provided to the beneficiaries on the 9th day of every month at the Pradhan Mantri Surakshit Matritva Clinics to ensure that every pregnant woman receives at least one checkup in the 2nd/3rd trimester of pregnancy (If the 9th day of the month is a Sunday/a holiday, then the Clinic should be organized on the next working day)
- PMSM clinics consists of Private Practitioners
- All the investigations will be done before seeing the obstetrician
- *Lab Investigations:* USG & all basic investigations (Hb, Urine Albumin, RBS Dip stick, Rapid Malaria test, Rapid VDRL test, Blood Grouping, CBC, ESR)
- The Obstetrician will do the complete examination
- This scheme is under MoHFW
- Public Health Facilities to access services under PMSMA
  – *Rural Areas:* Primary Health Centers, Community Health Centers, Rural Hospitals, SubDistrict Hospital, District Hospital, Medical College Hospital
  – *Urban Areas:* Urban Dispensaries, Urban Health Posts, Maternity Homes

PMMVY 2017

- *PMMVY:* Pradhan Mantri Matru Vandana Yojana
- *Description:* Centrally Sponsored DBT scheme with the cash incentive of ₹ 5000/- (in three instalments) being provided directly in the bank/post office account of Pregnant Women and Lactating Mothers

- It is a conditional cash transfer scheme for pregnant and lactating women of 19 years of age or above for the first live birth
- Objectives of PMMVY:
  - Providing partial compensation for the wage loss in terms of cash incentives so that the woman can take adequate rest before and after delivery of the first living child
  - The cash incentive provided would lead to improved health seeking behaviour amongst the Pregnant Women and Lactating Mothers (PW&LM)
- Cash Incentives Distribution:
  - *First Instalment:* Early Registration of pregnancy (Rs 1,000/-)
  - *Second Instalment:* Received at least one ANC/can be claimed after 6 months of pregnancy (Rs 2,000/-)
  - *Third Instalment:* Child Birth is registered, Child has received first cycle of BCG, OPV, DPT and Hepatitis-B or its equivalent/substitute (Rs 2,000/-)

DAKSHTA 2015

- *Description:* To empower providers for improved maternal & neonatal health care during institutional deliveries
- *Aim:* To reduce Maternal & neonatal Mortality
- *Implementation:* 98 districts of Madhya Pradesh, Maharashtra, Odisha, Andhra Pradesh, Jharkhand, Telangana
- 4 Pause Points has been identified: At the time of admission, Before pushing or CS, Soon after delivery (1 hour), After discharge
- Target population: Medical officers, Nurses, Auxilliary nursing Midwife

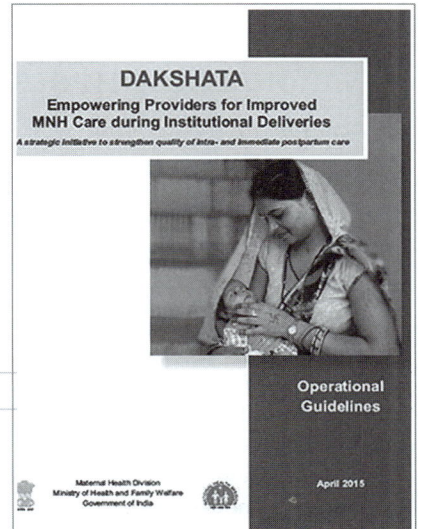

SAANS 2019

- *SAANS:* Social Awareness and action plan to neutralise pneumonia successfully
- *Target:* To reduce Childhood mortality due to Pneumonia to less than 3 per 1000 Live Birth by 2025
- *Objectives:*
  - Awareness in community
  - Awareness of care gives to identify early
  - Dispels myths and notions and trigger behaviour change
- *Target beneficiaries:*
  - *Primary beneficiaries:* All care givers, Mothers, Fathers
  - *Secondary beneficiaries:* Key Opinion Leaders (Gram Panchayat Leaders, Local Administration, Religious Leaders, Village Health Sanitation and Nutrition Committee Members, ICDS, Private practitioners)

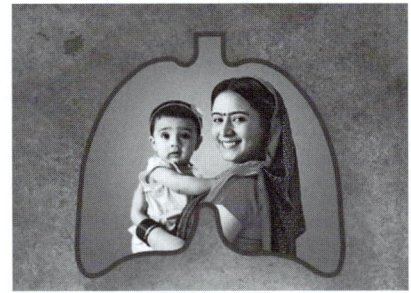

PRADHAN MANTRI JAN DHAN YOJANA (PMJDY) 2014^Q

- *Launched*: 15th August, 2014
- *Description*: "National Mission for Financial Inclusion "to ensure access to financial services, namely, Banking/Savings & Deposit Accounts, Remittance Credit, Insurance, Pension in an affordable manner.
- *Objectives*:
  - To ensure access to various financial services like availability of basic savings bank account, access to need based credit, remittances facility, insurance and pension to excluded sections (weaker sections & low income groups)
  - Effective use of technology to allow deep penetration at affordable cost

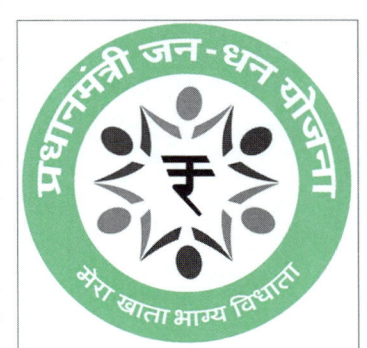

PMJDY

PRADHAN MANTRI SWASTHYA SURAKSHA YOJANA (PMSSY) 2006[Q]

- *Importance*: Aims at correcting the imbalances in the availability of affordable healthcare facilities in the different parts of the country in general, and augmenting facilities for quality medical education in the under-served States in particular
- *Components of first phase*:
  - Setting up 6 AIIMS institutions at Bhopal, Bhubaneswar, Jodhpur, Patna, Raipur and Rishikesh
  - Upgradation of 13 existing medical institutions at Jammu, Srinagar, Kolkata, Lucknow, Varanasi, Hyderabad, Tirupati, Salem, Ranchi, Ahmedabad, Bangalore, Mumbai, Thiruvananthapuram
- *Components of Second phase*:
  - Setting up 2 AIIMS institutions at Raebareli, Raigunj (Dinajpur)
  - Upgradation of 6 medical institutions at Rohtak, Tanda, Amritsar, Nagpur, Madurai, Aligarh
- *Components of Third phase*:
  - Upgradation of 39 more medical institutions

NATIONAL HEALTH POLICY (NHP) 2017

See Annexure 10

NATIONAL POPULATION POLICY 2000 (NPP 2000)

- *Immediate objective:* To address the unmet needs for contraception, health care infrastructure, and health personnel, and to provide integrated service delivery for basic reproductive and child health care
- *Mid-term objective:* To bring the TFR to replacement levels (TFR = 2.1) by 2010[Q]
- *Long term objective:* To achieve a stable population by 2045[Q]
- *National Socio-demographic goals for 2010:*
  - Address the unmet needs for basic reproductive and child health services, supplies and infrastructure
  - Make school education up to age 14 free and compulsory, and reduce drop outs at primary and secondary school levels to <20% for both boys and girls
  - Reduce IMR to <30 per 1000 live births[Q]
  - Reduce MMR to <100 per 100,000 live births[Q]
  - Achieve universal immunization of children against all VPDs
  - Promote delayed marriage for girls (not <18y and preferably >20y[Q]).
  - Achieve 80% institutional deliveries and 100% by trained persons[Q]
  - Achieve universal access to information/counseling, and services for fertility regulation and contraception with a wide basket of choices
  - Achieve 100% registration of births, deaths, marriage & pregnancy[Q]
  - Contain the spread of AIDS, and promote greater integration between the management of RTI and STI and the NACO
  - Prevent and control communicable diseases
  - Integrate Indian Systems of Medicine (ISM) in RCH services
  - Promote vigorously the small family norm to achieve replacement levels of TFR (i.e., TFR = 2.1[Q])
  - Bring about convergence in implementation of related social sector programmes so that family welfare becomes people centred programme.

NATIONAL MENTAL HEALTH POLICY 2014

- *Vision*: Promote mental health, prevent mental illness, enable recovery from mental illness and ensure accessible & affordable quality health and social care
- *Goals*[Q]:
  - To reduce distress, disability, exclusion morbidity and premature mortality associated with MH disorders

- To enhance understanding of MH in country
- To strengthen leadership in MH at district, state and national levels

Values and principles:	Objectives[a]:
Equity	To provide universal access to MH care
Justice	To increase access to MH services for vulnerable groups
Integrated care	To reduce prevalence & impact of risk factors
Evidence based care	To reduce risk & incidence of suicide
Quality	To ensure respect for right of persons with MH disorders
Participatory and rights based approach	To reduce associated stigma
Governance and effective delivery	To enhance availability & equity of human resources
Value base in teaching & training prog	To enhance financial allocation and improve utilization
Holistic approach to mental health	To identify social, biological & behavioral determinants

INTEGRATED CHILD PROTECTION SCHEME (ICPS 2009–10)

- Beneficiaries: Children in need of care and protection, Children in conflict, Children in contact with law, Children of migrant families, Children of prisoners/prostitutes, Working children, Street children, Trafficked children, Sexually-exploited children, Child drug abusers, Child beggars
- Objectives of ICPS: [**Mnemonic: S**uch **I**mportant **R**elease **E**merged **R**esponsibly]
  - **S**tructures establishment at all government levels for children in difficult circumstances
  - **I**mprove access to and quality of CPS
  - **R**aise public awareness about rights of children
  - **E**vidence based monitoring and evaluation system
  - **R**esponsibility and accountability of child protection articulated
- Services under ICPS: [**Mnemonic: Emergency WINGS**]
  - **Emergency** outreach service (Helpline 1098: 24-hour)
  - **W**eb-enabled child protection management system
  - **I**nstitutional services (Shelter home, Child home, Observation home)
  - **N**on-institutional family-based care (sponsors, adoption, foster-care, cradle-baby centres, after care)
  - **G**eneral grant-in-aid for need based interventions
  - **S**helters (open) for children in need in urban, semi-urban areas

NATIONAL FAMILY PLANNING INDEMNITY SCHEME

- Description: States/UTs to process and make payments to claims to acceptors of sterilization in cases of death/failure/complications/indemnity cover to doctors/health facilities

Category	Event	Amount (Rs.)
A	Death at hospital or <7 days of discharge	200,000/-
B	Death following sterilization (8–30 days)	50,000/-
C	Expense for treatment of medical complications	25,000/-
D	Failure of sterilization	30,000/-
E	Doctors/facilities coverage for litigations up to 4/year	200,000/-*

(* per case)
- Promotion of Small-family norm:
  - Central government employees get 1 increment after sterilization
  - State government employees get 2 increments (after 2 children) or 1 increment (after 3 children) after sterilization
  - Special leave (14 days for women, 7 days for men)
- Green cards issued to individual acceptors after 2 children, for recognition and priority attention in schemes
- Cash awards for best performing states

FAMILY WELFARE LINKED HEALTH INSURANCE SCHEME

- Description: FP Insurance scheme for acceptors of sterilization and indemnity cover for doctors
- Coverage: Government facilities, Accredited Private/NGO/Corporate health facilities
- Cover: Rs. 200,000/- per doctor/health facility per case
- Operational responsibility: ICICI

SOME IMPORTANT HEALTH LEGISLATIONS PASSED IN INDIA

- The Quarantine Act, 1870^Q
- The Vaccination Act, 1880
- The Child Marriage Restraint (SARDA) Act, 1929^Q
- The Employees State Insurance (ESI) Act, 1948^Q
- The Factories Act, 1948^Q
- The Prevention of Food Adulteration (PFA) Act, 1954
- The Immoral Traffic (Prevention) Act, 1956
- The Indian Medical Council (Prof. Conduct and Ethics) Act 1956
- The Children's Act 1960
- The Dowry Prohibition Act, 1961
- The Maternity Benefit Act, 1961
- The Registration of Births and Deaths Act, 1969^Q
- The Medical Termination of Pregnancy (MTP) Act, 1971^Q
- The Narcotic Drugs and Psychotropic Substances Act, 1985^Q
- The Consumer Protection Act (COPRA), 1986^Q
- The Environmental Protection Act (EPA), 1986
- The Mental Health Act, 1987^Q (Now, The Mental Health Case Act, 2017)
- The Infant Milk Substitutes, Feeding Bottles and Infant Food (Regulation of production, supply and distribution) Act, 1992^Q
- The Protection of Human Rights Act, 1993
- The Pre-conception and Pre-natal Diagnostic Techniques (Prohibition of Sex Selection) [PNDT] Act, 1994^Q
- The Transplantation of Human Organs Act, 1994^Q
- The Biomedical Waste (Management and Handling) Rules, 1998
- The National Rural Employment Guarantee Act (NREGA), 2005^Q
- The Protection of Women from Domestic Violence Act, 2005^Q
- The Right to Information (RTI) Act, 2005^Q.

OT ACT, 1994

- *The Transplantation of Human Organs Act* was passed by Government of India in 1994.
  - It is an act to provide for the regulation of removal, storage and transplantation of human organs for therapeutic purposes and for the prevention of commercial dealings in human organs and for matters connected therewith or incidental thereto
- Any person 18 years age or more can authorize, any of his near relatives (spouse, son, daughter, father, mother, brother or sister), for removal of organs from his/her body after death (parents can authorize in case of minors)
- No donor and no person shall authorize the removal of any human organ for any purpose other than therapeutic purposes
- Before removal of body organs, atleast RMPs should certify *that life or brain-stem function have ceased*
- *Punishments under Organ Transplantation Act 1994*:
  - *New Modification in 2011:* Punishment for persons involved to be increased to up to 10 years imprisonment^Q + fine up to ₹ 20,00,000–1,00,00,000/–.

Key points
The Quarantine Act, 1870^Q.

Key points
- The Employees State Insurance (ESI) Act, 1948^Q.
- The Factories Act, 1948^Q.

Key points
The Medical Termination of Pregnancy (MTP) Act, 1971^Q.

Key points
The Transplantation of Human Organs Act, 1994^Q.

Key points
The Right to Information (RTI) Act, 2005^Q.

Key points
The OT Act 1994 Punishment for persons involved to be increased to up to 10 years imprisonment^Q.

CBD REGISTRATION ACT, 1969

- According to *'The Registration of Births & Deaths Act 1969'*, both the births and deaths are to be registered within 21 days each^Q.

Time of registration	Additional Requirements
Within 21 days	None
Delay <30 days	Prescribed fee
Delay >30 days & <1 year	Late fee + affidavit from notary public
Delay >1 year	Late fee + order from Class I officer/magistrate

Key points

Both the births and deaths are to be registered within 21 days each^Q.

NATIONAL RURAL EMPLOYMENT GUARANTEE ACT (NREGA) 2005

- NREGA Act 2005 has been passed by the Parliament to provide for *'100 days of guaranteed wage employment in every year'*^{Q} to every household whose adult members volunteer to do *'unskilled manual work'*^{Q}
- Salient features:
  - A household is entitled for *'100 days of work in a year'*^{Q}
  - Rural Households to register to local gram panchayat. *'Job card'* to be given to every registered household (valid for 5 years)^Q
  - Registered adult must submit an application to gram panchayat (for at least 14 days of continuous work)
  - One-third of persons who are given employment will be women. Allotment for work: *'within 15 days'*^{Q}, else he/she shall be provided unemployment allowance
  - The statutory minimum wage applicable to agricultural workers in the state is to be paid
  - Work will be provided *'within 5 km'*^{Q} of applicant's residence, else he/she is entitled to 10 per cent additional wages towards transport and living expenses
  - Implementation of the Act: The *'gram sabha'* will identify works to be taken up. The *'panchayats'* have the principal responsibility for planning, implementation and monitoring
  - All agencies implementing NREGA will be accountable to the public for their work. Social audit and Right to Information will apply to each aspect of implementation.

NREGA

MCI ACT 1956

Professional Misconduct (Infamous Conducts) Under MCI Act^Q

- Non-maintenance of medical records of patients (for 3 years) and refusal to provide the same within 72 hours when the patient makes a request
- Non-display the registration number of State Medical Council or the Medical Council of India in his clinic, prescriptions and certificates
- Committing adultery or improper conduct with a patient
- Conviction by Court of Law
- Sex Determination Tests
- Signing professional Certificates, Reports and other Documents which are untrue, misleading or improper
- Contravening the provisions of the Drugs and Cosmetics Act and regulations
- Performing or enabling unqualified person to perform an abortion or any illegal operation for which there is no medical, surgical or psychological indication
- Issuing certificates of efficiency in modern medicine to unqualified or non-medical person
- Contributing to the lay press articles and give interviews regarding diseases and treatments which may have the effect of advertising himself or soliciting practices
- Advertisements of institution run by a physician containing anything more than the name of the institution, type of patients, type of training, other facilities and the fees
- Using an unusually large sign board and write on it anything other than his name, qualifications, titles and name of his specialty, registration number or affixing a sign-board on a chemist's shop or in places where he does not reside or work.

- Disclosing the secrets of a patient, except:
  - in a court of law under orders of the Presiding Judge.
  - in circumstances where there is a serious and identified risk to a specific person and/or community.
  - notifiable diseases.
- Refusal on religious grounds alone to give assistance in or conduct of sterility, birth control, circumcision and medical termination of Pregnancy.
- Not taking written consent.
- Publishing photographs or case reports of patients without their permission.
- Using touts or agents for procuring patients.
- Claiming to be specialist unless he has a special qualification in that branch.
- Undertaking act of in-vitro fertilization or artificial insemination without the informed consent of the female patient and her spouse as well as the donor.
- Violating existing ICMR guidelines in clinical drug trials or other research involving patients or volunteers.
- Physician posted in rural area found absent on >2 occasions during inspection by the Head of the District Health Authority or the Chairman, Zila Parishad.
- Physician posted in a medical college/institution both as teaching faculty or otherwise found absent on >2 occasions.

NATIONAL MEDICAL COMMISSION (NMC) 2020

- NMC National Medical Commission is an Indian regulatory body of 33 members which regulates medical education and medical professionals.
- NMC has replaced the Medical Council of India (MCI) on 25 September 2020
- Consists of 4 Autonomous Bodies: Under graduate Medical Education, Post Graduate Medical Education, Medical Assessment & Rating, Ethics & Medical Registration
- Common final year MBBS professional exam is being planned where the professional Exam will be replaced by NEXT (National Exit Exam)

THE NATIONAL MEDICAL COMMISSION BILL, 2017

- Bill to replace the apex medical education regulator—Medical Council of India (MCI) with a new body, to ensure transparency
- Introduced in Parliament in December 2017
  - GOI can dictate guidelines for fees up to 40% of seats in private medical colleges
  - Provision for a common entrance exam and licentiate (exit) exam that medical graduates have to pass before practising or pursuing PG courses
  - Recognized medical institutions don't need the regulator's permission to add more seats or start PG course
  - Fewer elected members to the new commission
  - Medical colleges get ease of establishment, recognition, renewal of the yearly permission or recognition of degrees, and even increase the number of students they admitted.

THE NARCOTIC DRUGS AND PSYCHOTROPIC SUBSTANCES ACT, 1985

- *Whosoever produce, manufacture, buy, sell, produce, transport, use, consume any narcotic drug (Opium/poppy) or psychotropic substance:* Shall be punished with imprisonment 10–20 years^Q + fine 1–2 lac rupees (5 years + 50000 rupees for Ganja).
  - Users, if not covered under Sections 15–25, will be sent for treatment/rehabilitation and not punished^Q.
- *Breach in licence for opium growth:* Shall be punished with imprisonment 3 years with or without fine.
- *Whosoever possess a small quantity for personal consumption:* Shall be punished with imprisonment 6 months + fine.
  - *Subsequent offences:* Death penalty.
- *Alcohol use:* IS NOT covered by this act^Q.

POCSO ACT (PREVENTION OF CHILDREN FROM SEXUAL OFFENCES ACT) 2012

- Child definition: Any person less than 18 years of age
- Includes: Sexual abuses and pornography
- Punishments under the act:

Offences (Section)	Punishment (Section)
Penetrative sexual assault (3)	7 years-Life imprisonment + Fine (4)
Aggravated penetrative sexual assault (5)	10 years-Life imprisonment + Fine (6)
Sexual assault (7)	3–5 years + Fine (8)
Aggravated sexual assault (9)	5–7 years + Fine (10)
Sexual harassment (11)	3 years + Fine (12)
Use of child for pornography (13)	5 years + Fine (14)

FOOD STANDARDS AND SAFETY ACT (FSSA) 2006[Q]

- *Ministry In-charge*: Ministry of Health and Family Welfare
- *Objectives*:
  - To introduce a single statute relating to food
  - To provide for scientific development of the food processing industry
- *Organization constituted*: Food Standards and Safety Association of India (FSSAI) 2008

The Rights of Persons with Disabilities Bill 2016 (21 Disabilities)

- Blindness
- Low-vision
- Leprosy Cured persons
- Hearing Impairment (deaf and hard of hearing)
- Locomotor Disability
- Dwarfism
- Intellectual Disability
- Mental Illness
- Autism Spectrum Disorder
- Cerebral Palsy
- Muscular Dystrophy
- Chronic Neurological conditions
- Specific Learning Disabilities
- Multiple Sclerosis
- Speech and Language disability
- Thalassemia
- Hemophilia
- Sickle Cell disease
- Multiple Disabilities including deaf blindness
- Acid Attack victim
- Parkinson's disease

THE HIV/AIDS (PREVENTION & CONTROL) ACT 2017

- Prevention of discrimination against HIV positive persons
- No test, treatment of medical research on any HIV patient without his/her consent
- Union and State Governments to take measures to prevent spread of HIV/AIDS, provide ART, provide for infections management and facilitate PLHA access to welfare schemes
- Ombudsman to look into complaints and provision of healthcare services
- A 12–18 years old mature enough to understand and handle HIV affected family shall be competent to act as guardian for sibling <18 months age
- Cases pertaining to PLHA shall be disposed off by Court on a priority basis; All proceedings to suppress identity, under camera trial and prevent publishing of information related to identity of person.

THE MENTAL HEALTH CARE ACT, 2017

- The Mental Health Care Act 2017 repeals the existing Mental Health Act 1987[Q]
- Formulated in line with the Convention on Rights of Persons with Disabilities and its Optional Protocol (United Nations)

- Definition of "Mental illness": Substantial disorder of thinking, mood, perception, orientation or memory that grossly impairs judgment, behaviour, capacity to recognize reality or ability to meet the ordinary demands of life, mental conditions associated with the abuse of alcohol and drugs
    - However, it does not include Mental retardation which is a condition of arrested or incomplete development of mind of a person, specially characterized by sub-normality of intelligence^Q
- Important components:
    - Right to access mental healthcare services run or funded by the Government
    - Mental health services of good quality at affordable cost, geographically accessible and without discrimination
    - Free legal services to exercise any of his rights
    - Person can specify type of treatment, person responsible
    - Medical practitioner/health professional shall not be held liable for any unforeseen consequences^Q
    - No use of electro-convulsive therapy without the use of muscle relaxants, anesthesia^Q
    - No seclusion or solitary confinement^Q
    - Government to plan, design and implement programmes for the promotion of mental health and prevention of mental illness in the country
    - Establishment of Central a State Mental Health Authority
    - State Mental Health Authority will constitute Mental Health Review Boards which will be chaired by a District Judge
    - Person who attempts suicide shall be presumed to be suffering from mental illness at that time and will not be punished under the Indian Penal Code^Q.

NATIONAL LISTS OF ESSENTIAL MEDICINES (NLEM) 2022

- 384 Drugs included in NLEM 2022; 34 new drugs added
- Criteria followed for inclusion in NLEM:
    - be useful in diseases which is a public health problem in India
    - be licensed/approved Drugs Controller General (India) (DCGI)
    - have proven efficacy and safety profile based on scientific evidence
    - be comparatively cost effective
    - be aligned with the current treatment guidelines
    - recommended under National Health Programs of India. (e.g. Ivermectin part of Accelerated Plan for Elimination of Lymphatic Filariasis 2018).
    - when more than one medicine are available from the same therapeutic class, one prototype/medically best suited medicine of that class to be included.
    - price of total treatment is considered and not the unit price of a medicine
    - fixed dose combinations are usually not included
    - vaccines as and when are included in Universal Immunization Program (e.g. Rotavirus vaccine).

PYQs: Quick Review for NEET

RNTCP

Under RNTCP, Case finding is	Passive as well as Active
In DOTS, diagnosis based on	Sputum smears, CBNAAT & other tests
DOTS Plus refers to	MDR TB treatment (Cat IV)
Diagnosis of TB in RNTCP	2 sputum smear examination (ZN Staining)
Sputum Smear +ve at or after 5 months defined as	ATT Failure
Only Bacteriostatic drug in Primary ATT Drugs	Ethambutol
Case finding Tool of choice in RNTCP is	Sputum Smear (ZN Staining)
DOTS is	Directly Observed Treatment, Short Course
'DOTS' indicates	Short-term treatment under supervision
Relapse/Defaulter/Failure in RNTCP DOTS is Category	Category II (8 Months treatment)
Sputum smear +ve on ZN Staining, if bacillary load	>10000 AFB per mL of sputum
Color blindness associated with Ethambutol	Red-green colour blindness
Anti-tubercular drug not given in children <6 years age	Ethambutol
As per RNTCP, DOTS Cat-1, should receive	4 drugs for 2 months, 2 drugs for 4 months
Nature of Category I TB treatment under DOTS is	Active
Nature of RNTCP case finding is	Passive
New change in RNTCP	Non-DOTS based therapy
Drug used only in RNTCP Category II is	Streptomycin
In the DOTS strategy under RNTCP, 'D' and 'O' stand for	Directly observed
Treatment of recently Sputum positive case of Pulmonary TB	RMP + INH + PZM + ETM
Tubercular pericarditis is treated with DOTS Category	Category I
Pediatric weight bands in RNTCP new guidelines	Six
DOTS provider gets honorarium on completion of treatment	Rupees 1000/- (Cat-1), 1500 (Cat-2), 5000/- (Cat-4/5)
Failure under RNTCP if sputum smear/culture if positive at or after	5 months of treatment
1 TB unit (RNTCP) is for a population of	2.0 Lac
RNTCP microscopic center is recommended for ____ population	100,000
Best indicator for spread of TB in a community	Annual infection rate
Role of ASHA in DOTS is	Providing DOTS

NPEP

Polio stool samples are transported in	Reverse Cold Chain (+ 2° to + 8° C)
In AFP, examination for residual paralysis should be done after	60 days
Target group for pulse polio immunization is	0–5 years

NVBDCP

Modified Plan Operation (1977) was based on	API (Annual parasitic incidence)
Indicator of operational efficiency in Malaria (NVBDCP)	ABER (Annual Blood Examination Rate)
In Malaria program, MPW does Active Surveillance once every	14 days (Fortnightly)
Health worker in Malaria control must visit all houses every	Fortnight
DOC for Kala Azar (Black sickness) in Indian program	Sodium Stibo-gluconate (Antimonials)
DOC for Filariasis	DEC
Index of Operational efficiency of the malaria control	Annual blood examination rate (ABER)
Treatment of Severe Falciparum malaria	Quinine
Blood smear must be made at night for	Filariasis

RCH Program

Under RCH Program, Kit A, B are kept at	Subcentre Level
Diagnosis of Severe Pneumonia in PHC is based on	Chest indrawing
Older name of Janani Suraksha Yojana	National Maternity Benefit Scheme
Pink colour in IMNCI indicate	Immediate referral
Green colour in IMNCI represent	Home based management

Contd...

Contd...

According to IMNCI, fast breathing in 5 month child is	>50 per minute
Patient treated at home according to IMNCI color coding	Green
IMNCI target group is	Up to 5 years
In CSSM Program drug of choice for Pneumonia	Cotrimoxazole
CSSM Program was started in year	1992
Eligible couple is defined as	Currently married couple, wife 15–45 years age
NPCB	
Main aim of Vision 2020	Eliminate avoidable blindness
In School eye-screening program, initial vision screening done by	School teachers
In SAFE strategy, S stands for	Surgery
In Vision 2020, target for Secondary service centres is one per	500,000 population
In vision 2020, recommended ophthalmic personnel per population ratio	1 per 500,000 population
NACP	
Nevirapine in MTCT given to child	Within 72 hours
Initiate ART in HIV+ve individuals if	Any CD4 count
HIV sentinel surveillance was started in 1994 with _____ sites	55
NLEP	
National Leprosy Eradication Program started in	1983
Multi drug therapy (MDT) is treatment for	Leprosy
Treatment duration of MBL	12 months (Surveillance 5 years)
Treatment duration of PBL	6 months (Surveillance 2 years)
Goal of NLEP is to bring Prevalence of leprosy to less than	1/10000 population
Other Programs	
National Rural Health Mission launched in	2005
ASHA full form is	Accredited Social Health Activist
First priority in Stroke Control Program	Control arterial hypertension
Functional unit of implementation in NMHP	District
National Mental Health Program (NMHP) launched in	1982
Amount of cereals in Mid-day meal program	100 grams
Midday meal program provides	1/3 calories and 1/2 proteins
Drug of choice for chemoprophylaxis of plague	Tetracycline
Swajaldhara Yojana is to provide	Water
Policies, Legislations, Schemes & Initiatives	
Baby Friendly Hospital Initiative (BFHI) launched in	1991
Jai Vigyan Mission is for control of	Rheumatic fever/RHD
Ujjwala scheme is related to	Human trafficking control & prevention
National Mental Health Act passed in year	1987 (Mental Health Care Act in 2017)
Eye donation fortnight	25th August – 6th September
Direct cash transfer scheme to pregnant lactating women is	Indira Gandhi Matritva Sahyog Yojana
National Population Policy was started from year	1976
RBD Act 1969, Birth and death are to be registered, respectively in	21 days, 21 days
MTP can be done by a RMP if gestation period is less than	24 weeks
Naranjo algorithms is used for calculating probability of	Adverse drug reaction
Elemental iron and folic acid contents of IFA adult tablet is	60 mg of iron, 500 mcg of folic acid
Narcotic drugs and psychotropic substances Act was passed in	1985
First National Population Policy was formulated in	1976
First National Health Policy was formulated in	1983

Multiple Choice Questions

NATIONAL TB ELIMINATION PROGRAM (NTEP)/RNTCP

1. A 35 years old male presented with fever, cough and chest symptom for last 2 months. His TB sputum samples turn out to be negative. Chest x-ray findings are suggestive of TB. Under NTEP, the next line of management is:
   [NEET PG Pattern 2023]
   (a) CBNAAT
   (b) Tuberculin testing
   (c) Repeat sputum samples testing
   (d) Start TB treatment

2. A patient having cough 3 weeks was started on ATT under NTEP. IP and CP were completed and then he tested smear negative for AFB on two samples. What's the status of patient? *[NEET PG Pattern 2022]*
   (a) Treatment completed
   (b) Cured
   (c) Improper follow-up
   (d) Failure

3. If someone has been diagnosed with TB and HIV both as coinfection, what should be the Treatment protocol?
   [INICET July 2021]
   (a) Give ART (antiretroviral therapy) once cd4 drops less than 200
   (b) Give ART first and then after 2 weeks treat with TB treatment
   (c) Give TB treatment first and then after 2 weeks treat with ART
   (d) Give both ART and TB treatments simultaneously

4. Sequence of AFB staining is: *[INICET July 2021]*
   (a) Carbol fuschin, Acid alcohol, Methylene blue
   (b) Hematoxylin, Alcoholic formalin, Methylene blue
   (c) Carbol fuschin, Acetic acid, Hematoxylin
   (d) Harris hematoxylin, Alcohol, Eosin

5. For sputum smear to come positive on ZN staining there should be minimum: *[AIIMS Nov 1999]*
   (a) 100 bacilli per mL sputum *[AIIMS Dec 1992]*
   (b) 1000 bacilli per mL sputum
   (c) 2000 bacilli per mL sputum
   (d) 10,000 bacilli per mL sputum

6. Best indicator of trend of Tuberculosis unaffected by current control measures is: *[AIIMS Nov 1993]*
   (a) Annual Risk of Infection
   (b) Prevalence of TB infection
   (c) % of primary drug resistance
   (d) % of Multidrug resistance

7. Multidrug resistance in TB is defined as resistance to:
   [AIIMS May 2004]
   (a) Streptomycin, Rifampicin and Isoniazid
   (b) Streptomycin and Rifampicin
   (c) Isoniazid and Rifampicin
   (d) Streptomycin and Isoniazid

8. Every TB sputum positive patient can infect up to:
   [AIIMS Dec 1995]
   (a) 1–2 persons per year
   (b) 5–6 persons per year
   (c) 10–15 persons per year
   (d) 100–200 persons per year

9. Anti-tubercular drug contraindicated during pregnancy is: *[AIIMS May 1994]*
   (a) Isoniazid (b) Rifampicin
   (c) Streptomycin (d) Ethambutol

10. True about revised National Tuberculosis programme (NTP): *[PGI June 03]*
    (a) Active case finding
    (b) DOTS applied
    (c) Treatment is given only in smear positive cases
    (d) General practitioners are restricted to give the treatment
    (e) It has replaced NTP

11. Which is included in RNTCP: *[PGI June 04]*
    (a) Active case finding *[NEET Pattern 2013]*
    (b) Directly observed
    (c) X-ray is diagnostic
    (d) Drugs given daily

12. True about DOTS: *[PGI June 2008]*
    (a) Drugs are given on supervision *[PGI Dec 08]*
    (b) Streptomycin always given in first two months
    (c) Intermittent regimen are used
    (d) Same regimen is given in all patient
    (e) In category – 1. new sputum positive cases sputum examined in 2.5 and 6 months

13. A person with tuberculosis on domiciliary treatment is expected to do all, *except*:
    (a) Dispose sputum safely
    (b) Use separate vessels
    (c) Collect drugs regularly
    (d) Report to PHC if new symptoms arise

14. Dose of Rifampicin in RNTCP is:
    [AIIMS November 2013] [NEET Pattern 2013]
    (a) 300 mg (b) 450 mg
    (c) 600 mg (d) 800 mg

15. Drugs are used in AKT-4 kit for TB as:
    [NEET Pattern 2013]
    (a) Decrease in resistance by mutation
    (b) Decrease in resistance by conjugation
    (c) To cure disease early
    (d) None

16. True about Category III RNCTP is/are:
    (a) Recently abolished [PGI November 2012]
    (b) Meant for MDR-TB treatment
    (c) Given for 6 months
    (d) Includes defaulters
    (e) Based on sputum culture findings

17. Why a TB patient is recommend a regimen of 4 drugs on 1st visit: [NEET Pattern 2013]
    (a) To avoid emergence of persistors
    (b) To avoid side effects
    (c) To cure early
    (d) None of the above

18. XDR-TB definition include resistance to:
    [PGI May 2014] [NEET Pattern 2014]
    (a) Rifampicin
    (b) Any one Fluoroquinolone
    (c) INH
    (d) Kanamycin
    (e) Ethionamide

19. Under RNCTP diagnosis, TB bacilli take up AFB stain faster showing 'Beaded appearance' due to presence of:
    (a) Palmitic acid [NEET Pattern 2014]
    (b) Wax-D
    (c) Cord-factor
    (d) Mycolic acid

20. Who cannot supervise DOTS under RNCTP?
    [NEET Pattern 2015]
    (a) Father   (b) Teacher
    (c) Health worker   (d) Social worker

21. Pitfalls of DOTS [NEET Pattern 2015]
    (a) High cost
    (b) De-stigmatization
    (c) High cure rate
    (d) Prevents failure and MDR

22. In a suspected TB patient, two boxes are given for sputum sample collection. They are labelled as
    [AIIMS May 2016]
    (a) a, b   (b) A, B
    (c) 1, 2   (d) Y, Z

23. A patient came to a private practitioner and was diagnosed Tuberculosis. Within how many days he has to inform or register to District Health Officer?
    [NEET Pattern 2016]
    (a) 1 day   (b) 7 days
    (c) 30 days (d) 1 year

24. A 45 years old male patient comes to OPD with cough and diarrhea since last 3 weeks. On diagnosis he is found to be HIV positive with Tuberculosis. Next line of management should be: [NEET Pattern 2017]
    (a) Start ATT followed by ART
    (b) Start ART followed by ATT
    (c) Start ATT
    (d) Start ART then start ATT after 6–8 weeks

25. For diagnosis of TB, Sputum microscopy has:
    [NEET Pattern 2017]
    (a) High sensitivity and high specificity
    (b) High sensitivity and low specificity
    (c) Low sensitivity and high specificity
    (d) Low sensitivity and low specificity

26. Not a component of DOTS [NEET Pattern 2017]
    (a) Political commitment
    (b) Uninterrupted supply of drugs
    (c) Medicine given for 1 month
    (d) Accountability

27. Objectives of RNTCP [NEET Pattern 2017]
    (a) Detects at least 85% of cases
    (b) Achieve at least 85% cure rate
    (c) No help from NGO
    (d) Achieve at least 90% cure rate

28. Which of the following is/are true about RNTCP?
    [PGI 2017]
    (a) TB is mandatory to notify
    (b) Suspicious TB patients are screened through 2 sputum smear examinations
    (c) MDR-TB is not included in RNTCP
    (d) Case finding is active
    (e) Covered the whole country since March 2006

29. IT based TB monitoring is known as
    [NEET Pattern 2018, 2019]
    (a) Nischay   (b) Nikshay
    (c) Nirbhay   (d) e-DOTS

30. Most peripheral Laboratory under RNTCP is
    [NEET Pattern 2018]
    (a) Tuberculosis unit
    (b) Peripheral reference laboratory
    (c) Intermediate reference laboratory
    (d) Designated microscopy centre

31. Minimum number of Sputum specimens required to confirm diagnosis TB according to RNTCP guidelines
    [NEET Pattern 2018]
    (a) One   (b) Two
    (c) Three (d) Four

Review Question

32. In revised National Tuberculosis Control Programme main objective is: [MP 2002]
    (a) To improve patient's compliance
    (b) Achievements of high cure rates through DOTS

(c) To decrease development of resistance against Antitubercular drugs
(d) To increase effectiveness

NATIONAL POLIO ELIMINATION PROGRAMME

33. TRUE/FALSE TYPE QUESTION: Which of the following is not done under AFP Surveillance? (True/False) [AIIMS May 2019]
    (a) AFP surveillance done in more than 15 years age
    (b) Stool sample of more than 15 years to be taken
    (c) Once diagnosed follow-up to be done after 60 days
    (d) Stool specimen should reach Laboratory in 72 hours
    (e) >1 case of non-polio AFP per 1 Lakh population be detected

34. Pulse polio immunization is administration of OPV to: [NEET Pattern 2012] [MP 2005] [AIIMS Nov 2007]
    (a) All children between 0–5 years of age on a single day, irrespective of their previous immunization status
    (b) Children in the age group of 0–1 year only who have not been immunized earlier
    (c) Children in the age group of 12–24 months only, as the booster dose
    (d) All children between 0–5 years of age, whenever there is an outbreak of poliomyelitis

35. Under AFP Surveillance, follow-up examination is done after (For residual paralysis): [AIPGME 2005, 2010] [AIIMS May 2012]
    (a) 15 days of onset of paralysis
    (b) 33 days of onset of paralysis
    (c) 60 days of onset of paralysis
    (d) 93 days of onset of paralysis

36. All are true regarding AFP Surveillance except: [AIPGME 2004]
    (a) WHO recommends it for age less than 15 yrs
    (b) Two stool samples are collected per case
    (c) Non-polio AFP rate should be >1 per 100000 among <15 years old
    (d) Adequate stool specimens should be taken from 100% AFP

37. Line listing of cases of Acute Flaccid Paralysis is done for all of the following reasons except: [NUPGET 2013]
    (a) To check for duplication
    (b) To document high risk groups
    (c) To confirm year of onset of illness
    (d) To identify high risk population

38. Under national polio eradication programme, a case of acute flaccid paralysis is confirmed as polio by surveillance after how many days? [DNB December 2009]
    (a) 15 days
    (b) 30 days
    (c) 60 days
    (d) 90 days

Review Question

39. All are true regarding Acute flaccid paralysis in National polio Eradication Programme, except: [UP 2008]
    (a) Acute flaccid paralysis in a child <15 years of age
    (b) All cases of AFP should be reported irrespective of diagnosis within 6 months of onset stool
    (c) Two specimens collected within 14 days of paralysis onset and at least 24 hours apart
    (d) 30 days follow up examination

RCH PROGRAMME

40. Improving Quality of Labour room is covered under which program? [AIIMS May 2019]
    (a) LaQshya
    (b) Improving care of newborn
    (c) Ayushman Bharat Scheme
    (d) JSSK

41. Integrated Management of Neonatal and Childhood Illness (IMNCI) includes all except: [AIPGME 09]
    (a) Malaria   (b) Respiratory infections
    (c) Diarrhoea   (d) Tuberculosis

42. Essential components of RCH Programme in India include all of the following except:
    (a) Prevention and management of unwanted pregnancies [AIPGME 04]
    (b) Maternal care including antenatal, delivery and postnatal services
    (c) Reduce the under five mortality to half
    (d) Management of reproductive tract infections and sexually transmitted infections

43. 'Seven Cleans' of safe and hygienic birth practices include: [AIIMS May 2007]
    (a) Clean walls and Clean floor
    (b) Clean towel and Clean water for hand washing
    (c) Clean birth canal and Clean cord surface
    (d) Clean mind and Clean environment

44. Elemental iron and folic acid contents of pediatric iron-folic acid tablets supplied under Reproductive and Child Health (RCH) Programme are: [AIPGME 03]
    (a) 20 mg iron and 100 micrograms folic acid
    (b) 40 mg iron and 100 micrograms folic acid
    (c) 40 mg iron and 50 micrograms folic acid
    (d) 60 mg iron and 100 micrograms folic acid

45. Copper-T with threads is visible in a case of early pregnancy. Treatment of choice is: [DPG 2011]
    (a) Remove CuT only
    (b) Suction evacuation with Copper-T removal
    (c) Reassurance and continue pregnancy
    (d) Laparotomy

46. Under RCH programme, intervention done in selected districts [NEET Pattern 2013]
    (a) Immunization
    (b) Treatment of STD
    (c) ORS therapy
    (d) Vitamin A supplementation

47. RCH programme includes [NEET Pattern 2013]
    (a) CSSM plus school health
    (b) CSSM plus family planning
    (c) CSSM plus ORS
    (d) CSSM plus pneumonia control

48. RCH phase 2 does not include [NEET Pattern 2012]
    (a) Immunization of pregnant women
    (b) Treatment of STD/RTI
    (c) Feed to malnourished children
    (d) Early registration of pregnancy up to 12–16 weeks

49. Components of RCH elaborated include [NEET Pattern 2013]
    (a) Prevention of STD
    (b) Family planning
    (c) Child survival
    (d) All of the above

50. Data regarding recent trends of Immunization in Community can be found by [AIIMS PG May 2015]
    (a) Census data
    (b) Rural survey
    (c) District level household survey
    (d) Sample registration system

51. A recently delivered woman with a 15-day old newborn suffering from Cough, sneezing and fever needs help. She has no money for transportation to nearby hospital. Which of the following National Health Programmes can help this woman? [AIIMS November 2015]
    (a) Facility based IMNCI
    (b) Janani Shishu Suraksha Karyakram
    (c) Navjat Shishu Suraksha Karyakram
    (d) Indira Gandhi Matritava Sahyog Karyakram

52. In RMNCH+A Strategy, what is Plus? [NEET Pattern 2015]
    (a) Adolescent health
    (b) Reproductive health
    (c) DPT vaccination
    (d) Newborn vaccination

53. Not done in RMNCH + A [NEET Pattern 2016]
    (a) Linking Maternal health to Reproductive health
    (b) Linking home & community based service to facility based care
    (c) Referral to PHC/CHC
    (d) Involvement of private organizations

54. RMNCH+A program related which is wrong for Adolescents [NEET Pattern 2016]
    (a) School health examinations
    (b) Iron supplementation
    (c) Nutritional education
    (d) Pneumonia treatment

55. All are true about IMNCI except: [NEET Pattern 2017]
    (a) Inclusion of early neonatal care
    (b) Inclusion of home based care
    (c) Dedication of 75% training the on younger infants
    (d) Pink color code represent urgent referral

56. Peripheral most unit for planning of Family planning and other services under RCH program is: [NEET Pattern 2019]
    (a) Sub-centre
    (b) Block/Taluka
    (c) PHC
    (d) District

Review Question

57. Recommended dose for treatment of pneumonia of 6 months old child is (1 tablet contains 100 mg of sulphamethoxazole and 20 mg of trimethoprim): [MP 2009]
    (a) ½ tablet twice daily
    (b) One tablet twice daily
    (c) Two tablets twice daily
    (d) Three tablets twice daily

NATIONAL BLINDNESS CONTROL PROGRAMME

58. Under the National Programme for Control of Blindness in India, medical colleges are classified as eye care centers of: [AIIMS Nov 2003]
    (a) Primary level   (b) Secondary level
    (c) Tertiary level   (d) Intermediate level

59. A 46 years old female presented at the eye OPD in a hospital. Her vision in the right eye was 6/60 and in left eye 3/60. Under the National Programme for Control of Blindness, she will be classified as: [AIIMS May 05] [AIIMS Nov 02]
    (a) Socially blind
    (b) Low vision
    (c) Economically blind
    (d) Normal vision

60. According to the World Health Organization, the definition of blindness is: [TNPG 1994, 2000] [AIPGME 06, AIPGME 2000, 01; AIIMS Nov 05]
    (a) Visual acuity <6/60 in the better eye with available correction
    (b) Visual acuity <3/60 in the better eye with available correction
    (c) Visual acuity <6/60 in the better eye with best correction
    (d) Visual acuity <3/60 in the better eye with best correction

61. According to the National Programme for Control of Blindness (NPCB) in India, the definition of blindness is: [AIPGME 1991]
    (a) Visual acuity <6/60 in the better eye with available correction
    (b) Visual acuity <3/60 in the better eye with available correction
    (c) Visual acuity <6/60 in the better eye with best correction
    (d) Visual acuity <3/60 in the better eye with best correction

62. The visual acuity used as cut off for differentiating "normal" from "abnormal" children in the School Vision Screening Programme in India is: [AIIMS Nov 02]
    (a) 6/6   (b) 6/9
    (c) 6/12   (d) 6/60

63. Revised strategies of National Programme for Control of Blindness include all except: [AIIMS Nov 2006]
    (a) To strengthen participation of voluntary organizations
    (b) To shift from fixed facility surgical approach to eye camp approach
    (c) To enhance coverage of eye care services in tribal and other under-served areas
    (d) To strengthen services for transplantation of cornea, treatment of glaucoma

64. Match the following NPCB categories of Visual impairment and Blindness: [AIPGME 1999]
    A <6/18 to 6/60, I - Economic Blindness
    B <6/60 to 3/60, II - Manifest Blindness
    C <3/60 to 1/60, III - Social Blindness
    D <1/60 to perception of light, IV - Low Vision
    (a) A-II, B-IV, C-III, D-I   (b) A-I, B-II, C-IV, D-IV
    (c) A-IV, B-I, C-III, D-II   (d) A-IV, B-II, C-III, D-I

65. All of the following are given global prominence in the VISION 2020 goals, except: [AIIMS May 07]
    (a) Refractive errors [AIIMS May 2010]
    (b) Cataract [NEET Pattern 2017]
    (c) Trachoma
    (d) Glaucoma

66. Target diseases for VISION 2020 in India does not include: [AIPGME 2012, AIIMS May 2007–2008]
    (a) Refractive errors and Low vision
    (b) Diabetic retinopathy
    (c) Trachoma
    (d) Xerophthalmia

67. The eye condition for which the World Bank assistance was provided to the National Programme for Control of Blindness (1994–2001) is: [AIIMS May 07]
    (a) Cataract   (b) Refractive errors
    (c) Trachoma   (d) Vitamin A deficiency

68. False about School Vision Screening Programme is:
    (a) Age group screened is 5–10 years [AIIMS Nov 2007]
    (b) Screening is done by Teacher
    (c) One teacher is for 150 students
    (d) Cut off for referral of a child is vision <6/9

69. SAFE strategy has been developed for the control of:
    (a) Onchocerciasis [AIPGME 07]
    (b) Trachoma
    (c) Refractive error
    (d) Ocular trauma

70. Which of the following Health organisation is not a part of Vision 2020? [AIIMS November 2011]
    (a) UNICEF
    (b) WHO
    (c) Orbis
    (d) International Agency for Prevention of Blindness

71. Number of Vision centers under Vision 2020, National Programme for Control of Blindness are: [AIIMS May 2013]
    (a) 20   (b) 200
    (c) 2000   (d) 20000

72. Follow-up of Cataract operations in National Blindness Control Programme is done by [AIIMS November 2013]
    (a) Active surveillance
    (b) Passive surveillance
    (c) Sentinel surveillance
    (d) Routine check-up

73. Under National Programme for Control of Blindness, District blindness control society is headed by: [AIIMS November 2014]
    (a) District programme manager [NEET Pattern 2014]
    (b) District eye surgeon
    (c) District collector
    (d) District health officer

74. Which of the following is NOT a criteria for diagnosing Blindness under NPCB? [NEET Pattern 2016]
    (a) Vision of 6/60 or less with best possible correction
    (b) Vision <4/60 in better eye
    (c) Diminution of Field of vision to 20 degrees
    (d) Inability of a person to count fingers from a distance of 20 feet

75. True statement(s) regarding National Program for Control of Blindness: [PGI November 2017]
    (a) Launched in 1962
    (b) Dr Rajendra Prasad Center for Ophthalmic Sciences AIIMS is apex body for implementation of NPCB
    (c) Promotion of eye camp and mobile unit
    (d) Intra-ocular lens implantation better than conventional surgery
    (e) NGOs are sidelined in this program

76. Vision 2020 includes all except [NEET Pattern 2018]
    (a) Onchocerciasis
    (b) Epidemic conjunctivitis
    (c) Cataract
    (d) Trachoma

NATIONAL HIV/AIDS CONTROL PROGRAMME

77. As per the NTEP, high priority TB-HIV district is defined as? [INICET May 2022]
    (a) >10% population of known HIV+ve among TB patients tested for HIV in the district
    (b) >12% population of known HIV+ve among TB patients tested for HIV in the district
    (c) >15% population of known HIV+ve among TB patients tested for HIV in the district
    (d) >20% population of known HIV+ve among TB patients tested for HIV in the district

78. While taking a blood sample of a HIV+ symptomatic patient, a resident doctor picks up Needle stick injury (NSI). Best regimen for Post-exposure prophylaxis for this resident doctor will be: [AIIMS June 2020]
    (a) Zidovudine + Lamivudine
    (b) Zidovudine + Lamivudine + Nevirapine
    (c) Tenofovir + Lamivudine + Lopinavir
    (d) Zidovudine + Stavudine + Nevirapine

79. Which of the following are not included in Sentinel surveillance of HIV in India?: [AIIMS June 2020]
    (a) Antenatal women
    (b) STD clinic attendees
    (c) Single male migrants
    (d) Long distance truckers

80. For diagnosis of HIV infection in asymptomatic, minimum number of tests required is/are:
    (a) 1   (b) 2   [AIIMS Nov 2003]
    (c) 3   (d) 4

81. Route for HIV transmission with maximum efficiency is:
    (a) Sexual   [AIIMS Nov 1999]
    (b) Transfusion of blood/blood products
    (c) Sharing needles/syringes
    (d) Mother to child transmission

82. CTL inducing vaccines, Recombinant Adeno-associated Virus Vaccine (rAAV) and Modified Vaccinia Ankara (MVA) are being developed for: [AIPGME 2002]
    (a) Tuberculosis   (b) Leprosy
    (c) Malaria   (d) HIV/AIDS

83. Targeted Interventions for HIV is done for all except:
    (a) Commercial sex workers   [AIIMS May 2009]
    (b) Migrant labourers
    (c) Street children
    (d) Industrial workers

84. According to CDC recommendations, HIV screening of pregnant women is: [AIIMS May 09]
    (a) Opt-in testing
    (b) Opt – out testing
    (c) Compulsory
    (d) Symptomatic

85. Drugs used to prevent Mother-to-child transmission of HIV in India is are [PGI November 2012]
    (a) Lamivudine   (b) Zidovudine
    (c) Nevirapine   (d) Ribavirin
    (e) Stavudine

86. Sentinel surveillance for HIV under National AIDS Control programme is used for all except: [AIIMS May 2014]
    (a) Estimation of total infection in community
    (b) Estimation of total cases in hospitals
    (c) Estimation of trend of the disease
    (d) Classification of districts

87. According to Suraksha Clinic in National AIDS Control Programme, infant coming with lower abdominal pain, the color code of kit in treatment is [NEET Pattern 2014]
    (a) White
    (b) Yellow
    (c) Green
    (d) Grey

88. NACO launched National Pediatrics AIDS Initiative on [NEET Pattern 2015]
    (a) 02 October 2005   (b) 30 November 2006
    (c) 30 October 2008   (d) 02 November 2010

89. For Post-exposure prophylaxis of HIV is [NEET Pattern 2016]
    (a) Zidovodine + Lamivudine for 4 weeks
    (b) Lamivudine + Ritonavir for 4 weeks
    (c) Zidovudine + Lamivudine + Indinavir for 4 weeks
    (d) Single dose Zidovudine + Lamivudine + Indinavir

90. Among the following Antiretroviral drugs, which one is most likely to be acceptable along with rifampicin based anti TB therapy? [NEET Pattern 2016]
    (a) Efavirenz   (b) Lopinavir/ritonavir
    (c) Nelfinavir   (d) Nevirapine

91. A pregnant lady was found to be HIV positive in First trimester. Next line of management is: [NEET Pattern 2018]
    (a) Start ART now, continue throughout pregnancy and till 6 weeks after delivery
    (b) Start ART now, continue throughout pregnancy and till lifelong
    (c) Start ART after First trimester, continue throughout pregnancy and till 6 weeks after delivery
    (d) Start ART after First trimester, continue throughout pregnancy and till lifelong

92. True about Sentinel surveillance of HIV/AIDS by NACO are all except: [JIPMER May 2018]
    (a) Yearly checkup is done
    (b) Pregnant females are included
    (c) Helps reduce antenatal HIV transmission
    (d) Target high risk population

NATIONAL VECTOR BORNE DISEASES CONTROL PROGRAMME

93. A 50-year-old male presents with fever for 3 weeks duration. Antibiotics and anti-malarials do not work. Abdomen distension present. rk39 dipstick test is positive. What will be the next management?
    [INICET May 2022]
    (a) Amphotericin B
    (b) Bedaquiline
    (c) Tigecycline
    (d) Fluconazole

94. Transmission assessment survey is for?
    [AIIMS May 2019]
    (a) Plasmodium vivax
    (b) Plasmodium falciparum
    (c) Leishmania donovani
    (d) Wuchereria bancrofti

95. Which of the following is not reported in India?
    [AIIMS Dec 1991]
    (a) Plasmodium vivax
    (b) Plasmodium falciparum
    (c) Plasmodium ovale
    (d) Plasmodium malariae

96. 'Dipstick Test' for rapid diagnosis of Plasmodium falciparum is based on: [AIIMS Nov 2004]
    (a) Arginine-rich protein
    (b) Histidine-rich protein
    (c) Tyrosine-rich protein
    (d) Serine-rich protein

97. Insecticide of choice for Phlebotamus argentipes is:
    (a) DDT [AIIMS Nov 2003]
    (b) BHC [NEET Pattern 2017]
    (c) Malathion
    (d) Pyrethrum

98. Measurement of operational efficiency of National Anti Malaria Programme (NAMP) is done by: [DPG 2006]
    (a) Annual parasite incidence (API) [Karnataka 2005]
    (b) Annual Blood Examination Rate (ABER)
    (c) Infant parasite rate [NEET Pattern 2017]
    (d) Slide positivity rate

99. Patient was given chloroquine and doxycycline for 7 days. Patients fever decreases in 4 days, but, peripheral smear showed occasional gametocytes of Plasmodium falciparum. This type of drug resistance:
    (a) R1 type
    (b) R2 type
    (c) R3 type
    (d) R4 type

100. In a town with population of 100,000 the number of slides examined is 5000. Out of these, 100 slides were positive for malaria. The API is: [DNB December 2010]
    (a) 2
    (b) 5
    (c) 1
    (d) 0.5

101. NVBDCP does not include [NEET Pattern 2013]
    (a) Malaria
    (b) Filariasis
    (c) Kala azar
    (d) Chikungunya fever

102. Urban malaria scheme is based on: [NEET Pattern 2012]
    (a) API levels
    (b) Anti-adult measures
    (c) Anti-larval measures
    (d) Drug based treatment

103. Most efficient anti-larval measure to prevent urban malaria is: [AIIMS November 2014]
    (a) Clean drainage and sewerage systems
    (b) Cover overhead tanks properly
    (c) Filling cesspools and ditches
    (d) Cover pits

104. Malaria Eradication Programme India based on use of Insecticides aims to reduce Lifespan of mosquito to less than [NEET Pattern 2015]
    (a) 1 day
    (b) 3 days
    (c) 6 days
    (d) 10 days

105. A pregnant woman in third trimester having fever was diagnosed as a case of Falciparum malaria. Under the National Health Programme, which drug is recommended?
    (a) ACT only [UPSC CMS 2015]
    (b) ACT accompanied by single dose of Primaquine on day 2
    (c) Only Quinine
    (d) Chloroquine

106. The causes for Resurgent malaria include following except: [ESI IMO 2014]
    (a) Inadequate vector control
    (b) Mosquito mutations
    (c) Improper use of drug treatment
    (d) Increase in the number Plasmodium species

107. According to Revise Malaria Drug Policy 2013, true is:
    [AIIMS November 2015]
    (a) Presumptive treatment with Chloroquine is given
    (b) ACT is not given in Falciparum
    (c) Primaquine is not given in Falciparum malaria
    (d) Primaquine contraindicated in infants and pregnant women

108. Not true about Strategic Plan for Malaria Control 2012–2017 [NEET Pattern 2016]
    (a) Objective is API <1 per 10,000
    (b) 50% reduction in mortality by 2017
    (c) Annual incidence <10 per 1000 by 2017
    (d) Complete treatment to at least 80% of patients

109. A patient was admitted to the govt. Hospital in Vijayawada with fever and microscopy of blood smear was positive

for P. falciparum. Which one of the following treatments is indicated as per the revised drug policy of India 2013?
[NEET Patterns 2016, 2017]
- (a) Artesunate 50mg for 3 days + Sulfadoxine - Pyremethamine (500 & 25 mg) single dose + Primaquine for 14 days [NEET Pattern 2017]
- (b) Artesunate alone 4 mg/kg if the patient were pregnant and in the 2 nd trimester
- (c) Artesunate 200 mg + Sulfadoxine -Pyremethamine (750 & 37.5 mg) daily for 3 days
- (d) Artesunate 4 mg/kg daily 3 days + Sulfadoxine - Pyremethamine (25/1.25 mg/kg) one dose + Primaquine 0.75 mg/kg single dose

110. A population of 100000 is under surveillance during a year. 100 cases were positive for malarial thick smear. 20 developed complications and 10 died among cases. What is the Annual parasite incidence? [NEET Pattern 2017]
- (a) 1 per 1000
- (b) 2 per 1000
- (c) 10 per 1000
- (d) 20 per 1000

Review Question

111. Plasmodium vivax malaria in pregnancy should be treated in pregnancy by: [Kolkata 2004]
- (a) Chloroquine
- (b) Quinine
- (c) Pyrimethamine
- (d) Mefloquine

NRHM, NUHM, NHM

112. For an Institutional delivery, ASHA worker motivated a woman in an Urban area of Madhya Pradesh. The ASHA worker and the Second gravida mother are given what amount (Rupees) under JSSK? [NEET PG Pattern 2022]
- (a) 1400 to mother and 1000 to ASHA
- (b) 1000 to mother and 400 to ASHA
- (c) 1400 to mother and 600 to ASHA
- (d) 700 to mother and 400 to ASHA

113. Mobile Medical Unit (MMU), Consider the following statements:
1. Government operated fully
2. CAPEX/Drugs/Medical supplies by Government, but Operations by Private
3. Drugs/Medical supplies by Govt, but Services/CAPEX/OPEX by Private
4. Private funded fully

Which of the following is correct combination?
[INICET July 2021]
- (a) 1,4
- (b) 2,4
- (c) 2,3
- (d) 1,2,3

114. All of the following health disorders are covered under Child Health Screening and Early Intervention Program (RBSK) except: [AIIMS June 2020]
- (a) Childhood cataract
- (b) Retinopathy of prematurity
- (c) Congenital glaucoma
- (d) Vitamin A deficiency

115. A 2-year-old child presents to PHC with fever and cough. He had Chest in-drawing and respiratory rate of 38 per minute, weight 11 kg. The next step in management according to IMNCI is: [NEET PG Pattern January 2020]
- (a) Only antipyretics are given
- (b) Refer to tertiary care
- (c) Give antibiotics and refer to tertiary centre
- (d) Give antibiotics and re-assess in 3 days

116. MULTIPLE COMPLETION TYPE QUESTION: Function/responsibility of ASHA worker
- A. Accompany pregnant females to hospital
- B. Help in completion of immunization as per schedule
- C. Spread awareness regarding contraception
- D. Malaria slide preparation

Use the following key to mark correct answer
[AIIMS May 2019]
- (a) If A, B, C are correct
- (b) If A and C are correct
- (c) If B and D are correct
- (d) If all four (A, B, C, & D) are correct

117. About ASHA (Accredited Social Health Activist) true is all except: [AIIMS Nov 06, AIIMS May 07]
- (a) They are preferably females
- (b) There is one ASHA worker per 1000 population
- (c) ASHA is skilled birth attendant
- (d) Provides primary medical care for minor ailments

118. Under National Rural Health Mission, ASHA stands for:
[AIIMS May 2007]
- (a) A Social Health Agent [NEET Pattern 2013]
- (b) A Specific Health Agent [DNB 2011]
- (c) Accredited Social Health Activist
- (d) Advanced Scientific Health Activist

119. Under National Rural Health Mission, lowest level at which Health Action Plan is prepared is:
[AIIMS Nov 2007]
- (a) State level
- (b) District Level
- (c) Subcentre Level
- (d) Village Level

120. Which of the following is the 'Impact indicator' for evaluation of ASHA's performance? [AIIMS November 09]
- (a) Number of meetings attended
- (b) Number of institutional deliveries
- (c) Reduction in infant mortality
- (d) Hours of training

121. **Which of the following is the ego-expansion of JSY?**
    (a) Janani Suraksha Yojana [AIPGME 2010]
    (b) Janani Samridhi Yojana
    (c) Janani Swarojgar Yojana
    (d) Janani Sampoorna Yojana

122. **Resource persons for training of ASHA:**
    (a) Medical officer and ANM [AIPGME 2012]
    (b) Medical officer and Anganwadi worker
    (c) ANM and Anganwadi worker
    (d) Medical officer

123. **ASHA is recruited under?** [NEET Pattern 2013]
    (a) NRHM
    (b) National urban health mission
    (c) ICDS
    (d) Village health system

124. **Janani Suraksha Yojana mainly focus on:**
    [DNB December 2011]
    (a) Tetanus immunization
    (b) Institutional deliveries
    (c) Iron supplementation
    (d) Abortions

125. **ASHA gets remuneration on all except:**
    (a) Institutional delivery [AIIMS May 2013]
    (b) Zero dose of OPV and BCG [AIIMS May 2014]
    (c) Recording birth weight
    (d) Birth registration

126. **All are true about Janani Shishu Suraksha Karyakram (JSSK), except:** [AIIMS May 2014]
    (a) Free diet to mother during hospital stay
    (b) Free delivery [NEET Pattern 2014]
    (c) Free transport from home to hospital and back
    (d) Free treatment of sick infants up to 1 year

127. **Asha worker works for …… population:**
    [NEET Pattern 2014]
    (a) 3000   (b) 1000
    (c) 5000   (d) 400

128. **Features of Janani Suraksha Yojana are the following except:** [UPSC CMS 2015]
    (a) 100% Centrally sponsored scheme
    (b) ASHA is a link between Woman and Government
    (c) Cash assistance is given to mothers for high and low performing states
    (d) It promotes institutional deliveries

129. **Village Health Nutrition Day is observed**
    [NEET Patterns 2016, 2017]
    (a) Every week   (b) Every month
    (c) Every six months (d) Every year

130. **ASHA is not a depot holder of** [NEET Pattern 2015]
    (a) ORS   (b) IFA
    (c) Contraceptives (d) OPV

131. **New born care corner is present in** [NEET Pattern 2016]
    (a) NICU
    (b) OPD
    (c) Labour room
    (d) Wards side room

132. **Function of ASHA** [NEET Pattern 2016]
    (a) Mobilization for institutional deliveries
    (b) Conduction of Home delivery
    (c) Give Immunization at birth
    (d) Provide DEC for filarial treatment

133. **Which of the following is not true for an ASHA worker?**
    [NEET Pattern 2016]
    (a) ASHA should be preferably in the age group of 25–45 years
    (b) She should be trained for a period of 21 days
    (c) Work with village health and sanitation committee (VHSC)
    (d) Act as depot holder for essential previsions ORS, iron and folic acid tablets

134. **Under National Health Mission which Committee is responsible for making plan for Village health?**
    [AIIMS May 2018]
    (a) Panchayat health committee (PHC)
    (b) Village health planning and management committee (VHPMC)
    (c) Village health sanitation and nutrition committee (VHSNC)
    (d) Rogi Kalyan Samiti

135. **Programs included in NHRM is/are:** [NEET Pattern 2017]
    (a) National Vector Borne Disease Control Program
    (b) Revised National Tuberculosis Control Program
    (c) National Program for the Control of Blindness
    (d) All of the above

136. **Which of the following is not the work responsibility of ASHA?** [NEET Pattern 2017]
    (a) Immunization and contraception counselling
    (b) Delivery at home
    (c) Provide primary medical care for minor ailments
    (d) Promote construction of household toilets

137. **True about incentives gives to ASHA worker in Janani Suraksha Yojana** [NEET Pattern 2017]
    (a) 400 INR to ASHA and 1000 INR to mother in rural area in high performing states
    (b) 400 INR to ASHA and 1000 INR to mother in rural area in low performing states
    (c) 400 INR to ASHA and 1000 INR to mother in urban area high performing states
    (d) 400 INR to ASHA and 1000 INR to mother in urban area low performing states

NATIONAL LEPROSY ELIMINATION PROGRAMME

138. Which of the following criteria should be satisfied to start MDT? *[INICET November 2022]*
    1. Hypopigmented patch with sensory loss
    2. Peripheral nerve thickening
    3. Peripheral nerve thickening with sensory loss
    4. Skin biopsy demonstrating bacilli
    (a) 1,4
    (b) 1,3
    (c) 1,3,4
    (d) 1,2,3,4

139. All of the following indicators can help in determining whether the health system is giving importance to identifying leprosy in the community, EXCEPT? *[INICET November 2022]*
    (a) Treatment completion rate
    (b) Annual new case detection rate per lac
    (c) Treatment initiation rate
    (d) Proportion of newly diagnosed patients with grade-2 disability

140. Leprosy prophylaxis for close contacts to be given if *[INICET May 2022]*
    (a) Sharing towels, clothes, etc.
    (b) Living together for 6 months since onset
    (c) Spending 20 hours or more a week in close contact
    (d) If age >2 years

141. A 26 years old pregnant lady on Leprosy treatment has type 2 Lepra reaction. Next line of management: *[INICET May 2022]*
    (a) Stop leprosy drugs and add steroids
    (b) Thalidomide
    (c) Thalidomide + steroids
    (d) Continue Anti leprosy drugs and add steroids
    (e) Antibiotics

142. Treatment for Paucibacillary Leprosy includes: *[AIIMS November 2019]*
    (a) Dapsone+Rifampicin+Clofazimine for 6 months
    (b) Dapsone+Rifampicin+Clofazimine for 12 months
    (c) Dapsone+Rifampicin for 6 months
    (d) Dapsone monotherapy

143. A leprosy case with a single anesthetic patch is treated with: *[AIIMS June 2000]*
    (a) Rifampicin + dapsone
    (b) Rifampicin + of loxacin + minocycline
    (c) Rifampicin + dapsone + clofazimine
    (d) Rifampicin + clofazimine

144. A 27- year-old patient was diagnosed to have borderline leprosy and started on multibacillary multi-drug therapy. Six weeks later, he developed pain in the nerves and redness and swelling of the skin lesions. The management of his illness should include all of the following, except: *[AIPGME 1992 and 2004]*
    (a) Stop anti-leprosy drugs
    (b) Systemic corticosteroids
    (c) Rest to the limbs affected
    (d) Analgesics

145. 'Accompanied MDT' in NLEP implies:
    (a) A patient will be given MDT only in the presence of a MDT provider *[AIPGME 2006]*
    (b) MDT should be accompanied with Steroids/Clofazimine to help fight Reversal reactions
    (c) Any responsible person from family or village can collect MDT, if patient is unable to come
    (d) MDT prescription should be accompanied by all the precautions to be observed by the patient

146. Multibacillary leprosy follow-up duration: *[DNB 2008]*
    (a) 12–18 months *[NEET Pattern 2012]*
    (b) 2 years
    (c) 5 years
    (d) 10 years

147. For treatment of paucibacillary leprosy drugs used are:
    (a) Dapsone *[NEET Pattern 2012]*
    (b) Dapsone, Rifampicin *[UP 2007]*
    (c) Rifampicin, Clofazimine
    (d) Dapsone, Rifampicin, Clofazimine

148. Two years duration in terms of leprosy is with regard to: *[NEET Pattern 2012]*
    (a) Treatment of paucibacillary leprosy
    (b) Treatment of multibacillary leprosy
    (c) Post-treatment surveillance of paucibacillary leprosy
    (d) Post-treatment surveillance of multibacillary leprosy

149. Which of the following Anti-leprotic drugs is not given in blister packs of NLEP? *[NEET Pattern 2014]*
    (a) Dapsone (b) Rifampicin
    (c) Clofazimine (d) Minocycline

150. In a case of Paucibacillary leprosy, treatment is considered adequate if the patient has received the six monthly doses of combined therapy within *[UPSC CMS 2015]*
    (a) 6 months (b) 9 months
    (c) 12 months (d) 15 months

OTHER PROGRAMMES

151. Under the Anemia Mukt Bharath initiative, mild to moderate anemia in pregnant women <34 weeks of gestation is treated using: *[INICET November 2022]*
    (a) 3 iron and folic acid (IFA) tablets, taken OD
    (b) IV iron sucrose for non-compliance with oral tablets
    (c) 2 iron and folic acid tablets OD + IV iron sucrose
    (d) IM ferric carboxy maltose (FCM)

152. For diagnosis of diabetes at a PHC, consider the following criteria:
    A. HbA1C
    B. Fasting blood sugar >/=126
    C. Random blood sugar >/= 200
    D. Capillary blood sugar post-prandial >/= 220
    Which of the following is the correct combination to be used? [INICET July 2021]
    (a) AB
    (b) BD
    (c) ABC
    (d) All of the above

153. IFA dose for Adolescent female under Anemia Mukt Bharat Program is: [AIIMS June 2020]
    (a) 100 mg Iron & 100 mcg Folic acid daily
    (b) 100 mg Iron & 100 mcg Folic acid weekly
    (c) 60 mg Iron & 500 mcg Folic acid daily
    (d) 60 mg Iron & 500 mcg Folic acid weekly

154. The Long term objective of National Programme for Prevention and Control of Deafness is:
    (a) To reduce disease burden by 25% by end of XI Five Year Plan [AIIMS May 2007]
    (b) To reduce disease burden by 50% by end of XI Five Year Plan
    (c) To reduce disease burden by 75% by end of XI Five Year Plan
    (d) To reduce disease burden by 100% by end of XI Five Year Plan

155. The best indicator for monitoring the impact of Iodine Deficiency Disorders control programme is:
    [DNB 2007, AIPGME 05, AIIMS Nov 2006, AIIMS May 2014, AIPGME 07]
    (a) Prevalence of goiter among school children
    (b) Urinary iodine levels among pregnant women
    (c) Neonatal Hypothyroidism
    (d) Iodine level in soil

156. Under National programme for prevention of nutritional blindness, a child in the age group of 6–11 months is given a mega dose of vitamin A equal to: [AIIMS Nov 05]
    (a) 50,000 IU (b) 1 lakh IU
    (c) 1.5 lakh IU (d) 2 lakh IU

157. The Vitamin A supplement administered in "Prevention of nutritional blindness in children programme" contains: [AIPGME 2003]
    (a) 25,000 IU/mL
    (b) 1 lakh IU/mL
    (c) 3 lakh IU/mL
    (d) 5 lakh IU/mL

158. Minimum level of iodine in iodized salt reaching the consumer level according to Iodine programme should be:
    [NEET Pattern 2013] [DPG 2006]
    (a) 15 ppm (b) 30 ppm
    (c) 5 ppm (d) 20 ppm

159. Effective Leprosy Control Programmes may be indicated by all *except*: [AIIMS Nov 09]
    (a) High new case detection rate
    (b) Increasing no. of children affected
    (c) Decreased type II disability
    (d) Proportion of multi-bacillary cases on treatment

160. Rashtriya Swasthya Bima Yojana is: [AIIMS May 2012]
    (a) Government run insurance scheme for its employees
    (b) Government run insurance scheme for all citizens
    (c) Government run insurance scheme for poor
    (d) Private insurance company run scheme for all poor

161. Which of the following diseases is not under surveillance in Integrated Disease Surveillance Project (P-FORM)?
    (a) Snake bite [AIIMS May 2013]
    (b) Acute Respiratory Tract Infections
    (c) Tuberculosis
    (d) Leptospirosis

162. Disease NOT covered under Integrated Disease Surveillance Project (IDSP) is [AIIMS November 2013]
    (a) Meningococcal disease
    (b) Tuberculosis
    (c) Herpes zoster
    (d) Cholera

163. National Programme for Prevention and Control of Cancer, Diabetes, Cardiovascular diseases and Stroke (NPCDCS), true is [AIIMS May 2013] [NEET Pattern 2017]
    (a) Separate centre for stroke, DM, cancer
    (b) Implementation in some 5 states over 10 districts
    (c) District hospital has specialised facilities
    (d) Subcentre has facility for diagnosis and treatment

164. True about National Programme for Prevention and Control of Cancer, Diabetes, Cardiovascular diseases and Stroke is [AIIMS November 2012]
    (a) Home based care is not given
    (b) Implementation in some 5 states over 10 districts
    (c) Separate centre for stroke, DM,
    (d) CHC has facilities for diagnosis and treatment of CVD, Diabetes

165. Type of surveillance included in integrated disease control programme for non-communicable disease is:
    [DNB December 2010]
    (a) Sentinel surveillance
    (b) Regular surveillance
    (c) Periodic regular survey
    (d) Additional state priority

166. What is the new change in National Programme on Prevention and Control of Diabetes, Cardiovascular diseases and Stroke? [NEET Pattern 2014]
    (a) Opportunistic screening
    (b) Awareness of lifestyle and behavior related diseases
    (c) Specialized units at Medical colleges
    (d) Integration with National Cancer Control Programme

167. In Integrated Disease Surveillance Project in India, which of the following type of diagnosis is done by PHC Medical Officer? [PGMCET 2015] [NEET Pattern 2015]
    (a) Syndromic
    (b) Presumptive
    (c) Confirmed
    (d) Laboratory

168. Not included in National Mental Health Programme 1982 [AIIMS November 2014]
    (a) Minimum mental health care for all
    (b) Application of mental health knowledge in general health care
    (c) Human rights of mentally ill
    (d) Community participation in mental health service development

169. All are true about Swajaldhara programme *except*: [NEET Pattern 2015]
    (a) Community led, participatory program
    (b) Provide drinking water in Rural areas
    (c) State Government maintain and manage all water supply
    (d) Encourage water harvesting practices

170. Which National Programme came into existence during 11th Five Year Plan? [UPSC CMS 2015]
    (a) National Cancer control programme
    (b) National Cardiovascular diseases & Stroke control programme
    (c) National Diabetes and Cancer control programme
    (d) National Programme for prevention and control of Cancer, Diabetes, Cardiovascular diseases and Stroke

171. Which of the following is not true for Steps wise approach developed by WHO wise approach developed by WHO for Non-communicable disease surveillance? [NEET Pattern 2016]
    (a) STEP 1 consists of interview for collecting relevant data
    (b) STEP 2 includes measurement of blood pressure and anthropometry
    (c) STEP 3 includes blood sample collection for estimation of blood sugar and cholesterol level
    (d) STEP 4 consists of treatment of NCD if found

172. IDSP is based on all types of Surveillance *except*: [NEET Pattern 2016]
    (a) Clinical
    (b) Geographical
    (c) Laboratory
    (d) Epidemiological

173. True regarding Total goitre rate (TGR) is [AIIMS May 2016]
    (a) Divided into three grades: Not visible, Palpable, Visible
    (b) Goitre is classified as endemic if TGR ≥ 10%
    (c) TGR reflects the current status of IDD in population
    (d) Field survey of TGR does not require doctors

Review Questions

174. True about Mid-day meal given in school is:

	Calories	Proteins	
			[DNB 2005]
(a)	1/3	1/2	[NEET Pattern 2017]
(b)	1/3	1/3	[AIIMS Nov 2018]
(c)	1/2	1/2	
(d)	1/2	1/3	

175. In leprosy mass survey is done if prevalence is (per 1000 person): [RJ 2003]
    (a) 1
    (b) 5
    (c) 7
    (d) 10

176. The multidrug regimen under the National Leprosy Eradication programme for the treatment of all multi-bacillary leprosy would include: [RJ 2007]
    (a) Clofazimine, thiacetazone and dapsone
    (b) Clofazimine, Rifampicin and dapsone
    (c) Ethionamide, Rifampicin and dapsone
    (d) Propionamide, Rifampicin and dapsone

177. All are true of Midday School Meal Programme *except*: [AP 2004]
    (a) Should supply ½ daily protein and ⅓ rd or daily calories
    (b) Is a substitute for regular food
    (c) Locally available foods are used
    (d) Cheap and easy to prepare

178. Single massive dose of vitamin A for preventing the deficiency in preschool children between the age of 1–6 years for every 6 months is: [MH 2007]
    (a) 2,000 IU
    (b) 20,000 IU
    (c) 2,00,000 IU
    (d) 20,00,000 IU

MISCELLANEOUS (H. PROGRAMMES)

179. Nikshay Poshan Yojana includes: [AIIMS June 2020]
    (a) 500 Rupees per month
    (b) 500 Rupees per week
    (c) Mid-day meal daily
    (d) Nutritional dietary advice/counselling

180. A young boy had a flea bite while working in a wheat grain godown. After 5 days he developed fever and had axillary lymphadenopathy. A smear was sent to the laboratory to perform a specific staining. Which one of the following staining methods would help in the identification of the suspected pathogen? [AIPGME 2006]
    (a) Albert staining
    (b) Ziehl-Neelsen staining
    (c) McFadyean's staining
    (d) Wayson's staining

181. Simplified Information System plays an important role as part of MIS in: [AIIMS Nov 2005]
    (a) RNTCP
    (b) National Leprosy Eradication Programme
    (c) National Vector Borne Disease Control Programme
    (d) National AIDS Control Programme

182. Which of the following drugs is not given as supervised regimen in National Health programmes of India:
    (a) Clofazimine [AIIMS Nov 09]
    (b) Dapsone
    (c) Rifampicin
    (d) Pyrazinamide

183. WHO funds which of the following programmes in India?
    (a) RNTCP [NEET Pattern 2013]
    (b) National Leprosy Eradication Programme
    (c) Janani Suraksha Yojna
    (d) National old age pension plan

184. Integrated Child Protection Scheme is under which ministry? [NEET Pattern 2012]
    (a) Health & Family Welfare
    (b) Women & Child Development
    (c) Home Affairs
    (d) Labour

185. 'NIKSHAY' is newly launched Central Government software. It is used for tracking [AIIMS PG May 2015]
    (a) High risk newborns
    (b) Malaria
    (c) Tuberculosis
    (d) High risk pregnancies

186. Link worker scheme are in which National health programme? [NEET Pattern 2015]
    (a) RNTCP
    (b) NACP
    (c) NLEP
    (d) ICDS

187. Behavioural surveillance survey is done in [NEET Pattern 2016]
    (a) Malaria   (b) Filariasis
    (c) AIDS   (d) TB

188. Not included not Empowered action group (EAG) states of India [NEET Pattern 2017]
    (a) UP
    (b) Bihar
    (c) Jharkhand
    (d) Maharashtra

RASHTRIYA SWASTHYA BIMA YOJANA

189. True regarding Rashtriya Swasthya Bima Yojana is [AIIMS November 2015]
    (a) Treatment provided only in Government hospitals
    (b) Valid for 4-member family only—Head, Spouse, 2 Children
    (c) Can avail facility in any hospital using his Smart card and Fingerprint
    (d) Cashless benefit in hospitals

NATIONAL HEALTH POLICY

190. 90:90:90 target in National Health Policy 2017 stand for [PGI November 2017]
    (a) 90% of all people living with HIV know their HIV status
    (b) 90% of all people diagnosed with HIV infection receive sustained antiretroviral therapy
    (c) 90% of all people living with HIV and TB know their HIV status
    (d) 90% of all people diagnosed with HIV infection and TB receive sustained antiretroviral therapy and ATT
    (e) 90% of all people receiving antiretroviral therapy will have effective viral suppression

NATIONAL POPULATION POLICY

191. 'Preferable' age for marriage for girls under National Population Policy 2000 is: [AIIMS Nov 2002]
    (a) 18 years
    (b) 19 years
    (c) 20 years
    (d) 21 years

192. National Population Policy 2000 has set a goal (by 2010) for 100 % Registration of all the following except:
    (a) Births and Deaths [AIIMS May 2003]
    (b) Marriages
    (c) Divorces
    (d) Pregnancies

193. National Population Policy 2000 aims to achieve all except: [Karnataka 2007]
    (a) Targets to be achieved by the year 2010
    (b) Reduction of IMR to less than 30 live births/1000 live births
    (c) Reduction of MMR to less than 1/1000 live births
    (d) Achieve 100% registration of births, deaths, marriage and pregnancy

194. Goals of national population policy are all except? [AIIMS May 2011]
    (a) Decrease IMR to below 30/1000 live births
    (b) Reduce MMR to below 100/100000 live births
    (c) Achieve 100% registration of births, deaths, marriage and pregnancy
    (d) Bring down TFR to replacement levels by 2015

NATIONAL MENTAL HEALTH POLICY

195. National Mental Health Policy of India was launched in [NEET Pattern 2015]
    (a) 1982   (b) 1987
    (c) 1994   (d) 2014

IT ACT

196. The information technology has revolutionized the world of medical sciences. In which of the following year the Information Technology Act was passed by the Government of India? [AIPGME 2005]
    (a) 1998
    (b) 2000
    (c) 2001
    (d) 2003

OT ACT

197. According to Organ Transplantation Act 1994, what is the punishment for doctor if found guilty?
    (a) 1 year [AIIMS November 2011]
    (b) 2 years
    (c) 2–5 years
    (d) More than 5 years

CBD REGISTRATION ACT

198. Birth and Death registration Act came into force on 1st April, [NEET Pattern 2015]
    (a) 1968
    (b) 1969
    (c) 1970
    (d) 1971

OTHER LEGISLATIONS

199. National Rural Employment Guarantee Act (NREGA) was passed in: [AIIMS May 2007]
    (a) 1947
    (b) 1991
    (c) 2005
    (d) 2008

200. 'Professional Misconduct' specified under MCI Act include all *except*: [AIPGME 1998]
    (a) Alcoholism
    (b) Smoking
    (c) Adultery
    (d) Human Rights Violation

201. Census 2001 Population Count was as on: [AIIMS May 2003]
    (a) 00.00 hrs 01 March
    (b) 06.00 hrs 01 March
    (c) 00.00 hrs 31 March
    (d) 00.00 hrs 01 April

202. Which act was passed before independence? [DPG 2008]
    (a) MTP
    (b) Indian factories act
    (c) Workman's compensation act
    (d) ESI

203. MTP Act of 1971 provides the following indications *except*: [Karnataka 2006]
    (a) Where continuation of pregnancy endangers mother's life
    (b) Where pregnancy is a result of rape
    (c) When acceptors requires incentives
    (d) Failure of contraceptive device

204. Licence to blood banks is given by: [AIIMS May 2009]
    (a) Drugs Controller General of India
    (b) Director Genera of Health Services
    (c) Director General, Indian Council of Medical Research
    (d) Director General, Blood Bank Services

205. What is correct for NDPS Act, 1985? [AIPGME 2012]
    (a) Drug users sent to treatment not jail if requested
    (b) Alcoholism is included in drugs
    (c) Farmers allowed to grow unlimited opium
    (d) Equal punishment for drug peddlers and drug users

206. Not included in NDPS Act is/are [PGI November 2012]
    (a) Alcohol
    (b) Opium
    (c) Cannabis
    (d) Nicotine
    (e) Morphine

207. Recent mental health act in India is designated as:
    (a) The Mental Health Act [AIIMS May 2013]
    (b) The Mental Health Care Act
    (c) The Mental Health Care and Rehabilitation Act
    (d) The Mental Health Treatment and Rehabilitation Act

208. Which of the following in NOT included in Mental Health Care Act 2011? [AIIMS November 2014]
    (a) Promotion of mental health and prevention of mental illness
    (b) Integration of mental health care system into all levels of health care
    (c) Fundamental rights of mentally retarded
    (d) Minimum mental health care for all

209. Central Drugs Standard Control Organisation Zonal Offices are located all of the following places *except*: [NEET Pattern 2014]
    (a) Mumbai
    (b) Chennai
    (c) Ahmedabad
    (d) Jaipur

210. Medical Termination of Pregnancy Act 1971, was amended in 2002 to include: [NEET Pattern 2014]
    (a) Risk to mother's life as an indication
    (b) Failure of contraception as an indication
    (c) 'Mentally ill' in place of lunatic
    (d) POG upto 20 weeks

211. Food Standards and Safety Authority of India comes under [AIIMS PG May 2015]
    (a) Ministry of Consumer Affairs
    (b) Ministry of Agriculture
    (c) Ministry of Health and Family Welfare
    (d) Ministry of Rural development

212. Regimen for Medical abortion upto 7 weeks of gestation as per Government of India guidelines includes
 [UPSC CMS 2015]
 (a) 200 mg of misfepristone on D_1 followed by 800 µg of misoprostol on D_3
 (b) 200 mg of misfepristone on D_1 followed by 400 µg of misoprostol on D_3
 (c) 400 mg of misfepristone on D_1 followed by 800 µg of misoprostol on D_3
 (d) 400 mg of misfepristone on D_1 followed by 400 µg of misoprostol on D_3

213. PCPNDT Act is regarding [NEET Pattern 2016]
 (a) Prevention of unauthorized kidney transplantation
 (b) Prevention of child trafficking
 (c) Prevention of female foeticides
 (d) Prevention of narcotics abuse

214. Right of consumers in Consumer Protection Act are all *except*: [NEET Pattern 2016]
 (a) Right to safety
 (b) Right of information
 (c) Right to choose
 (d) Right to reject

215. As per Consumer Protection Act in India, compensation claims entertained by National commission are in the range of Rupees _____ ? [NEET Pattern 2016]
 (a) 60–100 lakhs
 (b) More than 100 lakhs
 (c) 1–20 lakhs
 (d) 20–60 lakhs

216. As per "National Socio-demographic Goals for 2010" according to National Population Policy make school education up to age 14 years free and compulsory and reduce dropouts at primary school levels to below.....
 (a) 10% for both boys and girls [NEET Pattern 2016]
 (b) 30% for both boys and girls
 (c) 20% for both boys and girls
 (d) 90% for both boys and girls

217. Provisions of Mental Health Act 2017 based WHO Mental Action Gap Action Program (MHAGP) are all, except
 (a) Human rights [AIIMS November 2018]
 (b) Communication regarding care and career
 (c) Screening family members
 (d) Social support

218. Screening test commonly used for HIV is: [MP 2005]
 (a) Western Blot
 (b) Absolute CD4 count
 (c) ELISA
 (d) Viral load assay

Explanations

NATIONAL TB ELIMINATION PROGRAM (NTEP)/RNTCP

1. **Ans. (a) CBNAAT** [Ref. Park 27/e p220]
   - Suspected Pulmonary TB adult case with negative sputum samples but chest x-ray findings suggestive of TB are subjected to CBNAAT test under NTEP

2. **Ans. (b) Cured** [Ref. Park 26/e p209]
   TB patients is declared CURED
   - If a Pulmonary TB patient with bacteriologically confirmed TB at beginning of treatment who was smear or culture negative in last month of treatment and on at least one previous occasion

3. **Ans. (c) Give TB treatment first and then after 2 weeks treat with ART** [Ref. ART Guidelines. NACO. May 2013 p27]
   Patients with HIV and TB co-infection (Pulmonary/Extra-Pulmonary): Start ART irrespective of CD4 count and type of tuberculosis
   - Start ATT treatment immediately
   - Wait for ATT treatment to stabilize (Generally time required in 2 weeks to 2 months)
   - After stabilization, Start ATT

4. **Ans. (a) Carbol fuschin, Acid alcohol, Methylene blue** [Ref. Park 26/e p211–212]
   Ziehl-Neelsen Acid Fast Bacilli (ZN AFB) Staining
   - *Fix smear on slide:* Pass slide 3 times over flame (smear upside)
   - *Carbol Fuschin cover:* Steam gently for 5 minutes over direct flame
   - *Washing:* with de-ionised water
   - *Decolourisation:* 3% acid-alcohol (95% ethanol + 3% HCl)
   - *Washing:* With water
   - *Counter-staining:* 1 minute with Loeffler's methylene blue
   - *Washing:* With de-ionised water
   - Dry the slide

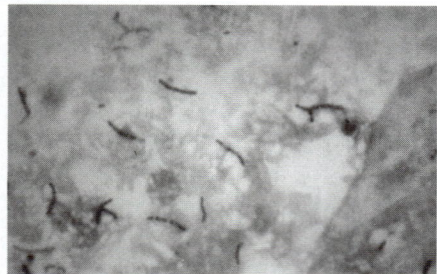

5. **Ans. (d) 10,000 bacilli per mL sputum**
   [Ref. National Health Programmes of India by Dr. J. Kishore, 8/e p205, Park 27/e p215]
   - *Zeihl Neelsen (ZN) Staining IN RNTCP:*
     - Sputum smear of a suspected TB patient is used for the diagnosis
     - Decolourizer: 25% sulphuric acid
   - Acid Fast Bacilli (AFB) of TB: 'Rod shaped' with 'beaded appearance' (Beads: Mycolic Acid)
   - >10,000 bacilli per mL sputum must be present for a positive result
   - Results of ZN staining: Minimum 100 fields examined

Grading of smears	Criterion
0	No bacilli per 100 oil immersion fields
Scanty	1–9 bacilli per 100 oil immersion fields
1+ grading	10–99 bacilli per 100 oil immersion fields
2+ grading	1–10 bacilli per oil immersion field
3+ grading	>10 bacilli per oil immersion field

ALSO REMEMBER
Other Tests in Tuberculosis:
- *Auramine-rhodamine stain (AR):* More sensitive than ZN staining
- *Culture (IUAT – LJ Medium/Kirchner Medium/Middlebrook 7H10 or 7H11 media):* Very sensitive; +ve even with '10–100 bacilli per mL sputum'
- *Chest radiography:* Findings suggestive of but not diagnostic of TB
- *Abreugraphy (Mass Miniature Radiography – MMR):* Sufficiently accurate for diagnosis of TB
- *BACTEC Radiometric System:* C14 radio-labelled with palmitic acid
  - Detect as early as 7–14 days
  - 95% sensitivity
- *Microscopic Observation Drug Susceptibility assay (MODS):*
  - Direct observation of TB and simultaneously yields drug-resistance
- *ELISA Test:*
  - A60 antigen
  - Nor sufficiently sensitive nor specific
  - Supportive value for diagnosis of extra-pulmonary TB
- *PCR Test (Nucleic acid amplification tests – NAAT):*
  - Detect within 1 day
  - Extremely sensitive; +ve even with '1–10 bacilli per mL sputum'
- *Restriction Fragment Length Polymorphism (RFLP):* Combines Southern blotting and hybridization with DNA probes
- *Fast Plaque TB (FTB):* Sputum, aspirates, pus, blood
  - Detect within 48–72 hours
  - 90% sensitivity and 100% specificity
- *Quantiferon TB Gold (QTG) (Interferon a–release assay):*
  - Detect within 3–5 days
  - Higher sensitivity
- *Adenosine Deaminase (ADA):*
  - Highest sensitivity in both pleural TB and TB meningitis
- *Tuberculin Test and Mantoux Test (Pirquet test or PPD Test):* Tool for detecting TB infection

6. **Ans. (a) Annual Risk of Infection** [Ref. National Health Programmes of India by Dr. J. Kishore, 8/e p196]
   - *Annual Risk of Infection (ARI):* Is the proportion of population which will be primarily infected with tuberculosis in course of 1 year
     - Is incidence of infection of TB
     - Is known as 'Tuberculin Conversion Index'
     - Best indicator of trend of TB unaffected by current control measures
     - Most informative index of magnitude of problem of TB
   - *ARI (India):* 1–2% (average ARI = 1.5%)
     - For every 1% rise of ARI, there are 50 SS +ve cases/lac population
   - *Key epidemiological indices for TB (India):*

Index	Situation in India	Remark
Incidence of Infection	1–2% (~1.5%)	ARI – Tuberculin Conversion Index
Prevalence of Infection	40%	Standard Tuberculin Test
Incidence of Disease	1.7 per 1000	New cases (culture +ve)
Prevalence of Disease	0.2%	Sputum positive

7. **Ans. (c) Isoniazid & Rifampicin**
   [Ref. National Health Programmes of India by Dr. J. Kishore, 8/e p197, Park 27/e p222]
   - *Multidrug Resistant TB (MDR-TB):* Resistance to Isoniazid and Rifampicin "with or without resistance to other drugs"
     - Treatment of MDR-TB must be done on the basis of sensitivity testing
     - Directly observed therapy certainly helps to improve outcomes and should be considered an integral part of the treatment of MDR-TB.
   - *Extensive Drug Resistant TB (XDR–TB):* Resistance to rifampicin and isoniazid as well as to any member of the quinolone family and at least one of the following second-line TB treatments: kanamycin, capreomycin, or amikacin
     - XDR-TB is MDR TB with further resistance to 3–6 classes of second line drugs (older definition)
     - Principles of treatment for MDR-TB and for XDR-TB are same.
     - XDR-TB does not transmit easily in healthy populations, yet is capable of causing 'epidemics in populations which are already stricken by HIV'
   - *Management of MDR – TB (DOTS – PLUS):* Refers to DOTS programmes that add components for MDR-TB diagnosis, management and treatment
     - Initiated as Category IV pilot projects (Gujarat)
     - Target: management of 5000 new MDR – TB cases per year

Category	Type of patient	Regimens		Duration (months)
		IP	CP	
Cat IV	MDR – TB	6–9 (KLCZEEt)	18 (LCEEt)	18–24

- [Letters: E – Ethambutol, Z – Pyrazinamide, K – Kanamycin, L – Levofloxacin, Et – Ethionamide, C – Cycloserine; Numbers: The numbers before letters refer to months of treatment (4 imply four months of treatment)]

8. **Ans. (c) 10–15 persons per year** [Ref. National Health Programmes of India by Dr. J. Kishore, 8/e p195]

Every TB sputum positive patient can infect up to 10–15 individuals in a year.

> **ALSO REMEMBER**
> - TB is 'Barometer of Social Welfare in India'
> - TB (AFB) Bacillus discovered by: Robert Koch
> - World TB Day: 24th March
> - TB was declared as 'Global emergency in 1983' by WHO
> - TB is the MC Opportunistic Infection (OI) in HIV in India
> - TB bacteria remain alive: in sputum for 1 day and in droplet nuclei for 10 days
> - *Elimination level for Tuberculosis (WHO and STOP TB Strategy):* <1 case per million population (to eliminate TB as a public health problem)
> - *TB Institutes of importance in India:*
>   - National Tuberculosis Institute (NTI) – Bangalore
>   - Tuberculosis Research Centre – Chennai
>   - LRS Institute of TB and Respiratory Diseases – New Delhi

9. **Ans. (c) Streptomycin** [Ref. RNTCP Technical Guidelines for Tuberculosis Control, DGHS; p16]
   - Pregnant women with active TB: Should start or continue their anti-TB treatment
   - Streptomycin should not be given during pregnancy as it crosses the placenta and may cause damage to the fetus (ototoxicity)
   - Breastfeeding of infants should continue irrespective of the TB status of mother
     - If mother SS +ve: Chemoprophylaxis to child for 3 months, then
       1. If child is Tuberculin –ve: Vaccinate child with BCG
       2. If child is Tuberculin +ve: Chemoprophylaxis continued for a total duration of 6 months
     - If mother SS –ve: Vaccinate child with BCG (No chemoprophylaxis)

10. **Ans. (b) DOTS applied; (e) It has replaced NTP**
    [Ref. Park 27/e p485–494]

11. **Ans. (a) Active case finding; (b) Directly observed; (c) X-ray is diagnostic; (d) Drugs given daily**
    [Ref. Park 27/e p485–494]

12. **Ans. (a) and (c) Drugs are given on supervision and Intermitten regimen used.** [Ref. Park 27/e p485–489]

    DOTS
    - DOTS is directly observed treatment short course.
    - In DOTS during the intensive phase of treatment a health worker are other trained person watches as the patients swallows the drugs in his presence.

- During continuation phase the patient is issued medicine for one week in multiblister combipack of which the first dose is swallowed by the patient in the presence of health worker or trained person.
- The consumption of medicine in the continuation phase is also checked by return of empty multiblister combipack when patient come to collect medicine for the next week.
- In this programme attemate day treatment is used.
- Patient compliance is critically important throughout the prescribed period of treatment. All other consideration are secondary.
- Drugs are given category wise, same regimen is not given to all patient.
- Streptomycin is given in category II only.
- In category-1 new sputum smear, positive cases sputum examination is done in 2, 4 and 6 months.

13. **Ans. (b) Use separate vessels**

[Ref. Park 21/e p119, 172–75]

Domiciliary Treatment
- Domiciliary/Ambulatory treatment: Self-administration of (oral) drugs by patients themselves without recourse to hospitalization
- Studies have shown that 'hospital treatment has no advantage over domiciliary treatment'
- Guidelines for patients on domiciliary treatment:
  - Collect drugs regularly
  - Dispose sputum safely (burning/5% cresol/boiling/autoclaving)
  - Report to PHC if new symptoms arise

14. **Ans. (b) 450 mg** [Ref. RNTCP Document, GOI]
- Thrice weekly dosages of Antitubercular drugs in RNTCP:
  - Pyrazinamide: 35 mg/kg (1500 mg)
  - Isoniazid: 10 mg/kg (600 mg)
  - Rifampicin: 10 mg/kg (450 mg; 600 mg IF weight >60 kg)
  - Ethambutol: 30 mg/kg (1200 mg)
  - Streptomycin: 15 mg/kg (750 mg)

15. **Ans. (a) Decrease in resistance by mutation**

[Ref. Park, 22/e p173]

16. **Ans. (a) Recently abolished; (c) Given for 6 months**

[Ref. Park 27/e p221]

17. **Ans. (a) To avoid emergence of persistors**

[Ref. Park 27/e p220]

18. **Ans. (a) Rifampicin; (b) Any one Fluoroquinolone; (c) INH; (d) Kanamycin** [Ref. Park 27/e p226]

19. **Ans. (d) Mycolic acid** [Ref. Short Textbook of Medical Microbiology by Satish Gupte, 1/e p153]

20. **Ans. (a) Father** [Ref. Park 27/e p486–487]

SUPERVISORS OF DOTS
- Peripheral health workers: MPWs
- Voluntary workers: Teachers, Anganwadi workers, Dais, Social workers, Ex-patients

21. **Ans. (a) High cost** [Ref. Comparison of DOTS with Self-Administered Therapy by Parida, Journal of Clinical and Diagnostic Research. 2014 Aug, Vol-8(8): HC29-HC31]

DOTS INDIAN EXPERIENCE

Advantages	Disadvantages
Doubles the accuracy of TB diagnosis	High cost
Success rates of up to 95%	Stigmatization
Cuts down TB deaths by seven fold	
Doubles the cure rate	
Reduces incidence and prevalence of TB	
Reduce duration of illness	
Prevent new infectious cases	
Improves the quality of care	
Prevents treatment failure	
Prevents emergence of MDR TB	

22. **Ans. (a) a, b** [Ref. Module for Laboratory Technicians. RNTCP. MOHFW. GOI 2005 p15]

LABELLING OF SPUTUM SAMPLES IN RNTCP
A new Laboratory Serial Number (LSN) is assigned to each of the chest-symptomatics whose sputum is examined beginning with 1 on 1 January each year and increases by one with each patient until 31 December of the same year
Each set of samples (2 for Diagnosis, 2 for each follow-up examination) is given one LSN
Diagnosis as well as follow-up samples are labelled with a single LSN with a suffix 'a' for the spot sample and 'b' for morning sample
LSN is given to a set of slides, and not to individual slides
- LSN is labelled on the side of the sputum container and the Laboratory Form

23. **Ans. (c) 30 days** [Ref. Guidelines for Tuberculosis Notification, NIKSHAY, GOI]
- All stakeholders, both public and private, are required to notify TB cases when patients have been diagnosed or when anti-TB treatment has already been initiated
- Report the cases to the nodal public health authority "at least on monthly basis,"
- "All cases diagnosed/treated since April 7, 2012 may be notified," states the TB notification module of NIKSHAY
- Notification methods: Hard copy by post, courier or by hand to the nodal officer/Soft copy by email from persons or institutes to nodal officer/Using authorized mobile numbers by phone call, IVRS or SMS/Uploading of information directly on to Nikshay portal/Direct online information transmission from newer diagnostic machines like CBNAAT or MGIT

24. **Ans. (a) Start ATT followed by ART**

[Ref. Park 27/e p235–236]

GUIDELINES FOR TREATMENT OF HIV+ TB PATIENTS
- ART offered to all HIV-TB and HIV-MDR TB patients irrespective of CD4 count
- Start ATT first, and allow it to be tolerated (2 weeks - 2 months), then start ART
- Start ATT as per RNTCP guidelines at ART Centre itself
- ATT treatment id same but treatment is more difficult and adverse reactions are more common

25. **Ans. (c) Low sensitivity and high specificity**
    [Ref. Expert Guide to Infectious Diseases, 2/e p500]

    MICROBIOLOGICAL TESTS FOR TB DIAGNOSIS

	Sputum smear	One culture	Three cultures	PCR
Sensitivity	60–70%	80–85%	80–100%	80–100%
Specificity	95%	98%	98%	98%

    ALSO REMEMBER
    - Overnight sputum collection for TB diagnosis has higher sensitivity
    - Sensitivity of TB sputum microscopy can be increased by fluorescence microscopy using an acid-fast fluorochrome dye (Auramine O or Auramine-rhodamine)
    - Result of smear microscopy in TB diagnosis is influenced by several variables like type of the specimen, thickness of the smear, technical preparation of the smear and experience of laboratory staff.

26. **Ans. (c) Medicine given for 1 month** *[Ref. Tuberculosis Control by Shrivastava, 1/e p3]*
    - Success of DOTS depend upon 5 components: [Mnemonic: **A G**ood **P**olitician **U**nderstands **D**evelopment]
        - **A**ccountability
        - **G**ood quality sputum microscopy
        - **P**olitical commitment
        - **U**ninterrupted supply of good quality drugs
        - **D**irectly observed treatment

27. **Ans. (d) Achieve at least 90% cure rate**
    [Ref. National Health Programmes in India by Dr Jugal Kishore, 8/e p202]

28. **Ans. (a) TB is mandatory to notify; (b) Suspicious TB patients are screened through 2 sputum smear examinations; (d) Case finding is active; (e) Covered the whole country since March 2006**
    [Ref. Park 27/e p220-222, 489]
    - India finally declared TB a notifiable disease in 2012: All private doctors, caregivers and clinics treating a patient suffering from TB now have to report every single case to the government
    - Suspicious TB patients are screened through 2 sputum smear examinations; Recently CBNAAT test has been added to comfort TB if Sputum smear results are inconclusive or not available
    - MDR-TB is included as Category 4 DOTS and XDR-TB as Category 5 DOTS
    - Case finding is mainly passive but now Systematic Active TB case finding strategy has been adopted too
    - Covered the whole country since March 2006

29. **Ans. (b) Nikshay** *[Ref. Park 27/e p222]*

30. **Ans. (d) Designated microscopy centre**
    [Ref. Park 27/e p487, 488]

    Designated Microscopy Centre (DMC) Under RNTCP
    - Most peripheral unit under RNTCP
    - Population covered: 100,000 in plains (50,000 in hilly/tribal areas)
    - DMCs are manned by a trained laboratory technician (LT) of the State health system
    - 1 TB Unit (each for 500,000 population) covers 5 DMCs

31. **Ans. (b) Two** *[Ref. Park 27/e p214-215]*

    Sputum Specimens to Confirm Diagnosis TB (RNTCP)
    - Two on 2 days: Spot sample (Day 1), Morning sample (Day 2)
    - Two on 1 day (If patient is from long distance): Spot sample (Day 1), Spot sample (Day 1 after gap of 1 hour)

Review Question

32. **Ans. (b) Achievements of high cure rates through DOTS**
    [Ref. Park 27/e p219]

NATIONAL POLIO ELIMINATION – PROGRAMME

33. **Ans. (c) TRUE, (d) TRUE, (e) TRUE**
    [Ref. Park 25/e p223-224]

    Polio AFP Surveillance
    - Age group: 0–15 years
    - Stool specimen should reach Laboratory in 72 hours (2 samples, 24–48 hours apart, within 14 days of onset of paralysis, transported to lab in Reverse cold chain)
    - Once diagnosed follow-up to be done after 60 days
    - >1 case of non-polio AFP per 1 Lakh population be detected [Now, New guideline for >2]

34. **Ans. (a) All children between 0–5 years of age on a single day, irrespective of their previous immunization status**
    [Ref. National Health Programmes of India by Dr. J. Kishore, 8/e p152 and Park 27/e p247]

    Pulse Polio Immunization (PPI) Programme in India
    - Launched in India: 1995–96 (1st round on 9th Dec 1995 and 20th Jan 1996)
        - First PPI targeted children <3 years age
        - Later on WHO recommended age group be 0–5 years (1996–97)
    - Meaning of 'Pulse': Sudden, simultaneous mass administration of Oral Polio Vaccine (OPV) on a single day to 'all children 0–5 years age', irrespective of their previous immunization status
        - PPI replaces wild virus with vaccine virus from the community
        - PPI is over and above routine immunization.

35. **Ans. (c) 60 days of onset of paralysis** *[Ref. Surveillance of Acute Flaccid Paralysis – Field Guide, MoHFW, 2/e p9]*
    - 60-day follow-up in a case of Acute Flaccid Paralysis (AFP): The District Immunization Officer (DIO) must visit every case of AFP 60 days after onset of paralysis 'to confirm the presence or absence of residual weakness'
        - Activity completed before 70th day
    - *Minimal levels of residual weakness can usually be detected by:*
        - Mid-arm or mid-thigh circumference: reveal wasting on one side.
        - Asymmetry in the skin folds on medial aspects of thigh.

ALSO REMEMBER

- All reported cases of AFP should be investigated by DIO 'within 48 hours' after notification
- 2 stool samples, atleast 24 hours apart, are collected within 14 days of onset of paralysis (maximum within 8 weeks)
- *Outbreak response immunization (ORI):* Following the AFP case investigation and stool specimen collection, ORI is organized in the community and performed as soon as possible
  - Children aged 0–59 months are given one dose of OPV regardless of previous immunization (in the village/locality of the AFP case)
  - The travel history of the child with AFP may suggest additional places of stay where ORI should also be conducted
- *Active case search in the community:* In the community where an AFP case resides or where an AFP case has visited during the incubation period for polio (4–25 days before paralysis onset), a house-to-house active case search is conducted to find additional AFP cases that may have occurred
  - This activity is carried out immediately along with ORI
  - A search is conducted for any children <15 years who have had the onset of AFP within the preceding 60 days
  - All cases that are found are investigated immediately, with collection from the case of two stool specimens before administration of OPV

36. **Ans. (c) Non-polio AFP rate should be >1 per 100000 among <15 years old; (d) Adequate stool specimens should be taken from 100% AFP** *[Ref. WHO Field Guide for supplementary activities aimed at achieving polio eradication, Geneva 1997; Park 27/e p247]*

    WHO Indicators of AFP Surveillance and Lab Performance: Two most critical indicators:
    - Non-polio AFP rate in children <15 years of age (Target ≥2/100,000): The non-polio AFP rate is an indicator of surveillance sensitivity; If it is ≥2/100,000 then the surveillance system is probably missing cases of AFP
    - Reported AFP cases with 2 stool specimens collected <14 days since paralysis onset (Target >80%)

37. **Ans. (d) To identify high risk population** *[Ref. Park 27/e p242]*

38. **Ans. (d) 90 days** *[Ref. Red Book: Field Immunization Guide, NPSP GOI document]*

Review Question

39. **Ans. (d) 30 days follow up examination** *[Ref. Park 27/e p247]*

RCH PROGRAMME

40. **Ans. (a) LaQshya** *[Ref. nhsrcindia.org]*

    Labor Room Quality Improvement Initiative—LaQshya
    - MoHFW launched LaQshya to improve the quality of care that is being provided to the pregnant mother in the Labor Room and Maternity Operation Theaters, thereby preventing the undesirable adverse outcomes associated with childbirth
    - *Aim:* To reduce Maternal and newborn mortality & morbidity and stillbirths
    - *Coverage:* Govt Medical colleges & hospitals/District hospitals/FRU >100 deliveries/month, High load CHC (>60 deliveries/month)

41. **Ans. (d) Tuberculosis** *[Ref. Textbook of Community Medicine by Sunder Lal, 2/e p135–36, Park 27/e p525]*

    Integrated Management of Neonatal and Childness illness (IMNCI):
    - IMNCI is a 'strategy for reducing morbidity and mortality associated with major causes of childhood illness'
      - *Curative component includes management of:*
        1. Diarrhoea
        2. Measles
        3. Pneumonia
        4. Malaria
        5. Severe malnutrition and nutritional counseling
    - *Case management process:* Is presented in a series of charts (**Mnemonic: A C**ase **I**s **T**reated **& C**are **G**iven)
      - **A**ssess the young infant or child
      - **C**lassify the illness
      - **I**dentify the treatment
      - **T**reat the infant or child
      - **C**ounsel the mother
      - **G**ive follow-up care

ALSO REMEMBER

- IMNCI is the Indian adaptation of IMCI (Integrated Management of Childhood Illness); major highlights of Indian adaptation are,
  - Inclusion of early neonatal age (0–7 days age) in programme
  - Incorporating national guidelines on malaria, anemia, Vitamin-A supplementation and immunization schedule
  - Training of health workers begin with sick young infants up to 2 months
  - Proportion of training time devoted to sick young infant and sick child is almost equal
  - Is skill based

42. **Ans. (c) Reduce the under five mortality to half** *[Ref. Textbook of Community Medicine by Sunder Lal, 2/e p202; Park 27/e p518–520]*
    - *Components of Reproductive and Child Health Programme:*
      - Community Needs Assessment Approach (CNAA)
      - Integrated packages of services for mother and child
      - MTP services at PHC and safe abortion
      - Control and prevention of RTI/STI
      - Adolescent health
      - Services in urban slums
      - Improving quality of services

- Unmet needs and sub-centre action plans
- Communication strategy
- Gender sensitiveness
- Greater involvement of Panchayati Raj Institutions (PRIs), NGOs and community.

43. **Ans. (b) Clean towel & Clean water for hand washing**
 [Ref. National Health Programmes of India by Dr. J. Kishore, 7/e p161]

- *'Five cleans'* (practices) under strategies for elimination of neonatal tetanus include,
  - Clean delivery surface
  - Clean hands (of birth attendants)
  - Clean cord cut (blade or instrument)
  - Clean cord tie
  - Clean cord stump (no applicant)
- Suggested *'Seven cleans'* include five cleans and
  - Clean water, and
  - Clean towel, for hand washing.

> **ALSO REMEMBER**
> - *Procedures undertaken to ensure 5 cleans:*
>   - Clean delivery surface: A clean plastic sheet
>   - Clean hands: Soap and clean water
>   - Clean cord cut: A new razor blade
>   - Clean cord tie: A clean piece of thread
>   - Clean cord stump: Nothing to be applied to cord
> - *Sometimes these practices are called as '3 cleans':*
>   - Clean delivery surface
>   - Clean hands
>   - Clean cord care (cut, tie and stump)
> - *Neonatal Tetanus Elimination:*
>   - Rate <0.1 per 1000 LB
>   - Attended deliveries >75%
>   - TT2 coverage >90%

44. **Ans. (a) 20 mg iron & 100 micrograms folic acid**
 [Ref. National Health Programmes of India by Dr. J. Kishore, 8/e p413]

- Iron and Folic Acid content per IFA tablet:
  - *Adult tablet:* 100 mg elemental iron and 500 mcg folic acid
  - *Pediatric tablet:* 20 mg elemental iron and 100 mcg folic acid

45. **Ans. (a) Remove CuT only** *[Ref. Park 27/e p573]*

Pregnancy with IUD-IN-SITU:
- If women requests termination of pregnancy: Legally induced abortion should be carried out
- If women wishes continuation of pregnancy + threads are visible: Remove IUD by gently pulling the threads
- If women wishes continuation of pregnancy + threads are NOT visible: Carefully examine for any complication; If there are sign of intrauterine infection and sepsis, evacuation of the uterus under broad spectrum antibiotic cover is mandatory.

46. **Ans. (b) Treatment of STD** *[Ref. Park 27/e p518–520]*
47. **Ans. (b) CSSM plus family planning** *[Ref. Park 27/e p518]*
48. **Ans. (c) Feed to malnourished children** *[Ref. Park 27/e p520]*
49. **Ans. (d) All of the above** *[Ref. Park 27/e p518–520]*
50. **Ans. (c) District level household survey**
 [Ref. DLHS, RCHIPS, MOHFW, GOI 2015]

DISTRICT LEVEL HOUSEHOLD AND FACILITY SURVEY (DLHS), MOHFW

- *Sample size:* 7 lakh households covering all districts of India
- *Importance:* Provide district level estimates on health indicators to assist policy makers and programme administrators in decentralized planning, monitoring and evaluation
- Main objective of the survey was to estimate the service coverage of the following:
  - Ante Natal Care (ANC) and Immunization services
  - Extent of safe deliveries
  - Contraceptive prevalence
  - Unmet need for family planning
  - Awareness about RTI/STI and HIV/AIDS
  - Utilization of government health services and users' satisfaction
- *Frequency:* Once every 5 years
  - DLHS-1: 1998–99
  - DLHS-2: 2002–04
  - DLHS-3: 2007–08
  - DLHS-4: 2012–13
- *DLHS-3 Key Data India:*
  - Literacy rate: 72%
  - Mean household size: 5.1
  - Improved source of drinking water: 84%
  - Mean age of marriage: 24 years (Boys), 19.8 years (Girls)
  - Family planning usage: 54%
  - Unmet need for Family planning: 21.3%
  - Institutional delivery: 47%
  - Fully immunize children (12–23 months): 54%
  - Exclusive breast feeding: 47%

51. **Ans. (b) Janani Shishu Suraksha Karyakram**
 [Ref. Park 27/e p522]

- Under JSSK, just like provision of services to Mothers, their sick newborns accessing public health institutions for treatment, have been given similar entitlements till 30 days after birth

52. **Ans. (a) Adolescent health** *[Ref. Park 27/e p531]*

'PLUS' IN RMNCH+A STRATEGIC APPROACH DENOTES

- Inclusion of adolescence as a distinct 'life stage' in the overall strategy
- Linking of maternal and child health to reproductive health and other components (like Family planning, Adolescent health, HIV, Gender and Preconception & Prenatal Diagnostic Techniques)
- Linking of home/community based care to and facility-based care
- Ensure linkages, referrals between various levels of health care system to create a "Continuous care pathway"

53. **Ans. (d) Involvement of private organizations**
 [Ref. Park 27/e p530–535]
54. **Ans. (d) Pneumonia treatment** *[Ref. Park 27/e p532]*
    - **PRIORITY INTERVENTIONS FOR ADOLESCENTS UNDER RMNCH+A**
    - Adolescent nutrition; iron and folic acid supplementation
    - Facility-based adolescent reproductive and sexual health services (Adolescent health clinics)
    - Information and counselling on adolescent sexual reproductive health and other health issues
    - Menstrual hygiene
    - Preventive health checkups (School health examination)
55. **Ans. (c) Dedication of 75% training the on younger infants** *[Ref. Park 27/e p528]*
    - Under IMNCI, the proportion of training time devoted to sick young infant and sick child is almost equal.
56. **Ans. (a) Sub-centre** *[Ref. Park 27/e p518]*
    - Sub-centre is the peripheral most post for delivery of health care in Rural areas of India
    - Under RCH program, Type B Sub centres conduct deliveries and Type A/B subcentre both provide antenatal/intranatal/postnatal services, child health care, family planning and contraceptive services along with adolescent health care

Review Question

57. **Ans. (c) Two tablets twice daily** *[Ref. Park 27/e p189]*

NATIONAL BLINDNESS CONTROL PROGRAMME

58. **Ans. (c) Tertiary level** *[Ref. Park 27/e p503–505]*
    Refer to theory.
59. **Ans. (b) Low vision**
    [Ref. National Health Programmes of India by Dr. J. Kishore, 8/e p422; Park 27/e p456]
    - WHO defines Blindness as 'visual acuity of <3/60 in better eye with best possible correction'
    - National Programme for Control of Blindness (NPCB), India defines Blindness as 'visual acuity of <6/60 in better eye with best possible correction'
    [New Guideline 2017–18]
    - *Comparison of WHO and NPCB definitions:*

WHO – ICD	Visual Acuity	NPCB, India
Low Vision		
Category 1	<6/18–6/60	Low Vision
Category 2	<6/60–3/60	Economic Blindness
Blindness		
Category 3	<3/60–1/60	Social Blindness
Category 4	<1/60 – PL+	Manifest Blindness
Category 5	PL–	Absolute Blindness

(PL+: Perception of Light; PL–: No perception of light)

60. **Ans. (d) Visual acuity <3/60 in the better eye with best correction** *[Ref. National Health Programmes of India by Dr. J. Kishore, 8/e p422, Park 27/e p456]*
61. **Ans. (d) Visual acuity <3/60 in the better eye with best correction** *[Ref. NPCB New Guideline 2017–18]*
62. **Ans. (b) 6/9** *[Ref. The Principles and Practice of Community Ophthalmology, NPCB, Govt. of India, 2002; p119]*
    - WHO defines Blindness as 'visual acuity of <3/60 in better eye with best possible correction'
    - National Programme for Control of Blindness (NPCB), India defines Blindness as 'visual acuity of <3/60 in better eye with best possible correction'
63. **Ans. (b) To shift from fixed facility surgical approach to eye camp approach** *[Ref. National Health Programmes of India by Dr. J. Kishore, 8/e p425]*
    - **Revised strategies of NPCB:**
      - To make NPCB more comprehensive by,
        1. Strengthening services for other causes of blindness like corneal blindness and refractive errors in school children
        2. Improving followup services of cataract operated persons
        3. Treating other causes of blindness like glaucoma.
      - To strengthen participation of voluntary organizations
      - To shift from eye camp approach to fixed facility surgical approach
      - To enhance coverage of eye services in tribal & underserved areas
      - To expand World Bank project activities
        1. Construction of dedicated eye OTs and eye wards
        2. Training of eye surgeons
        3. Modern cataract surgery
        4. Supply of ophthalmic equipment.
64. **Ans. (c) A-IV, B-I, C-III, D-II** *[Ref. National Health Programmes of India by Dr. J. Kishore, 8/e p422]*
65. **Ans. (d) Glaucoma** *[Ref. National Health Programmes of India by Dr. J. Kishore, 7/e p368 and The Principles and Practice of Community Ophthalmology, NPCB, Govt. of India, 2002; p234–45]*
    - *Vision 2020 – The Right To Sight:* A global initiative by WHO and International NGOs to reduce avoidable (preventable and curable) blindness by 2020.

Global Vision 2020 (5 diseases)	Indian Vision 2020 (7 diseases)
Cataract	Cataract
Refractive errors and low vision	Refractive errors and low vision
Childhood blindness	Childhood blindness
Trachoma	Focal trachoma
Onchocerciasis	Glaucoma
	Diabetic retinopathy
	Corneal blindness

National Health Programmes, Policies and Legislations in India | 477

66. Ans. (d) Xerophthalmia [Ref. National Health Programmes of India by Dr. J. Kishore, 8/e p428, Park 21/e p403]

ALSO REMEMBER
- *World Sight Day:* 2nd Thursday of October.

67. Ans. (a) Cataract [Ref. The Principles and Practice of Community Ophthalmology, NPCB, Govt. of India, 2002; p158]
- *MC cause of blindness in India:* Cataract
- Cataract is included among target diseases in Vision 2020 (both Global and Indian)
- National Programme for Control of Blindness (NPCB) was started in 1976 as a 100% centrally sponsored scheme
- Strategies of NPCB include establishing 'one eye care facility per 5 lac persons'
- Rate of cataract surgery required to clear backlog of cataract blindness in India: 400 operations per lac population

68. Ans. (a) Age group screened is 5–10 years [Ref. The Principles and Practice of Community Ophthalmology, NPCB, Govt. of India, 2002; p119 and Park 20/e p376]

69. Ans. (b) Trachoma [Ref. National Health Programmes of India by Dr. J. Kishore, 8/e p428–29]
- WHO has recommended '**SAFE** Strategy' for global elimination of blinding trachoma in the remaining countries
  - **S**urgery
  - **A**ntibiotic use
  - **F**acial cleanliness
  - **E**nvironmental improvement.

ALSO REMEMBER
- *Blinding trachoma:* Is found in countries with prevalence of blindness >0.5%. Is indicated by the presence of:
  - Corneal blindness
  - Trachomatous trichiasis and entropion
  - Moderate and severe trachomatous inflammation
- *Mass (Blanket) treatment of trachoma:*
  - Given where prevalence of moderate and severe trachoma in 0–10 years age group is >10%
  - Azithromycin is DOC
  - Treatment consists of 1% tetracycline (for 5 consecutive days each month or once daily for 10 days each month for 6 consecutive months, or for 60 days) or alternatively erythromycin
- *WHO recommended strategy for measles elimination:* 'Catch up – Keep up – Follow up strategy' & AMMRS strategy
- *WHO recommended strategy for polio eradication:* 'PULSE strategy'.

70. Ans. (a) UNICEF [Ref. www.who.int]

71. Ans. (d) 20000 [Ref. Park 27/e p504]
- Proposed Structure for Vision 2020, NPCB:
  - Vision centres 20,000 (Primary level)
  - Service centres 2,000 (Secondary level)
  - Training centres 200 (Tertiary level)
  - Centres for Excellence 20 (Tertiary level)

72. Ans. (c) Sentinel surveillance [Ref. NPCB Document, GOI]
- 25 Sentinel surveillance units have been established in Departments of Ophthalmology and PSM in Medical Colleges in India for assessment of,
  - Beneficiary profiles
  - Visual outcomes based on cataract surgery records
  - Follow-up of operated cases
  - Ocular morbidity data

73. Ans. (c) District collector [Ref. Park, 22/e p406; Guidelines for State Health Society and District Health Society, NPCB document, 11th FYP 2009, Pg 6]
- Composition of District Blindness Control Society (DBCS)/District Health Society: 15 members (7 member team plus 8 ex-officio members)

Chairman	District Collector/District Mission Director
Vice-Chairman	Chief Medical & Health Officer/District Health Officer
Member Secretary	District Programme Manager (Deputy CMO Ophthalmologist)
Technical Advisor	Chief Ophthalmic Surgeon of District hospital/HOD Ophthalmology
Other members	Medical Superintendent/Civil Surgeon of District Hospital/District Education Officer Representatives from NGOs/District Mass media (IEC) officer Prominent practicing eye surgeons

74. Ans. ALL CHOICES [Ref. New Guideline, NPCB, GOI 2017-18]

DEFINITION OF BLINDNESS UNDER NPCB
- Simple definition: Inability of a person to count fingers from a distance of 3 meters or 10 feet
- Technical definitions:
  - Vision 3/60 or less with the best possible spectacle correction
  - Diminution of field vision to 10° or less in better eye

75. Ans. (b) Dr Rajendra Prasad Center for Ophthalmic Sciences AIIMS is apex body for implementation of NPCB; (c) Promotion of eye camp and mobile unit; (d) Intra ocular lens implantation better than convention conventional surgery [Ref. Park 27/e p503–505]
- National Program for Control of Blindness (NPCB) was launched in the year 1976
- 100% Centrally sponsored program
- NPCB now renamed as National Program for Control of Blindness & Visual Impairment (NPCBVI)

76. Ans. (b) Epidemic conjunctivitis [Ref. Park 27/e p504]

NATIONAL HIV/AIDS CONTROL PROGRAMME

77. Ans. (a) >10% population of known HIV+ve among TB patients tested for HIV in the district [Ref. NACO Website]

Categorisation of Districts under NTEP (for HIV-TB Co-infection)

Category	Categorisation	Criteria
A	High TB	TB case notification rate >180/Lac population
B	High TB-HIV	>10% known HIV+ among TB patients tested
C	High DR-TB	>25% relapses among SS+ve incident TB cases
D	Very low case finding effort	Annual suspect TB examination rate <400/Lac population
E	Average	None of the above
F	High case finding but Low TCNR	Annual suspect TB examination rate >1200/Lac population AND TB case notification rate <80/Lac population

78. **Ans. (c) Tenofovir + Lamivudine + Lopinavir**
    [Ref. Park 26/e p399]

    OLDER GUIDELINES PEP for HIV (WHO 2016)
    - Initiated ideally within 72 hours
    - Wound/skin site should be washed immediately with soap and water, and exposed mucous membranes should be flushed with water (Use of caustic agents or antiseptics or disinfectants at the wound site is not recommended)
    - 3-drug regimen is preferably used (Lamivudine + Tenofovir + Efavirenz) for 4 weeks
    - HIV status assessment of exposed person should not be a barrier for initiating PEP

    NEW GUIDELINES PEP for HIV (2020)
    - Three drug regimen is preferred – Raltegravir 400 mg BD + Tenofovir disoproxil fumarate 300 mg OD + Emtricitabine 200 mg OD
    - Raltegravir could be replaced by a once-daily alternative "Dolutegravir"
    - Regimen should continue for 28 days
    - Similar regimen is suitable for children 2–12 years too, with each drug dosed to age and weight

79. **Ans. (b) STD clinic attendees**
    [Ref. HIV Behavior Sentinel Surveillance BSS 2021, NACP. NACO 2021]

    HIV Behavior Sentinel Surveillance BSS 2021
    - The yearly HIV surveillance system under NACP gradually evolved into biennial HIV sentinel surveillance (HSS) plus
    - The 17th round 2021, will be implemented among 8 population groups (Pregnant women, Single male migrants SMM, Long-distance truckers LDT, Inmates at central prison sites, Female sex workers FSW, Men who have sex with men MSM, Hijra/transgender H/TG people and Injecting drug users IDU)
    - Blood specimen will be tested for four biomarkers - HIV, Syphilis, HBV, HCV

80. **Ans. (c) 3** *[Ref. Project document: National AIDS Control Programme – II, NACO]*
    - Under National AIDS Control Programme (India):
      - *Screening of HIV:* E/R/S
        1. ELISA (E) Test
        2. RAPID (R) Test
        3. SIMPLE (S) Test
      - *Confirmatory diagnosis of HIV:* Western Blot Assay

- *Screening of HIV:*
  - *Strategy I:* One out of three screening tests (E/R/S) are used
    1. Done for screening every blood unit before transfusion
    2. Does not recommend its use for diagnosis of HIV in a person
  - *Strategy II:* Two out of three screening tests (E/R/S) are used
    1. Done for screening person who is symptomatic with any one of AIDS defining illness (NACO guidelines)
  - *Strategy III:* All three screening tests (E/R/S) are used
    1. Done for screening person who is asymptomatic

81. **Ans. (b) Transfusion of blood/blood products**
    [Ref. National Health Programmes of India by Dr. J. Kishore, 8/e p237; Park 21/e p321, Park 22/e p320, 24/e p364]
    - Risk of HIV transmission through different modes (Efficiency of routes):

Route of transmission	Efficiency
Sexual	0.01–1%
Blood and blood products transfusion	>90%
Sharing needle/syringes	0.1–0.3%
Mother to child transmission (MTCT)	25–30%
Per-cutaneous exposure	0.4%
Muco-cutaneous exposure	0.05%

- AIDS is known as 'Slim's Disease' in Africa
- Risk of Mother to child transmission (MTCT) of HIV:
  - Developing countries: 30%
  - Developed countries: 25%
- *Risk of HIV transmission with prolonged breast feeding:* 12–15%
- *Risk of HIV transmission in presence of other STD:* Increases 8–10 times.

82. **Ans. (d) HIV/AIDS** *[Ref. National Health Programmes of India by Dr. J. Kishore, 8/e p271]*
    - Since 1987, more than 30 HIV candidate vaccines have been tested in Clinical trials Phases I/II; Some of them are: **[Mnemonic: CRAMS]**
      - **C**ytotoxic T-Lymphocytes (CTL) Inducing vaccine
      - **R**ecombinant adeno- associated virus (rAAV) vaccine
      - **A**IDSVAX (gp 120 based vaccine): only vaccine in Phase III trials
      - **M**odified Vaccinia ankara (mVA) vaccine
      - **S**ubunit vaccine

83. **Ans. (d) Industrial workers** *[Ref. Park 27/e p500]*

    Targeted Interventions in NACP
    - *Basic purpose:* To reduce transmission of HIV amongst most vulnerable populations
    - *Approach:* Combines a comprehensive and integrated approach to vulnerable segments of population
      - Main activities:
      - Behaviour change

- Communication
- Treatment of STD
- Create enabling environment to facilitate behaviour change.

Segments of population covered:
- Sex workers
- Injecting Drug Users
- Truckers
- Homosexual men (MSM-Men having sex with men)
- Migrant labourers
- Transgenders & Hijra

84. **Ans. (b) Opt-out testing**
    [Ref. HIV testing guidelines, CDC Atlanta]

- *Opt-in testing:* testing is offered and the patient is required to actively give permission before it can occur
- *Opt-out testing:* means performing an HIV test after notifying the patient that the test is normally performed, but that the patient may elect to decline or defer testing; assent is then assumed unless the patient declines testing
- WHO and CDC recommends opt-out testing policies in health care settings
- Opt-out testing has a higher (85–98%) testing rate than opt-in testing (25–83%)
- It does NOT eliminate the need for informed consent.

85. **Ans. (a) Lamivudine; (b) Zidovudine and (c) Nevirapine**
    [Ref. Park 27/e p498]

86. **Ans. (b) Estimation of total cases in hospitals**
    [Ref. Park 27/e p496]

    Sentinel Surveillance under NACP
    - Basis for classification of districts
    - Monitoring trend of HIV in different age groups
    - Estimation of HIV infected persons in county

87. **Ans. (b) Yellow** *[Ref. Park 27/e p501]*
88. **Ans. (b) 30 November 2006** *[Ref. Park 27/e p500]*
89. **Ans. NONE** *[Ref. Park 27/e p402]*
- New Post-Exposure Guidelines for HIV 2014–15 for Adolescents and Adults:
  - Preferred backbone regimen: Tenofovir + Lamivudine
  - Preferred third drug: Lopinavir/Ritonavir OR Atazanavir/Ritonavir

90. **Ans. (a) Efavirenz** *[Ref. Pulmonary Complications of HIV by Feldman 1/e p118]*
- Based on pharmacokinetic studies and a substantial number of clinical studies, Efavirenz is the antiretroviral drug of choice to be used with a rifampicin-based anti-tuberculosis therapy
- Nevirapine based ART regimen is Second line of choice when Efavirenz cannot be used.

91. **Ans. (b) Start ART now, continue throughout pregnancy and till lifelong** *[Ref. Park 27/e p498]*

ART HIV+ Pregnant women and women doing Breastfeeding
- Should be initiated regardless of WHO clinical stage and at any CD4 count
- Continue lifelong

92. **Ans. (a) Yearly checkup is done** *[Ref. NACO Website]*

    HIV Sentinel Surveillance (HSS) system in India
    - Cross-sectional facility and Targeted Intervention (TI) based HIV sero-prevalence surveys at regular intervals among selected population groups (Sentinel groups)
    - Trends in HIV infection are monitored over the period of time by group and by site
    - Proxy for general population in HSS: Pregnant females attending AN clinics
    - During NACP-IV, HIV Sentinel Surveillance will be conducted once in two years (**"Biennial surveillance"**) so that adequate time is spent on in-depth analysis and modeling, epidemiological research and use of surveillance data for programmatic purposes

NATIONAL VECTOR BORNE DISEASES CONTROL PROGRAMME

93. **Ans. (a) Amphotericin B** *[Ref. Park 26/e p350]*
- rk39 dipstick test positive is serological test for Kala azar
- Treatment of choice for Kala-azar:
  - *First line:* Liposomal Amphotericin B (LAMB) Single dose 10 mg/kg
  - *Second line:* Paromomycin + Inj. Miltefosine (Combination regimens)
  - *Third line:* Amphotericin B emulsion
  - *Fourth line:* Miltefosine capsules
  - *Fifth line:* Inj. Amphotericin B deoxycholate (Multiple doses)

94. **Ans. (d) Wuchereria bancrofti**
    [Ref. WHO Lymphatic Filariasis: Monitoring and Epidemiological Assessment of Mass Drug Administration]

    Transmission assessment survey (TAS) for Filariasis
    - *Importance:* Helps us evaluate if transmission is not sustainable (at a quite low level) enough guiding us to stop MDA, To check for recrudescence
    - *Criteria:* Mf prevalence <1% even after 5th MDA, >65% in coverage in each MDA
    - *TAS carried out at:* **Schools** 1st/2nd year primary children (If enrolment is >75%), **Community** 6–7 years old children (If enrolment is <75%)
    - *Methods used:* Cluster survey, Systematic sampling
    - *Major diagnostic tools:* Immunochromatographic test (ICT), Brugia rapid (and Blood films, PCR)

95. **Ans. None** *[Ref. National Health Programmes of India by Dr. J. Kishore, 8/e p287K. 24/e p272]*
- In India, Plasmodium Falciparum is the commonest (51%), followed by P. vivax, P. malariae is rarely found and P. ovale has recently been reported in India
  - Recent trends have shown that P. falciparum is becoming most common cause of Malaria in India

- P. vivax is the most widely distributed and the most common species observed in temperate regions of the world, while P. falciparum is the most widespread throughout the world's tropics
- The occurrence of P. ovale has not been very common in India and till date only 4 reports of P. ovale are available from Kolkata, Orissa, Delhi and more recently from Gujarat
- Malaria is the commonest vector borne parasitic disease of the globe
- Malaria prevention and control is a component of 'National Vector Borne Diseases Control Programme' (NVBDCP);
 NVBDCP covers 6 vector borne diseases of public health importance in India:

Disease	Main vector
Malaria	Female Anopheles
Filariasis	Culex quinquefasciatus (C. fatigans)
Dengue	Aedes aegypti
Kala Azar	Sandfly (Phlebotamus)
Japanese Encephalitis	Culex tritaeniorhynchus
Chikungunya fever	Aedes aegypti

96. Ans. (b) Histidine-rich protein [Ref. National Health Programmes of India by Dr. J. Kishore, 8/e p289]

- 'Dipstick Test' is used for the rapid diagnosis of Plasmodium falciparum (Pf)
    - Is a 'rapid whole blood immuno-chromatographic test'
    - Uses 2 antibodies specific for 'Pf Histidine Rich Protein II Antigen'
    - Is a 'antigen capture assay'

> **ALSO REMEMBER**
> - *Optimal test (Parasite-specific lactic dehydrogenase (LDH dipstick test)):* Positive in P.falciparum and P.vivax parasitaemia; It is a simple and rapid, and superior to HRP II.
> - *K-39 Dipstick test:* Is for Visceral Leishmaniasis (Kala Azar).

97. Ans. (a) DDT [Ref. National Health Programmes of India by Dr. J. Kishore, 8/e p326; Park 21/e p281, Park 22/e p280]

- Insecticide of choice: DDT
    - 2 rounds of spray per year
    - Spray up to 6 feet height on walls
    - If DDT–resistant, use BHC

> **ALSO REMEMBER**
> - *Sandfly is the vector of:*
>   - Visceral Leishmaniasis (Kala azar)
>   - Cutaneous Leishmaniasis (Oriental Sore)
>   - Sandfly Fever
>   - Oroya Fever
> - Sandflies inject the infective stage, metacyclic promastigotes, during blood meals.
> - *DDT (Dichloro-Diphenyl-Trichloroethane):*
>   - *Synthesized by:* Othmar Zeidler (1874)
>   - *Insecticidal properties discovered by:* Swiss scientist Paul H. Müller (1939) (awarded the 1948 Nobel Prize in Physiology and Medicine)
>   - *Positive association found with:* Liver, biliary tract and breast cancers.

98. Ans. (b) Annual Blood Examination Rate (ABER) [Ref. Park 25/e p278]

99. Ans. (b) R2 type [Ref. Medical Entomology- A textbook on Public health and Veterinary Problems by Eldridge & Edman, 1/e p213]

Types of Drug Resistance in Malaria
- R1 resistance: Recrudescence of infection between 7–28 days of treatment completion following initial resolution of symptoms and parasite clearance.
- R2 resistance: Patients with marked reduction of parasitemia (parasite count reduced by more than 75%) at 48 h but failed to clear parasites by day 7.

100. Ans. (c) 1 [Park 27/e p474–479]
101. Ans. NONE [IT INCLUDES ALL] [Ref. Park 27/e p472]
102. Ans. (c) Anti-larval measures [Ref. Park 27/e p474–479]
103. Ans. (b) Cover overhead tanks properly [Ref. Guidelines for Source Reduction, NVBDCP, Government of India]

- In urban areas, Malaria is mainly transmitted by Anopheles stephensi
    - Breeds in man-made water containers in domestic/peridomestic situations such as tanks, wells, cisterns, which are of permanent nature and hence can malaria transmission throughout the year
- Recommended measures for Urban Malaria control:
    - Lids of overhead tanks must be checked and maintained monthly basis; any leakage be repaired immediately (most effective)
    - Cover-up of underground and open tanks
    - Open tanks used for animals be dead dried once in week
    - Never to throw any containers in open capable of holding water
    - Construction sites: Building bye-laws be implemented to prevent fault in designs, water flow on roof, gully traps open tanks for curing be treated with larvicides on weekly basis
    - Unused wells either be closed or treated with larvicides

- Ornamental tanks, fountains be checked periodically and larvivorous fish be introduced
- Public health engineers be involved for proper drainage, building designs, periodic flushing of water logged areas and drainage

104. **Ans. (d) 10 days**   *[Ref. New Scientist, Volume 97 p733]*
- 10 days is the minimum time required for reproductive cycle of parasite within the vector

105. **Ans. (a) ACT only**   *[Ref. Park 27/e p307]*

106. **Ans. (d) Increase in the number Plasmodium species**
[Ref. Short Textbook of PSM by Prabhakara, 1/e p147]
- There was a Malaria resurgence in India in Early 1970's due to:
  - Operational failure
  - Administrative failure
  - Technical failure: Insecticidal resistance, Drug resistance, population movements

107. **Ans. (d) Primaquine contraindicated in infants and pregnant women**   *[Ref. Park 27/e p307]*
- Presumptive treatment is not used in NVBDCP (Malaria) currently
- ACT is the DOC in P. falciparum and P. malariae
- Primaquine is given in all cases of malaria
- Primaquine contraindicated in infants and pregnant women

108. **Ans. (c) Annual incidence <10 per 1000 by 2017**

109. **Ans. (d) Artesunate 4 mg/kg daily 3 days + Sulfadoxine – Pyremethamine (25/1.25 mg/kg) one dose + Primaquine 0.7 5 mg/kg single dose**   *[Ref. Dte. of NVBDCP. Diagnosis and Treatment of Malaria 2013 Guidelines. GOI. p8]*

110. **Ans. (a) 1 per 1000**   *[Ref. Park 27/e p306]*
- API = Confirmed cases in 1 year/Population under surveillance × 1000
  In the given question, API = 100/100000 × 1000 = 1 per 1000

Review Question

111. **Ans. (a) Chloroquine**   *[Ref. Park 27/e p308–310]*

NRHM, NUHM, NHM

112. **Ans. (b) 1000 to mother and 400 to ASHA**
[Ref. Park 26/e p510]

Incentives under JSSK (NHM)

Category	Rural areas			Urban areas		
	Mother's package	ASHA's package	Total package	Mother's package	ASHA's package	Total package
LPS	1400	600	2000	1000	400	1400
HPS	700	600	1300	600	400	1000

(LPS: Low performing states; HPS: High performing states) (LPS include UP, Uttarakhand, MP, Jharkhand, Bihar, Chhattisgarh, Odisha, Assam, Jammu & Kashmir, Rajasthan)

113. **Ans. (d) 1, 2, 3**   *[Ref. Operational Guidelines for MMUs. NHM. MoHFW, GOI]*

Mobile Medical Units (MMUs)
- MMUs provide a range of health care services for populations living in remote, inaccessible, unserved and underserved areas mainly with the objective of taking healthcare service delivery to the doorsteps of these populations under NRHM and NUHM

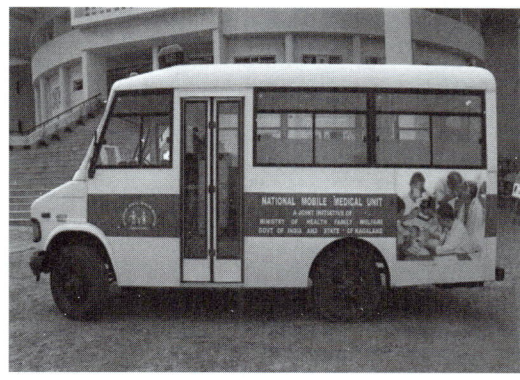

- Norms for Deployment of MMUs: One MMU per district (population of 10 lakhs, with a cap of five MMUs per district):
- District with population 10 lakhs: 1 MMU
- District with population of between 10 lakhs and 20 lakhs: 2 MMUs.
- District with population of between 20 lakhs and 30 lakhs: 3 MMUs
- District with population of between 30 lakhs and 40 lakhs: 4 MMUs
- District with population of over 40 lakhs: 5 MMUs
- Type of Service Provided through MMUs
- Primary care services for common communicable and non-communicable diseases, RCH services, carry out screening activities and provide referral linkage to appropriate higher faculties
- Provide point of care diagnostics: Blood glucose, pregnancy testing, urine microscopy, albumin and sugar, Hb, Height/Weight, vision testing, RDT
- Collect sputum samples
- Screen populations over 35 for Hypertension, Diabetes and Cancers annually and undertake follow-up checks including providing drugs with a monthly supply (Hypertension, Diabetes, Epilepsy)
- Undertake IEC sessions
- Suggested models of MMUs:
- Government operated MMU
- Operation of MMU on Out sourcing basis—CAPEX & drugs and supplies provided by Government
- Out sourcing of MMU services including CAPEX and OPEX (Drugs and supplies to be provided by the Govt)
- Suggested Human resources for an MMU include 1 MO (MBBS only, preferably women), 1 GNM, 1 Lab Technician, 1 Pharmacist cum Administrative Assistant, 1 Driver cum Support Staff

114. **Ans. (c) Congenital glaucoma** [Ref. Park 26/e p506]

Selected 34 diseases under RBSK:

Diseases in children	Deficiency conditions
• Skin conditions (Eczema, Fungal, Scabies) • Otitis media • Rheumatic heart disease • Reactive airway disease • Dental conditions • Convulsive disorders	• Anemia (especially severe) • Vitamin A deficiency (Bitot spots) • Vitamin D deficiency (Rickets) • Severe acute malnutrition • Goitre
Defects at birth	Developmental delays including disabilities
• Neural tube defects • Down's syndrome • Cleft lip/palate • Talipes • Dysplasia of hip • Congenital cataract • Congenital deafness • Congenital heart disease • Retinopathy of prematurity	• Vision impairment • Hearing impairment • Neuro-motor impairment • Motor delay • Cognitive delay • Language delay • Behaviour disorder (Autism) • Learning disorder • Attention deficit hyperactivity disorder • Congenital hypothyroidism • Sickle cell anemia • Beta thalassemia

115. **Ans. (d) Give antibiotics and re-assess in 3 days** [Ref. Park 25/e p656]
   - Pneumonia (Not severe) YELLOW is classified if there is Chest indrawing, Fast breathing present (RR >50 in 2–12 months; >40 in 12 months-5 years)
   - *Management is at PHC:* Oral Amoxycillin × 5 days, Inhaled bronchodilator × 5 days, Soothe throat with safe remedy, If cough >14 days, refer for TB assessment, If recurrent wheeze, refer for Asthma assessment, Follow-up in 3 days, Advise mother when to return immediately

116. **Ans. (a) If A, B, C are correct** [Ref. Park 25/e p486]
   - **Roles and responsibilities of ASHA** include Accompany pregnant females to hospital (JSSK), Help in completion of immunization as per schedule, Spread awareness regarding contraception, Counselling, Facilitate access to health care, Development of Village health plan VHP (with Village health and sanitation committee VHSC), Organize Village health days VHD, Accompany mother/child to health centre for health care, Provide primary medical care for minor ailments to community, Act as Depot holder for ORS/Chloroquine/IFA/Contraceptives/DDK/Share data and info on births/deaths in village
   - Malaria slide preparation is the responsibility of Multipurpose health worker (Male) at Sub Centre

117. **Ans. (c) ASHA is skilled birth attendant**
   [Ref. National Health Programmes of India by Dr. J. Kishore, 8/e p85–86, Park 21/e p407, Park 27/e p515]

118. **Ans. (c) Accredited Social Health Activist**
   [Ref. National Health Programmes of India by Dr. J. Kishore, 8/e p69, 79, 80 Park 21/e p405, Park 27/e p515]
   - *National Rural Health Mission (NRHM) 2005–12:* One of the key components of the is to provide every village in the country with a trained female community health activist – ASHA (Accredited Social Health Activist)
   - *Proposed population norm:* 2 ASHA worker per 1000 population (Village Level)

119. **Ans. (d) Village Level** [Ref. National Health Programmes of India by Dr. J. Kishore, 8/e p85; Park 23/e 24/e p470]
   - A core strategy of National Rural Health Mission (NRHM) is to develop 'Health Plan (VHP) for each village' through Village Health Samiti of Panchayat (PHS)
     – ASHA will make VHP: ASHA along with ANM, Aanganwadi Workers and community workers under the leadership of PHS.

120. **Ans. (c) Reduction in infant mortality** [Ref. Park 21/e p408, Park 22/e p414]

   Impact Indicators for Monitoring and Evaluation of Asha's Work:
   - Infant mortality rate (IMR)
   - Child malnutrition rates
   - No. of cases of TB/Leprosy detected as compared to last year

121. **Ans. (a) Janani Suraksha Yojana** [Ref. Park 27/e p521]

   Janani Suraksha Yojana (JSY)
   - Launched on 12th April 2005
   - Is 'modification of National Maternity Benefit Scheme
   - *Objectives of JSY:* Reduction of maternal mortality and infant mortality (through institutional deliveries and care especially for poor women)
   - *Salient features of JSY:*
     – Is 100% centrally sponsored
     – Combines 'benefit of cash assistance with institutional care'.

122. **Ans. (c) ANM and Anganwadi worker** [Ref. Park 27/e p701]
   - *Resource person for training of ASHA:* ANM and Anganwadi worker.

123. **Ans. (a) NRHM** [Ref. Park 27/e p515]

124. **Ans. (b) Institutional deliveries** [Ref. Park 27/e p521]

125. **Ans. (b) Zero dose of OPV and BCG** [Ref. Operational Guidelines for ASHA, NHRSC]

ASHA payments under JSY: On 45th Day	Other ASHA payments:
• 6 visits in Institutional deliveries (Day 3,7,14,21, 28,42) • 7 visits in home deliveries (Day 1,3,7,14,21,28,42) • Birth weight record • Immunized with BCG, First dose of OPV & DPT • Birth registration • Mother and child are safe	• Institutional deliveries • Arrange transport of AN mother • Escort AN mother to facility • Completed immunization upto 1 & 2 yrs age • Pulse Polio immunization • Family planning services • Sanitary napkins to adolescent girls • Promote use of sanitary toilets • DOTS provider • Leprosy treatment • P/S for Malaria • Malaria treatment

126. **Ans. (d) Free treatment of sick infants up to 1 year**
    [Ref. Park 27/e p522]

    PREGNANT WOMEN COMPONENTS IN JANANI-SHISHU SURAKSHA KARYAKRAM (JSSK)
    - Free deliveries (including caesarean section) in public health institutions
    - Free drugs and consumables
    - Free diet (Normal delivery: 3 days; Caesarean section: 7 days)
    - Free diagnostics
    - Free blood transfusion (whenever required)
    - Free transport from home to institution

127. **Ans. None (2 ASHA per 1000 population)**

128. **Ans. None (All are features of JSY)**
    [Ref. Park 27/e p521]
    - ASHA is designated Link worker between pregnant woman and Health care institution (Government) in JSY
    - Cash assistance is given to mothers for high and low performing states: Only for BPL family women, aged 19 years and above, upto first two live births

129. **Ans. (b) Every month**
    [Ref. Park 27/e p510, 700]

    VILLAGE HEALTH AND NUTRITION DAY (VHND)
    - Under NRHM, VHND is observed 'Once every month' in every village
    - Usually organized at Anganwadi centre (ICDS)
    - Purpose: To improve access to maternal, newborn, child health and nutrition (MNCHN) services at the village level
    - ASHA, AWW & ANM organize VHND and mobilize women, adolescents, children

130. **Ans. (d) OPV**
    [Ref. Park 27/e p700]
    - ASHA act as a depot holder for essential provisions like ORS, IFA tablets, Chloroquine, Disposable delivery kits, OCPs & Condoms
    - ASHA also carry a Drug-kit (AYUSH + Allopathic drugs)

131. **Ans. (c) Labour room**
    [Ref. Park 27/e p522]

    NEWBORN CARE CORNER (NBCC)
    - Component of JSSK
    - Level: All 3 levels MCH – I, MCH-II, MCH-III
    - Space within delivery room for immediate care to newborns mandatory for all health facilities where deliveries are conducted

132. **Ans. (a) Mobilization for institutional deliveries**
    [Ref. Park 27/e p700]
    - ASHA have to conduct home visits of pregnant women/mother/newborn under Home Based Post Natal Care (HBPNC), and counsel pregnant women on birth preparedness, importance of safe delivery, breast-feeding and complementary feeding, immunization, contraception and prevention of common infections including RTIs/STIs and care of young child
    - ASHA have to mobilize community and facilitate them in accessing health services available at public health facilities, such as Routine Immunization (RI), AN check-ups, Post Natal Check-ups (PNCs), sanitation and other services

133. **Ans. (b) She should be trained for a period of 21 days**
    [Ref. India 2010 by Dwivedi p15-8]
    - The induction training of ASHA would be completed in 23 days spread in five rounds over a period of 12 months to be followed by periodic re-training for about 2 days every alternate month

    RESPONSIBILITIES OF ASHA
    - Create awareness on health and its social determinants
    - Mobilize community towards health planning
    - Promote good health practices and provide a minimum package of curative care
    - Provide information on determinants of health, health services and timely utilization
    - Counsel women on aspects of reproductive and child health
    - Mobilise the community and facilitate them in accessing health services
    - Act as a Depot holder (ORS, IFA tablets, chloroquine, DDK, OCPS, condoms)
    - Provide primary medical care and act as DOTS provider
    - Help develop a comprehensive village health plan
    - Arrange escort/accompany pregnant women and children requiring treatment/admission to nearest health facility
    - Be a part of JSY (Janani Suraksha Yojana) and help reduce MMR

134. **Ans. (c) Village health sanitation and nutrition committee (VHSNC)**
    [Ref. Park 27/e p515]
    - A core strategy of National Rural Health Mission (NRHM) is to develop 'Health Plan (VHP) for each village' through Village Health Samiti
    - ASHA will make VHP: ASHA along with ANM, Aanganwadi Workers and community workers

135. **Ans. (d) All of the above**
    [Ref. Park 25/e p465; NHM website, GOI]

    National Health Mission (NHM) Components
    - **Reproductive and Child Health (RCH) Program - Reproductive, Maternal, Newborn, Child Health and Adolescent (RMNCH+A) Services:** Maternal Health, Access to safe abortion services, Prevention and Management of RTI & STI, Gender Based Violence, Newborn and Child Health, Universal Immunization, Rashtriya Bal Swasthya Karyakram (RBSK) - Child Health Screening and Early Intervention Services, Rashtriya Bal Swasthya Karyakram (RKSK) - Adolescent Health, Family Planning, Addressing the Declining Sex Ratio, Cross cutting areas
    - **Control of Communicable Diseases:** National Vector Borne Diseases Control Program (NVBDCP), Revised National Tuberculosis Control Program (RNTCP), National Leprosy Control Program (NLEP), Integrated Disease Surveillance Program (IDSP),
    - **Control of Non Communicable Diseases (NCD):** National Program for Prevention and Control of Cancer, Diabetes, Cardiovascular Diseases and Stroke

(NPCDCS), National Program for the Control of Blindness (NPCB), National Mental Health Program (NMHP), National Program for the Healthcare of the Elderly (NPHCE), National Program for the Prevention and Control of Deafness (NPPCD), National Tobacco Control Program (NTCP), National Oral Health Program (NOHP), National Program for Palliative Care (NPPC), National Program for the Prevention and Management of Burn Injuries (NPPMBI), National Program for Prevention and Control of Fluorosis (NPPCF), National Organ Transplant and Tissue Organization (NOTTO)

136. **Ans. (b) Delivery at home** [Ref. Park 27/e p700]

137. **Ans. (b) 400 INR to ASHA and 1000 INR to mother in rural area in low performing states** [Ref. Park 27/e p521]

Janani Suraksha Yojana (JSY) Incentives/NEWER Janani Shishu Suraksha Karyakram (JSSK) Incentives

Category	Rural Area		Urban Area	
	Mother's package	ASHA's package	Mother's package	ASHA's package
LPS	1400	600	1000	400
HPS	700	600	600	400

(LPS: Low performing states; HPS: High performing states)

NATIONAL LEPROSY ELIMINATION PROGRAMME

138. **Ans. (b) 1,3** [Ref. Park 27/e p370]
     - To start multidrug therapy (MDT), the criteria that should be satisfied are a hypopigmented patch with sensory loss and/or peripheral nerve thickening with sensory loss
       – Paucibacillary leprosy has sensory loss (hypoanesthesia) but may or may not have nerve involvement
       – Multibacillary leprosy has sensory loss (hypo-anesthesia) and nerve involvement

139. **Ans. (c) Treatment initiation rate** [Ref. Park 27/e p 377]

     Main/Core Indicators for NLEP: Monitor functioning of control activities
     - No. of new cases detected per 1 Lac population per year
     - New cases with Grade-2 disability 1 Lac population per year
     - Treatment completion/cure rate
     - Prevalence rate

140. **Ans. (c) Spending 20 hours or more a week in close contact; (d) If age >2 years**
     Post-exposure Prophylaxis (PEP) Leprosy
     [Ref. Leprosy/Hansen disease: Contact tracing and post-exposure prophylaxis – Technical Guidance. WHO]
     - Post-exposure prophylaxis for leprosy is given as chemoprophylaxis, where Rifampicin single dose is given
     - Inclusion Criteria for PEP Leprosy:
       – Being identified as a contact, i.e. a person who has been in close contact with the index case for 20 hours or more per week for more than 3 months
       – Age: more than 2 years; if younger than 2 years, the child can be given SDR at the age of 2, in follow up visits of contacts (if meeting all other inclusion criteria)

141. **Ans. (d) Continue Anti leprosy drugs and add steroids** [Ref. Park 26/e p367]
     - If patient of leprosy on treatment develops Lepra reaction, do not stop MDT. Rather complete the course of MDT.
     - Bed rest, rest to affected nerves (use splint), analgesics, prednisolone should be used

142. **Ans. (c) Dapsone+Rifampicin for 6 months** [Ref. Park 25/e p351]
     - Multidrug therapy (MDT) in NLEP: PBL (6 months) - Rifampicin 600 mg OAMS + Dapsone 100 mg daily; MBL (12 months) - Rifampicin 600 mg OAMS + Dapsone 100 mg daily + Clofazimine 300 mg OAMS, 50 mg daily

143. **Ans. (a) Rifampicin + dapsone** [Ref. National Health Programmes of India by Dr. J. Kishore, 8/e p361, Park 27/e p371]
     - Treatment of Single Skin Lesion (SSL) of Leprosy:
       – Previously: ROM therapy
         1. Rifampicin 600 mg
         2. Ofloxacin 400 mg
         3. Minocycline 100 mg
       – CURRENTLY: 6 month treatment as for Paucibacillary (PBL) Leprosy (Rifampicin and dapsone for 6 months)

> **ALSO REMEMBER**
> - Level of Leprosy for declaring it as a Public Health Problem: >1/10,000
> - Elimination Level of Leprosy: <1/10,000
> - Goal for Leprosy under National Health Policy (NHP) 2002: Elimination of Leprosy by 2005
> - India eliminated Leprosy in December 2005 (India has so far eliminated 4 diseases, namely, Guineaworm – 2000, Leprosy – 2005, Yaws – May 2016 (Free) and NNT – 2015).

144. **Ans. (a) Stop anti-leprosy drugs** [Ref. Park 27/e p372–373]
     - Lepra Reactions: Is an inflammation that can affect skin patches, nerves, eyes and in few case, internal organs They can occur anytime in a leprosy patient
       – Before diagnosis
       – At time of diagnosis
       – During treatment
       – After treatment has finished
     - There is no need to stop antiperosy drugs during MDT.

145. **Ans. (c) Any responsible person from family or village can collect MDT, if patient is unable to come** [Ref. Guide to eliminate Leprosy as a Public Health Problem, WHO & NLEP; p25]
     - Accompanied MDT: If patient is unable to come to collect his/her MDT from clinic, any responsible person from family or village can collect it
       – Designed to help patients who have to interrupt their treatment due to any avoidable reason

- Especially useful for irregular patients
- Gives patients a choice: Patients can collect entire MDT course when diagnosed after proper counseling.

146. **Ans. (c) 5 years** *[Ref. Park 27/e p374]*
147. **Ans. (b) Dapsone, Rifampicin** *[Ref. Park 27/e p371]*
148. **Ans. (c) Post-treatment surveillance of paucibacillary leprosy** *[Ref. Park 27/e p374]*
149. **Ans. (d) Minocycline** *[Ref. Park 22/e p296–97, 24/e p341]*
150. **Ans. (b) 9 months** *[Ref. Park 27/e p371]*
    - *Adequate treatment*: Patient has received 6 months of therapy in 9 months (for PBL) or 12 months of therapy within 18 months (for MBL)^Q
    - *Regular treatment*: Received MDT for two-thirds of total duration of therapy, i.e. 4 months for PBL (out of 6 months of duration of therapy) and 8 months for MBL (out of 12 months of duration of therapy)

OTHER PROGRAMMES

151. **Ans. (b) IV iron sucrose for non-compliance with oral tablets** *[Ref. AMB Document, NHM, MoHFW, GOI]*

    Under Anaemia Mukt Bharat
    - If Haemoglobin is 10–10.9 g/dl (mild anemia)
      - Two tablets of Iron and Folic Acid tablet (60 mg elemental Iron and 500 mcg Folic Acid) daily, orally given by the health provider during the ANC contact
      - Parental iron (IV Iron Sucrose or Ferric Carboxy Maltose (FCM) may be considered as the first line of management in pregnant women who are detected to be anemic late in pregnancy or in whom compliance is likely to be low (high chance of lost to follow-up)
    - If Haemoglobin is 7–9.9 g/dl (moderate anemia)
      - Two tablets of Iron and Folic Acid tablet (60 mg elemental Iron and 500 mcg Folic Acid) daily, orally given by the health provider during the ANC contact
      - Parental iron (IV Iron Sucrose or FCM) may be considered as the first line of management in pregnant women who are detected to be anemic late in pregnancy or in whom compliance is likely to be low (high chance of lost to follow-up)

152. **Ans. (b) BD** *[Ref. Training Module for Medical Officers for Prevention, Control and Population Level Screening of Hypertension, Diabetes and Common Cancer (Oral, Breast & Cervical) NPCDCS MoHFW 2017 p25]*

    Diabetes Diagnosis & Management under NPCDCS Program at PHC LEVEL: Random capillary blood sample is used for Screening of adults >30 years age
    1. If RCBS ≤100 mg/dl: Person is non-diabetic, Repeat after 3 years
    2. If RCBS 100–140 mg/dl: Suggest life style modification, Repeat after 1 year
    3. If RCBS >140 mg/dl: Refer to Health care facility
    - FBS <110 AND PPBS <140 (Capillary/Venous): Suggest life style modification, Repeat after 1 year
    - FBS 110–125 AND/OR PPBS 140–199 (Capillary/Venous): Suggest life style modification, Repeat after 1 year
    - FBS >126 (Capillary/Venous) OR 2 hour PPBS >200 (V)/>220 (C) OR 2 hour after 75 grams glucose >200 (V): Lifestyle modification, Metformin 500 mg BD, Baseline evaluations (BP, Fundus exam, S. creatinine, Urine albumin, Lipoid profile, ECG, Foot care), Repeat testing after 1 year or as required
      - Repeat after 4 weeks: If RBS <120 then repeat every 3 months OR If RBS ≥120 then refer to a specialist

153. **Ans. (d) 60 mg Iron & 500 mcg Folic acid weekly** *[Ref. Park 26/e p511]*

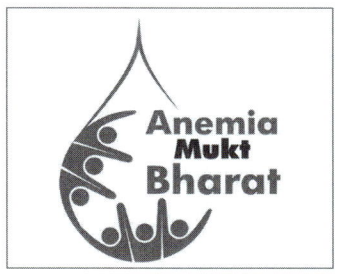

- Under Anemia Mukt Bharat, 10–19 years Adolescents get IFA supplementation as 60 mg elemental Iron + 500 mcg Folic acid on a Weekly basis through a Blue color tablet

Refer to Annexure 21

154. **Ans. (a) To reduce disease burden by 25% by end of XI Five Year Plan** *[Ref. National Health Programmes of India by Dr. J. Kishore, 8/e p490]*
    - *National Programme for Prevention and Control of Deafness:*
      - Long term objective: To reduce disease burden by 25% by end of XI Five Year Plan.

155. **Ans. (b) Urinary iodine levels among pregnant women** *[Ref. WHO-UNICEF-ICCIDD. Assessment of Iodine Deficiency Disorders and Monitoring their Elimination – A guide for programme managers, 2/e p5]*

    Indicators to Monitor Success of Idd Control Programme:
    - *Impact Indicators:* Indicators to assess baseline (Iodine Deficiency Disorders) IDD status and to monitor and evaluate the impact of salt iodization on the target population
    - *Urinary Iodine Levels:* The 'principal impact indicator' recommended once a salt iodization programme has been initiated (changes in goitre prevalence lag behind changes in iodine status and therefore cannot be relied upon to reflect accurately current iodine intake, although they may be useful in following trends)
    - *Goitre assessment:* (by palpation or by ultrasound) should remain a component of surveys to establish the baseline severity of IDD
    - *Neonatal thyroid stimulating hormone (TSH) levels:* may also play a role here if a country already has in place a screening programme for hypothyroidism.

> **ALSO REMEMBER**
> - *Criteria for tracking progress towards IDD elimination:*
>
> | Indicator | Goal |
> |---|---|
> | Proportion with enlarged thyroid (age 6–12 years) | <5% |
> | Urinary Iodine Excretion below 100 mcg/litre | <50% |
> | Urinary Iodine Excretion below 50 mcg/litre | <20% |
> | % houses consuming adequately iodised salt | >90% |
>
> - *Some noteworthy daily requirements:*
>
> | Nutrient | Recommended daily requirement |
> |---|---|
> | Calcium | 600 mg |
> | Iron | 17 mg (males); 21 mg (females) |
> | Iodine | 150 mg |
> | Fluorine | 0.5–0.8 mg/litre. |

156. **Ans. (b) 1 lakh IU**   *[Ref. Park 27/e p731]*
    - *National Programme for Prophylaxis against Blindness in Children caused by Vitamin A Deficiency:* Prophylaxis against Vitamin-A deficiency is provided in form of oral 5 doses of Vitamin-A
        - 1st dose (1 lac IU) at 9 months age (along with measles vaccine)
        - 2nd dose (2 lac IU) at 15 months age
        - then a dose (2 lac IU) every 6 months till the age of 3 years
    - *Vitamin A supplement administered in Prevention of Nutritional Blindness in Children Programme contain:* 1 Lac IU per mL

157. **Ans. (b) 1 lakh IU/mL**   *[Ref. Textbook of Community Medicine by Sunder Lal, 2/e p202; Park 27/e p731]*
    - Vitamin A solution contains 1 lac IU per mL solution
    - Vitamin A is given in NIS of India till 5 years age (Recent guidelines)
        - At 9 months age: 1 lac IU (1 mL)
        - Every 6 months, till 5 years age: 2 lac IU (2 mL) each
        - Total dose given: 17 lac IU (9 doses).

158. **Ans. (a) 15 ppm**   *[Ref. Assessment of IDD and monitoring their elimination, WHO, 3/e Park 27/e p739]*
    - Criteria for Sustainable Elimination of IDD:
        - Median Urinary Iodine Excretion 100 mcg/l
        - Level of iodization:
            1. 30 ppm at production level
            2. 15 ppm at consumer level
        - Total Goitre Rate (TGR) <5%

159. **Ans. (b) Increasing no. of children affected**   *[Ref. Park 27/e p369–371]*

    INDICATORS IN LEPROSY CONTROL
    Case detection indicators
    - % of children (0–14 yrs) among new detected cases: A high prevalence of infection among children indicate that Leprosy is a active and spreading
    - % of females among new detected cases
    - % of Multi-bacillary cases on regular treatment
    - % of new cases with grade 2 disability.

160. **Ans. (c) Government run insurance scheme for poor**   *[Ref. RSBY Document, Government of India]*

161. **Ans. (a) Snake bite**   *[Ref. Park 27/e p545–546]*

    Diseases covered under IDSP (P-FORM)
    - Acute Diarrhoea Disease (including acute gastroenteritis, Cholera)
    - Bacillary Dysentery
    - Viral Hepatitis
    - Enteric Fever
    - Malaria
    - Dengue/DHF/DSS
    - Chikungunya
    - Acute Encephalitis Syndrome
    - Meningitis
    - Measles
    - Diphtheria
    - Pertussis
    - Chicken Pox
    - Fever of Unknow Origin (PUO)
    - Acute Respiratory Infection (ARI) Influenza Like Illness (ILI)
    - Pneumonia
    - Leptospirosis
    - Acute Flaccid Paralysis <15 year of Age
    - Anthrax
    - Plague
    - Any other State Specific Disease
    - Unusual Syndromes NOT Captured Above

162. **Ans. (c) Herpes zoster**   *[Ref. Park 27/e p545–546]*

    Diseases Covered Under Idsp

Regular surveillance:	Sentinel surveillance:
Malaria	HIV, HBV, HCV
Cholera, Typhoid	Water quality
Tuberculosis	Air quality (outdoor)
Measles	Regular periodic surveys:
Poliomyelitis	Anthropometry
Road traffic accidents	Physical activity
Plague	Blood pressure
Unusual disease syndromes: Meningoencephalitis, Hemorrhagic fevers, Respiratory distress	Tobacco Nutrition
	Additional state priorities

163. **Ans. (c) District hospital has specialised facilities**   *[Ref. Park 27/e p541–544]*

164. **Ans. (d) CHC has facilities for diagnosis and treatment of CVD, Diabetes**   *[Ref. Park 27/e p541–544]*

165. **Ans. (c) Periodic regular survey**   *[Ref. Park 27/e p545]*

166. **Ans. (d) Integration with National Cancer Control Programme**   *[Ref. Park 23/e p471–473, 24/e p493]*

167. **Ans. (b) Presumptive**   *[Ref. Park 27/e p545–547]*

TYPES OF SURVEILLANCE IN IDSP

- *Syndromic*: Diagnosis made on the basis of clinical pattern by paramedical personnel and members of the community
  - Fever
  - Cough more than three weeks duration
  - Acute Flaccid Paralysis
  - Diarrhoea
  - Jaundice
  - Unusual events causing death or hospitalization
- *Presumptive*: Diagnosis made on typical history and clinical examination by Medical Officers
  - Validity of presumptive diagnosis will be higher than Syndromic
- *Confirmed*: Clinical diagnosis confirmed by an appropriate laboratory test

168. **Ans. (c) Human rights of mentally ill**
     [Ref. NMHP 1987, MOHFW, GOI]

- GOI launched National Mental Health Programme (NMHP) in 1982, with objectives:
  - To ensure the availability and accessibility of minimum mental healthcare for all in the foreseeable future, particularly to the most vulnerable and underprivileged sections of the population
  - To encourage the application of mental health knowledge in general healthcare and in social development; and
  - To promote community participation in the mental health service development and to stimulate efforts towards self-help in the community.

169. **Ans. (c) State Government maintain and manage all water supply** *[Ref. Park 27/e p549–550]*

SWAJALDHARA PROGRAMME

- *Launched*: 25 December 2002
- *Current status*: Renamed as National Rural Drinking Water Programme (2009), a component of Bharat Nirman
- *Description*: Community led, participatory programme with aim of providing drinking water in rural areas though community participation
  - Swajaldhara I (First dhara): Gram panchayat/Group of panchayats (Block/Tehsil level)
  - Swajaldhara II (Second dhara): District level
- *Key features/components*:
  - Government: planning, policy, monitoring, evaluation
  - Panchayat/Village water & Sanitation committee: Plan, implement, operate, maintain, manage project
  - Integrated service delivery mechanisms: Water conservation (rain water harvesting, Ground water recharge

170. **Ans. (d) National Programme for prevention and control of Cancer, Diabetes, Cardiovascular diseases and Stroke**
     [Ref. Park 27/e p541–543]

171. **Ans. (d) STEP 4 consists of treatment of NCD if found**
     [Ref. WHO STEPwise Surveillance]

172. **Ans. (b) Geographical** *[Ref. IDSP Manual. GOI p4]*

IDSP SURVEILLANCE SYSTEMS - 6 KEY ELEMENTS

- Detection and notification of health event
- Investigation and confirmation (Epidemiological, clinical, laboratory)
- Collection of data
- Analysis and interpretation of data
- Feed-back and dissemination of results
- Response – a link to public health program specially actions for prevention and control

173. **Ans. (b) Goitre is Classified as Endemic if TGR ≥ 10%**

DISTRICT IDD SURVEY

- Age group: 6–12 years old children
- Sampling: Systematic sampling, Probability proportionate to size (PPS)
- Grading of Goitre (WHO):
- Grade 0: No palpable or visible goitre (No goitre)
- Grade 1: Palpable BUT not visible
- Grade 2: Palpable AND visible
- Total goitre rate (TGR) classified as None (0–4.9%), Mild (5–19.9%), Moderate (20–29.9%), Severe (>30%)
- Goitre is Public health problem (Endemic) if: TGR >5%

> **ALSO REMEMBER**
> - Goitre is a 'Historic marker' of Iodine deficiency: measurement of goitre in a population does not reflect the current status of Iodine nutrition in population

Review Questions

174. **Ans. (a) 1/3 1/2**

175. **Ans. (d) 10** *[Ref. Park 27/e p364]*

176. **Ans. (b) Clofazimine, Rifampicin and dapsone**
     [Ref. Park 27/e p370–371]

177. **Ans. (b) Is a substitute for regular food**
     [Ref. Park 27/e p776]

178. **Ans. (c) 2,00,000 IU** *[Ref. Park 27/e p731]*

MISCELLANEOUS (H. PROGRAMMES)

179. **Ans. (a) 500 Rupees per month** *[Ref. Bhalwar, 4/e p770]*

Nikshay Poshan Yojana

- Financial incentive of Rs.500/- per month for each notified TB patient for duration for which the patient is on anti-TB treatment
- All TB patients notified on or after 1st April 2018 including all existing TB patients under treatment are eligible to receive incentives

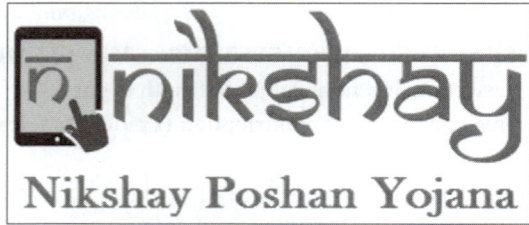

180. **Ans. (d) Wayson's staining**
     [Ref. Dr J. Kishore 8/e p258; Park 27/e p342]
     - **In the given question,** a young boy had a flea bite while working in a wheat grain godown and after 5 days he developed fever and had axillary lymphadenopathy
     - Thus most likely it is Plague which is transmitted by Rat flea (Xenopsylla cheopsis)
     - So the stain used will be Wayson's staining, which will show 'Bipolar appearance' or 'Safety pin appearance' of Yersinia pestis
     - *Stains commonly used in Public Health:*

Disease (organism)	Stain(s) used
TB (Mycobacterium tuberculosis)	Ziehl-Neelsen (ZN) stain (RNTCP) Auramine Rhodamine stain
Leprosy (Mycobacterium leprae)	Modifed Ziehl-Neelsen (Modified ZN) stain
Malaria (Plasmodium)	Jaswant Singh Bhattacharya (JSB) stain
Plague (Yersinia pestis)	Wayson's stain Giemsa stain
Diphtheria (Corynebacterium diphtheriae)	Albert's stain Neisser's stain Ponder's stain

181. **Ans. (b) National Leprosy Eradication Programme**
     [Ref. National Health Programmes of India by Dr. J. Kishore, 7/e p311, 8/e p366–67]
     - *Simplified Information System:* Is the Management and Information System (MIS) essential for the monitoring and evaluation of National Leprosy Eradication Programme (NLEP); It was started in 2002.

182. **Ans. (b) Dapsone** [Ref. National Health programmes of India by Dr. J. Kishore, 8/e p203 and Park 27/e p370–371]

183. **Ans. (a) RNTCP** [Ref. Park 27/e p485]

184. **Ans. (b) Women & Child Development**
     [Ref. ICPS Document, GOI]

185. **Ans. (c) Tuberculosis** [Ref. Park 27/e p488]
     NIKSHAY
     - *Description:* A web enabled application, which facilitates the monitoring of universal access to TB patients' data by all stakeholders at different tiers of the Healthcare Delivery System
       – SMS based communication: With TB patients, Grassroot level healthcare service providers, Policy makers, Health managers/administrators
       – Launched by: Central TB Division (MOHFW) & National Informatics Centre (NIC) on 4th June 2012
     - *Broad Objectives:* For the eradication of TB effectively in India,
       – To create a database of all TB patients including MDR cases across the country
       – Use this database for monitoring and for research purposes at all levels

186. **Ans. (b) NACP** [Ref. Park 27/e p500]
     LINK WORKER SCHEME
     - *Programme:* National AIDS Control Programme III
     - *Main objective:* To address populations with highrisk behaviours (including High Risk
     - Groups and Bridge Populations) with the premise that there are significant numbers in Rural areas and to reach out to them in order to saturate the coverage of these groups
     - *Link Worker:* Someone who is not "alien" to the neighbourhood, is accepted by the village community, and who can discuss intimate human relations and practices of sex and sexuality and help equip highrisk individuals and vulnerable young people with information and skills to combat the pandemic
     - *Population norm:* One link worker per 5000+ village population

     > **ALSO REMEMBER**
     > - Link workers have also been part of Enhanced Malaria Control Project
     > - ASHA worker is also called as Link worker

187. **Ans. (c) AIDS** [Ref. Park 27/e p496]
     - In order to design evidence-based interventions among the young people, it is essential to understand the levels of knowledge about HIV/AIDS, attitude and sexual behaviour of young people
     - Behavioural Surveillance Surveys (BSS) are internationally standardised tools used for understanding the knowledge, attitude and behaviour of populations
     - Undertaking BSS among Youth is an important effort by NACO and UNICEF to monitor changes in behavioural aspects of young people who are vulnerable to HIV infection

188. **Ans. (d) Maharashtra** [Ref. Park 25/e p473]
     - Eight socioeconomically backward states of Bihar, Chhattisgarh, Jharkhand, Madhya Pradesh, Orissa, Rajasthan, Uttaranchal and Uttar Pradesh are referred to as the Empowered Action Group (EAG) states

RASHTRIYA SWASTHYA BIMA YOJANA

189. **Ans. (d) Cashless benefit in hospitals**
     [Ref. RSBY Document, Government of India]

NATIONAL HEALTH POLICY

190. **Ans. (a) 90% of all people living with HIV know their HIV status; (b) 90% of all people diagnosed with HIV infection receive sustained antiretroviral therapy; (e) 90% of all people receiving antiretroviral therapy will have effective viral suppression** [Ref. Park 27/e p502]

National Strategic Plan for HIV/AIDS and STI, 2017–24
- **90-90-90** (Targets by 2020): 90% of those who are HIV positive in the country know their status, 90% of those who know their status are on treatment and 90% of those who are on treatment experience effective viral load suppression
- **95-95-95** (Targets by 2024): Ensuring that 95% of those who are HIV positive in the country know their status, 95% of those who know their status are on treatment and 95% of those who are on treatment experience effective viral load suppression

NATIONAL POPULATION POLICY

191. Ans. (c) 20 years [Ref. National Health Programmes of India by Dr. J. Kishore, 7/e p491, Park 27/e p568]

192. Ans. (c) Divorces [Ref. National Health Programmes of India by Dr. J. Kishore, 7/e p491, Park 27/e p568]
- According to National Population Policy 2000 (NPP 2000), one of the national socio-demographic goals is 'to achieve 100% registration of births, deaths, marriage & pregnancy by 2010'.
- According to 'The Registration of Births and Deaths Act 1969', both the births and deaths are to be registered within 21 days each.

Time of registration	Additional Requirements
Within 21 days	None
Delay <30 days	Prescribed fee
Delay >30 days & <1 year	Late fee + affidavit from notary public
Delay >1 year	Late fee + order from Class I officer/magistrate

Marriage registration has to be done within 30 days.

193. Ans. (c) Reduction of MMR to less than 1/1000 live births [Ref. Park 27/e p568]

194. Ans. (d) Bring down TFR to replacement levels by 2015 [Ref. Park 27/e p568]

NATIONAL MENTAL HEALTH POLICY

195. Ans. (d) 2014 [Ref. NMHP document, Ministry of Health & Family Welfare, Government of India 2014]

MILESTONES OF MENTAL HEALTH IN INDIA
- National Mental Health Programme (NMHP): 1982
- National Mental Health Act (NMHA): 1987
- District Mental Health Programme (Under NMHP): 1996
- National Mental Health Care Bill (NMHCB): 2013
- National Mental Health Policy (NMHP): 2014
- The Mental Health Case Act, 2017

IT ACT

196. Ans. (b) 2000 [Ref. Gazette of India – Extraordinary, Part II; Section 1]
- *The Information Technology Act:* was passed by the Government of India in 2000; it deals with:
  - Legal Recognition of Electronic Documents
  - Legal Recognition of Digital Signatures
  - Offenses and Contraventions
  - Justice Dispensation System for Cybercrimes.

> **ALSO REMEMBER**
> - *Some Important Health Legislations Passed in India:*
> - The Employees State Insurance (ESI) Act, 1948
> - The Factories Act, 1948
> - The Medical Termination of Pregnancy (MTP) Act, 1971
> - The Organ transplantation Act, 1994
> - The Pre-conception and Pre-natal Diagnostic Techniques (Prohibition of Sex Selection) (PNDT) Act, 1994
> - Information Technology Act, 2000
> - The National Rural Employment Guarantee Act (NREGA), 2005
> - The Right to Information (RTI) Act, 2005.

OT ACT

197. Ans. (d) More than 5 years [Ref. National Health Programmes of India by Dr. J. Kishore, 9/e p696]
- *Punishments under Organ Transplantation Act 1994:*
  - For medical practitioners involved: Removal of name for 2 years from Medical register (and permanent removal for any subsequent offence)
  - For other persons involved: Five years imprisonment + Fine up to ₹ 10,000/-
- *New Modification in 2011:* Punishment for persons involved to be increased to up to 10 years imprisonment + fine up to ₹ 20,00,000–1,00,00,000/-.

CBD REGISTRATION ACT

198. Ans. (c) 1970 [Ref. Park 25/e p877]
- Central Birth and Death Registration Act 1969 came into force on: 1st April 1970

OTHER LEGISLATIONS

199. Ans. (c) 2005 [Ref. National Health Programmes of India by Dr. J. Kishore, 8/e p712]

National Rural Employment Guarantee Act (NREGA) 2005:
- The NREGA Act 2005 has been passed by the Parliament to provide for '100 days of guaranteed wage employment in every year' to every household whose adult members volunteer to do 'unskilled manual work'; Salient features:
  - A household is entitled for '100 days of work in a year' (Minimum `130/- per day).

200. Ans. (b) Smoking [Ref. National Health Programmes of India by Dr. J. Kishore, 8/e p654]
- The Indian Medical Council Act, 1956; (Professional Conduct and Ethics) & Regulations, 2002: May remove name of physician or publicize his/her name in press on violation of code of conduct and ethics.

201. Ans. (a) 00.00 hrs 01 March [Ref. National Health Programmes of India by Dr. J. Kishore, 8/e p662]
- *Census Stop (India):* 01 March 00.00 Hours (First year of each decade) (Ist time and date on which population count is done).

202. **Ans. (c) Workman's compensation act** [Ref. Park 20/e p613]
- Workman's compensation act 1923
- MTP Act 1971
- Indian factories act 1948
- ESI Act 1948

203. **Ans. (c) When acceptors requires incentives**
[Ref. Park 27/e p580]

204. **Ans. (a) Drugs Controller General of India**
[Ref. National Health Programmes of India by Dr. J. Kishore, 8/e p587; Park 21/e p442, Park 22/e p440]

205. **Ans. (a) Drug users sent to treatment not jail if requested**
[Ref. National Health Programmes of India by Dr. J. Kishore, 9/e p690–692]

The Narcotic Drugs and Psychotropic Substances Act, 1985
- Whosoever produce, manufacture, buy, sell, produce, transport, use, consume any narcotic drug (Opium/poppy) or psychotropic substance: Shall be punished with imprisonment 10–20 years + fine 1–2 lac rupees (5 years + 50000 rupees for Ganja).
  – Users, if not covered under Sections 15–25, will be sent for treatment/rehabilitation and not punished
- Breach in licence for opium growth: Shall be punished with imprisonment 3 years with or without fine
- Whosoever possess a small quantity for personal consumption: Shall be punished with imprisonment 6 months + fine
- Subsequent offences: Death penalty
- Alcohol use: IS NOT covered by this act.

> **ALSO REMEMBER**
> - **ESSENTIAL MEDICINES**
> - **Essential medicines:** Those which satisfy the priority health care needs of the population (Mnemonic: 6A's)
>   – Available
>   – Adequate amounts
>   – Appropriate dosage forms
>   – Assured quality
>   – Adequate information
>   – Affordable (at a cost community/country can afford)
> - **WHO MODEL LIST OF ESSENTIAL MEDICINES**
> - *WHO Model List:*
>   – First drawn up in 1977
>   – Revised and updated at an interval of 2 years
>   – Latest list: 15th March 2007
>   – Not designed as a global standard; but many organisations have modelled their medicine supply system on this list
> - *Selection criteria:*
>   – Public health relevance
>   – Evidence of efficacy and safety
>   – Comparative cost effectiveness
>
> *Contd...*
>
> - *Core list:* List of minimum medicine needs for a basic health care system, listing most safe, efficacious and cost-effectiveness medicines of priority conditions
> - *Complementary list:* Essential medicines for priority diseases, for which specialised diagnostic or care facilities are needed
> - *Key notable points:*
>   – Brackets: To mention the strength of selected salt or ester
>   – When it refers to active moiety, the name of salt or ester in brackets is preceded by "as"
>   – Oral liquids: To mention suspension, solution or any other liquid
>   – Tablets: Allow forms of immediate-release tablets
>   – Enteric coated: Modified release dosage
>   – Square box symbol (%): Indicate similar clinical performance within a pharmacological class
> - *Dosage forms:* listed in alphabetical order.
> - **COUNTERFEIT MEDICINES:**
> - WHO definition: A drug/medication which is produced with intention to cheat
>   – Mislabelling (including fudging expiry date)
>   – No active ingredients
>   – Wrong ingredient
>   – Right ingredient in insufficient quantity
> - **Types of counterfeit medicines:**
>   – In developed countries: New expensive lifestyle medicines (hormones, steroids, antihistamines)
>   – In developing countries: Medications to treat life threatening conditions (HIV/AIDS, TB, Malaria)
> - Global burden: More than 10% of global medicines
>   – 25% of medicines in developing countries
> - QUALITY CONTROL IN DRUG SECTOR IN INDIA
> - *Quality control of drugs in India:*
>   – Drugs and Cosmetics Act 1940
>   – Drugs and Cosmetics Rules 1945
> - *Central Drugs Standard Control Organisation (CDSCO):*
>   – Headed by:
>   1. Central level: Drugs Controller General, India (DGHS, MOHFW)
>   2. State level: State Drugs Controllers
>   – Main functions:
>   1. Quality control of imported drugs
>   2. Coordination of activities under State Drugs Control Authorities
>   3. Approval for importation/manufacture of new drugs
>   4. Laying standards for and act as 'Central Licensing Authority for blood and blood products, iv fluids, sera, vaccines, r-DNA products'
> - *Zonal offices:* Mumbai, Kolkata, Ghaziabad, Chennai.

206. **Ans. (a) Alcohol; (d) Nicotine**
[Ref. Narcotics Control Bureau, India]

207. Ans. (b) The Mental Health Care Act
[Ref. Ministry of Health and Family Welfare, Government of India, 2013]

MENTAL HEALTH CARE ACT, 2011
Recognizing That
Persons with mental illness constitute a vulnerable section, and are subject to discrimination; Families bear disproportionate financial, physical, mental, emotional and social burden of providing treatment and care; Persons with mental illness should be treated like other persons with health problems. The Mental Health Act, 1987 has not been able to adequately protect the rights of persons with mental illness and promote access to mental health care in the country

And in Order to:
- Protect, promote and fulfill the rights of persons with mental illness during the delivery of health care in institutions and in the community; Ensure health care, treatment and rehabilitation to persons with mental illness is provided in the least restrictive environment possible, and in a manner that does not intrudes on their rights and dignity. Community-based solutions in the vicinity of the person's usual place of residence, are preferred to institutional solutions; Provide treatment, care and rehabilitation to improve the capacity of the person to develop his or her full potential and to facilitate his or her integration into community life; Fulfill obligations under the Constitution of India and obligations under various International Conventions ratified by India; Regulate the public and private mental health sectors within a rights framework to achieve the greatest public health good; Improve accessibility to mental health care by mandating sufficient provision of quality public mental health services and non-discrimination in health insurance; Establish a mental health care system integrated into all levels of general health care; Promote principles of equity, efficiency and active participation of all stakeholders in decision making;
- This Act may be called the Mental Health Care Act, 2011.

208. Ans. (c) Fundamental rights of mentally retarded
[Ref. The Mental Health Care Bill 2011 DRAFT, MOHFW, Government of India p6]

- Under Mental Health Care Act of India 2011, Mental retardation has been EXCLUDED from definition of mental illness

209. Ans. (d) Jaipur *[Ref. CDSCO Website]*

CDSCO (Central Drugs Standards Control Organization) Offices
- Ghaziabad (North Zone)
- Mumbai (West Zone)
- Chennai (South Zone)
- Kolkata (East Zone)
- Ahmedabad (Zone)
- Hyderabad (Zone)
- Bangalore (Subzone)
- Chandigarh (Subzone)
- Jammu (Subzone)
- Goa (Subzone)

210. Ans. (c) 'Mentally ill' in place of lunatic
[Ref. MTP Act 1971 Amendment 2002 document]

211. Ans. (c) Ministry of Health and Family Welfare
[Ref. FSSAI, MOHFW, GOI]

FOOD SAFETY AND STANDARDS AUTHORITY OF INDIA (FSSAI)
- *Background*: Established under Food Safety and Standards Act, 2006
- *Head office*: New Delhi
- *Function*:
  - Lay down Science-based standards for articles of food and to regulate their manufacture, storage, distribution, sale and import to ensure availability of safe and wholesome food for human consumption
  - Various Central Acts like Prevention of Food Adulteration Act 1954, Milk and Milk Products Order 1992, etc. to be repealed
  - Single reference point for all matters relating to food safety and standards
- Establishment of the Authority: Ministry of Health & Family Welfare, Government of India is the Administrative Ministry for the implementation of FSSAI

212. Ans. (b) 200 mg of mifepristone on D_1 followed by 400 μg of misoprostol on D_3
[Ref. Medical Methods of Abortion, GOI 2013 Guidelines, p13]

PROTOCOL FOR MEDICAL METHODS OF ABORTION (GOI)

Visit	Day	Drug(s) used
First	Day 1	200 mg Mifepristone orally\ Anti D, if Rh negative
Second	Day 2 or Day 3	For gestation upto 49 days 400 mcg Misoprostol orally or vaginally For gestation upto 63 days 800 mcg Misoprostol sublingually or vaginally Analgesics Home administration by woman may be tried in few cases
Third	Day 15	Confirm and ensure completion of procedure Contraceptives

213. Ans. (c) Prevention of female foeticides
[Ref. Principles of FMT by Bardale 1/e p362]

PRE-CONCEPTION AND PRE-NATAL DIAGNOSTIC TECHNIQUES (PCPNDT) ACT, 1994
- Prohibition of sex selection, before or after conception
- Regulation of prenatal diagnostic techniques for the purposes of detecting genetic abnormalities or metabolic disorders or chromosomal abnormalities or certain congenital malformations or sex-linked disorders
- Prevention of misuse of prenatal diagnostic techniques for sex determination leading to female foeticide

214. Ans. (d) Right to reject *[Ref. Park 27/e p809–810]*

RIGHTS OF PATIENT UNDER COPRA (Consumer Protection Act 1986)
- Right to Information
  - On health care services available for diagnosis & treatment
  - On professionals involved in patient care
  - On rules and regulations of hospital applicable to patient

- Right to informed consent
- Right to safety from errors and malpractice
- Right to confidentiality and privacy
- Right to prompt treatment in emergency
- Right to get copies of medical records
- Right to refuse to participate in human experimentation and research
- Right to choose and seek second opinion
- Right to complain and have compensation in short time

215. **Ans. (b) More than 100 lakhs**

[Ref. Private International Law in India by Agrawal 1/e p113]

THREE-TIER COMPENSATION SYSTEM UNDER COPRA 1986
- District forum: Less than 20 Lacs
- State forum: 20 Lacs – 1 Crore
- National commission: More than 1 Crore

216. **Ans. (c) 20% for both boys and girls**

[Ref. India's Journey Towards Sustainable Population by SyamRoyn 1/e p158]

217. **Ans. (c) Screening family members** [Ref. The Mental Health Care Act 2017 document, GOI]

THE MENTAL HEALTH CARE ACT, 2017
- Right to access Government provided mental health-care services
- Good quality, affordable, accessible, non-discriminatory Mental health services
- Free legal services to exercise any of his rights
- Medical practitioner shall not be held liable for any unforeseen consequences
- No use of ECT without the use of muscle relaxants, anesthesia
- No seclusion or solitary confinement
- Decriminalization of suicide attempt
- Establishment of Central a State Mental Health Authority
- Government to plan, design and implement programmes
- Mental Health Review Boards to be chaired by a District Judge

Review Question

218. **Ans. (c) ELISA** [Ref. Park 27/e p400]

CHAPTER 7

Demography, Family Planning and Contraception

DEMOGRAPHY

DEMOGRAPHIC CYCLE AND PROCESSES

Demography and Demographic Processes

- *Demography*: Is the scientific study of human population; It focuses attention on[Q],
  - Changes in population size
  - Composition of population
  - Distribution of population in space
- *Types of demography*:
  - *Formal demography*: Measurement of populations processes
  - *Social demography*: Also analyze relationships between economic, social, cultural and biological processes influencing a population
- *Basic demographic equation*: If a country has Population 't' persons at the time 't', then size of population at time 't + 1' will be, (Natural increase t = Births t – Deaths t; Net migration t = Immigration t – Emigration t)

  Population t + 1 = Population t + Natural increase t + Net migration t

- *Demographic Processes:* 5 processes continuously on work in a population, thus determining its' size, composition and distribution[Q]
  - Fertility
  - Marriage
  - Mortality
  - Migration
  - Social mobility

Key points

Demographic Processes:
- Fertility
- Marriage
- Mortality
- Migration
- Social mobility

Key points

General fertility rate (GFR): Annual number of live births per 1000 women of childbearing age (15–49 years old, or 15–44 years old) mid-year population[Q] (77.6 GFR India)

Important Definitions in Demography

- *Crude birth rate (CBR):* Annual number of live births per 1000 mid year population[Q]
- *General fertility rate (GFR):* Annual number of live births per 1000 women of childbearing age (15–49 years old, or 15–44 years old) mid-year population[Q]
- *General marital fertility rate (GMFR):* Annual number of live births per 1000 married women of childbearing age (15–49 years old, or 15–44 years old) mid-year population
- *Age-specific fertility rates (ASFR):* Annual number of live births per 1000 women in particular age groups (usually age 15–19 years, 20–24 years have higher)
- *Crude death rate (CDR):* Annual number of deaths per 1000 mid year population[Q]
- *Infant mortality rate (IMR):* Annual number of deaths of children less than 1 year old per 1000 live births[Q]
- *Expectation of life (Life expectancy):* The number of years which an individual at a given age could expect to live at present mortality levels
- *Total fertility rate (TFR):* Number of live births per woman completing her reproductive life, if her childbearing at each age reflected current ASFRs[Q]
- *Gross reproduction rate (GRR):* Number of daughters who would be born to a woman completing her reproductive life at current ASFRs[Q] (GRR 1.1 India 2016)

- *Net reproduction rate (NRR):* Expected number of daughters, per newborn prospective mother, who may or may not survive to and through the ages of childbearing[Q]

Demographic Cycle and Concepts

- *Demographic cycle is closely related to:* Socio-economic progress of a country
- 5 stages (phases) of demographic cycle through which a nation passes:

	Phase I	Phase II	Phase III[Q]	Phase IV	Phase V
Birth rate	High	High	Declining	Low	Declining
Death rate	High	Declining	Declining	Low	Low
DG	Narrow	Increasing	Decreasing	Narrow	Reversal
Population	Stationary	Growing*	Growing$	Stationary	Decreasing
Composition	Young	Young	Young	Mixed	Ageing
Age pyramid	Pyramidal	Losing pyramidal shape	Globular	Cylindrical	Losing cylindrical shape

(*: Increasing rate; $ Decreasing rate)

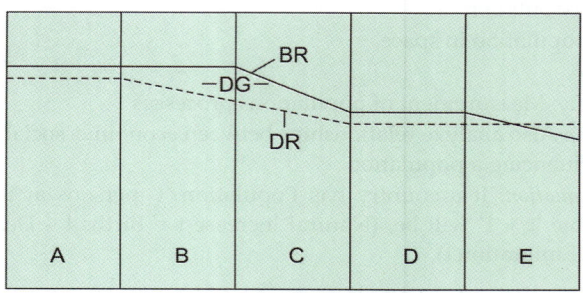

Stages of demographic cycle

[BR-birth rate, DR-death rate, DG-demographic gap, A-high stationary stage, B-early expanding stage, C-late expanding stage, D-low stationary stage, E-declining stage]

- *India is in Stage III (Late Expanding Phase) of Demographic cycle*[Q]
- *Stage V (Decline Phase):* Germany, Italy, Spain, Portugal, Greece, United Kingdom and Japan (populations are reproducing well < replacement levels)
- *Demographic transition:* is a model used to explain the process of transition from high BR and high DR to low BR and low DR as part of the economic development of a country from a pre-industrial to an industrialized economy
- *Demographic Window:* Period of time in a nation's demographic evolution when 'proportion of population of working age group is particularly prominent'
  - Typically, demographic window of opportunity lasts 30–40 years
  - UN Population Department definition: Period when the proportion of children and youth under 15 years falls <30% and proportion of people 65 years and older is still <15%
  - Countries status of demographic window:
    - *Europe:* 1950–2000
    - *China:* 1990–2015
    - *India:* 2010–2050 (expected)
    - *Africa:* 2045–? (expected)
- *Demographic dividend:* A rise in the rate of economic growth due to a rising share of working age people in a population
  - It usually occurs late in the demographic transition when the fertility rate falls and the youth DR declines
  - In this demographic window opportunity, output per capita rises
- *Demographic gift:* The initially favorable effect of falling fertility rates on the ratio of the working population to the dependent population

> **Key points**
>
> *India is in Stage III (Late Expanding Phase) of Demographic cycle*[Q]

- *Demographic trap:* Applies to a country whose population is growing rapidly due to a high BR and low DR^Q
- *Epidemiological transition:* A change in the pattern of disease in a country away from infectious diseases towards degenerative diseases

BIRTH RATE, DEATH RATE AND GROWTH RATE

Crude Birth Rate (CBR) and Crude Death Rate (CDR)

- *Crude birth rate (CBR):* is the natality or childbirths per 1,000 mid-year population^Q
  - CBR (World): 17.4 per 1000 population [2023]
  - CBR (India): 19.5 per 1000 population [2023]^Q
  - Is a measure of fertility
- *Crude Death Rate (CDR):* is the mortality per 1,000 mid-year population^Q
  - CDR (World): 7.64 per 1000 population [2023]
  - CDR (India): 6.0 per 1000 population [2023]^Q
  - CRUDE means it includes all causes and all ages – It is independent of age of population^Q

> **Key points**
> *Crude birth rate (CBR):* is the natality or childbirths per 1,000 mid-year population^Q

Growth Rate

- *Growth rate (GR):* Is the change in population overtime, and can be quantified as the 'change in the number of individuals in a population per unit time'
  - *Annual growth rate (AGR):* Crude birth rate (BR) minus crude death rate (DR)^Q
  - *Decadal growth rate (DGR):* Change in population over a decade
- *Growth rate (India):* [Census 2011]
  - *Annual growth rate (AGR):* 1.64%^Q
    - Since India's AGR is 1.64%, it is in very rapid growth phase; Population of India will double in 35–47 years
  - *Decadal growth rate (DGR):* 17.64%
    - Highest DGR: Dadra and Nagra Haveli (55.5%)
    - Lowest DGR: Nagaland (–0.47%)
- *Growth rate (World):* 1.05% (CIA 2019)
  - *Growth rates of countries:* [UN World's Population Prospects Report 2006]
    - South Sudan (3.83%) Highest growth rate^Q
    - India (1.17%)
    - Cook islands (–2.79%) Lowest growth rate
- *Relation between annual growth rate (AGR) and population:*

> **Key points**
> India's AGR is 1.64%

Rating	Annual GR (%)	Population doubling time
Stationary population	None	-
Slow growth	<0.5	>139 years
Moderate growth	0.5–1.0	139–70
Rapid growth	1.0–1.5	70–47
Very rapid growth^{Q*}	**1.5–2.0**	**47–35**^Q
Explosive growth	2.0–2.5	35–28
Explosive growth	2.5–3.0	28–23
Explosive growth	3.0–3.5	23–20
Explosive growth	3.5–4.0	20–18

(*India)

- *Growth ratio* = Growth rate × 100%
  - *Positive growth ratio:* Population is increasing
  - *Negative growth ratio:* Population is declining
  - *Growth ratio of zero:* There were the same number of people at the two times (or net difference between births, deaths and migration is zero)

Population Growth Models

- *Malthusian Growth Model:* (Simple exponential growth model)
  - Essentially exponential growth based on a constant rate of compound interest
  - RULE OF 70: explains the time periods involved in exponential growth at a constant rate. For example, if growth is measured annually then a 1% growth rate results in a doubling every 70 years. At 2% doubling occurs every 35 years.
- *Logistic growth model:* The Malthusian growth model is the direct ancestor of the logistic function.

POPULATION PYRAMID

Carrying Capacity

- *Carrying capacity:* The supportable population of an organism, given the food, habitat, water and other necessities available within an ecosystem is known as the ecosystem's *carrying capacity* for that organism
  - Refers to the number of individuals who can be supported in a given area *within natural resource limits*, and without degrading the natural social, cultural and economic environment for present and future generations
  - For human population more complex variables (sanitation, medical care) are sometimes considered as part of necessary infrastructure
  - Below carrying capacity, populations typically increase; while above, they typically decrease
  - May depend on a variety of factors including food availability; water supply, environmental conditions and living space

Population Pyramid (Age-Sex Pyramid)

- *Population composition of India^Q:* [SRS, 2017]
  - *0–14 years:* 27% (Children)
  - *15–49 years:* 56–6% (Reproductive age group)
  - *50–59 years:* 7.97%
  - *>60 years:* 8.5% (Geriatric age group)
- *Population pyramid:* (age-sex pyramid and age structure diagram^Q) Is a graphical illustration that shows the distribution of various age groups in a population which normally forms the shape of a pyramid
  - *Double Histogram^Q:* 2 back-to-back histograms
    - One showing the number of males and
    - One showing females in a particular population (Males are conventionally shown on left and females on right)
  - Population (%) is plotted on the X-axis and age on the Y-axis (in 5-year age group intervals)
- *Types of Population pyramid:*
  - *Stationary pyramid:* A population pyramid showing an unchanging pattern of fertility and mortality
  - *Expansive pyramid^Q:* A population pyramid showing a broad base, indicating a high proportion of children, a rapid rate of population growth, and a low proportion of older people
    - Indicates a population in which there is a high birth rate, a high death rate and a short life expectancy
    - Typical pattern for less economically developed countries
  - *Constrictive pyramid:* A population pyramid showing lower numbers or percentages of younger people
    - Country will have a greying population which means that people are generally older
- *Utility of Population pyramid:*
  - Shape of population pyramid indicates fertility pattern
    - *Broad base, Narrow top (upright triangle):* High proportion of younger population (developing countries^Q)
    - *Bulge in Middle, Spindle shape:* High proportion of adults (developed countries^Q)
  - Span (height) of population pyramid indicates life expectancy
    - *Taller pyramid:* Higher life expectancy (developed countries^Q)
    - *Shorter pyramid:* Lower life expectancy (developing countries^Q)

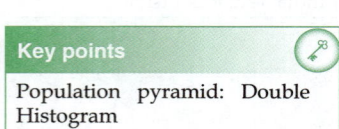

Key points

Population pyramid: Double Histogram

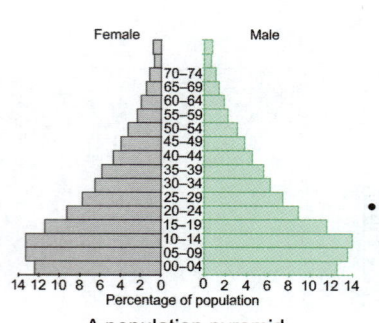

A population pyramid

- *Symmetry of population pyramid indicates sex ratio*
  - *Symmetric pyramid:* Ideal sex ratio (developed countries)^Q
  - *Asymmetric pyramid:* Unfavourable sex ratio <1000 (developing countries)^Q

SEX RATIO AND DEPENDENCY RATIO

Sex Ratio

- Sex Ratio: Is defined as number of females per thousand males^Q

$$\text{Sex Ratio} = \frac{\text{No. of Females}}{\text{No. of Males}} \times 1000$$

- *Sex Ratio (India):* [Census 2011]
  - **Sex ratio (India): 943**^{Q} *(Highly unfavourable)*
    - *Sex ratio (Rural India):* 947
    - *Sex ratio (Urban India):* 926
  - *Favourable sex ratio in India:*
    - *Kerala:* 1084^Q
    - *Puducherry:* 1038
- *Census 2011 data for sex ratio (India):*

> **Key points**
>
> Sex ratio (India): 943

Census 2011		Sex ratio
State with Highest Sex Ratio	Kerala^Q	1084
State with Lowest Sex Ratio	Haryana^Q	877
UT with Highest Sex Ratio	Puducherry	1038
UT with Lowest Sex Ratio	Daman & Diu^Q	618
District with Highest Sex Ratio	Mahe (Puducherry)	1176
District with Lowest Sex Ratio	Daman (Daman & Diu)	533

- *Types of sex ratio:*
  - *Primary sex ratio:* Ratio at the time of conception
  - *Secondary sex ratio:* Ratio at time of birth
  - *Tertiary sex ratio:* Ratio of mature organisms^Q
- *Interpretation of Sex ratio:*
  - *Ideal Sex Ratio:* Sex ratio of 1000 (equal no. of males & females)
  - *Favourable Sex Ratio:* Sex ratio >1000 (Females > Males)
  - *Unfavourable Sex Ratio:* Sex ratio <1000 (Females < Males)
- *Natural sex ratio at birth (estimated):* 950 [887 in India 2016]
- *Evolutionary stable sex ratio:* Ideal sex ratio (= 1000 or 50:50 males : females)
- *Sex ratio is an important and sensitive indicator of status of women*^{Q}

Child Sex Ratio (CSR)

- *Child Sex Ratio:* Is defined as number of female children 0–6 years age per thousand male children 0–6 years age^Q
  - **Child Sex Ratio (India): 919**^{Q} [Census 2011] (Highly unfavourable)
  - *Highest:* Mizoram; *Lowest:* Haryana

> **Key points**
>
> **Child Sex Ratio (India): 919**

Dependency Ratio

- *Dependency Ratio (DR):* The proportion of persons above 65 years of age and children below 15 years of age are considered to be dependent on economically productive age group (15–64 years) ^{Q}
  - DR is ratio dof the economically dependent part of the population to the productive part
  - DR is the 'age-wise' ratio of non-earning to earning population.
  - DR is also known as *'Societal Dependency ratio (SDR)'*

$$\frac{\text{Population} < 15 \text{ years} + \text{Population} > 65 \text{ years}}{\text{Population } 15\text{-}65 \text{ years}}$$

- *DR is of two types:*
  - Young age DR (0–14 years)
  - Old age DR (>65 years)
- *Importance of DR:* As DR increases, there is increased strain on the productive part of the population to support the upbringing and pensions of the economically dependent
  - *DR is CRUDE:* It fails to take into account the earning population in numerator and non-earning population in denominator
- *DR (India) is 53 per 100 or 0.53:* It implies 100 earning people in India are supporting 153 people (100 themselves and 53 non-earning dependents on them) (2017)
- *DR (India) projected in forthcoming years:*
  - DR will decrease
  - Young age DR will decrease
  - Old age DR will increase

LITERACY AND LIFE EXPECTANCY

Literacy

- *Literate (India)^Q:* Any person who can read AND write, WITH understanding, IN ANY ONE language of India AND who is >7 years if age (definition used in 1991 & 2001 Censuses)
  - *Literacy Rate:* Denominator is population >7 years age^Q
  - *Crude Literacy Rate:* Denominator is total population (used earlier) ^{Q}
  - *UN definition of Literacy:* Ability to read and write a simple sentence in any language^Q
- *Literacy Rate (India)^Q:* 74.04% [Census 2011]
  - *Literacy rate by sex^Q:* Males – 82% & Females – 65%
  - *Literacy rate by state^Q:* Maximum 94% (Kerala) & Least 64% (Bihar)
  - A Recent report suggest Tripura (94.6%) may have become most literate state in India
- *Literacy Rate (World):* 86% [CIA World Factbook 2015]
  - *Rank 1:* North Korea (100%)
  - Chad Niger (22%)
- *Indian Government Schemes for Literacy:*
  - *Sarva Siksha Abhiyan (2001):* All children in the age 6–14 years attend school and complete 8 years of schooling by 2010^Q
  - *District Primary Education Programme (1994):* Centrally sponsored; has so far opened more than 160,000 new schools, including almost 84,000 alternative schools.
  - *Mid day meal programme (1995)^Q*
  - *National Literacy Mission (1988):* Aims at attaining a literacy rate of 75% by 2007
- *International Literacy Day^Q:* 8th September (every year)
- *Threshold level of literacy:* 75%
- *Types of Literacy:*
  - *Functional Literacy:* Ability of an individual to use reading, writing, and computational skills efficiently in everyday life situations^Q
  - *Transliteracy:* The ability to read, write and interact across a range of platforms, tools and media from signing and orality through handwriting, print, TV, radio and film, to digital social networks
  - *Alliteracy:* The state of being able to read but being uninterested in doing so

> **Key points**
> Literacy Rate (India)^Q: 74.04% [Census 2011]

FERTILITY

Total Fertility Rate (TFR)

- Is STANDARDIZED INDEX FOR FERTILITY LEVEL^Q
- Average no. of children a woman would bear in her reproductive life span; Also known as 'Period Total Fertility Rate'
- Gives magnitude of approximately 'completed family size'^{Q} – no. of alive children in a family
- Obtained by summing single-year age-specific rates (ASFRs) at a given time^Q
- *TFR is a synthetic rate^Q:* Is not actually counted, as this would involve waiting until women complete childbearing
- *TFR (India):* 2.0 (2019–21, NFHS-5)

> **Key points**
> Total Fertility Rate (TFR) Gives magnitude of approximately 'completed family size'

- *Replacement level of fertility (TFR = 2.1)^Q:* TFR at which newborn girls would have an average of exactly 1 daughter over their lifetimes (women have just enough babies to replace themselves)
  - Replacement TFR (industrialized countries) = 2.1
  - Replacement TFR (developing countries) = 2.5–3.3
  - Replacement TFR (globally) = 2.33
- *Total cohort fertility rate (TCFR) is a better estimate of completed family size than TFR*

Fertility Rates

- *GFR is a better measure of fertility than CBR:* Number of live births per 1000 women in reproductive age group (15–49 years)^Q (77.6 GFR India 2016)
  - Major weakness of GFR: Not all women are exposed to risk of child birth
- *Total Fertility Rate (TFR):* Average no. of children a woman would bear in her reproductive life span. Also known as 'Period Total Fertility Rate'
  - Gives magnitude of approximately '*completed family size*' – no. of alive children in a family^Q
  - Obtained by summing single-year age-specific rates (ASFRs) at a given time^Q
  - TFR is a synthetic rate: Is not actually counted, as this would involve waiting until women complete childbearing^Q
- *Gross Reproduction Rate (GRR):* Measures the no. of daughters a woman would have in her lifetime if she experiences prevailing age-specific fertility, 'assuming no mortality'^{Q} (GRR 1.1 India 2016)
  - GRR is same as the NRR, except that, like the TFR, it ignores life expectancy
- *Net Reproduction Rate (NRR):* Number of daughters a newborn girl will bear during her lifetime assuming fixed age-specific fertility and mortality rates.
  - NRR = 1: Each generation of women is exactly reproducing itself^Q
  - To achieve NRR =1^Q: Couple Protection Rate (CPR) should be >60%
  - GRR or NRR = ½ TFR (approximately)^Q

> **Key points**
> To achieve NRR =1^Q: Couple Protection Rate (CPR) should be >60%

MISCELLANEOUS (DEMOGRAPHY)

Uses of Regular Reporting of Health Statistics^Q

- To measure health status of population
- To quantify health related problems
- To evaluate trends of disease in a population
- To compare health data locally, nationally and internationally
- To effective plan health programs, policies, services
- To monitor and evaluate health programs
- To evaluate satisfaction among population
- To appreciate health personnel's efforts
- To promote epidemiological research

Sample Registration System

- *Sample Registration System (SRS)* was initiated in 1964–65 (on a pilot basis; full scale from 1969–70) to provide national as well as state level reliable estimates of fertility and mortality
- *SRS is a dual record system:*^{Q}
  - *Field Investigation:* continuous enumeration of births and deaths by an enumerator
  - *Independent retrospective survey:* every 6 months by an investigator-supervisor^Q
- *Advantages of SRS as a dual record system:*
  - Elimination of errors of duplication
  - Leads to a quantitative assessment of the sources of distortion in the t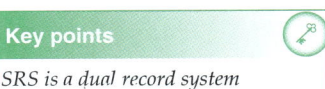 of records making it a self evaluating technique.
- *Primary objective:* To build up statistics on '*Most Probable Causes of Death*' for rural and urban areas using *lay diagnosis reporting (Post Death Verbal Autopsy^Q)*' method
- *Main objective of SRS:* To provide reliable estimates of BR, DR and IMR at the natural division level for rural areas and at the state level for urban areas^Q
- *Main components of SRS:*
  - Base-line survey of the sample units to obtain usual resident population of the sample areas
  - Continuous (longitudinal) enumeration of vital events pertaining to usual resident population by the enumerator

> **Key points**
> SRS is a dual record system

- Independent retrospective half-yearly surveys for recording births and deaths which occurred during the half-year under reference and updating the Houselist, Household schedule and the list of women in the reproductive age group along with their pregnancy status by the Supervisor
- Matching of events recorded during continuous enumeration and those listed in course of half-yearly survey
- Field verification of unmatched and partially matched events
- Filling of Verbal Autopsy forms for finalized deaths
- *Sample design adopted for SRS:* A unistage stratified simple random sample^Q
  - Infant Mortality is the decisive indicator for estimation of sample size at Natural Division
- SRS now covers the entire country
- *Findings of SRS Bulletin: [2022]:*
  - Crude Birth Rate (CBR): 19.5 per 1000 mid-year population
  - Crude Death Rate (CDR): 6.0 per 1000 mid-year population
  - Natural Growth Rate: 13.5%
  - Infant Mortality Rate (IMR): 28 per 1000 live births

Civil Registration System

> **Key points**
> - Births must be registered within: 21 days
> - Deaths must be registered within: 21 days

- *Civil Registration System (CRS):* Birth and death registration system is technically known as CRS^Q
- Registration of births and deaths (Birth and Death Registration Act, 1969) and marriages is compulsory at their place of occurrence with local registrar in India
  - *Births must be registered within:* 21 days^Q
  - *Deaths must be registered within:* 21 days^Q
  - *Marriages must be registered within:* Variable limits within India
- *In cases of delayed registration for birth/death:*
  - *After 21 days till 30 days:* Late fee
  - *After 30 days till 1 year:* Late fee + Written permission from district registrar (vide an affidavit)
  - *After 1 year:* Late fee + Order of executive magistrate
- *Registration of name of the child:*
  - *Within 12 months of birth registration:* Free of charge
  - *After 12 months of birth registration till 15 years:* ₹ 5.00
- Coverage of registration of births and deaths in India
  - *Coverage of births registration in India:* 89%
  - *Coverage of deaths registration in India:* 74%

Key Facts of Census (India) 2011

- *Frequency of census in India^Q:* Every 10 years (decadal)
- *Legal basis of conducting census:* The Census Act, 1948^Q
- *The census organization set up and working under:* Ministry of Home Affairs^Q
- *Head of census organization:* Registrar General and Census Commissioner^Q
- *Population enumeration:* 9th–28th February 2011
- *Revisional round:* 1st–5th March 2011
- *Houseless population enumeration:* Night of 28th February 2011
- *Districts covered:* 640^Q
- *Census Stop* (Census Movement)^Q: 00.00 hrs 01 March 2011 (The referral time and date at which snapshot of the population is taken)
- FIRST TIME ACTIVITIES EVER DONE: BIOMETRY^Q
  - Finger prints – 10
  - Iris scan
  - National population register (NPR)
  - UID – Unique identification number
  - Photograph

> **Key points**
> **Census Stop** (Census Movement^Q: 00.00 hrs 01 March 2011

Key Findings of Census of India 2011

- 35 States & UTs; 640 districts; 6.41 lac villages
- Total population — 1210.1 million (M : F = 51.4 : 48.6)
  - Highest population — Uttar Pradesh (199 million)
  - Lowest population — Lakshadweep (64000)
- **Sex ratio** — **943**

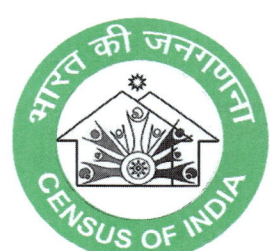

2011
Census of India

- Highest sex ratio — Kerala (1084)^Q; Puducherry (1038)
- Lowest sex ratio — Daman & Diu (618)^Q; Dadra & Nagar Haveli (775); Chandigarh (818); Delhi (866); Haryana (877)^Q
- **Child Sex Ratio (0–6 y)** — 919^Q
  - Highest CSR — Mizoram (971)
  - Lowest CSR — Haryana (830)
- **Literacy rate** — **74.04%^Q**
  - LR Males — 82.14%^Q
  - LR Females — 65.46%^Q
  - LR Highest — Kerala (93.9%)^Q
  - LR Lowest — Bihar (63.8%)
- **Density of population** — 382^Q
  - Highest density — Delhi (11,297)
  - Lowest density — Arunachal Pradesh (17)
- **Growth rate annual** — **1.64%^Q**
- Growth rate decadal — 17.64%
  - Highest DGR — Dadra & Nagar Haveli (55.5%)
  - Lowest DGR — Nagaland (–0.47%)

National Family Health Survey (NFHS)

Is a large-scale, multi-round survey conducted in a representative sample of households throughout India

- 4 rounds of the NFHS survey have been conducted till date^Q
  - NFHS–1: 1992–93
  - NFHS–2: 1998–99
  - NFHS–3: 2005–06
  - NFHS–4: 2015–16
- *Goals of NFHS survey:*
  - To provide essential data needed by Ministry of Health & Family Welfare and other agencies for policy and programme purposes
  - To provide information on important emerging health and family welfare issues
- *Main objective of NFHS survey:* To provide state and national information for India on fertility, infant and child mortality, the practice of family planning, maternal and child health, reproductive health, nutrition, anaemia, utilization and quality of health and family planning services
- *Nodal agency for NFHS:* International Institute for Population Sciences (IIPS), Mumbai^Q
- NFHS-5 2019–21, India: Key Parameters

> **Key points**
> 4 rounds of the NFHS survey have been conducted till date

Parameter	Value(s)
Population below age 15 years (%)	26.5%
Sex ratio of the total population (females per 1,000 males)	1,020
Sex ratio at birth (females per 1,000 males)	929
Births registered with the civil authority	89%
Deaths registered with the civil authority	71%
Households with an improved drinking-water source	96%
Households that use an improved sanitation facility	70%
Households using clean fuel for cooking	59%
Literacy levels (male, female)	84% (M), 71% (F)
Ever used Internet (male, female)	57% (M), 33% (F)
Total fertility rate (children per woman)	2.0
Infant mortality rate (IMR)	35
Neonatal mortality rate (NNMR)	25
Under-five mortality rate (U5MR)	42
Any method use for Family planning	66.7%
Total unmet need for Family planning	9.4%

Key Age-group Definitions

- *Ovum:* 0–2 weeks
- *Embryo:* 2–9 weeks
- *Fetus:* 9 weeks – delivery
- *Period of viability^Q:* POG >28 weeks
- *Perinatal period^Q:* 28 weeks POG – 7 days post-delivery
- *Neonatal period^Q:* 0–28 days after birth (0–4 weeks post-delivery)
    - *Early neonatal period:* 0–7 days after birth (1st week)
    - *Late neonatal period:* 8–28 days after birth (2–4 week)
    - *Post neonatal period:* 29 days – 365 days after birth (1 month – 1 year)
- *Infancy^Q:* Birth – 365 days (1st year of life)
- *Toddler:* 1–3 years age
- *Preschool child:* 3–6 years age
- *Puberty:* Is the stage of the lifespan in which a child develops secondary sex characteristics as his/her hormonal balance shifts strongly towards an adult state
    - *Average age for onset in girls:* 10–12 years^Q
    - *Average age for onset in boys:* 12–14 years^Q
- *Adolescent:* 10–19 years age (WHO definition^Q)
    - *Early adolescence:* 10–13 years
    - *Mid adolescence:* 14–16 years
    - *Late adolescence:* 17–19 years
- *Youth:* 15–24 years age group (UN definition^Q)
- *Reproductive age group:* 15–44 years or 15–49 years age
- *Geriatric age (India):* >60 years^Q
- *Legal age of marriage in India:* 18 years for girls and 21 years for boys^Q
- *Legal age for voting in India:* 18 years for both boys and girls
- *Legal age for employment in India:* >14 years^Q
- *Legal age of consent by a girl for sexual intercourse in India:* 18 years^Q [NEW GUIDELINE 2012]
- *Juvenile in India:* Boy less than 18 years and girl less than 18 years [NEW GUIDELINE 2011]
- *Major in India:* 18 years and above
- *Tobacco products cannot be sold in India:* To age below 18 years^Q
- *Alcohol cannot be sold in India:* To age below 25 years^Q

> **Key points**
> **Perinatal period^Q:** 28 weeks POG – 7 days post-delivery

> **Key points**
> **Adolescent:** 10–19 years age

> **Key points**
> **Legal age for employment in India:** >14 years^Q

> **Key points**
> **Juvenile in India:** Boy less than 18 years and girl less than 18 years

FAMILY PLANNING AND CONTRACEPTION

CONCEPTS OF FAMILY PLANNING

Definitions and Concepts

- *Birth control (contraception):* Is a regimen of one or more actions, devices, or medications followed in order to deliberately prevent or reduce the likelihood of pregnancy or childbirth. It is commonly used as part of family planning
- *Contraception:* May refer specifically to mechanisms which are intended to reduce the likelihood of the fertilization of an ovum by a spermatozoon
- *Family planning:* A couple plans when to have children, using birth control and other techniques (sexual education, prevention and management of STIs, preconceptional counselling & management, and infertility management).
- *Modern concept of family planning:* Family planning is not synonymous with birth control only. A WHO Expert Committee (1970) recommends that family planning includes in its' purview^Q:
    - Proper spacing and limitation of births
    - Advice on sterility
    - Education for parenthood
    - Sex education
    - Screening for pathological conditions related to reproductive system (e.g., Cervical cancer)
    - Genetic counseling
    - Marriage counseling

- Premarital consultation and examination
- Carrying out pregnancy tests
- Preparation of couples for arrival of their 1st child
- Providing services for unmarried mothers
- Teaching home economics and nutrition
- Providing adoption services

Contraceptive Efficacy

- *Contraceptive Efficacy:* Is assessed by measuring the number of unplanned pregnancies that occur during a specified period of exposure and use of a contraceptive method. Two methods used are^Q:
  - Pearl Index^Q
  - Life table analysis^Q

Pearl Index (PI)

- *PI or Pearl rate:* MC technique used in clinical trials for measuring the effectiveness of a birth control method
  - **PI is no. of failures per 100 woman years (HWY) of exposure**^{Q}

$$\text{Pearl Index (PI)} = \frac{\text{Total accidental pregnancy}^Q}{\text{Total months of exposure}} \times 1200$$

> **Key points**
> PI is no. of failures per 100 woman years (HWY) of exposure

- In designing a use-effectiveness trial, a 'minimum of 600 months of exposure' is required for a firm conclusion
- *Disadvantages for PI:*
  - PI assumes a constant failure rate over time
  - PI also provides no information on factors other than accidental pregnancy which may influence effectiveness calculations, viz. dissatisfaction with the method, trying to achieve pregnancy, medical side effects, lost to follow up
  - PI is only accurate as a statistical estimation of per-year risk of pregnancy if the pregnancy rate was very low
- *Pearl Indices for few contraceptive methods:*

Contraceptive Method	Pearl Index (per HWY)
No method used	80
Rhythm (calendar) Method	24
Coitus interruptus	18
Male condoms	2–14^Q
Female condoms	5–21
Diaphragm	12
Vaginal sponge	
Parous women	20–40
Nulliparous women	9–20
IUD	1–5^Q
Oral pill	0.1–2^Q
Centchroman (Saheli)	1.83–2.84

- *Second method for calculation of PI:* The number of pregnancies in the study is divided by the number of menstrual cycles experienced by women in the study, and then multiplied by 1300
  - 1300 instead of 1200 is used on the basis that the length of the average menstrual cycle is 28 days, or 13 cycles per year

$$\text{Pearl Index (PI)} = \frac{\text{Total accidental pregnancies}}{\text{Total no. of menstrual cycles experienced}} \times 1300$$

Life Table Analysis (LTA)

- *LTA as measure of contraceptive efficacy:* LTA calculates a failure rate per month of use^Q
  - Better measure than PI^Q

Eligible Couples

> **Key points**
>
> **EC register** is maintained at Subcentre^Q

- *Eligible couples (ECs):* A currently married couple with wife in reproductive age group (15–45 years age)^Q
  - There are 150–180 ECs per 1000 population in India^Q
  - ECs are in need of family planning services
  - 20% ECs are in age group 20–24 years
- EC register, a basic document for organizing family planning work, is maintained at Subcentre^Q

Couple Protection Rate (CPR) and Effective CPR

- *Couple Protection Rate (CPR):* Is an indicator of prevalence of contraceptive practice in a community^Q
  - CPR is percent of eligible couples (ECs) protected against one or the other approved methods of family planning, viz. condoms, OCPs, IUDs, sterilization^Q
  - NRR = 1 can be achieved if: CPR >60%^{Q}
  - CPR (India): 54% [2018]
  - Goal for CPR in RCH – II (2004–09): >65% [Goal by 2020 FP vision 2020: 63.7%]

$$CPR = \frac{\text{Total no. of ECs protected by any of 4 approved methods}}{\text{Total no. of ECs in the community}} \times 100$$

- *Effective Couple Protection rate (ECPR):*
  - ECPR is percent of eligible couples (ECs) protected against one or the other approved methods of family planning, viz. condoms, OCPs, IUDs, sterilization TAKING INTO ACCOUNT THEIR EFFECTIVITY^Q
  - *Effectivity of approved contraceptive methods^Q:*
    - Condoms: 50%
    - IUDs: 95%
    - OCPs: 100%
    - Sterilization (Vasectomy or Tubectomy): 100%

NATURAL METHODS

Natural Family Planning Methods

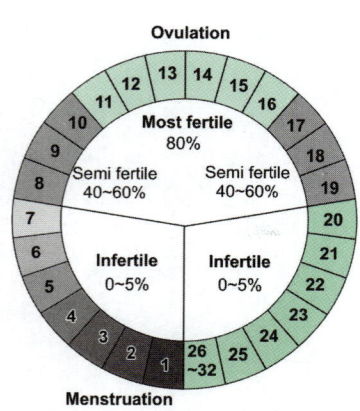

Fertile period method

> **Key points**
>
> **BBT Method:** Rise of temperature (0.3°–0.5°C) at ovulation^Q

- *Safe period (Rhythm method/Calendar method):*
  - *Fertile period:* Shortest cycle minus 18 days (Last day of fertile period: Longest cycle *minus* 10 days)^Q
  - *Drawbacks:*
    - Difficult to predict safe period in irregular cycles
    - Only suitable for educated couples with high motivation
    - PROGRAMMED SEX: Abstinence required for ½ month^Q
    - Not useful in postnatal period
    - High failure rate: 9 per HWY^Q
    - Medical complications: Ectopic pregnancies and embryonic abnormalities
- *Basal Body Temperature (BBT) Method:*
  - *Depends on:* Rise of temperature (0.3°–0.5°C) at ovulation^Q
  - *Occurs due to:* Increased progesterone production^Q
  - *Measurement:* Before getting out of bed in morning (preferably)
  - *Reliable if:* Intercourse restricted to post-ovulatory infertile period
  - *Drawback:* Abstinence necessary for entire pre-ovulatory period
- *Cervical Mucus Method:*
  - Also known as 'Billing's Method'^{Q} or 'Ovulation Method'^{Q}
  - *Based on:* Changes in characteristics of cervical mucus
  - *At ovulation:* Watery, clear, smooth, slippery, profuse (like Egg white)

- After ovulation: Thickens and lessens in quantity
- Method: Tissue paper to wipe off inside of vagina
- Drawback: Requires high degree of motivation
- *Symptothermic Method:*
  - Combines temperature, cervical mucus and calendar techniques[Q]
  - More effective than Billing's method[Q]
- *Sexual abstinence:*
  - Only method of birth control which is completely effective: Sexual abstinence[Q]
- *Coitus interruptus/Withdrawal method:*
  - Oldest method of voluntary fertility control: Coitus interruptus[Q]
- *Lactation amenorrhoea method (LAM):* A good method for natural conception under exclusive breast feeding

BARRIER METHODS

Condoms

- *Major advantage:* Protection against HIV and other sexually transmitted infections (STIs)
- *Male condoms versus female condoms:*

Characteristic	Male condoms	Female condoms
Material commonly used	Latex	Polyurethane/Nitrile
Pearl Index (failure rate)	2–14 per HWY[Q]	5–21 per HWY
No. of rings	1	2 (outer & inner)
Reusable	No	Yes
Covering skin around external genitals	No	Yes[Q]
Compatible with oil based lubricants	No	Yes
Insertion requires male erection	Yes	No
Prevention of pregnancy	Yes	Yes
Prevention of STIs	Yes[Q]	Yes[Q]

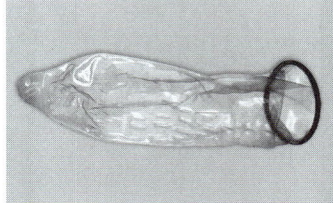

Male condom

Female Condoms

- *Female condoms:* A device that is used during sexual intercourse
- *Invented by Danish MD Lasse Hessel*[Q]
- It is worn internally by the receptive partner and physically blocks ejaculated semen from entering that person's body
- Prevent pregnancy and transmission of STIs
- *Three types:*
  - FC Female condom: made of polyurethane
  - FC2: made of nitrile polymer
  - Latex
- Only tool for HIV prevention that women can initiate & control[Q]

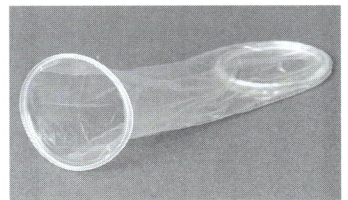

Female condom

Vaginal Sponge (TODAY)

- *VAGINAL SPONGE:* TODAY[Q] (brand name)
- *Sponge a barrier method of contraception:* It actually combines barrier and spermicidal methods to prevent conception[Q]
  - Is a small polyurethane sponge 5 cm × 2.5 cm
  - Saturated with 1000 mg of spermicide *'Non-oxynol-9'*[Q]
  - Today must be run under water till thoroughly wet before insertion
  - Sponges is *'inserted vaginally'* prior to intercourse and must be *'placed over the cervix to be effective'*[Q]
  - Sponge must be left in place for 6 hours after ejaculation[Q]: All sponges must be removed within the time limits specified by the manufacturer (24 hours for Today)
- *Disadvantages of sponge:*
  - Sponge provide no protection from STIs
  - Can lead to Toxic Shock Syndrome[Q]
  - Increased risk of yeast infection and UTI

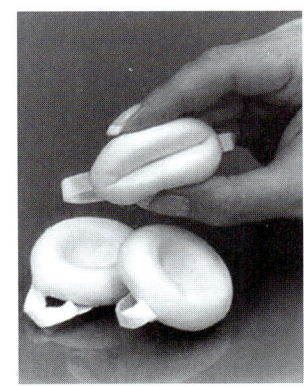

Vaginal sponge

- *Failure rate (Pearl Index):*
  - Parous women: 20–40 per HWY[Q]
  - Nulliparous women: 9–20 per HWY[Q]

Diaphragm

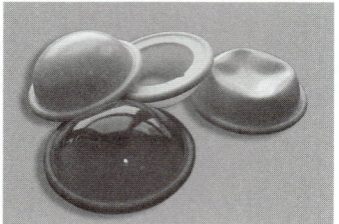

Diaphragm

- *DIAPHRAGM:* Is a cervical barrier type of birth control
- *Mechanism of action:* It is a soft latex or silicone dome with a spring molded into the rim; the spring creates a seal against the walls of the vagina and blocks sperm from entering the female reproductive tract
- One teaspoon (5 mL) of *spermicide* may be placed in the dome of the diaphragm before insertion, or with an applicator after insertion[Q]
- It must be inserted sometime before sexual intercourse, and remain in the vagina for 6–8 hours after a man's last ejaculation[Q]
- *Protection against:* PID and Human Papilloma Virus (HPV)[Q]
- *Disadvantages:*
  - Increased risk of UTI, yeast infection & bacterial vaginosis
  - Toxic Shock Syndrome (if left in-situ >24 hours)[Q]

IUDs

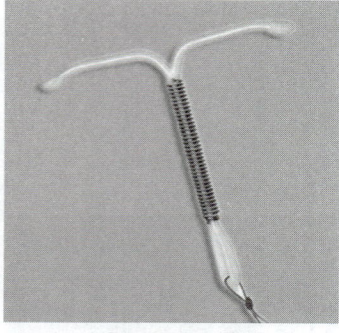

Copper T (IUD)

> **Key points**
> Numbers (7, 220, 380) in IUD represent[Q]: Surface area of copper (in sq. mm)

Types of Intrauterine Devices (IUDs)

- *Numbers (7, 220, 380) represent[Q]:* Surface area of copper (in sq. mm) on the device
- *B in CuT 220 B represent:* Size of IUD (IUDs were earlier available in different sizes – A, B, C and D; D was the largest size)
- *A or Ag in CuT 380 A represent[Q]:* Silver or Gold (with copper)

1st Generation IUDs[Q]	2nd Generation IUDs[Q]	3rd Generation IUDs[Q]
Non-medicated IUDs Inert IUDs[Q]	Medicated IUDs Bio-active IUDs[Q]	
No medication is added to the IUD	Metallic ions (Copper) are added to IUD	Hormones are added to IUD
Lippes Loop Grafenberg's Ring	CuT 7 CuT 220 B CuT 380 A/Ag	Progestasert LNG – IUD

Shelf-life of IUDs

IUD	Approved years of use
Copper IUDs[Q]	3–5
Progestasert[Q]	1
CuT 200	4
NOVA T	5
LNG IUD	7–10
CuT 380 A[Q]	10

Mechanisms of Action of Intrauterine Devices (IUDs) [Q]

- *'Foreign body reaction':*
  - Cellular/biochemical changes in endometrium/uterine fluids
  - Impair viability of gamete
  - Reduces chances of fertilization, rather than implantation
- *Copper in IUD:*
  - Enhances cellular response in endometrium
  - Affects enzymes in uterus
  - Alter cervical mucus thus affecting sperm motility, capacitation & survival
- *Hormones in IUD:*
  - Increase viscosity of cervical mucus

- Prevent sperm from entering cervix
- Make endometrium unfavorable to implantation (high progesterone & low estrogen)

Side Effects of IUD (Intrauterine Device) Insertion

- *Bleeding:*
    - MC side effect of woman with IUD: Increased vaginal bleeding^Q
    - Usually disappear by: 1–2 months
    - Leads to: 10–20% of all IUD removals (MCC removal: Pain^Q)
    - Greater bleeding with: Non-medicated (Inert) IUDs
    - Management of bleeding^Q:
        - Re-assure the female (DO NOT REMOVE IUD^Q)
        - Ferrous sulphate 200 mg TDS × 1–2 months
        - If bleeding is heavy or persistent: REMOVE IUD
- *Pain:*
    - Second major side effect of IUD insertion^Q
    - MCC requiring removal of IUDs^Q: Pain (15–40% removals)
    - Usually disappear by: 3 months
    - Pain is more common in:
        - Nullipara
        - Those who have not had child for many years
    - Management of Pain^Q:
        - Slight pain: Analgesics like Aspirin or Codeine
        - Intolerable pain: Remove the IUD, insert a copper based device or advise other contraceptives
- *Pelvic infection (Pelvic Inflammatory Disease–PID):*
    - Prompt treatment with broad spectrum antibiotics
    - If no response to antibiotics in 24–48 hours: Remove IUD
- *Uterine perforation:*
    - Management: Removal of IUD
- *Pregnancy with IUD-in-situ:*
    - Management:
        - If woman requests: Legally induced abortion
        - If woman wants to continue pregnancy and threads are visible: Remove IUD gently by pulling the threads
        - If woman wants to continue pregnancy and threads are NOT visible: Carefully examine for possible complications. If any sign of intrauterine infection – evacuation of uterus under broad spectrum antibiotic cover
- *Ectopic pregnancy with IUD-in-situ:*
- *Spontaneous expulsion:*
    - Expulsion rate: 12–20%
    - Usually occurs in: first few weeks following insertion or during menstruation
    - Higher risk of expulsion^Q:
        - Young women
        - Nullipara women
        - Women who have had a postpartum insertion
        - Inert (Non-medicated IUDs)
- *Mortality associated with IUD use:*
    - Very low: ~1 death per 1,00,000 years of use
    - Safer than OCPs

> **Key points**
>
> MC side effect of woman with IUD: Increased vaginal bleeding

IUDs Associated with Side-effects/Complications

Side effects or complications	IUD most commonly associated
Highest pregnancy rate^Q	Lippes Loop
Lowest pregnancy rate^Q	LNG – IUD
Highest expulsion rate^Q	Lippes Loop
Lowest expulsion rate^Q	Progestatsert
Highest removal rate^Q	LNG – IUD
Lowest removal rate^Q	Progestatsert

Contraindications for IUDs Use

> **Key points**
>
> **Absolute contraindications^Q for IUDs:**
> - Suspected pregnancy
> - PID
> - Vaginal bleeding of undiagnosed etiology
> - Cancer of cervix, uterus or adnexa and other pelvic tumors
> - Previous ectopic pregnancy

- *Absolute contraindications^Q:*
  - Suspected pregnancy
  - PID
  - Vaginal bleeding of undiagnosed etiology
  - Cancer of cervix, uterus or adnexa and other pelvic tumors
  - Previous ectopic pregnancy
- *Relative contraindications:*
  - Anemia
  - Menorrhagia
  - History of PID since last pregnancy
  - Purulent cervical discharge
  - Distortions of uterine cavity due to congenital malformations, fibroids
  - Unmotivated persons
- *The WHO Medical Eligibility Criteria for Contraceptive Use:*
  - *Category 3 (CuT NOT RECOMMENDED):*
    - Postpartum between 48 hours and 4 weeks
    - Benign gestational trophoblastic disease
    - Ovarian cancer
    - High likelihood of exposure to gonorrhea/chlamydial STIs
    - AIDS (unless clinically well on anti-retroviral therapy)
- *Category 4 (CuT CONTRAINDICATED^Q):*
  - Pregnancy
  - Postpartum puerperal sepsis
  - Immediately post-septic abortion
  - Before evaluation of unexplained vaginal bleeding suspected of being a serious condition
  - Malignant gestational trophoblastic disease
  - Cervical cancer (awaiting treatment)
  - Endometrial cancer
  - Distortions of the uterine cavity by uterine fibroids or anatomical abnormalities
  - Current PID
  - Current purulent cervicitis, chlamydial infection, or gonorrheal STIs
  - Known pelvic tuberculosis

Ideal IUD Woman Candidate^Q
(Planned Parenthood Federation of America PPFA)

- Who has borne at least one child
- Has no history of pelvic disease
- Has normal menstrual periods
- Is willing to check the IUD tail
- Has access to follow-up and treatment of potential problems
- Is in a monogamous relationship
- American College of Obstetricians and Gynaecologists (1985) stated that *'IUDs are not recommended for women who have not had children or who have multiple partners, because of the risk of PID and possible infertility'*

Pregnancy Rates of IUDs (Clinical Experience)

Device	Pregnancy rate (%)	Expulsion rate (%)	Removal rate (%)
Lippes Loop^Q	3	12–60	12–15
CuT 7	3	6	11
CuT 200	3	8	11
CuT 380 A	0.5–0.8	5	14^Q
Progestasert	1.5	3	10
LNG IUD	0.2	6	17

Timings of IUD Insertion

- *During menstruation or within 10 days of beginning of menstrual period:*
  - Best time for IUD insertion^Q
  - Cervical canal diameter greatest, lesser expulsion, least risk of pregnancy
- *Immediate post-partum insertion:* During 1st week after delivery before woman leaves hospital^Q
  - High chance of perforation
  - High chance of expulsion
- *Post-puerperal insertion:* 6–8 weeks after delivery^Q
  - Can be combined with follow-up visit of mother and child
  - Not recommended after 2nd trimester abortion

IUDs as Emergency Contraceptives

- IUDs can be used as emergency contraception to prevent pregnancy *'up to 5 days after'* unprotected sexual intercourse, or sexual intercourse during which the primary contraception is believed to have failed^Q
- Insertion of a CuT as emergency contraception is *'more than 99% effective'* (more effective than emergency contraceptive pills)^Q

Key points

Insertion of a CuT as emergency contraception is *'more than 99% effective'*

Grafenberg's Ring

- *Grafenberg's ring:* 1st Generation (Non-medicated/Inert) IUD^Q
- A flexible ring of *'silver wire'* used as a birth control device
- It was a precursor to the IUD (inserted into the woman's uterus)

Progestasert

- *Progestasert is a 3rd Generation IUD* (Medicated/Bio-active IUD)^Q
- Progestasert was the *'first hormonal uterine device'*, developed in 1976
- T-shaped device filled with 38 mg progesterone^Q
- *Reservoir:* Silicon oil (in vertical stem)
- *Rate of hormone release:* 65 mcg per day^Q
- *Shelf life:* 1–1½ years^Q
- *Mechanism of action:*
  - Direct local effect on uterine lining
  - Effect on cervical mucus
  - Effect on sperms
- *Advantages of Progestasert:*
  - IUD with *'Lowest expulsion rate'*
  - IUD with *'Lowest removal rate'*
  - Lesser chances of dysmenorrhoea and menorrhagia
- *Disadvantages of Progestasert:*
  - Expensive
  - Requires yearly replacement
  - Highest rate of ectopic pregnancy: 9-fold higher
  - Failure rate of Progestasert: 2% per year

Key points

Progestasert's
Rate of hormone release: 65 mcg per day

HORMONAL METHODS

Types of Combined OCPs

- *Monophasic OCPs* deliver the same amount of estrogen and progestin every day
- *Biphasic OCPs* deliver the same amount of estrogen every day for the first 21 days of the cycle^Q
  - first half of the cycle: progestin/estrogen ratio is lower to allow the endometrium to thicken
  - second half of the cycle: progestin/estrogen ratio is higher to allow normal shedding of the lining of the uterus
- *Triphasic OCPs* have constant or changing estrogen concentrations and varying progestin concentrations throughout the cycle

> **Key points**
>
> **Composition of Combined OCP^Q: (MALA-N)**
> - Ethinyl estradiol: 0.03 mg (30 mcg)
> - Norgestrel: 0.15 mg (150 mcg)

Composition of Combined OCPs

- *Composition of Combined OCP^Q*: (MALA-N)
  - Ethinyl estradiol: 0.03 mg (30 mcg)
  - Norgestrel: 0.15 mg (150 mcg)
- *Composition of 'New Low dose OCP'^Q*: (Brand name: *Femilon/Elogen*)
  - Ethinyl estradiol: 0.02 mg (20 mcg)
  - Desogestrel: 0.15 mg (150 mcg)

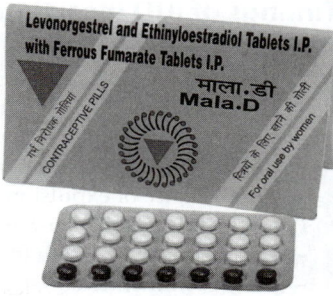

Mala-D

Combined OCPs under RCH Program

	MALA – N	MALA – D
Type of contraceptive	Combined OCP	Combined OCP
Estrogen^Q	Ethinyl estradiol (0.03 mg)	Ethinyl estradiol (0.03 mg)
Progesterone^Q	Norgestrel (0.15 mg)	Desogestrel (0.15 mg)
Status in RCH^Q	Provided free of cost	Provided at a subsidized cost (₹ 3/- per packet)

Adverse Effects of Combined Oral Contraceptive Pills (OCPs)^Q

- *Cardiovascular effects^Q*: (due to oestrogenic component)
  - Myocardial infarction
  - Cerebral thrombosis
  - Venous thrombosis (with or without pulmonary embolus)
  - Hypertension
- *Carcinogenesis:*^Q
  - Cervical cancer (increased risk)
  - Breast Cancer
- *Metabolic Effects^Q*: (due to progesterone component)
  - Elevated blood pressure (hypertension)
  - Altered lipid profile (reduced HDL)
  - Blood clotting
  - Hyperglycemia and increased plasma insulin
- *Hepatocellular adenoma^Q*
- *Gallbladder disease^Q*
- *Cholestatic jaundice^Q*
- *Monolial vaginitis (candidiasis)^Q*
- *Decline milk volume during lactation*
- *Slight delay in return of fertility (upon discontinuation)*
- *Depression*
- *Fetal birth defects (?)*
- *General effects:*
  - Breast tenderness
  - Weight gain^Q (due to water retention)
  - Headache & migraine^Q
  - Bleeding disturbances

Beneficial Effects of Combined Oral Contraceptive Pills (OCPs)^Q

- *Benign breast disorders (Fibrocystic disease, Fibroadenoma)*
- *Pelvic Inflammatory Disease (PID)*
- *Ectopic pregnancy*
- *Iron deficiency anemia*
- *Benign ovarian disease (Ovarian cysts)*
- *Malignant ovarian disease (Ovarian cancer^Q)*
- *Endometrial cancer^Q*
  - Combined oral contraceptive use *'reduces the risk of ovarian cancer by 40% and the risk of endometrial cancer by 50%'* compared to never users

- Risk reduction increases with duration of use (80% reduction in risk for both cancers with use >10 years)
- Risk reduction for both cancers persists for >20 years
- *Non-contraceptive benefits of combined OCPs:*
  - polycystic ovary syndrome (PCOS)
  - endometriosis
  - adenomyosis
  - anaemia related to menstruation
  - painful menstruation (dysmenorrhea)
  - mild or moderate acne
  - irregular menstrual cycles
  - dysfunctional uterine bleeding

Contraindications for Use of Combined Oral Contraceptive Pills (OCPs)

Absolute contraindications^Q	Relative contraindications*
1. Breast Cancer 2. Genital Cancer 3. Liver disease 4. History of thromboembolism 5. Cardiac abnormalities	1. Age >40 years^Q 2. Smoking and age >35 years^Q 3. Mild hypertension 4. Chronic renal disease 5. Epilepsy
6. Congenital hyperlipidemia 7. Undiagnosed abnormal uterine bleeding 8. Pregnancy	6. Migraine 7. Nursing mothers (0–6 months) 8. Diabetes mellitus 9. Gall bladder disease 10. History of infrequent bleeding 11. Amenorrhoea

(*require medical surveillance)

Centchroman (Saheli)

- *Synthetic NON-STEROIDAL oral contraceptive*^Q
- *Brand name:* Saheli
- *Chemical in Centchroman:* ORMELOXIFENE^Q
- *Mechanism of Action:* Selective estrogen receptor modulators (SERMs^Q) a class of medication which acts on the estrogen receptor
  - Works through a unique combination of weak estrogenic and potent anti-estrogenic properties
- *Developed by:* Central Drug Research Institute (CDRI), Lucknow, India^Q
- *Dosage & frequency:* 1 tablet (30 mg) twice a week × 3 months, then 1 tablet per week^Q
- *Failure rate (Pearl Index):* 1.83–2.84 per HWY^Q
- *Uses of Centchroman:*
  - As a contraceptive
  - Treatment of dysfunctional uterine bleeding
- *Contraindications of Centchroman:*
  - PCOD (Stein Leventhal Syndrome)^Q
  - Cervical hyperplasia
  - Recent history of jaundice
  - Severe allergic disease
- *Other features:*
  - Centchroman is also known as *'once-a-week pill'*^Q
  - Centchroman is the *'only anti-implantation agent approved for clinical use'* globally
  - Centchroman has also been found effective as an anti-breast cancer agent

> **Key points**
> Saheli
> *Synthetic NON-STEROIDAL oral contraceptive*

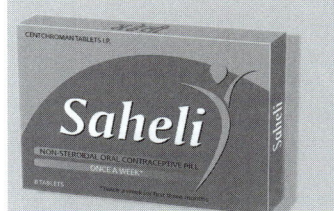
Centchroman (Saheli)

DEPOT Formulations (Injectable Hormones^Q)

- *DMPA (Depot Medroxy Progesterone Acetate):* a Progestogen only Injectable contraceptive (Depot formulation)^Q
  - *Dose:* 150 mg i/m every 3 months^Q
  - *Advantages:*
    - Highly effective

> **Key points**
> Side effects of DEPOT: Disruptions of normal menstrual cycles

- Long lasting and reversible
- Does not affect lactation
- Side effects:
  - Disruptions of normal menstrual cycles^Q
  - Amenorrhoea
- **NET–EN:** Norethisterone Enanthate, a Progestogen only Injectable contraceptive (Depot formulation)^Q
  - *Dose:* 200 mg i/m every 2 months^Q
  - *Advantages:*
    - Highly effective
    - Long lasting and reversible
  - *Side effects:*
    - Disruptions of normal menstrual cycles^Q
    - Amenorrhoea

Norplant

- *NORPLANT:* Subdermal implant contraceptive^Q
  - *6 silastic capsules containing 35 mg LNG each*^Q
  - Norplant R2: 2 capsules containing 75 mg LNG each
- *Mechanism of action:* Capsules or rods are inserted beneath skin of forearm; prevents ovulation
- *Effectiveness:* 5 years
- *Disadvantages:*
  - Irregularities of menstrual bleeding (MC)^Q
  - Surgical procedures require d for insertion and removal

> **Key points**
> **NORPLANT:** 6 silastic capsules containing 35 mg LNG each

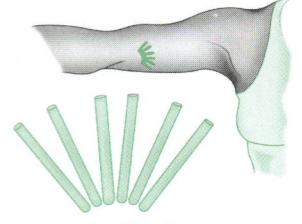

Norplant

EMERGENCY METHODS

Emergency Contraception (EC)

- *EC/Emergency postcoital contraception:* Contraceptive measures that, if taken after sex, may prevent pregnancy^Q
- *Yuzpe and Lancee Method*^Q: Combined oral pills are generally accepted as the preparation of choice for post-coital (emergency) contraception, as it is less likely to cause adverse side effects
  - *Regimens*^Q:
    - *Current recommendation*^Q *(pills with 30 mcg oestrogen):* 4 pills immediately followed by 4 pills 12 hours later
    - *Standard method (pills with 50 mcg oestrogen):* 2 pills immediately followed by 2 pills 12 hours later
    - *Pills with 200 mcg oestrogen:* 1 pill immediately followed by 1 pill 12 hours later
  - Regimens have to be *'completed within 72 hours of coitus'*^Q
    - The sooner started, the more effective it is and the effectiveness more than 72 hours after sexual intercourse is greatly reduced
  - *Method is not guaranteed to prevent pregnancy:*
    - A pregnancy test should be carried out if the period is >3 days late
    - The Regimen does not protect against STDs^Q
  - *Phrase 'morning-after pill' is figurative:* Combined OCPs can be used for up to 72 hours after sexual intercourse
  - *MC side effect reported by users of emergency contraceptive pills:* Nausea
- *Mini Pills (POP):* Progesterone only Pill (POP) 0.75 mg^Q
  - Pill has to be *'used within 72 hours of intercourse* (LNG oral tablet (0.75 mg): 1st tablet within 72 hours of intercourse and 2nd tablet after 12 hours of first dose)^Q
  - Reduces risk of pregnancy by 89%
  - Use in first 24 hours prevent 95% of expected pregnancies
  - POP as an Emergency Contraceptive has showed greater efficacy with reduced side effects and has therefore superseded Yuzpe & Lancee method (WHO)

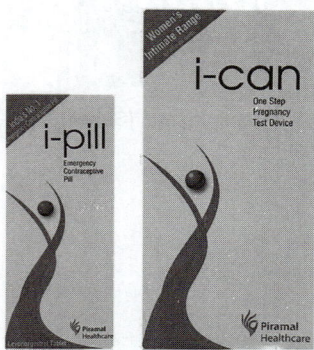

POP Emergency contraceptive

- IUD Insertion: Must be 'inserted within 5 days of coitus'^{Q}
  - Insertion of IUD is more effective than use of Emergency OCPs^Q
- High dose estrogens: Estrogen 5mg OD X 5 days^Q
- Antiprogestogen (Mifepristone RU 486): 600 mg stat within 72 hours of coitus^Q

> **Key points**
>
> **Mini Pills (POP):** Pill has to be *'used within 72 hours of intercourse* (LNG oral tablet (0.75 mg): 1st tablet within 72 hours of intercourse and 2nd tablet after 12 hours of first dose)

STERILIZATION

New Sterilization Guidelines in India 2014

- *Female sterilization:*
  - Married (or ever-married)
  - 22–49 years of age
  - At least one child >1 year age
  - No past history of sterilization of self/spouse
  - Sound mind
  - For mentally-ill:
    - Certified by Psychiatrist
    - Statement on soundness of mind by legal guardian/spouse
  - Service:
    - Minilap by Trained MBBS doctor/DGO/MD (Gynobs)/Surgeons
    - Laparoscopic sterilization by DGO, MD (GynObs) or MS (Surgery)
- *Male sterilization:*
  - Married (or ever-married)
  - <22–60 years of age
  - At least one child >1 year age
  - No past history of sterilization of self/spouse
  - Sound mind
  - For mentally-ill:
    - Certified by Psychiatrist
    - Statement on soundness of mind by legal guardian/spouse
  - Service:
    - Conventional vasectomy by Trained MBBS doctor
    - No-scalpel vasectomy (NSV) by Trained MBBS doctor

Vasectomy

- *Procedure of Vasectomy:*
  - Remove *'minimum 1 cm of vas deferens'*^{Q}
  - Ends are ligated and folded back to themselves
  - Person is NOT sterile UNTIL after 30 ejaculations (3 months) post-vasectomy^Q
  - Open ended Vasectomy:
    - Seals only top end of vas deferens
    - Sperms are free to spill out from the lower severed end of the vas
    - Likelihood of long-term testicular pain from *'backup pressure'* seems to be eliminated using this method
  - **No Scalpel Vasectomy (NSV):** vas is brought out through a tiny puncture which does not require any stitches
    - Also known as *'Key hole vasectomy'*^{Q}
    - Surgical hook (not scalpel) is used to enter the scrotum
    - New safer, convenient technique acceptable to males
    - Nearly painless, less invasive and faster

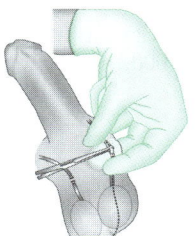
No-scalpel vasectomy

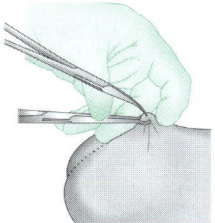
No-scalpel vasectomy

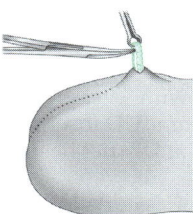
No-scalpel vasectomy

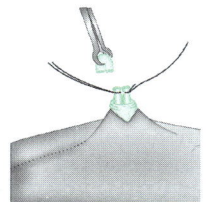
No-scalpel vasectomy

- *Post-operative advice:*
  - Patient need 30 ejaculations after vasectomy, before turning sterile^Q
  - Use of barriers methods till aspermia
  - Avoid bath for 24 hours after operation^Q
  - T-bandage for support for 15 days, keep site dry^Q
  - Avoid cycling, lifting heavy weights for 15 days^Q
  - Stitch removal on 5th day
- *After-effects of vasectomy^Q:*
  - *Operative*: Pain, scrotal hematoma, local infection
  - *Sperm granules*:
    - 7 mm painful mass
    - appears 10–14 days after vasectomy^Q
    - can provide a medium for re-anastomosis of vas
    - using metal clips reduce this problem
  - *Spontaneous recanalization*:
    - seen in 0–6% cases^Q
    - require regular follow-up for 3 years
  - *Autoimmune response*:
    - seen in 54% of vasectomised persons^Q
    - require regular follow-up for 3 years^Q
  - *Psychological*:
    - diminution of sex vigour, impotence,
    - fatigue, headache
  - *Post-Vasectomy Pain Syndrome*: primary long-term complication (permanent feeling)
- Sterilization is the most cost-effective contraceptive measure
  - Vasectomy is overall most cost-eefective: Cost wise ratio is 5 vasectomies to 1 tubectomy
- *Failure of vasectomy:*
  - *MCC in India:* Mistaken identification of vas deferens^Q
  - *Failure rate (Pearl Index):* 0.15 per HWY^Q
  - *Confirmation of successful vasectomy:*
    - Histological confirmation
    - Smear of squeeze of vas by Wright's stain^Q

> **Key points**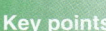
>
> **Failure of vasectomy:** *MCC in India:* Mistaken identification of vas deferens

Tubectomy

Refer to Obstetrics & Gynaecology book for Theory.

NEW INITIATIVES IN FAMILY PLANNING (FP)

Home Delivery of Contraceptives (HDC)

- *Key health functionary*: ASHA worker
- *Delivery charges by ASHA*: ₹ 1/- (3 condom pack), ₹ 1/- (A OCP cycle), ₹ 2/- (A pack of one tablet of Emergency contraceptive pill)

Mission Parivar Vikas (MPV)

- Program to accelerate the use and awareness of FP methods in 146 high TFR districts

Ensuring Spacing at Birth (ESB)

- *Key health functionary*: ASHA worker
- *Counselling charges by ASHA Worker*: ₹ 500/- (Delaying 1st child birth by 2 years after marriage), ₹ 500/- (Ensuring spacing of 3 years after the birth of 1st child), ₹ 1000/- (If couple opts for sterilization up to 2 children)
- *CuT 375*: Short term IUD with 5 years effectivity launched
- Introduction of Post-partum IUD insertion
- Promotion of FP services at District hospitals

Newer Contraceptives

- *Antara*: Injectable Hormonal contraceptive DMPA (Depot medroxyprogesterone acetate)
- *Chhaya*: Oral contraceptive pill 'Centchroman'

Fixed Day Static Services Approach
- Frequency of Sterilization services to be Twice-a-week (District hospital)/Weekly basis (Sub-district hospital), Fortnightly (CHC/Block PHC)/Monthly (24X7 PHC/PHC)

Pregnancy Testing Kits (PTKs)
- *NISCHAY*: Home-based pregnancy testing kits
- *Availability*: Subcentres, ASHA workers

MISCELLANEOUS (FAMILY PLANNING AND CONTRACEPTION)

Non-contraceptive Benefits of Contraceptives
- *Non-contraceptive benefit of Male Condom and Female condom:* Prevention of HIV and STI transmission^Q
- *Non-contraceptive benefit of Combined OCP^Q:*
  - Regularization of irregular menstrual cycles esp. in Stein-Leventhal Syndrome (Polycystic Ovarian Disease – PCOD)
  - *Reduced incidence or improvements in*:
    - Dysmenorrhoea
    - Anemia
    - Acne
    - Hirsutism
    - Ectopic pregnancy
    - Benign breast disease
    - Endometrial cancer
    - Ovarian cysts
    - Ovarian cancer
    - Colorectal cancer
    - Pelvic inflammatory disease (PID)
    - Osteopenia, osteoporosis
- *Non-contraceptive benefit of Centchroman:* Treatment of dysfunctional uterine bleeding (DUB)^Q
- *Non-contraceptive benefit of IUDs^Q:*
  - Synechiolysis in Asherman's Syndrome^Q
  - Reduction of risk of Endometrial cancer
  - Treatment of anemia
  - Treatment of menorrhagia (LNG IUD)
  - Hormone replacement therapy – HRT (LNG IUD)
  - Adjuvant therapy to tamoxifen (LNG IUD)

Medical Termination of Pregnancy Act, 1971^Q
- *Passed in:* April 1972^Q
- *Indications for MTP^Q:*
  - *Humanitarian:* If pregnancy is as a result of rape/sexual assault
  - *Eugenic:^{Q}* Any genetic/chromosomal anomaly detected in fetus
  - *Therapeutic^Q:* If carrying out full term pregnancy poses a risk to life of mother
  - *Social:^{Q}* If pregnancy is a result of contraceptive failure
- *Written consent of guardians:*
  - If woman is a lunatic^Q
  - If woman is less than 18 years age^Q
- *Period of gestation must be 'less than 24 weeks':* ^{Q}
  - 0–20 weeks: Opinion of one doctor is sufficient^Q
  - 20–24 weeks: Opinions of 2 doctors required^Q
- *Who can perform MTP^Q:*
  - *Qualification:* MD (Gyn-Obs) or DGO or 6-months Housemanship in Gyn-Obs
  - *Experience:* At least carried out 20–25 supervised MTPs^Q
- *Where MTP can be done:* At a place authorised by Government of India

> **Key points**
> Medical Termination of Pregnancy Act, 1971^Q
> *Period of gestation must be 'less than 20 weeks'*

MTP Amendment 2020–21
- Rajya Sabha passed the bill that **allows abortion up to 24 weeks** 'for special categories of women', from the existing 20 weeks gestation period (March 2021)
- The upper limit of termination of pregnancy to 20–24 weeks has been extended for 'special categories of women' which will include 'vulnerable women' such as survivors of rape and incest, women with disabilities, minors, etc.
- The bill allows abortion to be done on the advice of one doctor up to 20 weeks (low-risk), and two doctors in the case of certain categories of women between 20 and 24 weeks (high-risk).

Newer Contraceptives
- *Essure:* A permanent sterilization procedure for women (USA)
  - *Mechanism of action:*
    - Micro-inserts are placed into fallopian tubes by a catheter passed from vagina through cervix and uterus
    - Once in place, the device is designed to elicit tissue growth (scarring) in & around micro-insert to form over a period of 3 months an occlusion/blockage in fallopian tubes
    - Tissue barrier formed prevents sperm from reaching an egg
    - Occlusion confirmed by Hysterosalpingogram
    - No general anaesthetic nor incision through the abdomen required
  - *Effectiveness:* 99.80% effective based on 4 years of follow-up
  - *Disadvantages:*
    - Micro-inserts do not prevent the transmission of STIs
    - Ectopic pregnancy
    - Expulsion, perforation of uterus
- *Contraceptive patch: Is a 'transdermal patch'* applied to the skin that releases synthetic estrogen and progestin hormones to prevent pregnancy^Q
  - Have the same effectiveness as the combined OCPs
  - *Composition:* ethinyl estradiol (an estrogen) and norelgestromin (a progestin)
  - 1 patch is applied for 7 days; 3 such patches are applied successively, No patch is applied in the 4th week
  - *Mechanism of action:* Prevention of ovulation
- *Combined hormonal contraceptive vaginal ring:*
  - *Composition:* etonogestrel (a progestin) and ethinyl estradiol
  - *Mechanism of action:* Prevention of ovulation
  - Ring is inserted into vagina for a 3 week period, then removal of the ring for 1 week, during which user will experience menstrual period
  - Muscles of the vagina keep ring securely in place, even during exercise or sex
  - *Benefits of the ring include:*
    - Once-a-month self-administered use offering convenience, ease of use and privacy
    - Lower estrogen exposure than with OCPs or patch
    - Low incidence of estrogenic side effects such as nausea and breast tenderness
    - Low incidence of irregular bleeding.

Newer Contraceptives Introduced under RCH Program^Q
- DMPA 3-monthly Injectable contraceptive (**Antara** Program)
- Centchroman once-a-week non-hormonal contraceptive pill (**Chhaya** Program)
- POP Progesterone only pills for Lactating mothers

Contraception and Adolescence
- Barrier Methods
  - Male condoms give dual protection, against pregnancy as well as STDs (including HIV)
  - Cervical caps and Diaphragms: Not recommended

- Hormonal Contraception:
  - Perfectly suitable, if no cardiovascular problems
  - Completely reversible, No effect on future fertility
  - Developed nations: Pills preferred, Hormonal injections acceptable
- IUD: Theoretically contraindicated
- Other methods: Abstinence, Withdrawal methods, Spermicides not useful

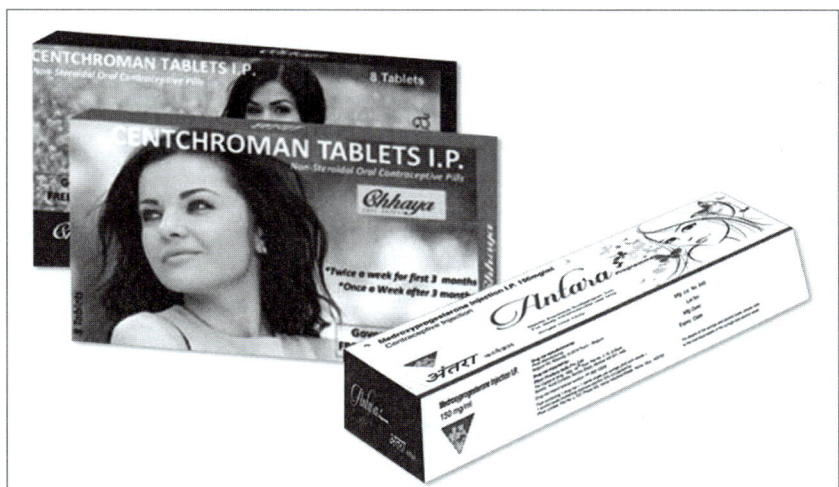

CHAYYA/ANTARA

PYQs: Quick Review for NEET

Demographic Cycle	
In a demographic cycle low stationary phase corresponds to	Fourth stage
India is in Demographic cycle stage	Stage 3 (Declining BR and declining DR)
India is passing through stage of Demographic cycle	III (Late expanding) stage
Census of India	
Census takes place every	10 years
Annual growth rate for India	1.64%
Sex ratio is defined as	No. of females/1000 males (943 in 2011)
Highest Growth Rate in India (Census 2011)	4.51% Dadra & Nagar Haveli
Last Census Stop of India	1st March 2011
Sex ratio of India (Census 2011)	943
First Disability Census in India	1881
The Great Demographic Divide in India	1921
Child sex ratio of India (Census 2011) is	919
State in India with lowest Sex ratio	Haryana
First census in India was done in	1871
First Disability census was done in the year	1881
Literacy rate of India as per Census 2011 is	74.04%
Sex ratio as per 2011 Census	943

Contd...

Contd...

Fertility/Demographic Indices	
Completed family Size represents	TFR (Total Fertility Rate)
2 child norm means	NRR = 1
No. of Eligible Couples in India	150–180 ECs/1000 population
Denominator of Crude birth rate	Mid-year population
Country with Highest Life Expectancy	Japan 83.7 (M: 80 years; F: 87 years)
Life expectancy in India	68.3 years (M: 67 years; F: 70 years)
% Geriatric population in India	8.1%
If annual growth rate is 1.5–2%, population doubles in	35–47 years
Birth rate is	Live birth/1000 mid-year population
Infant Mortality rate formula	No. of infant deaths per 1000 Live births
IMR of Japan	2 per 1000 LB
Mortality is included in TFR/ GRR/ NRR	NRR (Net reproduction rate)
Population growth is 'Explosive' if Annual growth rate is	>2.0%
Growth rate proportional to functions' current value	Exponential growth
Denominator of GFR	Women in reproductive age group (15–49 years)
Spindle-shaped Age pyramid denotes	Developed country
Denominator age group for calculation of Dependency ratio	15–65 years
Approximate magnitude of Completed family size is	Total fertility rate (TFR)
Children borne by female at the end of reproductive period	TFR
Best indicator of fertility	Net reproduction rate (NRR)
NFHS-3 was carried out in	2005
National family health survey is done once every	5 years
Second National Family Health Survey was done in	1998–99
SRS for both death and birth enumeration is once every	6 months
Mid-year population is estimated on	1st July
Mid-year population is calculated by	Arithmetic mean of population at 1st and 31st December
Family planning and Contraception	
Conventional Contraceptives include	Condoms/Spermicides
Progestasert (3rd gen IUD) releases	65 mcg/day Progesterone
MC complaint of IUD insertion is	Bleeding
Only Non-steroidal OCP	Centchroman (Saheli)
MTP Act, 1971 was passed in	April 1972
For sterilization, age of Husband should be	22–60 years
Contraceptive Efficacy/failure is measured by	Pearl index (____/HWY)
Failure rate of condoms	2–14 per HWY
WHO Oligospermia Sperm Count	Less than 15 million/mL
Unmet need for Family planning in India is highest for	Adolescents
MC side effect of Depot contraceptives	Irregular menstrual bleeding
Carcinoma protected by OCPs	Ovarian carcinoma
Numerator of Pearl Index	No. of accidental gestations
Condom failure occurs due to mainly	Incorrect use
Shelf life of CuT 380 A	10 years
Ideal contraceptive for newly married couple	Combined OCPs
Combined OCPs increase risk of carcinoma of	Breasts

Contd...

Contd...

Couple with wife 15–49 years is	Eligible couple
To achieve NRR = 1, CPR must be raised above	60%
Combined OCPs contain	Ethinyl estradiol + Norgestrel
Pearl Index is	Failures per 100 women-years of exposure
"Pearl Index" Is normally used for studying the	Failure rate/ Efficacy of contraceptive
TODAY, failure rate is	9–20/100 women year
Radio-opaque material in Copper-T	Barium sulphate
Minipill is contraceptive of choice for	Lactating females
Depot contraceptive DMPA is to be given every	3 months
Dose of Ethinyl estradiol in Mala-N	30 mcg
Dose of Levonorgestrel estradiol in Mala-N	150 mcg
MC sterilization practiced in India	Female sterilization
Failure rate of Pomeroy's technique of sterilization	0.1–0.5%
Family planning services were voluntary in India from	1977
Spermicide used in the contraceptive "TODAY"	Non-oxynol-9
IUD with maximum expulsion rate	Lippes loop
Least failure rate is seen in _____ IUD	LNG-IUD

Multiple Choice Questions

DEMOGRAPHY

DEMOGRAPHIC CYCLE AND PROCESSES

1. Demographic Gap attains its maximum limit in: [AIIMS May 2005]
   (a) Early Stage I
   (b) Late Stage II
   (c) Late Stage III
   (d) Early Stage IV

2. True about late expanding phase of demographic cycle: [NEET Pattern 2013] [AIPGME, 2004–09]
   (a) Birth rate is lower than the death rate
   (b) Death rate begins to decline, while the birth rate remains unchanged
   (c) Death rate declines still further, and the birth rate tends to fall
   (d) High birth rate and high death rate

3. Contraction of Demographic-Gap starts in: [AIIMS Nov 2005, Nov 05]
   (a) Stage I
   (b) Late Stage II
   (c) Early Stage III
   (d) Stage IV

4. In which stage of the demographic cycle is India currently? [NEET Pattern 2013] [AIIMS Dec 1997] [Karnataka 2004] [MP 2002, MH 2007, RJ 2002]
   (a) High stationary
   (b) Late expanding
   (c) Early stationary
   (d) Low stationary

5. 'Demographic Processes' does not include: [AIIMS Sep 1996]
   (a) Fertility
   (b) Morbidity
   (c) Mortality
   (d) Social mobility

6. Movement at socio-economic level is: [AIPGME 2010] [NEET Patterns 2013, 2017]
   (a) Social equality
   (b) Social mobility
   (c) Socio-economic upliftment
   (d) Social mobilization

7. Late expanding stage of population in India is due to? [AIIMS May 2011]
   (a) Birth rate stationary death rate continues to fall
   (b) Death rate declines faster than birth rate
   (c) Birth rate declines, death rate same
   (d) Birth rate is less than birth rate

8. True about Demographic cycle of India is/are: [PGI 2017]
   (a) Entered into low stationary phase
   (b) Dependency ratio <40%
   (c) Year of Big divide is 1921 AD
   (d) Population pyramid has a broad base and a tapering top
   (e) First regular census in India was carried in 1881

BIRTH RATE, DEATH RATE AND GROWTH RATE

9. At current growth rate, India's population will double in: [AIPGME 1992–1997]
   (a) 23–28 years
   (b) 28–35 years
   (c) 35–47 years
   (d) 47–70 years

10. Current annual growth rate of a population can be calculated by: [AIIMS Dec 1995]
    (a) Crude birth rate (CBR) minus Crude death rate (CDR)
    (b) Crude death rate (CDR) minus Crude birth rate (CBR)
    (c) Decadal growth rate/10
    (d) Crude birth rate (CBR) plus Crude death rate (CDR)

11. Crude birth rate is a simplest measure of fertility because it includes: [Karnataka 2006]
    (a) Total population
    (b) Mid year population
    (c) Live births only
    (d) Pre-term births

12. Which countries have a higher growth rate than India? [PGI June 08]
    (a) Myanmar
    (b) Nepal
    (c) Sri Lanka
    (d) Bangladesh

13. Crude birth rate – NOT true is: [AIIMS May 2010]
    (a) It is a measure of fertility
    (b) It is actually a ratio not a rate
    (c) It is independent of age of population
    (d) Numerator does not include still births

14. In a community of 5000 people, the crude birth rate is 30 per 1000 people. The number of pregnant females is? [NEET Pattern 2013, 2016]
    (a) 150
    (b) 165
    (c) 175
    (d) 200

15. What is exponential growth? [NEET Pattern 2013]
    (a) Rapid growth in population that leads to misbalance in birth and deaths
    (b) Slow growth rate
    (c) Growth limited by limiting factors
    (d) None of the above

Review Questions

16. Denominator of crude birth rate is: [UP 2000, MP 2000]
    (a) Mid year population
    (b) Number of living children
    (c) Number of death children
    (d) Total number of crude birth

17. Age pyramid of India is: [NEET Pattern 2012] [MH 2000]
    (a) Broad at base and narrow at apex
    (b) Broad from base to apex
    (c) Broad at apex and narrow at base
    (d) All

POPULATION PYRAMID

18. In India women in child-bearing (15–44 years) age group constitute …% of the population: [AIIMS Dec 1997]
    (a) 10   (b) 15
    (c) 22   (d) 35

19. The carrying capacity of any given population is determined by its: [AIIMS May 05]
    (a) Population growth rate
    (b) Birth rate
    (c) Death rate
    (d) Limiting resource

20. Reproductive age group in India contributes to total population as about: [AIIMS June 1997]
    (a) 26%   (b) 37%
    (c) 51%   (d) 66%

SEX RATIO AND DEPENDENCY RATIO

21. As per 2011 census, sex ratio is: [NEET Pattern 2014]
    (a) 940   (b) 933
    (c) 927   (d) 104

22. For a population of 10000, sex ratio of more than 1000 means: [AIIMS Nov 2003]
    (a) Males are less than 500
    (b) Females are less than 500
    (c) Males are less than 5000
    (d) Females are less than 5000

23. Community X has 30% below 15 yrs of age and 10% over 65 years of age. Dependency ratio for community X is: [AIIMS May 2002][NEET Pattern 2012, 2015]
    (a) 20%   (b) 40%
    (c) 66.6%   (d) 3%

24. Dependency ratio includes: [PGI June 05]
    (a) 0–5 yrs age   (b) 6–14 yrs age
    (c) 15–45 yrs age (d) >65 yrs

25. Potential Support Ratio (PSR) is defined as: [AP 2014]
    (a) Number of persons aged 15 to 65 per children below 15 years
    (b) Number of persons aged 15 to 65 per one older person aged >/= 65 years
    (c) Number of person aged 15 to 65 per one older person aged >65 and younger person <15 years
    (d) Number of persons aged 15 to 65 persons older person aged >60 and younger person <15 years

Review Question

26. All are true about sex ratio *except*: [MP 2001]
    (a) Kerala is the state where it is not adverse for women
    (b) Since 1901 it is unfavourable for women
    (c) Since 1901 there is steadily decreasing trend
    (d) It is determined by sex composition of population affected by differentials in mortality conditions of male and females, sex selective migration and sex ratio at birth

LITERACY AND LIFE EXPECTANCY

27. The denominator used for calculating literacy rate of Indian population (Census 2001) is: [DPG 2005] [AIIMS Nov 2003]
    (a) Total mid-year population
    (b) Population age 7 years or more
    (c) School going population
    (d) Population age 18 years or more

28. Effective literacy rate is calculated from: [AIIMS PGMEE November 2013]
    (a) Those above age of 7 years
    (b) Those who have completed 10 year schooling
    (c) Those who have completed 15 year schooling
    (d) Total population

29. A community has total population 10000. Children ranging 0–6 years are 2000. Literate persons among >7 years old are 4000. What is effective literacy rate? [NEET Pattern 2016]
    (a) 20%   (b) 40%
    (c) 50%   (d) 60%

FERTILITY

30. If the total fertility rate in India is 2.2, the crude birth rate would be: [AIPGME 1996]
    (a) 18.6 per 1000 population
    (b) 19.2 per 1000 population
    (c) 22.4 per 1000 population
    (d) 26.2 per 1000 population

31. Which of the following is the national level system that provides annual national as well as state level reliable estimates of fertility and mortality?
 [AIIMS Nov 96, 03, AIIMS May 05]
   (a) Civil registration system
   (b) Census
   (c) Ad-hoc survey
   (d) Sample registration system

32. The number of live birth per 1000 women in the reproductive age group in a year refers to:
 [AIIMS Nov 03, Dec 1997]
 [NEET Pattern 2012, 2014, 2018]
   (a) Total fertility rate
   (b) Gross Reproduction Rate
   (c) Net Reproduction Rate
   (d) General Fertility Rate

33. If TFR in a population is 4 per woman, the GRR approx. would be: [AIIMS Dec 1991, RJ 2006]
   (a) 2
   (b) 4
   (c) 8
   (d) 16

34. Total fertility rate: [PGI Dec 2K]
   (a) Total no. of children born to a woman in a given yr
   (b) Measure of completed family size
   (c) Sum of fertility of all age
   (d) No of female child born to mother
   (e) Total no of child born to mother

35. Population growth is said to be less than adequate requirement when NRR is: [PGI June 03]
   (a) <1
   (b) = 1
   (c) >1
   (d) = 0

36. Which of the following indicators involve reproductive woman: [PGI June 04]
   (a) Birth Rate
   (b) G.F.R.
   (c) T.F.R
   (d) Maternal mortality rate

37. Demographers are of the view that the demographic goal of NRR = 1 can be achieved only if the couple protection rate exceeds: [Karnataka 2011]
 [DNB 2011, MH 2008]
 [NEET Pattern 2018]
   (a) 40%
   (b) 50%
   (c) 60%
   (d) 70%

38. General fertility rate is: [NEET Pattern 2013]
   (a) Indicator of complete family size
   (b) Measure of fertility
   (c) Not better than crude birth rate
   (d) All of the above

39. Which of the following includes mortality rate in it?
 [PGI 1998, UP 2004, NEET Pattern 2012]
   (a) TFR
   (b) GFR
   (c) NRR
   (d) GRR

40. What is net reproduction rate? [NEET Pattern 2013, 2015]
   (a) No. of children a newborn girl has in her left time
   (b) No. of female children a newborn girl has in her life time
   (c) No. of male children a newborn girl has in her life time
   (d) No. of female children a newborn girl has in her life time taking into account mortality

41. Average number of girls that would be born to a woman if she experiences the current fertility pattern throughout her reproductive span assuming no mortality' is known as [PGMCET 2015]
   (a) General Fertility Rate
   (b) Total Fertility Rate
   (c) Gross Reproduction Rate
   (d) Net Reproduction Rate

Review Question

42. General fertility rate:
 [NEET Pattern 2013, Bihar 2003, UP 2004]
   (a) It is the number of live births per 1000 women in the reproductive age group in a given year
   (b) It is a better measure of fertility than crude birth rate
   (c) The major weakness of this rate is that not all women in the denominator are exposed to the risk of child birth
   (d) All of the above

MISCELLANEOUS (DEMOGRAPHY)

43. MULTIPLE RESPONSE TYPE QUESTION: The source for causes of Death data in India include
   1. Sample registration system
   2. Census
   3. Death declaration and Medical certification
   4. Lay information

   Use the following key to mark correct answer
 [AIIMS May 2019]
   (a) 1, 3
   (b) 2, 4
   (c) 1, 2, 3, 4
   (d) 1, 3, 4

44. Births in India must be registered within:
 [AIPGME 1994]
   (a) 7 days
   (b) 14 days
   (c) 21 days
   (d) 1 month

45. Percentage of people below poverty line in India:
   (a) 14%
   (b) 22% [AIIMS May 05]
   (c) 29%
   (d) 72%

46. National Family Health Survey has successfully completed: [AIIMS May 05]
    (a) One rounds
    (b) Two rounds
    (c) Three rounds
    (d) Four rounds

47. The age and sex structure of a population may be described by a: [AIIMS Nov 03, AIIMS May 05]
    (a) Life table
    (b) Correlation coefficient
    (c) Population pyramid
    (d) Bar chart

48. What is the best determinant of the health status of a country? [AIIMS May 94, 2001]
    (a) CPR
    (b) IMR
    (c) MMR
    (d) CDR

49. By 2015, Indian city likely to join group of Mega cities (Delhi, Mumbai, Kolkata) is: [AIPGME 2002]
    (a) Chennai
    (b) Ahmedabad
    (c) Hyderabad
    (d) Pune

50. WHO defines adolescent age between: [AIPGME 2005] [PGI November 2014]
    (a) 10–19 years of age
    (b) 10–14 years of age
    (c) 10–25 years of age
    (d) 9–14 years of age

51. Which is/are true for Kerala in relation to India?
    (a) High literacy rate [PGI May 2012]
    (b) High Doctor: Population ratio
    (c) High growth rate
    (d) Older age of marriage
    (e) Higher Life expectancy

52. A child is born to an Indian couple outside India. Birth registration must be done: [NEET Pattern 2014]
    (a) Within 21 days
    (b) Within 21 days of arrival into India
    (c) Within 60 days
    (d) Within 60 days of arrival into India

53. State used as Yardstick-of-health in India is [NEET Pattern 2015]
    (a) Tamil Nadu
    (b) Kerala
    (c) Andhra Pradesh
    (d) Gujarat

54. Vital statistics in a population include [NEET Pattern 2016]
    (a) Sex ratio
    (b) Age composition
    (c) Birth rate
    (d) Dependency ratio

55. National population stabilization fund is aimed at achieving population stabilization at a level consistent with the needs of sustainable economic growth, social development and environment protection by: [NEET Pattern 2016]
    (a) 2030
    (b) 2015
    (c) 2040
    (d) 2045

56. Dual record system is useful for estimation of: [NEET Pattern 2017]
    (a) Literacy
    (b) Fertility
    (c) Population density
    (d) Sex ratio

57. Sample registration is done [NEET Pattern 2017]
    (a) Every 3 months
    (b) Every 6 months
    (c) Every 9 months
    (d) Every 12 months

Review Questions

58. Which of the following year in the history of demography of India is India is known as the year of big divide: [NEET Pattern 2012] [MP 2002] [NEET Pattern 2014, 2016]
    (a) 1881
    (b) 1921
    (c) 1947
    (d) 1978

59. The system of collection of data to give national and sub-national estimate of vital indicators consist of continuous enumeration backed by 6 months survey is: [MH 2003]
    (a) Model registration survey
    (b) National sample survey
    (c) Sample registration survey
    (d) National family health survey

60. Which one of the following is a DUAL RECORD SYSTEM consisting of continuous enumeration of birth and death by numerator and which indicates survey every 6 months? [MH 2008]
    (a) Sample registration system
    (b) Civil registration system
    (c) Census
    (d) Model registration system

FAMILY PLANNING AND CONTRACEPTION

CONCEPTS OF FAMILY PLANNING

61. Contraceptive of choice for a Newly married couple is [NEET PG Pattern 2023]
    (a) Condoms
    (b) Combined OCPs
    (c) CuT
    (d) DMPA

62. Contraceptive failure is assessed using which of the following methods? [INICET November 2022]
    (a) Pharmacological index
    (b) Pearl index
    (c) Performance index
    (d) Efficacy index

63. A contraceptive 'Z' is used by 100 couples for a continuous period of 2 years. During this period 20 women become pregnant despite using the contraceptive 'Z'. What is the Pearl Index of 'Z'? [AIPGME 1993] [NEET Pattern 2018]
    (a) 0.1 per HWY
    (b) 5 per HWY
    (c) 10 per HWY
    (d) 1000 per HWY

64. Contraceptive efficacy is measured by: [AIIMS Dec 1995, Nov 2008]
    (a) Pearl Index only
    (b) Pearl Index and Life table analysis
    (c) Life table analysis and Couple protection rate
    (d) Pearl Index and Couple protection rate

65. Eligible couples per 1000 population in India is: [AIPGME 2002]
    (a) 50–70
    (b) 100–120
    (c) 150–180
    (d) 200–250

66. In a village with 180 eligible couples, Family Planning data of contraceptive methods is:
    • Sterilization: Vasectomy - 3 and Tubectomy - 8
    • IUD users - 10
    • Orals pills users - 10
    • Condom users - 29
    Effective CPR in the village is: [AIPGME 2004]
    (a) 60%
    (b) 33%
    (c) 25%
    (d) 10%

67. Which of the following is important in calculation of pearl index:
    (a) Number of abortions
    (b) Total accidental pregnancy
    (c) Socioeconomic status
    (d) Total gestational period

68. Pearl index is defined as: [NEET Pattern 2012, 2013]
    (a) Accidental pregnancies per 1000 women-years of exposure
    (b) Accidental pregnancies per 100 women-years of exposure
    (c) Accidental pregnancies per 10 women-years of exposure
    (d) Accidental pregnancies per women-years of exposure

69. Unmet need for contraception in a 35-year-old female is for [NEET Pattern 2016]
    (a) Spacing birth
    (b) Limiting birth
    (c) Improve maternal health
    (d) Improve family health

70. Pearl Index of 10 per HWY for a Contraceptive 'C' in a population. An average woman in this population is expected to have how many accidental pregnancies in her reproductive life span? [NEET Pattern 2017]
    (a) 1.5
    (b) 2.5
    (c) 3.5
    (d) 4.5

71. If 100 women experience 20 accidental pregnancies after using a contraceptive method for 2 years each, Pearl index is: [JIPMER November 2017]
    (a) 0.1 per 100 women years
    (b) 100 per 1000 woman years
    (c) 10 accidental pregnancies per 1000 woman years using contraceptives
    (d) 10 accidental pregnancies per 100 woman years using contraceptives

72. Contraceptive failure 10/100 women years means [JIPMER November 2017]
    (a) 0.1 accidental pregnancy per 100 woman year using contraceptives
    (b) 100 accidental pregnancy per 1000 woman years using contraceptives
    (c) 10 accidental pregnancy per 1000 woman year using contraceptives
    (d) 10 accidental pregnancy per 100 woman year using contraceptives

Review Questions

73. All parameters are used by epidemiologist in evaluation of the efficacy of acceptance of family planning method except: [DNB 2002]
    (a) Annual general marriage rate
    (b) Spacing between first and second child
    (c) Annual birth rate
    (d) Number of children born

74. Population control can be achieved by: [MP 2002]
    (a) By spacing between the pregnancies
    (b) By promoting infanticide
    (c) By prohibiting infanticide
    (d) Securing maximum involvement of non-governmental agencies

75. The couple protection rate (CPR) to bring within normal range in India, which of the following contraceptive measure is used? [MH 2005]
    (a) Sterilization
    (b) IUCD
    (c) Condom
    (d) All of the above

NATURAL METHODS

76. Natural Family Planning does not include:
    (a) Terminal methods [AIPGME 1994]
    (b) Basal Body Temperature Method
    (c) Cervical Mucus Method
    (d) Symptothermic Method

77. False regarding Calendar method of contraception is [NEET Pattern 2016]
    (a) Abstinence required only for few days of month
    (b) Associated with no costs
    (c) Safe period can also be observed using temperature rhythm or cervical mucus method
    (d) Ectopic pregnancy is a reported complication

Review Question

78. Which of the following Natural method of contraception is most effective? [MPSC 2006; MH 2008]
    (a) Calendar method
    (b) Billing method
    (c) Symptothermic method
    (d) Basal body temperature method

BARRIER METHODS

79. Match the contraceptive and its type:

Contraceptive		Type of contraceptive
A.	Vaginal Sponge	I. Subdermal implant
B.	Norplant	II. Barrier Method
C.	NET–EN	III. IUD
D.	Grafenberg's Ring	IV. Depot formulation

(a) A - IV, B - II, C - III, D - I [AIIMS Dec 1995]
(b) A - II, B - I, C - IV, D – III
(c) A - II, B - IV, C - I, D – III
(d) A - III, B - II, C - I, D – IV

80. Condom vending machine at petrol pump in high prevalence area is example of: [NEET Pattern 2016]
(a) Appropriate technology
(b) Social marketing
(c) Socialization
(d) Community participation

Review Question

81. 'Today' – a contraceptive contains: [DNB 2003, 2004]
(a) Prestaglandin F_2
(b) Norethisterone
(c) 9-Nonoxynol
(d) Cu releasing mesh

IUDs

82. Copper-T is contraindicated in [NEET PG Pattern 2022]
(a) Menstruation
(b) Broken condom
(c) Trophoblastic disease
(d) Post-partum immediately after delivery

83. Choice of contraception in women with heart disease is: [AIIMS June 2020]
(a) IUCD
(b) Mala N
(c) Inj. DMPA
(d) Condom

84. In Cu-T 380 A, 380 represents: [AIGPME 1997, PGI 2006]
(a) No. of turns of copper wire
(b) Surface area of Cu-T in sq. mm
(c) Surface area of copper in sq. mm
(d) Effective Life of Cu-T in quarters

85. The most common side effect of IUD insertion is: [AIPGME 2005] [NEET PATTERN 2018]
(a) Bleeding
(b) Pain
(c) Pelvic infection
(d) Ectopic pregnancy

86. All are true about Progestasert except: [AIPGME 2004]
(a) Progestasert releases 65 mcg progesterone per day
(b) Progestasert contains 38 mg progesterone
(c) Progestasert is implanted subdermally
(d) Progestasert is a T-shaped device

87. The most common side effect of IUD insertion, which requires its removal is: [AIIMS Nov 1992, 1996]
(a) Bleeding [AIIMS Sep 1997]
(b) Pain
(c) Pelvic infection
(d) Ectopic pregnancy

88. Characteristics of an ideal candidate for copper–T insertion include all of the following except: [AIIMS Nov 2005, Nov 02]
(a) Has borne at least one child
(b) Is willing to check IUD tail
(c) Has a history of ectopic pregnancy
(d) Has normal menstrual periods

89. Copper–T is preferably inserted postnatal, after: [Karnataka 2005]
(a) 2 weeks
(b) 4 weeks
(c) 5 weeks
(d) 8 weeks

90. Cu T 380A IUD should be replaced once in: [DNB 2008] [DNB June 2010] [NEET Pattern 2013, UPSC CMS 2015]
(a) 4 yrs
(b) 6 yrs
(c) 8 yrs
(d) 10 yrs

91. IUD 'Mirena' release Levonorgestrel for ………. years: [NEET Pattern 2014]
(a) 3
(b) 5
(c) 7
(d) 10

92. Mechanism of action of IUD is: [CGPG 2015]
(a) Prevent fertilization
(b) Prevention ovulation
(c) Prevent implantation
(d) Spermicidal

93. Third generation IUCD is: [NEET Pattern 2015]
(a) ML CuT 250
(b) MIRENA
(c) CuT 380 A
(d) Copper -7

94. Ideal candidate for IUCD include all except:
(a) Willing to check thread [NEET Pattern 2015]
(b) Have normal menstrual cycle
(c) No history of PID
(d) Who have minimum 2 children

95. Mechanism of IUCD all except: [NEET Pattern 2015]
(a) Increase cervical mucus
(b) Local foreign body like reaction
(c) Decrease diameter of fallopian tube
(d) Make endometrium unfavourable for implantation

Review Questions

96. True statements of Nova-T: [Kerala 2003, UP 2004]
(a) Effective for 10 years [Bihar 2003]
(b) Silver core
(c) More copper content
(d) More chances of perforation

97. All of the following are the advantages of 3rd generation IUD's *except*: [AP 2007]
    (a) High efficacy
    (b) Low expulsion rates
    (c) Long acting
    (d) Low risk of ectopic pregnancy

98. Third generation IUCD acts by: [MP 2003]
    (a) Strong anti-fertility effect of metallic copper
    (b) By altering the composition of cervical mucous
    (c) Hormonal effect on mucosa of endometrium
    (d) Enhanced cellular response on endometrium

99. Absolute contraindication of IUCD is: [RJ 2001]
    (a) Anemia   (b) Diabetes
    (c) PID   (d) Hemorrhage

100. Multi load device refers to: [RJ 2008]
    (a) First generation IUCD
    (b) Second generation IUCD
    (c) Oral contraceptive pills
    (d) Barrier contraceptives

HORMONAL METHODS

101. A 24-year-old female with 18 months baby on breast feed has heavy irregular bleeding on mensuration. What is best contraception advisable? [NEET PG Pattern 2022]
    (a) Mala N
    (b) Progestasert
    (c) CuT 380 A
    (d) Depot formulation

102. A 25-year-old female patient is started on ATT under RNTCP. She was currently using Combined OCPs as a Contraceptive method. Doctor advises her to add barrier method as an additional precaution. What is the underlying reason? [NEET PG Pattern September 2021]
    (a) Isoniazid induces OCP metabolism
    (b) Isoniazid failure is caused by OCP
    (c) Rifampicin induces OCP metabolism
    (d) OCP induces Rifampicin action

103. A 25-year-old woman has been taking OCPs gave a history of 4 missed pills on different days over last 7 weeks. Next line of management is [NEET PG Pattern September 2021]
    (a) Take next pill as soon as possible and consider barrier method/emergency contraception if had intercourse in last 72 hours
    (b) Take 4 pills as soon as possible and consider barrier method/emergency contraception if had intercourse in last 72 hours
    (c) Adopt another method of contraception
    (d) Disregard the current pack and start a new cycle of pack

104. Consider the following sentence:
    Use of oral contraceptive pills confers additional protection against [AIIMS Nov 2005]
    I. Fibroadenoma
    II. Ectopic pregnancy
    III. Ovarian cysts and iron deficiency anemia
    Which of these statements are correct?
    (a) I and II   (b) I and III
    (c) II and III   (d) I, II and III

105. If a women was taking oral contraceptive pill, then which of the following investigation would be related to the long term consumption of steroidal contraceptives?
    1. Liver functions test [AIIMS Nov 2002]
    2. Cervical pap smear
    3. Wet smear of vaginal secretions for monilial
    4. Endometrial biopsy
    (a) 2, 3 and 4   (b) 1, 3 and 4
    (c) 1, 2 and 4   (d) 1, 2 and 3

106. Besides pregnancy the oral contraceptive protect against all *except*: [AIPGME 1995] [NEET Pattern 2019]
    (a) Fibroadenoma breast
    (b) Iron deficiency anemia
    (c) Ovarian cancer
    (d) Hepatocellular adenoma
    (e) Thromboembolism

107. How much ethinyl estradiol does the new low dose oral contraceptive pill contain (IN MICROGRAMS)? [AIPGME 2005]
    (a) 20   (b) 25
    (c) 30   (d) 35

108. Which one of the following is NOT an absolute contraindication for oral contraceptive pills? [AIPGME 2008]
    (a) Nursing mothers
    (b) Cancer of breasts
    (c) Cardiac abnormalities
    (d) History of thromboembolism

109. Mala – N oral contraceptive pill differs from Mala–D, in terms of: [Karnataka 2005]
    (a) Norgestrol dosage
    (b) Oestradiol dosage
    (c) Sold under social marketing scheme
    (d) Supplied free of cost

110. Contraindication of OCP: [PGI June 04]
    (a) Liver disease   (b) PID
    (c) Renal disease   (d) Epilepsy (A, C, D)

111. Which of the following is/are benefits of combined OCPs use? [PGI November 2013]
    (a) Hepatocellular adenoma
    (b) PID
    (c) Ovarian cysts
    (d) Fibrocystic disease of breast
    (e) Ectopic pregnancy

112. A woman using combined oral contraceptive has the following non-contraceptive benefits except: [UPSC CMS 2015]
    (a) Protection against PID
    (b) Prevention of colorectal malignancy
    (c) Protection against ovarian cancer
    (d) Protection against cervical cancer

113. A woman on combined OCPs forgot taking them on 2 successive doses. Next line of management is: [NEET Pattern 2015]
    (a) Continue next pill next day onwards
    (b) Take 3 pills next day, then shift to one pill per day
    (c) Shift to barrier methods of contraception
    (d) Take 2 pills each for rest of the cycle

Review Questions

114. Oral contraceptive cause: [DNB 2001]
    (a) Monilial vaginitis
    (b) Pituitary adenoma
    (c) Ca uterus
    (d) Ovarian cysts

115. Non-contraceptive effect of oral contraceptive pills is all except: [UP 2001]
    (a) Protection against benign breast disease
    (b) Prevention of ectopic pregnancy
    (c) Dysmenorrhoea protection
    (d) Iron-deficiency anemia

116. Serious complication of oral contraceptive is: [UP 2006]
    (a) Leg vein thrombosis
    (b) Headache
    (c) Break through bleeding
    (d) Breast tenderness

117. A health worker who distributes OC pills — checks all of the following except: [AP 2001]
    (a) Headache
    (b) Weight gain
    (c) Breast tenderness
    (d) Pervaginal bleeding

118. The absolute contraindication for prescribing normal contraceptive pills in a woman of reproductive age group is: [MP 2008]
    (a) Epilepsy
    (b) Diabetes mellitus
    (c) Milk hypertension
    (d) Congenital hyperlipidemia

119. Minipills contain: [RJ 2006]
    (a) Only progesterone is small quantity
    (b) Progesterone and estrogen
    (c) Estrogen in small quantity and progesterone in large
    (d) Estrogen

120. DMPA is an injectable contraceptive given every: [RJ 2007] [DNB 2004]
    (a) Three weeks
    (b) Two months
    (c) Three months
    (d) Two years

EMERGENCY METHODS

121. Emergency contraception commonly used in India [INICET November 2021]
    (a) Levonorgestrel dose 1.5 mg
    (b) Ulipristal acetate 30 mg
    (c) Combined OCPs
    (d) Oestrogen dose 1 mcg

122. Which of the following cannot be used as Post-coital contraceptive? [NEET PG Pattern January 2020]
    (a) Danazol
    (b) CuT 200
    (c) RU 486
    (d) High dose estrogens

123. All of the following can be used as emergency contraceptive measures except: [AIIMS Nov 1992]
    (a) Female condoms
    (b) IUD
    (c) Minipill
    (d) Yuzpe and Lancee

124. Yuzpe and Lancee Method is used for: [AIIMS May 1992]
    (a) Sterilization with 'No Scalpel Technique'
    (b) Emergency contraception with OCPs
    (c) Emergency contraception with IUDs
    (d) Evaluation of newer contraceptives

125. Which of the following is not used as an emergency contraceptive?
    (a) LNG- Intrauterine device
    (b) Oral LNG
    (c) CuT-Intrauterine device
    (d) Oral Mifepristone

126. Yuzpee and Lancee regimen must be administered within maximum [NEET Pattern 2015]
    (a) 3 hours
    (b) 12 hours
    (c) 24 hours
    (d) 72 hours

127. What is the Drug of choice for Emergency contraception? [ESI IMO 2014]
    (a) Yuzpe regimen (combined oral pill)
    (b) High dose oestrogen alone
    (c) Levonorgestrel only pill
    (d) Danazol

Review Question

128. Post coital contraceptives are all except: [MP 2000]
    (a) Norgestrel
    (b) OCPs
    (c) RU-486
    (d) Copper-T

STERILIZATION

129. Following vasectomy for family planning. A patient should be advised to use some other method of contraception, till: [RJ 2007]
    (a) Removal of all sutures
    (b) Pain completely sutures
    (c) Two weeks
    (d) Eight weeks

130. A case of vasectomy is said to have failed as the vasectomised person's wife gives birth to a child ten months after the operation. Which one of the following is the most probable cause? [DPG 2011]
    (a) Failure of the husband to use condom after vasectomy
    (b) Surgical failure
    (c) Recanalisation
    (d) Wife had extramarital contact

131. Ideal time to perform post partum sterilization as per Government of India guidelines is: [UPSC CMS 2015]
    (a) From 12 hours to 7 days of delivery
    (b) From 24 hours to 7 days of delivery
    (c) From 48 hours to 7 days of delivery
    (d) Within 7 days of delivery

MISCELLANEOUS (FAMILY PLANNING AND CONTRACEPTION)

132. All are long-term and reversible contraceptive except: [INICET November 2021]
    (a) Tubal sterilization
    (b) Implanon
    (c) IUCD
    (d) LNG IUD

133. Which of the following statements is incorrect? [AIIMS May 1992]
    (a) IUDs predispose to PID and Actinomycosis
    (b) OCPs protect against Candidiasis
    (c) Condoms are protective against PID
    (d) Female condoms protect against STDs and HIV

134. Increased incidence of ectopic is associated with all except: [AIPGME 1995]
    (a) IUD
    (b) Combined oral pills
    (c) Menstrual regulation
    (d) Safe period method

135. Conventional Contraceptives are those which: [AIPGME 1996]
    (a) Were discovered before 1960
    (b) Require action after intercourse
    (c) Require action at time of intercourse
    (d) Require action before intercourse

136. All are Socio-demographic Goals of National Population Policy except: [AIIMS Nov 2004]
    (a) Achieve 100% institutional deliveries
    (b) Reduce MMR to <100 per Lac LBs
    (c) Achieve 100% registration of births, deaths, marriages and pregnancies
    (d) Prevent and control communicable diseases

137. The National Population Policy of India has set the following goals except: [AIIMS Nov 2008]
    (a) To bring down Total Fertility Rate (TFR) to replacement levels by 2015
    (b) To reduce the Infant Mortality Rate to 30 per 1000 live births
    (c) To reduce the Maternal Mortality Rate to 100 per 100,000 live births
    (d) 100 percent registration of births, deaths, marriages and pregnancies

138. Conventional contraceptive includes one of the following: [AIIMS May 1994]
    (a) Condom
    (b) Copper-T
    (c) Oral pills
    (d) Tubectomy

139. The Medical Termination of Pregnancy Act does not protect act of termination of pregnancies after: [Karnataka 2005] [NEET Pattern 2014]
    (a) 20 weeks
    (b) 24 weeks
    (c) 28 weeks
    (d) 30 weeks

140. Best contraceptive for a newly married healthy couple:
    (a) Barrier method [AIIMS May 2009]
    (b) IUCD [NEET Pattern 2013]
    (c) Oral contraceptive pills [UPSC CMS 2015]
    (d) Natural methods

141. Regular reporting of health statistics is done for: [AIPGME 2012]
    (a) To evaluate trends of a disease
    (b) To appreciate health personnel's efforts
    (c) For epidemiological research
    (d) All of the above

142. Ideal Contraceptive for lactating women:
    (a) POP [AIIMS May 2011]
    (b) IUCD
    (c) Lactation amenorrhoea
    (d) Barrier methods

143. Ideal contraceptive for a couple who are living separately in two cities and meets only occasionally:
    (a) Barrier methods [AIIMS May 2011]
    (b) OCP's
    (c) IUCD
    (d) Inj. DMPA

144. Under Medical Termination of Pregnancy Act (MTP) Act 1971 of India, permission for MTP has to be given by:
    (a) Wife only [AIPGME 2012]
    (b) Husband only
    (c) Both wife and husband
    (d) Guardian

145. Tubal block constitutes what proportion of female infertility? [NEET Pattern 2014]
    (a) 5–7% (b) 15–20%
    (c) 30–35% (d) 90–95%

146. Contraceptive options for a 28-year-old woman who is breastfeeding a 6-week-old baby, wanting to avoid pregnancy for a longer interval are the following *except*:
    (a) LNG-IUD [UPSC CMS 2015]
    (b) IUD- 380A
    (c) Implanon
    (d) Combined oral contraceptives

Review Questions

147. The contraceptive method of choice (temporary) for 37-year-old well educated woman: [DNB 2002]
    (a) Mala-N
    (b) Mala-D
    (c) I.U.D.
    (d) Diaphragm

148. True regarding MTP act is: [TN 2000]
    (a) MTP act was passed in 1971
    (b) MTP act has brought down the incidence of illegal abortions
    (c) In an emergency, pregnancy can be terminated by a single doctor even after 20 weeks without consulting a second doctor
    (d) MTP can be done after 20 weeks of gestation, if the two doctors agree together

Explanations

DEMOGRAPHY

DEMOGRAPHIC CYCLE AND PROCESSES

1. **Ans. (b) Late Stage II**
   [Ref. Foundations of Community Medicine, GM Dhaar & I Robbani, 1/e p156 and Park 27/e p554]

   DEMOGRAPHIC CYCLE
   - Demographic cycle is closely related to: Socio-economic progress of a country
   - There are 5 stages (phases) of demographic cycle through which a nation passes

Demographic cycle		Parameters	
Stages	Phases	CBR	CDR
Stage I	High Stationary	High	High
Stage II	Early expanding	High	Starts declining
Stage III	Late expanding	Starts declining	Continue declining
Stage IV	Low stationary	Low	Low
Stage V	Declining	CDR > CBR	

   - *Demographic cycle is based on*: Demographic gap:
     – DG = Crude Birth Rate (CBR) – Crude Death Rate
     – DG starts increasing: Early Stage II (early expanding phase)
     – DG is Maximum: Late Stage II (early expanding phase)
     – DG starts declining: Early Stage III (late expanding phase)
     – DG is Negative: Stage V (Declining phase)
     – DG is Narrow: Stage I (high stationary); Stage IV (low stationary)

   > **ALSO REMEMBER**
   > - *India is in Stage III (Late Expanding Phase)* of Demographic cycle
   > - *Stage V (Decline Phase)*: Germany, Italy, Spain, Portugal, Greece, United Kingdom and Japan (populations are reproducing well < replacement levels)

2. **Ans. (c) Death rate declines still further, and till birth rate tends to fall** [Ref. Foundations of Community Medicine, GM Dhaar & I Robbani, 1/e p156 and Park 27/e p554]

3. **Ans. (c) Early Stage III** [Ref. Foundations of Community Medicine, GM Dhaar & I Robbani, 1/e p156 and Park 27/e p554]

4. **Ans. (b) Late expanding** [Ref. Park 27/e p554]

5. **Ans. (b) Morbidity** [Ref. Park 25/e p530]
   - *Demographic Processes*: 5 processes continuously on work in a population, thus determining its' size, composition and distribution
     – Fertility
     – Marriage
     – Mortality
     – Migration
     – Social mobility

   > **ALSO REMEMBER**
   > **IMPORTANT DEFINITIONS IN DEMOGRAPHY:**
   > - *Crude birth rate (CBR):* Annual number of live births per 1000 mid year population
   > - *General fertility rate (GFR):* Annual number of live births per 1000 women of childbearing age (15–49 years old, or 15–44 years old) mid-year population
   > - *General marital fertility rate (GMFR):* Annual number of live births per 1000 married women of childbearing age (15–49 years old, or 15–44 years old) mid-year population
   > - *Age-specific fertility rates (ASFR):* Annual number of live births per 1000 women in particular age groups (usually age 15–19 years, 20–24 years, etc.)
   > - *Crude death rate (CDR):* Annual number of deaths per 1000 people
   > - *Infant mortality rate (IMR):* Annual number of deaths of children less than 1 year old per 1000 live births
   > - *Expectation of life (Life expectancy):* The number of years which an individual at a given age could expect to live at present mortality levels
   > - *Total fertility rate (TFR):* Number of live births per woman completing her reproductive life, if her childbearing at each age reflected current ASFRs
   > - *Gross reproduction rate (GRR):* Number of daughters who would be born to a woman completing her reproductive life at current ASFRs
   > - *Net reproduction rate (NRR):* Expected number of daughters, per newborn prospective mother, who may or may not survive to and through the ages of childbearing

6. **Ans. (b) Social mobility** [Ref. Textbook of Community Medicine by Sunder Lal, 2/e p18]
   - *Social mobility:* Socio-economic status of an individual/family ca change/advance over a period of time due to any reason (s), viz attainment of literacy, change in occupation, income change, etc.
   - Stories of 'Rags to riches' are common examples.

7. **Ans. (b) Death rate declines faster than birth rate**
   [Ref. Park 27/e p554]

8. **Ans. (c) Year of Big divide is 1921 AD; (d) Population pyramid has a broad base and a tapering top**
   [Ref. Park 27/e p554–558]

   ### Demographics of India
   - India is currently in Late expanding stage (Stage III) of Demographic cycle: Both Birth rate and Death rate are declining
   - Dependency ratio of India is 0.524 (52.4%): Young age DR 43.9%, Old age DR 8.6%
   - Year of Big divide in Census was year 1921: Population actually reduced from previous census
   - Population pyramid has a broad base and a tapering top: Typical of developing countries
   - Indian census operations began in 1871; the first synchronic census covering almost the whole of the territory of India.

BIRTH RATE, DEATH RATE AND GROWTH RATE

9. **Ans. (c) 35–47 years** [Ref. Park 27/e p556]
   - *Growth rate (GR)*: Is the change in population overtime, and can be quantified as the 'change in the number of individuals in a population per unit time'
     - Annual growth rate (AGR): Crude birth rate (BR) minus crude death rate (DR)
     - Decadal growth rate (DGR): Change in population over a decade
   - *Growth rate (India)*: [Census 2011]
     - Annual growth rate (AGR): 1.64%
     - Decadal growth rate (DGR): 17.64%
   - Relation between annual growth rate (AGR) and population:

Rating	Annual GR (%)	Population doubling time
Stationary population	None	–
Slow growth	<0.5	>139 years
Moderate growth	0.5–1.0	139–70
Rapid growth	1.0–1.5	70–47
Very rapid growth	1.5–2.0	47–35
Explosive growth	2.0–2.5	35–28
Explosive growth	2.5–3.0	28–23
Explosive growth	3.0–3.5	23–20
Explosive growth	3.5–4.0	20–18

   - Since India's AGR is 1.64%, it is in very rapid growth phase; Population of India will double in 35–47 years.

> **ALSO REMEMBER**
> - *Population growth models*: *Malthusian Growth Model*: (Simple exponential growth model)
>   1. Essentially exponential growth based on a constant rate of compound interest
>   2. RULE OF 70: explains the time periods involved in exponential growth at a constant rate. For example, if growth is measured annually then a 1% growth rate results in a doubling every 70 years. At 2% doubling occurs every 35 years.
>   - *Logistic growth model:* The Malthusian growth model is the direct ancestor of the logistic function

10. **Ans. (a) Crude birth rate (CBR) minus Crude death rate (CDR)** [Ref. Park 27/e p556]

11. **Ans. (b) Mid year population** [Ref. Park 27/e p563]
    - *Crude birth rate*: Number of live births in a year per 1000 mid-year population
    - *CBR is simplest indicator of fertility*: Total mid-year population is not exposed to child bearing thus it does not give true idea of fertility of a population

12. **Ans. None of the Choices** [Ref. UNDP, Website]
    - *Growth rate of Countries (UN 2017]*

Country	Population growth rate (%)
Lebanon	5.99 (Highest)
Nepal	1.18
Bangladesh	1.20
Pakistan	2.4
India	1.26
Myanmar	0.82
Sri Lanka	0.50
Andorra	– 3.61 (Lowest)

13. **Ans. (b) It is actually a ratio not a rate**
    [Ref. Park 23/e 24/e p514, 539]
    - *Crude birth rate (CBR)*: is the natality or childbirths per 1,000 people per year
      - CBR (World): 18.6 per 1000 population (Max 50 Niger; Min 9 Monaco) [2017]
      - CBR (India): 20.4 per 1000 population [2017]
      - Is a measure of fertility
      - CRUDE means it includes all causes and all ages. It is independent of age of population

14. **Ans. (b) 165 [Hint: Add 10% pregnancy wastage also]**
    [Ref. Kamalam, 1/e p288]

15. **Ans. (a) Rapid growth in population that leads to misbalance in birth and deaths**
    [Ref. Rotifera Nine by Shiel, 1/e p103]

Review Questions

16. **Ans. (a) Mid year population** [Ref. Gupta & Mahajan 3/e p408; Park 21/e p451, Park 23/e 25/e p539]

17. **Ans. (a) Broad at base and narrow at apex**
    [Ref. Park 27/e p554–562]

POPULATION PYRAMID

18. **Ans. (c) 22** *[Ref. NFHS – 3, 2005–06; Park 27/e p557]*
    - *Population composition of India*: [SRS 2017]
      – 0–14 years: 27% (Children)
      – 15–49 years: 56% (Reproductive age group)
      – 50–59 years: 8%
      – >60 years: 8.5% (Geriatric age group)
    - Women in child-bearing (15–44 years) age group constitute 22–25% of population

19. **Ans. (d) Limiting resource** *[Ref. Wikipedia]*
    - *Carrying capacity*: The supportable population of an organism, given the food, habitat, water and other necessities available within an ecosystem is known as the ecosystem's *carrying capacity* for that organism
      – Refers to the number of individuals who can be supported in a given area within natural resource limits, and without degrading the natural social, cultural and economic environment for present and future generations
      – For human population more complex variables (sanitation, medical care) are sometimes considered as part of necessary infrastructure
      – Below carrying capacity, populations typically increase; while above, they typically decrease
      – May depend on a variety of factors including food availability; water supply, environmental conditions and living space

20. **Ans. (c) None [NOW 56%]** *[Ref. Park 27/e p557]*

> **ALSO REMEMBER**
> - *Population pyramid*: (age-sex pyramid and age structure diagram) Is a graphical illustration that shows the distribution of various age groups in a population which normally forms the shape of a pyramid
>   – *Double Histogram*: 2 back-to-back bar graphs
>   – *Double Histogram*: 2 back-to-back bar graphs
>   1. One showing the number of males and
>   2. One showing females in a particular population (Males are conventionally shown on left and females on right)
>   – The population (%) is plotted on the X-axis and age on the Y-axis (in 5-year age group intervals)

SEX RATIO AND DEPENDENCY RATIO

21. **Ans. NONE [Now 943 in Census 2011]** *[Ref. Park 27/e p558]*
    Sex Ratio
    - *Sex Ratio*: Is defined as number of females per thousand males

- Sex Ratio = $\dfrac{\text{No. of Female}}{\text{No. of Male}} \times 1000$

- *Sex Ratio* (*India*): [Census 2011]

CENSUS 2001		SR
State with Highest Sex Ratio	Kerala	1084
State with Lowest Sex Ratio	Haryana	877
UT with Highest Sex Ratio	Puducherry	1038
UT with Lowest Sex Ratio	Daman & Diu	618
District with Highest Sex Ratio	Mahe (Puducherry)	1176
District with Lowest Sex Ratio	Daman (Daman & Diu)	533

> **ALSO REMEMBER**
> - *Interpretation of Sex ratio*:
>   – Ideal Sex Ratio: Sex ratio of 1000 (equal no. of males & females)
>   – Favourable Sex Ratio: Sex ratio >1000 (Females > Males)
>   – Unfavourable Sex Ratio: Sex ratio <1000 (Females < Males)
> - *Child Sex Ratio*: Is defined as number of female children 0–6 years age per thousand male children 0–6 years age
>   – Child Sex Ratio (India): 919 [Census 2011] (Highly unfavourable)

22. **Ans. (c) Males are less than 5000** *[Ref. Park 27/e p558]*
    In the given question
    - Total population is 10,000.
    - Also, Ideal sex ratio implies 5000 females for 5000 males
    - So, Sex ratio is more than 1000, it implies, Females are more than 1000 per 1000 males
    - Thus, females are >5000 and males are <5000

23. **Ans. (c) 66.6%** *[Ref. Park 27/e p559]*
    Thus, DR = $\dfrac{30\% + 10\%}{60\%}$ = 0.66 or 66.6% or 66 per 100
    - *DR of 0.66 or 66/100 or 66% implies*: 100 earning people in that community will have to support 166 people (100 themselves and 66 non-earning dependents on them)

24. **Ans. (a) 0–5 yrs age; (b) 6–14 yrs age; (c) 15–45 yrs age; (d) >65 yrs** *[Ref. Park 27/e p559]*

25. **Ans. (b) Number of persons aged 15 to 65 per one older person aged >/= 65 years** *[Ref. Population and Development: Selected Issues, United Nations Series 161, p115]*
    Potential support ratio PSR
    - Number of persons aged 15 to 65 per one older person aged more than or equal to 65 years
    - It gives burden placed on working population
    - Is inverse of old age dependency

Review Question

26. **Ans. (c) Since 1901 there is steadily decreasing trend**
    [Ref. Park 27/e p559]

LITERACY AND LIFE EXPECTANCY

27. **Ans. (b) Population age 7 years or more**
    [Ref. Park 27/e p560-561]
    - *Literate* (India): Any person who can read AND write, WITH understanding, IN ANY ONE language of India AND who is >7 years if age (definition used in 1991 & 2001 Censuses)
        - Literacy Rate: Denominator is population >7 years age
        - Crude Literacy Rate: Denominator is total population (used earlier)
    - *Literacy Rate* (India): 75.04% [Census 2011]
        - Literacy rate by sex: Males – 82% & Females – 65%
        - Literacy rate by state: Maximum 94% (Kerala) & Least 64% (Bihar)

> **ALSO REMEMBER**
> - *International Literacy Day*: 8th September (every year)
> - *UN definition of Literacy*: Ability to read and write a simple sentence in any language
> - *Functional Literacy*: Ability of an individual to use reading, writing, and computational skills efficiently in everyday life situations
> - *Transliteracy*: The ability to read, write and interact across a range of platforms, tools and media from signing and orality through handwriting, print, TV, radio and film, to digital social networks
> - *Alliteracy*: The state of being able to read but being uninterested in doing so

28. **Ans. (a) Those above age of 7 years**
    [Ref. Park 27/e p560-561]

29. **Ans. (c) 50%**
    [Ref. Park 27/e p560-561]
    Effective literacy rate (ELR) = No. of literates/Total population >7 years age × 100

    In the given question,
    Total population =10000, Population 0–6 years age = 2000
    So Population >7 years age = 10000–2000 = 8000
    So ELR = 4000/8000 × 100 = 50%

FERTILITY

30. **Ans. (a) 18.6 per 1000 population**
    [Ref. Internet]
    - Relationship between Crude birth rate (CBR) and Total fertility rate (TFR):
    - CBR = (8 × TFR) + 1 [approx.]
    - **In the given question,** the total fertility rate in India is 2.2
    - Thus, CBR = (8 × 2.2) + 1 = 17.6 + 1 = 18.6

31. **Ans. (d) Sample registration system**
    [Ref. Park 27/e p969]
    - Sample Registration System (SRS) was initiated in 1964–65 (on a pilot basis; full scale from 1969–70) to provide national as well as state level reliable estimates of fertility and mortality
    - SRS is a dual record system:
        - *Field Investigation:* Continuous enumeration of births and deaths by an enumerator
        - *Independent retrospective survey:* every 6 months by an investigator-supervisor
    - Findings of SRS Bulletin: 2017
        - Crude Birth Rate (CBR): 20.4 per 1000 mid-year population
        - Crude Death Rate (CDR): 6.4 per 1000 mid-year population
        - Natural Growth Rate: 14%
        - Infant Mortality Rate (IMR): 34 per 1000 live births

> **ALSO REMEMBER**
> - *Civil Registration System (CRS)*: Birth and death registration system is technically known as CRS
>   - Births, deaths and still-births are required to be each registered to the concerned Registrar within 21 days of its occurrence
> - *Census*: Total process of collecting, compiling, analyzing or otherwise disseminating demographic, economic and social data pertaining, at a specific time, of all persons in a country or a well-defined part of a country
>   - Provides snapshot of the country's population and housing at a given point of time
> - *Ad-hoc survey*: Is a survey without any plan for repetition

32. **Ans. (d) General Fertility Rate** *[Ref. Park 27/e p562-563]*

> **ALSO REMEMBER**
> - *GFR is a better measure of fertility than CBR*: as denominator is restricted to no. of women in child-bearing age, rather than the whole population
> - *Major weakness of GFR*: Not all women are exposed to risk of child birth
> - *Measurements of birth rates*:
>   - Crude birth rate (CBR)
>   - General fertility rate (GFR)
>   - Standardized birth rate
>   - Total fertility rate (TFR)

33. **Ans. (a) 2** *[Ref. Park 27/e p562-563]*
    - GRR or NRR = ½ TFR (approximately)

34. **Ans. (b) Measure of completed family size; (c) Sum of fertility of all age; (e) Total no. of children born to a mother** *[Ref. Park 27/e p562-563]*

35. **Ans. (a) <1** *[Ref. Park 27/e p562-563]*
    - *Replacement level of fertility (TFR = 2.1, i.e. NRR = 1)*: TFR at which newborn girls would have an average of exactly 1 daughter over their lifetimes (women have just enough babies to replace themselves)
        - Is also known as 'Adequate level'

36. **Ans. (b) G.F.R.; (c) T.F.R. (d) Maternal mortality rate**
    [Ref. Park 27/e p562-563]

37. **Ans. (c) 60%** *[Ref. Park 27/e p564]*
    - To achieve NRR = 1, CPR >60%
    - Then population will stabilize by 2045

38. Ans. (b) Measure of fertility [Ref. Park 27/e p562]
39. Ans. (c) NRR [Ref. Park 27/e p564]
40. Ans. (d) No. of female children a newborn girl has in her life time taking into account mortality [Ref. Park 27/e p564]
41. Ans. (c) Gross Reproduction Rate [Ref. Park 27/e p564]

Review Question

42. Ans. (d) All of the above [Ref. Park 27/e p562]

MISCELLANEOUS (DEMOGRAPHY)

43. Ans. (d) 1, 3, 4 [Ref. Park 25/e p903]
    - Vital Statistics Data Sources: Census, Sample Registration System (SRS), Demographic Surveys (NSSO), Civil Registration System, Health Surveys (NFHS, DLHS)
    - Sources for Causes of Death: SRS (IMR, NNMR, MMR, U5MR), Death declaration and Medical certification, Lay information (Through First line health workers)
44. Ans. (c) 21 days [Ref. Textbook of Community Medicine by Sunder Lal, 2/e p330]
    - Civil Registration System (CRS): Birth and death registration system is technically known as CRS

> **ALSO REMEMBER**
> - Registration of name of the child:
>   – Within 12 months of birth registration: Free of charge
>   – After 12 months of birth registration till 15 years: ₹ 5.00
> - Coverage of registration of births and deaths in India:
>   – Coverage of births registration in India: 89%
>   – Coverage of deaths registration in India: 74%

45. Ans. (c) 29% [Ref. Park 27/e p815]
    - *Poverty:* Deprivation of those things that determine the quality of life, including food, clothing, shelter and safe drinking water, but also such 'intangibles' as the opportunity to learn, to engage in meaningful employment, and to enjoy the respect of fellow citizens
      – *Absolute poverty:* a set standard which is consistent over time and between countries
      – *Relative poverty:* as being below some relative poverty threshold
    - *Poverty threshold (poverty line):* Is the minimum level of income deemed necessary to achieve an adequate standard of living
    - Definitions of Below Poverty Line (BPL):
      – Based on per capita caloric intake per day:
        1. *Rural areas:* per capita daily caloric intake <2400 kcal
        2. *Urban areas:* per capita daily caloric intake <2100 kcal
      – Based on per capita expenditure per month: [New Guideline Tendulkar Committee 2011–12]
        1. *Rural areas:* Per capita expenditure per day INR 27/- [INR 32 - Rangarajan Committee]
        2. *Urban areas:* Per capita expenditure per day INR 33/- [INR 47 - Rangarajan Committee]
      – Based on criteria for International comparisons (World Bank):
        1. *Extreme poverty:* Living on <1.90 $ per person per day
        2. *Moderate poverty:* Living on <3.10 $ per person per day
    - Poverty in India:
      – Most obvious problem of India
      – Population living BPL in India: 22% [2013] [29.5% Rangarajan Committee 2014]

46. Ans. (d) Four rounds [Ref. National Health Programs of India by Dr. J. Kishore, 8/e p37]

National Family Health Survey (NFHS)
- Is a large-scale, multi-round survey conducted in a representative sample of households throughout India
- 4 rounds of the survey have been conducted till date,
  – NFHS–1: 1992–93
  – NFHS–2: 1998–99
  – NFHS–3: 2005–06
  – NFHS–4: 2015–16

47. Ans. (c) Population pyramid [Ref. Park 27/e p567–568]
    - *Population pyramid:* (age-sex pyramid or age-structure diagram) Is a graphical illustration that shows the distribution of various age groups in a population which normally forms the shape of a pyramid
      – *Double Histogram:* 2 back-to-back histogram graphs
        1. One showing the number of males and
        2. One showing females in a particular population (Males are conventionally shown on left and females on right)
      – The population (%) is plotted on the X-axis and age on the Y-axis (in 5-year age group intervals)

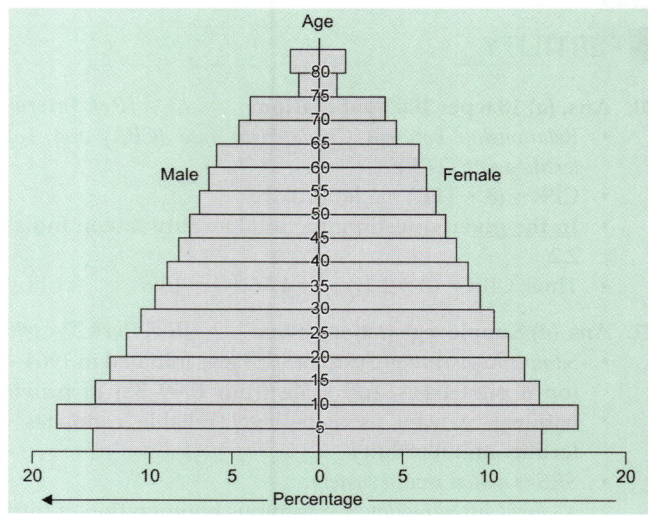

Age and sex pyramid

> **ALSO REMEMBER**
> - *Life table analysis:* Biometer of Population
>   - Core demographic technique to analyze mortality and other non-renewable processes
>   - Is a special type of 'Cohort Analysis'
>   - Is an example of 'Indirect Standardization'
>   - Used for:
>   1. Mortality (Life expectancy)
>   2. Natality
>   3. Reproduction (Contraceptive use/failure rates)
>   4. Chances of survival (Survival curves)
> - *Correlation coefficient (r):* indicates the strength and direction of a linear relationship between two random variables
>   - *Correlation coefficient (r) lies between –1 and +1 (–1 < r < +1)*
> - *Bar chart:* is a chart with rectangular bars of lengths proportional to that value that they represent
>   - Bar chart is for *'non-continuous qualitative data'*
>   - Bar charts are used for comparing two or more values
>   - Bars can be horizontally or vertically oriented

48. Ans. (b) IMR *[Ref. Park 27/e p646]*
- Most important indicator of health status of a country: IMR

> **ALSO REMEMBER**
> - *Couple Protection rate* (CPR):
>   - CPR is percent of eligible couples effectively protected against one or the other approved methods of family planning, viz. condoms, OCPs, IUDs, sterilization

49. Ans. (c) Hyderabad *[Ref. Park 21/e p448, Park 22/e p446]*
- *UN Classification of urban agglomerations:*

Classification	Population count
Mega city	>10 millions
Million-plus city	1–10 millions
Major city	0.1–1 million (1–10 Lac)
Town	<0.1 million (<1 Lac)

- *Megacity:* Is defined as a metropolitan area with
  - Total population: in excess of 10 million people
  - A minimum level for population density: 2,000 persons/square km
- In World (2005), there were 25 megacities
- *Urban area with maximum population the world:* Tokyo
- *Largest mega city in the world:* Tokyo

50. Ans. (a) 10–19 years of age *[Ref. A Picture of Health – A Review and Annotated Bibliography of the Health of Young People in Developing Countries by Goodburn, Elizabeth and Ross (WHO & UNICEF) 1995]*
- *Adolescence:* Is a transitional stage of physical and mental human development that occurs between childhood and adulthood
- The World Health Organization (WHO) defines adolescence as the period of life between 10 and 19 years of age

51. Ans. (a) High literacy rate; (d) Older age of marriage; (e) Higher Life expectancy *[Ref. Multiple documents]*

52. Ans. (d) Within 60 days of arrival into India *[Ref. Handbook of Civil Registration, Government of India, p49]*

53. Ans. (b) Kerala *[Ref. Park 27/e p23]*
- *Kerala is considered 'Yardstick for judging health status in India':* Kerala has achieved high levels of health (similar to Develop countries) even on moderate levels of income through Strong political commitment to equitable socio-economic development.

	Kerala	India
Birth rate (per 1000 MYP)	14.3	20.4
Death rate (per 1000 MYP)	7.6	6.4
IMR (per 1000 LB)	12	34
Annual growth rate	0.6%	1.40%
Life expectancy at birth	73 (M), 77 (F)	67 (M), 69 (F)
Literacy rate	90%	74%
Per capita income (2016)	₹ 196,842	₹ 112,432
Mean age at marriage (F)	23 years	22 years

54. Ans. (c) Birth rate *[Ref. Park 27/e p563]*

Population statistics	Vital statistics
Population size	Birth rate, Death rate
Sex ratio	Natural growth rate
Density of population	Life expectancy at birth
Dependency ratio	Mortality rates
	Fertility rates

55. Ans. (d) 2045 *[Ref. Population Stabilization Through District Action Plans 1/e Chap 4]*

AIMS & OBJECTIVES OF JANSANKHYA STHRITHA KOSH (NATIONAL POPULATION STABILIZATION FUND)
- To provide or undertake activities aimed to achieve population stabilization, at a level consistent with the needs of sustainable economic growth, social development and environment protection, by 2045
- To promote and support schemes, programs, projects and initiatives for meeting the unmet needs for contraception and reproductive and child health care
- To promote and support innovative ideas in the Government, private and voluntary sector with a view to achieve the objectives of the National Population Policy 2000
- To facilitate the development of a vigorous people's movement in favour of the national effort for population stabilization
- To provide a window for canalizing contributions from individuals, trade organizations and others within the country and outside, in furtherance of the national cause of population stabilization

56. **Ans. (b) Fertility**
    [Ref. Handbook on the Collection of Fertility and Mortality Data— United Nations, 1/e p10]

    Dual-Records System
    - Devised to obtain further refinements in the measurement of fertility and mortality and thus of the natural population growth rate
    - Data on vital events are obtained in a defined area by two independent data collection methods, a periodic household survey and a separate reporting method
    - Separate reporting method records vital events on a current basis in the sample households, which may involve regular visits to the household, or it may rely on a network of informers, the recorder verifying the occurrence of the events.

    > **ALSO REMEMBER**
    > - Sample Registration System of India is a 'Dual record system':
    >   – Field investigation: continuous enumeration of births and deaths by an enumerator
    >   – Independent retrospective survey: every 6 months by an investigator-supervisor.

57. **Ans. (b) Every 6 months** *[Ref. Park 27/e p969]*

Review Questions

58. **Ans. (b) 1921** *[Ref. Park 27/e p556]*
59. **Ans. (c) Sample registration Survey** *[Ref. Park 27/e p969]*
60. **Ans. (a) Sample registration system** *[Ref. Park 27/e p969]*

FAMILY PLANNING AND CONTRACEPTION

CONCEPTS OF FAMILY PLANNING

61. **Ans. (b) Combined OCPs** *[Ref. Park 27/e p575]*
    - Contraceptive of choice for a Newly married couple is Combined OCPs
    - Mala-N or Mala-D are available under RCH Program

62. **Ans. (b) Pearl index** *[Ref. Park 27/e p585]*
    - Pearl index is the common method used to measure contraceptive failure rate.
    - It is defined as the number of failures per 100 woman-years of exposure (HWY)
    - Pearl index = Total accidental pregnancies/Total months of exposure × 1200

63. **Ans. (c) 10 per HWY** *[Ref. Park 27/e p584]*
    - *PEARL INDEX (PI) as measure of contraceptive efficacy*
      – PI or Pearl rate: MC technique used in clinical trials for measuring the effectiveness of a birth control method
      – PI is no. of failures per 100 woman years (HWY) of exposure
      – Pearl Index (PI)

    $$= \frac{\text{Total accidental pregnancy}}{\text{Total months of exposure}} \times 1200$$

    - **In the given question,**
      – Total accidental pregnancies = 20
      – Total months of exposure = 100 couples × 24 months each = 2400 months
      – Thus, $PI = \frac{20}{2400} \times 1200 = 10$ per HWY

64. **Ans. (b) Pearl Index and Life table analysis**
    [Ref. Park 27/e p585]
    - *Contraceptive Efficacy*: Is assessed by measuring the number of unplanned pregnancies that occur during a specified period of exposure and use of a contraceptive method. Two methods used are:
      – Pearl index
      – Life table analysis
    - *Life Table Analysis (LTA) as measure of contraceptive efficacy*:
      – LTA calculates a failure rate per month of use
      – Better measure than PI

    > **ALSO REMEMBER**
    > - *Couple Protection Rate (CPR)*: Is an indicator of prevalence of contraceptive practice in a community
    >
    > $$CPR = \frac{\text{Total no. of ECs protected by any of 4 approved methods}}{\text{Total no. of ECs in the community}} \times 100$$

65. **Ans. (c) 150–180** *[Ref. Park 27/e p567]*
    - *Eligible couples (ECs)*: A currently married couple with wife in reproductive age group (15–45 years age)
      – ECs are in need of family planning services
      – There are 150–180 ECs per 1000 population in India
      – 20% ECs are in age group 20–24 years
      – EC register, a basic document for organizing family planning work, is maintained at Subcentre
      – Total no. of ECs in a community is used (as a denominator) in the calculation of Couple Protection Rate (CPR)

66. **Ans. (c) 25%** *[Ref. Internet; Park 27/e p567]*
    - *Couple Protection rate (CPR)*:
      – CPR is percent of eligible couples (ECs) protected against one or the other approved methods of family planning, viz. condoms, OCPs, IUDs, sterilization
      – NRR = 1 can be achieved if: CPR >60%
      – CPR (India): 54% (2018)
      – Goal for CPR in RCH – II (2004–09): >65% (Goal of CPR in A vision 2020: 63.7%)
      – CPR is an indicator of prevalence of contraceptive practice in a community
    - *Effective Couple Protection rate (ECPR)*:
      – ECPR is percent of eligible couples (ECs) protected against one or the other approved methods of family planning, viz. condoms, OCPs, IUDs, sterilization Taking into Account Their Effectivity

– *Effectivity of approved contraceptive methods*:
  1. Condoms: 50%
  2. IUDs: 95%
  3. OCPs: 100%
  4. Sterilization (Vasectomy or Tubectomy): 100%
- **In the given question**, ECs = 180

Contraceptive methods used	No. of couples using contraception	Effectivity of contraceptive methods	Effectively protected couples
Condoms	29	50%	14.5
IUDs	10	95%	9.5
Oral Pills	10	100%	10
Vasectomy	03	100%	03
Tubectomy	08	100%	08
Total	60	–	45

$CPR = \frac{60}{180} = 33.3\%$ and $ECPR = \frac{45}{180} \times 100 = 25\%$

67. **Ans. (b) Total accidental pregnancy** *[Ref. Park 27/e p585]*
68. **Ans. (b) Accidental pregnancies per 100 women-years of exposure** *[Ref. Park 27/e p585]*
69. **Ans. (b) Limiting birth** *[Ref. Park 27/e p585]*

    Unmet need of family planning
    - Unmet need for family planning: Percentage of women of reproductive age, either married or in a union, who have an unmet need for family planning
      – Women with unmet need are those who are want to stop or delay childbearing but are not using any method of contraception
    - Unmet need in India:
      – Unmet need in <20 years old women: Spacing the births
      – Unmet need in 20–24 years old women: Spacing the births
      – Unmet need in >30 years old women: Limiting the births
    - NFHS-4 India data:
      – Total unmet need in India: 12.9%
      – Total unmet need for spacing births in India: 5.7%

70. **Ans. (b) 2.5** *[Ref. Park 27/e p585]*
    - Pearl Index of contraceptive 'C' is 10 per hundred women years.

    It implies,
    - If 100 women use 'C' for one year continuously then 10 of them will get pregnant despite using the contraceptive, OR
    - If a woman use 'C' for 100 years continuously then she is likely to get pregnant 10 times despite using the contraceptive.

    Now considering reproductive life-span of a woman is around 25 years, she's likely to get pregnant total = 25/100 × 10 = 2.5 times!

71. **Ans. (d) 10 accidental pregnancies per 100 woman years using contraceptives** *[Ref. Park 27/e p585]*

- Pearl Index = No of accidental pregnancies/Total months of exposure × 1200
- **In the given question,** Total accidental pregnancies = 20 and Total months of exposure = 2400 (100 women for 2 years each)
- **So,** Pearl Index = 20/2400 × 1200 = 10 per HWY

72. **Ans. (d) 10 accidental pregnancy per 100 woman year using contraceptives** *[Ref. Park 27/e p585]*
    - Pearl index is expressed as Failure per Hundred women years
    - It implies Failure among 100 women using contractive for 1 year each
    - **So, PI 10/HWY means** if 100 women use the given contraceptive for 1 year each, then 10 of them will become pregnant despite using the contraceptive (accidental pregnancies)

Review Questions

73. **Ans. (a) Annual general marriage rate** *[Ref. Park 27/e p566–568]*
74. **Ans. (a) By spacing between the pregnancies** *[Ref. Park 27/e p568]*
75. **Ans. (d) All of the above** *[Ref. Park 27/e p567]*

NATURAL METHODS

76. **Ans. (a) Terminal Methods** *[Ref. Park 27/e p581]*

    Natural Family Planning Methods:
    - *Basal Body Temperature (BBT) Method*:
      – *Depends on*: Rise of temperature (0.3°–0.5°C) at ovulation
      – *Occurs due to*: Increased progesterone production
    - *Cervical Mucus Method*:
      – *Also known as 'Billing's Method' or 'Ovulation Method'*
      – *Based on*: Changes in characteristics of cervical mucus
        1. At ovulation: Watery, clear, smooth, slippery, profuse (like Egg white)
        2. After ovulation: Thickens and lessens in quantity
    - *Symptothermic Method*:
      – Combines temperature, cervical mucus and calendar techniques

> **ALSO REMEMBER**
> - *Only method of birth control which is completely effective*: Sexual abstinence
> - *Oldest method of voluntary fertility control*: Coitus interruptus
> - *Safe period (Rhythm method/Calendar method)*:
>   – *Fertile period*: Shortest cycle *minus* 18 days (Last day of fertile period: Longest cycle *minus* 10 days)
>   – *Drawbacks*: PROGRAMMED SEX: Abstinence required for ½ month

77. Ans. (a) Abstinence required only for few days of month
[Ref. Park 27/e p581]

Calendar Method
- Compulsory abstinence for nearly half of the month – Programmed sex
- Known complications: Ectopic pregnancy, Embryonic abnormalities
- Not useful in post-natal period, irregular cycles
- Need educated couples with high degree of motivation
- High failure rate PI = 24/HWY

Review Question

78. Ans. (c) Symptothermic method [Ref. Park 27/e p582]

BARRIER METHODS

79. Ans. (b) A - II, B - I, C - IV, D – III
[Ref. Park 27/e p569–570]

- *Vaginal Sponge*: Today (brand name)
  - *Sponge a barrier method of contraception:* It actually combines barrier and spermicidal methods to prevent conception
  - Saturated with 1000 mg of spermicide 'Non-oxynol–9'
  - *Disadvantages of sponge:*
    1. Sponge provide no protection from STIs
    2. Can lead to Toxic Shock Syndrome
- *Norplant*: Subdermal implant (Depot formulation)
  - 6 silastic capsules containing 35 mg LNG each
    1. Norplant R2: 2 capsules containing 75 mg LNG each
  - *Disadvantages:* Irregularities of menstrual bleeding
- *NET–EN*: Norethisterone Enanthate, a Progestogen only Injectable contraceptive (Depot formulation)
  - *Dose:* 200 mg i/m every 2 months
  - *Side effects:* Disruptions of normal menstrual cycles
- *Grafenberg's ring*: 1st Generation (Non-medicated/Inert) IUD [Similar to Lippes loop]

ALSO REMEMBER
- *DIAPHRAGM*: Is a cervical barrier type of birth control
  - It must be inserted sometime before sexual intercourse, and remain in the vagina for 6–8 hours after a man's last ejaculation
  - *Disadvantages*:
    1. Increased risk of UTI, yeast infection & bacterial vaginosis
    2. Toxic Shock Syndrome (if left in-situ >24 hours)
- *DMPA (Depot Medroxy Progesterone Acetate)*: A progestogen only Injectable contraceptive (Depot formulation)
  - *Dose*: 150 mg i/m every 3 months

80. Ans. (b) Social marketing
[Ref. Social Marketing in India by Deshpande 1/e p263]

Social Marketing
- Concept: Seeks to develop and integrate marketing concepts with other approaches to influence behaviors that benefit individuals and communities for the greater social good
- Social marketing seeks to influence social behaviors not to benefit the marketer, but to benefit the target audience and the general society
- Example: Installation of Condom vending machines (CVM)s at parks, pay and use toilets, railway stations, bus stations, petrol pumps, wine shops, bars, restaurants, STD/PCO booths, tea-shops, paan-shops

Review Question

81. Ans. (c) 9-Nonoxynol [Ref. Park 27/e p570]

IUDs

82. Ans. (c) Trophoblastic disease
[Ref. IUCD Reference Manual for Medical Officers, MOHFW 2007 p21]

CuT CONTRAINDICATED
- Pregnancy
- Postpartum puerperal sepsis
- Immediately post-septic abortion
- Before evaluation of unexplained vaginal bleeding suspected of being a serious condition
- Malignant gestational trophoblastic disease
- Cervical cancer (awaiting treatment)
- Endometrial cancer
- Distortions of the uterine cavity by uterine fibroids or anatomical abnormalities
- Current PID
- Current purulent cervicitis, chlamydial infection, or gonorrheal STIs
- Known pelvic tuberculosis

83. Ans. (a) IUCD
[Ref. Textbook of Family Medicine by Arulrhaj 3/e p477]
- IUDs are an excellent and safe contraceptive option for women with cardiovascular ailments
- Barrier methods are good too but carry high risk of failure

84. Ans. (c) Surface area of copper in sq. mm
[Ref. Park 27/e p571–572]

- In CuT 7, CuT 220 B and CuT 380 A or Ag,
  - *Numbers (7, 220, 380) represent:* Surface area of copper (in sq. mm) on the device
  - *B in CuT 220 B represent:* Size of IUD (IUDs were earlier available in different sizes – A, B, C and D; D was the largest size)
  - *A or Ag in CuT 380 A represent:* Silver or Gold (with copper)
- IUDs are world's most widely used method of reversible birth control
- Change of IUD: (Shelf life of copper IUDs)

IUD	Approved years of use
Copper IUDs	3–5
Progestasert	1
CuT 200	4
NOVA T	5
LNG IUD	7–10
CuT 380 A	10

- Non-hormonal (copper) IUDs are considered safe to use while breastfeeding
- All 2nd generation copper-T IUDs have failure rates of less than 1% per year

85. Ans. (a) Bleeding [Ref. Park 27/e p572–574]

ALSO REMEMBER
- IUDs associated with side effects or complications:

Side effects or complications	IUD most commonly associated
Highest pregnancy rate	Lippes Loop
Lowest pregnancy rate	LNG – IUD
Highest expulsion rate	Lippes Loop
Lowest expulsion rate	Progestasert
Highest removal rate	LNG – IUD
Lowest removal rate	Progestasert

86. Ans. (c) Progestasert is implanted subdermally [Ref. Park 27/e p571]

Progestasert
- *Progestasert is a 3rd Generation IUD* (Medicated/Bioactive IUD)
- Progestasert was the *'first hormonal uterine device'*, developed in 1976
- *T-shaped device filled with 38 mg progesterone*
- *Rate of hormone release*: 65 mcg per day
- *Shelf life*: 1–1½ years
- *Advantages of Progestasert*:
  - IUD with *'Lowest expulsion rate'*
  - IUD with *'Lowest removal rate'*

87. Ans. (b) Pain [Ref. Park 27/e p572–574]

88. Ans. (c) Has a history of ectopic pregnancy [Ref. Park 27/e p572]
- Ideal IUD woman candidate (Planned Parenthood Federation of America PPFA):
  - Who has borne at least one child
  - Has no history of pelvic disease
  - Has normal menstrual periods
  - Is willing to check the IUD tail
  - Has access to follow-up and treatment of potential problems
  - Is in a monogamous relationship
- However, the federation does not rule out women who do not conform to this profile
- American College of Obstetricians and Gynaecologists (1985) stated that 'IUDs are not recommended for women who have not had children or who have multiple partners, because of the risk of PID and possible infertility'

ALSO REMEMBER
- *Contraindications for IUDs use:*
  - *Absolute contraindications*:
    1. Suspected pregnancy
    2. PID
    3. Vaginal bleeding of undiagnosed etiology
    4. Cancer of cervix, uterus or adnexa and other pelvic tumors
    5. Previous ectopic pregnancy
  - *Relative contraindications*:
    1. Anemia
    2. Menorrhagia
    3. History of PID since last pregnancy
    4. Purulent cervical discharge
    5. Distortions of uterine cavity due to congenital malformations, fibroids
    6. Unmotivated persons

89. Ans. (d) 8 weeks [Ref. Park 27/e p572]

Timings of Iud Insertion
- *During menstruation or within 10 days of beginning of menstrual period*:
  - Best time for IUD insertion
  - Cervical canal diameter greatest, lesser expulsion, least risk of pregnancy
- *Immediate post-partum insertion*: During 1st week after delivery before woman leaves hospital
  - High chance of perforation
  - High chance of expulsion
- *Post-puerperal insertion*: 6–8 weeks after delivery
  - Can be combined with follow-up visit of mother and child
  - Not recommended after 2nd trimester abortion

90. Ans. (d) 10 yrs [Ref. Park 27/e p571]

91. Ans. (b) 5 [Ref. Park 27/e p571]

92. Ans. (a) Prevent fertilization [Ref. Park 27/e p571]
- IUD cause a foreign body reaction:
  - Cellular and biochemical reaction in endometrial and uterine fluids
  - Impaired viability of gamete reduces chances of fertilization

93. Ans. (b) MIRENA [Ref. Family Medicine by Rakel, 9/e p614]
- *Mirena IUD*: Levonorgestrel-releasing intrauterine contraceptive system measuring 32 × 32 mm placed for up to 5 years

94. Ans. (d) Who have minimum 2 children [Ref. Park 27/e p572]

95. Ans. (c) Decrease diameter of fallopian tube [Ref. Park 27/e p571]

Mechanism of Action Iuds
- Intrauterine device: Foreign body reaction in uterus
  - Cellular and biochemical changes in endometrium and uterine fluids
  - Impaired viability of gamete
  - Reduced chances of fertilization

- Copper ions:
  - Alter biochemical composition of cervical mucus
  - Affect sperm motility/capacitation/survival
- Hormones in IUD
  - Increase cervical mucus viscosity, preventing sperm from entering cervix
  - Sustain unfavorable endometrium for implantation by maintaining high level of progesterone

Review Questions

96. Ans. (b) Silver core [Ref. Park 27/e p571]
97. Ans. (d) Low risk of ectopic pregnancy [Ref. Park 27/e p571]
98. Ans. (c) Hormonal effect on mucosa of endometrium [Ref. Park 27/e p571]
99. Ans. (c) PID [Ref. Park 27/e p572]
100. Ans. (b) Second generation IUCD [Ref. Park 27/e p570]

HORMONAL METHODS

101. Ans. (b) Progestasert [Ref. Park 26/e p577]
- Third generation hormonal bio-active IUDs (Progestasert, LNG IUD) are associated with fewer days of bleeding and lesser blood loss
- Mala N is a combined OCP where estrogen content may suppress lactation; there is a chance of lactation failure hence its not useful during lactation

102. Ans. (c) Rifampicin induces OCP metabolism [Ref. Park 26/e p582]
- Rifampicin leads to Induction of cytochrome P450 group of hepatic microsomal enzymes
- It increases metabolism of both estrogen and progesterone component, reducing their blood levels and increased clearance

103. Ans. (a) Take next pill as soon as possible and consider barrier method/emergency contraception if had intercourse in last 72 hours
[Ref. Reference Manual for Oral Contraceptive Pills. MOHFW GOI p30]

MOHFW Guidelines in case of Missed OCPS
- Missed 1 or 2 pills/started new pack 1 or 2 days late: Take one hormonal pill as soon as possible or two pills at scheduled time. There is little or no risk of pregnancy.
- Missed 3 or more pills in the first or second week/started new pack 3 or more days late: Take one hormonal pill as soon as possible and continue the scheduled pill. Use a backup method for the next 7 days. Also can consider taking ECPs, if she had sex in the past 72 hours.
- Missed 3 or more pills in the third week: Take one hormonal pill as soon as possible and finish all hormonal pills in the pack as scheduled. Throw away the 7 non-hormonal pills in a 28-pill pack. Start a new pack the next day. Use a backup method for the next 7 days. Also can consider taking ECPs, if she had sex in the past 72 hours
- Missed any nonhormonal pills? (last 7 pills in 28-pill pack): Discard the missed non-hormonal pill(s). Keep taking COCs, one each day. Start the new pack as usual.
- Severe vomiting or diarrhoea: If she vomits within 2 hours after taking a pill, she should take another pill from pack as soon as possible and continue taking the scheduled pills. If she has vomiting or diarrhoea for more than 2 days, follow instructions for 1 or 2 missed pills above.

104. Ans. (d) I, II and III [Ref. Park 27/e p576–577]
- *Adverse effects of Combined Oral Contraceptive Pills (OCPs):*
  - *Cardiovascular effects:* (due to oestrogenic component)
    1. Myocardial infarction
    2. Cerebral thrombosis
    3. Venous thrombosis (with or without pulmonary embolus)
    4. Hypertension
  - *Carcinogenesis:*
    1. Cervical cancer (increased risk)
    2. Breast cancer
  - *Metabolic effects:* (due to progesterone component)
    1. Elevated blood pressure (hypertension)
    2. Altered lipid profile (reduced HDL)
    3. Blood clotting
    4. Hyperglycemia and increased plasma insulin
  - *Hepatocellular adenoma*
  - *Gallbladder disease*
  - *Cholestatic jaundice*
  - *Monolial vaginitis (candidiasis)*
  - *Decline milk volume during lactation*
  - *General effects:*
    1. Breast tenderness
    2. Weight gain (due to water retention)
    3. Headache & migraine
    4. Bleeding disturbances
- *Beneficial effects of Combined Oral Contraceptive Pills (OCPs):*
  - Benign breast disorders (Fibrocystic disease, Fibroadenoma)
  - Benign ovarian disease (Ovarian cysts)
  - Malignant ovarian disease (Ovarian cancer)
  - Pelvic Inflammatory Disease (PID)
  - Ectopic pregnancy
  - Iron deficiency anemia
  - Endometrial cancer

105. Ans. (d) 1, 2 and 3 [Ref. Park 25/e p535–536]
106. Ans. (d) Hepatocellular adenoma; (e) Thromboembolism [Ref. Park 27/e p577]
107. Ans. (a) 20 [Ref. Internet, Organon-India website]
- *Composition of 'New Low dose OCP':* (Brand name: *Femilon/Elogen*)
  - Ethinyl estradiol: 0.02 mg (20 mcg)
  - Desogestrel: 0.15 mg (150 mcg)
- *Composition of Combined OCP:* (*MALA-N*)
  - Ethinyl estradiol: 0.03 mg (30 mcg)
  - Norgestrel: 0.15 mg (150 mcg)

ALSO REMEMBER
- *Composition of few contraceptives:*
    - *Centchroman* (Brand name: *Saheli*): Ormeloxifene
    - *TODAY* (vaginal sponge): Non-oxynol–9
    - *Male condom* (common): Latex
    - *Female condom* (common): Polyurethane
    - *Norplant*: Levonorgestrel (LNG)
    - *CuT 380 A or Ag*: Copper + Silver or Copper + Gold
    - *Minipill* (Brand name: *Cerazette*): Progesterone

108. Ans. (a) Nursing mothers *[Ref. Park 27/e p577]*
- Contraindications for use of oral contraceptive pills (OCPs):

Absolute contraindications:	Relative contraindications: (require medical surveillance)
1. Breast cancer 2. Genital cancer 3. Liver disease 4. H/o thromboembolism 5. Cardiac abnormalities 6. Cong.hyperlipidemia 7. Undiagnosed abnormal uterine bleeding 8. Pregnancy	1. Age >40 years 2. Smoking and age >35 years 3. Mild hypertension 4. Chronic renal disease 5. Epilepsy 6. Migraine 7. Nursing mothers (0–6 m) 8. Diabetes mellitus 9. Gall bladder disease 10. History of infrequent bleeding 11. Amenorrhoea

109. Ans. (d) Supplied free of cost *[Ref. Park 27/e p575]*

	MALA – N	MALA – D
Type of contraceptive	Combined OCP	Combined OCP
Estrogen	Ethinyl estradiol (0.03 mg)	Ethinyl estradiol (0.03 mg)
Progesterone	Norgestrel (0.15 mg)	Desogestrel (0.15 mg)
Status in RCH	Provided free of cost	Provided at a subsidized cost (₹ 3/- per packet)

110. Ans. (a) Liver disease; (c) Renal disease; (d) Epilepsy *[Ref. Park 27/e p577]*

111. Ans. (b) PID; (c) Ovarian cysts; (d) Fibrocystic disease of breast; (e) Ectopic pregnancy *[Ref. Park 27/e p577]*

112. Ans. (d) Protection against cervical cancer *[Ref. Park 27/e p577]*

COMBINED OCPS AND CARCINOGENESIS
- Reduction in cancers: Ovarian cancer, Endometrial cancer, Fibrocystic disease of breast, Cystic disease of ovary
- Increase in cancers: Breast cancer, Cervical cancer

113. Ans. (c) Shift to barrier methods of contraception
[Ref. Missed Pill Recommendations. Faculty of Sexual and Reproductive Healthcare, CDC Guidelines]

Recommendation on Missed OCPs:
- 1 pill missed:
    - Take missed as soon as possible OR 2 pills next days
    - Then continue with one pill per day
- 2 pills missed:
    - Stop current pack of OCPs
    - Continue with barrier methods for rest of the cycle
    - Test for pregnancy towards end of cycle

Review Questions
114. Ans. (a) Monolial vaginitis *[Ref. Park 27/e p576–577]*
115. Ans. None *[Ref. Park 27/e p577]*
116. Ans. (a) Leg vein thrombosis *[Ref. Dutta 6/e p 543, 546; Park 27/e p577]*
117. Ans. (d) Pervaginal bleeding *[Ref. Park 27/e p576–577]*
118. Ans. (d) Congenital hyperlipidemia *[Ref. Park 27/e p577]*
119. Ans. (a) Only progesterone is small quantity *[Ref. Park 27/e p575]*
120. Ans. (c) Three months *[Ref. Park 27/e p577–578]*

EMERGENCY METHODS

121. Ans. (a) Levonorgestrel dose 1.5 mg *[Ref. Park 26/e p581]*
- The Drug Controller General of India approved levonorgestrel; a progestin only pill, as a dedicated product for Emergency Contraception in 2001 and it has been introduced in the Family Welfare Program since 2003
- Under the National Reproductive and Child Health Programme, the Drug Controller of India has only approved Levonorgestrel (LNG) 0.75mg tablets for use as ECP (One tablet + One tablet at gap of 12 hours, both completed within 72 hours)

122. Ans. (a) Danazol *[Ref. Park 25/e p552]*
- Post-coital contraceptives recommended include Combined POPs, POPs (RCH Program), CuT, RU 486 (Mifepristone), High dose estrogens

123. Ans. (a) Female condoms *[Ref. National Health Programs of India by Dr. J. Kishore, 8/e p120–22]*

ALSO REMEMBER
- *Female condoms*: A device that is used during sexual intercourse
    - Invented by Danish MD Lasse Hessel
    - It is worn internally by the receptive partner and physically blocks ejaculated semen from entering that person's body
    - Prevent pregnancy and transmission of STIs
    - Three types:
        1. FC Female condom: made of polyurethane
        2. FC2: made of nitrile polymer
        3. Latex
    - Only tool for HIV prevention that women can initiate & control

Contd...

Contd...

- *Male condoms versus female condoms:*

Characteristic	Male condoms	Female condoms
Material commonly used	Latex	Polyurethane*
Pearl Index (failure rate)	2–14 per HWY	5–21 per HWY
No. of rings	1	2 (outer & inner)
Reusable	No	Yes
Covering skin around external genitals	No	Yes
Compatible with oil based lubricants	No	Yes
Insertion requires male erection	Yes	No
Prevention of pregnancy	Yes	Yes
Prevention of STIs	Yes	Yes

(* Now also made of nitrile polymers, known as FC2)

124. **Ans. (b) Emergency contraception with OCPs**
 [Ref. National Health programs of India by Dr J. Kishore, 8/e p121]
 - *Phrase 'morning-after pill' is figurative*: Combined OCPs can be used for up to 72 hours after sexual intercourse
 - Insertion of an IUD is more effective than use of Emergency Contraceptive Pills
 - POP as an Emergency Contraceptive has showed greater efficacy with reduced side effects and has therefore superseded Yuzpe & Lancee method (WHO)
   - A single dose of 100 mg mifepristone is also more effective than the Yuzpe regime
 - MC side effect reported by users of emergency contraceptive pills: Nausea

125. **Ans. (a) LNG- Intrauterine device**
 [Ref. Park 27/e p579–580]

 Recommended Methods of Post Coital (Emergency) Contraception
 - *Intra-uterine devices (IUDs)*:
   - *CuT within 5 days*
 - *Hormonal*:
   - *LNG oral tablet (0.75 mg)*: 1st tablet within 72 hours of intercourse and 2nd tablet after 12 hours of first dose
   - *Combined OCPs (high estrogen 50 mcg)*: 2 pills within 72 hours of intercour + 2 pills after 12 hours
   - *Combined OCPs (low estrogen 30 mcg)*: 4 pills within 72 hours of intercour + 4 pills after 12 hours
 - Oral Mifespristone 10 mg once within 72 hours

126. **Ans. (d) 72 hours** *[Ref. Park 25/e p535]*

 Yuzpe and Lancee Method
 - Method: Combined oral pills are generally accepted as the preparation of choice for Post-coital (Emergency) contraception
 - Regimens have to be 'completed within 72 hours of coitus': Sooner started, the more effective it is
 - Regimens:
   - *Current recommendation (pills with 30 mcg oestrogen Mala-N/Mala-D)*: 4 pills immediately followed by 4 pills 12 hours later
   - *Standard method (pills with 50 mcg oestrogen)*: 2 pills immediately followed by 2 pills 12 hours later
   - Pills with 200 mcg estrogen: 1 pill immediately followed by 1 pill 12 hours later

127. **Ans. (c) Levonorgestrel only pill** *[Ref. Research on Reproductive Health at WHO, Biennial Report 2000–2001 Chapter 1]*

Review Question

128. **Ans. (a) Norgestrel** *[Ref. Park 25/e p535]*

STERILIZATION

129. **Ans. (d) Eight weeks [correct answer is three months]** *[Ref. Park 27/e p583]*

130. **Ans. (b) Surgical failure** *[Ref. Park 27/e p584]*

131. **Ans. (b) From 24 hours to 7 days of delivery** *[Ref. Standards for Female and Male Sterilization Services, MOHFW, GOI, p6]*

 Surgical Procedure Timings for Female Sterilization (GoI)
 - Interval sterilization: Within 7 days of the menstrual period (in the follicular phase of the menstrual cycle).
 - Post-partum sterilization: After 24 hours up to 7 days of delivery
 - Sterilization with medical termination of pregnancy (MTP): Performed concurrently
 - Sterilization following spontaneous abortion: Performed provided the client fulfils the medical eligibility criteria

> **ALSO REMEMBER**
> - Laparoscopic tubal ligation should not be done concurrently with second-trimester abortion and in the post-partum period

MISCELLANEOUS (FAMILY PLANNING AND CONTRACEPTION)

132. **Ans. (a) Tubal sterilization** *[Ref. Park 26/e p589]*
 - Vasectomy and Tubectomy are permanent methods (one time) for contraception

133. **Ans. (b) OCPs protect against Candidiasis** *[Ref. Shaw's Textbook of Gynaecology, 14/e p208; Park 27/e p576]*
 - Oral pills are associated with monolial vaginitis (candidiasis)

> **ALSO REMEMBER**
> - *IUDs and Actinomycosis*: Actinomyces is a normal commensal of vagina. In presence of an IUD, it can cause an *'ascending Infection'* through threads of the device.
>   - If actinomycosis occurs in a female with IUD-in-situ: Remove IUD and cut and send its threads for culture; Antibiotics should be given to control the infection.

134. **Ans. (b) Combined oral pills** *[Ref. Shaw's Textbook of Gynaecology, 14/e p208–09; Park 27/e p576]*
- *Increased incidence of ectopic is associated with*:
  - Previous salpingitis due to STD (MCC)
  - Congenital defects ion fallopian tubes
  - Transperitoneal migration of fertilized ovum to other side tube
  - Pelvic abnormalities
  - Tubal reconstructive surgery
  - Tubectomy operation
  - In-vitro fertilization
  - Rapid development of trophoblast
  - Extraneous events like appendicitis & endometriosis
  - IUDs (Progestagen containing IUDs have 9-fold higher risk)
  - Induction of ovulation by gonadotropins
  - Others: advancing age, smoking, vaginal douching, exposure to diethylstilbestrol (DES) in utero
- *Combined oral pills lead to reduced incidence of ectopic pregnancy*, due to
  - Suppression of ovulation
  - Reduction in PID

> **ALSO REMEMBER**
> - *MC type of ectopic pregnancy*: Tubal pregnancy (Fallopian Tubes)
> - *MC site of implantation*: Ampulla (tubal pregnancy)
> - *Threshold of discrimination of intrauterine pregnancy*: 1500 IU/mL of α-hCG
> - *Cullen's sign* can indicate a ruptured ectopic pregnancy
> - *Non-surgical treatment of ectopic pregnancy*: Methotrexate

135. **Ans. (c) Require action at time of intercourse**
[Ref. Park 27/e p568]
- *Conventional Contraceptives*: Methods that require action at the time of coitus
  - Condoms
  - Spermicides
  - Jellies
- *Conventional Contraceptives does not mean older contraceptives*

> **ALSO REMEMBER**
> - *Oldest methods of contraception* (aside from sexual abstinence):
>   - coitus interruptus
>   - lactational
>   - certain barrier methods
>   - herbal methods (ammenagogues and abortifacients)

136. **Ans. (a) Achieve 100% institutional deliveries**
[Ref. Park 27/e p568]

> **ALSO REMEMBER**
> **Key ANC–Related Findings of NFHS-4, India (2015–16)**
> - *No. of AN visits* (≥ 4): 51%
> - *Took IFA for 100 days or more*: 30%
> - *Received >2 TT injections*: 89%
> - *Home delivery*: 21% (Delivery at health facility: 79%)
> - *Delivery conducted by a skilled provider*: 81%

137. **Ans. (a) To bring down Total Fertility Rate (TFR) to replacement levels by 2015** *[Ref. Park 27/e p568]*
138. **Ans. (a) Condom** *[Ref. Park 27/e p569]*
- *Condom fatigue*: Is a term used by medical professionals and safer sex educators to refer to the phenomenon of decreased condom use
  - Also be used to describe a general weariness of and decreased effectiveness of safer sex messages (prevention fatigue)
  - The term has particularly been used to describe men who have sex with men (MSM), though the term applies to people of all genders and sexual orientations
  - Condom fatigue has been partially blamed for an increase in HIV infection rates, though this has not been substantiated in any study

> **ALSO REMEMBER**
> - *Male contraceptives under trials*:
>   - *Gossypol* (Chinese cotton derivative; research suspended due to 10–20% permanent azoospermia)
>   - *Reversible inhibition of sperm under guidance (RISUG)* consists of injecting 'styrene maleic anhydride in dimethyl sulfoxide' into the vas deferens and leads to long lasting sterility (Phase III trial)
>   - *Vas-occlusive contraception* consists of partially or completely blocking the vas deferens, the tubes connecting the epididymis to the urethra (intra-vas device IVD and other injectable plugs)
>   - *Heat-based contraception*: heating the testicles to high temperature for a short period of time to prevent the formation of sperm.
>   - *Adjudin*: A non-toxic analog of 'lonidamine' disrupts the junctions between nurse cells (Sertoli cells) in the testes and forming spermatids; the sperm are released prematurely and never become functional gametes
>   - *A male hormonal contraceptive combination protocol* has been developed, involving injections of Depo-Provera to prevent spermatogenesis, combined with the topical application of testosterone gel to provide hormonal support
>   - *Interference with the maturation of sperm in the epididymis* (under research)

139. **Ans. (a) 20 weeks** *[Ref. Park 27/e p580]*
Medical Termination of Pregnancy Act, 1971
- *Passed in*: April 1972
- *Indications for MTP*:
  - Humanitarian: If pregnancy is as a result of rape/sexual assault

- Eugenic: Any genetic/chromosomal anomaly detected in fetus
- Therapeutic: If carrying out full term pregnancy poses a risk to life of mother
- Social: If pregnancy is a result of contraceptive failure
- *Written consent of guardians*:
  - If woman is a lunatic
  - If woman is less than 18 years age
- *Period of gestation must be 'less than 20 weeks'*:
  - 0–12 weeks: Opinion of one doctor is sufficient
  - 12–20 weeks: Opinions of 2 doctors required
- *Who can perform MTP*:
  - Qualification: MD (Gyn-Obs) or DGO or 6-months Housemanship in Gyn-Obs
  - Experience: At least carried out 20–25 supervised MTPs
- *Where MTP can be done*: At a place authorised by Government of India

140. **Ans. (c) Oral contraceptive pills**
 [Ref. RCH- II Programme document]
- Contraceptive choices for a newly married healthy couple
- *Barrier method*:
  - Has a high failure rate; only consistent use for 2 years reduce it
  - Has advantage of HIV/STI protection but a 'healthy' couple may not need it
- *IUCD*
  - Is not a method of first choice for nulliparous female
- *Oral contraceptive pills*
  - Low failure rate
  - Ideal method of choice for newly married healthy couple
- *Natural methods*
  - Has a high failure rate

141. **Ans. (d) All of the above**
 [Ref. Park 21/e p778, Park 22/e p772]

Uses of Regular Reporting of Health Statistics
- To measure health status of population
- To quantify health related problems
- To evaluate trends of disease in a population
- To compare health data locally, nationally and internationally
- To effective plan health programs, policies, services
- To monitor and evaluate health programs
- To evaluate satisfaction among population
- To appreciate health personnel's efforts
- To promote epidemiological research

142. **Ans. (b) IUCD** [Ref. Post-puerperal Cu-T insertion: A prospective study. J Postgrad Med. 1989; 35:70–73]

WHO Guidelines for Contraceptive use in Lactating Women
- Progestin-only methods of contraception (i.e., oral contraceptives, levonorgestrel-IUDs, levonorgestrel implant, Depo-Provera injection) are not usually recommended before 6 weeks postpartum unless other more appropriate methods are not available or not acceptable
- Progestin-only methods can be used in any circumstances after 6 weeks postpartum
- Combined estrogen-progestin contraceptives (i.e., oral contraceptives, transdermal path, or vaginal ring) are not to be used before 6 weeks postpartum
- Combined estrogen-progestin contraceptives are not usually recommended between 6 weeks and 6 months postpartum unless other more appropriate methods are not available or not acceptable
- Combined estrogen-progestin contraceptives can be generally used after 6 months postpartum

An IUD is an ideal contraceptive for lactating women because it has no effect on the quality or composition of breast milk:
- A post-partum IUD is generally inserted 6–8 weeks after delivery
- IUD is an effective method for long term contraception

143. **Ans. (a) Barrier methods** [Ref. Park 27/e p569]
- Ideal contraceptive for a couple who are living separately in two cities and meets only occasionally is Condom as long term contraception is not desirable
  - Also OCPs, Barrier methods are required for long term contraception and both of them have few side effects too; so they are not desirable in this case
  - Inj. DMPA is an injectable (DEPOT) hormonal formulation which given contraception for 3 months which is not desirable here.

144. **Ans. (a) Wife only** [Ref. MTP Act, GoI]

Consent Under MTP Act, 1972
- *If pregnant female is 18 years or above*: Consent of woman alone is required
- *If pregnant female is less than 18 years*: Consent of guardian is required
- *If pregnant female is lunatic*: Consent of guardian is required

Also Refer to Ans. 173

145. **Ans. (c) 30–35%** [Ref. Human Reproductive Biology by Lopez & Jones, 4/e p286]

146. **Ans. (d) Combined oral contraceptives** [Ref. Park 27/e p575]

COMBINED OCPs CONTRAINDICATED DURING LACTATION
- Estrogen adversely affect quantity and constituents of breast milk
- Estrogen cause premature cessation of lactation
- Hormones excretions occur in breast milk

Review Questions

147. **Ans. (d) Diaphragm** [Ref. Park 27/e p569]
148. **Ans. None** [Ref. Park 27/e p580]

CHAPTER 8

Preventive Obstetrics, Pediatrics and Geriatrics

MCH

Ante-natal and Post-natal Visits (RCH Program)

- *Ideal recommended ante-natal visits^Q*: 13–14

Period of gestation	Frequency of visit^Q
0–7 months	Once every month
8th month	Twice a month
9th month onwards	Once a week

- *Minimum recommended ante-natal visits^Q*: 4

Visit	Period of gestation^Q
First AN visit	Early registration
Second AN visit	14–26 weeks POG
Third AN visit	28–34 weeks POG
Fourth AN visit	36 weeks POG - Term

> **Key points**
> Minimum recommended antenatal visits^Q: 4

- *Minimum recommended post-natal visits^Q*: 3–4

Visit	Time
First PN visit	Day 0*
Second PN visit	Day 3
Third PN visit	Day 7
Fourth PN visit	Day 42

> **Key points**
> Minimum recommended postnatal visits^Q: 3–4

(* Day 0 visit only for deliveries at home and sub-centres)
(All visits undertaken post-delivery by HWF/ANM to the home of female)

Nutritional Requirements

- *Recommended daily energy intake*: [NEW GUIDELINES 2011]

Group	Energy Allowance per day (kcal)
Infancy 0–6 months^Q 6–12 months^Q	 92 kcal/kg/day 80 kcal/kg/day
Adult Reference Male (Wt: 60 kg) Sedentary/Light work^Q Moderate work Heavy work	 2320 2730 3490
Adult Reference Female (Wt: 55 kg) Sedentary/Light work^Q Moderate work Heavy work	 1900 2230 2850
Pregnancy^Q	+ 350

> **Key points**
> Pregnancy^Q additional energy: + 350 kcal/day

Group	Energy Allowance per day (kcal)
Lactation	
First 6 months[Q]	+ 600
6–12 months	+ 520

(+ indicates 'over and above the daily requirement')

- *Requirements in pregnancy and lactation:*

	Requirement per day	
Group	Energy (kcal/day)[Q]	Proteins (g/day)
Woman		
Sedentary work[Q]	1900	55
Moderate work	2230	55
Heavy work	2850	55
Pregnancy[Q]	+ 350	+23
Lactation		
0–6 months[Q]	+600	+19
6–12 months	+520	+13

(+ indicates 'over and above the daily requirement')

> **Key points**
> Lactation additional energy
> First 6 months[Q]: + 600 kcal/day

> **Key points**
> *Five cleans*
> - Clean delivery surface
> - Clean hands (of birth attendants)
> - Clean cord cut (blade or instrument)
> - Clean cord tie
> - Clean cord stump

- *Other requirements in pregnancy and lactation:*

	Pregnancy	Lactation	
		0–6 months	6–12 months
Proteins	+23 g/day[Q]	+19 g/day	+13 g/day
Calcium	1200 mg/day[Q]	1200 mg/day[Q]	1200 mg/day
Iron	35 mg/day[Q]	21 mg/day	21 mg/day
Vitamin A	800 mcg/day[Q]	950 mcg/day	950 mcg/day

(+ indicates 'over and above the daily requirement')

Cleans of Safe Delivery

- *'Five cleans'* (practices) under strategies for elimination of neonatal tetanus include[Q],
  - Clean delivery surface
  - Clean hands (of birth attendants)
  - Clean cord cut (blade or instrument)
  - Clean cord tie
  - Clean cord stump (no applicant)
- *Procedures undertaken to ensure 5 cleans*:
  - *Clean delivery surface:* A clean plastic sheet
  - *Clean hands:* Soap and clean water
  - *Clean cord cut:* A new razor blade
  - *Clean cord tie:* A clean piece of thread
  - *Clean cord stump:* Nothing to be applied to cord
- Sometimes these practices are called as '*3 cleans*':
  - Clean delivery surface
  - Clean hands
  - Clean cord care (cut, tie and stump)
- Suggested '*Seven cleans*'[Q] (include five cleans)
  - Clean delivery surface
  - Clean hands (of birth attendants)
  - Clean cord cut (blade or instrument)
  - Clean cord tie
  - Clean cord stump (no applicant)
  - Clean water, and
  - Clean towel, for hand washing

IFA Tablets

- *An adult tablet of IFA contains*[Q]: 100 mg elemental Iron and 500 mcg Folic acid (to be given for 100 days minimum in pregnancy) and 100 days post-delivery
  - Schedule: 1 Tablet per day in 4–5–6 month POG (Total 100 tablets)
- *A pediatric tablet of IFA contains*[Q]: 20 mg elemental Iron and 100 mcg Folic acid (to be given for 100 days minimum every year till 5 years age of child)
  For New guidelines, see Annexure 21 (AMB)

> **Key points**
> Adult tablet of IFA contains[Q]: 100 mg elemental Iron and 500 mcg Folic acid

TT in Pregnancy
Refer to Chapter 3, Theory

Mother to Child Transmission (MTCT)
Refer to Chapter 5, Theory

Birth Weight

- Birth weight of an infant is the '*single most important determinant of its chances of survival, healthy growth and development*'[Q]
- Single best measure to assess physical growth: Weight[Q]
- Birth weight preferably be measured within: 1st hour of life[Q]
- Average birth weight in India: 2.8 kg (2.7–2.9 kg) [Q]
- Majority of LBW in India is due to: Maternal malnutrition associated with fetal growth retardation
- Relationship between maternal nutrition and birth weight of babies: Linear[Q]
- Smoking during pregnancy reduces birth weight by an average: 170 grams
- LBW is not a contraindication for any vaccination EXCEPT Hepatitis B: Hepatitis B vaccine is contraindicated in preterm children with birth weight <2.0 kg[Q]
- Field instrument for measurement of birth weight: Salter's Scale[Q]
- Growth chart is plotted between: Weight and Age[Q]
- Birth weight doubles at 5 months age, triples at 1 year and quadruples at 2 years age[Q]
- Birth weight increments:

> **Key points**
> Single best measure to assess physical growth: Weight

Age	Weight increments
0–3 months	200 grams per week
4–6 months	150 grams per week
7–9 months	100 grams per week
10–12 months	50 grams per week
1–2 years	2.5 kg per year
3–5 years	2.0 kg per year

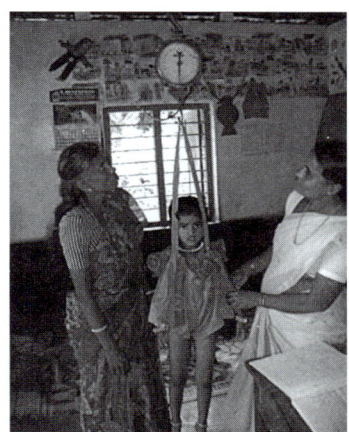
Salter Scale

Low Birth Weight (LBW)

- *Low Birth Weight (LBW)* [Q]: Birth weight less than 2500 grams (<2.5 kg) [WHO]. It includes both pre-term (<37 weeks POG) and full-term (>37 weeks POG) babies
- *Prevalence of LBW*: 15% (World); 18% (India[Q])
  - If cutoff for LBW is reduced to 2.0 kg, expected prevalence of LBW in India will be 5.5%[Q]
- LBW is regardless of gestational age[Q]
- Depending on the population, the percentage of LBW be based on measurements of at least 500 babies[Q]
- 3 inter-related risk factors for LBW: Malnutrition, Infection and Unregulated fertility
- Babies according to gestational age:

> **Key points**
> LBW[Q]: Birth weight less than 2500 grams (<2.5 kg)

Type	Gestational age[Q]
Pre-term babies	<37 weeks (<259 days)
Term babies	37–42 weeks (259–293 days)
Post-term babies	>42 weeks (>294 days)

- Low birth weight: 'Less than 2500 grams IRRESPECTIVE of gestational age'

- *Pre-term babies:* Born at <37 weeks POG
- *Small-for-date (SFD) babies^Q:* Born at term or post-term
  - Weigh *'less than 10th percentile for gestational age'^{Q}*
  - As a result of IUGR^Q
  - High risk of dying in neonatal and infancy period

MCH INDICATORS

Infant Mortality Rate (IMR)

> **Key points**
> IMR is usually expressed as a rate per 1000 live births (LB)^Q

> **Key points**
> MCC of IMR in India: Low birth weight and prematurity^Q

- *Infant mortality rate (IMR):* Is the ratio of infant deaths registered in a given year to the total number of live births registered in the same year; IMR is usually expressed as a rate per 1000 live births (LB)^Q
- IMR = $\dfrac{\text{No. of infant deaths in a given year}}{\text{Total no. of live births in the same year}} \times 1000$
- *Infant Mortality Rate (IMR) is the SECOND best indicator of socio-economic development of a country^Q*
  - *Best indicator of SE development^Q:* Under 5 mortality rate (U5MR)
- IMR is most important indicator of
  - Health status of a community
  - Level of living and
  - Effectiveness of MCH services in general
- The infant mortality rate is among *'the best predictors of state failure'^{Q}*
- Infant Mortality Rate (IMR):
  - *Infant Mortality Rate (IMR) is a rate*
  - Infant mortality accounts for 18% of total deaths in India
  - *MCC of IMR in India:* Low birth weight and prematurity^Q
  - *MCC of IMR in World:* Pneumonia^Q
- *IMR (World):* 26 per 1000 LB [2023]
- *IMR (India):* 28 per 1000 LB [2022]

Factors Affecting IMR

- Likely factor affecting infant mortality in contemporary India is inadequate prenatal care and infrequent attendance at delivery
- *Factors affecting Infant Mortality Rate (IMR):*
  - Biological factors:
    - *Birth weight (BW):* IMR greater in BW <2.5 kg and >4.0 kg
    - *Age of mother:* IMR is greater in age <19 and >35 years
  - *Birth order:* Infant mortality is greatest for birth order 1 and least for 2; It increases from birth order 3 onwards^Q
    - *Birth spacing:* IMR reduces with wider birth spacing
    - *Multiple births:* IMR increases in multiple births
    - *Family size:* IMR increases as family size increases
    - *High fertility:* IMR increases with high fertility
  - Economic factors:
    - *Socio-economic status (SES):* IMR higher in lower SES
  - Cultural and social factors:
    - *Breastfeeding:* IMR higher in early weaning and bottle fed infants living in poor hygienic conditions
    - *Religion and caste:* IMR is affected by patterns, habits, customs, child care, etc.
    - *Early marriages:* IMR higher in teen age pregnancy
  - Other factors:
    - *Sex of the child:* IMRgirls >IMRboys^Q
    - *Quality of mothering:* IMR low in good quality of mothering
    - *Quality of health care:* IMR high in improper obstetric and pediatric care
    - *Maternal education:* IMR low in mother with high literacy rate
    - *Broken family:* IMR higher
    - *Illegitimacy:* IMR higher
    - *Brutal habits and customs:* IMR high (Not feeding colostrum, applying cow-dung to umbilical-stump, faulty feeding practices)

- *Untrained dai:* High IMR
- *Bad environmental sanitation:* High IMR

Neonatal Mortality Rate (NNMR)

- *Neonatal mortality rate (NNMR):* Is the number of neonatal deaths (deaths within completed 28 days after birth) per 1000 live births in that year^Q
- NNMR = $\dfrac{\text{No. of neonatal deaths in a given year}}{\text{Total no. of live births in the same year}} \times 1000$
  - *Early neonatal mortality (ENNM):* Neonatal mortality in first week (1–7 days) of life^Q
  - *Late neonatal mortality (LNNM):* Neonatal mortality in first to fourth week (8–28 days) of life
- *NNMR (India):* 20 per 1000 LB [2019]^Q
- NNMR is directly related with birth weight and gestational age
- NNMRboys >NNMRgirls^Q
- *MCC of NNMR in India is preterm birth*
  - *MCC of ENNMR:* Prematurity and congenital anomalies^Q
  - *MCC of LNNMR:* Infections (diarrhea and tetanus)^Q
- *Causes of Neonatal mortality (0–4 weeks):*
  - Low birth weight and prematurity
  - Birth injury and difficult labour
  - Sepsis
  - Congenital anomalies
  - Hemolytic diseases of newborn
  - Conditions of placenta and cord
  - Diarrhoeal diseases
  - Acute respiratory infections
  - Tetanus

> **Key points**
> MCC of NNMR in India is Preterm birth

Maternal Mortality Ratio (MMR)

- *Maternal Mortality Ratio (MMR):* Maternal deaths expressed as per 100,000 live births, where a 'maternal death' is defined as 'death of a woman while pregnant or during delivery or within 42 days (6 weeks) of termination of pregnancy, irrespective of duration or site of pregnancy, from any cause related to or aggravated by the pregnancy or its management but not from accidental or incidental causes'^{Q}
  - *Maternal deaths expressed as per 100,000 live births* (earlier it was expressed per 1000 live births but that yielded fractions like 4.08 maternal deaths per 1000 LB; so denominator was extrapolated to 100,000 to make MMR value more sensible) ^{Q}
  - *MMR is a ratio*^{Q}
  - MMR = $\dfrac{\text{No. of maternal deaths in a given year}}{\text{Total no. of live births in the same year}} \times 100{,}000$

> **Key points**
> (MMR): Maternal deaths expressed as per 100,000 live births

- *MMR World:* 216 per 100,000 live births; *Causes of MMR (globally):*
  - *Hemorrhage (25%)*^{Q}
  - *Indirect causes (20%)*
  - *Infection (15%)*
  - *Unsafe abortion (13%)*
  - *Eclampsia (12%)*
  - *Obstructed labour (8%)*
- *MMR India:* 97 per 100,000 live births [2023]^Q; *Causes of MMR (India) [SRS 2023]:*
  - *Hemorrhage (38%)*^{Q}
  - *Other conditions (34%)*
  - *Sepsis (11%)*
  - *Abortion (8%)*
  - *Obstructed labour (5%)*
  - *Hypertensive disorders (5%)*
- *RHIME*^{Q} - '*Representative, re-sampled, routine household interview of mortality, with medical evaluation*': Is a new method for MMR estimation introduced in India from 2003 SRS
  - RHIME is an enhanced form of *verbal autopsy*^{Q}

> **Key points**
> MMR is a ratio

Maternal Mortality Rate
- *Maternal mortality rate (MMRate):* Dividing the average annual number of maternal deaths in a population by the average number of women of reproductive age (typically those aged 15 to 49 years) who are alive during the observation period
- MMRate reflects not only the risk of maternal death per pregnancy or per birth, but also the level of fertility in a population

NEW Initiatives in MCH

Labor Room Quality Improvement Initiative – LaQshya
- MoHFW launched LaQshya to improve the quality of care that is being provided to the pregnant mother in the Labor Room and Maternity Operation Theaters, thereby preventing the undesirable adverse outcomes associated with childbirth

Pradhan Mantri Surakshit Matritva Abhiyan (PMSMA)
- To provide assured, comprehensive and quality antenatal care, free of cost, universally to all pregnant women on the 9th of every month
- Guarantees a minimum package of antenatal care services to women in their 2nd/3rd trimesters of pregnancy at designated government health facilities.

Child Mortality Rate, CMR (Under 5 Mortality Rate, U5MR)

$$CMR = \frac{\text{No. of deaths of children less than 5 years age in a year}}{\text{No. of live births in a year}} \times 1000$$

- *U5MR (India):* 32 per 1000 LB [2022]^Q
- *U5MR (World):* 38 per 1000 LB [2021]
- *Single MCC of U5MR or CMR is Prematurity*
- *Neonatal conditions lead to 47% of total U5MR or CMR^Q:*
  - Prematurity (MCC)
  - Infections
  - Preterm births
  - Asphyxia

Child Death Rate, CDR (1–4 year Mortality Rate)

$$CDR = \frac{\text{No. of deaths of children aged 1-4 years in a year}}{\text{Mid year population of children aged 1-4 years}} \times 1000$$

- *CDR is a more refined indicator of social situation in a country than infant mortality*
- *Highest risk of death in 1–4 years age:* 2nd year of life
- *CDR (India):* 2.8% of total deaths [2014]^Q
- *MCC CDR (Developing countries):* Diarrhoeal diseases and respiratory infections^Q
- *MCC CDR (Developed countries):* Accidents
- *Millennium Development Goal (MDG) 4:* Reduce child mortality by two-thirds by 2015
- UNICEF considers U5MR or CMR as '*single best indicator of socio-economic development and well being*'^{Q}

Child Survival Rate (CSR) [Child Survival Index]^Q

$$CSR = \frac{1000 - U5MR}{10}$$

- *CSR (India):* 97 [2022]

Post Neonatal Mortality Rate (PNNMR)
- *Post-neonatal mortality rate (PNNMR):* Is the number of infant deaths after Neonatal period (deaths within completed 28 days after birth) per 1000 live births in that year^Q [PNNMR India 2018 = 11 per 1000 LB]

$$\text{PNMR} = \frac{\text{No. of deaths between age 28 days to 1 year in a given year}}{\text{Total no. of live births in the same year}} \times 1000$$

Perinatal Mortality Rate (PNMR)

- *Perinatal mortality rate (PNMR)*: Includes both late fetal deaths (stillbirths) and early neonatal deaths^Q

$$\text{PNMR} = \frac{\text{Late fetal deaths and early neonatal deaths in a given year}}{\text{Total no. of live births in the same year}} \times 1000$$

- Perinatal period is from 28 weeks period of gestation to 7th completed days of life (But the *WHO definition of perinatal period* is from 22 completed weeks gestation to 7th completed days of life^Q)
    - PNMR is the sum of the fetal mortality and the neonatal mortality
- *PNMR is a major marker to assess the quality of healthcare delivery^Q*
- *PNMR (India): 18 per 1000 LB [2022]*
- *P List^Q (ICD 10):* 100 causes of perinatal mortality and morbidity

> **IMA Guidelines on Period of Viability**
> - **Born >28 weeks POG and >1000 grams:** Viable child
> - **Born 20–24 weeks POG:** Not viable child; it is not advisable to resuscitate him or her but the child should be given comfort care
> - **Born 24–28 weeks POG:** Chances of survival is less and should be decided on case to case basis, and >28 weeks every effort should be made to ensure the child survives
>   - Anything less than viability (28 weeks and 1000 gram), level of treatment has to be decided on case to cases basis on chances of intact survival, informed consent taking into consideration social determinants of health; Basic care should not be compromised
>   - Non-initiation of resuscitation may be considered appropriate in confirmed gestation <25 weeks, anencephaly and confirmed lethal genetic malformation disorder

BREASTFEEDING

WHO Guidelines for India

- WHO recommends, in developing countries, *exclusive breastfeeding till 6 months age^Q*
- WHO recommends, in developing countries, *breastfeeding till minimum 2 years age^Q*

Nutritional Importance of Breast Milk

- *Energy content of breast milk: 65 kcal/100 mL^Q*
- *Protein content of breast milk: 1.1 grams/100 mL^Q*
- Mean output of breast milk per day (mL):

Months of lactation	Mean output (mL)
0–2	530
3–4	640
5–6	730^Q
7–8	660
9–10	600
11–12	525

> **Key points**
> **Perinatal period** is from 28 weeks period of gestation to 7th completed days of life

> **Key points**
> *Exclusive breastfeeding* till 6 months age^Q

> **Key points**
> *Energy content of breast milk: 65 kcal/100 mL*
> *Protein content of breast milk: 1.1 grams/100 mL*

- Nutritive values of milk (per 100 gm):

	Cow's milk	Human milk
Lactose (g)	4.4	7.4
Proteins (g)	3.2	1.1
Fat (g)	4.1	3.4
Calcium (mg)	120	28
Iron (mg)	0.2	0.35
Water (g)	87	88
Energy (kcal)	67	65
Casein: Whey ratio	80:20	40:60

- *Human Milk is richer in Carbohydrate (lactose), Iron and Water content* WHILE Cow's milk is richer in Fat, Protein, Calcium and energy content[Q]
    - *Human milk proteins:* More cystine and taurine; less methionine; better digested than cow's milk proteins[Q]
    - *Human milk fats:* Higher levels of PUFAs, esp., linoleic acid and -linoleic acid; better digested and absorbed; low calcium content but better absorbed than cow's milk[Q]
    - *Human milk vitamins and minerals:* Human milk is richer in Vitamin A, C; richer in copper, cobalt and selenium; richer in iron and higher bioavailability; high calcium/phosphorus ratio; Human milk has lesser sodium[Q]
- *Comparative contents of nutrients in different types of milk:*
    - *Fat content of milk:* Buffalo > Goat > Cow > Human
    - *Protein content of milk:* Buffalo > Goat > Cow > Human
    - *Energy content of milk:* Buffalo > Goat > Cow > Human
    - *Lactose content of milk[Q]:* Human > Buffalo > Goat > Cow

Colostrum

- Is the most suitable food immediately after birth of the baby; Regular milk comes 3–6 days after birth
- Also known as '*Beestings*', '*First milk*' or '*Immune Milk*'[Q]
- High in carbohydrates, protein, and antibodies and low in fat
- Contains all five immunoglobulins found in all mammals, IgA, IgD, IgE, IgG and IgM[Q]
- *Few occasions when breastfeeding might harm the infant[Q]:*
    - Infants with classic galactosemia
    - Mother has untreated pulmonary tuberculosis
    - Mother is taking certain medications that suppress the immune system
    - Mother has had unusually excessive exposure to heavy metals such as mercury
    - Mother has HIV
    - Mother uses potentially harmful substances such as cocaine, heroin, and amphetamines

GROWTH AND DEVELOPMENT

Indicators of Malnutrition

> **Key points**
> '*Underweight*' is Acute + Chronic Malnutrition

- *Indicators of malnutrition:*
    - *Single best parameter for assessment of physical growth:* Weight (and rate of weight gain)[Q]
    - *Single most sensitive measure of growth:* Weight[Q]
    - *Single most reliable criterion of assessment of health and nutritional status:* Weight[Q]
    - *Weight for height is considered more important than weight alone,* for the measurement of physical growth
    - Height is a stable measurement of growth as opposed to body weight[Q]
    - *Weight:* Reflects only present health status
    - *Height:* Indicates events in past also
- *Acute and Chronic Malnutrition[Q]:*
    - *Low weight for age:* Is known as '*Underweight*'[Q] (Acute on Chronic Malnutrition[Q])

> **Key points**
> *Wasting is Acute Malnutrition[Q]*

- Low weight for height: Is known as 'Nutritional wasting'^Q or 'Emaciation' (Acute Malnutrition^Q)
- Low height for age: Is known as 'Nutritional stunting'^Q or 'Dwarfing' (Chronic malnutrition^Q)
- *Age independent parameters for growth assessment:*
  - Weight for height
  - Mid arm circumference (MAC)
  - Thickness of subcutaneous fat
  - Body ratios
  - Weight: Height
  - MAC: Head circumference
- *Gomez Classification of malnutrition:* Is based on 'weight for age'

Weight for age*	Grade of malnutrition
90–110%	Normal
75–89%	1st degree (MILD)
60–74%	2nd degree (MODERATE)
<60%	3rd degree (SEVERE)

> **Key points**
> *Stunting* is *Chronic malnutrition*^Q

- *Waterlow classification:*

Weight/height Height/age	>Mean – 2SD	<Mean – 2SD
>Mean – 2SD	Normal	Wasted
<Mean – 2SD	Stunted	Wasted & Stunted

- *Welcome trust classification:*

Weight for age	With oedema	Without oedema
60–80%	Kwashiorkar	Undernutrition
<60%	Marasmic-kwashiorkar	Marasmus

Milestones of Development^Q

Age	Motor development	Language development	Adaptive development	Socio-personal development
6–8 wks	–	–	–	look/smiles at mother
3 m	holds head erect	–	–	–
4–5 m	–	listening	reach for objects	recognizes mother
6–8 m	sits without support	experiment with noises	hand-transfer object	enjoys hide & seek
9–10 m	crawls	increase sound-range	releases objects	stranger suspicion
10–11 m	stands with support	first words	–	–
12–14 m	walks wide base	–	builds	–
18–21 m	walks narrow base	joining words	begins to explore	–
24 m	runs	short sentences	–	dry by day

Birth Weight

- *Average birth weight in India:* 2.8 kg (2.7–2.9 kg)^Q
  - Low Birth Weight (LBW): BW <2.5 kg^Q
  - LBW in India: 18%^Q

> **Key points**
> - LBW in India: 18%
> - BW doubles at 5 months, triples by 1 year

- BW doubles at 5 months, triples by 1 year and quadruples by 2 years age^Q
  - Minimum expected weight gain per month: 500 grams
- Weight gain pattern in children:

Age	Weight increments
0–3 months	200 grams per week
4–6 months	150 grams per week
7–9 months	100 grams per week
10–12 months	50 grams per week
1–2 years	2.5 kg per year
3–5 years	2.0 kg per year

Birth Length/Height

- *Average birth length in India:* 50 cms^Q
- *BL doubles at:* 4 years age^Q
- Height increase pattern in children:

Age	Height increments
1st year	25 cm per year^Q
2nd year	12 cm per year
3rd year	9 cm per year
4th year	7 cm per year
5th year	6 cm per year

- *Near-final height attainment^Q:*
  - Indian boys attain 98% of final height by 17.75 years
  - Indian girls attain 98% of final height by 16.5 years

Growth Charts

- *Growth Chart (Road-to-health chart):* Is a visible display of child's physical growth and development
  - *Growth chart was developed by:* David Morley^Q
  - *Growth chart is designed for:* Longitudinal follow-up (growth monitoring) of a child
  - *Growth chart is generally plotted between:* Weight and Age^Q
- *Growth chart provides information on^Q:*
  - Identification and registration
  - Birth date and birth weight
  - Chronological age
  - Weight-for-age
  - Developmental milestones
  - History of sibling health
  - Immunization procedures
  - Introduction of supplementary foods
  - Episodes of sickness
  - Child spacing (Contraceptive/family planning methods used)
  - Reasons for special care

WHO Home Based Growth Chart (Same for Both Sexes)

- *WHO growth chart has 2 reference curves^Q:*
  - *Upper Reference Curve (URC):* 50th percentile for boys^Q
  - *Lower Reference Curve (LRC):* 3rd percentile for girls
- *Road to Health:* Is the space between two growth curves (weight channel). It includes zone of normality for most populations, i.e. 95% of healthy normal children used as a reference fall in this area^Q
- *WHO reference curves are based on^Q:* NCHS Standards (National Centre for Health Statistics, USA)

Key points
- BL doubles at: 4 years age

Key points
Growth chart was developed by: David Morley

Key points
WHO growth chart
Upper Reference Curve (URC): 50th percentile for boys

- *The 3rd percentile (LRC) corresponds to approximately 2 SD below the median of weight-for-age reference value (URC)^Q*

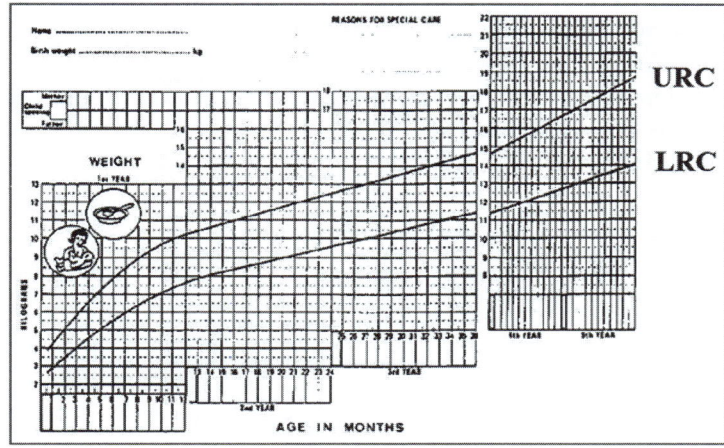

Growth chart (WHO)

WHO Service Growth Chart (Separate for Both Sexes)

- *Has 5 reference curves:*
  - *97th percentile of standard reference population*
  - *50th percentile of standard reference population*
  - *3rd percentile of standard reference population*
  - *3rd SD value of standard median population*
  - *4th SD value of standard median population*

Government of India (GOI) recommended Growth Chart (used in Anganwadis)

- *GOI recommended growth chart has 4 reference curves:*
  - *80% of median (50th percentile or URC) of WHO reference standard*
  - *70% of median (50th percentile or URC) of WHO reference standard*
  - *60% of median (50th percentile or URC) of WHO reference standard*
  - *50% of median (50th percentile or URC) of WHO reference standard*
    - *The 80% of median corresponds to approximately 2 SD below the median of weight-for-age reference value (i.e., URC)^Q*
- *Interpretation of plot of weight on GOI recommended growth chart:*
  - *Between 80% and 70% lines: 1st degree or Mild malnutrition*
  - *Between 70% and 60% lines: 2nd degree or Moderate malnutrition*
  - *Between 60% and 50% lines: 3rd degree or Severe malnutrition*
  - *Below 50% line: 4th degree or IV grade malnutrition*

ICDS Growth Chart (Based on WHO MGRS Child Growth Standards 2006) (used in Anganwadis)

- *ICDS Growth chart has 3 reference curves^Q:*
  - *Reference standard*
  - *2SD below of reference standard*
  - *3SD below reference standard*

Key Facts about Growth Charts

- Growth chart was first designed by *'David Morley'* (and later modified by WHO)
- Growth chart is the *'passport to child's health care'*^{Q}

> **Key points**
> *WHO reference curves are based on: NCHS Standards*

> **Key points**
> Growth chart is the 'passport to child's health care'

- *Best original available standards of growth:* NCHS standards^Q
- *Direction of growth in a growth chart is more important* than the position of dots
  - Periodic weight record is more useful than a single weight plot
- *Objective in child care:* To keep the child above 3rd percentile^Q
- *Flattening of a child's plot:* indicates malnutrition
- During states of under-nutrition, weight, height and brain growth are affected in that order
- There are 49 types of growth charts used in India
- *Uses of growth chart:*^{Q}
  - Growth monitoring tool
  - Diagnostic tool for identifying high risk children
  - Planning and policy making
  - Educational tool
  - Tool for action
  - Evaluation of corrective measures and impact of a programme
  - Tool for teaching
- *Reference or standard values of growth:*
  - Harvard (Boston) standards
  - NCHS standards (WHO reference values)
  - Indian standards (ICMR values)
  - MGRS (WHO 2006 values)

> **Key points**
> School Health Exam
> NRHM [New Guidelines] recommendation: Once every 6 months^Q

SCHOOL HEALTH

Health Disorders among School Children

- *Commonly detected morbidities in school children (in decreasing order of prevalence):*
  - Dental defects^Q (180.3 per 1000)
  - Goiter (123.8 per 1000)
  - Malnutrition (123.5 per 1000)

School Health Examination

- In 1961, 'Rennuka Roy School Health Committee' laid the foundations for a comprehensive school health programme in India
  - Recommendation: Medical examination of children *'at the time of entry and thereafter every 4 years'*
  - NRHM [New Guidelines] recommendation: Once every 6 months^Q
- *School Eye Screening Programme:*
  - Focus on middle schools (V–VIII classes: 10–14 years age group)
  - Teachers to do screening: 1 teacher per 150 students^Q
  - Visual acuity cutoff for referral to PHC: <6/9^Q

> **Key points**
> Visual acuity cutoff for referral to PHC: <6/9

Healthful School Environment

- *Healthful school environment:* Suggested minimum standards for sanitation of schools and its environs in India include,
  - *Location:* Away from noisy surroundings; kept fenced
  - *Site:* 5 acres for primary schools; 10 acres for higher elementary schools
  - *Structure:* Exterior walls 10 inch thick and heat resistant
  - *Class room:* 1 class room per 40 students maximum^Q
  - *Per capita space:* >10 sq. feet^Q
  - *Furniture:* Single desks of 'minus (–) type'^{Q}
  - *Doors and windows:* Doors and windows area >25% of floor area^Q
  - *Color:* Inside color of walls should be white
  - *Lighting:* Natural light from left side
  - *Water supply:* Safe and potable and continuous supply through taps
  - *Lavatory:* 1 urinal per 60 students and 1 latrine per 100 students^Q

> **Key points**
> School Health:
> - Desks of 'minus (–) type'
> - Doors and windows area >25% of floor area

ICDS, IMNCI AND BFHI

NEW WHO/UNICEF Baby Friendly Hospital Initiative (BFHI) 2018 Guidelines

A package of policies and procedures that facilitates providing maternity and newborn services should implement to support breastfeeding. Ten steps to successful breastfeeding:

Critical Management Procedures

1a. Comply fully with the International Code of Marketing of Breast-milk Substitutes and relevant World Health Assembly resolutions
1b. Have a written infant feeding policy that is routinely communicated to staff and parents.
1c. Establish ongoing monitoring and data-management systems
2. Ensure that staff have sufficient knowledge, competence and skills to support breastfeeding.

Key Clinical Practices

3. Discuss the importance and management of breastfeeding with pregnant women and their families
4. Facilitate immediate and uninterrupted skin-to-skin contact and support mothers to **initiate breastfeeding as soon as possible after birth**
5. Support mothers to initiate and maintain breastfeeding and manage common difficulties
6. Do not provide breastfed newborns any food or fluids other than breast milk, unless medically indicated
7. Enable mothers and their infants to remain together and to practice **rooming-in 24 hours a day**
8. Support mothers to recognize and respond to their infants' cues for feeding
9. Counsel mothers on the use and risks of feeding bottles, teats and pacifiers
10. Coordinate discharge so that parents and their infants have timely access to ongoing support and care.

Key points
School Health:
1 urinal per 60 students
1 latrine per 100 students

Integrated Management of Neonatal and Childhood Illness (IMNCI)

Refer to Theory, Chapter 6

Integrated Child Development Services (ICDS)

- *Integrated Child Development Services (ICDS), 1975:* ICDS aims at providing services to pre-school children in an integrated manner so as to ensure proper growth and development of children in rural, tribal and slum areas
  - ICDS is one of the world's largest programmes for early childhood development^Q
- *ICDS is a centrally sponsored scheme^Q*
- *ICDS provides an integrated package of services^Q:*
  - Supplementary nutrition
  - Immunization
  - Health check-up
  - Medical referral services
  - Nutrition and health education for women
  - Non-formal education for children aged 3–6 years, and pregnant and nursing mothers in rural, urban and tribal areas
- *ICDS Beneficiaries (Irrespective of income of family)^Q*
  - Children 0–6 years age
  - Pregnant and lactating mothers
  - Women in reproductive age group
  - Adolescent girls 11–18 years
- **Heart of ICDS system: Anganwadi^Q**
- *Focal point for ICDS services delivery is Anganwadi Worker^Q*; Each Anganwadi has 1 Anganwadi worker and 1 helper
  - 1 Anganwadi centre per 400–800 population in rural and urban projects^Q
  - 1 Anganwadi centre per 300–800 population in tribal projects^Q
  - 1 Mini-Anganwadi centre per 150–300 population
  - 1 Anganwadi on Demand (AOD) for settlement ≥ 40 children under 6 years age

Key points
Heart of ICDS system: Anganwadi

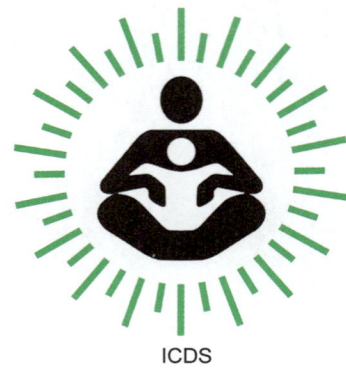

ICDS

- *Supplemental nutrition given through ICDS:* 300 feeding days in a year [NEW 2014 GUIDELINES]

Category	Older		New revised^Q	
	Calories (kcal)	Protein (g)	Calories (kcal)	Protein (g)
Children (6–72 months)	300	8–10	500	12–15
Severely malnourished children (6–72 m)	600	20	800	20–25
Pregnant women and Nursing mothers	500	15–20	600	18–20

- *Administrative unit of ICDS:* 'Community Development Block^Q'; each project covering a population of 1,00,000 (rural/urban) or 35,000 (tribal)^Q
  - 1 CDPO (Community Development Project Officer) is in charge of 4 supervisors (*Mukhyasevikas*) and 100 Anganwadis (each supervisor for 25 Anganwadis)^Q
- *Kishori Shakti Yojana:* Scheme for adolescent girls in ICDS
- *ICDS in India:* Implementation by Ministry of Women and Child Development
  - ICDS projects sanctioned: 7076
  - Anganwadis functioning: 13.46 lacs
  - MiniAWCs: 1.13 lacs

Kishori Shakti Yojana (KSY)

- KSY is rename of 'Adolescent Girl's Scheme' under ICDS (Integrated Child Development Services)^Q
- *Aim of KSY:*
  - To improve the nutritional and health status of adolescent girls
  - To promote self-development, awareness of health, hygiene, nutrition, and family life and child care
- KSY covers 2000 ICDS projects
- *Options for interventions under KSY:*

Options for intervention	Activities
Adolescent girls scheme-I^Q *'Girl-to-girl Approach'* 11–15 years old girls	– Preventive health, hygiene & nutrition education – Working on Anganwadi centre – Family life education – Participate in creative activities – Skill development or vocational training – Learn about significance of education & life skills, personal hygiene, environmental sanitation, nutrition, home nursing, first aid, communicable diseases, VPDs, family life, child care and development, constitutional rights & their impact on quality of life
Adolescent girls scheme-II^Q *'Balika Mandals'* 11–18 years old girls	

NEONATAL SCREENING

Neonatal Screening

- *Neonatal Screening:* Secondary Level of Prevention
  - *MC neonatal disorder screened:* Neonatal hypothyroidism (NNH)^Q
- *Disorders screened among neonates:*
  - Neonatal hypothyroidism
  - Phenylketonuria
  - Sickle cell anemia
  - Thalassemia
  - Congenital dislocation of hip
  - Other disorders: G6PD deficiency

Phenylketonuria and Guthrie Test^Q

- *PKU is an autosomal recessive trait^Q* with a frequency of 1 in 10,000 births
  - *Enzyme deficient in PKU:* Phenylalanine hydroxylase^Q
  - *Treatment of PKU:* restricting or eliminating foods high in phenylalanine, such as breast milk, meat, chicken, fish, nuts, cheese, legumes and other dairy products
- *Guthrie Test:* Is done in neonates for mass screening of Phenylketonuria (PKU)
  - *Guthrie test was the first screening test used in neonates^Q*
  - *Blood sample* is collected by heel prick of the baby 7-10 days after birth^Q
  - *Guthrie Test is negative* in first 2–3 days of life
  - *Guthrie test can detect* PKU, Galactosemia and Maple syrup urine disease
  - *Chemicals detected:* Phenylalanine, Phenylpyruvate and Phenyllactate
  - *It is a semi-quantitative test*
  - Currently, Guthrie test has been replaced by *Tandem mass Spectrometry*

Neonatal Hypothyroidism

- *Most common neonatal disorder to be screened:* Neonatal *hypothyroidism (NNH)^Q*
  - NNH has a frequency of 1 in 4000 birth
  - *MCC of congenital hypothyroidism:* Iodine deficiency^Q
- *Blood sample collected from:* Cord's Blood^Q
- *Test involves measurement of:* T4 or TSH both simultaneously
  - As a single method, T4 is more useful (greater precision and reproducibility^Q
- *Treatment:* Daily dose of thyroid hormone (thyroxine) by mouth

Key points

Most common neonatal disorder to be screened: Neonatal hypothyroidism

GERIATRICS

- *Age group for geriatrics in India:* 60 years and above^Q
- *Geriatric age group among Indian population^Q:* 8.1%
- *MC health disorder among Indian geriatrics:* Visual impairment (Cataract) ^{Q}
- *MCC death among Indian geriatric aged above 70 years:* Cardiovascular disorders^Q

MISCELLANEOUS

Semen analysis [NEW WHO Guidelines 2022]

Parameter	Lower reference limit
Semen volume (mL)	1.4
Total sperm number	39×10^6 per ejaculate
Sperm concentration	16×10^6 per mL
Total motility	42%
Progressive motility	30%
Vitality (live spermatozoa)	54%
Sperm morphology (normal forms)	4%
pH	>7.2

Key points

Geriatric age group among Indian population^Q: 8.1%

- *Grading of sperm motility:*
  - *Grade I:* Immotile (no movement at all)
  - *Grade II:* Non-progressive motility (no movement but tails move)
  - *Grade III:* Non-linear motility, curved/crooked motility (type b)
  - *Grade IV:* Linear progressive motility (type a)

Child Placement

- *Orphanages:* For children who have no home or cannot be taken care of by their parents
- *Foster Homes:* Several types of facilities for rearing children other than in natural families
- *Adoption:* Legal adoption confers upon child and the adoptive parents, rights and responsibilities similar to that of natural parents

- *Borstals^Q:* Boys over 16 years who are too difficult to be handled in a certified school or have misbehaved there, are sent to a Borstal. Borstal, as an institution, falls between a certified school and an adult prison:
  - A borstal sentence is usually for 3 years, and is regarded as a method of training and reformation
- *Remand Homes:* Child is placed under the care of doctors, psychiatrists and other trained personnel to improve the mental and physical well being of the child

Borstals

- *Borstal:* Boys over 16 years who are too difficult to be handled in a certified school or have misbehaved there, are sent to a Borstal^Q
  - Borstal, as an institution, falls between a certified school and an adult prison
- *Primary objective of borstal:* Is to ensure care, welfare and rehabilitation of young offenders and to keep them away from the contaminating atmosphere of the prison
  - The emphasis is given on the education, training and moral influence, conducive for their reformation and prevention of crime
  - A borstal sentence is usually for 3 years, and is regarded as a method of training and reformation
- *Borstals in India:* Borstals do not come under the Children Act but are governed by the *'State Inspector General of Prisons'*
  - 12 Borstals in India [2005]
  - Total inmate capacity: 2260
  - Total inmate population: 1106 (Boys 970; Girls 136)
- *Bombay Borstal School Act, 1929:* It authorizes First Class Magistrate and Superior Courts to pass in lieu of imprisonment, an order for detention in a borstal school for not <3 or >5 years; It applies to young offenders^Q,
  - Boys: 16–21 years age
  - Girls: 18–21 years age

Congenital Disorders among Newborns

- *Congenital disorders:* Those diseases that are substantially determined before or during birth and which, in principle, are recognizable in early life
- *Incidence of congenital disorders (World):* 30–70 per 1000 live births
  - MC disorders are of cardiovascular system and nervous system
- *Birth defects in Indian newborns* are seen in 2.5%^{Q}. The figure rises to 4% if they are followed upto age of 5 years
  - MC birth defect in North India: Neural tube defects or spina bifida^Q
  - MC birth defect in rest of India: Musculoskeletal disorders^Q

> **Key points**
> Birth defects in Indian newborns are seen in 2.5%^{Q}

Children in Difficult Circumstances^Q

• Homeless children	• Children of prisoners
• Orphaned or abandoned children	• Children affected by conflicts
• Whose parents cannot take care of them	• Children affected by natural disasters
• Children separated from parents	• Children affected by HIV/AIDS
• Migrant or refugee children	• Children suffering from terminal diseases
• Street children	• Girl child
• Trafficked children	• Children with disabilities and special needs
• Working children	• Children belonging to minorities, SC, ST
• Children in prostitution	• Children in institutional care
• Children in bondage	• Children in conflict with law
• Children of sex workers/prostitutes	• Children who are victims of crime

PYQs: Quick Review for NEET

Preventive Obstetrics and Pediatrics

3 most important MCH problems	Malnutrition, Infection and Unregulated fertility
MC disorder to be screened in neonates	Neonatal Hypothyroidism
World's greatest Public Health Tool is	Immunization
Juvenile is age	Less than 18 years age
Juvenile definition in Juvenile Justice Act 1986	Boy <16, Girl <18 years
Normal respiratory rate in a newborn	40–60 breaths per minute
National Maternity Benefit Scheme	500/- per birth to poor women (first 2 births)
MDG Goal 4 was	Reduce child mortality by 2/3rd by 2015
1 Community Development Block population	100,000 population (100 villages)
TT doses for a primigravida	2 doses
In Indian laws, Child age is	0–18 years
WHO gave idea of "Safe Motherhood Initiative" in	1987 (Nairobi, Kenya)
Protective shield is made up of	Lead
Daily need of calories in pregnancy	2250 kcal/ day
Boys >16 years difficult to be handled in a certified school are sent to	Borstal

BreastfEeding

Exclusive breastfeeding recommended till	6 months age
Most abundant Ig in breast milk	IgA
Mean output of breast milk per day is maximum during	5–6 months of lactation
Amount of calcium in human milk in 100 mL	28 mg
Whey: Casein ratio in breast milk	7:3
World breastfeeding week is celebrated in	1–7 August
MAA (Mother's Absolute Affection) program is related to	Promotion of breastfeeding
Innocenti Declaration is for promotion of	Breastfeeding

MCH Indicators

Apart from IMR other important indicator for socioeconomic health	Under-5 mortality rate
Maternal mortality ratio (MMR) is expressed as	Maternal deaths per 100,000 live births
Extended definition perinatal mortality includes crown heel length of	>35 cm at birth
Postnatal period extends for	6 weeks
Current neonatal mortality rate of India is	20 per 1000 LB (2019)
Denominator of perinatal mortality rate	Total live births >1000 grams at birth
Denominator of stillbirth rate	Live births + Still births (>1000 gm)
MC indirect cause of maternal mortality	Anemia
Global burden of child mortality	6.3 millions
Denominator for MMR	Live Births
MCC of MMR is	Hemorrhage
MCC of neonatal mortality in India	LBW and prematurity
Effectiveness of MCH services is given by	IMR
Denominator in MMR is	1000 live birth (Expressed per 100,000 LB)

Contd...

Contd...

Growth and Development	
Low Birth Weight is Birth Weight	Less than 2.5 kg
Most sensitive indicator of growth among children	Weight
Best parameter for assessment of chronic malnutrition	Height for age
Low birth weight incidence in India	18%
Weight of a newborn triples in	1 year
A child draws triangle by age	5 years
Preterm birth takes place before	37 weeks POG
Preterm babies are those born	Before 37 weeks
In WHO growth chart 'Lower reference curve' represents	3rd percentile for girls
Best indicator for growth measurement is	Weight
According to NFHS 3, percentage of wasting in India is	20% (21% in NFHS-4)
Best parameter for assessment of chronic malnutrition	Height for age
Best parameter for assessment of Acute malnutrition	Weight for height
Mid-arm circumference is constant during age	6m - 5y
Extremely low birth weight is	<1000 gram
ICDS	
One community development bock equals	100 Villages (100,000 population)
Uppermost curve in ICDS growth chart is	50th percentile for boys
ICDS covered under Ministry	Women and Child Development
Anganwadi worker covered under Ministry	Women and Child Development
Integrated Child Development Services (ICDS) launched in year	1975
Child age under ICDS covered	Up to 6 years age
'Heart of ICDS system'	Anganwadi
Population covered by Anganwadi in tribal area	300–800
Population covered by Anganwadi in plains area	400–800
School Health	
Recommended frequency of school health examination	Once every 6 months
Doors + windows area in a school class	>25% of floor area
Maximum recommended students in a school class room	40
Ideal desk recommended for a school child	'Minus' desk

Multiple Choice Questions

MCH

1. A 27 years old pregnant woman presented to a PHC antenatal clinic with Hemoglobin level of 9 gm/dL. Iron folic acid tablets are advisable to start
   [NEET PG Pattern 2023]
   (a) Immediately
   (b) At 10–12 weeks POG
   (c) After 14 weeks POG
   (d) After 20 weeks POG

2. Which of the following should be considered a 'High risk infant'? [AIIMS November 2019]
   (a) Mal-presentation
   (b) Folic acid tablet not consumed
   (c) Working mother
   (d) Antenatal preeclampsia

3. The extra energy allowances needed per day during pregnancy is: [AIPGME 2006, NEET Pattern 2012]
   (a) 150 KCals
   (b) 200 KCals
   (c) 300 KCals
   (d) 350 KCals

4. Additional daily energy requirement during the first 6 months for a lactating woman is: [AIIMS Nov 03] [UP 2005]
   (a) 350 K calories
   (b) 450 K calories
   (c) 550 K calories
   (d) 650 K calories

5. Under MCH programme, iron and folic acid tablets to be given daily to mother has:
   [AIPGME 2003, AIIMS May 04]
   (a) 60 mg iron + 500 mcg folic acid
   (b) 100 mg iron + 500 mcg folic acid
   (c) 60 mg iron + 100 mcg folic acid
   (d) 100 mg iron + 100 mcg folic acid

6. Which of the following is not included in '5 cleans' in conduct of delivery? [AIIMS, May Dec 1994]
   (a) Clean hands
   (b) Clean perineum
   (c) Clean cutting and care of cord
   (d) Clean surface for delivery

7. A 37 weeks pregnant woman attends an antenatal clinic at a Primary Health Centre. She has not had any antenatal care till now. The best approach regarding tetanus immunization in this case would be to: [AIPGME 04]
   (a) Give a dose of Tetanus Toxoid (TT) and explain to her that it will not protect the newborn and she should take the second dose after four weeks even if she delivers in the meantime
   (b) Do not waste the TT vaccine as it would anyhow be of no use in this pregnancy
   (c) Given one dose of TT and explain that it will not be useful for this pregnancy
   (d) Give her anti-Tetanus Immunoglobulin along with the TT vaccine

8. All are criteria for identifying 'at risk' infants except: [AIPGME 1996]
   (a) Birth weight less than 2.8 kg
   (b) Birth order 5 or more
   (c) PEM, diarrhoea
   (d) Working mother

9. All are true regarding Congenital Syphilis except: [AIIMS Dec 1995]
   (a) Procaine Penicillin can prevent it satisfactorily
   (b) Infection of the fetus most commonly occurs in 1st trimester
   (c) Neurological damage with mental retardation can be a serious consequence
   (d) If mother has Late syphilis, chances of transmission decreases

10. A 24-year-old primigravida wt 57 kg, Hb 11.0 gm% visits an antenatal clinic during 2nd trimester of pregnancy seeking advice on dietary intake. She should be advised: [DPG 2011]
    (a) Additional intake of 300 kcal
    (b) Additional intake of 500 kcal
    (c) Additional intake of 650 kcal
    (d) No extra kcal

11. The daily extra calorie requirement in first trimester of pregnancy is: [DNB 2007]
    (a) 50
    (b) 150
    (c) 350
    (d) 450

12. Recommended dose of folic acid during pregnancy is [PGMCET 2015]
    (a) 200 mcg/day
    (b) 300 mcg/day
    (c) 400 mcg/day
    (d) 500 mcg/day

13. What is the best indicator to evaluate obstetric and neonatal care given at around the time of birth?
    [NEET Pattern 2015]
    (a) IMR
    (b) Perinatal mortality rate
    (c) U5MR
    (d) Still birth rate

14. State with lowest IMR is: [NEET Pattern 2015]
    (a) Uttar Pradesh
    (b) Kerala
    (c) Maharashtra
    (d) Tamil Nadu

15. In a town there are 2500 live birth within 6 months. During same period, 5 women died due to peripartum infection, 5 died due to electrocution, 2 died due to obstructed labor and 3 died due to PPH. What is the MMR? [NEET Pattern 2016]
    (a) 4 per 1000 LB
    (b) 6 per 1000 LB
    (c) 40 per 1000 LB
    (d) 60 per 1000 LB

16. In a Subcenter population, Crude birth rate (CBR) is 20. What is the minimum expected number of pregnancies registered with ANM? [AIIMS November 2017]
    (a) 110
    (b) 120
    (c) 55
    (d) 100

LBW

17. Mean Birth weight of Indian babies is [AIPGME 2001] [NEET Pattern 2013]
    (a) 2.5 kg
    (b) 2.8 kg
    (c) 3.1 kg
    (d) 3.5 kg

18. As per WHO low birth weight is defined as: [PGI Dec 03]
    (a) Birth weight less than 2.5 kg [NEET Pattern 2012, 2013]
    (b) Birth weight <10th percentile [Karnataka 2004]
    (c) Gestational age <34 weeks
    (d) Gestational age <28 weeks

19. Which of the following advise should be given for an infant suffering from mild diarrhea? [DPG 2007]
    (a) Continue breastfeeding
    (b) Antibiotics
    (c) Stop all breast feed and start ORS
    (d) Intravenous fluid administration

20. The term used for babies born as a result of retarded intrauterine fetal growth is: [Karnataka 2005]
    (a) Pre-term babies
    (b) Low birth weight babies
    (c) Small-for-date babies
    (d) Retarded babies

21. Minimum antenatal visit as per MCH is: [PGI Dec 03]
    (a) 1
    (b) 2 [MH 2000]
    (c) 3
    (d) 4
    (e) 5

22. Very low birth weight is less than: [NEET Pattern 2018]
    (a) <1000 g
    (b) <1500 g
    (c) <2000 g
    (d) <2500 g

Review Questions

23. The outer line of under-5 clinic which touches all others is: [DNB 2002]
    (a) Preventive care
    (b) Growth monitoring
    (c) Health education to mother
    (d) Immunisation

24. Essential criteria for K washiorkor is: [UP 2002]
    (a) Body weight is less than 60%
    (b) Thin dry brittle hair
    (c) Vocarious appetite
    (d) Edema in dependent part

25. Elemental iron supplementation in Iron deficiency anemia is: [UP 2008]
    (a) 300–400 mg
    (b) 150–200 mg
    (c) 100–150 mg
    (d) <100 mg

26. Which of the following is age independent indicator of malnutrition? [MP 2006]
    (a) Underweight
    (b) Stunting
    (c) Wasting
    (d) MAC

27. Osteomalacia in pregnancy and lactation is best treated by: [MH 2000]
    (a) Vitamin D
    (b) Vitamin D and calcium
    (c) Calcium
    (d) Vitamin D-calcium and phosphorous

28. The average weight of newborn in South India is: [TN 2000]
    (a) 2.2 kg
    (b) 2.5 kg
    (c) 3.0 kg
    (d) 3.5 kg

29. Most common cause of low birth wt baby is: [RJ 2004]
    (a) Prematurity
    (b) Infection
    (c) Anemia
    (d) Diabetes

MCH INDICATORS

30. Best option for feeding a preterm baby if mother has no breast milk production [INICET May 2022]
    (a) Donor mother's milk
    (b) Preterm formula
    (c) Cow's milk
    (d) Standard term formula

31. Causes of mortality in neonates in descending order (according to 2013 data) as based on verbal autopsy data for India is: [INICET November 2021]
    1. Prematurity
    2. Birth asphyxia
    3. Sepsis
    4. Congenital anomalies
    (a) 1 3 2 4
    (b) 2 1 3 4
    (c) 3 4 2 1
    (d) 1 2 3 4

32. Sequential Arrangement Question – Consider the following causes of death in 1–4 years old children in India.
    1. Diarrhoea
    2. Injury
    3. Malaria
    4. Pneumonia
    Now arrange the following in reducing order: [INICET July 2021]
    (a) 1 2 3 4
    (b) 1 4 2 3
    (c) 4 1 2 3
    (d) 4 1 3 2

33. **Definition of Maternal mortality ratio is:** *[AIIMS June 2020]*
    (a) Dividing average annual number of maternal deaths in a population by the average number of married women who are alive during observation period
    (b) Maternal deaths expressed as per 100,000 live births, where a 'maternal death' is defined as 'death of a woman while pregnant or during delivery or within 14 days (2 weeks) of termination of pregnancy
    (c) Dividing average annual number of maternal deaths in a population by average number of women of reproductive age (aged 15–49 years) who are alive during observation period
    (d) Maternal deaths expressed as per 100,000 live births, where a 'maternal death' is defined as 'death of a woman while pregnant or during delivery or within 42 days (6 weeks) of termination of pregnancy

34. **Numerator in Perinatal mortality is:** *[AIIMS November 2019]*
    (a) Post neonate death with weight 2.5 kg
    (b) Early neonatal death with weight >1000 grams
    (c) Abortion of <500 grams foetus
    (d) Still birth of fetus >500 grams

35. **In a town of 20,000 population, total 456 births were there in a year out of which 56 were dead born. The total deaths were 247 out of which 56 deaths were within first 28 days of life and another 34 had died after 28 days and before completing the first birthday. Calculate the Infant mortality rate of the area.** *[AIIMS May 2019]*
    (a) 197
    (b) 225
    (c) 392
    (d) 344

36. **All of the following are common cause of post neonatal infant mortality in India, *except*:** *[MP 01, AIPGME 02]*
    (a) Tetanus
    (b) Malnutrition
    (c) Diarrhoeal diseases
    (d) Acute respiratory infection

37. **Which one of the following is the leading cause of mortality in under five children in developing countries?**
    (a) Malaria *[AIPGME 2004]*
    (b) Acute lower respiratory tract infections
    (c) Hepatitis
    (d) Pre-maturity

38. **All of the following deaths are included in as causes of maternal death except:** *[AIIMS June 1997]*
    (a) Following abortion
    (b) During lactation 1st month
    (c) During lactation 8th month
    (d) During the last trimester due to APH

39. **Among the following the best indicator of health in a community is:** *[AIIMS Dec 1994]*
    (a) Maternal mortality rate
    (b) Infant mortality rate
    (c) Life expectancy
    (d) Neonatal mortality rate

40. **Leading Cause of maternal deaths in India is:**
    (a) Anemia *[AIIMS May Nov 02- 04, 05,*
    (b) Hemorrhage *May 08, Nov 02 AIPGME 08]*
    (c) Sepsis *[AIIMS 2011, MP 2005]*
    (d) Obstructed labour

41. **Of total deaths in India per year, infant deaths contribute about:** *[AIIMS Dec 1994]*
    (a) 6%
    (b) 13%
    (c) 19%
    (d) 44%

42. **Infant mortality does not include:** *[AIPGME 2005]*
    (a) Early neonatal mortality *[AIIMS November 2014]*
    (b) Perinatal mortality *[DNB 2007]*
    (c) Post neonatal mortality *[NEET Pattern 2017]*
    (d) Late neonatal mortality

43. **Sensitivity parameter of combined pediatric and obstetric care in our country is:**
    [NEET Pattern 2018, AIPGME 2006]
    (a) IMR
    (b) PNMR
    (c) NNMR
    (d) NMR

44. **Late foetal deaths and early neonatal deaths are considered in which of the following indices?**
    (a) Infant mortality rate *[Karnataka 2007]*
    (b) Perinatal mortality rate
    (c) Still birth rate
    (d) Post neonatal mortality rate

45. **The highest rate of infant mortality in India is reported from:** *[Karnataka 2008]*
    (a) Madhya Pradesh
    (b) Bihar
    (c) Uttar Pradesh
    (d) Orissa

46. **Mainly included in child survival index:** *[PGI June 01]*
    (a) MMR
    (b) IMR
    (c) Mortality between 1 to 4 yr. age
    (d) Under 5 mortality

47. **Perinatal mortality rate includes:** *[NEET Pattern 2013]*
    (a) Deaths within first week of life
       [NEET Pattern 2012, DNB 2010, UP 2001]
    (b) Abortions, Stillbirths, deaths within first week of life
       [DNB 2001, 2005, AIPGME 2010]
    (c) Deaths from 28 weeks to with first week of life
    (d) Deaths within one month of life

48. **In a given population, total births in a year are 4050. There are 50 still births. 50 neonates die within first 7 days of life whereas the number of deaths within 8–28 days of life is 150. What is the Neonatal mortality rate in the population?** *[AIIMS Nov 2010]*
    (a) 12.5
    (b) 50 *[AIIMS 2012, 2014]*
    (c) 49.4
    (d) 62.5

49. Which of the following is the least likely cause of Neonatal mortality in India? [AIIMS Nov 2010]
    (a) Severe infections [NEET Pattern 2013]
    (b) Congenital malformations
    (c) Prematurity
    (d) Birth asphyxia

50. Annual Under-five deaths globally reported are:
    (a) 6 million [AIIMS November 2013]
    (b) 8 million
    (c) 10 million
    (d) 12 million

51. Most common cause of infant mortality in India is?
    (a) Low birth weight [NEET Pattern, 2012, 2013]
    (b) Respiratory disease
    (c) Diarrhoeal diseases
    (d) Congenital anomalies

52. Child survival index is calculated by? [NEET Pattern 2013]
    (a) 1000-IMR/10
    (b) IMR-1000/10
    (c) 1000-U5MR/10
    (d) U5MR-1000/10

53. Maternal mortality is maximum in ……….. period:
    (a) Antepartum [NEET Pattern 2012, 2013]
    (b) Peripartum
    (c) Postpartum
    (d) None

54. Maternal mortality rate definition include all *except*:
    (a) Death in pregnancy [NIMHANS 2014, DNB 2001]
    (b) Death during delivery
    (c) Death within 6 weeks post delivery
    (d) Death within 6 months post delivery

55. Maternal death is defined as, when mother dies during pregnancy or at the time of delivery or after delivery upto [PGMCET 2015]
    (a) 4 weeks (b) 6 weeks
    (c) 8 weeks (d) 10 weeks

56. Acute Respiratory Infections (ARI) are important causes of under-five mortality in India. In remote areas, Children develop frequent episodes of ARI. What measures will you take for prevention and control of ARI amongst under-five children in that area? [UPSC CMS 2015]
    (a) Case management and Health education to mothers
    (b) Vaccination
    (c) Controlling malnutrition, Promoting breastfeeding, Vitamin A supplementation
    (d) All of these

57. Which does not have Live Birth as denominator?
    [NEET Pattern 2017]
    (a) Infant mortality rate
    (b) Neonatal mortality rate
    (c) Child mortality rate
    (d) Child death rate

Review Questions

58. Denominator in, under 5 proportionate mortality rate is:
    (a) Mid year population [UP 2002]
    (b) Mid year population in 5 years age
    (c) Number of live birth in same year
    (d) Total death in same year

59. The following does not suggest Under Five Care in the community: [AP 2005]
    (a) Infant mortality rate
    (b) 1–4 year mortality
    (c) Neonatal tetanus
    (d) Deaths due to diarrhoeal disease between 1–5 years

60. In a population of 5000, with birth rate of 30/1000 population, 15 children died during first year life in one year: of these 9 died during first month of life. What is the infant mortality rate in this population? [MP 2006]
    (a) 100 (b) 60
    (c) 150 (d) 45

61. In India, approximately 50% of maternal deaths are caused by: [MP 2009]
    (a) Sepsis and abortion
    (b) Sepsis and obstructed labour
    (c) Sepsis and Hypertension
    (d) Sepsis and hemorrhage

62. Commonest cause of perinatal mortality in India: [RJ 2001]
    (a) Prematurity (b) Birth injury
    (c) Metabolic (d) Congenital

BREASTFEEDING

63. Which of the following are Key features of Kangaroo mother care? [INICET July 2021]
    (a) Skin to skin contact, exclusive breastfeeding, prevention of infection
    (b) Skin to skin contact, exclusive breastfeeding, early discharge
    (c) Skin to skin contact, prevention of infection, early discharge
    (d) Skin to skin contact, prevention of early infections

64. The following statements about breast milk are true *except*: [AIPGME 2004]
    (a) The maximum milk output is seen at 12 months
    (b) The coefficient of uptake of iron in breast milk is 70%
    (c) Calcium absorption of human milk is better than that of cow's milk
    (d) It provides about 70 K cals per 100 mL

65. The current recommendation for breastfeeding is that:
    [AIPGME 1999, 2004]
    (a) Exclusive breastfeeding should be continued till 6 months of age followed by supplementation with additional foods
    (b) Exclusive breast-feeding should be continued till 4 months of age followed by supplementation with additional foods

(c) Colostrum is the most suitable food for a new born baby but it is best avoided in first 2 days
(d) The baby should be allowed to breast-feed till one year of age

66. As compared to cow milk, breast milk contains more: *[DPG 2005]*
    (a) Energy
    (b) Fat
    (c) Lactose
    (d) Proteins

67. Not true about breast milk is: *[AIIMS May 2011]*
    (a) Maximum output is at 12 months of lactation
    (b) Coefficient of iron absorption is 70%
    (c) Calcium utilization more than cows milk
    (d) Breast milk contains high amounts of lactose

68. Human breast milk has more of: *[PGI May 2011]*
    (a) Lipids   *[Karnataka 2011, NEET Pattern 2012]*
    (b) Carbohydrates
    (c) Proteins
    (d) Iron
    (e) Calcium

69. In normal delivery, breastfeeding should be started within: *[NEET Pattern 2012]*
    (a) ½ hour of delivery
    (b) 1 hour of delivery
    (c) 4 hour of delivery
    (d) 6 hour of deliver

70. A woman suffering from active tuberculosis not on ATT has a full term vaginal delivery. All the following should be done *except*: *[UPSC CMS 2015]*
    (a) Breastfeed the neonate
    (b) BCG should be given to the neonate
    (c) Neonate should be given INH
    (d) Neonate should be isolated from mother

71. Breast milk contains? *[PGI May 2018]*
    (a) Fat
    (b) Protein
    (c) Vitamin A
    (d) Vitamin C
    (e) Vitamin K

GROWTH AND DEVELOPMENT

72. An Anganwadi worker takes measurements for weight and height for a child. Height for age in the child is less than -2SD. It signifies: *[NEET PG Pattern September 2021]*
    (a) Acute weight loss
    (b) Acute infection
    (c) Chronic malnutrition
    (d) No malnutrition

73. Severe acute malnutrition (SAM) criteria *except*: *[AIIMS June 2020]*
    (a) Mid arm circumference <115 mm
    (b) Weight for age below 3 SD
    (c) Weight for height below 3 SD
    (d) Bipedal edema

74. The uppermost line of the 'road to health card' is equivalent to: *[AIIMS Jan 1998]*
    (a) 80% for boys   *[DNB 2001, 2005, MH 2006]*
    (b) 50% for girls
    (c) 50th percentile for boys
    (d) 3rd percentile for girls

75. Wasting represents: *[AIPGME 2006]*
    (a) Acute malnutrition
    (b) Chronic malnutrition
    (c) Normal child
    (d) Overweight child

76. If the birth weight is 3 kg by the end of one year of age it should become: *[AIIMS May 2001]*
    (a) 6 kg
    (b) 9 kg
    (c) 12 kg
    (d) 15 kg

77. At birth head circumference is about: *[AIIMS May 1994]*
    (a) 32 cm
    (b) 34 cm
    (c) 36 cm
    (d) 38 cm

78. WHO Growth Chart has got information for all *except*:
    (a) Immunisation procedures   *[AIIMS Nov 1992]*
    (b) Child spacing
    (c) History of sibling health
    (d) History of maternal health

79. Around whole symbol for Under-five's clinic there is a border touching all other areas. This border represents:
    (a) Preventive care   *[AIPGME 1994]*
    (b) Care in illness
    (c) Growth monitoring
    (d) Health education

80. All are true about growth chart *except*: *[AIIMS Nov 09]*
    (a) It is a tool for educating mothers
    (b) The position of dots is more important than direction
    (c) Between top 2 lines, it shows 'Road-to-Health' or 'zone of normality'
    (d) Lowermost line corresponds to children below 3 percentile

81. Which of the following does not indicate poor nutrition in children? *[AIPGME 2010]*
    (a) Low birth weight   *[NEET Pattern 2012]*
    (b) Infection
    (c) Hemoglobin >11 gm%
    (d) Malnutrition

82. Age independent anthropometric measure of malnutrition is: *[DNB June 2009]*
    (a) Weight/height
    (b) Mid arm circumference
    (c) Head circumference
    (d) Mid arm circumference/height

83. The best parameter for assessment of chronic malnutrition is: *[DNB 2006, 2007]*
    (a) Weight for age
    (b) Weight for height
    (c) Height for age
    (d) Any of the above

84. In WHO "Road to Health" chart, upper and lower limit of represents: [AIIMS May 2012]
    (a) 30 percentile for boys and 3 percentile for girls
    (b) 50 percentile for boys and 3 percentile for girls
    (c) 30 percentile for boys and 5 percentile for girls
    (d) 50 percentile for boys and 5 percentile for girls

85. Height of a Newborn doubles by the age of [NEET Pattern 2015]
    (a) 5 months   (b) 1 year
    (c) 4 years   (d) 5 years

86. In 'Milestones of Development' 'Listening' refers to which type of development? [PGMCET 2015]
    (a) Motor   (b) Language
    (c) Adaptive   (d) Sociopersonal

87. Which of the milestone develops first? [ESI IMO 2014]
    (a) Mirror play (b) Crawling
    (c) Creeping   (d) Pincer grasp

88. A 2-year-old boy is being evaluated for severity of malnutrition. The child weighs 7 kg and measures 74 cm in length. Expected (median) weight for height, and height for age for this child are 9 kg and 86 cm respectively. According to WHO classification of undernutrition, which of the following is the correct category for this child? [UPSC CMS 2015]
    (a) Wasted, stunted
    (b) Wasted, severely stunted
    (c) Severely wasted, stunted
    (d) Severely wasted, severely stunted

89. Multicenter growth reference study (MGRS) all are true except: [NEET Pattern 2015]
    (a) Participating countries were India, Brazil, Ghana, Oman, USA, Norway
    (b) Done by case control study
    (c) Age group 1–10 years was used
    (d) Total 8500 breast fed infants and young children participated

90. Which of the following indicator is used for growth monitoring at Anganwadi centre? [AIIMS May 2016]
    (a) Height for age
    (b) Mid arm circumference
    (c) Weight for age
    (d) Height for weight

91. Gomez classification is based on: [NEET Pattern 2017]
    (a) Weight retardation
    (b) Height retardation
    (c) Mid arm circumference
    (d) Stunting

Review Questions

92. WHO growth chart is: [UP 2005]
    (a) International based
    (b) National based
    (c) Home based
    (d) Community based

93. Bad prognosis in PEM is indicated by all except: [AP 2008]
    (a) Keratomalacia   (b) Hypothermia
    (c) Hepatomegaly   (d) Hypoalbuminemia

94. Road to health card or the growth chart was first designed by: [NEET Pattern 2013] [MP 2003]
    (a) Edwin Chadwick (b) David Morley
    (c) C. Gopalan   (d) C.E. Winslow

95. True about WHO growth chart is: [MH 2000]
    (a) Used for monitoring growth and development of child
    (b) Has 3 lines
    (c) Highest line corresponds to 80th percentile and above
    (d) Lowest line corresponds to 50th percentile and above

SCHOOL HEALTH

96. The commonest morbidity in schools is: [AIIMS Jan 1998]
    (a) Dental ailments   (b) Worm infestations
    (c) Malnutrition   (d) Skin diseases

97. All of the following are minimum standards for sanitation of schools and its environs in India except: [AIPGME 2003]
    (a) Desks to be of 'Minus type'
    (b) Combined doors + windows area minimum 25% of floor space area
    (c) Maximum 40 students per classroom
    (d) One urinal for 10 students and one latrine for 25 students

98. With reference to school health, which one of the following statements is NOT correct? [AIPGME 2004]
    (a) Per capita space for students in classroom should not be less than 10 sq ft.
    (b) Desks should be of plus type
    (c) Classroom should have sufficient natural light preferably from the left
    (d) There should be one urinal for 60 students and one latrine for 100 students

99. Which of the following is not emphasized in School health services [NEET Pattern 2017]
    (a) Dental caries
    (b) Infectious diseases
    (c) Malnutrition
    (d) Lung infections

Review Questions

100. A – Sex education should not be given in school R – It will lead to increased incidence of sexual promiscuity: [DNB 2000]
     (a) A and R correct and R explains A
     (b) A and R correct and R does not explain A
     (c) A is correct, R is incorrect
     (d) A is incorrect, R is correct

101. True about Mid-day meal given in school is: *[DNB 2006]*

	Calories	Proteins
(a)	1/3	1/2
(b)	1/3	1/3
(c)	1/2	1/2
(d)	1/2	1/3

ICDS, IMNCI AND BFHI

102. Which of the following is the nodal ministry for Integrated Child Development Services (ICDS)? *[AIIMS May 04]*
    (a) Ministry for Human Resource Development
    (b) Ministry for Rural Development
    (c) Ministry for Health and Family Welfare
    (d) Ministry for Social Justice

103. Integrated Management of Childhood Illness (IMCI) was taken to prevent morbidity and mortality from all *except*: *[WB 2009] [AIPGME 2008]*
    (a) Malaria   (b) Malnutrition
    (c) Otitis media   (d) Neonatal tetanus

104. Administrative unit of the ICDS project in rural areas is: *[NEET Pattern 2013] [Karnataka 2007]*
    (a) PHC
    (b) Community development block
    (c) Zilla parishad
    (d) Gram panchayat

105. Mother friendly childbirth initiative was launched in: *[NEET Pattern 2014]*
    (a) India   (b) Britain
    (c) Australia   (d) USA

106. Diet given to a pregnant lady under ICDS is: *[AIIMS November 2014] [AIIMS 2001]*
    (a) 200 kcal + 10 grams proteins
    (b) 250 kcal + 12 grams proteins
    (c) 300 kcal + 15 grams proteins
    (d) 350 kcal + 15 grams proteins

107. Population covered under one community development block is: *[NEET Pattern 2017]*
    (a) 10,000   (b) 30,000
    (c) 50,000   (d) 100,000

108. Who looks after the work of Anganwadi worker? *[NEET Pattern 2017]*
    (a) Auxiliary nurse midwife
    (b) Mukhyasevika
    (c) Village health guide
    (d) ASHA

Review Questions

109. All are true about Anganwadi workers *except*: *[UP 2002]*
    (a) Covers population of 5000
    (b) Time part workers
    (c) Supply nutrition, educate to vaccination
    (d) Under controls ICDS

110. ICDS does not cover: *[Kolkata 2005]*
    (a) Nutritional supplementation
    (b) Formal education
    (c) Health education
    (d) Immunization

111. According to ICDS programme, children should be supplemented with which of the following? *[MH 2002] [AIIMS 2000, 2001]*
    (a) 200 cal + 20 g proteins
    (b) 300 cal + 15 g proteins
    (c) 500 cal + 25 g proteins
    (d) 300 cal + 10 g proteins

112. According to IMNCI Programme the term "YOUNG INFANTS" includes children below the what age? *[MH 2008]*
    (a) Seven days   (b) 28 days
    (c) Two months   (d) Six months

NEONATAL SCREENING

113. 'Guthrie Test' is done in neonates for mass screening of: *[AIPGME 1999]*
    (a) Neonatal hypothyroidism
    (b) Phenylketonuria
    (c) Hemoglobinopathies
    (d) Congenital Dislocation of Hip

114. Most common neonatal disorder screened is:
    (a) Neonatal hypothyroidism *[AIPGME 1998]*
    (b) Phenylketonuria
    (c) Hemoglobinopathies
    (d) Congenital Dislocation of Hip

MISCELLANEOUS

115. To promote healthspan, the best recommendation is *[NEET PG Pattern 2022]*
    (a) Restrict caloric intake
    (b) Exercise
    (c) Reduce stress levels
    (d) Restrict caloric intake and exercise

116. According to WHO criteria, all are true in a normal person *except*: *[AIIMS May 08]*
    (a) Sperm count >20 million
    (b) Volume >1 mL
    (c) Normal morphology in >15% (strict criteria)
    (d) Aggressive forward motility in >25%

117. Kishori Shakti Yojana (KSY) is: *[AIIMS Nov 2006]*
    (a) Empowerment of females under Maternity Benefit Scheme
    (b) Adolescent girl's scheme under ICDS
    (c) Free and compulsory education for girl child
    (d) Child care home scheme for female juvenile delinquents

118. At PHC level, a women who complains of spotting following IUCD insertion should be advised:
    [AIPGME 2006]
    (a) Analgesic and observation
    (b) Antibiotic and observation
    (c) Iron supplements and observation
    (d) Removal of IUCD

119. Hb of less than what value is the cut off used by WHO guidelines to label an infant under 6 months of age as being anemic? [AIIMS Nov 01]
    (a) 100 g/L   (b) 105 g/L
    (c) 110 g/L   (d) 115 g/L

120. In which one of the following situations is Amniocentesis NOT called for? [AIIMS Nov 1999]
    (a) Mother's age is 35 year or more
    (b) Parents who are known to have chromosomal translocation
    (c) Raised alpha fetoprotein in amniotic fluid during earlier pregnancy
    (d) A Rh –ve multipara mother aged 30 years with two live healthy boys

121. When an abandoned child is legally accepted by a couple, it is called as: [AIIMS Nov 2000]
    (a) Remand home placement and Foster home placement
    (b) Remand home placement and Borstal placement
    (c) Adoption and Foster home placement
    (d) Adoption and Remand home placement

122. Boys over 16 years who are difficult to be handled in a certified school are sent for training and reformation, for 3 yrs, to a: [AIIMS Nov 1993, DPG 2005]
    (a) Orphanage   (b) Foster home
    (c) Borstal   (d) Remand home

123. Birth defects in Indian newborns are seen in: [AIPGME 2003]
    (a) 2–3% of newborns
    (b) 5% of newborns
    (c) 8% of newborns
    (d) 12–14% of newborns

124. Child rights are guaranteed in which article of the constitution: [PGI Dec 01]
    (a) Article 24
    (b) Article 28
    (c) Article 35
    (d) Article 42
    (e) Article 45

125. A place where children are kept in care of doctor and psychiatrist is: [NEET Pattern 2012]
    (a) Borstal
    (b) Foster home
    (c) Remand home
    (d) Orphangae

126. All are included in Kangaroo Mother Care except: [AIIMS May 2014]
    (a) Skin to skin contact
    (b) Early discharge and follow up
    (c) Free nutritional supplements
    (d) Exclusive Breastfeeding

127. Ujjwala Scheme include all except: [NEET Pattern 2015]
    (a) Rescue
    (b) Rehabilitation
    (c) Remuneration
    (d) Repatriation

Explanations

MCH

1. **Ans. (a) Immediately** [Ref. Park 27/e p522]

   If Haemoglobin is 7–9.9 g/dL (moderate anemia) under AMB
   - First level of treatment (at all levels of care) includes 2 tablets of IFA (60 mg elemental Iron and 500 mcg Folic Acid) daily, orally given by the health provider during the ANC contact
   - Parental iron (IV Iron Sucrose or FCM) may be considered as the first line of management in pregnant women who are detected to be anemic late in pregnancy or in whom compliance is likely to be low (high chance of lost to follow-up)

2. **Ans. (c) Working mother** [Ref. Park 25/e p587]
   - "At risk infants" include Birth weight <2.5 kg (low birth weight), Twin, Birth order >5, Artificial feeding, Weight <70% of expected (II and III degrees of malnutrition), Failure to thrive (failure to gain weight in 3 successive months), Children with PEM/ diarrhea, Working mother/single parent

3. **Ans. (d) 350 KCals** [Ref. Park 27/e p748]
   - *The recommended daily energy intake:*
     [NEW GUIDELINES 2021–22]

Group	Energy Allowance per day (kcal)
Infancy	
0–6 months	550 kcal/day
6–12 months	670 kcal/day
Adult Reference Male (Wt: 60 Kg)	
Sedentary/Light work	2110
Moderate Work	2710
Heavy Work	3470
Adult Reference Female (Wt: 55 kg)	
Sedentary/Light work	1660
Moderate Work	2130
Heavy Work	2720
Pregnancy	+ 350
Lactation	
First 6 months	+ 600
6–12 months	+ 520

   (+ indicates 'over and above the daily requirement')

4. **Ans. NONE [Its 600 kcalories]** [Ref. Park 27/e p748]

5. **Ans. (a) 60 mg iron + 500 mcg folic acid** [Ref. Park 25/e p562]
   - *An adult tablet of IFA contains*: 60 mg elemental Iron and 500 mcg Folic acid (to be given for 180 days minimum in pregnancy/lactation)
   - *A pediatric tablet of IFA contains*: 20 mg elemental Iron and 100 mcg Folic acid (to be given for 100 days minimum every year till 5 years age of child)

   > **ALSO REMEMBER**
   > - At MCH centres several supplements are provided free of cost to expectant mothers:
   >   - IFA tablets
   >   - 2 doses of tetanus toxoid
   >   - Fresh milk (or skimmed milk)
   >   - Capsules of Vitamin A and D
   > - Requirement of Iron and Folic Acid: Pregnancy > Lactation

   - Recommended daily intake values of folate:

Group	Intake per day
Healthy adults	200 mcg
Pregnancy	500 mcg
Lactation	300 mcg
Children	100 mcg

6. **Ans. (b) Clean perineum** [National Health Programs of India by Dr. J. Kishore, 7/e p108 and 8/e p128, Park 21/e p287, Park 22/e p286]

   - **CLEANS OF SAFE DELIVERY:**
   - *'Five cleans'* (practices) under strategies for elimination of neonatal tetanus include,
     - *Clean delivery surface*
     - *Clean hands (of birth attendants)*
     - *Clean cord cut (blade or instrument)*
     - *Clean cord tie*
     - *Clean cord stump (no applicant)*

   > **ALSO REMEMBER**
   > - *6 F's of Sanitation Barrier:*
   >   - Fingers
   >   - Flies
   >   - Fomites
   >   - Food
   >   - Faeces
   >   - Fluids
   >
   > - *4 D's of Pellagra:*
   >   - Diarrhoea
   >   - Dermatitis
   >   - Dementia
   >   - Death
   >
   >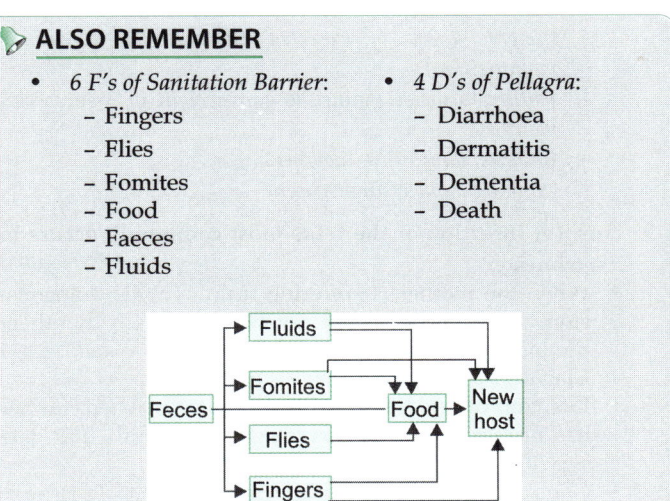

Contd...

Contd...

- **5 D's of Ill-health:**
  - Disease
  - Discomfort
  - Disability
  - Dissatisfaction
  - Death
- **5 I's of Ageing (old age):**
  - Impairment
  - Instability
  - Incontinence
  - Immobility
  - Isolation

7. **Ans. (a) Give a dose of Tetanus Toxoid (TT) and explain to her that it will not protect the newborn and she should take the second dose after four weeks even if she delivers in the meantime** *[Ref. Park 27/e p604]*

> **ALSO REMEMBER**
> - In developing countries, antenatal mothers should be given TT irrespective of period of gestation (as she may not return); There is no evidence to suggest that TT is dangerous or harmful to fetus
> - Infants born to unimmunized mothers or partially immunized mothers should be given: 750 IU antitoxin (heterologous serum) within 6 hours of birth (for prevention of neonatal tetanus)

8. **Ans. (a) Birth weight less than 2.8 kg** *[Ref. Park 27/e p611]*
   - *At risk approach*: Central purpose is to identify high risk cases (as early as possible) from a large group of all antenatal mothers/infants, and *provide specialized care to them, while continuing to provide appropriate care to all antenatal mothers/infants*
   - *At risk infants*: Contribute to perinatal, neonatal and infant mortality; so they have to be provided with special intensive care; Basic criteria for identifying these babies include:
     - *Birth weight <2.5 kg (low birth weight)*
     - *Twins*
     - *Birth order >5*
     - *Artificial feeding*
     - *Weight <70% of expected (II and III degrees of malnutrition)*
     - *Failure to thrive (failure to gain weight in 3 successive months)*
     - *Children with PEM, diarrhea*
     - *Working mother/single parent*

9. **Ans. (b) Infection of the fetus most commonly occurs in 1st trimester** *[Ref. Park 27/e p604]*
   - When the mother is suffering from syphilis, transmission occurs to fetus, but not before the 4th month of pregnancy; It is most likely to occur after 6th month, when Langhan's cell layer has completely atrophied
   - Infection of fetus is most likely to occur when mother has primary or secondary stages of syphilis than late syphilis
   - Clinical features include *Hutchinson's Triad* (deafness, Hutchinson's teeth – centrally notched, widely-spaced peg-shaped upper central incisors and interstitial keratitis), *snuffles* (rhinitis) and *Mulberry Molars* (sixth year molars with multiple poorly developed cusps)
   - Neurological damage with mental retardation is one of the most serious consequences of congenital syphilis
   - Ten daily injections of Procaine Penicillin (600,000 Units) are almost adequate.
   - According to the CDC, 40% of births to syphilitic mothers are stillborn and 30% are infected

> **ALSO REMEMBER**
> **MOTHER TO CHILD TRANSMISSION (MTCT):**
> - *Rubella:* Any trimester; MC and most serious in I trimester
> - *Varicella:* Any trimester; MC and most serious in I trimester
> - *Syphilis:* Any trimester; More common in Late II trimester or III trimester
> - *Toxoplasmosis:* Any trimester; MC in III trimester; Most serious in I trimester
> - *Herpes simplex:* During delivery (from infected genital secretions)
> - *HIV:* during delivery (30% chance in developing countries, 20% in developed countries), breastfeeding (16%)
> - *Hepatitis B:* 90% (in presence of HBeAg); 20% (in presence of HBsAg); MC in III trimester and through breastfeeding
> - *Cytomegalovirus:* Any trimester (MC third trimester)

10. **Ans. NONE [new guidelines 350 + kcal/d]** *[Ref. Park 27/e p602]*

11. **Ans. (b) 150** *[Ref. Manual of Nutritional Therapeutics by Alpers, Taylor, Bier & Stenson, 5/e p90]*

12. **Ans. (d) 500 mcg/day** *[Ref. Park 27/e p603]*

13. **Ans. (b) Perinatal mortality rate** *[Ref. Park 27/e p642–643]*
    - PNMR is a 'Yardstick of Obstetric and Pediatric acre before and around the time of birth'

14. **Ans. NONE** *[Ref. SRS Bulletin, July 2016. Registrar General of India. GOI]*
    IMR SRS BULLETIN 2023
    - IMR Overall India: 28 per 1000 LB
    - IMR Rural India: 31 per 1000 LB
    - IMR Urban India: 19 per 1000 LB
    - Highest IMR: MP (43 per 1000 LB)
    - Lowest IMR: Mizoram (3 per 1000 LB)

15. **Ans. (a) 4 per 1000 LB** *[Ref. Park 27/e p635]*
    MMR = Total maternal deaths/Total Live births × 100,000
    - Maternal deaths include deaths during pregnancy, labor/delivery or <42 days of birth provided it is related to pregnancy or its complications.
    In the given question,
    - Total LB = 2500
    - Total maternal deaths = 5 + 2 + 3 = 10 (Electrocution deaths would not be included as they are accidental)
    - So, MMR = 10/ 2500 × 100, 000 = 400 per 100,000 LB = 4 per 1000 LB

16. **Ans. (c) 55** *[Ref. Park 25/e p559]*
    - Total subcenter population = 5000

Preventive Obstetrics, Pediatrics and Geriatrics

In the given question,
- Total CBR = 20 per 1000 mid-year population
- So, for 5000 population, expected number of births in a year = 20/1000 × 5000 = 100 births.

Now since,
- Abortions and still births account for 10% of wasted pregnancies
- So, expected number of total pregnancies in 1 year = 100 + (10% of 100) = 100 + 10 = 110 pregnancies.

As per thumb rule, ANM should have at least 50% pregnancies registered with her
- Hence, total minimum expected registered pregnancies with ANM = 50% of 110 = 55.

LBW

17. **Ans. (b) 2.8 kg** [Ref. Park 23/e p536]
    - *Average birth weight in India*: 2.8 kg (2.7–2.9 kg)
    - *Prevalence of LBW (BW <2.5 kg) in India*: 18%

18. **Ans. (a) Birth weight less than 2.5 kg**
    [Ref. Park 27/e p611]

19. **Ans. (a) Continue breastfeeding** [Ref. Park 27/e p684]
    - *Breastfeeding during diarrhoea*:
      – Newborns with diarrhoea who have little or no signs of dehydration can be treated by breastfeeding alone
      – Newborns with diarrhoea who have moderate or severe dehydration should be given ORS; breastfeeding is continued along with ORS given after each liquid stool
      – Breastfeeding rehydrates, provides nutrients to help recovery and prevents further infection

20. **Ans. (c) Small-for-date babies** [Ref. Park 27/e p612–613]
    - Babies according to gestational age:

Type	Gestational age
Pre-term babies	<37 weeks (<259 days)
Term babies	37–42 weeks (259–293 days)
Post-term babies	>42 weeks (≥294 days)

    - Low birth weight:'Less than 2500 grams IRRESPECTIVE of gestational age'
      – Pre-term babies: Born at <37 weeks POG
      – Small-for-date babies: Born at term or post-term
        1. Weigh 'less than 10th percentile for gestational age'
        2. As a result of IUGR
        3. High risk of dying in neonatal and infancy period

21. **Ans. (d) 4** [Ref. Park 27/e p599]
    - *Minimum recommended ante-natal visits*: 4

Visit	Period of gestation^a
First AN visit	Early registration
Second AN visit	14–26 weeks POG
Third AN visit	28–34 weeks POG
Fourth AN visit	36 weeks POG - Term

22. **Ans. (b) <1500 g** [Ref. Surgery by Norton 2/e p650]
    Newborn Classification of Birth Weight
    - Low birth weight (LBW): <2500 grams
    - Moderately Low birth weight (MLBW): 1501–2500 grams
    - Very Low birth weight (VLBW): 1001–1500 grams
    - Extremely Low birth weight (ELBW): <1000 grams

Review Questions

23. **Ans. (c) Health education to mother** [Other components are: Family Planning, Preventive care, Care in Illness, Growth monitoring] [Ref. Park 17/e p383]
24. **Ans. (d) Edema in dependent part** [Ref. Park 27/e p755]
25. **Ans. (c) 100–150 mg** [Ref. Park 27/e p757]
26. **Ans. (d) MAC** [Ref. Internet, Park 21/e p600, Park 22/e p602]
27. **Ans. (b) Vitamin D and calcium** [Ref. Park 27/e p603]
28. **Ans. (b) 2.5 kg** [Ref. Park 23/e p536]
29. **Ans. (a) Prematurity** [Ref. Park 27/e p611–612]

MCH INDICATORS

30. **Ans. (a) Donor mother's milk**
    [Ref. Gelano, T.F., Bacha, Y.D., Assefa, N. et al. Acceptability of donor breast milk banking, its use for feeding infants, and associated factors among mothers in eastern Ethiopia. Int Breastfeed J 13, 23 (2018)]
    - If a mother's own breast milk is not available, the second choice should be donor breast milk
    - Studies have indicated that donor breast milk has short- and long-term benefits as compared to preterm formula (WHO)

31. **Ans. (d) 1 2 3 4** [Ref. Park 26/e p651]
    Causes of Neonatal Death in India 2017
    - Prematurity and LBW (48%)
    - Birth asphyxia and Birth trauma (12.9%)
    - Neonatal pneumonia (12%)
    - Other NCDs (7%)
    - Sepsis (5)
    - *Others:* Congenital anomalies, Diarrhoea

32. **Ans. (c) 4 1 2 3** [Ref. Park 26/e p658]
    - Under-5 deaths causes (Developing nations): Preterm birth complications > Pneumonia > Diarrhoea > Injury > Malaria
    - Under-5 deaths causes (Developed nations): Accident injury > Congenital anomaly > Neoplasms > Influenza > Pneumonia

33. **Ans. (d) Maternal deaths expressed as per 100,000 live births, where a 'maternal death' is defined as 'death of a woman while pregnant or during delivery or within 42 days (6 weeks) of termination of pregnancy**
    [Ref. Park 27/e p635]
    - *Maternal Mortality Ratio (MMR):* Maternal deaths expressed as per 100,000 live births, where a 'maternal death' is defined as 'death of a woman while pregnant or during delivery or within 42 days (6 weeks) of

termination of pregnancy, irrespective of duration or site of pregnancy, from any cause related to or aggravated by the pregnancy or its management but not from accidental or incidental causes. Current MMR India is 113 (SRS 2018)
- *Maternal mortality rate (MMRate):* Dividing the average annual number of maternal deaths in a population by the average number of women of reproductive age (typically those aged 15 to 49 years) who are alive during the observation period

34. **Ans. (b) Early neonatal death with weight 1000 grams**
    [Ref. Park 25/e p617]
    - Perinatal Mortality includes Late fetal deaths/live births/early neonatal deaths (>1000 grams at birth equivalent or >28 weeks POG or >35 cms body length

35. **Ans. (b) 225** *[Ref. Park 25/e p622]*
    - IMR = Infant deaths/Live births × 1000
    - So, IMR = (56 + 34)/(456–56) × 1000 = 225 per 1000 LB

36. **Ans. (a) Tetanus** *[Ref. Park 27/e p643–646]*
    NEONATAL MORTALITY RATE (NNMR):
    - Neonatal mortality is the 'most difficult' part of IMR to alter
    - *NNMR (India):* 24 per 1000 LB [2019]
    - MCC of NNMR in India is preterm birth
    - MCC of ENNMR: Prematurity and congenital anomalies
    - MCC of LNNMR: Infections (diarrhea and tetanus)
    - $NNMR_{boys} > NNMR_{girls}$
    - *Causes of Neonatal mortality (0–4 weeks):*
      – Low birth weight and prematurity
      – Birth injury and difficult labour
      – Sepsis
      – Congenital anomalies
      – Hemolytic diseases of newborn
      – Conditions of placenta and cord
      – Diarrhoeal diseases
      – Acute respiratory infections
      – Tetanus

37. **Ans. (b) Acute lower respiratory tract infections**
    [Ref. Park 27/e p651–654]
    - *Child mortality rate, CMR (Under 5 mortality rate, U5MR):*
      – $CMR = \dfrac{\text{No. of deaths of children less than}}{\text{No. of live births in a year}} \times 1000$
      – U5MR (India): 39.4 per 1000 LB [2019]
      – U5MR (World): 39.1 per 1000 LB [2019]
      – Single MCC of U5MR or CMR is Prematurity
    - *Child death rate, CDR (1–4 year mortality rate):*
      – $CDR = \dfrac{\text{No. of deaths of children aged 1-4 years in a year}}{\text{Mid year population of children aged 1-4 years}} \times 1000$
      – CDR is a more refined indicator of social situation in a country than infant mortality
      – Highest risk of death in 1–4 years age: 2nd year of life
      – CDR (India): 2.8% of total deaths [2014]
      – MCC CDR (Developing countries): Diarrhoel diseases and respiratory infections
      – MCC CDR (Developed countries): Accidents

> **ALSO REMEMBER**
> - *Millennium Development Goal (MDG) 4:* Reduce child mortality by two-thirds by 2015
> - UNICEF considers U5MR or CMR as *'single best indicator of socio-economic development and well being'*
> - *Child Survival Rate (CSR) [Child Survival Index]:*
> $CSR = \dfrac{1000 - U5MR}{10}$
> - *CSR (India):* 96% [2018]

38. **Ans. (c) During lactation 8th month**
    [Ref. Park 27/e p637–639]
    - *Maternal death:* Is defined as 'Death of a woman while pregnant or during delivery or within 42 days (6 weeks) of termination of pregnancy, irrespective of duration or site of pregnancy, from any cause related to or aggravated by the pregnancy or its management but not from accidental or incidental causes'
    - *Late maternal death:* If death due to obstetric or related complication(s) occurs after 42 days of delivery but within 1 year
      – Late maternal death is not included in MMR
    - So a mother dying due to any cause at 8 months lactation will not be included in Maternal Mortality Rate (MMR), since it occurs after 6 weeks of delivery

39. **Ans. (b) Infant mortality rate**
    [Ref. Textbook of Community Medicine by Sunder Lal, 2/e p276, Park 27/e p646]
    - Infant Mortality Rate (IMR) is the second best indicator of socio-economic development of a country
      – Ultimate solution for lowering IMR lies in socio-economic development [U5MR is even better]
    - IMR is most important indicator of
      – health status of a community
      – level of living and
      – effectiveness of MCH services in general
    - The infant mortality rate is among *'the best predictors of state failure'*
    - IMR in India:
      – Infant Mortality Rate (IMR) is a rate
      – MCC of IMR in India: Low birth rate and prematurity (57%)
      – MCC of IMR in World: Pneumonia
      – IMR (India): 28 per 1000 LB [2023]

40. **Ans. (b) Hemorrhage** *[Ref. Park 27/e p636–637]*
    - *MCC of Maternal Mortality Rate (MMR in World):* Obstetric hemorrhage (25%)
    - *MCC of MMR in India:* Obstetric hemorrhage (38%)

ALSO REMEMBER

- *Maternal Mortality Ratio (MMR)*: Maternal deaths expressed as per 100,000 live births, where a 'maternal death' is defined as 'death of a woman while pregnant or during delivery or within 42 days (6 weeks) of termination of pregnancy, irrespective of duration or site of pregnancy, from any cause related to or aggravated by the pregnancy or its management but not from accidental or incidental causes'

$$MMR = \frac{\text{No. of maternal deaths in a given year}}{\text{Total no. of live births in the same year}} \times 100{,}000$$

41. Ans. (b) 13% [Ref. Park 27/e p634]

- Deaths in the age group 0–1 year (infants) account for 12.3% of total deaths in the country
- About 68% of infant deaths occur in neonatal period. Of these three-fourths 75% occur in first week of life (early neonatal period)
- The risk of death in infancy is greatest during the first 24 – 48 hours after birth

ALSO REMEMBER

- *Infant Mortality Rate (IMR)*:
  - Infant Mortality Rate (IMR) is a rate
  - Is the second best indicator of socio-economic development of a country [BEST : U5MR]
  - Is most important indicator of health status of a community, level of living and effectiveness of MCH services in general
  - The infant mortality rate is among *'the best predictors of state failure'*
  - *MCC of IMR in India*: Low birth rate and prematurity (57%)
  - *MCC of IMR in World*: Pneumonia

42. Ans. (b) Perinatal mortality [Ref. Park 27/e p642]

- *Infant mortality rate (IMR)*: Is the ratio of infant deaths registered in a given year to the total number of live births registered in the same year; IMR is usually expressed as a rate per 1000 live births (LB)

$$IMR = \frac{\text{No. of neonatal deaths in a given year}}{\text{Total no. of live births in the same year}} \times 1000$$

- *Neonatal mortality rate (NNMR)*: Is the number of neonatal deaths (deaths within completed 28 days after birth) per 1000 live births in that year

$$IMR = \frac{\text{No. of neonatal deaths in a given year}}{\text{Total no. of live births in the same year}} \times 1000$$

  - Early neonatal mortality (ENNM): Neonatal mortality in first week (1–7 days) of life
  - Late neonatal mortality (LNNM): Neonatal mortality in first to fourth week (8–28 days) of life

- *Post-neonatal mortality rate (PNNMR)*: Is the number of neonatal deaths (deaths within completed 28 days after birth) per 1000 live births in that year

$$PNNMR = \frac{\text{No. of deaths between age 28 days to 1 year in a given year}}{\text{Total no. of live births in the same year}} \times 1000$$

  - Thus, IMR = NNMR + PNNMR = ENNMR + LNNMR + PNNMR

- *Perinatal Mortality rate (PNMR)*: Includes both late fetal deaths (stillbirths) and early neonatal deaths

$$PNMR = \frac{\text{Late fetal deaths and early neonatal deaths in a given year}}{\text{Total no. of live births in the same year}} \times 10000$$

- Perinatal period is from 28 weeks period of gestation to 7th completed days of life (But the *WHO definition of perinatal period* is from 22 completed weeks gestation to 7th completed days of life)

ALSO REMEMBER

- *Perinatal Mortality rate (PNMR)*:
  - PNMR is the sum of the fetal mortality and the neonatal mortality
  - PNMR is usually reported on an annual basis
  - PNMR is a major marker to assess the quality of health care delivery
  - *PNMR (India)*: 23 per 1000 LB [2019]
  - *P List (ICD 10)*: 100 causes of perinatal mortality and morbidity

43. Ans. (b) PNMR [Ref. Textbook of Community Medicine by Sunder Lal, 2/e p92, Park 27/e p642–643]

- Likely factor affecting infant mortality in contemporary India is inadequate prenatal care and infrequent attendance at delivery
  1. *Sex of the child*: $IMR_{girls} > IMR_{boys}$
     $NNMR_{boys} > NNMR_{girls}$
     $PNNMR_{girls} > PNNMR_{boys}$
  2. *Quality of mothering*: IMR low in good quality of mothering
  3. *Quality of health care*: IMR high in improper obstetric and pediatric care

44. Ans. (b) Perinatal mortality rate [Ref. Park 27/e p642]

45. Ans. (a) Madhya Pradesh [Ref. Park 27/e p648]

- *IMR of few states in India*: [2023]

State	IMR (per 100 live births)
Madhya Pradesh	43
Odisha	36
Uttar Pradesh	38
Assam	36
Bihar	27
Kerala	6
Mizoram	3

46. Ans. (d) Under 5 mortality [Ref. Park 27/e p651–654]

47. Ans. (c) Deaths from 28 weeks to with first week of life
[Ref. Park 27/e p642]

48. Ans. (b) 50 [Ref. Park 27/e p643]
    - In the given question,
    - Total neonatal deaths = Total early neonatal deaths + Total late neonatal deaths = 50 + 150 = 200
    - Total live births = Total births – Total stillbirths = 4050 – 50 = 4000
    - Thus, Neonatal mortality rate, NNMR = 200/4000 × 1000 = 50 per 1000 live births

49. Ans. (b) Congenital malformations [Ref. Park 27/e p643]
    - Congenital malformations are most common cause of Neonatal mortality in developed countries

50. Ans. (a) 6 million [Ref. WHO Population data, WHO website, 24/e p609]

Under-five Deaths
- Burden: 6.3 million Under-five child deaths in world [2014]
- Leading causes of deaths: [45% associated with PEM]
    - Pneumonia
    - Low birth weigh and Prematurity
    - Birth asphyxia
    - Diarrhoea
    - Malaria

51. Ans. (a) Low birth weight [Ref. Park 27/e p648]
52. Ans. (c) 1000-U5MR/10 [Ref. Park 27/e p651]
53. Ans. (c) Postpartum [Ref. Park 27/e p636–637]
54. Ans. (d) Death within 6 months post delivery [Ref. Park 27/e p635]
55. Ans. (b) 6 weeks [Ref. Park 27/e p635]
    - *Maternal death (WHO):* Death of a woman while pregnant or within 42 days of termination of pregnancy, irrespective of the duration and site of the pregnancy, from any cause related to or aggravated by the pregnancy or its management but not from accidental or incidental causes

56. Ans. (d) All of these [Ref. Park 27/e p652–653]
57. Ans. (d) Child death rate [Ref. Park 27/e p650]
    - Child death rate (1–4 year mortality rate) = No. of deaths of children aged 1–4 years in a year/Mid-year population of children aged 1–4 years × 1000.

Review Questions

58. Ans. (d) Total death in same year [Ref. Park 27/e p651]
59. Ans. (b) 1–4 year mortality [Ref. Park 27/e p650]
60. Ans. (a) 100 [Ref. Park 27/e p646]
61. Ans. (d) Sepsis and hemorrhage [Ref. Park 27/e p637]
62. Ans. (a) Prematurity [Ref. Park 27/e p642]

BREASTFEEDING

63. Ans. (b) Skin to skin contact, exclusive breastfeeding, early discharge [Ref. Park 26/e p622]

    KANGAROO MOTHER CARE for prevention of neonatal hypothermia in low birth weight/premature newborns:
    - Skin-to-skin positioning of newborn on mother's chest
    - Adequate nutrition through breastfeeding
    - Early discharge and ambulatory care
    - Support for mother and family for child care

64. Ans. (a) The maximum milk output is seen at 12 months [Ref. Park 27/e p615]
    - Mean output of breast milk per day (mL) is maximum towards the end of 1st half of lactation (5–6 months)

Months of lactation	Mean output (mL)
0–2	530
3–4	640
5–6	730 (Maximum)
7–8	660
9–10	600
11–12	525

    - *Human Milk is richer in iron and has better bioavailability than cow's milk.* Human milk has coefficient of iron uptake around 70%; It is only 30% in cow's milk and infant formulas

> **ALSO REMEMBER**
> - *Nutritive values of milk (per 100 gm):*
>
> | | Cow's milk | Human milk |
> |---|---|---|
> | Lactose (g) | 4.4 | 7.4 |
> | Proteins (g) | 3.2 | 1.1 |
> | Fat (g) | 4.1 | 3.4 |
> | Calcium (mg) | 120 | 28 |
> | Iron (mg) | 0.2 | 0.35 |
> | Water (g) | 87 | 88 |
> | Energy (kcal) | 67 | 65 |
>
> - *Human Milk is richer in Carbohydrate (lactose), Iron and Water content* WHILE Cow's milk is richer in Fat, Protein, Calcium and energy content
>   - *Human milk proteins*: More cystine and taurine; less methionine; better digested than cow's milk proteins
>   - *Human milk fats*: Higher levels of PUFAs, esp., linoleic acid and a-linoleic acid; better digested and absorbed; low calcium content but better absorbed than cow's milk
>   - *Human milk vitamins and minerals*: Human milk is richer in Vitamin A, C; richer in copper, cobalt and selenium; richer in iron and higher bioavailability; high calcium/phosphorus ratio. Human milk has lesser sodium

65. Ans. (a) Exclusive breastfeeding should be continued till 6 months of age followed by supplementation with additional foods [Ref. Park 27/e p615, 616]
    - WHO recommends, in developing countries, *excluive breastfeeding till 6 months age*
    - WHO recommends, in developing countries, *breastfeeding till minimum 2 years age*

ALSO REMEMBER
COLOSTRUM:
- Is the most suitable food immediately after birth of the baby; Regular milk comes 3–6 days afterbirth
- Also known as *'Beestings'*, *'First milk'* or *'Immune Milk'*
- High in carbohydrates, protein, and antibodies and low in fat
- Contains all five immunoglobulins found in all mammals, IgA, IgD, IgE, IgG and IgM
- *Few occasions when breastfeeding might harm the infant:*
  - Infants with classic galactosemia
  - Mother has untreated pulmonary tuberculosis
  - Mother is taking certain medications that suppress the immune system
  - Mother has had unusually excessive exposure to heavy metals such as mercury
  - Mother has HIV
  - Mother uses potentially harmful substances such as cocaine, heroin, and amphetamines

66. Ans. (c) Lactose   [Ref. Park 27/e p616]
67. Ans. (a) Maximum output is at 12 months of lactation   [Ref. Park 27/e p615]
68. Ans. (b) Carbohydrates; (d) Iron   [Ref. Park 27/e p616]
69. Ans. (b) 1 hour of delivery   [Ref. Park 27/e p615]
70. Ans. (d) Neonate should be isolated from mother
    [Ref. Management of newborn infant born to mother suffering from tuberculosis: Current recommendations & gaps in knowledge by Mittal, p34]
    - In Tuberculosis of Mother, WHO recommends feeding under all circumstances, however, close contact with the baby should be reduced
    - TB WOMAN CASE WITH NVD
    - Start ATT of mother immediately
    - Start Exclusive breastfeeding of newborn
    - Start INH prophylaxis 5 mg/kg of newborn for 6 months
71. Ans. ALL OF THE CHOICES   [Ref. Park 27/e p616]
    - Breast milk contain all nutrients but its' deficient in Vitamins D & B

GROWTH AND DEVELOPMENT

72. Ans. (c) Chronic malnutrition   [Ref. Park 26/e p730]
    Acute and Chronic Malnutrition Indicators:
    - *Low weight for age*: Is known as 'Underweight' (Acute on Chronic Malnutrition)
    - *Low weight for height*: Is known as 'Nutritional wasting' or 'Emaciation' (Acute Malnutrition)
    - *Low height for age*: Is known as 'Nutritional stunting' or 'Dwarfing' (Chronic malnutrition)
73. Ans. (b) Weight for age below 3 SD
    [Ref. Partha's Fundamental of Paediatrics, 2/e p69]
    WHO & UNICEF's Acute Malnutrition Criteria
    - Presence of Bipedal edema
    - Visible severe wasting
    - Mid arm circumference below 115 mm
    - Weight for height below 3SD of WHO Growth Standards 2006
74. Ans. (c) 50th percentile for boys   [Ref. Park 27/e p622]

75. Ans. (a) Acute malnutrition   [Ref. Park 27/e p754]
    - *Low weight for age*: Is known as 'Underweight' [Acute and Chronic Malnutrition]
    - *Low weight for height*: Is known as 'Nutritional wasting' or 'Emaciation' (Acute Malnutrition)
    - *Low height for age*: Is known as 'Nutritional stunting' or 'Dwarfing' (Chronic malnutrition)

ALSO REMEMBER
FOR CHILDREN
- *Single best parameter for assessment of physical growth*: Weight (and rate of weight gain)
- *Single most sensitive measure of growth*: Weight
- *Single most reliable criterion of assessment of health and nutritional status*: Weight
- *Single most reliable criterion of assessment of health and nutritional status*: Weight
- Height is a stable measurement of growth as opposed to body weight
  - *Weight*: reflects only present health status
  - *Height*: indicates events in past also
  - *Age independent parameters for growth assessment*:
  - Weight for height
  - Mid arm circumference (MAC)
  - Thickness of subcutaneous fat
  - Body ratios
    1. *Weight*: Height
    2. MAC: Head circumference

76. Ans. (b) 9 kg   [Ref. Park 27/e p620]
    - *Average birth weight in India*: 2.8 kg (2.7–2.9 kg)
    - BW doubles at 5 months, triples by 1 year and quadruples by 2 years age
      - So BW of 3 kg will become 6 kg, 9 kg and 12 kg at 5 months, 1 year and 2 years age respectively
    - *Weight gain pattern in children*:

Age	Weight increments
0–3 months	200 grams per week
4–6 months	150 grams per week
7–9 months	100 grams per week
10–12 months	50–75 grams per week
0–1 year	7.0 kg per year
1–2 year	2.5 kg per year
3–5 year	2.0 kg per year

ALSO REMEMBER
- Weight reflects only present status of the child, whereas height indicates events in the past also
- *Height increase pattern in children*:

Age	Height increments
1st year	25 cm per year
2nd year	12 cm per year
3rd year	9 cm per year
4th year	7 cm per year
5th year	6 cm per year

- *Near-final height attainment*:
  - Indian boys attain 98% of final height by 17.75 years
  - Indian girls attain 98% of final height by 16.5 years

77. Ans. (b) 34 cm [Ref. Park 27/e p621]
- At birth the head circumference is about 34 cms, about 2 cms more than the chest circumference
- By 6–9 months, Head circumference (HC) = Chest circumference (CC)
- Normal children: CC overtakes HC at around 1 year age
  - Malnourished children: CC may overtake HC at around 3–4 years age

> **ALSO REMEMBER**
> - *HC should be measured in Occipito-frontal diameter*, with a fibre-glass tape
> - *HC growth velocity in 0–3 months age*: 2 cms per month
> - *During 1st year there is increase in HC by 12 cms*; Adult head size is achieved by 5–6 years age

78. Ans. (d) History of maternal health [Ref. Park 27/e p622]

GROWTH CHART:
- *Growth Chart (Road-to-health chart)*: Is a visible display of child's physical growth and development
- *Growth chart is designed for*: Longitudinal follow-up (growth monitoring) of a child
- *Growth chart is generally plotted between*: Weight and Age
- *Growth chart provides information on*:
  - Identification and registration
  - Birth date and birth weight
  - Chronological age
  - Weight-for-age
  - Developmental milestones
  - History of sibling health
  - Immunization procedures
  - Introduction of supplementary foods
  - Episodes of sickness
  - Child spacing (Contraceptive/family planning methods used)
  - Reasons for special care

WHO HOME BASED GROWTH CHART:
- *WHO growth chart has 2 reference curves*:
  - *Upper Reference Curve (URC)*: 50th percentile for boys
  - *Lower Reference Curve (LRC)*: 3rd percentile for girls
- *Road to Health*: Is the space between two growth curves (weight channel). It includes zone of normality for most populations, i.e. 95% of healthy normal children used as a reference fall in this area
- *WHO reference curves are based on*: NCHS Standards (National Centre for Health Statistics, USA)
- *The 3rd percentile (LRC) corresponds to approximately 2 SD below the median of weight-for-age reference value (i.e. URC)*

> **ALSO REMEMBER**
> - Growth chart was first designed by *'David Morley'* (and later modified by WHO).
> - Growth chart is the *'passport to child's health care'*
> - *Best available standards of growth*: NCHS standards

Contd...

Contd...
- *Direction of growth in a growth chart is more important* than the position of dots
- *Periodic weight record is more useful than a single weight plot*
- *Objective in child care*: To keep the child above 3rd percentile
- *Flattening of a child's plot*: indicates malnutrition
- REFERENCE OR STANDARD VALUES OF GROWTH:
  - WHO 2006 (MGRS) Child Growth Standards
  - Harvard (Boston) standards
  - NCHS standards (WHO reference values)
  - Indian standards (ICMR values)

79. Ans. (d) Health education [Ref. K. Park 17/e p383]
- *Under fives clinic concept*: Includes
  - Preventive care
  - Care in illness
  - Growth monitoring
  - Family planning (Centre)
  - Health education (Border covering all 4 components)

80. Ans. (b) The position of dots is more important than direction [Ref. Park 27/e p622–624]

81. Ans. (a) Low birth weight [Ref. Park 27/e p611–613]
- Low birth weight is associated with 'Maternal malnutrition'

82. Ans. (b) Mid arm circumference
[Ref. Nutrition in Children in Developing Countries by P Choudhary, 1/e p190]

83. Ans. (c) Height for age [Ref. Park 27/e p620]

84. Ans. (b) 50 percentile for boys and 3 percentile for girls [Ref. Park 27/e p624–625]

85. Ans. (c) 4 years
[Ref. Pediatric Board Review by Naga, 1/e p1]

HEIGHT CHANGES POST BIRTH
- Average birth length of an Indian newborn: 50 cm
- Increase of height in 1st year of life: 25 cm
- Height doubles (Become 100 cm) by: 4 years age

86. Ans. (b) Language [Ref. Park 27/e p621]

87. Ans. (a) Mirror play [Ref. Physical Therapy by Kessler, 3/e p67, 24/e p580]
- Mirror play milestone is see at age around 6 months+
- Crawling, Creeping, Pincer grasp are seen in age above 9 months

88. Ans. (a) Wasted, stunted [Ref. Park 27/e p626]

WHO CLASSIFICATION OF MALNUTRITION

	Moderate malnutrition	Severe malnutrition
Weight for Height (Wasting)	Wasting 70–79% of expected –2 to –3 SD score	Severe wasting <70% of expected <–3 SD score
Height for Age (Stunting)	Stunting 85–89% of expected –2 to –3 SD score	Severe stunting <85% of expected <–3 SD score

In the given question,
- W for H (%) = Weight of child/Weight of normal child at that age × 100 = 7/9 × 100 = 77.7%

- H for Age (%) = Height of child/Height of normal child at that age × 100 = 74/86 × 100 = 86%
- So it's a case of wasting plus stunting.

89. **Ans. (b) Done by case control study** [Ref. Park 27/e p622]

    MULTICENTER GROWTH REFERENCE STUDY (MGRS) 1997–2003
    - Type: Population based study
    - Countries: Brazil, Ghana, India, Oman, Norway, USA
    - Primary growth data and related information gathered form 8440 healthy breast-fed infants and children (0–60 months age)
    - Mother followed breastfeeding and not smoking during and after pregnancy
    - New standards generated: Percentile and Z-scores for H for age, W for age, W for L, W for H and BMI for age
    - A key component of the MGRS design was a longitudinal cohort of children who were examined in a sequence of 21 visits starting at birth and ending at 24 months of age: Principal rationale for the longitudinal component was to allow for the development of growth velocity standards.

90. **Ans. (c) Weight for age** [Ref. Park 27/e p623]

    ANGANWADI CENTRE ICDS GROWTH CHART
    - Nutritional status of the child is assessed against weight for age
    - Separate charts for girls and boys
    - 3 zones: Normal zone (grey), Undernutrition below –2 SD (light grey), Severe underweight below –3 SD (dark grey).

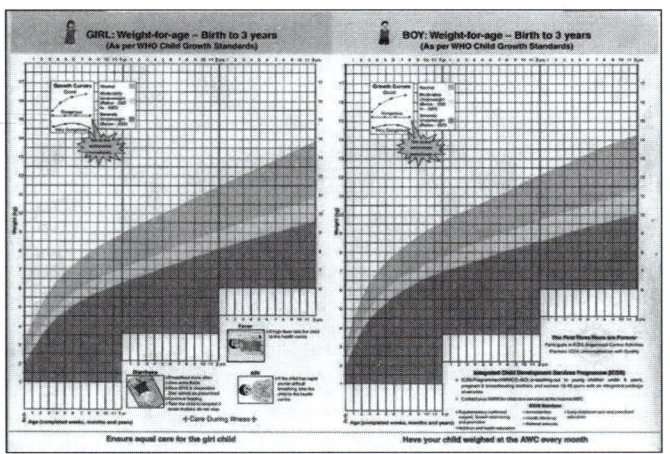

91. **Ans. (a) Weight retardation**
    [Ref. Achars Textbook of Pediatrics, 4/e p46]

    Gomez Classification of malnutrition: It is based on 'weight for age'

Weight for age	Grade of malnutrition
90–110%	Normal
75–89%	1st degree (Mild)
60–74%	2nd degree (Moderate)
<60%	3rd degree (Severe)

Review Questions

92. **Ans. (c) Home based** [Ref. Park 27/e p622]
93. **Ans. (a) Keratomalacia** [Ref. Park 21/e p590–92, Park 22/e p592–94, 24/e p576–678]
94. **Ans. (b) David Morley** [Ref. Park 27/e p622]
95. **Ans. (a) Used for monitoring growth and development of a child** [Ref. Park 27/e p622]

SCHOOL HEALTH

96. **Ans. (a) Dental ailments** [Ref. Evaluation Study of Government of India's Intensive Pilot Project of School Health Services, 1980 by Sapru, R, and Pandey, D.C.]
    - *Commonly detected morbidities in school children (in decreasing order of prevalence):*
      – Dental defects (180.3 per 1000)
      – Goiter (123.8 per 1000)
      – Malnutrition (123.5 per 1000)

> **ALSO REMEMBER**
> - School age children represent >25% of total Indian population
> - School health committee (1961) in India recommended medical examination of children *'at the time of entry and thereafter every 4 years'* [New NRHM guideline: Once every 6 months]
> - *School Eye Screening Programme*:
>   – Focus on middle schools (V–VIII classes: 10–14 years age group)
>   – Teachers to do screening: 1 teacher per 150 students
>   – Visual acuity cutoff for referral to PHC: <6/9
> - In 1961, *'Rennuka Roy School Health Committee'* laid the foundations for a comprehensive school health programme in India

97. **Ans. (d) One urinal for 10 students and one latrine for 25 students** [Ref. Park 27/e p659]
    - *Healthful school environment:* Suggested minimum standards for sanitation of schools and its environs in India include,
      – *Location:* Away from noisy surroundings; kept fenced
      – *Site:* 5 acres for primary schools; 10 acres for higher elementary schools
      – *Structure:* Exterior walls 10 inch thick and heat resistant
      – *Class room:* 1 class room per 40 students maximum; Per capita space >10 sq. feet
      – *Furniture:* Single desks of 'minus (–) type'
      – *Doors and windows:* Doors and windows area >25% of floor area
      – *Color:* Inside color of walls should be white
      – *Lighting:* Natural light from left side
      – *Water supply:* Safe and potable and continuous supply through taps
      – *Lavatory:* 1 urinal per 60 students and 1 latrine per 100 students

98. **Ans. (b) Desks should be of plus type**
 [Ref. Park 27/e p659]

> **ALSO REMEMBER**
> - *Minus (-) type desks*: Desks where sitting table slides under the front portion (writing board)

99. **Ans. (d) Lung infections** [Ref. Park 27/e p658]
   - School health services emphasize on Malnutrition, Infectious diseases, Intestinal parasites, Diseases of skin/eye/ear, Dental caries.

Review Questions

100. **Ans. None (Both are incorrect statements)**
 [Ref. Logical reasoning]

101. **Ans. (a) 1/3; 1/2** [Ref. Park 27/e p776]

ICDS, IMNCI AND BFHI

102. **Ans. None** [Ref. Park 27/e p673–677]
   - *Ministries to combat malnutrition*:

Programme	Ministry
Vitamin A prophylaxis programme	Ministry of Health and Family Welfare
Prophylaxis against nutritional anemia	Ministry of Health and Family Welfare
Iodine deficiency disorders control programme	Ministry of Health and Family Welfare
Special nutrition programme	Ministry of Social Welfare
Balwadi nutrition programme	Ministry of Social Welfare
ICDS programme	Ministry of Women and Child Development
Midday meal programme	Ministry of Human Resource Development

> **ALSO REMEMBER**
> - *Employees State Insurance (ESI) Scheme is under*: 'Ministry of Labour'

103. **Ans. (d) Neonatal tetanus** [Ref. Textbook of Community Medicine by Sunder Lal, 2/e p135–36, Park 27/e p655–656]
   - **INTEGRATED MANAGEMENT OF NEONATAL AND CHILDHOOD ILLNESS (IMNCI):**
   - IMNCI is a '*strategy for reducing morbidity and mortality associated with major causes of childhood illness*'
     – Curative component includes management of:
       1. Diarrhoea
       2. Measles
       3. Pneumonia
       4. Malaria
       5. Severe malnutrition and nutritional counseling

> **ALSO REMEMBER**
> - IMNCI is the Indian adaptation of IMCI; major highlights of Indian adaptation are,
>   – Inclusion of early neonatal age (0–7 days age) in programme
>   – Incorporating national guidelines on malaria, anemia, Vitamin-A supplementation and immunization schedule
>   – Training of health workers begin with sick young infants up to 2 months
>   – Proportion of training time devoted to sick young infant and sick child is almost equal
>   – Is skill based
> - Currently ICDS is the '*most important scheme in field of child welfare*'; It is '*both a preventive and a developmental effort*'
> - *1 Mini-Anganwadi Centre* is for population of 150–500 population (rural/urban) or 150–300 population (tribal)
> - *Kishori Shakti Yojana*: Scheme for adolescent girls in ICDS
> - *Wheat Based Nutrition Programme (WBNP)*: The Government of India allocates food grains (wheat and rice) at BPL rates to the States for providing supplementary nutrition to beneficiaries under the ICDS Scheme
> - *UDISHA*: A World Bank assisted countrywide training programme for all ICDS functionaries; 3 main components:
>   – Regular training
>   – Other training
>   – IEC
> - *ICDS in India*: Implementation by Ministry of Women and Child Development:
>   – ICDS projects sanctioned: 5671
>   – ICDS projects functioning: 5422
>   – Anganwadis functioning: 578,457

104. **Ans. (b) Community development block**
 [Ref. Park 27/e p673–677]
   - Administrative unit of an ICDS project is '*Community Development Block*'; each project covering a population of 1,00,000 (rural/urban) or 35,000 (tribal)
     – 1 CDPO (Community Development Project Officer) is in charge of 4 supervisors (Mukhyasevikas) and 100 Anganwadis (each supervisor for 25 Anganwadis)

105. **Ans. (d) USA** [Ref. Birthing Normally After A Caesarean or Two, H Vadeboncoeur, 2/e, 21]

MOTHER FRIENDLY CHILDBIRTH INITIATIVE (MFCI)

Description: To improve care throughout the childbearing continuum in order to save lives, prevent illness and harm from the overuse of obstetric technologies, and promote health for mothers and babies around the world
   - *Launched*: 1996, USA

10 Steps of MFCI:

Step 1: Treat every woman with respect and dignity, providing her right to informed consent and refusal

Step 2: Possess and routinely apply midwifery knowledge and skills related to normal physiology

Step 3: Inform the mother of the benefits of continuous support during labour and birth,

Step 4: Provide drug-free comfort and pain-relief methods during labour

Step 5: Provide specific evidence-based practices proven to be beneficial

Step 6: Avoid potentially harmful procedures and practices that have no scientific support

Step 7: Implement measures that enhance wellness and prevent emergencies, illness, and death of Mother and Baby

Step 8: Provide access to evidence-based skilled emergency treatment for life-threatening complications

Step 9: Provide a continuum of collaborative maternal and newborn care with all relevant health care providers, institutions and organizations

Step 10: Strive to achieve the 10 Steps to Successful Breast-feeding (WHO/UNICEF Baby-friendly Hospital Initiative BFHI)

106. **Ans. NONE OF THE CHOICES**
[Ref. ICDS document, Ministry of Women & Child Development, Government of India]
- Revised norms for free food supplementation under ICDS:

Category	Older		NEW REVISED	
	Calories (kcal)	Protein (g)	Calories (kcal)	Protein (g)
Children (6–72 months)	300	8–10	500	12–15
Severely malnourished children (6–72 m)	600	20	800	20–25
Pregnant women and Nursing mothers	500	15–20	600	18–20

107. **Ans. (d) 100,000** *[Ref. Park 27/e p674]*
- One Community Development Block (ICDS) comprises of:
  – Rural/Urban areas: 1,00,000 population (100 villages)
  – Tribal areas: 35,000 population (550 villages).

108. **Ans. (b) Mukhyasevika** *[Ref. Park 27/e p701]*
- Administrative unit of ICDS, Community Development Block, each project covers population of 1,00,000 (rural/urban) or 35,000 (tribal)
- 1 CDPO (Community Development Project Officer) is in charge of 4 supervisors (Mukhyasevikas) and 100 Anganwadis (each supervisor for 25 Anganwadis).

Review Questions

109. **Ans. (a) Covers population of 5000** *[Ref. Park 27/e p701]*
110. **Ans. (b) Formal education** *[Ref. Park 27/e p673–677]*
111. **Ans. None [Now 500 kcal + 12–15 g proteins]** *[Ref. Park 27/e p674]*
112. **Ans. (c) Two months** *[Ref. Park 25/e p612–613]*

NEONATAL SCREENING

113. **Ans. (b) Phenylketonuria** *[Ref. Park 27/e p611]*

    GUTHRIE TEST:
    - *Guthrie Test*: Is done in neonates for mass screening of Phenylketonuria (PKU)
    - *Guthrie test was the first screening test used in neonates*
    - *Blood sample* is collected by heel prick of the baby 7–10 days after birth
    - *Guthrie Test is negative* in first 2–3 days of life
    - *Guthrie test can detect* PKU, Galactosemia and Maple syrup urine disease
    - *Chemicals detected*: Phenylalanine, Phenylpyruvate and Phenyllactate
    - *It is a semi-quantitative test*

ALSO REMEMBER
- Neonatal Screening is primarily a Secondary Level of Prevention
- *Most common neonatal disorder to be screened is Neonatal hypothyroidism (NNH)*
- *PKU is an autosomal recessive trait* with a frequency of 1 in 10,000 births
- *Enzyme deficient in PKU*: Phenylalanine hydroxylase
- *Treatment of PKU*: restricting or eliminating foods high in phenylalanine, such as breast milk, meat, chicken, fish, nuts, cheese, legumes and other dairy products
- Currently, Guthrie test has been replaced by *Tandem mass Spectrometry*

114. **Ans. (a) Neonatal hypothyroidism** *[Ref. Park 27/e p611]*
- *Most common neonatal disorder to be screened is Neonatal hypothyroidism (NNH)*
- *Blood sample* is collected from Cord's Blood
- *Test involves measurement of* T_4 or TSH both simultaneously. As a single method, T_4 is more useful (greater precision and reproducibility)

ALSO REMEMBER
- NNH has a frequency of 1 in 4000 births
- *The most common cause of congenital hypothyroidism is iodine deficiency*
- Treatment of NNH consists of a daily dose of thyroid hormone (thyroxine) by mouth

MISCELLANEOUS

115. **Ans. (d) Restrict caloric intake and exercise**
[Ref. Broskey NT, Marlatt KL, Most J, Erickson ML, Irving BA, Redman LM. The Panacea of Human Aging: Calorie Restriction Versus Exercise. Exerc Sport Sci Rev. 2019 Jul;47(3):169–175]
- Primary aging (Normal aging) refers to the maximum lifespan of a species
- Secondary aging refers to the life expectancy of a population, or the amount of time an individual is expected to live. It's affected by genetics and environmental factors.
- To improve human lifespan, successful anti-aging interventions need to counteract both primary and secondary causes of aging
- Calorie restriction and exercise both extend healthspan; however, calorie restriction is superior to exercise because of the additional attenuation of primary aging.

116. **Ans. (b) Volume >1 mL [NEW GUIDELINES >1.5 mL]**
    [Ref. Internet; www.who.int]

> **ALSO REMEMBER**
> - *Aspermia*: Absence of semen
> - *Azoospermia*: Absence of sperms
> - *Oligospermia*: Low no. of sperms
> - *Asthenozoospermia*: Poor sperm motility
> - *Teratozoospermia*: Sperms carry more morphological defects than usual

117. **Ans. (b) Adolescent girl's scheme under ICDS**
    [Ref. Textbook of Community Medicine by Sunder Lal, 2/e p17 and Park 21/e p545, Park 22/e p443, 24/e p629]

    KISHORI SHAKTI YOJANA (KSY):
    - KSY is rename of *'Adolescent Girl's Scheme'* under ICDS (Integrated Child Development Services)
    - Aim of KSY:
        - To improve the nutritional and health status of adolescent girls
        - To promote self-development, awareness of health, hygiene, nutrition, and family life and child care
        - KSY covers 2000 ICDS projects

118. **Ans. (c) Iron supplements and observation**
    [Ref. Park 27/e p572-573]

> **ALSO REMEMBER**
> - *Bleeding on IUD insertion*: Reassure + Iron supplementation
> - *Pain on IUD insertion*: Remove the IUD
> - *Pregnancy with IUD-in-situ*:
>   - Legally induced abortion
>   - If woman wants to continue pregnancy: Remove IUD by pulling threads
>   - If signs of intra-uterine infection: Evacuation under broad spectrum antibiotic cover

119. **Ans. (b) 105 g/L** [Ref. Internet]

> **ALSO REMEMBER**
> - *Cut-off points for diagnosis of anemia (WHO)*:
>
> | Group | Hb (g/dL) | MCHC (%) |
> | --- | --- | --- |
> | Adult males | 13 | 34 |
> | Adult females, non-pregnant | 12 | 34 |
> | Adult females, pregnant | 11 | 34 |
> | Children, 6 m–6 y | 11 | 34 |
> | Children, 6–14 y | 12 | 34 |
>
> - *12 by 12 Initiative*: The initiative was launched by MoHFW, GOI; FOGSI and UNICEF on April 24, 2007
>   - *Main Objective*: To ensure that every child have a healthy hemoglobin of 12 gm% by the age of 12 years

120. **Ans. (d) A Rh –ve multipara mother aged 30 years with two live healthy boys** [Ref. Park 27/e p955–956]

- *Amniocentesis*: Amniotic Fluid Test or AFT is a medical procedure used in prenatal diagnosis of genetic risk factors; In AFT, a small amount of amniotic fluid, which contains fetal tissues, is extracted from the amnion or amniotic sac surrounding a developing fetus, and the fetal DNA is examined for genetic abnormalities
- Amniocentesis can be performed *'usually after the 14th week of pregnancy'* (and not before 12 weeks of POG)
- Indications for Amniocentesis:
    - *Advanced maternal age (>35 years) for risk of Down's Syndrome*
    - *Previous child with Down's Syndrome or other chromosomal anomalies*
    - *Parents with known chromosomal translocation*
    - *Previous child with a metabolic defect (neural tube defects, anencephaly and spina bifida) – raised alpha fetoprotein*
    - *Sex determination is warranted (history of sex linked genetic diseases)*

> **ALSO REMEMBER**
> - Through amniocentesis, the *'three most common abnormalities tested'* for are:
>   - Down's syndrome
>   - Trisomy 18
>   - Spina bifida

121. **Ans. (c) Adoption and Foster home placement**
    [Ref. Park 27/e p672]

    CHILD PLACEMENT:
    - *Orphanages*: For children who have no home or cannot be taken care of by their parents
    - *Foster Homes*: Several types of facilities for rearing children other than in natural families
    - *Adoption*: Legal adoption confers upon child and the adoptive parents, rights and responsibilities similar to that of natural parents
    - *Borstals*: Borstal: Boys over 16 years who are too difficult to be handled in a certified school or have misbehaved there, are sent to a Borstal. Borstal, as an institution, falls between a certified school and an adult prison
        - *A borstal sentence is usually for 3 years, and is regarded as a method of training and reformation*
    - *Remand Homes*: Child is placed under the care of doctors, psychiatrists and other trained personnel to improve the mental and physical well being of the child

> **ALSO REMEMBER**
> - Law relevant to adoption in India: *'The Hindu Adoptions and Maintenance Act, 1956'*

122. **Ans. (c) Borstal** [Ref. Park 27/e p672]

123. **Ans. (a) 2–3% of newborns**
    [Ref. Park 21/e p531, Park 22/e p533]

- *Congenital disorders*: Those diseases that are substantially determined before or during birth and which, in principle, are recognizable in early life
- *Incidence of congenital disorders (World)*: 30–70 per 1000 live births
  - MC disorders are of cardiovascular system and nervous system
- Birth defects in Indian newborns are seen in 2.5%. The figure rises to 4% if they are followed upto age of 5 years
  - MC birth defect in North India: Neural tube defects or spina bifida
  - MC birth defect in rest of India: Musculoskeletal disorders

124. Ans. (a) Article 24; (e) Article 45
[Ref. Park 21/e p508, Park 22/e p510]

- Articles on Child rights in our Constitution:

Article	Details
Article 24	Prohibits employment of children below 14 years in factories
Article 24	Prevents abuse of children at tender age
Article 24	Provides for free and compulsory education for all children till 14 yrs age

> **ALSO REMEMBER**
> - *NPAC 2005 definition of Child (adopted by India)*:
>   - All persons upto the age of 18 years
>   - All rights apply to all age-groups, including before birth
> - *National Policy 1974 mandate*: State takes responsibility for children 'both before and after birth'
>
> **HEALTH OF ADOLESCENTS:**
> - *Definitions*:
>   - *Adolescents*: 10–19 years age
>   - *Youth*: 15–24 years age
>   - *Young people*: 10–24 years age

125. Ans. (c) Remand home *[Ref. Park 27/e p672]*

126. Ans. (c) Free nutritional supplements *[Ref. Park 27/e p615]*
- KANGAROO MOTHER CARE for prevention of neonatal hypothermia in low birth weight/premature newborns:
  - *Skin-to-skin positioning of newborn on mother's chest*
  - *Adequate nutrition through breastfeeding*
  - *Early discharge and ambulatory care*
  - *Support for mother and family for child care*

127. Ans. (c) Remuneration *[Ref. Park 27/e p670]*

CHAPTER 9

Nutrition and Health

NEW NUTRITION GUIDELINES 2021–22

- These guidelines are devised by:
  - Indian Council of Medical Research, (ICMR), New Delhi
  - National Institute of Nutrition (NIN), Hyderabad
  - Department of Health Research, New Delhi
  - Ministry of Health & Family Welfare, New Delhi

Reference Indian Man Woman

	Reference Indian Man	Reference Indian Woman
Age	19–39 years	19–39 years
Weight	65 kg	55 kg
Height	95th centile for adult male	95th centile for adult female
BMI	18.5–22.9	18.5–22.9
Others	95th centile values of heights and weights for a given age and gender which are representative of well-nourished population of India were considered for calculations	

(Table © Dr Vivek Jain 2022–23)

RDA Energy Requirements

	Adult Man	Adult Woman
Sedentary	2110	1660
Moderate	2710	2130
Heavy	3470	2720

- Pregnancy Additional Energy Requirements:
  - +350 kcal/day
- Lactation Additional Energy Requirements:
  - 0–6 m: +600 kcal/day
  - 6–12 m: +520 kcal/day
- Infant Energy Requirements:
  - 0–6 m: 550 kcal/day
  - 6–12 m: 670 kcal/day
- Children Energy Requirements:
  - 1–3 y: 1000 kcal/day
  - 4–6 y: 1400 kcal/day
  - 7–9 y: 1700 kcal day

RDA for Important Nutrients

	Iron	Folate	Calcium	Vitamin A	Vitamin C	Vitamin D	Iodine
	mg/d	mcg/d	mg/d	mcg/d RE	mg/d	IU/d	mcg/d
Man	19	300	1000	1000	80	600	150
Woman	29	220	1000	840	65	600	150
Pregnancy	40	570	1000	900	+15	600	250
Lactation	23	330	1200	950	+50	600	280

(Table © Dr Vivek Jain 2022–23)

Recommended Intake for Minerals/Trace Elements

Nutrient	Requirement
Phosphorous	1000 mg/day
Sodium	2000 mg/day
Potassium	3500 mg/day
Copper	2 mg/day
Manganese	4 mg/day
Chromium	50 µg/day
Selenium	40 µg/day

(Table © Dr Vivek Jain 2022–23)

Recommendations in New Nutrition Guidelines 2020–21

- Energy: A reduction in the BMR to 10% and 9% for males and females respectively with simultaneous reduction in PAL values is proposed
  - New Energy requirements Adults: Males (Sedentary, Moderate, Heavy work - 2110, 2710, 3470 kcal per day) and Females (Sedentary, Moderate, Heavy work - 1660, 2130, 2720 kcal per day)
  - Energy requirements Infants: 550 kcal per day (0–6 months age) and 670 kcal per day (6–12 months age)
- Proteins: A median obligatory nitrogen loss of 48 mg/kg (WHO, 2007) has been used to compute mean (0.66 g/kg/day) and safe protein requirements (0.83 g/kg/day) for healthy Indian adults
- Fats and oils: Visible fat intake for sedentary, moderate and heavy activity has been set at 25, 30 and 40 g/d for adult man and 20, 25 and 30 g/d for adult women
- Fibre: Based on energy intake, fibre intake level of about 40 g/2000 kcal has been considered as safe
- Water: The water required from beverages for adult man ranges from 32 to 58 mL per kg body mass and for woman, it ranges from 27 to 52 mL per kg body mass

CONCEPTS IN NUTRITION

Nutrients in Diet

- *Macronutrients*: Proximate principles which form the bulk of the diet^Q
  - Carbohydrates
  - Fats
  - Proteins
- *Micronutrients*: Vitamin and Minerals (which are required in small quantities).
  - *Major minerals*: Sodium, Potassium, Magnesium, Calcium, Phosphorus
  - *Trace elements*: Iron, Iodine, Fluorine, Zinc, Copper, Cobalt, Selenium, Chromium, Manganese, Molybdenum, Nickel, Tin, Silicon, Vanadium
  - *Trace contaminants (no known function in body)*: Lead, Mercury, Barium, Boron, Aluminium^Q.

> **Key points**
> **Proximate principles:**
> - Carbohydrates
> - Fats
> - Proteins

Proximate Principles of Diet

- *Energy yield of macro-nutrients (Proximate principles):*^{Q}

Nutrient	Energy yield
Carbohydrates	4 kcal per gram (17 KJ)
Proteins	4 kcal per gram (17 KJ)
Fats	9 kcal per gram (37 KJ)

- Carbohydrates, fats and proteins form the main bulk of food; thus they are known as *'Macronutrients'* or *'Proximate principles'*
- In *'Balanced Diet'*,
    - Proteins should constitute 10–15% of total daily energy intake^Q
    - Fats should constitute 15–30% of total daily energy intake^Q
    - Carbohydrates constitute remaining 50–70% of energy.

> **Key points**
> **Energy:** Pregnancy + 350 kcal/d
> Lactation (0–6 m) + 600 kcal/d

Consumption Units

- *Definition*: A 'Consumption Unit' is a coefficient of dietary intake, which varies between individuals based on the basis of their age, sex and physical activity^Q
    - Appraisal of dietary intake of very family by weighment method is worked out in terms of consumption units
- *Consumption Unit Coefficients (CUC):*

Group	Particulars	CUC
Adult Male	Sedentary worker^Q	1.0
	Moderate worker	1.2
	Heavy worker	1.6
Adult Female	Sedentary worker^Q	0.8
	Moderate worker	0.9
	Heavy worker	1.2
Adolescents	12–21 years	1.0
Children	9–12 years	0.8
	7–9 years	0.7
	5–7 years	0.6
	3–5 years	0.5
	1–3 years	0.4

Recommended Dietary Allowance (RDA)

> **Key points**
> RDA covers requirement of 97.5%

- *Definition*^{Q}: Recommended Dietary Allowance (RDA): Is a level of intake corresponding to Mean + 2 Standard Deviation, which covers requirement of 97.5% of population
    - RDA is safe level of intake which is likely to be inadequate in not more than 2.5% population
    - RDA is decided by a panel of experts and is based on scientific research
- *RDA is often higher than the recommended minimum requirement*: RDA includes both daily requirement and some additional requirement for periods of growth or illness
    - RDA is based on Estimated Average Requirement
- RDA 'safe level approach' is not used for energy since excess energy intake is undesirable^Q
    - *For energy*: only mean or average requirement is defined as RDA.

> **Key points**
> RDA 'safe level approach' is not used for energy

PROTEINS

Protein Quantity of Food Items

Food Item	Protein content (gm % per 100 gm)
Soyabean[Q]	43
Pulses	22–25
Fish	21
Meat	20
Egg (hen)	13
Wheat	12
Rice	7
Milk (cow)	3

Protein Energy Ratio (PE Ratio)

- Assessment of protein quantity is done by 'Protein-Energy Ratio' (PE)[Q]

$$PE\ percent = \frac{Energy\ from\ protein}{Total\ energy\ in\ diet} \times 100$$

  - It is recommended that protein should account for approximately 15–20% of total daily energy intake
  - If PE is less than 4 percent, then the subject will be unable to eat enough to satisfy protein requirements.
- *Recommended PE Ratios:*

Group	PE Ratio (%)
Reference adult man	8.3
Reference adult woman	9.1
Pregnant woman	10.4
Lactating woman	10.9
Adolescent 16–18 yr boys	11.4
Adolescent 16–18 yr girls	11.7

- *PE Ratios of food items:*

Food Item	PE % (kcal)
Fish[Q]	80
Milk (cow)	20
Dal (pulses)	24
Rice	8

Methods of Assessing Protein Quality

- Digestible Indispensable Amino Acid Score (DIAAS):
  - FAO has recommended DIAAS replace PDCAAS as preferred method of measuring protein quality[Q]

$$DIAAS\ \% = \frac{Digestible\ dietary\ indispensable\ amino\ acid\ mg\ in\ 1\ g\ of\ dietary\ protein}{Same\ dietary\ indispensable\ amino\ acid\ mg\ in\ 1\ g\ of\ reference\ protein} \times 100$$

- *Protein Digestibility Corrected Amino Acid Score (PDCAAS):*
  - PDCAAS is Amino Acid Score with an added digestibility component
  - PDCAAS is closely compares to determinations done with animals[Q]
- *Amino Acid Score (AAS):*
  - A chemical technique considered fast, consistent, and inexpensive
  - It measures the indispensable amino acids present in a protein and compares the values with a reference protein
  - The protein is rated based upon the most limiting indispensable amino acid

> **Key points**
>
> **DIAAS** is the 'current accepted measure of protein quality'

- *Protein Efficiency Ratio (PER)*:
  - It represents the ratio of weight gain to the amount of protein consumed
  - This method may not be applied to growing infants and children
  - Also PER measures growth but not maintenance so it may be of limited use in determining the protein needs of adults
- *Biological Value (BV)*:
  - Measures the amount of nitrogen retained in comparison to the amount of nitrogen absorbed
  - The BV and the NPU methods reflect both availability and digestibility and they give an accurate appraisal of maintenance needs
- *Net Protein Utilization (NPU)*: The ratio of the nitrogen used for tissue formation versus the amount of nitrogen digested.

Net Protein Utilization

> **Key points**
> NPU is a good indicator of protein quality

- *Net Protein Utilization*: Is the proportion of ingested proteins that is retained in the body under specified conditions for the maintenance and/or growth of the tissues
  - In calculating protein quality, *1 gram of nitrogen is assumed to be equivalent to 6.25 grams of proteins*^{Q}
- *Importance*: NPU is the best indicator of protein quality for recommending the dietary protein requirement^Q
  - *Net Protein Utilization*: Provides a complete expression of *'protein quality'*

$$NPU = \frac{\text{Nitrogen retained by body}}{\text{Nitrogen intake}} \times 100$$

> **Key points**
> $NPU = \frac{BV \times DC}{100}$

$$NPU = \frac{\text{Biological value} \times \text{Digestibility coefficient}}{100}$$

- NPU of selected food items:

Food Item	Net Protein Utilization
Egg (hen)	96*
Milk (cow)	81
Meat	79
Fish	77
Rice	65
Soyabean	55
Wheat	51
Grams (pulses)	45–50
Groundnut	50

> **Key points**
> NPU of egg is 96. **Egg is 'reference protein'**

(*NPU of egg is 96. Since egg is *'reference protein'*, its NPU is taken as 100 for comparison)

Limiting Amino Acids

- *Definition*: Amino acids most deficient in proteins of a food item are 'Limiting amino acids'

Food Item	Limiting Amino Acid(s)
Cereals^Q	Threonine (& Lysine)
Pulses^Q	Methionine (& Cysteine)
Maize^Q	Tryptophan (& Lysine)

- *Supplementary action of proteins*^{Q}: Deficiency develops due to only consumption of a particular type of food item with limiting amino acids (e.g. wheat); Thus two or more food items are eaten together so that their proteins supplement one another; this is known as 'Supplementary Action of Proteins'.

Essential Amino Acids

- *Essential Amino Acids (EAA):* Amino acids which are not synthesized in adequate amounts in the human body; so they have to be supplemented in diet from outside to prevent deficiency^Q
- 10 EAA [**Mnemonic: PVT TIM HALL** or *Any Help In Learning These Little Molecules Proves Truly Valuable*]^Q
  - **P**henylalanine
  - **V**aline
  - **T**hreonine
  - **T**ryptophan
  - **I**soleucine
  - **M**ethionine
  - **H**istidine (Semi-essential)
  - **A**rginine (Semi-essential)
  - **L**eucine
  - **L**ysine

> **Key points**
> 10 EAA [**Mnemonic: PVT TIM HALL**]

FATS AND CARBOHYDRATES

Essential Fatty Acids (EFA)

- *Essential Fatty Acids (EFA):* Are those that cannot be synthesized completely in human body; they can only be supplemented from the food^Q
  - Most important EFA: Linoleic Acid, which serves as a basis for production of other EFA^Q
  - EFA deficiency lead to 'Phrenoderma' (Toad Skin)^Q: Rough rash like eruptions on back and sides of arms and legs, back, and buttocks
- *Types of EFAs:*

Type of fatty acids	Type of chain	Examples
ω-3 Fatty Acids	Short chain	α-Linolenic acid
	Long chain	Eicosapentaenoic acid Docosahexaenoic acid
ω-6 Fatty Acids	Short chain	Linoleic Acid
	Long chain	Arachidonic acid γ-Linolenic acid Dihomo-γ-Linolenic acid

  - *ω-9 Fatty Acids* are non-essential in human beings
  - *ω-3 Fatty Acids* are derived from α-Linolenic acid; *ω-6 Fatty Acids* are derived from Linoleic Acid and *ω-9 Fatty Acids* are derived from Oleic Acid^Q
  - EFA were earlier known as *'Vitamin F'*
  - *ω-3 Fatty Acids* have been shown to reduce the incidence of Coronary Heart Disease
  - *ω-6: ω-3 Fatty Acids* ratio in diet is ideally recommended to be 1:1 to 4:1 (IDEAL FAT^Q)
- *Dietary sources of EFA:*

EFA	Dietary source	% Content
Linoleic Acid	Safflower oil Corn oil Sunflower oil Soyabean oil	73 57 56 51
Arachidonic Acid	Meat, Eggs	0.5
	Milk (fat)	0.5
Linolenic Acid	Soyabean oil	7
Eicosapentaenoic Acid	Fish oil	10

> **Key points**
> **Richest source of EFA:** Safflower Oil

- *Fatty acid content of different fats (%)*^{Q}:

Fats	SFA*	MUFA*	PUFA*
Safflower oil	10	15	75
Sunflower seed oil	8	27	65
Soya bean oil	14	24	62

Contd...

Contd...

Fats	SFA*	MUFA*	PUFA*
Margarine	25	25	50
Groundnut oil	19	50	31
Palm oil	46	44	10
Butter	60	37	3
Coconut oil	92	6	2

VITAMINS

Vitamins and Vitamin Deficiencies

Vitamins	Chemical Name(s)	Deficiency^Q
Vitamin A	Retinol, Retinoid, Carotenoid	Xerophthalmia^Q
Vitamin B_1	Thiamine	Beri-beri^Q, Wernickes Korasoff Psychosis^Q
Vitamin B_2	Riboflavin	Ariboflavinosis
Vitamin B_3	Niacin, Niacinamide	Pellagra^Q
Vitamin B_5	Pantothenic Acid	Burning feet Syndrome^Q
Vitamin B_6	Pyridoxine, Pyridoxamine, Pyridoxal	Anemia
Vitamin B_7	Biotin	Dermatitis, Enteritis
Vitamin B_9	Folic Acid, Folinic Acid	Megaloblatic Anemia^Q, Neural tube defects^Q
Vitamin B_{12}	Cyanocobalamin, Hydroxocobalamin, Methylcobalamin	Megaloblastic Anemia^Q
Vitamin C	Ascorbic Acid	Scurvy^Q
Vitamin D	Ergocalciferol, Cholecalciferol	Rickets^Q, Osteomalcia
Vitamin E	Tocopherols, Tocotrienols	Hemolytic anemia in newborn^Q
Vitamin K	Phylloquinone, Menaquinone, Menadione	Hemorrhagic disease of new born^Q

Recommended Daily Requirements of Vitamins

Vitamin	Recommended daily requirement
Vitamin A^Q	600 mcg retinol
Vitamin B_1 (Thiamine)	0.5 mg per 1000 kcal of energy intake
Vitamin B_2 (Riboflavin)	0.5 mg per 1000 kcal of energy intake
Vitamin B_3 (Niacin)	6.6 mg per 1000 kcal of energy intake
Vitamin B_5 (Pantothenic Acid)	10 mg
Vitamin B_6 (Pyridoxine)	2 mg
Vitamin B_9 (Folic Acid)	100 mcg
Vitamin B_{12} (Cobalamin)	1 mcg
Vitamin D^Q	100 IU (2.5 mcg calciferol)
Vitamin E (Tocopherol)	0.8 mg per gm of essential fatty acids
Vitamin K^Q	0.03 mg per kg

> **Key points**
>
> **RDA**
> **Vitamin A^Q:** 600 mcg retinol

Vitamin A

- *Recommended daily requirement of Vitamin-A*:

Group		Retinol (mcg) OR	β-carotene (mcg)
Adults	Man^Q	600	4800
	Woman	600	4800
	Pregnancy^Q	800	6400
	Lactation	950	7600
Infants	0–12 months	350	2800
Children	1–6 years	400	3200
	7–12 years	600	4800
Adolescents	13–19 years	600	4800

> **Key points**
> **Strength of Vitamin-A solution:** 1 lac IU per mL

- *Under National Immunization Schedule (NIS), Vitamin-A is given;*^{Q}
  - 1 lac IU at 9 months age (along with measles vaccine),
  - 2 lac IU every 6 months thereafter, till the age of 5 years (at 18, 24, 30, 36, 42, 48, 54, 60 months of age)
  - A total of 17 lac IU is given^Q
  - Vitamin-A is administered by a '2 mL spoon'^{Q}
  - Strength of Vitamin-A solution: 1 lac IU per mL^Q

Vitamin A Deficiency: Xerophthalmia

Bitot spot

- *Ocular manifestations of Vitamin-A deficiency*^{Q}: 'Xerophthalmia' (Dry Eye)
- Xerophthalmia is most common in children aged 1–3 years
  - 'First clinical sign' of Vitamin-A deficiency^Q: Conjunctival xerosis
    *Conjunctival xerosis in Xerophthalmia has a characteristic appearance of 'emerging like sand banks at receding tide'
  - 'First clinical symptom' of Vitamin-A deficiency^Q: Night blindness
  - 'Bitot's Spots' are triangular, pearly-white or yellowish, foamy spots on bulbar conjunctiva, on either side of cornea; In young children they indicate Vitamin-A deficiency, whereas in adults they are often inactive sequelae of earlier disease
  - Corneal xerosis is a serious manifestation of Vitamin-A deficiency
  - Keratomalacia (liquefaction of corne(a) is a 'grave medical emergency'
- *Extraocular manifestations of Vitamin-A deficiency*: Follicular hyperkeratosis, anorexia, growth retardation, etc.
- *Prevalence criteria for determining the Xerophthalmia problem in a community*: (Preschool children 6 months- 6 years).

Criteria	Prevalence
Night blindness^Q	>1.0%
Bitot's spots^Q	>0.5%
Corneal xerosis/corneal ulceration/keratomalacia	>0.01%
Corneal ulcer	>0.05%
Serum retinol (<10 mcg/dL)	>5.0%

> **Key points**
> 'First clinical sign' of Vitamin-A deficiency^Q: Conjunctival xerosis

> **Key points**
> 'First clinical symptom' of Vitamin-A deficiency^Q: Night blindness

- *WHO recommended strategy for prevention of Xerophthalmia*:
  - *Short term action*: Vitamin-A prophylaxis to vulnerable groups.

Individual	Dose* (IU)	Timing
Child <12 months age	1,00,000	Once every 4–6 months
Child >12 months age	2,00,000	Once every 4–6 months
Newborn	50,000	At birth
Women 15–49 years	3,00,000	Within 1 month of delivery
Pregnancy and Lactation	5000 OR	Every day
	20,000	Once every week

(* Oral dose of *retinol palmitate*, where 55 mg = 1,00,000 IU)

  - *Medium term action*: Fortification of certain foods with Vitamin-A.

- *Long term action*: Promotion of consumption of green leafy vegetables, promotion of breast feeding for as long as possible, improvements in environmental health, immunization against measles, prompt treatment of diarrhoel infections, social and health education, etc.

Vitamin B3 (Niacin) Deficiency: Pellagra

- Pellagra occurs due to Vitamin B3 (Niacin) deficiency^Q
- Pellagra is characterized by 4 D's^Q:
    - Diarrhoea
    - Dementia
    - Death
    - Dermatitis
        *Skin rash in pellagra may appear as pigmented and scaly in areas exposed to sunlight. Esp. neck when it is known as 'Casal's Necklace'^{Q}
- *Pellagra is common in maize/jowar eating populations*:
    - Limiting amino acid in maize is Tryptophan^Q
    - 60 mg Tryptophan is converted to 1 mg Niacin in the body^Q
    - 'Excess of leucine' in such populations appears to interfere in conversion of tryptophan to niacin^Q

> **Key points**
> Pellagra is characterized by 4 D's:
> - Diarrhoea
> - Dementia
> - Death
> - Dermatitis

Vitamin B9 (Folic Acid)

- Body stores of folate are not large (about 5–10 mg), therefore folate deficiency can develop quickly
- *Recommended daily intake values of folate*:

Group	Intake per day
Healthy adults	200 mcg
Pregnancy^Q	500 mcg
Lactation	300 mcg
Children	100 mcg

> **Key points**
> An adult tablet of IFA contains^Q: 100 mg elemental Iron and 500 mcg Folic acid

- *An adult tablet of IFA contains^Q*: 100 mg elemental Iron and 500 mcg Folic acid (to be given for 100 days minimum in pregnancy)
- *A pediatric tablet of IFA contains^Q*: 20 mg elemental Iron and 100 mcg Folic acid (to be given for 100 days minimum every year till 5 years age of child)

IRON

Iron Status Evaluation

- *Hemoglobin concentration*: A relatively insensitive index of nutrient depletion
- *Serum iron concentration*: Normal range is 0.80–1.80 mg/L
- *Serum ferritin^Q*: 'Most sensitive tool for evaluation of iron status', especially in populations with low prevalence of anemia
- *Serum transferrin saturation*: Normal value is 30%

> **Key points**
> Serum ferritin^Q: 'Most sensitive tool for evaluation of iron status'

Cut-off for Diagnosis of Anemia (WHO)^Q

Group	Hb (g/dL)	MCHC (%)
Adult males	13	34
Adult females, non-pregnant	12	34
Adult females, pregnant	11	34
Children, 6 m–6 y	11	34
Children, 6–14 y	12	34

Intensified Iron-plus Initiative

See Anemia Mukt Bharat Annexure 21

IODINE AND FLUORINE

Fluorine
- *Recommended level in drinking water in India^Q*: 0.5–0.8 mg/litre (ppm)
  - In temperate countries where water intake is low, the optimum level of fluorides in drinking water is accepted as 1–2 mg/litre
  - *Major source of fluorine to man^Q*: Drinking water
- 'Fluorine is a double edged sword': Inadequate intake is associated with 'dental caries' whereas excess intake with 'dental and skeletal fluorosis'
  - *Level >1.5 ppm*: Dental fluorosis (mottling^Q)
  - *Level 3.0–6.0 ppm*: Skeletal fluorosis
  - *Level >10.0 ppm*: Crippling fluorosis

Key points

Recommended level of fluorine in drinking water in India^Q: 0.5–0.8 mg/litre (ppm)

Key points

'Fluorine is a double edged sword'

Fluorosis
- Dental fluorosis occurs when excess fluoride is ingested during first 7 years of life (years of tooth calcification)
  - It occurs at levels above 1.5 mg/litre intake
  - It is characterized by 'Mottling', which is best seen on incisors of upper jaw^Q
- Fluorosis endemic area: Habitation/village/town having fluoride level >1.5 ppm in drinking water^Q
- Villages classification based on the level of fluoride content^Q:

Strata	Fluoride Level
I	1.0–3.0 ppm
II	3.1–5.0 ppm
III	>5.0 ppm

Nalgonda Technique
- 'Nalgonda Technique' has been developed by National Environmental Engineering Research Institute (NEERI), Nagpur for defluoridation of water^Q
- It involves addition of (in sequence^Q):
  - Lime^Q
  - Alum (major role)^Q
  - Bleaching powder
  - Flocculation,
  - Sedimentation
  - Filtration
- *Household level de-fluoridation can be done by*:
  - Nalgonda Technique
  - Alumina
  - Phosphates

Key points

NALGONDA Technique Involves addition of:
- Lime^Q
- Alum (major role)^Q
- Bleaching powder

Iodine
- *Iodine requirement^Q*: 150 mcg per day (<1 teaspoon over lifetime)
- *WHO/UNICEF/ICCIDD recommended daily iodine intake*:

Group	Recommended daily intake
Preschool children (0–59 months)	90 mcg
School children (6–12 years)	120 mcg
Adults (>12 years)	150 mcg
Pregnancy and lactation	250 mcg

Key points

Iodine requirement^Q: 150 mcg per day

Iodised Salt
- Iodisation of salt is the 'most widely used prophylactic measure against prevention of goiter'
- Iodised salt is most convenient, effective and economical method of mass prophylaxis in endemic areas

Key points

Level of iodisation in salt:
- *30 ppm at production level
- *15 ppm at consumer level

- *According to Prevention of Food Adulteration (PFA) Act' 1954*:
  - Level of iodisation in salt (PFA Act' 1954)^Q:
    - *30 ppm at production level
    - *15 ppm at consumer level
  - *Moisture content*: <6.0% by weight
  - *Sodium chloride*: >96.0% by weight

Double Fortified/Twin Fortified Salt (DFS/TFS)
- *Developed by*: National Institute of Nutrition (Hyderabad)
- *DFS contains Iron and Iodine*:
  - DFS provides 40 mcg Iodine and 1 mg Iron per gram of salt^Q
  - DFS contains salt, potassium iodate, ferrous sulphate and sodium hexa meta phosphate

District IDD/Goitre Survey
- *Age group*: 6–12 years age group^Q
- *Sampling*:
  - 30 villages/wards or schools are selected from district by 'Cluster Sampling Technique'^{Q}
  - Proportionate to Size Sampling (PPS)
  - Sample of 90 children (45 boys and 45 girls) from school
  - Salt sample collection: From the house of every 5th child selected in earlier steps for goiter survey
  - Sample collection for urinary iodine excretion (UIE): Every alternate child out of those selected earlier for salt samples has to be taken
- *Monitoring*: 50 salt samples per month, 25 UIE samples per month
- *Classification of Goitre*:
  - *Grade 0*: No palpable or visible goiter (No Goitre)
  - *Grade I*: A mass in neck that is consistent with enlarged thyroid, that is 'palpable but not visible'; moves up in neck as one swallows (Goitre palpable but not visible)
  - *Grade II*: A swelling in neck that is visible when the neck is in a normal position, and is consistent with an enlarged thyroid when neck is palpated (Goitre visible and palpable)

Criteria & Indicators in IDD Control and Elimination
- *IDD Elimination criteria*^{Q}:

Indicator	Goal
Proportion with enlarged thyroid (age 6–12 years)	<5%
Urinary Iodine Excretion below 100 mcg/litre	<50%
Urinary Iodine Excretion below 50 mcg/litre	<20%
Proportion of houses consuming adequately iodised salt	>90%

- *Indicators for epidemiological assessment of iodine deficiency*:
  - Prevalence of goitre
  - Prevalence of cretinism
  - Urinary iodine excretion
  - Measurement of thyroid function (T4, TSH)
  - Prevalence of neonatal hypothyroidism
- *Epidemiological criteria for assessing severity of IDD*:
  - Total Goitre Rate (TGR) - Grade I + Grade II
  - Median Urinary Iodine Excretion
  - Thyroid volume (ultrasound)
  - Salt iodine content
- *Criteria for Sustainable Elimination of IDD*:
  - Median Urinary Iodine Excretion 100 mcg/l
  - Level of iodization^Q:
    - 30 ppm at production level
    - 15 ppm at consumer level
  - Total Goitre Rate (TGR) <5%

- *Indicators to monitor success of IDD control programme*:
  - *Process Indicators*: Indicators to monitor and evaluate the salt iodization process
    - Salt iodine content at the production site
    - Salt iodine content at point of packaging
    - Salt iodine content at wholesale and retail levels
    - Salt iodine content in households
  - *Impact Indicators*: Indicators to assess baseline (Iodine Deficiency Disorders) IDD status and to monitor and evaluate the impact of salt iodization on the target population
    - Urinary Iodine Levels^Q: The *'principal impact indicator'* recommended once a salt iodization programme has been initiated (changes in goitre prevalence lag behind changes in iodine status and therefore cannot be relied upon to reflect accurately current iodine intake, although they may be useful in following trends)
    - Goitre assessment: (by palpation or by ultrasound) should remain a component of surveys to establish the baseline severity of IDD
    - Neonatal thyroid stimulating hormone (TSH) levels: may also play a role here if a country already has in place a screening programme for hypothyroidism
  - *Sustainability Indicators:* Indicators to assess whether iodine deficiency has been successfully eliminated and to judge whether achievements can be sustained and maintained for the decades to come
    - Median urinary iodine levels in the target population
    - Availability of adequately iodized salt at the household level
    - Set of programmatic indicators (as evidence of sustainability)

> **Key points**
> Urinary Iodine Levels^Q: 'principal impact indicator'

OTHER NUTRIENTS

Dietary Fibre

- *Description*: Dietary fibre is a non-starch polysaccharide and a physiologically important component of diet; there are two types of dietary fibres:
  - Insoluble fibres: Cellulose, hemi-cellulose and lignin
  - Soluble fibres: Pectins, gums and mucilages
- *Recommended intake*: A daily intake of about 40 grams of fibre is desirable^Q
  - Indian diets provide about 50–100 grams of fibre per day
  - Cereals and pulses are good sources of fibre (>10 gm fibre per 100 gm)
- *Functions/uses of dietary fibre^Q*:
  - Forms bulk of stool; reduces tendency of constipation
  - By reducing intestinal transit time of stools, it reduces toxicity
  - Inhibits fecal mutagen synthesis
  - Reduces incidence of colonic polyps and invasive colon cancer
  - Reduces incidence of stomach, breast and prostate cancers
  - Reduces incidence of coronary heart disease
  - Reduces blood levels of glucose and cholesterol
  - Used in the management of irritable bowel syndrome and recurrent diverticulitis

> **Key points**
> Daily intake of about 40 grams of fibre is desirable

Zinc Deficiency^Q

- Growth failure
- Sexual infantilism
- Impaired immunity
- Decreased insulin synthesis
- Delayed wound healing
- Loss of taste (Aguesia)
- Liver disease (Hepatomegaly + Splenomegaly), Pernicious anemia, Thalassemia, Myocardial infarction
- Megaloblastic anemia (due to reduced absorption of Folyl-glutamates)
- *Maternal zinc deficiency*: Spontaneous abortion, Congenital malformation (Anencephaly), Low birth weight, IUGR, Preterm delivery

EGG

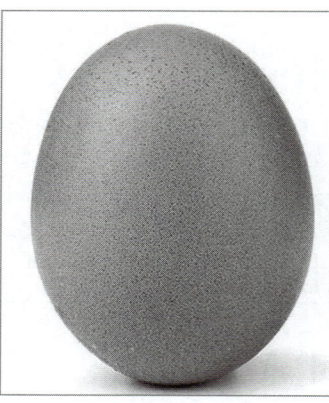

Egg

Egg

- An egg (60 grams) contain^Q:
  - 6 gm proteins
  - 6 gm fat
  - 30 mg calcium
  - 1.5 mg iron
  - 250 mg cholesterol
  - 70 kcal energy
- Egg protein is best among proteins (NPU = 96), thereby making it *'Reference Protein'*^{Q}
- Egg is a poor source of Vitamin C and Carbohydrates^Q

MILK

Types of Milk

- *Fat content of milk*: Buffalo > Goat > Cow > Human
- *Protein content of milk*: Buffalo > Goat > Cow > Human
- *Lactose content of milk*: Human > Buffalo > Goat > Cow
- *Energy content of milk*: Buffalo > Goat > Cow > Human

> **Key points**
>
> *Lactose content of milk:* Human > Buffalo > Goat > Cow

Types of Commercially Available Milk in India

Milk type	Fat content	SNF (Solid-not-fat) content
Full cream	6.0%	9.0%
Standardised	4.5%	8.5%
Toned	3.0%	8.5%
Double toned	1.5%	9.0%
Skimmed^Q	0.5%	8.7%

Methods of Pasteurization

Method	Temp	Time	Remarks
Holder/Vat Method^Q	63–66°C	>30 min	For small and rural communities
HTST Method*^{Q}	72°C	>15 sec	Most widely used; for large quantities
HHST Method	68°C	30 min	'Batch Pasteurization'
UHT Method	125°C	Few sec	Heating in 2 stages; 2nd stage under pressure

(*Flash Pasteurization)

Tests of Pasteurized Milk (for Adequacy/Sufficiency of Pasteurization)^Q

- *Phosphatase Test*: Widely used test^Q
- *Standard Plate Count*: Enforced limit is 30,000 bacterial count per mL of pasteurized milk
- *Coliform Count*: Standard is coliforms be absent in 1 mL of milk.

Milk Borne Diseases

Infections of animals transmitted to man^Q	
Primary importance^Q	*Lesser importance*
Tuberculosis	Anthrax
Brucellosis	Cow pox
Streptococcal infections	Foot and mouth disease
Staphylococcal poisoning	Leptospirosis
Salmonellosis	Tick-borne encephalitis
Q fever	

Contd...

Contd...

Infections primary to man	
Diarrhoeal diseases	*Non-diarrhoeal diseases*
Typhoid and para-typhoid fevers	Tuberculosis
Shigellosis	Diphtheria
Cholera	Streptococcal infections
E. coli	Staphylococcal food poisoning
	Enteroviral infections
	Hepatitis viral

OTHER FOOD ITEMS

Foods as Sources of Nutrients

- Food Items as Poor Sources of nutrients[Q]:
  - Milk is a poor source of Vitamin C and Iron
  - Meat is a poor source of Calcium
  - Fish is a poor source of Carbohydrates
  - Egg is a poor source of Vitamin C and Carbohydrates
- Food Items as Rich Sources of nutrients[Q]:
  - Halibut Liver Oil is richest source of Vitamin A and Vitamin D
  - Indian Gooseberry (amla) is richest source of Vitamin C
  - Gingelly seeds are richest source of Vitamin B1 (Thiamine)
  - Sheep liver is richest source of Vitamin B2 (Riboflavin)
  - Ragi (millet) is a rich source of calcium
  - Dried pumpkin seeds > Pistachio is the richest source of iron

> **Key points**
> Halibut Liver Oil is richest source of Vitamin A and Vitamin D

Pulses

Pulse	Energy (kcal)	Proteins (g)	Fats (g)	Calcium (mg)	Iron (mg)
Bengal Gram	360	17	5	202	5
Black Gram	347	24	1	154	4
Red Gram	335	22	2	73	3
Soya Bean[Q]	432	43	20	240	10

> **Key points**
> Limiting amino acid in soya bean is Methionine

Soyabean

- Soya bean is richest among pulses
  - It contains 43.2% proteins[Q], 20% fats and 4% of minerals
  - Proteins of soya bean are of high nutritive value
- Soya bean is also relatively richer in Calcium, Iron and Vitamin B as compared to other pulses[Q]
- NPU of Soya bean is 55[Q]
- Limiting amino acid in soya bean is Methionine[Q]

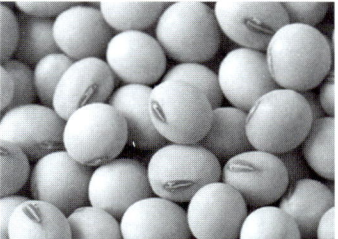

Soyabean

Fish

- Richest source of Vitamin A and D is fish liver oils (especially Halibut fish)[Q]
- Rich source of proteins (15–20%)
- Rich source of Calcium, phosphorus, fluorides
- Good source of iron
- Poor source of Carbohydrates[Q]
- Poor source of iodine (barring few sea fish)[Q]

FOOD ADULTERATION

Food Adulteration Diseases

Disease	Toxin^Q	Adulterant
Lathyrism^Q	BOAA	Khesari Dal (Lathyrus sativus)
Epidemic Dropsy^Q	Sanguinarine	Argemone mexicana (oil)
Endemic Ascites^Q	Pyrrolizidine alkaloids	Crotolaria seeds (Jhunjhunia)
Aflatoxicosis^Q	Aflatoxin	Aspergillus flavus/parasiticus
Ergotism^Q	Clavine alkaloids	Claviceps fusiformis

> **Key points**
> Toxin: Present in lathyrus seeds is 'Beta oxalyl amino alanine (BOAA)'

Lathyrism

- *Lathyrism is of two types*:
  - Neurolathyrism^Q: In human beings
  - Osteolathyrism (Odoratism^Q): In animals
    - Neurolathyrism is caused by eating the pulse 'Khesari Dal (Lathyrus sativus)'. Diets containing over 30% of this dal consumed over a period of 2–6 months result in neurolathyrism
    - Lathyrism affects 15–45 years of age
- *Toxin*: present in lathyrus seeds is 'Beta oxalyl amino alanine (BOAA)'^Q
- *It manifests as following stages*:
  - Latent stage
  - No-stick stage
  - One-stick stage
  - Two-stick stage
  - Crawler stage
- *Interventions for prevention and control of Lathyrism*:
  - Vitamin C prophylaxis^Q
  - Banning the crop
  - *Removal of toxin*: Steeping method and Parboiling^Q
  - Education
  - Genetic approach
  - Socio-economic changes.

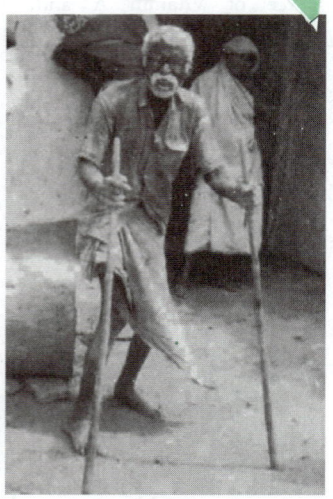

Lathyrism

> **Key points**
> 'Sanguinarine' is the toxin contained in argemone oil

Epidemic Dropsy

- *Description*: Is caused by contamination of mustard oil with 'Argemone oil'^Q
- *Toxin*: 'Sanguinarine' is the toxin contained in argemone oil^Q
- *Mechanism^Q*: Sanguinarine interferes with oxidation of 'pyruvic acid', which accumulates in blood: It may lead to sudden non-inflammatory edema of bilateral lower limbs, diarrhea, dyspnoea, cardiac failure and death; It can also lead to glaucoma; It may sometimes manifest as 'Sarcoids' (dilatation of skin capillaries)
  - Epidemic dropsy may occur in all ages except breast-fed infants
  - The mortality of epidemic dropsy varies from 5 to 50%
  - Edema in Epidemic dropsy occurs due to proteinuria (specifically loss of albumin).
- *Argemone oil may be detected by following tests^Q*:
  - Nitric acid test
  - Paper chromatography test: Most sensitive test

> **Key points**
> Toxin^Q: Pyrrolizidine alkaloids in Endemic Ascites

Endemic Ascites

- *Toxin^Q*: Pyrrolizidine alkaloids (Hepatotoxins)
- *Adulterant^Q*: Crotolaria plant (Jhunjhunia)

> **Key points**
> Food toxicant - ergot fungus 'Claviceps fusiformis'^Q

Ergotism

- *Description*: Occurs due to food toxicant - ergot fungus 'Claviceps fusiformis'^Q
- *Food items having a tendency for ergotism^Q*:
  - Bajra^Q
  - Rye

- Sorghum
- Wheat
- *Removal of ergot*:
  - Float them in 20% salt water
  - Hand-picking
  - Air-floatation
- *Upper safe limit for ergot*: 0.05 mg per 100 grams food material

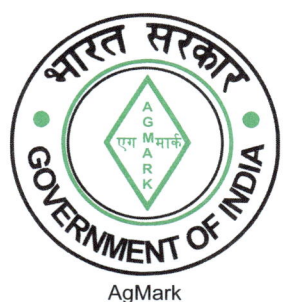
AgMark

MISCELLANEOUS

Food Standards

- *Codex Alimentarius*: Joint FAO/WHO standards for international markets; Food standards in India are based on Codex Alimentarius[Q]
- *PFA standards*: Laid under 'Prevention of Food Adulteration Act 1954'; to obtain a minimum level of quality of food stuffs attainable under Indian conditions
- *Bureau of Indian Standards*: Purely voluntary; express degree of excellence above PFA standards
- *Agmark standards*: Purely voluntary; express degree of excellence above PFA standards.

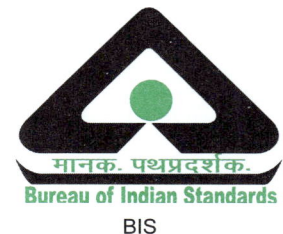
BIS

Mid-day Meal Programme (MDMP) & Scheme (MDMS)

- *Mid-day meal programme (MDMP)*: Also known as 'School Lunch Programme', it has been in operation since 1961
  - *The major objective of MDMP*[Q]: To attract more children for admission to schools and retain them so that literacy improvement of children could be brought about.
  - The meal is a supplement and not a substitute to the home diet[Q]
  - The meal should supply 1/3 of the total energy requirement and 1/2 of the total protein requirement[Q]
  - MDMP is being operationalised under the Ministry of Human Resource & Development [Q]
  - National Institute of Nutrition, Hyderabad is of the view that minimum number of feeding days in year be 250 to have the desired impact on children
- *Mid-day meal scheme (MDMS) (National Programme of Nutritional Support to Primary Education)*: Launched in 1995
  - *Main objective*: Universalisation of primary education by increasing enrolment, retention and attendance and simultaneously impacting on nutrition of students in primary classes
  - The mid-day meal should supply 1/3 of the total energy requirement and 1/2 of the total protein requirement[Q]
  - A model menu for mid-day school meal[Q]:

> **Key points**
>
> Mid day Meal should supply 1/3 of the total energy requirement and 1/2 of the total protein requirement[Q]

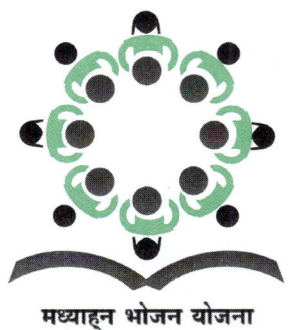
MDMP

Item	Quantity per child per day	
	Primary	Upper primary
Food grains	100 grams	150 grams
Pulses	20 grams	30 grams
Vegetables	50 grams	75 grams
Oils & fats	5 grams	7.5 grams
Salt	As per need	As per need
TOTAL calories	450 kcal	700 kcal
TOTAL proteins	12 grams	20 grams

- *Principles for formulating mid-day meals*:[Q]
  - Meal should be a supplement only not a substitute for home diet
  - Meal should provide 1/3 calories and 1/2 proteins
  - Meal cost should be low
  - Complicated cooking process must not be involved
  - Use locally available foods
  - Keep changing menu frequently

Prudent Diet

Refer to Chapter 5, Theory.

Nutritional Status Assessment

- Assessment of dietary intake (Diet Survey): Dietary Cycle[Q] (weighment of raw foods done over a period of 7 days)
- Assessment of nutritional status: **[Mnemonic: CABFAVE]**
  - **C**linical examination
  - **A**nthropometry
  - **B**aboratory and **B**iochemical evaluation
    - Laboratory tests
      1. Hemoglobin
      2. Stools and urine
    - Biochemical tests
  - **F**unctional assessment
  - **A**ssessment of dietary intake
    - Weighment of raw foods (Dietary cycle - 7 days[Q])
    - Weighment of cooked foods
    - Oral questionnaire method
  - **V**ital and health statistics
  - **E**cological studies
    - Food balance sheet
    - Socio-economic factors
    - Health and educational services
    - Conditioning influences

> **Key points**
> Dietary Cycle[Q] (weighment of raw foods done over a period of 7 days)

Food Fortification

- *Food fortification*: Is a public health, measure where nutrients are added to food (in relatively small quantities), to maintain/improve the quality of diet of a group, community or a population[Q]
- *Examples of Food Fortification[Q]*:
  - Iodisation of salt
  - Vitamin A and Vitamin D in Vanaspati
    - Vanaspati is fortified with '2500 IU Vitamin A and 175 IU Vitamin D' per 100 grams
  - Fluoridation of water
- Food Fortification is an example of 'Primary Level of Prevention'
- *Criteria for food fortification*:
  - Vehicle to be fortified must be consumed regularly in diet by populations
  - Amount of nutrient added must not cause deficiency or toxicity in consumers
  - On addition of nutrient, there should be no change in taste, odour, consistency or appearance
  - Cost of fortification must be affordable by consumers

Mid-arm Circumference (MAC)

- MAC is measured for age group 6 months-5 years (as it remains practically constant during this age)[Q]
- *Shakir's Tape[Q]*: A useful field instrument for measurement of nourishment status of a child, through measurement of MAC
- *Interpretation of Shakir's tape findings*:

MAC (cms)	Color Zone	Interpretation	Management
>13.5[Q]	Green	Satisfactory nutritional status	-
12.5–13.5	Yellow	Mild-moderate malnutrition	At home; through diet
<12.5	Red	Severe malnutrition	Refer; Institutional

- WHO use MUAC <11.5 cm as a marker of severe acute malnutrition.

> **Key points**
> Shakir's Tape[Q]: A useful field instrument of MAC

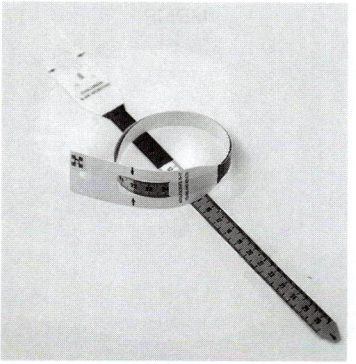

Shakirs tape

Nutritional Surveillance

- *Nutritional surveillance*: Keeping a watch over nutrition, in order to make decisions that will lead to improvement in nutrition of population
- *Main strategy*: Detection of malnutrition (nutritional survey)

- *Approach*: Diagnostic-interventional
- *Sample*: Representative, 50–100 size group
- *Objectives*:
  - To aid health and development
  - To provide input for program management and evaluation (to policy makers)
  - To give timely warning and intervention (to prevent short-term food crises).

National Nutrition Mission (NNM) 2017–18

Syn. Poshan Abhiyan

Description: Apex body to monitor, supervise, fix targets and guide the nutrition related interventions across the Ministries.

- Major impact: To reduce the level of stunting, under-nutrition, anemia and low birth weight babies
- Components: Mapping of various Schemes contributing towards addressing malnutrition, Introducing a very robust convergence mechanism, ICT based Real Time Monitoring system, Incentivizing States/UTs for meeting the targets, Incentivizing Anganwadi Workers (AWWs) for using IT based tools, Eliminating registers used by AWWs, Introducing measurement of height of children at the Anganwadi Centres (AWCs), Social Audits, Setting-up Nutrition Resource Centres, involving masses through Jan Andolan
- NNM vision: To ensure attainment of malnutrition-free India by 2022
- NNM targets:
  - To reduce stunting, under- nutrition, anemia (among young children, women and adolescent girls) and reduce low birth weight by 2%, 2%, 3% and 2% per annum respectively
  - Although the target to reduce Stunting is at least 2% p.a., Mission would strive to achieve reduction in Stunting from 38.4% (NFHS-4) to 25% by 2022 (Mission 25 by 2022)

Global Hunger Index (GHI)

- The Global Hunger Index is a tool designed to comprehensively measure and track hunger at the global, regional, and country levels
- The International Food Policy Research Institute (IFPRI) calculates GHI scores each year to assess progress, or the lack thereof, in combating hunger
- To capture the multidimensional nature of hunger, GHI scores are based on the following indicators:

2014 Guidelines	2016 Guidelines
• Child undernourishment • Child underweight • Child mortality	• Undernourishment • Child Wasting (Acute undernutrition) • Child Stunting (Chronic undernutrition) • Child mortality (Under 5 age)

- GHI Classification and Interpretation:

GHI Value	Interpretation for Level of Hunger
≤9.9	Low
10–19.9	Moderate
20–34.9	Serious
35–49.9	Alarming
≥50	Extremely alarming

- India, Global Hunger Index GHI 2021: Score 27.5, Serious level of hunger (Rank 101st out of the 116 countries)

PYQs: Quick Review for NEET

Basic Principles

Most important essential fatty acid is	Linoleic acid
Tocopherols are	Vitamin-E
Amino acid converted in body to Niacin	Tryptophan
Best indicator of protein quality	NPU
Most essential fatty acid is	Linoleic acid
Pyridoxine is vitamin	B_6
Protein quality indicator adopted by ICMR for RDA	NPU
Vitamin-A solution contains	1,00,000 IU per mL
Most sensitive tool for evaluating iron status of body	Serum ferritin
Trace element is what percent of body weight	0.01%
Trace element having vitamin E like action	Selenium
Exclusive breast feeding must be given up to	6 months
Food standards in India are based on the standards of	Codex alimentarius
Carbohydrate reserve of human body	340 grams

Nutritional Requirements

RDA of proteins for adult Indian	0.83 gm/kg/day
Iodine dose in pregnancy	250 mcg per day
Recommended daily energy intake adult woman (Heavy work)	2720 kcal per day
13–15 year female child, recommended daily protein intake	0.86 gm/kg/day
Energy requirement in late pregnancy for a moderate worker	2500 kcal/day
Reference weight of Indian men and women	65 kg and 55 kg
Energy requirement of a sedentary female	1660 kcal
Calories required for 0–6 m infant is	550 kcal/d
Semi essential amino acids are	Histidine, Arginine
Daily requirement of vitamin K	55 mcg/d
Vitamin A requirement in infant is	350 mcg
Vitamin A requirement in adult male	1000 mcg/d
Total Iron requirement in pregnancy	1000 mg
Daily dose of Iron for adult man	19 mg per day
Acceptable fluoride concentration in drinking water	1 ppm
Expected level of iodine in iodized salt at production level is	>30 ppm
Expected level of iodine in iodized salt at consumer level is	>15 ppm
RDA of calcium in normal adult male	1000 mg/d
Iron recommended intake of adult woman per day	29 mg per day

Food Items

Richest source of vitamin-A and D is	Halibut liver oil
Richest source of vitamin-C	Amla (Indian Gooseberry)
Adult pregnant females are anemic, if hemoglobin level	Less than 11 gm%
Optimum level of fluorine intake	0.5–0.8 ppm (mg/L)
Soybean contains _____ proteins	43.2% proteins
Best among food proteins	Egg
Indian reference man weighs	60 kg
Richest source of vitamin D	Halibut liver oil

Contd...

Contd...

Richest source of Iron among nuts	Pistachio
Two-in-one salt contains	Iron + Iodine
Phosphatase test is done for	Efficiency of pasteurization
Golden rice is rich in	Beta-carotene and Iron
Milk is poor in	Vitamin C and Iron
Pulse with highest protein content	Soybean (43%)
Reference protein	Egg (NPU 96)
Toxin in Lathyrism	BOAA
No plant source for vitamins	B_{12} and D
Methionine is limiting amino acid is	Pulses
Highest content of saturated fatty acids is in	Coconut oil
Highest content of vitamin D is in	Halibut fish liver oil
Sufficiency of pasteurization is tested by	Phosphatase test
Maize is pellagrogenic due to excess of	Leucine
Tests of pasteurization of milk	Phosphatase test (MC), Coliform count, Standard plate count
Halibut liver oil rich in	Vitamin A, D
Known as "Poor man's meat"	Pulses
Pulse proteins are poor in	Methionine
NPU is highest in	Egg (NPU 96)
Biological value of rice protein	67
Amount of cereals provided in mid-day meal program	100 grams primary (150 grams upper primary)
Richest source of cholesterol	Egg
Maximum amount of essential fatty acids is found in	Safflower oil
1 gram of 'Twin fortified salt' provides	40 mcg Iodine + 1 mg Iron
Vitamin lacking gin egg	C
In egg, egg white contributes	58%
One egg yield about kcal of energy	70 kcal
Level of proteins in human milk (per 100 mL)	1.1 grams
Pasteurized milk is most commonly tested by	Phosphatase test
Highest protein content is in food item	Soyabean
An amino acid found in excess in some strains of maize	Leucine
Pulses are deficient in amino acid	Methionine
Limiting amino acid in cereals	Lysine
One egg yields _____ energy [kcal]	70 kcal
Ragi is rich in	Calcium
White polished rice is deficient in	Thiamine & Riboflavin
Richest source of Vitamin B12 is	Liver (Meat)
Human milk Calories [per 100 gm] content	65 kcal/100 mL
Lactose in per 100 grams of breast milk	7.4 grams
Nutritional disorders	
First clinical sign of Xerophthalmia	Conjunctival xerosis
First Indicator of PEM	Under-weight for age
Toxin in Lathyrism	BOAA
Pellagra occurs due to	Niacin (B_3) deficiency
Order in Nalgonda technique for defluoridation	Lime + Alum

Contd...

Contd...

Acrodermatitis enteropathica is due to deficiency of	Zinc
Pellagra occurs due to	Vitamin B_3 (niacin) deficiency
Maize-eaters are prone to	Pellagra
Amino acid deficient in wheat	Threonine & Lysine
Milk reduces absorption of	Iron
Acrodermatitis enteropathica is due to	Zinc deficiency
Fluorosis is not seen in	Free flowing surface waters
Xerophthalmia is public health problem, if Bitot spots	>0.5%
Mild degree of malnutrition is Serum albumin level	3.0–3.5 gm/dL
Besides diarrhoea, dermatitis and dementia in pellagra, 4th D is	Death
Avidin has affinity for	Biotin
Earliest feature of vitamin A deficiency	Dryness of conjunctiva
Papilledema is caused by nutritional toxicity of	Vitamin A
In Measles which vitamin deficiency occurs	Vitamin A
Defluoridation of water is done by technique	Nalgonda technique
Micronutrient deficiency associated with rash and diarrhea	Zinc
Parboiling of rice reduces disease	Beriberi
BOAA toxin responsible for Neurolathyrism, contains amino acid	Alanine
Lathyrism is due to consumption of	Khesari dhal
Cause of endemic ascites	Pyrrolizidine alkaloids
Dental caries is due to deficiency of	Fluorine
First sign of vitamin A deficiency is	Conjunctival xerosis (Dry eye)
First symptom of vitamin A deficiency is	Night blindness
Vitamin A requirement in 1–6 years old child is	400 mcg
Phrynoderma is due to deficiency of	Essential fatty acids
Kanawati index is used for	Protein energy malnutrition
Most common nutritional problem in India	Iron deficiency anaemia
Endemic ascites is caused by	Crotalaria seeds

Multiple Choice Questions

ENERGY AND PROTEIN REQUIREMENTS

1. Correct about additional nutritional caloric in pregnancy is: [NEET PG Pattern 2022]
   (a) 300 kcal throughout pregnancy
   (b) 400 kcal in second trimester
   (c) 400 kcal in third trimester
   (d) 200 kcal in second trimester

2. Among the following nutrients, lactating mothers needs more as compared to a pregnant female: [INICET July 2021]
   (a) Calcium
   (b) Iron
   (c) Vitamin A
   (d) Folic acid

3. The recommended daily energy intake of an adult pregnant woman with heavy work is: [AIPGME 05]
   (a) 2100 kcal
   (b) 2500 kcal
   (c) 3200 kcal
   (d) 2900 kcal

4. Extra calories required by lactating mother during first six months over and above daily requirement is: [AIIMS Nov 2003, Dec 1997, AIPGME 2000] [NEET Pattern 2012] [AP 2007, RJ 2009]
   (a) 550 kcal
   (b) 400 kcal
   (c) 300 kcal
   (d) 250 kcal

5. Consumption Unit, the coefficient of Dietary Intake, for an adolescent is of value: [AIIMS Dec 1994]
   (a) 0.9
   (b) 1.0
   (c) 1.2
   (d) 1.7

6. Protein requirement of an adult is: [AIPGME 2001]
   (a) 0.7 gm/kg in terms of Egg protein & 0.7 gm/kg in terms of mixed vegetable protein
   (b) 1.0 gm/kg in terms of Egg protein & 1.0 gm/kg in terms of mixed vegetable protein
   (c) 1.0 gm/kg in terms of Egg protein & 0.7 gm/kg in terms of mixed vegetable protein
   (d) 0.7 gm/kg in terms of Egg protein & 1.0 gm/kg in terms of mixed vegetable protein

7. In calculating RDA for a particular nutrient, 2 SD are not added for: [AIIMS Nov 2006]
   (a) Iron
   (b) Calcium
   (c) Energy
   (d) Vitamin A

8. For a 60 kg Indian male, the minimum daily protein requirement has been calculated to be 40 g (mean) ± 10 (Standard deviation). The recommended daily allowance of protein would be: [AIPGME 2002]
   (a) 60 g/day
   (b) 70 g/day
   (c) 40 g/day
   (d) 50 g/day

9. False regarding Indian Reference Woman:
   (a) 18–29 years age
   (b) 50 kg weight
   (c) 1.61 meters height
   (d) 21.2 BMI

10. A 70 kg farmer is consuming 56 grams proteins, 275 grams carbohydrate and 60 grams lipids. He is consuming: [NEET Pattern 2017]
    (a) Less calories
    (b) More calories
    (c) Adequate calories
    (d) Cannot be commented upon

Review Questions

11. The daily extra colorie requirement is first trimester of pregnancy is: [DNB 2000]
    (a) 50
    (b) 150
    (c) 350
    (d) 450

12. Which of the following trace element cannot be Completely supplemented by diet during pregnancy:
    (a) Fe
    (b) Ca++ [UP 2000]
    (c) Zn
    (d) Mn

13. According to ICMR the 'Cereals and pulses' requirement for a sedentary strict vegetarian male is? [MH 2008]
    (a) 200 and 50 grams
    (b) 300 and 60 grams
    (c) 460 and 40 grams
    (d) 560 and 50 grams

PROTEINS

14. Highest Thermic effect is seen in: [INICET May 2023, November 2020]
    (a) Carbohydrate diet
    (b) Protein diet
    (c) Fat diet
    (d) Vitamin diet

15. Which one of the following is the best indicator of protein quality for recommending the dietary protein requirement? [AIIMS Nov 2005]
    (a) Protein-efficiency ratio
    (b) Biological value
    (c) Digestibility coefficient
    (d) Net protein utilization

16. The optimum calories to be provided by proteins should be: [A 1999]
    (a) 5–10%
    (b) 10–15%
    (c) 15–20%
    (d) 20–30%
17. Conditionally Essential amino acids are:
    (a) Leucine & Lysine [AIIMS Nov 2005]
    (b) Histidine & Arginine
    (c) Tyrosine & Cysteine
    (d) Phenylalanine & Tryptophan
18. The Protein Efficiency Ratio (PER) is defined as: [AIPGME 1994, AIPGME 2003]
    (a) The gain in weight of young animals per unit weight of protein-consumed
    (b) The product of digestibility coefficient and biological value
    (c) The percentage of protein absorbed into the blood
    (d) The percentage of nitrogen absorbed from the protein absorbed from the diet
19. Highest protein content is in: [AIIMS May 2005]
    (a) Red gram [BIHAR 2001, DNB 2008, WB 2002]
    (b) Black gram
    (c) Bengal gram
    (d) Soya bean
20. Limiting Amino acids in wheat are: [AIPGME 1997]
    (a) Methionine and lysine [UP 2004, 2005, 2007]
    (b) Lysine and threonine
    (c) Threonine and methionine
    (d) Arginine and lysine
21. Pulse protein is deficient in which of the following Essential Amino Acid? [Karnataka 2009]
    (a) Lysine [NEET Pattern 2013]
    (b) Methionine
    (c) Threonine
    (d) Tryptophan
22. All are true about Net protein utilization (NPU) except: [AIIMS May 2011]
    (a) Defined as Nitrogen retained by Nitrogen consumed × 100
    (b) Good for estimating protein quality
    (c) Egg has the highest NPU value
    (d) 1 gram protein is equivalent to 1 gram Nitrogen
23. Lysine is deficient in: [DNB 2007] [DNB December 2011]
    (a) Pulse (b) Wheat [DNB 2001]
    (c) Both of the above (d) None of the above
24. Biological value is maximum of:
    (a) Egg [DNB, 2000, 2003, 2007]
    (b) Milk [NEET Pattern 2018]
    (c) Soyabean
    (d) Pulses
25. The protein quality indicator adopted by ICMR in recommending dietary protein requirement is: [DNB 2007]
    (a) Amino acid score
    (b) Net protein utilization
    (c) Biological value
    (d) Protein efficiency ratio
26. Limiting amino acids in Cereals & Pulses respectively:
    (a) Lysine & Threonine [NEET Pattern 2015]
    (b) Lysine & Cysteine
    (c) Threonine & Methionine
    (d) Lysine & Methionine
27. Recommended Protein intake (high quality) of an Indian adult man according to 2010 Guidelines is:
    (a) 0.2 g/kg/d [NEET Pattern 2015, 2017]
    (b) 0.83 g/kg/d [DNB 2007]
    (c) 1.0 g/kg/d
    (d) 1.2 g/kg/d
28. Protein requirement of a Neonate is: [CGPG 2015]
    (a) 1.5 grams (b) 2.5 grams
    (c) 3.5 grams (d) 4.5 grams
29. Pulses requirement of an adult male person with sedentary lifestyle is: [NEET Pattern 2016]
    (a) 40 grams (b) 60 grams
    (c) 100 grams (d) 160 grams

Review Questions

30. Which of the following has highest protein content:
    (a) Mutton (b) Soyabean [DNB 2000]
    (c) Egg (d) Milk
31. Amino acid lesser in rice is: [DNB 2001]
    [NEET Pattern 2017]
    (a) Lysine (b) Methionine
    (c) Both (d) None
32. Maize is deficient in: [MH 2000, MH 2002]
    (a) Methionine (b) Lysine
    (c) Lucine (d) All
33. Which method of assessment of quality of proteins gives more complete assessment of protein quality?
    (a) Biological value [MH 2007]
    (b) Net protein utilization
    (c) Digestibility coefficient
    (d) Amino acid score

FATS AND CARBOHYDRATES

34. True about FDA approved high fat-diet is:
    [INICET May 2023]
    (a) >80% should be contribution by fat
    (b) Fat content should be >2000 kcal
    (c) Total carbohydrates should be 400 kcal
    (d) Total calorie content should be 800–1000 kcal

35. Which of the following is a w-3 Fatty Acid?
    [AIPGME 1993, 2002]
    (a) Linoleic Acid
    (b) α-Linolenic acid
    (c) Arachidonic acid
    (d) γ-Linolenic acid

36. The highest percentage of polyunsaturated fatty acids is present in: [AIIMS May 06; AIPGME 07, 08]
    (a) Groundnut oil
    (b) Soya bean oil
    (c) Margarine
    (d) Palm oil

37. Suggested intake of dietary fat per day in pregnancy is:
    [AIIMS May 1999]
    (a) 20 gm
    (b) 22 gm
    (c) 30 gm
    (d) 45 gm

38. Most important Essential Fatty Acid is: [AIIMS Nov 2006]
    (a) Linoleic Acid [NEET Pattern 2012]
    (b) Linolenic Acid
    (c) Arachidonic Acid
    (d) Eicosapentarnoic Acid

39. Rank the food items in descending order of their energy yield per 100 grams Carbohydrate – A, Fats – B, Alcohol – C:
    [AIIMS May 2001] [NEET Pattern 2012]
    (a) A B C
    (b) B C A
    (c) C A B
    (d) C B A

40. Highest fat content is present in: [DPG 2008]
    (a) Rice
    (b) Wheat
    (c) Bajra
    (d) Jowar

41. The highest content of saturated fatty acid is in:
    [Karnataka 2008]
    (a) Palm oil
    (b) Butter
    (c) Coconut oil
    (d) Margarine

42. Which among the following is a cardio-protective fatty acid? [AIPGME 2011]
    (a) Palmitic acid
    (b) Stearic acid
    (c) Omega-3 fatty acids
    (d) Oleic acid

43. Low glycemic index is for: [NEET Pattern 2012]
    (a) Sucrose
    (b) Potato
    (c) White bread
    (d) Fruits

44. Consider the following:
    1. Coconut oil
    2. Groundnut oil
    3. Mustard oil
    Which of the above is/are dietary sources of linoleic acid?
    [UPSC CMS 2015]
    (a) 1 and 2 only
    (b) 1, 2 and 3
    (c) 3 only
    (d) 2 and 3 only

45. Low glycemic index is seen in: [NEET Pattern 2015]
    (a) Corn flakes
    (b) Brown rice
    (c) Lentils
    (d) White bread

46. Vanaspati Ghee is fortified with: [NEET Pattern 2016]
    (a) Iodine
    (b) Vitamin A
    (c) Iron
    (d) Calcium

Review Questions

47. Linoleic acid/EFA's is maximum in: [DNB 2000, 2004]
    (a) Groundnut oil [WB 2002, RJ 2004, MP 1998]
    (b) Safflower oil [AP 2001, UPSC 1990, PGMCET 2015]
    (c) Mustard oil
    (d) Coconut oil

48. What % of total calorie should be from Fat & EFA:
    (a) 10–30
    (b) 7–15 [RJ 2009]
    (c) 65–80
    (d) 1–7

VITAMINS

49. Vitamin deficiency which may lead to the triad of diarrhoea, dermatitis and dementia is: [NEET PG Pattern 2023]
    (a) Thiamine
    (b) Riboflavin
    (c) Niacin
    (d) Folic acid

50. A 32-year-old alcoholic patient presented to Medicine OPD at a medical college with confusion, ataxia and visual impairment. Most likely cause is: [NEET PG Pattern 2023]
    (a) Niacin deficiency
    (b) Biotin deficiency
    (c) Vitamin A deficiency
    (d) Thiamine deficiency

51. Vitamin deficiency which may lead to bleeding tendency (hemorrhages, ecchymosis) is:
    (a) A [NEET PG Pattern 2023]
    (b) B3
    (c) C
    (d) B12

52. In which of the following deficiency there is collagen maturation defect? [INICET November 2021]
    (a) Beri beri
    (b) Vitamin A deficiency
    (c) Scurvy
    (d) Rickets

53. Maize diet consumption is associated with _____ vitamin deficiency: [NEET PG Pattern September 2021]
    (a) Pyridoxine (B6)
    (b) Thiamine (B1)
    (c) Niacin (B3)
    (d) Cyanocobalamin (B12)

54. A patient presented with diminishing of vision in low light. On examination there are dry eyes and roughening of corneal surface. Most likely deficiency associated is:
    [NEET PG Pattern September 2021]
    (a) Iron
    (b) Proteins
    (c) Retinoic acid
    (d) Niacin

55. Neonatal seizure due to deficiency of which vitamin: [AIIMS June 2020]
    (a) Riboflavin
    (b) Pantothenic Acid
    (c) Pyridoxine
    (d) Thiamine

56. A child was fed on staple diet of Maize for a long time. Which of the following vitamins may get deficient in his body? [NEET PG Pattern January 2020]
    (a) Vitamin B1
    (b) Vitamin B12
    (c) Niacin
    (d) Pyridoxine

57. Major source of Cyanocobalamin vitamin is: [NEET PG Pattern January 2020]
    (a) Animal only diet
    (b) Plant only diet
    (c) Sunlight
    (d) None

58. Casal's Necklace is seen in deficiency of: [AIIMS Nov 1999]
    (a) Vitamin A
    (b) Vitamin B3
    (c) Vitamin B6
    (d) Vitamin D

59. Vitamin A deficiency is considered a public health problem if prevalence rate of night blindness in children between 6 months to 6 years is more than: [AIIMS May 2006]
    (a) 0.01%
    (b) 0.05%
    (c) 0.1%
    (d) 1.0%

60. Recommended Daily Allowance of free folate in pregnancy is: [AIIMS Feb 1997]
    (a) 500 mcg
    (b) 150 mcg
    (c) 300 mcg
    (d) 400 mcg

61. First clinical sign of Vitamin-A deficiency is: [AIIMS May 2007]
    (a) Night blindness
    (b) Conjunctival xerosis
    (c) Bitot's spots
    (d) Keratomalacia

62. Under National Immunisation Schedule, total dose of Vitamin-A given to a child is: [AIPGME 1992]
    (a) 5 lac IU
    (b) 6 lac IU
    (c) 9 lac IU
    (d) 13.5 lac IU

63. Minimum amount of sunlight exposure necessary for adequate synthesis of Vitamin-D in the human body is: [AIIMS Dec 1994]
    (a) 5 min
    (b) 30 min
    (c) 2 hrs
    (d) 5 hrs

64. 'Burning Sole Syndrome' is seen in deficiency of: [AIIMS May 1995]
    (a) Riboflavin
    (b) Pyridoxine
    (c) Pantothenic acid
    (d) Vitamin B12

65. Dose of vitamin A prophylaxis in 6–11 months old child is: [DPG 2005]
    (a) 2,00,000 IU
    (b) 30,000 IU
    (c) 60,000 IU
    (d) 1,00,000 IU

66. Incidence of Bitot spots to label it as a public health problem is: [DPG 2007]
    (a) 0.1% [AIIMS 1998]
    (b) 0.5% [NEET Pattern 2013, 2014, 2016]
    (c) 1%
    (d) 5%

67. Vitamin D is maximum in: [NEET Pattern 2012]
    (a) Milk [NEET Pattern 2013]
    (b) Fish fat
    (c) Eggs
    (d) Cod liver oil

68. False statement regarding folic acid supplementation? [AIIMS November 2013]
    (a) Fortified in all wheat products in India like as in USA
    (b) Preconceptionally given for prevention of neural tube defects
    (c) It is present in leafy vegetables, spinach, paneer
    (d) Requirement per day in pregnancy is 500 mcg

69. Pellagra in Jowar eating population is due to:
    (a) Niacin in bound form [NUPGET 2013]
    (b) Deficiency of Tryptophan
    (c) Excess of Leucine
    (d) High consumption of milk and milk products

70. In Xeropthalmia, what is X1B: [NEET Pattern 2014]
    (a) Conjunctival xerosis
    (b) Bitot's spot
    (c) Corneal xerosis
    (d) Corneal ulcer

71. Disease which is characterized by three D's – Diarrhoea, Dermatitis and Dementia is due to deficiency of: [PGMCET 2015]
    (a) Vitamin A
    (b) Niacin
    (c) Folate
    (d) Vitamin C

72. No. of doses for treatment of Vitamin A deficiency:
    (a) 1
    (b) 2 [NEET Pattern 2015]
    (c) 3
    (d) 4

73. Highest amount of Vitamin D is contained in [NEET Pattern 2015]
    (a) Sunlight
    (b) Shark liver oil
    (c) Cod liver oil
    (d) Halibut fish liver oil

74. Which Vitamin RDA is related to Daily requirement for Proteins? [JIPMER 2015]
    (a) B1
    (b) B2
    (c) B3
    (d) B6

75. Highest thiamine content is found in: [NEET Pattern 2015]
    (a) Whole wheat
    (b) Milled rice
    (c) Ground nut
    (d) Gingelly seeds

Review Questions

76. Prevalence of Vitamin A deficiency in a community is assessed as cutoff: [DNB 2000]
    (a) Night blindness-10%
    (b) Corneal ulcer-0.01%
    (c) Bitot spots-0.5%
    (d) Decreased serum retinol level-0.05%

77. Vitamin E rich foods are: [UP 2002]
    (a) Sunflower oil
    (b) Wheat germ oil
    (c) Soya bean
    (d) All of the above

78. Vitamin C content of which of the following is >5 mg per 100 grams? [AP 2005]
    (a) Human milk
    (b) Dates
    (c) Egg
    (d) Sitaphal

79. Vitamin D is least in: [AP 2007]
    (a) Milk
    (b) Eggs
    (c) Fish fat
    (d) Shark liver oil

80. Deficiency of folic acid produces: [TN 1999, TN 2000]
    (a) Carcinoma stomach
    (b) Spinal degeneration
    (c) Changes in central nervous system
    (d) Megaloblastic anaemia

81. Richest source of vitamin B1: [Kolkata 2008]
    (a) Rice
    (b) Milk
    (c) Egg
    (d) Groundnut

82. Which of the following is NOT a criteria for determining xerophthalmia problem in the community? [MP 2008]
    (a) Bitot's spots 0.05%
    (b) Corneal xerosis 0.01%
    (c) Corneal ulcer 0.05%
    (d) Serum retinol level less than 10 mcg/dL 10%

83. Highest amount of vit. C is found in: [RJ 2004]
    (a) Orange
    (b) Lemon
    (c) Indian goose berry
    (d) Grapes

IRON

84. You are Medical officer at PHC. What will be your advice regarding an economical method for Mass drug administration for Iron deficiency anemia in the catchment population? [INICET November 2020]
    (a) Ferrous sulphate
    (b) Intravenous iron
    (c) Ferrous fumarate + Folic acid + Vitamin B12 + Vitamin C
    (d) Iron (III)-hydroxide polymaltose complex

85. Best test to detect iron deficiency in community is: [AIPGME 2001, 1995]
    (a) Serum transferrin
    (b) Serum ferritin
    (c) Serum iron
    (d) Hemoglobin

86. An adult pregnant female is termed anemic if her hemoglobin (venous blood) is: [AIIMS Nov 1999]
    (a) Less than 11 g/dL
    (b) Less than 12 g/dL
    (c) Less than 13 g/dL
    (d) Less than 14 g/dL

87. Which one of the following pulses has the highest content of iron? [AIPGME 2006]
    (a) Bengal gram
    (b) Black gram
    (c) Red gram
    (d) Soya bean

88. Iron absorption from habitual Indian diets is approx: [AIPGME 1992]
    (a) <5 %
    (b) 15–20%
    (c) 40–50%
    (d) 70–80%

89. Lowest iron content is present in: [DPG 2008]
    (a) Milk
    (b) Liver
    (c) Meat
    (d) Fist

90. Oral iron pills or iron injections must be taken along with: [AIPGME 2012]
    (a) High doses of Vitamin A
    (b) High doses of Vitamin C
    (c) High doses of Essential fatty acids
    (d) High doses of Vitamin D

91. Poor man's iron source is: [DNB June 2009] [NEET Pattern 2017]
    (a) Almond
    (b) Grapes
    (c) Soya
    (d) Jaggery

92. National iron plus initiative includes: [NEET Pattern 2016]
    (a) Biweekly supplementation of iron & FA to 6–60 months of age
    (b) Biweekly supplementation of iron & FA to pregnant & lactating woman
    (c) Biweekly supplementation of iron & FA to adolescent girls
    (d) All of the above are parts of initiative

93. Which of the following is true for iron prophylaxis as per National iron plus initiative? [AIIMS May 2016]
    (a) A tablet containing 100 mg elemental iron and 500 mcg of folic acid weekly for aged 10–19 years
    (b) A syrup containing 20 mg of elemental iron and 100 mcg of folic acid weekly for children less than 5 years
    (c) A tablet containing 100 mg elemental iron and 500 mcg of folic acid biweekly for adults
    (d) A tablet containing 45 mg of iron and 400 mcg of folic acid for biweekly for children from age 6–10

94. Which of the following is/are true about National Iron Plus Initiative? [PGI 2017]
    (a) Only school going adolescents are covered
    (b) Adolescents of age group 10–19 years are covered
    (c) Preschool children are covered through Anganwadi center
    (d) Biannual deworming through Albendazole tablet
    (e) Screening of target groups for moderate/severe anaemia and referring these cases to an appropriate health facility

95. Total Iron required per day for Pregnancy period: [NEET Pattern 2018]
    (a) 65 mg/day   (b) 35 mg/day
    (c) 25 mg/day   (d) 70 mg/day

IODINE AND FLUORINE

96. Fluoride content in drinking H_2O normally safe is:
    (a) 0.5–0.8 mg/l   [NEET Pattern 2015, AIPGME 1994]
    (b) 0.8–1.0 mg/l   [TN 2003, MH 2008, RJ 2002]
    (c) 0.2–0.8 mg/l
    (d) 0.2–0.5 mg/l

97. Dental fluorosis is best seen in: [AIIMS Nov 2007]
    (a) Central & Lateral Incisors
    (b) Central Incisors & 1st Molars
    (c) 1st & 2nd Molars
    (d) Canines

98. PFA Act' 1954 has laid down standard for level of Iodisation of salt: [DNB 2001] [AIIMS June 1997]
    (a) 90 ppm at Production level & 60 ppm at Consumer level [Karnataka 2011] [UP 2008]
    (b) 60 ppm at Production level & 15 ppm at Consumer level [NEET Pattern 2013]
    (c) 30 ppm at Production level & 60 ppm at Consumer level
    (d) 30 ppm at Production level & 15 ppm at Consumer level

99. Iodised oil (usual dose of 1 mL i/m) gives protection for: [AIPGME 2005]
    (a) 3–4 weeks   (b) 3–4 months
    (c) 3–4 years   (d) 10–12 years

100. Daily requirement of Iodine in adults is:
    (a) 50 mcg   [AIIMS Sep 1996, RJ 2001, 2008]
    (b) 100 mcg   [NEET Pattern 2013, TN 1997, 2003]
    (c) 150 mcg
    (d) 200 mcg

101. As per the World Health Organization guidelines, iodine deficiency disorders are endemic in a community if the prevalence of goiter in school age children is more than: [AIIMS Nov 02]
    (a) 1%   (b) 5%
    (c) 10%   (d) 15%

102. Recommended Iodine dose in pregnancy is: [AIIMS November 2013]
    (a) 15 mcg   (b) 100 mcg
    (c) 150 mcg   (d) 250 mcg

103. Endemic cretinism is seen when iodine uptake is less than: [DNB December 2011]
    (a) 5 micro gram/day   (b) 20 micro gram/day
    (c) 50 micro gram/day   (d) 75 micro gram/day

104. Prevalence of iodine deficiency in India: [NEET Pattern 2012]
    (a) 1:100   (b) 1:10
    (c) 3:100   (d) 3:10

105. Fluorine levels intake required for development of Skeletal fluorosis [NEET Pattern 2015]
    (a) 1.0–1.5 ppm   (b) 1.5–3.0 ppm
    (c) 3.0–6.0 ppm   (d) >10 ppm

106. Fluorine levels intake required for development of Crippling fluorosis [NEET Pattern 2015]
    (a) 1.0–1.5 ppm   (b) 1.5–3.0 ppm
    (c) 3.0–6.0 ppm   (d) >10 ppm

107. Iodine requirement during Lactation is: [NEET Pattern 2018]
    (a) 100 mcg per day
    (b) 150 mcg per day
    (c) 220 mcg per day
    (d) 290 mcg per day

108. True statement about Iodine deficiency disorder [PGI November 2017]
    (a) Exclusively found in Himalayan goiter belt
    (b) Goiter prevalence of 10% is cut-off value for endemicity
    (c) Strabismus is also a manifestation
    (d) Only monitored by blood thyroid test
    (e) Include only Goitre

Review Questions

109. Maximum Permitted level of fluoride in drinking water is – – mEq/L: [DNB 2000]
    (a) 0.5   (b) 0.8
    (c) 1.0   (d) 1.5

110. In Iron deficiency anemia, after haemoglobin level has returned to normal so that iron stores are replenished. The Iron tablets should be recommended for: [UP 2008]
    (a) 0–3 months   (b) 3–6 months
    (c) 6–12 months   (d) 12–24 months

111. Poor source of Iron is in: [AP 2002]
    (a) Butter   (b) Green leafy vegetable
    (c) Jaggery   (d) Meat

OTHER NUTRIENTS

112. Deficiency of a nutrient led to poor wound healing and erythematous scaly pustular lesions in perioral region and diarrhoea. Most likely it is: [NEET PG Pattern 2023]
    (a) Selenium   (b) Zinc
    (c) Iodine   (d) Copper

113. **Daily requirement for Dietary Fibre by an adult is approx:**
     [AIIMS Nov 2005]
     (a) 1 gm   (b) 4 gm
     (c) 40 gm   (d) 100 gm

114. **Which of the following is the non-essential micronutrient?** [AIIMS Nov 2010]
     (a) Iron   (b) Manganese
     (c) Lead   (d) Sodium

115. **One of the following is not reported to be a clinical manifestation of Zinc deficiency in children:**
     (a) Dwarfism and hypogonadism   [NEET Pattern 2013]
     (b) Liver and spleen enlargement
     (c) Impaired cell-mediated immunity
     (d) Macrocytic anaemia

116. **Zinc supplement given in 12 month baby:**
     [NEET Pattern 2013]
     (a) 20 mg/day
     (b) 10 mg/day
     (c) 5 mg/day
     (d) 15 mg/day

117. **Adult non-pregnant female requires, calcium per day:**
     [NEET Pattern 2013]
     (a) 400 mg   (b) 600 mg
     (c) 800 mg   (d) 1000 mg

118. **Daily calcium requirement of infants is:**
     [NEET Pattern 2012]
     (a) 300 mg   (b) 500 mg
     (c) 600 mg   (d) 1200 mg

119. **Keshan cardiomegaly occur due to deficiency of:**
     [NEET Pattern 2013]
     (a) Selenium   (b) Copper
     (c) Zinc   (d) Iron

120. **Acrodermatitis enteropathica is:** [NEET Pattern 2014]
     (a) Inherited disorder of excessive excretion of zinc from body
     (b) Inherited disorder of impaired uptake of zinc from body
     (c) Inherited disorder of excessive excretion of copper from body
     (d) Inherited disorder of impaired uptake of copper from body

121. **Zinc deficiency leads to all *except*:** [PGMCET 2015]
     (a) Delayed Sexual Maturation
     (b) Impaired Immune function
     (c) Skeletal Abnormalities
     (d) Excessive Appetite

122. **Rich source of fiber:**   [NEET Pattern 2015]
     (a) Spinach   (b) Wheat
     (c) Green gram   (d) Ragi

123. **Fibers are maximum in:**   [NEET Pattern 2016]
     (a) Wheat   (b) Oat
     (c) Rice   (d) Corn

Review Questions

124. **Spectrum of IDD cretin does not include:** [AP 2005]
     (a) Still births (b) Hyperactivity
     (c) Deafness   (d) Delayed development

125. **The level of fluorine in drinking water highly associated with dental fluorosis is:** [MP 2008]
     (a) 0.5 mg/L   (b) 1.0 mg/L
     (c) 1.5 mg/L   (d) 2.0 mg/L

126. **Highest calcium concentration is present in:**
     [Kolkata 2007]
     (a) Dates   (b) Guava
     (c) Amla   (d) Mango

127. **Copper deficiency is characterized by:** [RJ 2009]
     (a) Myelopathy   (b) Neutropenia
     (c) Anemia   (d) All of the above

128. **Egg are "reference protein" because:** [UP 2004]
     (a) High caloric content
     (b) Increased protein/100 gm
     (c) Increased biological value and +NPU
     (d) Decreased digestibility coefficient

EGG

129. **Consumption of raw egg is associated with deficiency of:**
     [NEET PG Pattern 2023]
     (a) Thiamine   (b) Niacin
     (c) Biotin   (d) Folic acid

130. **Egg is poor in:**   [AIIMS Dec 1998]
     (a) Proteins
     (b) Carbohydrate & Vitamin C
     (c) Calcium & Iron
     (d) Fats

131. **NPU value for Egg is:**   [AIIMS Sep 1996]
     (a) 140   (b) 96
     (c) 81   (d) 52

132. **True about egg:**   [NEET Pattern 2015]
     (a) NPU is 70
     (b) Rich in all vitamin including vitamin C
     (c) 60 gm of egg contain 6 gm protein, 6 gm fat, 30 mg calcium
     (d) Deficient in essential amino acids

Review Questions

133. **Egg is deficient in which of the following:**
     (a) Fat   [AP 2005] [Bihar 2004]
     (b) Protein
     (c) Carbohydrate
     (d) Vitamin

134. Egg is ideal protein because it has: [AP 2002]
    (a) High digestibility
    (b) It has best quality of protein
    (c) High proteins
    (d) High protein and fats

MILK

135. Pasteurization test done for milk *except*:
    [INICET November 2021]
    (a) Phosphatase test
    (b) Standard plate count
    (c) Methylene blue reduction test
    (d) Iodine test

136. Pasteurization by Holder method is heating milk at:
    (a) 60°C for 45 minutes [AIPGME 2000]
    (b) 65°C for 30 minutes
    (c) 100°C for 15 minutes
    (d) 136°C for 15 minutes

137. Which one of the following is NOT used in testing for adequate pasteurization of milk?
    (a) Phosphatase test [AIPGME 2005, AIIMS Nov 2008]
    (b) Coliform count   [NEET Pattern 2013, 2014]
    (c) Standard plate count
    (d) Methylene blue reduction test

138. Milk is a good source of all vitamins *except*:
    [AIIMS Jan 1998]
    (a) Vitamin A   (b) Vitamin B
    (c) Vitamin C   (d) Vitamin D

139. Milk is rich in all *except*: [PGI Dec 01]
    (a) Vitamin A
    (b) Vitamin D
    (c) Iron
    (d) Vitamin E
    (e) Vitamin C

140. True about cow's milk are all *except*: [AIIMS May 2010]
    (a) Cow's milk contains 80% whey protein and not casein
    (b) Has more protein than breast milk
    (c) Has more K+ and Na+ than breast milk
    (d) Has less carbohydrates than mothers milk

141. Arrange the following milk/milk products in term of increasing content of Fat (per 100 grams or 100 mL)
    [NEET Pattern 2015]
    (a) Human milk, Buffalo milk, Curd (Cow's milk), Cheese
    (b) Cheese, Human milk, Curd (Cow's milk), Buffalo milk
    (c) Human milk, Curd (Cow's milk), Buffalo milk, Cheese
    (d) Curd (Cow's milk), Human milk, Cheese, Buffalo milk

142. Consider the following milk borne diseases,
    1. Brucellosis
    2. Listeriosis
    3. Salmonellosis

Which of the above can be controlled by Pasteurization?
    [UPSC CMS 2015]
    (a) 1 only   (b) 2 and 3 only
    (c) 3 only   (d) 1, 2 and 3

143. Human's breast milk is essential for the newborn as it contains: [AIIMS November 2011]
    (a) Linoleic acid
    (b) Linolenic acid
    (c) Docosahexaenoic acid
    (d) Arachidonic acid

144. Colostrum has in compared to normal milk:
    (a) Decreased Vitamin A [NEET Pattern 2012]
    (b) Decreased Na+
    (c) Increased proteins
    (d) Increased calories

145. What is absent in breast milk? [DNB December 2011]
    [NEET Pattern 2013]
    (a) Vitamin K   (b) Vitamin C
    (c) Vitamin D   (d) Vitamin A

146. Phosphatase test in milk is done to know: [DNB 2007]
    (a) Quality of pasteurization
    (b) Contamination of milk
    (c) Nutritive value
    (d) Coliform count

147. Pasteurization of milk is achieved by boiling at:
    [NEET Pattern 2013]
    (a) 65°C for 30 min   (b) 72° for 10 sec
    (c) 100° for 20 sec   (d) 136° for 30 sec

148. Which one of the following bacteria can survive in Holder method of pasteurization? [NEET Pattern 2016]
    (a) Salmonella typhi   (b) Mycobacterium bovis
    (c) Coxiella burnetii   (d) Brucella melitensis

Review Questions

149. A child is exclusively fed on cow's milk, the deficiency seen in: [DNB 2002]
    (a) Iron   (b) Riboflavin
    (c) Vitamin A   (d) Thiamine

150. All are true about human milk *except*:
    (a) Low lactose   [Kerala 2001 UP 2004]
    (b) Contains more Vitamin-D
    (c) Higher percentage of linoleic acid and oleic acid
    (d) Better iron bioavailability

151. Milk transmits all *except*: [Kolkata 2008]
    (a) Q fever   (b) Typhoid fever
    (c) Brucellosis   (d) Endemic typhus

152. Which of the following contains least amount of protein in 100 gm of milk? [MP 2001]
    (a) Human milk   (b) Cow milk
    (c) Buffalo milk (d) Goat milk

153. Milk is deficient in the following: [MP 2007]
    (a) Tryptophan containing amino acids
    (b) Linoleic acid
    (c) Ascorbic acid
    (d) Calciferol

154. Compared with cow's milk, mother's milk has more: [RJ 2008]
    (a) Lactose
    (b) Vitamin D
    (c) Protein
    (d) Fat

OTHER FOOD ITEMS

155. Match List I correctly with List D and select your answer using the codes given below:

List I	List D
a. Papaya fruit	I. Calcium
b. Soya beans	II. Vitamin C
c. Ragi	III. Protein
d. Amla fruit	IV. Vitamin A

    (a) a-I, b-III, c-II, d-IV [AIPGME 1993]
    (b) a-IV, b-I, c-III, d-II
    (c) a-IV, b-III, c-I, d-II
    (d) a-I, b-III, c-IV, d-II

156. Rice is poor in all except: [AIIMS Sep 1996]
    (a) Calcium
    (b) Iron
    (c) Vitamins A, D, C
    (d) Lysine

157. Fish is the source of all except? [AIIMS May 2011]
    (a) Iron
    (b) Iodine
    (c) Vitamin A
    (d) Phosphorus

158. Nutritional value(s) of dates (per 100 grams) include:
    (a) Iron 10 mg [PGI May 2012]
    (b) Calcium 39 mg
    (c) Beta carotene 6 micrograms
    (d) Calories 280 kcal
    (e) Vitamin C 100 mg

159. Tomatoes are rich in: [DNB 2008]
    (a) Oxalic acid
    (b) Citric acid
    (c) Acetic acid
    (d) Formic acid

160. Banana is good source of: [PGI November 2014]
    (a) Calcium
    (b) Phosphorus
    (c) Vitamin B6
    (d) Vitamin C
    (e) Potassium

161. Fermentation of Pulses increase following except: [NEET Pattern 2015]
    (a) Thiamine
    (b) Riboflavin
    (c) Niacin
    (d) Ascorbic acid

162. White polished rice causes deficiency of: [NEET Pattern 2015]
    (a) Thiamine
    (b) Tryptophan
    (c) Riboflavin
    (d) Protein

163. Parboiling is done for: [NEET Pattern 2016]
    (a) Milling process
    (b) Polishing of rice
    (c) Preservation of nutrition
    (d) Storage of rice

Review Questions

164. One of the following contains maximum calcium:
    (a) Rice
    (b) Wheat [AP 2000]
    (c) Ragi
    (d) Jowar

165. Dates are rich source of: [AP 2004]
    (a) Calcium
    (b) Iron
    (c) Vitamin C
    (d) Carotene

166. Highest calorie content is found in: [MP 2002]
    (a) Banana
    (b) Apple
    (c) Guava
    (d) Orange

167. The food item rich in calcium is: [MP 2008]
    (a) Rice
    (b) Wheat
    (c) Jowar
    (d) Ragi

168. Lysine is deficient in: [MH 2000]
    (a) Cereals
    (b) Pulses
    (c) Jowar
    (d) Soyabean

169. Sorghum is pellagrogenic due to excess content of:
    (a) Lysine [MH 2006, 2007]
    (b) Threonine
    (c) Leucine
    (d) Tryptophan

FOOD ADULTERATION

170. A 38-year-old poor farmer has successive crop failures. He has currently progressive spastic paraparesis, upper motor neuron signs and instability in gait. Toxin responsible is: [NEET PG Pattern 2023]
    (a) BOAA
    (b) Aflatoxin
    (c) Ergot toxin
    (d) Sanguinarine

171. Vitamin useful in treatment of neuro-lathyrism is: [NEET PG Pattern 2023]
    (a) Niacin
    (b) Ascorbic acid
    (c) Cyanocobalamin
    (d) Vitamin D

172. A 55-year-old farmer from the State of Chhattisgarh presented with complaints of progressive muscle weakness, stiffness and pain in both legs. On examination, Pure motor paresis is present. What further history would you take? [NEET PG Pattern September 2021]
    (a) History of fever
    (b) History of vaccination
    (c) History of diet
    (d) History of similar events in the past

173. Endemic ascites is caused by: [AIIMS Nov 06, May 08]
    (a) Aflatoxin [UP 2001] [MP 2008] [NEET Pattern 2018]
    (b) Sanguinarine
    (c) Pyrrolizidine alkaloid
    (d) Ergot alkaloid

174. Epidemic dropsy is caused by:
    [NEET Pattern 2016, 2017, AIIMS Feb 1997]
    (a) Sanguinarine [June 1998, Nov 2007, Karnataka 1999]
    (b) BOAA [NEET Pattern 2012, Bihar 1999]
    (c) Pyruvic Acid [DNB 2011, UP 1998, 1999, DPG 2005]
    (d) Mustard oil [RJ 2000, 04, AP 02, MH 1995, 97, 02]

175. BOAA is the toxin responsible for:
    (a) Epidemic Dropsy [AIPGME 92, AIIMS June 1997]
    (b) Neurolathyrism [DNB 2000, 2005, 2006]
    (c) Endemic Ascitis [RJ 2000, MH 2003]
    (d) Fluorosis [NEET Pattern 2013]

176. Ingestion of which of the following can result in ergotism? [DPG 2007]
    (a) Bajra
    (b) Maize
    (c) Kesari dal
    (d) Mustard

177. Which of the following statement (s) is/are true about Lathyrism: [PGI May 2011]
    (a) Vitamin C prophylaxis
    (b) Banning of crop
    (c) Flaccid paralysis
    (d) Parboiling detoxicate pulses
    (e) BOAA is causative toxin

178. Manifestation(s) of Epidemic dropsy is/are:
    (a) Glaucoma [PGI May 2011]
    (b) CHF
    (c) GI bleed
    (d) Gut telangiectasia
    (e) Dyspnoea

179. Ergotism is due to toxic alkaloids produced by fungus:
    [DNB December 2011] [NUPGET 2013]
    (a) Trichophyton
    (b) Claviceps purpurea
    (c) Fusarium species
    (d) Absidia

180. Argemone oil contamination of mustard oil can be detected by: [NEET Pattern 2012]
    (a) Phosphatase test
    (b) Nitric acid test
    (c) Coliform test
    (d) Methylene blue test

181. Most sensitive test for sanguinarine is: [NEET Pattern 2013]
    (a) FeC13
    (b) Paper chromatography
    (c) HCl
    (d) Nitric Acid

182. A 42-year-old woman from a dry state who ingested rye for long time presented with complaints of weakness in both the lower limbs, nausea and fatigue. Over due course of time she is completely unable to walk. What is the likely cause? [AIIMS November 2016]
    (a) Lathyrus sativus
    (b) Amanita
    (c) Argemone mexicana
    (d) Ergot alkaloids

Review Questions

183. Lathyrism from Khesari dal can be prevented by which process: [MP 2003]
    (a) Parboiling
    (b) Heating
    (c) Soaking
    (d) Filtration

184. Test to detect contamination of mustard oil with argemone oil? [MH 2008]
    (a) Nitric acid test
    (b) Sulphuric acid test
    (c) Chromic acid test
    (d) All of the above

MISCELLANEOUS

185. Which is a 'conditioning factor' for Malnutrition – a man-made disease? [NEET PG Pattern September 2021]
    (a) Infectious disease
    (b) Socio-economic factors
    (c) Child rearing habits
    (d) Food habits

186. International Food Policy Research Institute calculated Global Hunger Index for a Country with given parameters:
    1. Proportion of undernourished population 27%
    2. Prevalence of underweight children 25%
    3. Mortality rate of Under-5 children 29%
    4. Infant mortality rate 20%
    Which of the following will not be used in calculation?
    [NEET PG Pattern September 2021]
    (a) IMR
    (b) Child mortality
    (c) Child undernourishment
    (d) Child underweight

187. Which of the following statements about Recommended Dietary Allowance is false?
    [AIIMS Nov 2007; AIPGME 2008]
    (a) RDA is decided by a panel of experts and is based on scientific research
    (b) RDA caters to dietary requirements of all people
    (c) RDA is often higher than the recommended minimum requirement
    (d) RDA is based on Estimated Average Requirement

188. A man weighing 68 kg, consumes 325 gm carbohydrate, 65 gm protein and 35 gms fat in his diet. The most applicable statement here is: [AIPGME 01]
    (a) His total calorie intake is 3000 kcal
    (b) The proportion of proteins, fats and carbohydrates is correct and in accordance with a balanced diet
    (c) He has a negative nitrogen balance
    (d) 30% of his total energy intake is derived from fat

189. Weight of an Indian reference woman is: [AIIMS Nov 04,08]
    (a) 45 kg
    (b) 50 kg
    (c) 55 kg
    (d) 60 kg

190. True about midday meal programme: [AIPGME 1997]
    (a) Provides 1/2 the total energy requirement & 1/3 the total protein requirement in a child
    (b) A substitute for home diet
    (c) Main objective of this scheme is to eliminate malnutrition
    (d) None of the above

191. Mid day meal contains proteins and calories in what proportions: [AIPGME 1997] [DNB 2000, 2007]
    (a) 1/2 proteins and 1/2 calories
    (b) 1/2 proteins and 1/3rd calories
    (c) 1/3rd proteins and 1/3rd calories
    (d) 2/3rd calories and 1/3rd proteins

192. Dietary changes advocated by WHO for prevention of heart diseases include all of the following except: [AIIMS Dec 1995]
    (a) A decrease in complex carbohydrate consumption.
    (b) Reduction in fat intake to 20–30 per cent of caloric intake.
    (c) Consumption of saturated fats be limited to less than 10% of total energy intake.
    (d) Reduction of cholesterol to below 100 mg per 1000 kcal per day.

193. 'One Dietary Cycle' comprises of: [AIIMS Dec 1992]
    (a) 24 hrs   (b) 48 hrs
    (c) 7 days   (d) 1 month

194. All are examples of Food Fortification except: [AIIMS May 1991]
    (a) Iodisation of salt
    (b) Vitamin A in Vanaspati
    (c) Fluoridation of water
    (d) Saffron colour in milk

195. Nalgonda Technique is used for: [AIPGME 1999]
    (a) Chlorination of water
    (b) Defluoridation of water
    (c) Iodisation of salt
    (d) Detoxification of contaminated mustard oil

196. Salter's Scale is a useful method employed in the field to measure: [AIIMS May 1994]
    (a) Mid arm Circumference
    (b) Length at birth
    (c) Skin fold thickness
    (d) Birth weight

197. What will be the BMI of a male whose weight is 89 kg and height is 172 cm? [AIIMS Nov 1993]
    (a) 27   (b) 30
    (c) 33   (d) 36

198. Which of the following poisonings can result in spastic paraplegia? [DPG 2005]
    (a) Lathyrus   (b) Strychnine
    (c) Sanguinarine   (d) Organophosphates

199. Pellagra: [Karnataka 2008]
    (a) Is due to pyridoxine deficiency
    (b) Occurs with diet chiefly on maize
    (c) Night blindness is a presenting feature
    (d) Causes high output cardiac failure

200. Why cereals and pulses are combined: [DPG 2006]
    (a) 10% cereals contain protein and pulses contain 40%
    (b) Cereals are deficient in methionine and lysine is deficient in pulses
    (c) Cereals are deficient in lysine and methionine is deficient in pulses
    (d) Cereals are rich in essential AA

201. What is/are components of Nutrition surveillance?
    (a) Policy maker   [PGI Nov 2010]
    (b) AFP surveillance
    (c) Nutritional survey
    (d) DOTS

202. Regular drinking of which of the following can help prevent Urinary tract infection (UTI)?
    (a) Grape juice   [AIIMS November 2011]
    (b) Orange juice
    (c) Cranberry juice
    (d) Raspberry juice

203. Common to both acute and chronic malnutrition is: [AIIMS May 2012]
    (a) Weight for age   (b) Weight for height
    (c) Height for age   (d) BMI

204. Food with maximum cholesterol content: [AIIMS May 2012]
    (a) Egg   (b) Coconut oil
    (c) Hydrogenated fats   (d) Ghee (hydrogenated)

205. True about Indian reference male is: [AIIMS May 2012] [NEET Pattern 2012]
    (a) Age 18–29 yrs
    (b) Weight 65 kg
    (c) Work is mainly sedentary
    (d) Works for 10 hrs

206. International food standards include: [JIPMER 2014]
    (a) BIS standards
    (b) Codex alimentarius standards
    (c) AgMark standards
    (d) PFA standards

207. Acute severe malnutrition diagnostic criteria include all except: [AIIMS May 2014] [NEET Pattern 2019]
    (a) Bipedal edema
    (b) Visible severe wasting
    (c) Mid arm circumference below 115 mm
    (d) Weight for height below 2SD of WHO Growth Standards 2006

208. Consider the following statements,
    1. In food preservation by irradiation, ionising rays are used.
    2. Irradiation does not affect the colour, odour, taste, pH and levels of vitamin contents in foods.
    Which of the statements given above is/are correct?
    (a) 1 only
    (b) 2 only   [UPSC CMS 2015]
    (c) Both 1 and 2
    (d) Neither 1 nor 2

209. Consider the following,
    1. Lactic acid
    2. Sorbic acid
    3. Sulphurous acid
    Which of the above are food preservatives?
    (a) 1 and 2 only   [UPSC CMS 2015]
    (b) 2 and 3 only
    (c) None of these
    (d) 1, 2 and 3

Review Questions

210. About protein energy malnutrition, following are true except: [DNB 2001]
    (a) Optimal protein supplementation is 1.5–2g/kg/day
    (b) Hepatomegaly is an essential feature
    (c) Hypothermia may be a cause of death
    (d) Common in developing countries

211. The best parameter for assessment of chronic malnutrition is: [DNB 2002]
    (a) Weight for age
    (b) Weight for height
    (c) Height for age
    (d) Any of the above

212. In assessing the nutritional status of community the following are used except: [UP 2002]
    (a) Mortality in 1–4 years age group
    (b) Low birth weight
    (c) Weight/height index in preschool children
    (d) Percentage of pregnant lady with less than 11.5% Hb

213. Vitamin A prophylaxis includes all except:
    (a) For infant 1,00,000 I.U. at 6 month interval
    (b) For more than 1 years 2,00,000 I.U at 6 month interval
    (c) For postpartum 3,00,000 I.U   [UP 2002]
    (d) 50,000 I.U at birth

214. Nutritional status of community is measured by all except: [AP 2007]
    (a) Mid-arm circumference in 0–1 year age group
    (b) Anemia detection in pregnancy
    (c) Child birth weight <2500 gm
    (d) Height and weight calculated in <5 years age group

215. Methylene blue test is used to detect: [Kolkata 2007]
    (a) Microorganisms
    (b) Lactose
    (c) Protein
    (d) Sugar

216. Calcium content is highest in: [MP 2001]
    (a) Jowar
    (b) Bajra
    (c) Ragi
    (d) Cereals

217. Standardization of food by the directorate of marketing and inspection of government of India is known as: [JIPMER 2005; MH 2006]
    (a) PFA standards
    (b) Codex Alimentarius
    (c) AGMARK standard
    (d) Bureau of India standards

218. A patient has microcytic Anemia, least likely diagnosis is: [RJ 2003]
    (a) Iron deficiency
    (b) Thalassemia
    (c) Sideroblastic anemia
    (d) B12 deficiency

Explanations

ENERGY AND PROTEIN REQUIREMENTS

1. **Ans. (a) 300 kcal throughout pregnancy**
   [Ref. Park 26/e p723]
   - Caloric intake should increase by approximately 300 kcal/day during pregnancy
   - New Nutrition guidelines mention that there should be an additional +350 kcal/day energy to be supplemented in pregnancy

2. **Ans. (c) Vitamin A; (a) Calcium**
   [Ref. Recommended Dietary Allowances & Estimated Average Requirements for Indians – 2020. A SHORT REPORT p7]

   Nutritional requirements: New Nutritional Guidelines 2020–21

	Iron	Folic Acid	Calcium	Vitamin A	Vitamin D
	mg/day	mcg/day	mg/day	mcg/day	IU/day
Man	19	300	1000	1000	600
Woman	29	220	1000	840	600
Pregnancy	40	570	1000	900	600
Lactation	23	330	1200	950	600

3. **Ans. NONE** *[Ref. Park 27/e p748, 751]*
   - *Recommended daily energy and protein intake: (New Guidelines 2021)*

Group	Particulars	Energy (kcal/(d)	Proteins (g/(d)
Adult Male	Sedentary worker	2100	54
	Moderate Worker	2700	54
	Heavy Worker	3500	54
Adult Female	Sedentary worker	1700	45.7
	Moderate Worker	2100	45.7
	Heavy Worker	2700	45.7
	Pregnancy	+350	+9.5, +22
	Lactation (0–6 m)	+600	+17
	Lactation (6–12 m)	+520	+13
Infants	0–6 months	550 kcal/d	8.1
	6–12 months	670 kcal/d	10.5

   In the given question, for an adult pregnant woman with heavy work recommended daily energy intake will be:
   2700 + 300 = 3000 kcal
   Similarly, daily protein intake for such a woman will be 78 gm

   - Total additional energy requirement in a pregnancy, over and above normal metabolic requirements is + 60,000 kcal
   - On an average a healthy adult woman gains 12 kg in pregnancy (6.5 kg in poor Indian women).

4. **Ans. NONE (Now 600 kcal)** *[Ref. Park 27/e p748]*

   > **ALSO REMEMBER**
   > - *Requirement of Iron and Folic Acid:* Pregnancy > Lactation
   > - *Requirement of Calcium and Pyridoxine:* Pregnancy = Lactation
   > - *Requirement of other Nutrients:* Pregnancy < Lactation
   > - *Requirement of Iron:* Non-pregnant state = Lactation
   > - *Requirement of Vitamin B12 and C:* Non-pregnant state = Pregnancy

5. **Ans. (b) 1.0**
   [Ref. Foundations of Community Medicine, 1/e p369]
   - A 'Consumption Unit' is a coefficient of dietary intake, which varies between individuals based on the basis of their age, sex and physical activity
   - Appraisal of dietary intake of very family by weighment method is worked out in terms of consumption units
   - Consumption Unit Coefficients (CUC) of an adolescent = 1.0

6. **Ans. (d) 0.7 gm/kg in terms of Egg protein & 1.0 gm/kg in terms of mixed vegetable protein** *[Ref. Foundations of Community Medicine, 1/e p369]*
   - *Protein requirement of an adult:*
     - 0.7 gm/kg/day in terms of Egg protein or
     - 1.0 gm/kg/day in terms of mixed vegetable protein (NEW GUIDELINE: 0.83 g/kg/d)
   - Egg protein has the highest NPU of 96
   - Indian Council of Medical Research (ICMR) has recommended 1.0 gm protein per kg of body weight for an Indian adult, assuming a NPU of 65 for dietary proteins.

7. **Ans. (c) Energy** *[Ref. Nutrient Requirements and RDAs for Indians, ICMR; p4; Park 21/e p585, Park 22/e p587]*
   - *Recommended Dietary Allowance (RDA):* Is a level of intake corresponding to Mean + 2 Standard Deviation, which covers requirement of 97.5% of population
   - RDA is safe level of intake which is likely to be inadequate in not more than 2.5% population
   - RDA 'safe level approach' is NOT USED FOR ENERGY since excess energy intake is undesirable; For energy only mean or average requirement is defined as RDA.

8. **Ans. (a) 60 g/day** *[Ref. Nutrient Requirements and RDAs for Indians, ICMR; p4; Park 21/e p583–84, Park 22/e p858–586]*
   In the given question, For a 60 kg Indian male, the minimum daily protein requirement with 40 g (mean) ± 10 (Standard deviation), will be:

Mean + 2 SD = 40 + 2(10) = 60 g/day
- RDA 'safe level approach' is Not used for energy since excess energy intake is undesirable; For energy only mean or average requirement is defined as RDA.

9. **Ans. (b) 50 kg weight** [Ref. Park 27/e p747]

   REFERENCE INDIAN WOMAN
   - Age 19–39 years, Weight 55 kg
   - Non-pregnant, Non-lactating, Free from disease, Fit for active work
   - Engaged in 8 hours of occupation (usually moderate activity), 8 hours in bed, 4–6 hours in sitting & moving about, 2 hours in walking and in active recreation or household duties

10. **Ans. (a) Less calories** [Ref. Park 27/e p748,750,751]
    - Energy requirements in kcal/kg/day:
      - *Sedentary worker: 39 kcal/kg/day*
      - *Moderate worker: 46 kcal/kg/day*
      - *Heavy worker: 58 kcal/kg/day*

    As per the given question,
    - Total energy requirement of Farmer (Heavy worker) = 70 kg × 58 kcal/kg/day = 4060 kcal/day
    - Actual consumption = 235 kcal (56 grams proteins @ 4.2 kcal/gram) + 1128 kcal (275 grams carbohydrates @ 4.1 kcal/gram) + 540 kcal (60 grams fats @ 9.0 kcal/gram) = 1903 kcal.

Review Questions

11. **Ans. (b) 150** [Ref. Park 21/e p585, Park 22/e p587]
12. **Ans. (a) Fe** [Ref. Gupta & Mahajan 3/e p 358; Park 21/e p575–76, Park 22/e p577–79]
13. **Ans. (c) 460 and 40 grams** [Ref. Park 21/e p613, Park 22/e p615]

PROTEINS

14. **Ans. (b) Protein diet**
    [Ref. Dietary Protein and Resistance Exercise by Antonio 1/e p127]

    Specific dynamic action (SDA) [Thermic effect of food (TEF)/Dietary induced thermogenesis (DIT)]
    - TEF is the amount of energy expenditure above the basal metabolic rate due to the cost of processing food for use and storage
    - TEF is the energy required for digestion, absorption, and disposal of ingested nutrients
    - TEF magnitude depends on the composition of food consumed: Proteins (20–30% of energy consumed) > Carbohydrates (5–15%) > Fats: (at most 5–15%)
    - A thermic effect of 30% for proteins means that 100 calories of protein only end up as 70 usable calories

15. **Ans. NONE** [Ref. Park 23/e p634]
    - *Net Protein Utilization (NPU):* Is the proportion of ingested proteins that is retained in the body under specified conditions for the maintenance and/or growth of the tissues
    - NPU is a good indicator of protein quality for recommending the dietary protein requirement.

> **ALSO REMEMBER**
> - *Methods of Assessing Protein Quality:* [NEW GUIDELINES 2014]
>   - Digestible indispensable Amino Acid Score (DIAAS) BEST indicator
>   - Protein Digestibility Corrected Amino Acid Score (PDCAAS)
>   - Amino Acid Score (AAS)
>   - Protein Efficiency Ratio (PER): It represents the ratio of weight gain to the amount of protein consumed
>   - Biological Value (BV): Measures the amount of nitrogen retained in comparison to the amount of nitrogen absorbed
>   - Net Protein Utilization (NPU): The ratio of the nitrogen used for tissue formation versus the amount of nitrogen digested.

16. **Ans. (b) 10–15%** [Ref. Park 27/e p749]
    - Assessment of protein quantity is done by 'Protein-Energy Ratio' (PE).

    $$\text{PE percent} = \frac{\text{Energy from protein}}{\text{Total energy in diet}} \times 100$$

    - It is recommended that protein should account for approximately 10–15% of total daily energy intake
    - If PE is less than 4 percent, then the subject will be unable to eat enough to satisfy protein requirements.

17. **Ans. (c) Tyrosine & Cysteine**
    [Ref. & Foundations of Community Medicine, 1/e p369]
    - Conditionally Essential Amino Acids (CEAA): Non-essential amino acids may turn essential if their precursors are limited in the body
      - *There are 2 CEAA, namely, Tyrosine (derived from Phenyaalanine) and Cysteine (derived from methionine)*

> **ALSO REMEMBER**
> - Other CEAA include Arginine, Glutamine, Taurine and Glycine.

18. **Ans. (a) The gain in weight of young animals per unit weight of protein-consumed** [Ref. Dictionary of Public Health, Dr. Jugal Kishore; p423–24, Park 23/e p634]
    - Protein efficiency ratio (PER) is based on the weight gain of a test subject divided by its intake of a particular food protein during the test period
      - *From 1919 until very recently, the PER had been a widely used method for evaluating the quality of protein in food*

19. **Ans. (d) Soya bean** [Ref. Park 27/e p743]
    - Soya bean is richest among pulses. It contains 43.2% proteins (other pulses contain 17–25% proteins)
    - 100 gms Soya bean contain 43 gms proteins, 20 gms fat and 4 gms minerals

- Limiting amino acid in soya bean is methionine
- NPU of soya bean is 55.
- Soyabean also has higher fats, calcium, iron, vitamin B1/B2/B3 than other pulses.

> **ALSO REMEMBER**
> - 'Egg is the reference protein' having NPU of 96.

20. **Ans. (b) Lysine and threonine** *[Ref. Park 27/e p725]*
    - Amino acids most deficient in proteins of a food item are 'Limiting amino acids'

Food Item	Limiting Amino Acid(s)
Cereals	Threonine (& Lysine)
Pulses	Methionine (& Cysteine)
Maize	Tryptophan (& Lysine)

    - Deficiency develops due to only consumption of a particular type of food item with limiting amino acids (e.g. wheat); Thus two or more food items are eaten together so that their proteins supplement one another; this is known as 'Supplementary Action of Proteins'

> **ALSO REMEMBER**
> - *Essential Amino Acids (EAA):* Amino acids which are not synthesized in adequate amounts in the human body; so they have to be supplemented in diet from outside to prevent deficiency.
>   - There are 10 EAA, namely, Phenylalanine, Valine, Threonine, Tryptophan, Isoleucine, Methionine, Histidine, Arginine, Leucine, Lysine
>   **Mnemonic: PVT TIM HALL** or Any Help In Learning These Little Molecules Proves Truly Valuable)
>   - Histidine and Arginine are semi-essential amino acids.

21. **Ans. (b) Methionine** *[Ref. Park 27/e p725]*
22. **Ans. (d) 1 gram protein is equivalent to 1 gram Nitrogen** *[Ref. Park 27/e p749]*
    - 1 gram of Nitrogen is equivalent to: 6.25 grams Proteins
    - NPU of India diets: 50–80
23. **Ans. (b) Wheat** *[Ref. Park 27/e p742]*
24. **Ans. (a) Egg** *[Ref. Park 27/e p745]*
25. **Ans. (b) Net protein utilization** *[Ref. Park 27/e p749]*
26. **Ans. (d) Lysine & Methionine** *[Ref. Park 27/e p725]*
27. **Ans. (b) 0.83 g/kg/d** *[Ref. RDA 2010 Draft Guidelines NIN, p109]*
    - RDA Safe Protein Requirement of High Quality Protein:
      - *1–5 years age: 0.94 g/kg/d*
      - *6–10 years old children: 0.91 g/kg/d*
      - *Adolescent boys: 0.88 g/kg/d*
      - *Adolescents girls: 0.86 g/kg/d*
      - *Adult man/woman: 0.83 g/kg/d*
28. **Ans. (a) 1.5 grams** *[Ref. RDA 2010 Draft, GOI p98]*
    - Protein requirement of infants:
      - *1 month age: 1.41 grams*
      - *2 month age: 1.23 grams*
      - *3 month age: 1.13 grams*
      - *4 month age: 1.07 grams*
      - *6 month age: 0.98 grams*
29. **Ans. (a) 40 grams** *[Ref. Park 27/e p778]*

BALANCED DIETS

Food item	Adult sedentary man	Adult sedentary woman
Cereals	460 g	410 g
Pulses	40 g	40 g
Leafy vegetables	40 g	100 g
Other vegetables	60 g	40 g
Roots and tubers	50 g	50 g
Milk	150 g	100 g
Oil and fat	40 g	20 g
Sugar/jaggery	30 g	20 g

Review Questions

30. **Ans. (b) Soyabean** *[Ref. Park 27/e p743]*
31. **Ans. (a) Lysine** *[Ref. Park 27/e p741]*
    - Rice is deficient in Lysine and Threonine
    - Rice contain higher quantity of Lysine only if compared to other cereals
    - Rice contain high quantities of sulfur-containing amino acids, Cysteine and Methionine
32. **Ans. (b) Lysine** *[Ref. Park 27/e p741]*
33. **Ans. (b) Net protein utilization** *[Ref. Park 27/e p749]*

FATS AND CARBOHYDRATES

34. **Ans. (d) Total calorie content should be 800–1000 kcal**
    [Ref. Assessing the Effects of Food on Drugs in INDs and NDAs FDA-CDER document p12]

    Composition of a High-Fat Meal (FDA)
    - Total Calories 800–1000
    - Calories from Protein 150 kcal
    - Calories from Carbohydrates 250 kcal
    - Calories from Fat 500–600 kcal
    - Percent Calories from Fat >50%

35. **Ans. (b) α-Linolenic acid** *[Ref. Internet 3]*
    - *Essential fatty Acids (EFA):*

Type of fatty acids	Type of chain	Examples
ω-3 Fatty Acids	Short chain Long chain	α-Linolenic acid Eicosapentaenoic acid Docosahexaenoic acid
ω-6 Fatty Acids	Short chain Long chain	Linoleic Acid Arachidonic acid γ-Linolenic acid Dihomo-γ-Linolenic acid

> **ALSO REMEMBER**
> - Safflower oil is the richest source of Linoleic acid, most important Essential fatty Acid
> - Flaxseed Oil is the richest source of Linolenic Acid
> - Fish is the richest source of Eicosapentaenoic acid.

36. Ans. (b) Soya bean oil [Ref. Park 27/e p726]

- Fatty acid content of different fats (%):

Fats	SFA*	MUFA*	PUFA*
Coconut oil	92	6	2
Safflower oil	10	15	75
Sunflower seed oil	8	27	65
Soya bean oil	14	24	62
Margarine	25	25	50
Groundnut oil	19	50	31
Palm oil	46	44	10
Butter	60	37	3

(*SFA: Saturated Fatty Acids; MUFA: Mono-unsaturated Fatty Acids; PUFA: Poly- unsaturated Fatty Acids)

37. Ans. (c) 30 gm [Ref. Park 27/e p750]

- Suggested intake of dietary fat:

Group	Fat intake (g/d)	EFA (energy %)
Adult (Man/Woman)	20	3
Pregnant woman	30	4.5
Lactating mother	45	5.7
Older children	22	3
Young children	25	3

38. Ans. (a) Linoleic Acid [Ref. Park 27/e p725]

- Essential Fatty Acids (EFA): Are those that cannot be synthesized in human body; they can only be derived from the food
- The most important EFA is Linoleic Acid, which serves as a basis for production of other EFA
- Dietary sources of EFA:

EFA	Dietary source	% Content
Linoleic Acid	Safflower Oil	73
	Corn Oil	57
	Sunflower Oil	56
	Soyabean oil	51
Arachidonic Acid	Meat, Eggs	0.5
	Milk (fat)	0.5
Linolenic Acid	Soyabean oil	7
Eicosapentaenoic Acid	Fish oil	10

> **ALSO REMEMBER**
> - EFA deficiency lead to 'Phrynoderma' (Toad Skin): It is characterized by rough rash like eruptions on the back and sides of arms and legs, the back, and the buttocks. It can be cured by giving 'linseed of safflower oil' which are rich in EFAs

39. Ans. (b) B C A [Ref. Park 21/e p585, Park 22/e p587, 24/e p672]

> **ALSO REMEMBER**
> - Energy yield of macro-nutrients (Proximate principles):

Nutrient	Energy yield
Carbohydrates	4 kcal per gram (17 KJ)
Proteins	4 kcal per gram (17 KJ)
Fats	9 kcal per gram (37 KJ)

- Alcohol yields 7 kcal per gram
- Carbohydrates, fats and proteins form the main bulk of food; thus they are known as 'Macronutrients' or 'Proximate principles'
- In 'Balanced Diet',
  - Proteins should constitute 10–15% of total daily energy intake
  - Fats should constitute 15–30% of total daily energy intake
  - Carbohydrates, rich in fibre, should constitute the remaining of energy.

40. Ans. (c) Bajra [Ref. Park 27/e p743]

- Fat content of food items:

Food item	Fat content (per 100 grams)
Jowar	1.9
Bajra	5.0
Ragi	1.3
Rice	0.5
Wheat	1.5
Maize	3.6

41. Ans. (c) Coconut oil [Ref. Park 27/e p726]

42. Ans. (c) Omega-3 fatty acids [Ref. Internet, Wikipedia]

- Omega-3 fatty acids reduce incidence of CHD.

43. Ans. (d) Fruits [Ref. Park 27/e p729]

44. Ans. (b) 1, 2 and 3 [Ref. Park 27/e p726]

45. Ans. (c) Lentils [Ref. Park 27/e p729]

GLYCEMIC INDEX OF FOOD ITEMS
- Low GI (GI ≤55): Most fruits and vegetables (EXCEPT potato/watermelon/sweet potato), Whole grains, Beans, Pasta, Lentils)
- Medium GI (GI 56–69): Sucrose, Basmati rice, Brown rice
- High GI (GI ≥70): Corn flakes, Baked potato, White bread, Candy bar, Syrupy food, Jasmine rice.

46. **Ans. (b) Vitamin A** [Ref. Park 25/e p696]
    - Vanaspati is fortified with '2500 IU vitamin A and 175 IU vitamin D' per 100 grams

Review Questions

47. **Ans. (b) Safflower oil** [Ref. Park 27/e p726]
48. **Ans. (a) 10–30** [Ref. Park 27/e p726, 750]

VITAMINS

49. **Ans. (c) Niacin** [Ref. Park 27/e p734]
    - Pellagra occurs due to Vitamin B3 (Niacin) deficiency
    - Pellagra is characterized by 4 D's: Diarrhoea, Dermatitis, Dementia, Death

50. **Ans. (d) Thiamine deficiency** [Ref. Park 27/e p733]
    - Wernicke-Korsakoff syndrome is caused by a deficiency of Thiamine (Vitamin B1)
    - Patients classically present with a "Clinical triad" of Ophthalmoplegia, Altered mental status, and Ataxia

51. **Ans. (c) C** [Ref. Park 27/e p736]
    - Classic constellation of corkscrew hairs, perifollicular hemorrhage, and gingival bleeding is highly suggestive of vitamin C deficiency (Scurvy)
    - Bleeding gums, conjunctival hemorrhages, most petechiae, and ecchymoses are nonspecific

52. **Ans. (c) Scurvy** [Ref. Park 26/e p711]
    - Vitamin C is functionally most relevant for the triple-helix formation of collagen
    - Vitamin C deficiency (Scurvy) results in impaired collagen synthesis (Delayed wound healing)

53. **Ans. (c) Niacin (B3)** [Ref. Park 26/e p709]
    - Pellagra is common in maize/jowar eating populations as the Limiting amino acid in maize is Tryptophan
    - 'Excess of Leucine' in such populations appears to interfere in conversion of Tryptophan to Niacin

54. **Ans. (c) Retinoic acid** [Ref. Park 26/e p705–706]
    - Xerophthalmia (Vitamin A deficiency) is associated with night blindness, dry conjunctiva, bitot spots, dull/dry cornea, corneal ulcer and keratomalacia
    - Extra-ocular manifestations include anorexia, growth retardation, hyperkeratosis, predisposition to respiratory/intestinal infections

55. **Ans. (c) Pyridoxine**
    [Ref. Pyridoxine-dependent Seizures: A Review by R Rajesh. Indian Paediatrics 2003; 40:633–638]
    - Pyridoxine-dependent epilepsy (PDE) is a rare cause of stubborn, difficult to control, (intractable) seizures appearing in newborns, infants and occasionally older children
    - Underlying cause: Inborn abnormality of the enzyme glutamic acid decarboxylase, which results in reduced pyridoxine-dependent synthesis of the inhibitory neurotransmitter gamma amino butyric acid (GABA)
    - Diagnosis: Parenteral pyridoxine injection test
    - Treatment: Loading dose B6 (50–100 mg) + Maintenance therapy (10–200 mg/day)

56. **Ans. (c) Niacin** [Ref. Park 25/e p676]
    - Pellagra is common in maize/jowar eating populations as the Limiting amino acid in maize is Tryptophan
    - 'Excess of Leucine' in such populations appears to interfere in conversion of Tryptophan to Niacin

57. **Ans. (a) Animal only diet** [Ref. Park 25/e p677]
    - No plant source is available for Vitamin B12 and Vitamin D

58. **Ans. (b) Vitamin B3** [Ref. Harrison, 15/e p463; Park 27/e p734]

    PELLAGRA
    - Pellagra occurs due to Vitamin B3 (Niacin) deficiency
    - Pellagra is characterized by 4 D's:
        - Diarrhoea
        - Dermatitis
        - Dementia
        - Death
    - Skin rash in pellagra may appear as pigmented and scaly in areas exposed to sunlight. Esp. neck when it is known as 'Casal's Necklace'

    > **ALSO REMEMBER**
    > - Pellagra is common in maize/jowar eating populations:
    >   - Limiting amino acid in maize is Tryptophan. 60 mg Tryptophan is converted to 1 mg Niacin in the body
    >   - Excess of leucine' in such populations appears to interfere in conversion of tryptophan to niacin

59. **Ans. (d) 1.0%** [Ref. Park 27/e p731]
    - *Prevalence criteria for determining the Xerophthalmia problem in a community*

Criteria	Prevalence
Night blindness	>1.0%
Bitot's spots	>0.5%
Corneal xerosis/corneal ulceration/keratomalacia	>0.01%
Corneal ulcer	>0.05%
Serum retinol (<10 mcg/dL)	>5.0%

    - Prevalence is measured in population at risk, i.e., preschool children 6 months - 6 years.

60. **Ans. (a) 500 mcg** [Ref. Park 27/e p751]
    - Body stores of folate are not large (about 5–10 mg), therefore folate deficiency can develop quickly
    - *Recommended daily intake values of folate:*

Group	Intake per day
Healthy adults	200 mcg
Pregnancy	500 mcg
Lactation	300 mcg
Children	100 mcg

    - *An adult tablet of IFA contains:* 100 mg elemental Iron and 500 mcg Folic acid (to be given for 100 days minimum in pregnancy)

- A pediatric tablet of IFA contains: 20 mg elemental Iron and 100 mcg Folic acid (to be given for 100 days minimum every year till 5 years age of child)

61. **Ans. (b) Conjunctival xerosis** [Ref. Park 27/e p730–731]
    - All the ocular manifestations of Vitamin-A deficiency are collectively known as 'Xerophthalmia' (Dry Eye)
      - Xerophthalmia is most common in children aged 1–3 years
    - 'First clinical sign' of Vitamin-A deficiency: Conjunctival xerosis
    - 'First clinical symptom' of Vitamin-A deficiency: Night blindness
    - Conjunctival xerosis in Xerophthalmia has a characteristic appearance of 'emerging like sand banks at receding tide
    - 'Bitot's Spots' are triangular, pearly-white or yellowish, foamy spots on bulbar conjunctiva, on either side of cornea; In young children they indicate Vitamin-A deficiency, whereas in adults they are often inactive sequelae of earlier disease

62. **Ans. NONE** [Ref. Park 23/e p616]
    - Under National Immunisation Schedule (NIS), Vitamin-A is given; (Older Guidelines)
      - 1 lac IU at 9 months age (along with measles vaccine),
      - 2 lac IU every six months thereafter, till the age of 3 years (at 18, 24, 30 and 36 months of age)
      - A total of 9 lac IU is given
    - Vitamin-A is administered by a '2 mL spoon'
    - Strength of Vitamin-A solution: 1 lac IU per mL
    - Under the New Guidelines in Nis, Vitamin-A is given;
      - 1 lac IU at 9 months age (along with measles vaccine),
      - 2 lac IU every six months thereafter, till the age of 5 years (at 18, 24, 30, 36, 42, 48, 54 and 60 months of age)
      - A total of 17 lac IU is given

63. **Ans. (a) 5 min** [Ref. Park 23/e p617]
    - Vitamin D can be synthesized in the body in adequate amounts by simple exposure to sunlight even for 5 minutes per day
    - Vitamin D is synthesized in sunlight when '7-dehydrocholesterol (present in abundance in skin) is converted to cholecalciferol'
    - 'UV-B rays' (wavelength 270–300 nm) play an important role in Vitamin D synthesis
    - Vitamin D is 'Kidney Hormone'
    - Two major forms of Vitamin D are D2 (Ergocalciferol/calciferol) and D3 (Cholecalciferol)
    - There is no plant source for Vitamin D (and Vitamin B12)
    - Vitamin D deficiency leads to rickets, osteomalacia, osteoporosis and colon cancer.

64. **Ans. (c) Pantothenic acid** [Ref. Harrison, 15/e p465]
    - Pantothenic acid deficiency was thought to be cause of 'Burning Feet/Sole Syndrome' among prisoners of World War II
    - Pantothenic acid is required by adrenal cortex.

65. **Ans. (d) 1,00,000 IU** [Ref. Park 27/e p731]
    - Community based intervention against nutritional blindness:
      - Evolved by National Institute of Nutrition (NIN), Hyderabad
    - Strategy:
      - Administer a single massive dose of 200,000 IU of Vitamin A (Retinol palmitate) orally every six months to pre-school children (1–6 years age)
      - Half that dose (100,000 IU) be administered to children between 6 months – 1 year age
      - Also known as 'Immunization against Xerophthalmia'
      - Incidence of Keratomalacia reduced by 80%.

66. **Ans. (b) 0.5%** [Ref. Park 27/e p731]

67. **Ans. (d) Cod liver oil [BUT overall Richest source is Halibut liver oil]** [Ref. Park 27/e p730]

68. **Ans. (a) Fortified in all wheat products in India like as in USA** [Ref. Park 27/e p735]
    FOLIC ACID
    - India has NOT YET adopted recommendation of fortification of all wheat products in India with Folic acid
    - Preconceptionally given for prevention of neural tube defects
    - It is present in leafy vegetables, spinach, paneer
    - Requirement per day in pregnancy is 500 mcg

69. **Ans. (c) Excess of Leucine** [Ref. Park 27/e p742]

70. **Ans. (b) Bitot's spot** [Ref. Postgraduate Xerophthalmia (Volume 2) by Zia Choudhary, 1/e p591]

WHO Classification of Xerophthalmia

Primary signs	Secondary signs
X1A Conjunctival xerosis	XN Night blindness
X1B Bitot spots	XF Xerophthalmic fundus
X2 Corneal xerosis	XS Xerophthalmic scarring
X3A Corneal ulceration	
X3B Keratomalacia	

71. **Ans. (b) Niacin** [Ref. Park 27/e p734]

72. **Ans. (c) 3** [Ref. Guidelines for the inpatient treatment of severely malnourished children, WHO p23]
    - Vitamin A deficiency treatment: Vitamin A on days 1, 2 and 14 each (for age >12 months, give 200,000 IU; for age 6–12 months, give 100,000 IU; for age 0–5 months, give 50,000 IU)

73. **Ans. (d) Halibut fish liver oil** [Ref. Park 27/e p730]

74. **Ans. (d) B6** [Ref. Encyclopedia of Aging and Public Health by Loue, 1/e p813]
    - Daily requirements of pyridoxine are directly related to protein intake
    - With a low protein diet, less vitamin is needed

75. **Ans. (d) Gingelly seeds** *[Ref. Park 27/e p733]*
    - Thiamine content of food items: Gingelly seeds (Highest) > Ground nut > Bengal gram > Whole wheat > Sheep liver > Raw rice

Review Questions

76. **Ans. (c) Bitot spots-0.5%** *[Ref. Park 27/e p731]*
77. **Ans. (d) All of the above** *[Ref. Gupta & Mahajan 3/e p335; Park 27/e p732]*
78. **Ans. (d) Sitaphal** *[Ref. Park 27/e p735–736]*
79. **Ans. (a) Milk** *[Ref. Park 27/e p732]*
80. **Ans. (d) Megaoblastic anaemia** *[Ref. Park 27/e p735]*
81. **Ans. (d) Groundnut** *[Ref. Park 27/e p733]*
82. **Ans. (a) Bitot's spots 0.05%** *[Ref. Park 27/e p731]*
83. **Ans. (c) Indian goose berry** *[Ref. Park 27/e p736]*

IRON

84. **Ans. (c) Ferrous fumarate + Folic acid + Vitamin B12 + Vitamin C** *[Ref. Park 26/e p732]*
    MC causes of Anaemia
    - Nutritional deficiencies: Iron, Folate, Vitamin B12 and Vitamin A
    - Haemoglobinopathies
    - Infectious diseases: Malaria, TB, HIV and Parasitic infections

85. **Ans. (b) Serum ferritin** *[Ref. Park 27/e p738]*
    - Evaluation of iron status in the body can be done by:
      – *Hemoglobin concentration:* A relatively insensitive index of nutrient depletion
      – *Serum iron concentration:* Normal range is 0.80 - 1.80 mg/L
      – *Serum ferritin:* 'Most sensitive tool for evaluation of iron status', especially in populations with low prevalence of anemia
      – *Serum transferring saturation:* Normal value is 30%

86. **Ans. (a) Less than 11 g/dL** *[Ref. Park 27/e p738]*
    - Cut-off points for diagnosis of anemia (WHO):

Group	Hb (g/dL)	MCHC (%)
Adult males	13	34
Adult females, non-pregnant	12	34
Adult females, pregnant	11	34
Children, 6 m - 6 y	11	34
Children, 6 y - 14 y	12	34

87. **Ans. (d) Soya bean** *[Ref. Park 27/e p738]*
    - Only Bengal gram contains Vitamin C among the common pulses
    - Iron absorption from Indian diets is less than 5%.

88. **Ans. (a) <5%** *[Ref. Park 27/e p737]*
    - Iron absorption from habitual Indian diets is less than 5%
    - Iron absorption is low in Indian diets due to presence of inhibitors (phytates, tannates, oxalates, calcium)
    - Vitamin C (Ascorbic acid) is a facilitator of iron absorption

89. **Ans. (a) Milk** *[Ref. Park 27/e p743]*
    - Iron content of food items:

Food item	Iron content (mg per 100 grams)
Jowar	4.1
Bajra	8.0
Ragi	3.9
Bengal gram	4.6
Horse gram	6.7
Peas dry	7.0
Soyabean	10.4
Banana	0.5
Mango	1.3
Sitaphal	4.3
Raisins	7.7
Dates	7.3
Milk	0.2–0.3

90. **Ans. (b) High doses of Vitamin C** *[Ref. Park 27/e p757–758]*
91. **Ans. (d) Jaggery** *[Ref. Multiple sources]*
92. **Ans. (a) Biweekly supplementation of iron & FA to 6–60 months of age** *[Ref. National Iron Plus Initiative Guidelines, MoHFW, GOI]*

    IFA SUPPLEMENTATION – NATIONAL IRON PLUS INITIATIVE
    - 6–60 months age: 20 mg of elemental iron and 100 mcg of folic acid, Biweekly (Syrup)
    - 5–10 years age: 45 mg elemental iron and 400 mcg of folic acid, Weekly
    - 10–19 years age: 100 mg elemental iron and 500 mcg of folic acid, Weekly
    - 10–19 years age: 100 mg elemental iron and 500 mcg of folic acid, 1 tablet daily for 100 days (starting after the first trimester), to be repeated for 100 days post-partum
    - Women in reproductive age (WRA) group: 100 mg elemental iron and 500 mcg of folic acid, Weekly

93. **Ans. (a) A tablet containing 100 mg elemental iron and 500 mcg of folic acid weekly for aged 10–19 years** *[Ref. National Iron Plus Initiative Guidelines, MoHFW, GOI]*

94. **Ans. (b) Adolescents of age group 10–19 years are covered; (d) Biannual deworming through Albendazole tablet; (e) Screening of target groups for moderate/severe anaemia and referring these cases to an appropriate health facility** *[Ref. National Iron Plus Initiative Guidelines, MoHFW, GOI]*

    National Iron+ Initiative
    - Target beneficiary groups:
      – *Preschool children (6 months-5 years)*

- School children (I-V class) in Govt. & Govt. Aided schools
- Out of school children (5–10 years) at Anganwadi centres
- Adolescents (10–19 years)
- Pregnant and lactating women
- Women in reproductive age (15–49 years)

- IFA supplement for 6–60 months aged children to be administered under the direct supervision of ANM/ASHA on fixed days on a biweekly basis; Micro plan for reaching out to these children to be worked out at village level
- Albendazole tablets will be provided to children for biannual de-worming; Half tablet between 1–2 years age and full tablet from the age >2 years
- Weekly dose of 100 mg elemental iron and 500 mcg folic acid with Biannual de-worming to be done in adolescents (10–19 years) under WIFS
  - WIFS program will be implemented in urban and rural areas for adolescent boys and girls in school (10–19 years) through the platform of Government/Government aided/Municipal schools
  - WIFS will also reach out-of-school girls in the age group 10–19 years through the platform of Anganwadi Kendras
- ASHAs and ANMs will screen children from 6–60 months for signs of Anaemia as per IMNCI Guidelines through opportunistic screening at (and referral if required)
  - VHNDs
  - Immunization sessions
  - House-to-house visits by ASHAs for biweekly IFA supplementation
  - Sick child coming to health facility (Sub-centre/PHC)

95. Ans. (b) 35 mg/day   [Ref. Park 27/e p757–758]

Iron in Pregnancy

- Iron requirement per day in Non-pregnant woman: 1.6 mg per day
- Iron intake (suggested) per day in Non-pregnant woman: 21 mg per day
- Iron requirement per day in Pregnant woman: 2.8 mg per day
- Iron intake (suggested) per day in Pregnant woman: 35 mg per day
- Iron content of IFA tablets in Pregnancy: 100 mg per day
- Total iron requirement in Pregnancy: 1000 mg

IODINE AND FLUORINE

96. Ans. (a) 0.5–0.8 mg/L   [Ref. Park 27/e p739]

- The recommended level of fluorides in drinking water in India is accepted as '0.5–0.8 mg/litre' (0.5–0.8 ppm)
- In temperate countries where water intake is low, the optimum level of fluorides in drinking water is accepted as 1–2 mg/litre
- 'Fluorine is a double edged sword: 'Inadequate intake is associated with 'dental caries' whereas excess intake with 'dental and skeletal fluorosis'.

> **ALSO REMEMBER**
> - Daily requirement for Iodine for adults: >150 mcg.

97. Ans. (b) Central Incisors & 1st Molars   [Ref. Park 27/e p739]

- Dental fluorosis occurs when excess fluoride is ingested during first 7 years of life (years of tooth calcification)
  - It occurs at levels above 1.5 mg/litre intake
  - It is characterized by 'Mottling', which is best seen on incisors of upper jaw.

> **ALSO REMEMBER**
> - *Major source of fluorine to man:* Drinking water
> - *Optimum level of fluorine in drinking water:* 0.5–0.8 ppm (0.5–0.8 mg/litre)
>   - *Level >1.5 ppm:* Dental fluorosis (mottling)
>   - *Level 3.0–6.0 ppm:* Skeletal fluorosis
>   - *Level >10.0 ppm:* Crippling fluorosis

98. Ans. (d) 30 ppm at Production level & 15 ppm at consumer level   [Ref. Park 27/e p738–739]

- Iodisation of salt is the 'most widely used prophylactic measure against prevention of goiter'
  - Iodised salt is most convenient, effective and economical method of mass prophylaxis in endemic areas
- According to Prevention of Food Adulteration (PFA) Act' 1954:
  - Level of iodisation: Minimum '30 ppm at production level and 15 ppm at consumer level'
  - Moisture content: <6.0% by weight
  - Sodium chloride: >96.0% by weight.

> **ALSO REMEMBER**
> - *Iodine requirement:* 150 mcg per day (<1 teaspoon over lifetime)
> - *Salt containing compound potassium iodide is termed 'Iodised salt' whereas salt containing compound potassium iodate is termed 'Iodated salt'*
> - *Global Iodine Deficiency Disorders (IDD) Day:* 21st October
> - *Criteria for tracking progress towards IDD elimination:*
>
> | Indicator | Goal |
> |---|---|
> | % with enlarged thyroid (age 6–12 years) | <5% |
> | Urinary Iodine Excretion below 100 mcg/litre | <50% |
> | Urinary Iodine Excretion below 50 mcg/litre | <20% |
> | % houses consuming adequately iodised salt | >90% |

99. Ans. (c) 3–4 years   [Ref. Park 27/e p 738–739]

- Intramuscular Iodised Oil (poppy-seed oil): Average dose 1 mL injection provided protection for 4 years
- Oral Iodised Oil: 2 mL dose is effective for 2 years

100. Ans. (c) 150 mcg   [Ref. Park 27/e p739]

- The daily requirement of iodine is 150 mcg supplied normally by well balanced diets and drinking water.

> **ALSO REMEMBER**
> - *Indicators for epidemiological assessment of iodine deficiency:*
>   - Prevalence of goitre
>   - Prevalence of cretinism
>   - Urinary iodine excretion
>   - Measurement of thyroid function (T4, TSH)
>   - Prevalence of neonatal hypothyroidism
> - *Some noteworthy daily requirements:*
>
> | Nutrient | Recommended daily requirement |
> |---|---|
> | Calcium | 400–500 mg |
> | Iron | 17 mg (males); 21 mg (females) |
> | Iodine | 150 mcg |
> | Fluorine | 0.5–0.8 mg/litre |

101. **Ans. (c) 10%** *[Ref. Assessment of IDD and monitoring their elimination, WHO, 3rd Ed.]*

    - Epidemiological criteria for assessing severity of IDD:
      - Total Goitre Rate (TGR) - Grade I + Grade II
      - Median Urinary Iodine Excretion
      - Thyroid volume (ultrasound)
      - Salt iodine content
    - Criteria for Sustainable Elimination of IDD:
      - Median Urinary Iodine Excretion 100 mcg/l
      - Level of iodization:
        1. 30 ppm at production level
        2. 15 ppm at consumer level
      - Total Goitre Rate (TGR) <5%.

102. **Ans. (d) 250 mcg** *[Ref. Park 27/e p751]*
    - India has recently adopted WHO guideline of 250 mcg per day in pregnancy
    - Iodine requirement in Adult: 150 mcg per day

103. **Ans. (b) 20 micro gram/day** *[Ref. Mechanism of Iodine Deficiency, UN System documents, Chapter 6]*

104. **Ans. (d) 3:10**
    [Ref. Fifth Report on the World Nutrition Situation: Nutrition for Improved Development Outcomes. 2004]

105. **Ans. (c) 3.0–6.0 ppm** *[Ref. Park 27/e p758–759]*

106. **Ans. (d) >10 ppm** *[Ref. Park 27/e p758–759]*

107. **Ans. (d) 290 mcg per day** *[Ref. Park 27/e p751]*

    Iodine Requirements
    - India had adopted WHO guideline of Iodine requirement 150 mcg per day in Adults, 250 mcg per day in Pregnancy and 280 mcg per day in Lactation
    - US recommended daily allowances (RDA) for iodine intake are 150 mcg in adults, 220–250 mcg in pregnant women, and 250–290 mcg in breastfeeding women.
    [PLEASE NOTE: Since 280 mcg is not mentioned in the choices, logically one should consider next higher value option 290 mcg, so as to prevent deficiency among lactating women].

108. **Ans. (b) Goiter prevalence of 10% is cut-off value for endemicity; (c) Strabismus is also a manifestation** *[Ref. Park 27/e p758]*
    - Iodine Deficiency Disorders (IDD)
    - IDD include Goitre, Hypothyroidism, Mental deficiency, Hearing/speech defects, Delayed motor milestones, Strabismus, Nystagmus, Spasticity, NM weakness, Cretinism, IUD
    - An area arbitrarily defined as Endemic If >10% of its population was found to be Goitrous on appropriate survey
    - Monitoring done by Urinary iodine excretion levels, Iodine in soil/food/water, Iodization level of salt

Review Questions

109. **Ans. (d) 1.5** *[Ref. Park 21/e p577, Park 22/e p579, 24/e p663]*
110. **Ans. (a) 0–3 months** *[Ref. Park 23/e p623]*
111. **Ans. (a) Butter** *[Ref. Park 23/e p628–629]*

OTHER NUTRIENTS

112. **Ans. (b) Zinc** *[Ref. Park 27/e p740]*
    - Zinc deficiency is Acrodermatitis enteropathica (ADE), a disorder of zinc absorption or acquired, usually described in alcoholics
    - Clinical triad of acral dermatitis, alopecia and diarrhea
    - Zinc deficiency may decrease rates of fibroplasia, epithelialization, and collagen synthesis and impaired wound healing

113. **Ans. (c) 40 gm** *Ref. Park 27/e p729]*
    - Dietary fibre is a non-starch polysaccharide and a physiologically important component of diet; there are two types of dietary fibres:
      - *Insoluble fibres: Cellulose, hemi-cellulose and lignin*
      - *Soluble fibres: Pectins, gums and mucilages*
    - A daily intake of about 40 grams of fibre is desirable
    - Indian diets provide about 50–100 grams of fibre per day
    - Cereals and pulses are good sources of fibre (>10 gm fibre per 100 gm).

114. **Ans. (c) Lead** *[Ref. Park 23/e p621–626]*
    - *Macronutrients:* Proximate Principles which form the bulk of the diet
      - *Carbohydrates*
      - *Fats*
      - *Proteins*
    - *Micronutrients:* Vitamin and Minerals (which are required in small quantities).
      - *Major minerals: Sodium, Potassium, Magnesium, Calcium, Phosphorus*
      - *Trace elements: Iron, Iodine, Fluorine, Zinc, Copper, Cobalt, Selenium, Chromium, Manganese, Molybdenum, Nickel, Tin, Silicon, Vanadium*
      - *Trace contaminant with no known function in body: Lead, Mercury, Barium, Boron, Aluminium.*

115. **Ans. None of the choices**
    [Ref. Vitamins-the fundamental aspects in nutrition and health by Gerald F. Combs, 3/e p 376]
    - Zinc deficiency

- Growth failure
- Sexual infantilism
- Impaired immunity
- Decreased insulin synthesis
- Delayed wound healing
- Loss of taste (Ageusia)
- Liver disease (Hepatomegaly + Splenomegaly), Pernicious anemia, Thalassemia, Myocardial infarction
- Megaloblastic anemia (due to reduced absorption of Folyl-glutamates)
- Maternal zinc deficiency: Spontaneous abortion, Congenital malformation (Anencephaly), Low birth weight, IUGR, Preterm delivery.

116. Ans. (a) 20 mg/day [Ref. Neonatal Formulary, 5/e p270]
117. Ans. (b) 600 mg [Ref. Park 27/e p751]
118. Ans. (b) 500 mg [Ref. Park 27/e p751]
119. Ans. (a) Selenium [Ref. Selenium in Food and Health by C Reilly, 5/e p91]
120. Ans. (b) Inherited disorder of impaired uptake of zinc from body [Ref. NUTR by Beerman, 1/e p217]
121. Ans. (d) Excessive Appetite [Ref. Park 27/e p739–740]
    - *Zinc deficiency:* Growth failure, Sexual infantilism, Loss of taste, Delayed wound healing, Loss of integrity of immune system, Spontaneous abortions, Congenital malformations, Low birth weight, IUGR, Preterm delivery, Skin lesions, Depressed appetite, Skeletal abnormalities
122. Ans. (d) Ragi [Ref. Park 27/e p729]
    - Dietary fibre content: Ragi > Cluster beans > Maize > Jowar > Bajra/Chick pea
    - Richest source of Dietary fibre: Miller's bran
123. Ans. (b) Oats [Ref. Park 27/e p729]

Review Questions

124. Ans. (b) Hyperactivity [Ref. Park 21/e p576, Park 22/e p578]
125. Ans. (d) 2.0 mg/L [Ref. Park 27/e p739]
126. Ans. (a) Dates [Ref. Park 21/e p581, Park 22/e p583]
127. Ans. (d) All of the above [Ref. Park 27/e p739–740]
128. Ans. (c) Increased biological value and +NPU [Ref. Park 27/e p745]

EGG

129. Ans. (c) Biotin [Ref. Nutrition by Webb 4/e p389]
    - Prolonged consumption of raw eggs may cause biotin deficiency because raw egg white contains an antimicrobial protein known as avidin that tightly binds biotin and prevents its absorption
130. Ans. (b) Carbohydrate & Vitamin C [Ref. Park 27/e p745]
    Food Items as Poor Sources of Nutrients:
    - Milk is a poor source of Vitamin C and Iron
    - Meat is a poor source of Calcium
    - Fish is a poor source of Carbohydrates
    - Egg is a poor source of Vitamin C and Carbohydrates

> **ALSO REMEMBER**
> - An egg (60 grams) contain: 6 gm proteins, 6 gm fat, 30 mg calcium, 1.5 mg iron, 250 mg cholesterol and 70 kcal energy
> - Egg protein is best among proteins (NPU = 96), thereby making it 'Reference Protein'

131. Ans. (b) 96 [Ref. Foundations of Community Medicine, 1/e p369; Park 25/e p648, 668]
    - *Net Protein Utilization (NPU):* Provides a complete expression of 'protein quality'

    $$NPU = \frac{\text{Nitrogen retained by body}}{\text{Nitrogen intake}} \times 100$$

    $$NPU = \frac{\text{Biological value} \times \text{Digestibility coefficient}}{100}$$

    - *NPU of selected food items:*

Food Item	Net Protein Utilization
Egg (hen)	96*
Milk (cow)	81
Meat	79
Fish	77
Rice	65
Soyabean	55
Wheat	51
Grams (pulses)	45–50
Groundnut	50

(*NPU of egg is 96. Since egg is 'reference protein', its NPU is taken as 100 for comparison)

132. Ans. (c) 60 gm of egg contain 6 gm protein, 6 gm fat, 30 mg calcium [Ref. Park 27/e p745]
    EGG AS A FOOD ITEM
    - 6 gm proteins, 6 gm fat, 30 mg calcium, 1.5 mg iron, 250 mg cholesterol and 70 kcal energy
    - Poor in Carbohydrates and Vitamin C
    - NPU is 96 (Highest NPU, Highest Quality of proteins)
    - Contains all essential amino acids in correct proportions

Review Questions

133. Ans. (c) Carbohydrate [Ref. Park 27/e p745]
134. Ans. (b) It has best quality of protein [Ref. Park 27/e p745]

MILK

135. Ans. (d) Iodine test [Ref. Park 26/e p744]
    - Methods of Pasteurization: Holder/Vat Method, HTST (Flash) Method, HHST Method, UHT Method

- Tests of Pasteurized Milk (for adequacy/sufficiency of pasteurization): Phosphatase Test, Standard Plate Count, Coliform Count
- Methylene Blue Reduction Test: An indirect method for detection of microorganisms in milk (Test for Contamination of milk)

136. **Ans. (b) 65°C for 30 minutes** [Ref. Park 27/e p744]

- *Methods of Pasteurization:*

Method	Temp	Time	Remarks
Holder/Vat Method	63–66°C	>30 min	For small and rural communities
HTST Method	72°C	>15 sec	Most widely used; for large quantities; 'Flash Pasteurization'
HHST Method	68°C	30 min	'Batch Pasteurization'
UHT Method	125°C	Few sec	Heating in 2 stages; 2nd stage under pressure

ALSO REMEMBER
- *Some other noteworthy temperatures:*

Method/Procedure	Temperature
Incineration	>1200 °C
Autoclave	121°C at 15 psi for 45–60 min 135°C at 3–10 psi for 30 min
Cold Chain	+2° to +8°C
OPV (Long term storage)	−15° to −25°C
Yellow fever vaccine	−30° to +5°C
Reverse Cold Chain	+2° to +8°C
Parboiling (Hot Soaking)	65°–70°C
Comfort Zone (Effective temp)	25–27°C
Heat exhaustion	>102°F
Heat hyperpyrexia	>106°F
Heat stroke	>110°F

137. **Ans. (d) Methylene blue reduction test** [Ref. Park 27/e p769]

- Tests of Pasteurized Milk (for adequacy/sufficiency of pasteurization):
  - Phosphatase Test: Widely used test
  - Standard Plate Count: Enforced limit is 30,000 bacterial count per mL of pasteurized milk
  - Coliform Count: Standard is coliforms be absent in 1 mL of milk
- 'Methylene Blue Reduction Test':
  - Is an indirect method for detection of microorganisms in milk
  - The test is 'carried out on milk accepted for pasteurization'
  - Blue colour disappears from milk when held at a uniform temperature of 37°C: Milk which remains blue the longest is of best quality

138. **Ans. (c) Vitamin C** [Ref. Park 27/e p744]
- Milk is a good source of all vitamins except Vitamin C.

ALSO REMEMBER
- *Milks available in India:*

Milk Type	Fat content	SNF (Solid-not-fat) content
Full cream	6.0%	9.0%
Standardised	4.5%	8.5%
Toned	3.0%	8.5%
Double toned	1.5%	9.0%
Skimmed	0.5%	8.7%

139. **Ans. (c) Iron; (e) Vitamin C** [Ref. Park 27/e p744]

140. **Ans. (a) Cow's milk contains 80% whey protein and not casein** [Ref. Park 27/e p744]

141. **Ans. (c) Human milk, Curd (Cow's milk), Buffalo milk, Cheese** [Ref. Park 27/e p744]
- Fat content of milk (gm per 100 mL): Human (3.3) < Cow (4.1) < Goat (4.5) < Buffalo (6.5) < Cheese (9–20)

142. **Ans. (d) 1, 2 and 3** [Ref. Milk Processing and Quality Management by Tamime, 1/e p54]

143. **Ans. (c) Docosahexaenoic acid** [Ref. Nutrition and Metabolism, 1/e, Section 8.5]
- Breast milk contains higher amounts of Docosahexaenoic acid (DHA)
  - DHA is an omega-3 fatty acid required for brain development
  - Levels in breast milk depend on mother's consumption of foods rich in omega-3 fatty acids namely, flax and fish
  - Longer the duration of breast feeding, higher the DHA levels in infants.

144. **Ans. (c) Increased proteins** [Ref. Nutrition through Life Cycle by Judith E Brown, 3/e p160]

145. **Ans. (c) Vitamin D [Vitamin D is in Least Quantity]** [Ref. Understanding Nutrition by Whitney & Rolfes, 12/e p533]

146. **Ans. (a) Quality of pasteurization** [Ref. Park 27/e p769–770]

147. **Ans. (a) 65°C for 30 min** [Ref. Park 27/e p769]

148. **Ans. (c) Coxiella burnetii** [Ref. Essentials of Microbiology by Kumar 1/e p27]
All non-sporing pathogens like Mycobacterium, Brucellae and Salmonellae are destroyed by Pasteurisation
Coxiella burnetii is relatively heat-resistant and may survive the Holder method

Review Questions

149. **Ans. (a) Iron** [Ref. Park 27/e p744]

150. **Ans. (a) Low lactose; (b) Contains more Vitamin-D**
 [Ref. Park 27/e p744]
151. **Ans. (d) Endemic typhus** [Ref. Park 27/e p769]
152. **Ans. (a) Human milk** [Ref. Park 27/e p744]
153. **Ans. (c) Ascorbic acid** [Ref. Park 27/e p744]
154. **Ans. (a) Lactose** [Ref. Park 27/e p744]

OTHER FOOD ITEMS

155. **Ans. (c) a-IV, b-III, c-I, d-II** [Ref. Park 23/e p615, 621, 634]

> **ALSO REMEMBER**
> - Among common vegetables, cabbage is the richest source of Vitamin C. (But also a Goitrogen)

156. **Ans. (d) Lysine** [Ref. Park 25/e p665]
  - Rice is a poor source of Thiamine, Calcium, Iron and Vitamins A, D, C
  - Protein content of rice varies from 6–9%
    - 'Rice proteins are better than other cereal proteins' as rice is richer in lysine
  - Rice is staple food of >50 % population globally.

> **ALSO REMEMBER**
> - Food Items as Rich Sources of nutrients:
>   - Halibut Liver Oil is richest source of Vitamin A and Vitamin D
>   - Indian Gooseberry (amla) is richest source of Vitamin C
>   - Gingelly seeds are richest source of Vitamin B1 (Thiamine)
>   - Sheep liver is richest source of Vitamin B2 (Riboflavin)
>   - Ragi (millet) is a rich source of calcium
>   - Dried pumpkin seeds > Pistachio is the richest source of iron.

157. **Ans. (b) Iodine** [Ref. Park 27/e p744]
  - Richest source of Vitamin A and D is fish liver oils (especially Halibut fish)
  - Rich source of proteins (15–20%)
  - Rich source of Calcium, phosphorus, fluorides
  - Good source of iron
  - Poor source of Carbohydrates
  - Poor source of iodine (barring few sea fish)

158. **Ans. (b) Calcium 39 mg; (c) Beta carotene 6 micrograms; (d) Calories 280 kcal** [Ref. Multiple sources]

159. **Ans. (b) Citric acid** [Ref. Food Processing by Arthur & Ashurst, 1/e p32]

160. **Ans. (b) Phosphorus; (c) Vitamin B6; (d) Vitamin C; (e) Potassium** [Ref. Encyclopedia of Foods: A Guide to Healthy Nutrition, 1/e p158]
  - Banana is a good source of:
    - Vitamins A, B6, C
    - Carbohydrates, Energy
    - Fibre
    - Potassium, Phosphorus
  - Banana is NOT a good source of:
    - Calcium, Iron (Due to presence of phytates)
    - Zinc

161. **Ans. (d) Ascorbic acid** [Ref. The Lentil by Erskine, 1/e p419]
  FERMENTATION OF PULSES
  - Increase content of B complex vitamins (Thiamine, Riboflavin, Niacin, Biotin, Cyanocobalamin)
  - Decrease phytate and trypsin inhibitors
  - Increase ionisable iron content

162. **Ans. (a) Thiamine** [Ref. Park 27/e p733]
  - Beriberi is caused by a pronounced deficiency of the antineuritic vitamin, vitamin B, or thiamine, which is required for utilization of carbohydrates
  - Up to 80 percent of Thiamine (B1 vitamin) is removed during the process of milling brown rice to white polished rice

> **ALSO REMEMBER**
> - Thiamine loss occur in: Polishing of rice, Milling of rice, Washing/cooking of rice, Toast, Cereals cooked with baking soda, Prolonged storage of fruits & vegetables

163. **Ans. (c) Preservation of nutrition** [Ref. Park 27/e p741]
  PARBOILING OF RICE (Partial cooking in steam process)
  - Major purpose: Preserving nutritive quality of rice
  - Method used: Hot soaking process (CFTRI, Mysore)
    - Vitamins/minerals in outer aleurone layer are driven into endosperm
    - Preservation of nutritive quality even during milling
    - Hardening of grain
    - Insect-resistant, improved storage quality
  - Disadvantage: Development of peculiar smell

Review Questions

164. **Ans. (c) Ragi** [Ref. Park 27/e p736]
165. **Ans. (b) Iron** [Ref. Park 23/e p629]
166. **Ans. (a) Banana** [Ref. Elizabeth's nutrition & child development 2/e p67; Park 27/e p780]
167. **Ans. (d) Ragi** [Ref. Park 27/e p736]
168. **Ans. (a) Cereals** [Ref. Park 27/e p725]
169. **Ans. (c) Leucine** [Ref. Park 27/e p742]

FOOD ADULTERATION

170. **Ans. (a) BOAA** [Ref. Park 27/e p759]
  - Human neurolathyrism (NL) is a self-limiting disease of the nervous system mainly affecting the upper motor neuron and causing degeneration of the distal

corticospinal tract in the spinal cord which results in a spastic paraparesis spastic paraparesis, instability in gait'
- Toxin in Lathyrism is BOAA (beta-oxalyl amino alanine)

171. **Ans. (b) Ascorbic acid**   *[Ref. Park 27/e p759]*
- Interventions for prevention and control of Lathyrism include Vitamin C prophylaxis, Banning the crop, Removal of toxin (Steeping method and Parboiling), Education, Genetic approach, Socio-economic changes

172. **Ans. (c) History of diet**   *[Ref. Park 26/e p734]*
- In Lathyrism, there is pain in lumbar region and stiffness and weakness of the lower extremities with paresthesias and weakness developing later
- Legs become spastic and exhibit clonic tremor
- In addition to the more common spastic paraplegia, polyneuropathy and peripheral mononeuropathy may be present
- **In the given question,** take Dietary history as Food adulteration disease - Lathyrism occurs due to consumption of Red gram contaminated with Lathyrus sativus (Khesari dal) that leads to production of toxin BOAA

173. **Ans. (c) Pyrrolizidine alkaloid**   *[Ref. Park 27/e p771]*
- Food Adulteration diseases:

Disease	Toxin	Adulterant
Lathyrism	BOAA	Khesari Dal (Lathyrus sativus)
Epidemic Dropsy	Sanguinarine	Argemone mexicana (oil)
Endemic Ascites	Pyrrolizidine alkaloids	Crotalaria seeds (Jhunjhunia)
Aflatoxicosis	Aflatoxin	Aspergillus flavus/parasiticus
Ergotism	Clavine alkaloids	Claviceps fusiformis

> **ALSO REMEMBER**
>
> **Lathyrism**
> - Lathyrism is of two types:
>   - Neurolathyrism: In human beings
>   - Osteolathyrism (Odoratism): In animals
> - Neurolathyrism is caused by eating the pulse 'Khesari Dal (Lathyrus sativus)'. Diets containing over 30% of this dal consumed over a period of 2–6 months result in neurolathyrism
> - Toxin: present in lathyrus seeds is 'Beta oxalyl amino alanine (BOAA)
> - Interventions for prevention and control of lathyrism:
>   - Vitamin C prophylaxis
>   - Banning the crop
>   - Removal of toxin: Steeping method and Parboiling
>   - Education
>   - Genetic approach
>   - Socio-economic changes
>
> *Contd...*

Contd...

> **Epidemic Dropsy**
> - Is caused by contamination of mustard oil with 'Argemone oil'
> - Toxin: 'Sanguinarine' is the toxin contained in argemone oil
> - Sanguinarine interferes with oxidation of 'pyruvic acid', which accumulates in blood: It may lead to sudden non-inflammatory edema of bilateral lower limbs, diarrhea, dyspnoea, cardiac failure and death; It can also lead to glaucoma; It may sometimes manifest as 'Sarcoids' (dilatation of skin capillaries)
> - Epidemic dropsy may occur in all ages except breast-fed infants.
>
> **Endemic Ascites:**
> - Toxin: Pyrrolizidine alkaloids (Hepatotoxins)
> - Adulterant: Crotalaria plant (Jhunjhunia)

174. **Ans. (a) Sanguinarine**   *[Ref. Park 27/e p771, 772]*
- Edema in Epidemic dropsy occurs due to proteinuria (specifically loss of albumin).
- Argemone oil may be detected by following tests:
  - *Nitric acid test*
  - *Paper chromatography test: Most sensitive test*

175. **Ans. (b) Neurolathyrism**   *[Ref. Park 27/e p771]*
- Neurolathyrism is caused by eating the pulse 'Khesari Dal (Lathyrus sativus)'; Diets containing over 30 % of this dal consumed over a period of 2–6 months result in neurolathyrism
- Toxin present in lathyrus seeds is 'Beta oxalyl amino alanine (BOAA)'

176. **Ans. (a) Bajra**   *[Ref. Park 27/e p772]*
- *Ergotism:*
  - *Occurs due to food toxicant - ergot fungus 'Claviceps fusiformis'*
  - *Food items having a tendency for ergotism:*
- Bajra
- Rye
- Sorghum
- Wheat
  - *Removal of ergot:*
- Float them in 20% salt water
- Hand-picking
- Air-floatation
  - *Upper safe limit for ergot: 0.05 mg per 100 grams food material*

177. **Ans. All Choice**   *[Ref. Park 27/e p771]*
178. **Ans. All Choices**   *[Ref. Park 27/e p772]*
179. **Ans. (b) Claviceps purpurea**   *[Ref. Park 27/e p772]*
180. **Ans. (b) Nitric acid test**   *[Ref. Park 27/e p772]*
181. **Ans. (b) Paper chromatography**   *[Ref. Park 27/e p772]*
182. **Ans. (a) Lathyrus sativus**   *[Ref. Park 27/e p771]*

LATHYRISM MANIFESTATIONS
- Latent stage: Ungainly gait when subjected to physical stress

- No-stick stage: Short jerky steps
- One-stick stage: Crossed gait, tendency to walk on toes; Requires stick to walk
- Two-stick stage: Excessive bending of knees, crossed legs, slow clumsy gait; Requires crutches to walk
- Crawler stage: Atrophy of thigh/leg muscles, erect posture is impossible; Patient reduced to crawling by throwing his weight on hands.

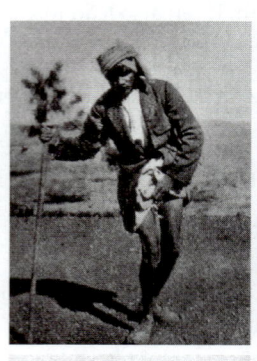
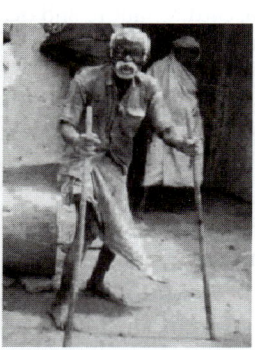
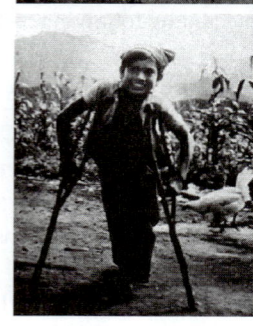
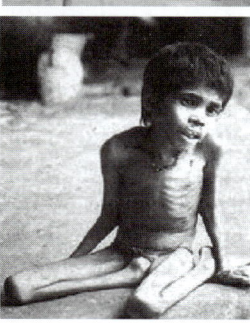

Review Questions

183. Ans. (a) Parboiling [Ref. Park 27/e p771]
184. Ans. (a) Nitric acid test [Ref. Park 27/e p772]

MISCELLANEOUS

185. **Ans. (a) Infectious disease** [Ref. Park 26/e p740]
     Ecological factors of Malnutrition
     - Food balance sheet: Food consumption
     - Socio-economic factors: Family size, income, occupation, education, customs and cultural patterns
     - Health and educational services: Primary health care services, feeding programs, Immunization programs
     - Conditioning influences: Parasitic, bacterial and viral infections that precipitate malnutrition

186. **Ans. (a) IMR** [Ref. Park 26/e p791]
     - The Global Hunger Index (GHI) is a tool designed to comprehensively measure and track hunger at the global, regional, and country levels
     - The International Food Policy Research Institute (IFPRI) calculates GHI scores each year to assess progress, or the lack thereof, in combating hunger
     - To capture the multidimensional nature of hunger, GHI scores are based on the following indicators:

2014 Guidelines	2016 Guidelines
• Child undernourishment • Child underweight • Child mortality	• Undernourishment • Child Wasting (Acute undernutrition) • Child Stunting (Chronic undernutrition) • Child mortality (Under 5 age)

187. **Ans. (b) RDA caters to dietary requirements of all people**
     [Ref. Nutrient Requirements and RDAs for Indians, ICMR; p4; Park 27/e p746]
     - RDA is often higher than the recommended minimum requirement: RDA includes both daily requirement and some additional requirement for periods of growth or illness.

> **ALSO REMEMBER**
> - RDA 'safe level approach' is not used for energy since excess energy intake is undesirable; for energy only mean or average requirement is defined as RDA

188. **Ans. (b) The proportion of proteins, fats and carbohydrates is correct and in accordance with a balanced diet**
     [Ref. Park 27/e p751–752]
     - In 'Balanced Diet',
       - Proteins should constitute 10–15% of total daily energy intake
       - Fats should constitute 15–30% of total daily energy intake
       - Carbohydrates, rich in fibre, should constitute the remaining of energy

     In the given question, a man weighing 68 kg, consumes 325 gm carbohydrate, 65 gm protein and 35 gms fat in his diet

	Energy (kcal per gram)	Amount consumed (grams)	Energy consumed (kcal)	% of total energy consumed
Carbohydrate	4	325	1300	68%
Fats	4.2	65	275	15%
Proteins	9.0	35	315	17%
Total				1890 kcal

His total energy intake is 1890 kcal
15% of his energy is derived from fats
Thus, the proportion of proteins, fats and carbohydrates is correct and in accordance with a balanced diet.

189. **Ans. (c) 55 kg** [Ref. Park 27/e p747]

> **ALSO REMEMBER**
> - Reference body weights of Infants (both male and female):
>   – 0–6 months: 5.4 kg
>   – 6–12 months: 8.4 kg

190. **Ans. (d) None of the above** [Ref. Park 27/e p776]
     - *Mid-day meal programme (MDMP):* Also known as 'School Lunch Programme', it has been in operation since 1961

- *The major objective of MDMP:* To attract more children for admission to schools and retain them so that literacy improvement of children could be brought about.
- The meal is a supplement and not a substitute to the home diet
- The meal should supply 1/3 of the total energy requirement and 1/2 of the total protein requirement.

> **ALSO REMEMBER**
> - MDMP is being operationalised under the Ministry of Human Resource & Development
> - National Institute of Nutrition, Hyderabad is of the view that minimum number of feeding days in year be 250 to have the desired impact on children
> - *Mid-day meal scheme (MDMS) (National Programme of Nutritional Support to Primary Education):* Launched in 1995 with the main objective universalisation of primary education by increasing enrolment, retention and attendance and simultaneously impacting on nutrition of students in primary classes
>   - It aims at providing 450–700 calories and 12–20 gm proteins per day to all children class I to VIII.

191. **Ans. (b) 1/2 proteins and 1/3rd calories** [Ref. Park 27/e p776]
     - The mid-day meal should supply 1/3 of the total energy requirement and 1/2 of the total protein requirement

Item	Quantity per child per day	
	Primary	Upper primary
Food grains	100 grams	150 grams
Pulses	20 grams	30 grams
Vegetables	50 grams	75 grams
Oils & fats	5 grams	7.5 grams
Salt	As per need	As per need
TOTAL calories	450 kcal	700 kcal
TOTAL proteins	12 grams	20 grams

192. **Ans. (a) A decrease in complex carbohydrate consumption** [Ref. Park 27/e p760–761]

193. **Ans. (c) 7 days** [Ref. Park 27/e p764]
     - Assessment of dietary intake (Diet Survey) can be carried out by 'Dietary Cycle', where 'weighment of raw foods is done over a period of 7 days'.

194. **Ans. (d) Saffron colour in milk** [Ref. Park 27/e p773]
     - Food fortification: Is a public health, measure where nutrients are added to food (in relatively small quantities), to maintain/improve the quality of diet of a group, community or a population
     - Examples of Food Fortification:
       - *Iodisation of salt*
       - *Vitamin A and Vitamin D in Vanaspati*
       - *Fluoridation of water*

> **ALSO REMEMBER**
> - Food Fortification is an example of 'Primary Level of Prevention'
> - Vanaspati is fortified with '2500 IU Vitamin A and 175 IU Vitamin D' per 100 grams.

195. **Ans. (b) Defluoridation of water** [Ref. Park 27/e p759]
     - 'Nalgonda Technique' has been developed by National Environmental Engineering Research Institute (NEERI), Nagpur for defluoridation of water. It involves 'addition of lime, alum and bleaching powder' followed by flocculation, sedimentation and filtration. In Nalgonda technique, aluminium is major de-fluoridating agent.
     - Household level de-fluoridation can be done by:
       - *Nalgonda Technique*
       - *Alumina*
       - *Phosphates*

> **ALSO REMEMBER**
> - 'Bangle Test' (4 cm diameter) is also used for quick assessment of MAC
> - 'Quac Stic' measures malnourishment by comparing MAC with height.

196. **Ans. (d) Birth weight** [Ref. Pediatric Clinic Methods by Meharban Singh, 2/e p51]
     - Bathroom weighing scale is unreliable instrument for measuring weight of children; For field conditions, Salter's Spring Scale is quite satisfactory as it is easy to carry.

197. **Ans. (b) 30** [Ref. Park 27/e p454]
     - Body Mass Index (BMI): A simple index of weight-for-height that is commonly used to classify under-weight, over-weight and obesity in adults.
       - BMI is also known as 'Quetelet's Index'
       - $BMI = \dfrac{Weight\ (Kg)}{Height^2\ (m^2)}$
       - In the given question, weight = 89 kg and height = 172 cm,
       - Thus, BMI = $89/(1.72)^2$ = 30.08.

198. **Ans. (a) Lathyrus** [Ref. Park 27/e p771]
     - Neurolathyrism is a crippling disease of nervous system, characterized by gradually developing spastic paralysis of lower limbs, occurring mostly in adults.

199. **Ans. (b) Occurs with diet chiefly on maize** [Ref. Park 27/e p742]

200. **Ans. (c) Cereals are deficient in lysine and methionine is deficient in pulses** [Ref. Park 27/e p725]

201. **Ans. (a) Policy maker; (c) Nutritional survey** [Ref. Park 27/e p765]
     - *Nutritional surveillance:* Keeping a watch over nutrition, in order to make decisions that will lead to improvement in nutrition of population
       - *Main strategy:* Detection of malnutrition (nutritional survey)
       - *Approach:* Diagnostic-interventional
       - *Sample:* Representative, 50–100 size group

- *Objectives:*
    1. To aid health and development
    2. To provide input for program management and evaluation (to policy makers)
    3. To give timely warning and intervention (to prevent short-term food crises)

202. **Ans. (c) Cranberry juice**
[Ref. How Cranberry Juice can prevent Urinary Tract Infections, Science Daily, July 21, 2008]
Cranberry Juice
- Mechanism for prevention of UTI: Proanthocyanidins in Cranberry juice prevent bacterial fimbriae from attaching to wall of urinary bladder and urinary tract.

203. **Ans. (a) Weight for age** *[Ref. WHO Malnutrition Document]*
204. **Ans. (a) Egg** *[Ref. Park 27/e p745]*
205. **Ans. (a) Age 18–29 yrs** *[Ref. Park 27/e p747]*
206. **Ans. (b) Codex alimentarius standards**
[Ref. Park 27/e p774]
207. **Ans. (d) Weight for height below 2SD of WHO Growth Standards 2006**
[Ref. Partha's Fundamental of Paediatrics, 2/e p69]
WHO & UNICEF's Acute Malnutrition Criteria
- Presence of Bipedal edema
- Visible severe wasting
- Mid arm circumference below 115 mm
- Weight for height below 3SD of WHO Growth Standards 2006

208. **Ans. (a) 1 only** *[Ref. Food Processing and Preservation by Sivasankar, 1/e p246]*

209. **Ans. (d) 1, 2 and 3** *[Ref. The PFA Act 1954, p91]*
Food Preservatives: Substances, which if added to food, are capable of inhibiting, retarding or arresting the process of fermentation, acidification or other decomposition of food

Class I preservatives	Class II preservatives
Common salt	Benzoic acid
Sugar, Dextrose, Glucose	Sulphuric acid
Spices	Sorbic acid, Lactic acid
Honey	Nicin
Vinegar, Acetic acid	Propionic acid

Review Questions

210. **Ans. (a) Optimal protein supplementation is 1.5–2 g/kg/day** *[Ref. Park 27/e p752]*
211. **Ans. (c) Height for age** *[Ref. Park 27/e p620]*
212. **Ans. (d) Percentage of pregnant lady with less than 11.5% haemoglobin** *[Ref. Gupta & Mahajan 3/e p362; Park 27/e p765]*
213. **Ans. (c) For postpartum 3,00,000 I.U; (d) 50,000 I.U at birth** *[Ref. Park 27/e p731]*
214. **Ans. (a) Mid-arm circumference in 0–1 year age group** *[Ref. Park 27/e p765]*
215. **Ans. (a) Microorganisms** *[Ref. Park 27/e p772]*
216. **Ans. (c) Ragi** *[Ref. Park 27/e p742]*
217. **Ans. (c) AGMARK standard** *[Ref. Park 27/e p774]*
218. **Ans. (d) B12 deficiency** *[Ref. Park 27/e p735]*

CHAPTER 10

Social Sciences and Health

CONCEPTS IN SOCIOLOGY

Definitions in Sociology

- *Society*^{Q}: Is a group of individuals who have organized themselves and follow a way of life
  - *Outstanding feature of society is a System*, a system of relationships between individuals
- *Community*^{Q}: A social group determined by geographical boundaries and/or common values or interests
- *Sociology*^{Q}: Study of individuals as well as groups in a society. It can be viewed as from 2 angles:
  - Study of relationships between human beings
  - Study of human behaviour
- *Socialisation*^{Q}: Process by which an individual gradually acquires culture and becomes member of a social group
- *Social structure*^{Q}: Patterns of inter-relationships between persons in a society
- *Medical sociology*^{Q}: Includes studies of medical profession, of the relationship of medicine to public, and of the social factors in the aetiology, prevalence, incidence and interpretation of disease
- *Socialism*^{Q}: Any economic doctrine that favours the use of property and resources of the country for public welfare
  - Based on social ownership for raising the living standard of working class
- *Social epidemiology:* When the objective of the research is to study the role of social factors in the etiology of the disease, epidemiological survey and social survey are merged together
- *Socialised medicine*^{Q}: Provision of medical service and professional education by the State (as in state medicine), but the programme is operated and regulated by professional groups rather than by government
- *Social medicine:* Study of the social, economical, environmental, cultural, psychological and genetic factors, which have a bearing on health
- *Social defence:* Covers preventive, therapeutic and rehabilitative services for the protection of society from antisocial, criminal or deviant conduct of man.

Key points

Social structure^Q: Patterns of inter-relationships between persons in a society

Key points

Socialised medicine^Q: Provision of medical service and professional education by the State (as in state medicine), but the programme is operated and regulated by professional groups rather than by government

Social and Behavioural Sciences

- *Social Sciences*^{Q}: Comprises of those disciplines which are committed to the scientific examination of human behaviour; these are economics, political science, sociology, social psychology and social anthropology
- '*Behavioural Sciences*'^{Q} is applied to last three, viz., sociology, social psychology and social anthropology, because they directly deal with human behaviour
  - *Economics:* Deals with human relationships in specific context of production, distribution, consumption and ownership of scarce resources, goods and services
  - *Political Science:* Study of systems of laws and institutions which constitute government of whole societies
  - *Sociology:* Study of human relationships and human behaviour for a better understanding of pattern of life
  - *Social psychology:* Concerned with psychology of individuals living in human society or groups
  - *Social anthropology:* Study of development and various types of social life.

Anthropology

- *Anthropology*^{Q}: Study of physical social and cultural history of man
  - *Physical (Biological) anthropology:* Study of human evolution, racial differences, inheritance of bodily traits, growth and decay

> **Key points**
>
> *Culture*^Q: Is the learned behaviour which is socially acquired
> *Acculturation*^Q: Is 'cultural contact' or mixing of two cultures. It can occur through

- *Social anthropology:* Study of development and various types of social life
- *Cultural anthropology:* Study of total way of life of contemporary primitive man, his ways of thinking, feelings and action
- *Medical anthropology:* Deals with cultural component in ecology of health and disease
- *Linguistic anthropology:* Seeks to understand the processes of human communications, verbal and non-verbal, including language.

Social Pathology

- *Social Pathology*[Q]: Is the study of social problems which undermine the social, psychological or economical health of the populations; it is used to describe relationship between disease and social conditions
- Social pathology is uncovered by 'Social Surveys'
- Social Problems studied under social pathology:
  - Social constraints:
    - Poverty and destitution
    - Illiteracy and ignorance
    - Migration and environmental crisis
    - Industrialization and Urbanization
  - Social evils:
    - Smoking and drinking
    - Caste and casteism
    - Gender bias and gender discrimination
    - Child neglect and child abuse
    - Child labour and child abandonment
    - Stress and stress behaviour
    - Crime and corruption
    - Prostitution and STDs
  - Social deviance:
    - Drug abuse
    - Juvenile delinquency
    - Suicide.

Culture and Acculturation

- *Culture*[Q]: Is the learned behaviour which is socially acquired
- *Acculturation*[Q]: Is 'cultural contact' or mixing of two cultures. It can occur through
  - Trade and commerce
  - Industrialization
  - Propagation of religion
  - Education
  - Conquest
- *Custom*[Q]: The established patterns of behavior that can be objectively verified within a particular social setting
  - *Folkways*[Q]: Right ways of doing things in less vital areas of human conduct
  - *Mores*[Q]: More stringent customs.

Theories in Sociology

- *Feminist Theory:* Focuses on how gender inequality has shaped social life
  - Disease is due to social role of women enforced by men
- *Parsonian Theory:* States that illness did not simply imply a 'biologically altered state, but also a socially altered state'
  - Disease is due to social strain caused by social demands
- *Marxist Theory:* Is concerned with the relationship between health and illness and capitalist social organization
  - Cause of disease is putting profit ahead of health[Q]
- *Foucauldian Theory:* medical discourse plays an important role in the management of individual bodies (anantomopolitics) and bodies en masse (biopolitics)
  - Disease is labels to segregate population to make it easier to control.

PSYCHOLOGY

Definitions and Concepts

- *Emotions:* Strong feelings of whole organism, which motivate human behaviour
- *Value:* The ideals, customs, institutions of a society toward which the people of the group have an affective regard
  - May be positive (cleanliness, freedom, or education) or negative (cruelty, crime, or blasphemy)
- *Opinions^Q:* Views held by people on a point of dispute
  - Are 'temporary, provisional'^{Q}
  - Is 'subjective in nature'^{Q}
- *Belief^Q:* Views derived from parents, grand parents and other people we respect
  - Are 'permanent, stable, almost unchanging'^{Q}
  - Is 'subjective in nature'^{Q}
- *Attitude^Q:* Relatively enduring organization of beliefs around an object or subject which predisposes one to respond in a preferential manner
  - Acquired characteristics of an individual
  - Is more or less 'permanent ways of behaving'^{Q}
  - Is 'caught, not taught'
  - Is 'objective in nature'^{Q}
- *Habits:* An accustomed way of doing things^Q
  - Habits are acquired through repetitions, are automatic and can be performed only under similar circumstances.

Key points

Opinions^Q: Views held by people on a point of dispute
Are 'temporary, provisional'^{Q}

Key points

Attitude^Q: Is more or less 'permanent ways of behaving'

Emotions

- *Definition:* Strong feelings of whole organism, which motivate human behaviour^Q
- *Types of emotions:*
  - *Fear:* MC emotion of man^Q
  - *Phobia:* when fear becomes exaggerated or unnecessary
  - *Anger (Rage):* Reaction of offensive type; destructive in nature
  - *Anxiety:* may lead to tension or pain
  - *Love:* Feeling of attachment to some person.

Key points

Fear: MC emotion of man^Q

Learning

- *Definition:* Any relative permanent change in behaviour that occurs as a result of practice or experience
- *Conditions affecting learning:*
  - Intelligence
  - Age
  - Learning situation
  - Motivation
  - Physical health
- *Types of learning:*

Type of learning^Q	Associations
Cognitive learning	Knowledge
Affective learning	Attitudes
Psychomotor learning	Skills

Intelligence Quotient (IQ)

- *Intelligence Quotient:* Is a score derived from one of several different standardized tests attempting to measure intelligence
- *First intelligence tests were developed by:* Binet and Simon (1896)
- *Stern's IQ Test ^{Q}:* Originally IQ was calculated for children

$$IQ = \frac{Mental\ age}{Chronological\ age} \times 100$$

- *Wechsler Adult Intelligence Scale (WAIS):* David Wechsler (1939) published the first intelligence test designed for an adult population; It was the *'first IQ test based on Normal/Gaussian distribution'*^{Q}

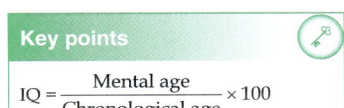

- *Levels of Intelligence based on IQ levels^Q*:

Levels of Intelligence	IQ range
Idiot	0–24
Imbecile^Q	25–49
Moron^Q	50–69
Borderline	70–79
Low normal	80–89
Normal^Q	90–109
Superior	110–119
Very superior	120–139
Near Genius^Q	140 and over

- *Categories of mental retardation based on IQ levels^Q*:

Mental status	IQ range^Q
Normal IQ^Q	70 and over
Mild mental retardation	50–69
Moderate mental retardation	35–49
Severe mental retardation	21–34
Profound mental retardation	20 or below

FAMILY

Family Cycle

A normal *family cycle is conceived as having 6 phases^Q*:

Phases of family life cycle		Events characterising	
No.	Description	Beginning of phase	End of phase
I	Formation	Marriage	Birth of 1st child
II	Extension	Birth of 1st child	Birth of last child
III	Complete extension	Birth of last child	1st child leaves home
IV	Contraction	1st child leaves home	Last child leaves home
V	Completed contraction	Last child leaves home	1st spouse dies
VI	Dissolution	1st spouse dies	Death of survivor (extinction)

Definitions and Concepts

- *Nuclear Family (Elementary/Unitary Family)^Q*: Consists of a married couple and their children while they are still regarded as dependents
- *Joint Family^Q*: Consists of no. of married couples and their children who live together in the same household
  - All males are related by blood while females are wives, daughters, sisters and widows
  - Property is held in common; there is a common family purse to which the all the family income goes and from which all the expenditures are met
  - All authority is vested in the senior male member of the family
  - Familial relations enjoys primacy over marital relations
- *3-Generation Family*: Consists of a household with representatives of three generations
- *Complex Family*: Is a generic term for any family structure involving more than two adults; term can refer to any extended family or to a polygamy of any type
- *Communal Family^Q*: Is a family where all of its members are playing a part in its management
  - Is a good example of 'division of labour', an important function of a family.
- *Conjugal Family^Q*: Is nuclear family of adult partners and their children (by birth or adoption) where the family relationship is principally focused inwardly and ties to extended kin are voluntary and based on emotional bonds, rather than strict duties and obligations; most common form is nuclear family

> **Key points**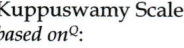
> Kuppuswamy Scale based on^Q:
> - Education status
> - Occupation
> - Income

- *Broken Family*^{Q}: Where both parents have separated or where death has occurred of one or both then parents
- *Problem Family*^{Q}: Is a family which lags behind rest of the community; underlying factors in most problem families are those of personality, relationships, backwardness, poverty, illness, mental and social instability, character defects and marital disharmony
    - Standards of life are generally far below the accepted minimum
    - Parents are unable to meet the physical and emotional needs of children
    - Home life is utterly unsatisfactory
- *Dysfunctional Family*: Is a family in which conflict, misbehavior and even abuse on the part of individual members of the family occur continually, leading other members to accommodate such actions
- *Consanguineal Family:* Consists of a mother and her children, and other people — usually the family of the mother, like her husband
- *Matrifocal Family:* Consists of a mother and her children
- *New Family*^{Q}: A family of less than 10 years duration and consists of parents and children
    - It is a variant of nuclear (elementary/unitary) family
    - New Family concept is important in view of studies related to family planning.

SOCIO-ECONOMIC STATUS

Socio-economic Status (SES) Scales^Q

Urban SES scales: Modified Kuppuswamy Scale^q Kulshreshtha Scale Srivastava Scale Jalota Scale	Rural SES scales: Udai Pareek Scale^q Modified B. G. Prasad Scale^q Radhukar Scale Shirpurkar Scale
Student's scale: Bhardwaj Scale	Non-Indian SES scales: Hollingshead (Occupation based) Scale Henderson Scale

Modified Kuppuswamy Scale
- Is used for Urban families
- *Is based on 3 parameters*^{Q}:
    - Education status of head of family (Score 1 to 7)
    - Occupation of head of family (Score 1 to 10)
    - Income of the family per month (Score 1 to 12)
- *Scoring:* Each component is given a weighted score and summed up
- *Socio-economic classes based on scores:*

Score	Socio-economic class
26–29	I. Upper
16–25	II. Upper - middle
11–15	III. Lower - middle
05–10	IV. Upper - lower
<05	V. Lower

(Minimum score 3; Maximum score 29)

Udai Pareek Scale
- Is for Rural families
- Is not dependent on income^Q
- Is based on 9 parameters:
    - Caste
    - Occupation
    - Education
    - Land
    - Social participation
    - Family members
    - House

- Farm power
- Material possession
- *Scoring:* Each component is given a weighted score and summed up
- *Socio-economic classes based on scores:*

Score	Socio-economic class
>43	I
33–42	II
24–32	III
13–23	IV
<13	V

BG Prasad Scale

- Is for Rural families
- Is based on per capita monthly income
- *Socio-economic classes based on scores:*

Per capita monthly income (INR)		Socio-economic class
BG Prasad's Classification (1961)	BG Prasad's Classification (2019) Updated	
≥100	≥7008	I
50–99	3504–7007	II
30–49	2102–3503	III
15–29	1051–2101	IV
<15	≤1050	V

ECONOMICS

Definitions

- *Gross National Income (GNI)/Gross National Product (GNP)^Q:* Is gross income generated from within the country as also net income received from abroad
- *Gross Domestic Product (GDP)^Q:* Gross income generated within a country (excludes net income received)
- *Net National Product (NNP):* GNP minus capital we consume
- *Net Domestic Product (NDP):* GDP minus value of depreciation on fixed assets
- *Purchasing Power Parity (PPP):* No. of units of a country's currency required to buy the same amount of goods and services in domestic market, as 1 dollar would buy in USA.

> **Key points**
> Rural areas poverty <2400 kcal per day

Health Expenditure in India (2014 World Bank)

Parameter	Value
Health expenditure, total (% of GDP)^Q	4.7%
Health expenditure, public (% of GDP)^Q	1.3%
Health expenditure, public (% of total health expenditure)	30%
Out-of-pocket health expenditure (% of total expenditure on health)	63%
Health expenditure per capita (current US$)	75 US$

Below Poverty Line (BPL)

- *Below Poverty Line (BPL) Criteria^Q:*

BPL Criteria	Rural areas	Urban areas
Per capita caloric intake	<2400 kcal per day	<2100 kcal per day
Per capita income (TC)	<27/- INR per day	<33/- INR per day
Per capita income (RC)	<32/- INR per day	<47/- INR per day
Per capita income (WHO)	<1.90 US$ per day	

(TC: Tendulkar Committee 2011–12; RC: Rangarajan Committee 2014)

- *Below Poverty Line (BPL) population in India^Q:*
  - 22% (Tendulkar Committee 2011–12)
  - 29.5% (Rangarajan Committee 2014).

Social Security and Social Safety Net

- *Social security^Q:* primarily refers to a social insurance program providing social protection, or protection against socially recognized conditions, including poverty, old age, disability, unemployment and others
  - *Bismarck introduced a system of social insurance in Germany in 1883^Q:* It became a model for other European countries to introduce similar social security systems
- *Approaches to social security system:*
  - *Social assistance^Q:* Non-contributory benefit extended to vulnerable groups
  - *Social insurance^Q:* Contributory benefit extended to individuals as a matter of right
- *Social Security measures for Industrial workers^Q:*
  - Workmen's Compensation Act 1923
  - The Factory's Act 1948
  - Employees State Insurance Act 1948 (including Disablement Benefit)
  - Central Maternity Benefit Act 1961
  - The Family Pension Scheme 1971
- *Social safety net^Q:* is a term used to describe a collection of services provided by the state, such as welfare, unemployment benefit, universal healthcare, homeless shelters, the minimum wage and sometimes subsidized services such as public transport, which prevent individuals from falling into poverty beyond a certain level.

> **Key points**
> Urban areas poverty <2100 kcal per day

INTERVIEWING

Interview

- *Interview:* A technique for investigation and an instrument for research
- *Types of Interview:*
  - *Direct (structured) Interview:* Pre-determined questions are asked
  - *Non directive (unstructured) Interview:* Collection of information by free discussion; no pre-determined questions
  - *Focussed Interview:* Focussing attention on a particular aspect of a problem
  - *Repetitive Interview:* To note the gradual influence of some social or psychological process.

Steps of Interview

- *Establishing contact:* First requisite before conducting an interview^Q
- Starting an interview
- Securing rapport
- Recall
- Probe questions
- Encouragement
- Guiding the interview
- Closing the interview
- Report.

> **Key points**
> *Establishing contact:* First requisite before conducting an interview

> **Key points**
> Family is the *'most powerful example of social cohesion'*

MISCELLANEOUS

Group Dynamics

- *Family^Q:* Is a group of biologically related individuals living together and eating from a common kitchen
  - Family is the primary unit of all societies
  - Family is the *'most powerful example of social cohesion'*^{Q}
- *Crowd^Q:* A group of people coming together temporarily for a short period, motivated by a common interest or curiosity
  - Crowd lacks internal organization and leadership^Q
- *Mob^Q:* A group of people coming together temporarily for a short period, having a leader who forces members into action
  - Mob is more emotional than crowd^Q
  - Like crowd, mob is unstable and lacks internal organization

- *Herd^Q:* Is a crowd with a leader, where members of the group have to follow the orders of the leader without question
- *Band:* Most elementary community of a few families living together
  - Group has organized itself and follows a pattern of life
- *Village:* A small collection of people permanently settled down in a locality with their homes and cultural equipments
- *Towns and Cities:* A relatively large, dense and permanent settlement of socially heterogeneous individuals
  - Community is subdivided into smaller groups on the basis of wealth and social class
- *State:* An ecological social group based on territory
  - State is more stabilised and formalized
  - State is heterogeneous in nature
  - Indian Union is a large state.

Global Hunger Index (GHI)

- *Description:* Tool designed to comprehensively measure and track hunger globally, by region and country
- *Agency involved:* International Food Policy Research Institute
- **GHI calculation:** Combination of 3 equally weighted indicators,
  - Undernourishment
  - Child underweight (<5 years age)
  - Child mortality (<5 years age)
- **Scale used:** 0–100 [Score 0: Best (No hunger), Score 100: Worst].

Hidden Hunger (Micronutrient Deficiency)

- A form of under nutrition occurring when intake and absorption of vitamins and minerals are too low to sustain development.

PYQs: Quick Review for NEET

Sociology	
Acculturation is	Cultural contact
Learned behavior which is socially acquired	Culture
Relationship between the disease and social conditions	Social pathology
Study of physical, social and cultural history of man is	Anthropology
Society is a	System of relations between individuals
Child's W for H >2SD of mean, H for age <2SD of mean	Stunted
Social psychology is	Psychology of individuals in society
Estimated children affected by trafficking every year	1.2 million
Poverty line can be defined in terms of	Daily calorie intake
In interview, first stage is to	Establish contact
Complete extension of family occurs when/at	1st child leave home
IQ level	
IQ formula	Mental Age/Chronological Age × 100
Mental retardation if IQ Level	Less than 70
Normal IQ is	90–109 IQ points
IQ level in severe mental retardation	21–34 IQ points
A person with an IQ of 55 is	Mild mental retardation
Severe mental retardation is	Intelligence quotient 20–34
IQ = 35–49 classified according to WHO is	Moderate mental retardation
Mild mental retardation is defined when IQ is	50–69 IQ points

Multiple Choice Questions

CONCEPTS IN SOCIOLOGY

1. India is a diverse country having a wealth of different cultures and languages. Correct statement is: [INICET May 2022]
    (a) Physician should emphasize on communication
    (b) Treat patients regardless of patient's perception
    (c) Due emphasis should be given in patient cultural extent
    (d) Leave communication to interpreter

2. Pattern of interrelationships between persons in a society is known as: [AIIMS June 1997] [AIPGME 1997]
    (a) Socialism   (b) Socialization
    (c) Social structure (d) Medical sociology

3. 'Learned behaviour which is socially acquired' is known as: [AIIMS Dec 1992, May 2000]
    (a) Customs   [NEET Pattern 2012]
    (b) Acculturation
    (c) Standard of living
    (d) Culture

4. The systematic study of human disease and social conditions/factors is known as: [AIIMS May 2001]
    (a) Social physiology   [AIPGME 1993]
    (b) Social pathology
    (c) Socialised medicine
    (d) Social medicine

5. All of the following social sciences deal directly with human behaviour except: [AIPGME 1993]
    (a) Political Science
    (b) Anthropology
    (c) Social Psychology
    (d) Sociology

6. Putting profit ahead of health as a cause of disease is provided by which theory of sociology: [AIIMS May 2009]
    (a) Feminist   (b) Parsonian
    (c) Marxist   (d) Foucauldian

7. Acculturation may take place by: [Karnataka 2011]
    (a) Education
    (b) Industrialization
    (c) Trade and commerce
    (d) All of the above

8. Social pathology is: [AIIMS PGMEE May 2013]
    (a) Change in disease pattern due to change in lifestyle
    (b) Study of social problems which cause disease in population
    (c) Conflicts arising from new opportunities in transitional societies
    (d) Study of human relationships and behaviour

9. An organized group of people with social relationship: [NEET Pattern 2013]
    (a) Community   [AP 2003]
    (b) Association
    (c) Society
    (d) Family

10. Acculturation is: [DNB June 2009]
    (a) Triage
    (b) Cultural change due to socialization
    (c) Attitude
    (d) Belief

Review Questions

11. Acculturation means: [MP 2003] [DNB 2004]
    (a) Culture contact [NEET Pattern 2012, 2017]
    (b) Study of the various cultures
    (c) Cultural history of health and disease
    (d) Exchange of Ideas

12. When there is contact between two people with different types of culture, there is diffusion of culture both ways which is called: [AP 2008]
    (a) Socialization   (b) Acculturation
    (c) Adjustment   (d) All of the above

13. Tendency of some members of a group to identify and interact with selected members only, leads to formation of a subgroup, this is called as: [MH 2003]
    (a) Cohesion   (b) Sociometry
    (c) Group structure (d) Group dynamics

14. Which of the following is an example of primary social relationship? [MH 2003]
    (a) Husband and wife (b) Author and publisher
    (c) Both   (d) None

15. Change in the affective level after communication and health education means change in: [MH 2006]
    (a) Knowledge   (b) Attitude
    (c) Skills   (d) All

PSYCHOLOGY

16. Phobia is exaggerated or unnecessary form of: [AIPGME 1995]
    (a) Fear   (b) Anger
    (c) Anxiety   (d) Love

17. Match the following types of learning: [AIPGME 1999]
    Type of learning   Associations
    I. Cognitive learning   A. Skills
    II. Affective learning   B. Knowledge
    III. Psychomotor learning C. Attitudes

(a) I – B, II – A, III – C
(b) I – B, II – C, III – A
(c) I – A, II – C, III – B
(d) I – A, II – B, III – C

18. Most important epidemiological tool used for assessing disability in children is: [AIPGME 2003]
    (a) Activities of Daily living (ADL) scale
    (b) Wing's Handicaps, Behavior and Skills (HBS) Schedule
    (c) Binet and Simon IQ tests
    (d) Physical Quality of Life Index (PQLI)

19. Inner subjective thought of a person towards an individual or a situation is best described as: [AIIMS May 2009]
    (a) Attitude
    (b) Value
    (c) Belief
    (d) Opinion

20. A temporary, provisional view held by people on a point of debate is: [AIIMS May 2009]
    (a) Opinion
    (b) Practice
    (c) Attitude
    (d) Belief

21. Learned behaviour which is permanent and consistent, but liable to change is: [AIIMS Nov 2009]
    (a) Cultural belief
    (b) Attitude
    (c) Knowledge
    (d) Practice

22. According to Maslow's hierarchy of needs, following is at the top of pyramid: [NUPGET 2013]
    (a) Physical needs
    (b) Self actualization
    (c) Safety
    (d) Esteem recognition

Review Questions

23. Not a method of learning: [DNB 2001]
    (a) Propaganda
    (b) Writing
    (c) Group discussion
    (d) Reading

24. A primitive man, feeling, thinking deals with: [UP 2003]
    (a) Social psychology
    (b) Sociometry
    (c) Sociopathy
    (d) Sociotherapy

IQ

25. 'Moron' is one with an IQ of: [AIIMS Nov 2003]
    (a) 0–24
    (b) 25–49
    (c) 50–69
    (d) 70–79

26. Average Mental IQ according to Wechsler's Scale is: [AIIMS PGMEE May 2013]
    (a) 70–79
    (b) 80–89
    (c) 90–109
    (d) 110–119

27. Mild mental retardation does not include IQ level(s): [PGI May 2012]
    (a) 45
    (b) 55
    (c) 65
    (d) 75
    (e) 85

28. IQ is calculated by: [NEET Pattern 2013]
    (a) Mental age/chronological age × 100
    (b) Mental age – chronological age × 100
    (c) Chronological age/mental age × 100
    (d) Chronological age – mental age × 100

29. Chronological age 10 yrs, mental age 4 yrs. What that person called as? [NEET Pattern 2012]
    (a) Idiot
    (b) Imbecile
    (c) Normal
    (d) Genius

30. Mental retardation term has been replaced by: [NEET Pattern 2018]
    (a) Mental deficiency
    (b) Mental lack
    (c) Mentally challenged
    (d) Intellectual disability

FAMILY

31. Arrange the following stages of family cycle in chronological sequence: [AIIMS Dec 1991] [NEET Pattern 2013]
    (a) Formation, Extension, Complete extension, Dissolution, Contraction, Complete contraction
    (b) Formation, Extension, Contraction, Complete extension, Complete contraction, Dissolution
    (c) Formation, Contraction, Complete contraction, Extension, Complete extension, Dissolution
    (d) Formation, Extension, Complete extension, Contraction, Complete contraction, Dissolution

32. A family where all of its members are playing a part in its management is known as: [AIIMS May 2006]
    (a) Elementary family
    (b) New family
    (c) 3-Generation family
    (d) Communal family

33. Family, which lags behind rest of the community, is known as: [AIIMS Nov 2003]
    (a) Communal family
    (b) Elementary family
    (c) Problem family
    (d) Broken family

34. The following is true about the term 'New Families': [AIIMS May 2003]
    (a) It is a variant of the 3-generation family
    (b) It is applied to all nuclear families of less then 10 years duration
    (c) It is a variant of the joint family
    (d) It is applied to all nuclear families of less then 2 years duration

35. Nuclear family consists of: [NEET Pattern 2012]
    (a) Husband, wife and son
    (b) Husband, wife and dependent children
    (c) Husband and wife only
    (d) Father mother husband and wife

36. ………………. is a bridge between generations, and a transfer point of civilization [NEET Pattern 2015]
    (a) School
    (b) Orphanage
    (c) Family
    (d) Recreational club

SOCIO-ECONOMIC STATUS

37. Kuppuswamy Scale for socio-economic status is based on [DNS 2011] [AIPGME 1994, AIIMS Nov 1999]
    (a) Income of the family, No. of livestock, No. of acres of farm land [MH 2000]
    (b) Income of the family, No. of members in the family, Education of head of family
    (c) No. of vehicles in family, Occupation of head of family, Education of head of family
    (d) Income, Occupation of head of family, Education of head of family

38. Upper class score in Kuppuswamy Socio-economic status scale is: [NEET Pattern 2014]
    (a) 5–10   (b) 11–15
    (c) 16–25   (d) 26–29

39. Scales used for assessing socio-economic status of populations are the following *except*:
    (a) Modified Udai Pareek scale [NEET Pattern 2016]
    (b) Modified Kuppuswamy scale
    (c) Likert scale
    (d) BG Prasad scale

Review Question

40. Socioeconomic status in urban areas is indicated by which of the following? [AP 2006]
    (a) Kuppuswamy scale
    (b) Sullivan index
    (c) Human development index
    (d) Physical quality of life index

SOCIAL PROBLEMS

41. The Children's Act was passed in: [AIIMS May 2000]
    (a) 1960   (b) 1969
    (c) 1971   (d) 1986

42. Which of the following is best suited for the role of social worker? [AIIMS PGMEE May 2012]
    (a) Health professional involved in physiotherapy
    (b) Health professional involved in coping strategies, interpersonal skills, adjustment with family
    (c) A person involved in finding jobs and economic support for disabled
    (d) Health professional involved in treatment of patients

43. Which of the following statement(s) is/are true about Women empowerment? [PGI May 2013]
    (a) Power over resources
    (b) Involvement in Political decision making
    (c) Involvement in economic decision making
    (d) Improved standard of living
    (e) Increased life expectancy

44. The 'Nirbhaya Fund' set up by the Government of India is for [UPSC CMS 2015]
    (a) Ensuring the safety of women
    (b) Promoting the financial literacy of rural poor
    (c) Promoting Self-Help Groups of women
    (d) Providing free education

ECONOMICS

45. Social insurance was introduced by: [AIPGME 2005]
    (a) Martin Luther King
    (b) Bismarck
    (c) Dr Watson
    (d) Baba Amte

46. Poverty line is defined as expenditure required for daily calorie consumption below (urban): [DPG 2007]
    (a) 1800   (b) 2000
    (c) 2100   (d) 2200

47. Total health expenditure as percentage of GDP in India is: [AIIMS PGMEE November 2013]
    (a) 1.2   (b) 12
    (c) 5   (d) 0.12

48. As current percent of Indian GDP, Public health expenditure is: [AIIMS PGMEE November 2012]
    (a) 1.2   (b) 2
    (c) 10   (d) 15

Review Question

49. In "poverty lines" the expenditure required for a daily calorie intake of ………….. in rural areas: [UP 2008]
    (a) 2200   (b) 2400
    (c) 2100   (d) 2300

INTERVIEWING

50. First requisite before conducting an interview is:
    (a) Securing rapport [AIIMS June 1998]
    (b) Probe questions [DNB 2011]
    (c) Establishing contact
    (d) Guiding the interview

MISCELLANEOUS

51. Increased Drug Compliance can be seen with:
    (a) Frequent dosing
    (b) Longer duration of treatment
    (c) Multiple drugs
    (d) Involving family members in observation

52. An unstable and emotional temporary social group with a leader is known as: *[Karnataka 2011]*
    (a) A band
    (b) A crowd
    (c) A herd
    (d) A mob

53. Study of designing equipment and devices that fit the human body, its movements, and its cognitive abilities is: *[DNB December 2009]*
    (a) Economics
    (b) Ergonomics
    (c) Bionomics
    (d) Socionomics

Review Question

54. All are included in 'High social safety net' *except*:
    (a) High birth rate *[Kolkata 2002]*
    (b) High MMR
    (c) Reduction in institutional delivery
    (d) High IMR

Explanations

CONCEPTS IN SOCIOLOGY

1. **Ans. (a) Physician should emphasize on communication; (c) Due emphasis should be given in patient cultural extent** [Ref. Park 26/e p783]
   - The communication skills of physicians are an effective step of making effective relationship between doctor and patient
   - Research has shown that the way patients perceive their connection with their physician significantly influences their sense of satisfaction and level of concern about their health
   - The goal of culturally competent health care services is to provide the highest quality of care to every patient, regardless of race, ethnicity, cultural background
   - Assume, and insist, that everything you say, everything the patient says, and everything that family members say is interpreted, and give short segments to interpreter

2. **Ans. (c) Social structure** [Ref. Park 27/e p786]
   - *Social structure:* Patterns of inter-relationships between persons in a society
   - *Socialism:* Is economic doctrine that favours the use of property and resources of the country for public welfare; it is a system of production and distribution based on social ownership
   - *Socialization:* Process by which an individual gradually acquires culture and becomes member of a social group
   - *Medical sociology:* Includes studies of medical profession, of the relationship of medicine to public, and of the social factors in the aetiology, prevalence, incidence and interpretation of disease
   - *Society:* Is a group of individuals who have organized themselves and follow a way of life
     - Outstanding feature of society is a System, a system of relationships between individuals
   - *Community:* A social group determined by geographical boundaries and/or common values or interests
   - *Sociology:* Study of individuals as well as groups in a society. It can be viewed as from 2 angles:
     - Study of relationships between human beings
     - Study of human behaviour

> **ALSO REMEMBER**
> - *Sociology:* Study of human relationships and human behaviour for a better understanding of pattern of life

3. **Ans. (d) Culture** [Ref. Park 27/e p787]
   - *Culture:* Is the learned behaviour which is socially acquired
   - *Acculturation:* Is 'cultural contact' or mixing of two cultures. It can occur through
     - Trade and commerce
     - Industrialization
     - Propagation of religion
     - Education
     - Conquest
   - *Custom:* The established patterns of behavior that can be objectively verified within a particular social setting
     - *Folkways:* Right ways of doing things in less vital areas of human conduct
     - *Mores:* More stringent customs
   - *Standard of Living:* Refers to the usual scale of our expenditure, goods we consume and services we enjoy. Standard of living (WHO) includes
     - Income and Occupation,
     - Standards of housing, sanitation and nutrition,
     - Level of provision of health, educational, recreational and other services.

> **ALSO REMEMBER**
> - *'Taboos are the most extreme form of mores'* as they forbid a society's most outrageous practices, such as incest and murder
> - Standard of living depends on *'Per capita GNP'*

4. **Ans. (b) Social pathology** [Ref. Park 27/e p788]
   SOCIAL PATHOLOGY:
   - *Social Pathology:* Is the study of social problems which undermine the social, psychological or economical health of the populations; it is used to describe relationship between disease and social conditions
   - *Social pathology is uncovered by 'Social Surveys'*

> **ALSO REMEMBER**
> - *Social surveys* disclose social pathology.
>   - *Social epidemiology:* When the objective of the research is to study the role of social factors in the etiology of the disease, epidemiological survey and social survey are merged together
> - *Socialised medicine:* Provision of medical service and professional education by the State (as in state medicine), but the programme is operated and regulated by professional groups rather than by government
> - *Social medicine:* Study of the social, economical, environmental, cultural, psychological and genetic factors, which have a bearing on health

5. **Ans. (a) Political Science** [Ref. Park 27/e p785]
   - *Social Sciences:* Comprises of those disciplines which are committed to the scientific examination of human behaviour; these are economics, political science, sociology, social psychology and social anthropology (*'Behavioural Sciences'* is applied to last three, viz., sociology, social psychology and social anthropology, because they directly deal with human behaviour)

- *Economics:* Deals with human relationships in specific context of production, distribution, consumption and ownership of scarce resources, goods and services
- *Political Science:* Study of systems of laws and institutions which constitute government of whole societies
- *Sociology:* Study of human relationships and human behaviour for a better understanding of pattern of life
- *Social psychology:* Concerned with psychology of individuals living in human society or groups
- *Social anthropology:* Study of development and various types of social life

> **ALSO REMEMBER**
> - *Social defence:* Covers preventive, therapeutic and rehabilitative services for the protection of society from antisocial, criminal or deviant conduct of man

6. **Ans. (c) Marxist** [Ref. An Introduction to Sociology, health and Illness by Kevin white; p7]

THEORIES IN SOCIOLOGY
1. *Feminist Theory:* Focuses on how gender inequality has shaped social life
   - Disease is due to social role of women enforced by men
2. *Parsonian Theory:* States that illness did not simply imply a 'biologically altered state, but also a socially altered state
   - Disease is due to social strain caused by social demainds
3. *Marxist Theory:* Is concerned with the relationship between health and illness and capitalist social organization
   - Cause of disease is putting profit ahead of health
4. *Foucauldian Theory:* medical discourse plays an important role in the management of individual bodies (anantomopolitics) and bodies en masse (biopolitics)
   - Diesease is labels to segregate population to make it easier to control

7. **Ans. (d) All of the above** [Ref. Park 27/e p787]
8. **Ans. (b) Study of social problems which cause disease in population** [Ref. Park 27/e p788]
9. **Ans. (c) Society** [Ref. Park 27/e p785]
10. **Ans. (b) Cultural change due to socialization** [Ref. Park 27/e p787]

Review Questions

11. **Ans. (a) Culture contact** [Ref. Park 27/e p787]
12. **Ans. (b) Acculturation** [Ref. Park 27/e p787]
13. **Ans. (b) Sociometry** [Ref. Internet]
14. **Ans. (a) Husband and wife** [Ref. Park 22/e p606]
15. **Ans. (b) Attitude** [Ref. Park 27/e p791]

PSYCHOLOGY

16. **Ans. (a) Fear** [Ref. Park 27/e p790]
    - *EMOTIONS:* Strong feelings of whole organism, which motivate human behaviour
    - *Fear:* MC emotion of man
      - *Phobia:* when fear becomes exaggerated or unnecessary
    - *Anger (Rage):* Reaction of offensive type; destructive in nature
    - *Anxiety:* may lead to tension or pain
    - *Love:* Feeling of attachment to some person

> **ALSO REMEMBER**
> - *Emotional Intelligence (EI) measured as Emotional quotient (EQ):* describes an ability, capacity, skill or a self-perceived ability, to identify, assess, and manage the emotions
> - *Alexithymia:* describe a state of deficiency in understanding, processing, or describing emotions

17. **Ans. (b) I – B, II – C, III – A** [Ref. Park 27/e p791]
    - *LEARNING:* Any relative permanent change in behaviour that occurs as a result of practice or experience
    - *Types of learning:*

Type of learning	Associations
Cognitive learning	Knowledge
Affective learning	Attitudes
Psychomotor learning	Skills

18. **Ans. (b) Wing's Handicaps, Behavior and Skills (HBS) Schedule** [Ref. Park 27/e p795]
    - *Wing's Handicaps, Behavior and Skills (HBS) Schedule:* One of the most important epidemiological tool used for assessing abilities and disabilities in children
      - Wing's HBS in not useful for those who are not retarded

MENTAL HEALTH RATING SCALES IN CHILDREN:
- *Adaptive Behaviour Scale (AAMR ABS):* To evaluate functional and behavioural disorder in children and adolescents with mental retardation, autism and other developmental disabilities
- *Child Behaviour Checklist (CBCL) Scale:* To evaluate pathological behaviours and social competence in children aged 1½ to 18 years.
- *Children's Depression Inventory (CDI) Scale:* To evaluate depression in children and adolescents
- *Children's Depression Rating Scale (CDRS):* To evaluate severity of depression in children
- *Comprehensive Behaviour Rating Scale for Children (CBRS(C):* To assess child's school functioning
- *Conners' Rating Scale (CRS):* To assess psychopathology and behavioural problems in children and adolescents

- *Diagnostic Interview Schedule for Children (DIS(C):* To diagnose mental disorders in children and adolescents
- *Revised Children's Manifest Anxiety Scale (RCMAS):* To evaluate anxiety in children
- *Reynolds Adolescent Depression Scale (RADS):* To screen for and measure depression in adolescents

ALSO REMEMBER
- **International Classification of Functioning, Disability and Health (ICF)** is a classification of the health components of functioning and disability
  - The ICF classification complements WHO's International Classification of Diseases-10th Revision (IC(D), which contains information on diagnosis and health condition, but not on functional status
  - The ICF is structured around the following broad components:
    1. Body functions and structure
    2. Activities (related to tasks and actions by an individual) and participation (involvement in a life situation)
    3. Additional information on severity and environmental factors

19. **Ans. (c) Belief**   *[Ref. Park 27/e p791]*
    - *Attitude:* Relatively enduring organization of beliefs around an object or subject which predisposes one to respond in a preferential manner
      - Acquired characteristics of an individual
      - Is more or less 'permanent ways of behaving'
      - Is 'caught, not taught'
      - Is 'objective in nature'
    - *Value:* The ideals, customs, institutions of a society toward which the people of the group have an affective regard
    - May be positive (cleanliness, freedom, or education) or negative (cruelty, crime, or blasphemy)
    - *Opinions:* Views held by people on a point of dispute
      - Are 'temporary, provisional'
      - Are 'Subjective in nature'
    - *Belief:* Views derived from parents, grand parents and other people we respect
      - Are 'permanent, unstable, almost unchanging'
      - Is 'subjective in nature'

20. **Ans. (a) Opinion**   *[Ref. Park 27/e p791]*
21. **Ans. (a) Cultural belief**   *[Ref. Park 27/e p787, 791]*
22. **Ans. (b) Self actualization**   *[Ref. Textbook of Basic Nursing by Rosdahl and Kowaiski, 9/e p44–45]*

Review Questions

23. **Ans. (a) Propaganda**   *[Ref. Park 27/e p792]*
24. **Ans. (a) Social psychology**   *[Ref. Park 27/e p785]*

IQ

25. **Ans. (c) 50–69**   *[Ref. Park 27/e p794]*
    - *Levels of intelligence based on IQ levels:*

Levels of Intelligence	IQ range
Idiot	0–24
Imbecile	25–49
Moron	50–69
Borderline	70–79
Low normal	80–89
Normal	90–109
Superior	110–119
Very superior	120–139
Near Genius	140 and over

    - *Categories of mental retardation based on IQ levels:*

Mental status	IQ range
Normal IQ	70 and over
Mild mental retardation	50–69
Moderate mental retardation	35–49
Severe mental retardation	21–34
Profound mental retardation	20 or below

ALSO REMEMBER
- **Sentience Quotient (SQ):** Is a measure of the efficiency of an individual brain, not its relative intelligence
- **Emotional Intelligence Quotient (EQ):** Describes an ability, capacity, or skill to perceive, assess, and manage the emotions of one's self, of others, and of groups
- **Social intelligence:** Is the ability to understand and manage men and women, boys and girls, to act wisely in human relations

26. **Ans. (c) 90–109**   *[Ref. Park 27/e p794]*
27. **Ans. (a) 45; (d) 75; (e) 85**   *[Ref. Park 23/e p679]*
28. **Ans. (a) Mental age/chronological age × 100**   *[Ref. Park 27/e p794]*
29. **Ans. (b) Imbecile**   *[Ref. Park 27/e p794]*
30. **Ans. (d) Intellectual disability**   *[Ref. DSM-V Updates by Wicks-Nelson 8/e p278]*
    - American Psychiatric Association (APA) is responsible for naming, defining, and describing mental disorders
    - In the fifth edition of the Diagnostic and Statistical Manual of Mental Disorders (DSM-5), the APA replaced "Mental retardation" with "Intellectual disability (intellectual developmental disorder)"

FAMILY

31. **Ans. (d) Formation, Extension, Complete extension, Contraction, Complete contraction, Dissolution**   *[Ref. Park 27/e p798]*

- A normal *family cycle* is conceived as having 6 phases:

	Phases of family life cycle	Events characterising	
	Description	Beginning of phase	End of phase
I	Formation	Marriage	Birth of 1st child
II	Extension	Birth of 1st child	Birth of last child
III	Complete extension	Birth of last child	1st child leaves home
IV	Contraction	1st child leaves home	Last child leaves home
V	Completed contraction	Last child leaves home	1st spouse dies
VI	Dissolution	1st spouse dies	Death of survivor (extinction)

32. **Ans. (d) Communal family**   [Ref. Park 27/e p799]
    - *Communal family:* Is a family where all of its members are playing a part in its management
      - Is a good example of 'division of labour', an important function of a family.

> **ALSO REMEMBER**
> - *Most powerful example of social cohesion:* Family

33. **Ans. (c) Problem family**   [Ref. Park 27/e p801]
    - *Problem Family:* Is a family which lags behind rest of the community; underlying factors in most problem families are those of personality, relationships, backwardness, poverty, illness, mental and social instability, character defects and marital disharmony
      - Standards of life are generally far below the accepted minimum
      - Parents are unable to meet the physical and emotional needs of children
      - Home life is utterly unsatisfactory

> **ALSO REMEMBER**
> - *Nuclear Family (Elementary/Unitary Family):* Consists of a married couple and their children while they are still regarded as dependents
> - *Broken Family:* Where both parents have separated or where death has occurred of one or both the parents
> - *Communal Family:* Is a family where all of its members are playing a part in its management

34. **Ans. (b) It is applied to all nuclear families of less then 10 years duration**   [Ref. Park 27/e p799]
    - *New Family:* A family of less than 10 years duration and consists of parents and children
      - It is a variant of nuclear (elementary/unitary) family
      - New Family concept is important in view of studies related to family planning

35. **Ans. (b) Husband, wife and dependent children**   [Ref. Park 27/e p798–799]

36. **Ans. (c) Family**   [Ref. Sociology by Basu, 1/e p24]
    - Goldenwiser speaks of family as a bridge between generations and between fathers and sons
    - It is a transfer point of civilization

SOCIO-ECONOMIC STATUS

37. **Ans. (d) Income, Occupation of head of family, Education of head of family**   [Ref. Textbook of Community Medicine by Sunder Lal, 2/e p17, Park 27/e p805]
    - *Modified Kuppuswamy Scale:* For socioeconomic status
      - Is used for Urban families
      - Is based on 3 parameters:
        1. Education status of head of family
        2. Occupation of head of family
        3. Income of the family per month
      - *Scoring:* Each component is given a weighted score and summed up
      - Socio-economic classes based on scores:

Score	Socio-economic class
26–29	I
16–25	II
11–15	III
05–10	IV
<05	V

- *Udai Pareek Scale:*
  - Is for Rural families
  - Is not dependent on income

> **ALSO REMEMBER**
> - *Socio-economic status (SES) scales:*
>
> | – Urban SES scales: | – Rural SES scales: |
> |---|---|
> | 1. Modified Kuppuswamy Scale | 1. Udai Pareek Scale |
> | 2. Kulshreshtha Scale | 2. Modified B. G. Prasad Scale |
> | 3. Srivastava Scale | 3. Radhukar Scale |
> | 4. Jalota Scale | 4. Shirpurkar Scale |
> | – Student's scale: | – Non-Indian SES scales: |
> | 1. Bhardwaj Scale | 1. Hollingshead (Occupation base(d) Scale |
> | | 2. Henderson Scale |

38. **Ans. (d) 26–29**   [Ref. Park 27/e p805]

    Socioeconomic classes under Modified Kuppuswamy Scale

Socioeconomic class	Total score
Upper	26–29
Upper middle	16–25
Lower middle	11–15
Upper lower	05–10
Lower	01–04

39. **Ans. (c) Likert scale** [Ref. Park 23/e p689]

LIKERT SCALE
- A psychometric response scale primarily used in questionnaires to obtain participant's preferences or degree of agreement with a statement or set of statements
- Likert scales are a non-comparative scaling technique and are unidimensional (only measure a single trait) in nature
- Respondents are asked to indicate their level of agreement with a given statement by way of an ordinal scale.

Review Question
40. **Ans. (a) Kuppuswamy scale** [Ref. Park 27/e p804–805]

SOCIAL PROBLEMS

41. **Ans. (a) 1960** [Ref. Park 23/e p697, 27/e p672]

IMPORTANT ACTS IN PUBLIC HEALTH: (Related to child health)	Year
The Vaccination Act	1880
The Child Marriage Restraint (SARD(A) Act	1929
The Children's Act	1960
The Registration of Births and Deaths Act	1969
The Infant Milk Substitutes, Feeding Bottles and Infant Food (Regulation of production, supply and distribution) Act	1992
The Pre-conception and Pre-natal Diagnostic Techniques (Prohibition of Sex Selection) [PNDT] Act	1994

42. **Ans. (b) Health professional involved in coping strategies, interpersonal skills, adjustment with family** [Ref. Logical Reasoning]

43. **Ans. (b) Involvement in Political decision making; (c) Involvement in economic decision making** [Ref. Women Empowerment Through Literacy Campaign by J Varghese, 1/e p120–21]

44. **Ans. (a) Ensuring the safety of women** [Ref. Current Affairs 2015, p107]
- Nirbhaya Fund is an Indian rupee 30 billion corpus (over first 2 years) announced by Government of India in February 2013
- This fund is expected to support initiatives by the government and NGOs working towards protecting the dignity and ensuring safety of women in India
- Nodal Ministry: Ministry of Women and Child Development.

ECONOMICS

45. **Ans. (b) Bismarck** [Ref. Foundations of Community Medicine, GM Dhaar and I Robbani, 1/e p25]
- *Social security:* primarily refers to a social insurance program providing social protection, or protection against socially recognized conditions, including poverty, old age, disability, unemployment and others
- *Approaches to social security system:*
  - *Social assistance:* Non-contributory benefit extended to vulnerable groups
  - *Social insurance:* Contributory benefit extended to individuals as a matter of right
- *Bismarck* introduced a system of social insurance in Germany in 1883: It became a model for other European countries to introduce similar social security systems.

> **ALSO REMEMBER**
> - *Social safety net:* is a term used to describe a collection of services provided by the state, such as welfare, unemployment benefit, universal healthcare, homeless shelters, the minimum wage and sometimes subsidized services such as public transport, which prevent individuals from falling into poverty beyond a certain level

46. **Ans. (c) 2100** [Ref. Park 23/e p702]
- Below Poverty Line (BPL) Criteria[Q]:

BPL Criteria	Rural areas	Urban areas
Per capita caloric intake	<2400 kcal/day	<2100 kcal/day
Per capita income (TC)	<27/- INR/day	<33/- INR/day
Per capita income (RC)	<32/- INR/day	<47/- INR/day
Per capita income (WHO)	<1.90 US$ per day	

(TC: Tendulkar Committee 2011–12; RC: Rangarajan Committee 2014)

- *Below Poverty Line (BPL) population in India[Q]:*
  - 22% (Tendulkar Committee 2011–12)
  - 29.5% (Rangarajan Committee 2014)

> **ALSO REMEMBER**
> - *World Bank definition of poverty:*
>   - Extreme poverty as living on less than US$ (PPP) 1 per day
>   - Moderate poverty as living on less than $2 a day
> - *'Eradication of extreme poverty and hunger by 2015'* is the first Millennium Development Goal (MDG)
> - *Diseases of poverty:* Diseases that are more prevalent among 'the poor' than among wealthier people
>   - *3 primary diseases of poverty:* AIDS, malaria, and tuberculosis
>   - *3 additional diseases of poverty:* measles, pneumonia and diarrheal diseases
> - *Gini coefficient:* A measure of statistical dispersion most prominently used as a measure of inequality of income distribution or inequality of wealth distribution
> - *Human Poverty Index (HPI):* Is an indication of the standard of living in a country, developed by the United Nations
>   - HDI is a measure of development, whereas HPI is a measure of its deprivation

47. **Ans. (c) 5** *[Ref. Annual Report 2013–14, MoHFW, Government of India]*
    - Current India's Total health expenditure is 4.7% of GDP (2014)

48. **Ans. (a) 1.2 [RECENT VALUE 1.3%]**
    [Ref. XIIth FYP document, Volume 3, Health, p2–3]

Review Question

49. **Ans. (b) 2400** *[Ref. Park 27/e p817]*

INTERVIEWING

50. **Ans. (c) Establishing contact** *[Ref. Park 27/e p812]*
    - *Steps of Interview:*
        – *Establishing contact:* First requisite before conducting an interview
        – Starting an interview
        – Securing rapport
        – Recall
        – Probe questions
        – Encouragement
        – Guiding the interview
        – Closing the interview
        – Report

MISCELLANEOUS

51. **Ans. (d) Involving family members in observation** *[Ref. Park 27/e p800]*

    In DOTS (RNTCP), several studies have shown improved compliance of treatment when family members are involved in observation

52. **Ans. (d) A mob** *[Ref. K. Park 27/e p797]*
53. **Ans. (b) Ergonomics** *[Ref. Park 27/e p930]*

Review Question

54. **Ans. (c) Reduction in institutional delivery** *[Ref. Internet]*

CHAPTER 11

Environment and Health

WATER

Safe and Wholesome Water
- *Safe and wholesome water*^Q: Has been defined as water that is
  - Free from pathogenic agents
  - Free from harmful chemical substances
  - Pleasant to taste (free from colour and odour)
  - Usable for domestic purposes
- Water is said to be *'polluted'* or *'contaminated'* if it does not fulfill above criteria.

Sources of Water
- *Rain*:
  - Is the prime source of all water^Q
  - Is the *'purest form of water in nature'*^Q
  - *Chemically, it is very soft water*: contains traces (0.0005%) of solids
  - Gibraltar depends on rain water as a source of supply
- *Surface water*:
  - Impounding reservoirs
    - Artificial lakes for storing large quantities
    - Mumbai, Chennai, Nagpur derive water from it
    - Next to rain water in purity
  - Rivers and streams
    - Grossly polluted; unfit for drinking without treatment
    - Delhi, Kolkata, Allahabad derive water from it
  - Tanks, ponds and lakes
- *Ground water*:
  - Shallow wells
    - Moderately hard, grossly contaminated water
    - Taps water from above 1st impervious layer^Q
  - Deep wells
    - Much hard, pure water; constant supply
    - Taps water from below 1st impervious layer^Q
  - Springs.

> **Key points**
>
> Rain: Is the *'purest form of water in nature'*

Criteria for Identification of 'Problem Habitations'
- *Not Covered (NC)/No Safe Source (NSS) Habitations*^Q:
  - Drinking water source point is not within 1.6 km in plains or 100 m elevation in hilly areas
  - Water source affected with quality problems like excess salinity, iron, fluoride, arsenic, or other toxic materials or biologically contaminated
  - Quantum of availability of safe water is not enough to meet drinking and cooking needs
- *Partially Covered (PC) Habitations*:
  - Drinking water source point is within 1.6 km in plains or 100 m elevation in hilly areas
  - Capacity of system is 10–40 lpcd
- *Fully Covered (FC) Habitations*: include all the remaining habitations.

Purification of Water

- *Purification of water on a large scale*:
  - *Storage of water*:
    - Physical
    - Chemical
    - Biological
  - *Filtration of water*:
    - Slow sand (Biological) filters
    - Rapid sand (Mechanical) filters
  - *Disinfection of water*:
    - Chlorination
    - Ozonation
    - Ultraviolet irradiation
- *Purification of water on a small scale*:
  - *Household purification of water*:
    - Boiling
    - *Chemical disinfection*: Bleaching powder, Chlorine solution, High test hypochlorite (HTH), Chlorine (Halozone) tablets, Iodine, Potassium permanganate
    - *Filtration*: Ceramic filters (Pasteur Chamberland filter, Berkefeld filter, Katadyn filter)
  - *Disinfection of wells*:
    - *Chemical*: Bleaching powder (Double pot method).

Comparison of Rapid and Slow Sand Filters[Q]

	Rapid Sand Filter	Slow Sand Filter
Space	Occupies very little space	Occupies large area
Rate of filtration	200 m.g.a.d.	2–3 m.g.a.d.
Effective size of sand[Q]	0.4–0.7 mm	0.2–0.3 mm
Preliminary treatment	Coagulation, sedimentation	Plain sedimentation
Washing[Q]	By back-washing	By scraping sand bed
Frequent washing[Q]	Required	Not required
Mechanism of action	Essentially physical	Both physical & mechanical
Operation	Highly skilled	Less skilled
Loss of head allowed[Q]	6–8 feet	4 feet
Removal of turbidity	Good	Good
Removal of colour	Good	Fair
Removal of bacteria[Q]	98–99 percent	99.9–99.99 percent
Suitability	For big cities	For small towns

Key Guideline Aspects Recommended Drinking Water Quality

- *Colour* <15 true colour units (TCU)[Q] [<5 Hazen units]
- *Turbidity* <1 nephlometric turbidity units (NTU)[Q]
- *Hardness* <100–300 mg/litre calcium ion
- *pH*: 6.5–8.5
- *Total dissolved solids (TDS)* <500 mg/litre[Q]*(BIS 2017)
- Zero pathogenic microorganisms
- Zero infectious viruses
- *Absence of pathogenic protozoa and infective stages of helminthes*
- *Fluoride* <1 ppm (0.5–0.8 ppm: Optimum level)
- *Nitrates* <45 mg/litre[Q]
- *Nitrites* <3 mg/litre[Q]
- *Gross alpha radiological activity* <0.5 Bq/litre [New Guideline — WHO][Q]
- *Gross beta radiological activity* <1.0 Bq/litre [New Guideline — WHO][Q]

Key Guideline Aspects of NPCB (India) Recommended Drinking Water Quality

	After disinfection (Class A)	After conventional treatment and disinfection (Class C)
Total coliforms organism MPN/100 mL	<50	<5000
pH	6.5–8.5	6.0–9.0
Dissolved oxygen	>6 mg/L	>4 mg/L
Biochemical oxygen Demand 5 days 20°C	<2 mg/L	<3 mg/L

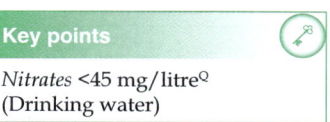

Key points

Nitrates <45 mg/litre^Q (Drinking water)

Chlorination of Water

- *Disinfecting action of chlorine in water is due to*:
  - Hypochlorous acid (HOCl)–Main role in disinfection^Q
  - Hypochlorite ions (OCl)–Minor role in disinfection
- *Chlorine has residual germicidal effect* (and not Ozone or UV rays): Provides a margin of safety against subsequent microbial contamination, as may occur during storage and distribution
- *Phases of Chlorination*:
  - Phase I: Formation of chloramines
  - Phase II: Destruction of chloramines
  - Phase III: Appearance of break-point
  - Phase IV: Accumulation of free residual chlorine.

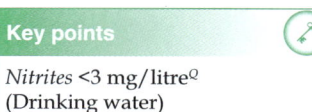

Key points

Nitrites <3 mg/litre^Q (Drinking water)

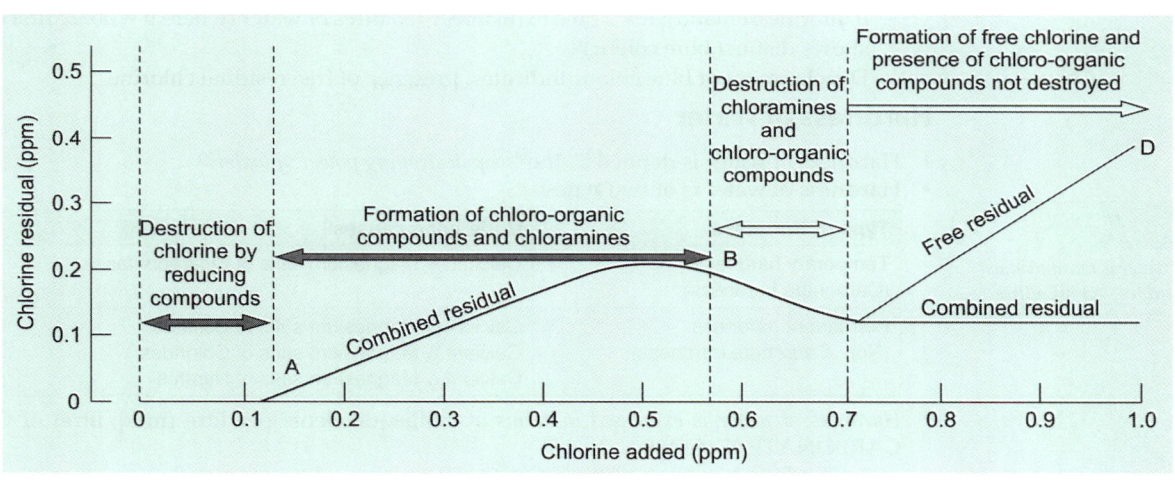

Phases of chlorination

- *Recommended contact period of free residual chlorine in water*: 1 hour^Q
- *Level of free residual chlorine (FRC) recommended*:

Water type	Recommended Residual chlorine level*	Contact period
Drinking water^Q	>0.5 mg per litre (ppm)	1 hour
Water bodies, post disaster	>0.7 mg per litre (ppm)	1 hour
Swimming pool sanitation^Q	>1.0 mg per litre (ppm)	1 hour

(*1 mg per litre = 1 ppm)

- *Instruments used in chlorination of water*:

Instrument	Utility
Horrock's Apparatus^Q	Chlorine demand estimation
Chlorinator/Chloronome	Mixing or regulating dose of chlorine
Chloroscope^Q	Measuring residual level of chlorine

> **Key points**
>
> Disinfecting action of chlorine in water is due to:
> Hypochlorous acid (HOCl)

- *Tests for chlorination of water*:
  - *Ortho-toluidine (OT) Test^Q*: Measure the levels of,
    - Free (residual) chlorine
    - Free & Combined chlorine
  - *Ortho-toluidine Arsenite (OTA) Test^Q*: Measure the levels of,
    - Free chlorine
    - Combined chlorine
  - OTA test is better than OT test as^Q:
    - Detects both free and combined chlorine separately
    - Not affected by interfering substances (nitrites, iron, manganese).

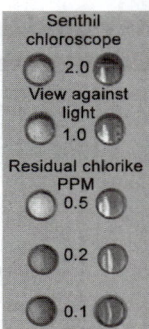

Horrock's Apparatus

> **Key points**
>
> Horrock's Apparatus
> 'Chlorine demand estimation of water'

- *Use*: To find out the dose of bleaching powder required for disinfection of water, i.e. 'Chlorine demand estimation of water'^{Q}
- *Contents*:
  - 6 white cups (200 mL capacity each)
  - 1 Black cup (with a circular mark inside)
  - 2 metal spoons
  - 7 glass stirring rods
- *Indicator*: Starch iodide (producing blue colour)^Q

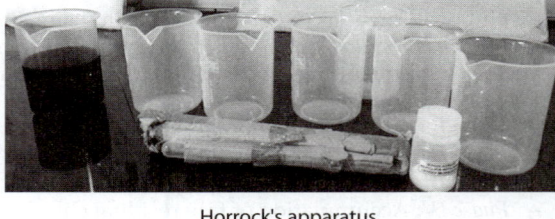

Horrock's apparatus

  - Dose of bleaching powder required (Chlorine demand): n × 2 gms to disinfect 455 litres of water (where n = no. of first cup which shows distinct blue colour)^Q
  - Development of blue colour indicates: presence of free residual chlorine.

Hardness of Water

- Hardness of water is defined as the *'soap destroying power of water'*^{Q}
- Hardness of water is of two types:

Type of Hardness	Underlying causes^Q
Temporary hardness (Carbonate hardness)	Calcium & Magnesium salts of Bicarbonates
Permanent hardness (Non- Carbonate hardness)	Calcium & Magnesium salts of Sulfates Calcium & Magnesium salts of Chlorides Calcium & Magnesium salts of Nitrates

> **Key points**
>
> Softening of water is recommended at level of hardness >3 mEq/litre

- *Hardness of water is expressed in terms of*: milliequivalents per litre (mEq/litre) of CALCIUM CARBONATE ($CaCO_3$)^Q
  - 1 mEq/litre hardness = 50 mg $CaCO_3$ (50 ppm) per litre of water^Q
- *Classification of hardness in water*:

Classification	Level of Hardness (mEq/litre)
Soft water	<1 (<50 mg/l)
Moderately Hard water	1–3 (50–150 mg/l)
Hard water	3–6 (150–300 mg/l)
Very Hard water	>6 (>300 mg/l)

  - *Softening of water is recommended at level of hardness >3 mEq/litre (>150 mg/litre of Calcium carbonate)*^{Q}
- *Methods of removal of hardness of water*:

Type of hardness	Methods of removal^Q
Temporary hardness	Boiling Addition of lime Addition of sodium carbonate Permutit process
Permanent hardness	Addition of sodium carbonate Base exchange process

Bacteriological Indicators of Water Quality[Q]

- *Coliform organisms*:
  - Primary & most reliable bacterial indicator for water quality[Q]
  - E. coli is most important coliform indicator[Q]
  - Reasons for choosing coliforms as indicators of fecal pollution Rather Than Water Borne Pathogens[Q]:
    - Constant presence in great abundance in human intestine; foreign to potable waters
    - Easily detectable by culture methods
    - Longer survival period
    - Greater resistance to forces of natural purification
- *Fecal streptococci*:
  - Indicate 'recent contamination of water'[Q]
- *Clostridium perfringens*:
  - Indicate 'remote contamination of water'[Q]

> **Key points**
>
> *Coliform organisms:*
> Primary & most reliable bacterial indicator for water quality

Presumptive Coliform Test

- *MPN Multiple Tube test*: Is based on estimating the most probable number (MPN) of coliform organisms in 100 mL of water[Q]
  - *Culture medium*: McConkey's Lactose Bile Salt broth[Q]
  - *Indicator*: Bromocresol purple[Q]
  - *Presumption*: Tubes showing fermentation (acid & gas) contain coliforms
  - *Method*: 4 tubes inoculated with 0.1, 1.0, 10, 50 mL of water & incubated for 48 hrs
  - *Confirmatory tests (EIKJMAN'S Tests[Q])*: Subculture each presumptive positive tube in 2 tubes of brilliant green bile broth.
    - Incubate one tube at 37 °C × 48 hrs: confirmation of presence of coliforms
    - Incubate second tube at 44° C × 6–24 hrs: confirmation of presence of E.coli
  - *True MPN Index*: Calculate revised MPN from McCrady's tables[Q]
- *Membrane Filtration Technique*:
  - *Membrane*: cellulose ester
  - *Method*: pass known volume of water through membrane, inoculate membrane on suitable media, count colonies in 20 hrs.

> **Key points**
>
> - *Fecal streptococci:* Indicate 'recent contamination of water'[Q]
> - *Clostridium perfringens:* Indicate 'remote contamination of water'[Q]

Public Health Classification of Water Borne Diseases

- *Water borne diseases*: Occur due to drinking contaminated water, transmitted by faeco-oral route
  - Examples: Typhoid, Cholera, Dysentery, Viral Hepatitis A
- *Water washed diseases*[Q]: Include infections of the outer body surface which occur due to inadequate use of water or improper hygiene
  - Examples: Scabies, Trachoma, Typhus, Bacillary dysentery, Amoebic dysentery
- *Water based diseases*[Q]: Refers to infections transmitted through an aquatic invertebrate animal
  - Examples: Schistosomiasis, Dracunculiasis (Guineaworm disease)
- *Water related diseases (Water breeding diseases)*: Are infections spread by insects that depend on water
  - Examples: Malaria, Filariasis, Dengue, Yellow fever, Onchocerciasis

AIR

Ventilation

- *Types of ventilation*:
  - *Natural ventilation*:
    - *Wind*: It blows through a room (*Perflation*) and may exert a suction at its tail end (*Aspiration*)
    - *Diffusion*: When passes through smallest openings
    - Inequality of temperature.
  - *Mechanical (artificial) ventilation*:
    - *Exhaust ventilation*: Air is extracted to outside by exhaust fans driven by electricity
    - *Plenum ventilation*[Q]: Fresh air is blown into rooms by centrifugal fans

> **Key points**
> Air change^Q: 2–3 changes per hour in living rooms

- *Balanced ventilation*: Combination of exhaust and plenum ventilation
- *Air conditioning*: Simultaneous control of all factors especially temperature, humidity and air movement
- *Standards of Ventilation*:
  - *Cubic space*: Fresh air supply of 3000 cu. ft. per hour per person
  - *Air change*^{Q}: 2–3 changes per hour in living rooms; 4–6 changes per hour in work rooms and assemblies
  - *Floor space*: Minimum 50–100 sq. ft. per person^Q

Air Humidity

- *Description*: Air humidity is moisture content of air
- *Air humidity can be measured by*^{Q}:
  - Dry and wet bulb thermometers
  - Hygrometer
  - Sling/Whirling Psychrometer
  - Assman Psychrometer.

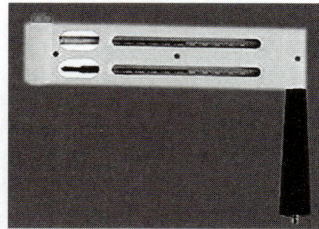
Sling psychrometer

Air Pollution

- *Primary pollutants*: are emitted directly (SO_2, NO_2, CO, Hydrocarbons, Particulate matter, CFCs, Ammonia, Radioactive materials, Metals like lead, cadmium, copper, Volatile organic compounds)
- *Secondary pollutants*: are formed by interaction between primary pollutants (Ground level ozone, Peroxyacetyl nitrate, Particulate matter formed from primary pollutants)
- *Chemical indicators of air pollution*^{Q}:
  - *Sulphur dioxide*: BEST INDICATOR of air pollution^Q
  - *Smoke or Soiling index*: Air strain on a filter paper measured through photoelectric meter
  - *Grit & dust measurement*
  - *Coefficient of haze*
  - *Air pollution index*
  - *Soiling Index*^{Q}
- *BEST Biological indicator of air pollution*: Lichens^Q

> **Key points**
> Sulphur dioxide: BEST INDICATOR of air pollution

National Air Quality Index (NAQI)

- *Description:* NAQI is a tool for effective communication of air quality status to people in terms, which are easy-to-understand. It transforms complex air quality data of various pollutants into a single number (index value), nomenclature and colour
- *NAQI monitoring is done by:* Central Pollution Control Board (CPCB)
- NAQI sub-index and health breakpoints are evolved for eight pollutants (PM10, PM2.5, NO_2, SO_2, CO, O_3, NH_3, and Pb) for which short-term (up to 24-hours) National Ambient Air Quality Standards are prescribed

AQI	Remark	Color Code	Possible Health Impacts
0–50	Good	Green	Minimal impact
51–100	Satisfactory	Light green	Minor breathing discomfort to sensitive people
101–200	Moderate	Yellow	Breathing discomfort to people with lungs, asthma, heart diseases
201–300	Poor	Orange	Breathing discomfort to most people on prolonged exposure
301–400	Very Poor	Red	Respiratory illness on prolonged exposure
401–500	Severe	Dark red	Affects healthy people & seriously impacts those with existing diseases

Sources of Indoor Air Pollution

Indoor air pollutant	Sources
Respirable particles	Tobacco smoke, Stove, Aerosols
Carbon monoxide	Combustion equipment, Stove, Gas heaters
Nitrogen dioxide	Gas cookers, Cigarettes
Sulphur dioxide	Coal combustion
Carbon dioxide	Combustion, Respiration
Formaldehyde	Particle board, Carpet adhesives, Insulation
Organic vapours (benzene, toluidine)	Solvents, Adhesives, Resins, Aerosols
Ozone	Electric arcing, UV light
Radon & daughters	Building materials^Q
Asbestos	Insulation, Fire-proofing
Mineral fibres	Appliances

Instruments used in Air Temperature^Q

Instrument	Measures^Q
Dry bulb thermometer	Air temperature
Wet bulb thermometer	Air temperature
Maximum thermometer	Air temperature
Minimum thermometer	Air temperature
Six's maximum & minimum thermometer	Air temperature
Silvered thermometer	Air temperature
Globe thermometer	Mean radiant temperature
Wet Globe thermometer	Environmental heat
Kata thermometer	Cooling power of Air; Low air velocity

Key points

Tolerable sound level to human ear 85–90 dB^Q

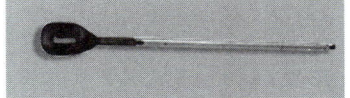

Kata thermometer

Global Warming

- *Greenhouse gases^Q*:
  - Water vapour (Highest contribution)
  - Carbon dioxide (Second highest contribution)
  - Methane
  - Ozone
    - *Ozone layer*: Is beneficial as it cuts down UV transmission
    - CFCs depletes ozone layer.
- *Kyoto Protocol^Q*:
  - *Entered into force*: 16th Feb 2005
  - *Signed and ratified by*: 187 countries
  - *Targeted reductions in transmissions^Q*:
    - Carbon dioxide
    - Methane
    - Nitrous oxide
    - Sulphurhexafluoride (SF6)
    - Perfluorocarbons (PFC)
    - Chlorofluorocarbons (CFC).

SOUND

Sound Levels

- *Human ear is sensitive to sound frequency*: 20–20,000 Hz^Q

- *Daily maximum tolerable sound level to human ear* (without substantial damage to their hearing): 85–90 dB^Q
- *Auditory fatigue appears in*: 90 dB region (greatest at 4000 Hz)^Q
- *Sound level above which tympanic membrane rupture* (permanent mechanical damage): 150–160 dB^Q.

Noise Levels

- *Whisper*: 20–30 dB
- *Normal conversation*: 60–70 dB
- *Mechanical damage*: 150–160 dB (e.g., Jet taking off).

Acceptable Noise Levels

Environment	Place	Acceptable noise level dB (A)
Residential	Bed room	25
	Living room	40
Commercial	Office	35–45
	Conference	40–45
	Restaurants	40–60
Industrial	Workshop	40–60
	Laboratory	40–50
Educational	Class room	30–40
	Library	35–40
Hospitals^Q	**Wards**	**20–35**

> **Key points**
> Hospitals^Q
> Wards noise levels: 20–35 dB

LIGHT

Illumination

- *Basic minimum illumination for satisfactory vision*: **15–20 foot candles**^Q
- *Reflection factors for efficient vision*:
  - Ceilings and roofs: 80%
  - Walls: 50–60%
  - Floor: 15–20%
  - Furniture: 30–40%
- *Daylight factor (D.F.)*^Q: Measures intensity of daylight illumination
  - Recommended D.F. for living rooms: ≥ 8%
  - Recommended D.F. for kitchens: ≥ **10%**.

HOUSING

Housing Standards in India

- *Site*: Elevated from surroundings; away from nuisances; subsoil water below 10 feet
- *Set back*: Built up area up to 2/3 of total area
- *Floor*: Pucca; height of plinth 2–3 feet
- *Walls*: 9-inch brick wall plastered; low heat capacity
- *Roof*: >10 feet in absence of air-conditioning; low heat transmittance coefficient
- *Rooms*: should be depending on family size
- **Floor area: 50–100 sq. ft. per person**^Q
- *Cubic space*: >500 cu. ft. per capita
- *Windows*: Windows area 1/5 of floor area (**Doors + windows area 2/5 of floor area**^Q); placed at height of not more than 3 ft from floor
- *Lighting*: Day light factor >1% over half of floor area^Q
- *Kitchen*: Separate; impervious floor; adequately lighted; provided with water supply and drainage
- *Privy*: Sanitary privy in each house
- *Garbage and refuse*: Sanitary disposal method
- *Bathing and washing*: Exclusive facilities
- *Water supply*: Safe and adequate water supply.

> **Key points**
> *Floor area in a house (recommended):*
> 50–100 sq. ft. per person

Rural Housing Standards in India

- Minimum 2 living rooms
- Ample verandah space
- Built up area up to 1/3 of total area
- Separate kitchen with paved sink/platform
- Sanitary latrine
- Windows area 10% of floor area
- Sanitary well/tube well within ¼ mile
- Cattle shed >25 ft away
- Adequate arrangement for disposal of waste water, refuse and garbage

> **Key points**
> *Sanitary Landfill (Controlled Tipping): Most Satisfactory Method^Q*
> For solid waste disposal

WASTE DISPOSAL

Types of Wastes

- *Refuse*: Solid waste generated
  - Street refuse
  - Market refuse
  - Stable refuse
  - Industrial refuse
  - Constructional refuse
  - Hospital refuse
  - Domestic refuse
    - *Ash*: Residue from fire used for cooking & heating
    - *Rubbish*: Paper, clothing, wood, metal, glass, dust
    - *Garbage*: Processed food waste generated from kitchen^Q
- *Sewage*: Liquid waste containing excreta^Q
- *Sullage*: Liquid waste without excreta^Q
- *Litter*: Waste disposed in wrong place by unlawful human action.

> **Key points**
> *Composition of sewage^Q*: 99.9% water + 0.1% solids

Methods of Refuse Disposal

Methods of refuse disposal	
Insanitary methods^Q	**Sanitary methods^Q**
Hog feeding	Composting
Stacking	Sanitary landfill
Salvaging	Incineration
Dumping	

- *Hog feeding*: Traditional way of refuse disposal by feeding to pigs
  - Insanitary method: Leads to soil pollution & water pollution
- *Stacking*: Piling up of refuse & cow dung
- *Salvaging*: Screening refuse dumps to recover objects that can be reclaimed & reused
- *Dumping*: Throwing refuse openly in an insanitary manner in periurban areas
- *Composting*: Integrated method of disposal of refuse & night soil
  - *Bangalore method^Q* (*Anaerobic hot fermentation process^Q*): Alternate layers of refuse & night soil in proportion 3:1, with refuse layer both as lowermost as well as topmost
  - *Indore Method* (*Aerobic process*)
- *Sanitary Landfill* (*Controlled Tipping*): Laying of dry & condensed refuse in layers with intervening earth partitions & coverings, followed by mechanical compression [*Most Satisfactory Method^Q*]
  - Trench Method
  - Ramp Method
  - Area Method
- *Incineration*: High temperature dry oxidation process which reduces waste volume & weight^Q.

Sewage

- *Sewage*: Is waste water from a community, containing solid and liquid excreta, derived from houses, street and yard washings, factories and industries
- *Composition of sewage^Q*: 99.9% water + 0.1% solids (organic & inorganic).

- *Amount of sewage that flows in sewers depends upon*:
  - Habits of people
  - Time of day
- *Dry weather flow*: Is the average amount of sewage that flows in sewerage system in 24 hours^Q
- **STRENGTH OF SEWAGE IS EXPRESSED IN TERMS OF**^{Q}:
  - *Biological Oxygen Demand* (**BOD**^{Q}): Is defined as 'amount of oxygen absorbed by a sample of sewage' during a specified period (Generally 5 days), at a specified temperature (generally 20°C) for aerobic destruction or use of organic matter by living organisms
    - BOD is most important test done on sewage (done through Dilution method and Manometric method)
    - Strong Sewage has BOD >300 g/litre and Weak Sewage has BOD <100 g/litre^Q
  - *Chemical Oxygen Demand (COD)*: Measures oxygen equivalent of that portion of organic matter in a sample, which is susceptible to oxidation by a strong chemical oxidizer
    - Potassium dichromate is best for COD estimation.
  - *Suspended solids*: Amount in domestic sewage varies from 100–500 mg/litre
    - Strong Sewage has suspended solids amount >500 mg/litre and Weak Sewage has suspended solids amount <100 mg/litre.

> **Key points**
> **Strong Sewage** has BOD > 300 g/litre

Methods of Sewage Disposal

- *Modern sewage treatment*:
  - Primary treatment:
    - Screening
    - Grit chamber
    - Primary sedimentation
  - Secondary treatment:
    - Aerobic oxidation (Trickling filter method; Activated sludge process)
    - Secondary sedimentation
    - Sludge digestion.
- *Sea outfall*
- *River outfall*
- *Land treatment* (*sewage farming/broad irrigation*)
- *Oxidation ponds* (*waste stabilization pond/redox pond/sewage lagoons*^{Q}): Predominantly organic during day and some part of night; only bottom layers have anaerobic digestion
- *Oxidation ditches*

Methods of Excreta Disposal in Unsewered Areas

- *Service type latrines* (*Conservancy system*):
  - Pail type latrine
  - Bucket type latrine
- *Non-service type latrines* (*Sanitary latrines*):
  - Bore hole latrine
  - Dug well or pit latrine
  - Water seal type latrines
    - P.R.A.I. type
    - R.C.A. type
    - Sulabh shauchalaya
  - Septic tank
  - Aqua privy
- *Latrines suitable for camps and temporary use*^{Q}:
  - Shallow trench latrine
  - Deep trench latrine
  - Pit latrine
  - Bore hole latrine

> **Key points**
> *Ideal retention period in Septic tank:* **24 hours**

Septic Tank

- *Description*: Is a water-tight masonary tank into which household sewage is admitted for treatment
  - Is a satisfactory method of disposing liquid and excreta wastes from individual dwellings, small groups of houses or institutions which have 'adequate water supply but do not have access to a public sewerage system'
- *Design features of a septic tank*:
  - *Capacity*: Minimum should be 500 gallons
  - *Length*: to be twice the breadth
  - *Depth*: 1.5–2 m
  - *Liquid depth*: 1.2 m
  - *Air space depth*: 30 cm
  - **Ideal retention period: 24 hours**[Q]
- *Steps of purification in a septic tank*[Q]:
  - *Anaerobic digestion*: takes place in septic tank proper
  - *Aerobic oxidation*: takes place in sub-soil (outside septic tank)
- *Process of purification in a septic tank*:
  - Solids settle down in tank to form '*Sludge*' whereas lighter solids (including grease and fat) rise to surface to form '*Scum*': Solids undergo anaerobic digestion; methane is formed
  - Liquid which passes out of outlet pipe is called '*Effluent*' (containing bacteriae, cysts, helminthic ova and organic matter) which is allowed to percolate in sub-soil: undergoes aerobic digestion by bacteria
- *Operation and maintenance of a septic tank*:
  - Avoid soap water and disinfectants (phenol) as they are injurious to bacterial flora
  - 'Desludging' should be carried out once a year
  - New tanks to be filled with water and seeded with ripe sludge from another septic tank (to provide right kind of bacteria).

MISCELLANEOUS (ENVIRONMENT)

Sanitation Measures for Swimming Pool Sanitation

- *Recommended area*: Recommended area is minimum 2.2 sq. metre (24 sq. ft.) per swimmer[Q]
- *Surveillance*: Rules and regulations to be posted in appropriate place
- *Filtration of water*: Water to be refiltered in less than 6 hours (rapid sand filters); 15% water to be replaced by fresh water everyday[Q]
- *Chlorination of water*: Residual level of free chlorine to be >1.0 ppm to protect against bacterial and viral agents[Q]
- *pH of water*: 7.4–7.8
- *Bacteriological quality of water*: To be as close to standards prescribed for drinking water.

Radiation

- *Sources of radiation exposure*:
  - *Natural sources*: (total exposure is 0.1 rad per person per year[Q])
    - Cosmic rays[Q]
    - Environmental
    - Internal
  - *Man-made sources*:
    - X-rays[Q]
    - Radioactive fall-out
- *Types of radiation*:
  - *Electromagnetic*:
    - X-rays
    - Gamma rays
  - *Corpuscular*:
    - Alpha particles

- Beta particles
- Protons
- *Biological effects of Radiation exposure*:
  - *Somatic effects*:
    - Immediate
      1. Radiation sickness
      2. Acute radiation syndrome
    - Delayed
      1. Leukaemia
      2. Carcinogenesis
      3. Foetal anomalies
      4. Shortening of life
  - *Genetic effects*:
    - Chromosomal mutations
    - Point mutations.

ENTOMOLOGY AND VECTOR CONTROL

Biological Transmission of Arthropod-borne Diseases

Transmission	Definition	Examples^Q
Propagative^Q	Disease agent only multiplies in the body of vector	Plague bacilli in rat fleas Yellow fever virus in Aedes mosquitoes
Cyclo-propagative^Q	Disease agent undergoes cyclical change and multiplies in the body of vector	Malarial parasite in anopheline mosquitoes
Cyclo-developmental^Q	Disease agent undergoes only cyclical change in the body of vector	Filarial parasite in culex mosquitoes Guineaworm embryo in cyclops

Vectors and Diseases Transmitted

Vector	Disease(s) transmitted^Q
Housefly (Musca domestica)^Q	Diarrhoeal & dysentrical diseases, Poliomyelitis, Yaws, Anthrax, Trachoma
Sandfly (Phlebotomus argentipes)^Q	Kala azar (Visceral Leishmaniasis), Oriental sore (Cutaneous Leishmaniasis), Sandfly fever, Oroya fever
Tse-Tse fly (Glossina palpalis)^Q	Sleeping sickness of Africa (African Trypanosomiasis)
Reduviid bug (Triatominae)^Q	Chagas Disease (Sleeping sickness of America- American Trypanosomiasis)
Black fly (Simulium)^Q	Onchocerciasis (River Blindness)
Soft tick^Q	Relapsing fever, Q fever, KFD (outside India)
Hard tick	Tularemia, Babesiosis, KFD (India), Tick paralysis, Tick encephalitis, Tick hemorrhagic fever, Indian Tick Typhus, RMSF
Louse^Q	Epidemic typhus, Trench fever, Relapsing fever
Mite	Scrub typhus, Rickettsial pox
Flea^Q	Plague, Murine typhus
Anopheles mosquito^Q	Malaria, Filaria (outside India)
Culex mosquito^Q	Bancroftian Filariasis, Japanese Encephalitis, West Nile fever, Viral arthritis
Aedes mosquito^Q	Yellow fever, Dengue, DHF, Chikungunya, Rift Valley fever, Filariasis (Outside India)
Mansonoides mosquito	Malayan (Brugian) filariasis, Chikungunya

> **Key points**
>
> *Life span of a mosquito varies from*: 8–34 days

Life Cycle of Mosquito

- *Life span of a mosquito varies from*: 8–34 days^Q
  - Males, as a rule, are short lived
  - Life of a mosquito is influenced by temperature & humidity
- *Life history of a mosquito*:
  - *Egg*: Laid on surface of water, 100–250 at a time

- Egg stage lasts for 1–2 days
- *Gonotrophic cycle*: Period that elapses from the moment a blood meal is taken until the eggs are laid; it is about 48 hours in hot & humid tropical areas
- *Larva*: Passes through 4 stages of growth called '*instars*', with moulting between each stage
  - Larval stage occupies 5–7 days^Q
  - Culicine larvae (Culex, Aedes, Mansonia) have a siphon tube^Q
- *Pupa*: Represents '*resting stage*' in life cycle of mosquito
  - Pupal stage lasts for 1–2 days
  - Have 2 respiratory tubes (trumpets) in thorax
  - Does not feed, prefers to stay quiet at the water surface
- *Adult*: Life cycle from egg to adult is complete in 7–10 days
  - Adult mosquito lives for about 2 weeks.

Important Mosquito Vectors in India^Q

	Anopheles	**Culex**	**Aedes**	**Mansonia**
Diseases transmitted^Q	Malaria	Bancroftian filariasis, Japanese encephalitis, West Nile fever	Dengue & DHF, Chikungunya, Yellow fever, Rift valley fever	Malayan (Brugian) filariasis
Breeding Habitat^Q	Clean water	Dirty, polluted water	**Artificial collections of water^Q**	Water bodies containing aquatic plants
Eggs	**Laid singly, Boat shaped with lateral floats^Q**	Laid in small clusters/rafts	Laid singly, cigar shaped^Q	Laid in star shaped clusters
Larvae	**No siphon tube; Rest parallel to undersurface of water^Q**	Siphon tube; Rest perpendicular to undersurface of water	Siphon tube; Rest in dark bottom corners	Siphon tube; Rest attached to rootlets of plants
Pupae	Broad & short siphon tube	Long & narrow siphon tube	Long & narrow siphon tube	Long & narrow siphon tube
Adults	Inclined at an angle to surface; Spotted wings	'Hunch back' rest^Q	Stripes on body & legs^Q	-
Flight range	3–5 km	11 km^Q	100 m^Q	-
Remark(s)	Sophisticated mosquito	Nuisance mosquito	**Tiger mosquito^Q**	-

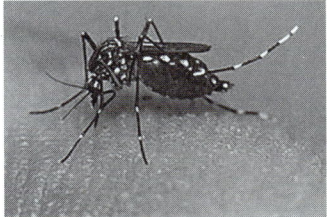

Aedes aegypti

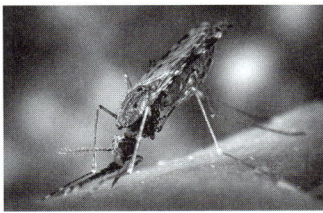

Anopheles

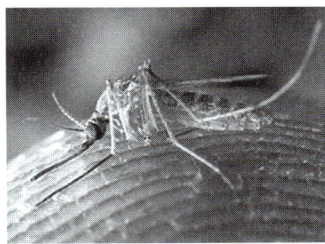

Culex mosquito

Hard Ticks Versus Soft Ticks

	Hard ticks	**Soft ticks**
Biological name	Ixodidae	Argasidae
Scutum	Present	Absent
Head	At anterior end	Lies ventrally
Spiracles	Behind IV coxa	Behind III and IV coxa
Eggs	Hundreds–thousands in 1 sitting	Batches of 20–100 over long period
Nymphal stages	1	5
Habits	Cannot stand starvation	Can stand starvation for ≥ 1 year
Diseases transmitted^Q	Tick typhus (RMSF); Viral encephalitis; Tick fevers; Hemorrhagic fevers (KFD in India); Tularaemia; Tick paralysis; Human babesiosis	Q fever (few animal cases); Relapsing fever; KFD (outside India)

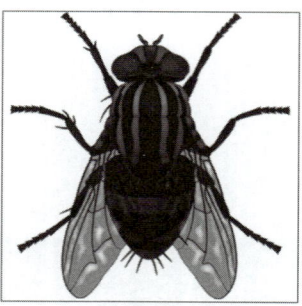
Housefly

Housefly

- *'Houseflies should be regarded as a sign of insanitation'* and their number as index of that sanitation^Q
- *Important species*: Musca domestica, M. vicinia, M. nebula, M. sorbens
- *Life span*: 15–25 days
  - Eggs: 8–24 hours
  - Larvae (maggots): 2–7 days
  - Pupae: 3–6 days
  - Adults: 5–20 days
- *Important breeding places (in order of importance)*^Q:
  - Fresh horse manure
  - Human excreta
  - Manure of other animals
  - Garbage
  - Decaying fruits and vegetables
  - Rubbish dumps containing organic matter
  - Grounds where liquid wastes are spilled
- *Feeding habits*:
  - *Housefly does not bite*: It cannot eat solid foods; it vomits on solid foods to make a solution of it, and sucks in a liquid state^Q
  - *Dispersal*: up to 4 miles
- *Modes of disease transmission*^Q:
  - Mechanical transmission: Houseflies are known as *'Porters of infection'*
  - Vomit-drop
  - Defecation
- *Houseflies in disease causation*:
  - *As vector of diseases*: Typhoid and paratyphoid fevers, diarrhoeas and dysenteries, cholera and gastroenteritis, amoebiasis, helminthic manifestations, Poliomyelitis, Yaws, Anthrax, Trachoma, conjunctivitis
  - *As causative agent of disease*: Myiasis^Q.

> **Key points**
> Phlebotomus argentipes^Q transmits Kala azar

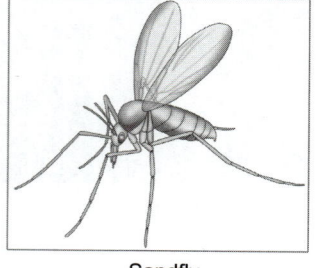
Sandfly

Sandfly

Sandfly species	Diseases transmitted
Phlebotomus argentipes^Q	Kala azar (Visceral Leishmaniasis)
Phlebotomus papatasii^Q	Sandfly fever, Oriental sore (Cutaneous Leishmaniasis)
Phlebotomus sergenti^Q	Oriental sore (Cutaneous Leishmaniasis)
Sergentomyia punjabensis	Sandfly fever

- *Habitats*^Q: Holes and crevices in walls, holes in trees, dark rooms, stables and store rooms
- *Sanitation measures are carried out for a distance of 50 feet*
- *Insecticide of choice*^Q: DDT (1–2 gm/m² single application)
- *DDT is sprayed up to height of 4–6 feet of walls*^Q: as Sandfly cannot fly; it only hops
- *Only female sandflies bite*: Require a blood meal every 3–4 days for oviposition.

> **Key points**
> Insecticide of choice for sandfly^Q: DDT

Rat Flea (Xenopsylla)

- *Rat flea acts as a vector for*^Q:
  - Bubonic plague
  - Murine (endemic/flea-borne) typhus
  - Chiggerosis
- *Rat flea acts as a host for*:
  - Hymenolepis diminuta (Rat tapeworm)
  - Hymenolepis nana (Dwarf tapeworm).

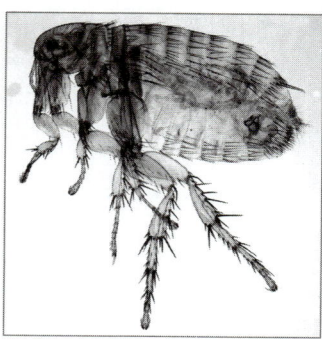
Xenopsylla cheopis

Diseases Associated with Rodents^Q

Bacterial: Plague Tularaemia Salmonellosis	Viral: Lassa fever Hemorrhagic fever Encephalitis
Rickettsial: Scrub typhus Murine (Flea-borne) typhus Rickettsial pox	Parasitic: Hymenolepis dimunita Leishmaniasis Amoebiasis Trichinosis Chagas disease
Others: Rat bite fever Leptospirosis Histoplasmosis	

Key points

Rat flea acts as a vector for^Q:
- Bubonic plague
- Murine (endemic/flea-borne) typhus
- Chiggerosis

General Principles of Arthropod Control

- *Environmental control*:
  - Best approach to control of arthropods, because results are likely to be permanent^Q
  - *Examples*: Elimination of breeding places (source reduction), filling & drainage operation, planned water management
- *Chemical control*:
  - *No longer fully effective if used alone*: Resistance has appeared in about 100 arthropods of public health importance
  - *Essential to use biodegradable, less toxic compounds*: Methoxychlor, Abate, Dursban
  - *Other examples*: Mosquito larvicidal oil (MLO), Paris green, Pyrethrum.
- *Biological control*:
  - Minimises environmental pollution
  - EXAMPLES^Q:
    - Larvivorous fishes (Gambusia affinis, Lebister reticulates, Poecilia reticulata)
    - Fungi (Coelomomyces)
    - Bacteria (Bacillus thuringiensis H14)
    - Predator mosquito (Toxorhynchitis splendens).
- *Genetic control*:
  - Techniques^Q: Sterile male technique, cytoplasmic incompatibility, chromosomal translocations
- *Newer methods*:
  - *Examples*: Insect growth regulators, chemosterilants, pheromones (sex attractants).

Key points

Environmental control: Best approach for arthropod control

Mosquito Control Measures

- *Anti-larval measures*:
  - *Environmental control*: Source reduction (minor engineering methods–filling, leveling & drainage of breeding places and water management–intermittent irrigation)
    - Filling & drainage of clean water collections–Anopheles
    - Abolition of domestic and peridomestic collections of polluted dirty water–Culex
    - Getting rid of artificial collections of water–Aedes
    - Aquatic plants removed or destroyed by herbicides–Mansonia
  - *Chemical control*:
    - *Mineral oils:* Applied once-a-week in dose of 40–90 litres per hectare; makes water unfit for human consumption and kills fish
    - *Paris green*^Q: 2 percent dust applied in dose of 1 kg per hectare; '*stomach poison*' to larvae but harmless to humans, animals or fish
    - *Synthetic insecticides:* Abate (very effective larvicide and least toxic at dose of 1 ppm), Malathion, Fenthion, Chlorpyrifos
  - *Biological control*^Q: through use of small fishes
    - Gambusia affinis
    - Lebister reticulata
    - Poecilia.
- *Anti-adult measures*:
  - *Residual sprays*:

Key points

Pyrethrum extract: 'nerve poison'

Toxicant	Dosage (gm per m²)	Average duration of effectiveness (months)
DDT	1–2	6–12
BHC (Lindane)	0.5	3
Malathion	2	3

- *Space sprays*:
    - *Pyrethrum extract*: 'nerve poison'; Active principal 'pyrethrin'; no residual action–short-lived effect^Q
    - *Residual insecticides*: Malathion and fenitrothion for ULV (Ultra low volume) fogging^Q
- *Genetic control*:
    - Sterile male technique
    - Cytoplasmic incompatibility
    - Chromosomal translocations
    - Sex distortion
    - Gene replacement
- *Personal protection measures (against mosquito bites)*:
    - *Mosquito nets*:
        - No. of holes per square inch: **150**^Q
        - Size of each hole diameter: **<0.0475 inch**^Q
        - *Screening*:
            1. Size: 16 meshes to inch
            2. Aperture size: <0.0475 inch
    - *Repellants*^Q:
        - Diethyltoluamide (DEET)
        - Ethyl hexanediol
    - *Pyrethrum*:
        - *Space spray for killing adult mosquitoes*^Q
        - **Contact poison**
        - *Knock-down effect with paralysis*^Q
        - Insecticide of plant origin: Flowers of Chrysanthemum
        - 5 active principles (all 'nerve poisons') ^Q:
            1. Pyrethrin I
            2. Pyrethrin II
            3. Cinerin I
            4. Cinerin II
            5. Jasmoline II
        - No residual effect: Short lived effect
        - Synthetic pyrethroids: permethrin, allethrin, furethrin, cyclethrin
        - Because of the natural insecticidal properties used as 'companion plants', to repel pest insects from nearby crops.
- *Common insect repellents*:
    - **DEET (*N,N*-diethyl-*m*-toluamide)** ^Q
    - **Allethrin**
    - Essential oil of the lemon eucalyptus [p-menthane-3,8-diol (PMD)]
    - Icaridin (picaridin)
    - Nepetalactone (catnip oil)
    - Citronella oil
    - Permethrin
    - Soyabean oil
    - Neem oil
- *Few uncommon insect repellants*:
    - Thiamine (vitamin B1)
    - Garlic
    - Incense
    - Ultrasonic devices

> **Key points**
>
> **Mosquito Nets:**
> - No. of holes per square inch: 150^Q
> - Size of each hole diameter: <0.0475 inch^Q

- *Bacillus thuringiensis H14^Q*: Spores and crystalline insecticidal proteins produced by B. thuringiensis are used as specific insecticides. Because of their specificity, these pesticides are regarded as environmentally friendly, with little or no effect on humans, wildlife, pollinators, and most other beneficial insects.
  - *Bacillus thuringiensis* serovar *israelensis* is widely used as a larvicide against mosquito larvae (Bt Toxin)
- *Insecticide treated bed nets (ITBN)*:
  - Chemicals used in ITBN Program: *Synthetic pyretheroids^Q*
    1. Deltamethrin: 2.5 % in dosage of 25 mg/m²
    2. Cyfluthrin: 5 % in dosage of 50 mg/m²
    3. Other insecticides used: Permethrin, Lambdacyhalothrin, Etofenprox, -cypermethrin
  - *Effectiveness of pyretheroids^Q*: 6–12 months (Retreatment every 6 months)
  - *Long-lasting insecticidal mosquito nets (LLINs)*: Also use pyrethroid insecticides, and a chemical binder that allows the nets to be washed ≥20 times, allowing use for ≥3 years.

> **Key points**
> Insecticide treated bed nets (ITBN): Synthetic pyretheroids^Q

Insecticides

Organo-phosphorus Insecticides^Q	Organo-chlorine Insecticides^Q	Carbamate Insecticides
Malathion	DDT	Carbaryl
Parathion	BHC (HCH)	Propoxur
Fenthion	Lindane	
Diazinon	Dieldrin	
Fenitrothion		
Chlorpyrifos		
Dioxathion		
Chlorthion		

> **Key points**
> Paris green is a 'stomach poison'

Paris Green (Copper Acetoarsenite)

- *Description*:
  - Emerald green, microcrystalline powder
  - Anti-larval measure, kills mainly Anopheles larvae as they are surface feeders^Q
  - Bottom feeding larvae can also be killed, when applied as a special granular formulation
  - Paris green is a 'stomach poison'^Q
  - Is most widely used larvicide for mosquito control
- *Recommended dose*: 1 kg paris green per hectare water surface
  - In dosage applied, paris green does not harm fish, man or domestic animals.

> **Key points**
> Paul Muller^Q (Nobel prize)
> - DDT properties

DDT (Dichloro-diphenyl-trichloro Ethane)

- *Type of insecticide*: Organochlorine compound^Q
  - *Synthesised by*: **Ziedler^Q**
  - *Properties discovered by*: **Paul Muller^Q** (Nobel prize)
  - *Most active form*: **Para-para isomer** (70–80% in DDT)^Q
- *Mechanism of action*:
  - *Contact poison*: Nerve poison which inhibits Acetylcholinesterase enzyme^Q
  - **Takes several hours to kill**^Q (No immediate death)
  - Residual action lasts for 18 months^Q
  - **No repellent action**^Q
- *Application*: 100–2000 mg per sq. foot
  - *Dosage*: 100–200 mg per sq.ft.
- *Technical DDT*: 70–80% para-para isomer (most active form)^Q
- Sandflies (Phlebotomus) have not demonstrated resistance to DDT^Q.

> **Key points**
> *Mechanism of action of DDT*:
> - Contact poison: (Nerve poison)
> - Takes several hours to kill^Q
> - Residual action for 18 months

Pyrethrum

- *Description*:
  - Insecticide of plant origin: Flowers of Chrysanthemum
  - *Space spray for killing 'adult mosquitoes'*^Q: Active principal *'pyrethrin'*; no residual action–short-lived effect

- *Mechanism of action*:
  - Contact 'nerve' poison^Q
  - Knock-down effect with paralysis
- 5 active principles (all *'nerve poisons'*):
  - Pyrethrin I
  - Pyrethrin II
  - Cinerin I
  - Cinerin II
  - Jasmoline II
- *No residual effect*: Short lived effect.

Malathion

- Is *'least toxic among Organophosphate compounds'*^Q
  - Because of its low toxicity, it is recommended as *'an alternative to DDT'*
  - *Dosage*: 100–200 mg per sq. ft. every 3 months
  - *ULV spray*: Used to kill adult mosquitoes
- *Mechanism of action*: Interfere with transmission of nerve impulses
  - Act by *'inhibiting Acetyl-cholinesterase'*^Q.

Scabies

- *Scabies*: Is a transmissible ectoparasite skin infection characterized by superficial burrows, intense pruritus (itching) and secondary infection^Q
  - Scabies is caused by the mite *Sarcoptes scabiei*, variety *hominis* (known as *'Itch mite'*)^Q
  - Scabies is usually transmitted by close contact with an infested person. Scabies is transmitted readily, often throughout an entire household, by skin-to-skin contact with an infected person and thus is sometimes classified as a sexually transmitted disease (STD)
- *Drug of Choice for scabies*: 5% Permethrin^Q
- *Other treatment modalities for Scabies*^Q:
  - 25% Benzyl benzoate (2 applications)
  - 1% HCH (*Gammaxene; lindane*) (2 applications)
  - 5% Tetmosol solution (3 daily applications)
  - 10% Sulphur ointment (4 daily applications)
  - Crotamiton lotion (3 applications)
  - Malathion (1 application)
  - Ivermectin (Single dose) — Oral/Systemic Drug of Choice^Q
  - Neem oil (for persistent cases).

> **Key points**
> *Technical DDT:* 70–80% para-para isomer

> **Key points**
> Malathion
> Is 'least toxic among Organophosphate compounds'

> **Key points**
> *Drug of Choice for scabies:* 5% Permethrin^Q

> **Key points**
> Ivermectin (Single dose) — Oral/Systemic Drug of Choice for scabies

PYQs: Quick Review for NEET

Water	
Disinfecting action of chlorine is due to	Hypochlorous acid
Residual level of chlorine in water	Minimum 0.5 mg × contact period 1 hour
Temporary hardness of water is due to	Ca^{++} and Mg^{++} Bicarbonates
Use of Horrock's Apparatus (Starch Iodide indicator)	Chlorine demand estimation
Level of residual level of chlorine in water	0.5 ppm (mg/litre) for contact period 1 hour
Maximum tolerable level of nitrates in water	50 mg/litre
Recommended residual Cl_2 level in Swimming pool	≥ 1 mg/L
Softening of water is recommended above hardness	>150 mg/litre
Main disinfection in chlorination of water is by	Hypochlorous acid
Clostridium perfringens cause _____ pollution	Water pollution
Standard for bacterial water quality in small community supplies	No coliforms
Bleaching powder required for disinfection of water is found by	Horrock's apparatus

Contd...

Contd...

In slow sand filter, responsible for yielding bacteria free water is	Vital layer
Process of defluoridation of water is	Nalgonda technique
Chloride level_____ is said to be accepted by WHO	200 mg/L
Bacterial indicator of recent contamination of water	Faecal streptococci
Confirmatory test for coliform count in drinking water	Eijkman test
Fresh bleaching powder contains	33% chlorine
Contact time for chlorination of water	1 hour
Vital layer of slow sand filter is	Schmutzdecke (Zoogleal layer)
1 Chlorine tablet is efficient to chlorinate __ liters of water	20 litres
Instrument used for recording very low air velocities	Kata thermometer
Upper limit of Fluoride in drinking water should be	1.5 ppm (WHO)
As per Indian standards for drinking water, desirable pH is	6.5–8.5
Presumptive coliform count includes_____ bacteria	All coliform bacteria
Air	
Anemometer measures	Air velocity
Kata thermometer measures	Low air velocity (Earlier cooling power of air)
Maximum allowable sweat rate	4.5 litres per 4 hours
Recommended air changes/hour in a living room	2–3
Cooling curve of body follows _____ shape	Sigmoid shape
Settle plate culture method is used to assess	Air quality in hospital wards/OTs
Acceptable level for physical comfort	Corrected effective temperature 77–80°F
Carbon dioxide in air is measured by	Kieffer test
Maximum contribution to atmospheric air	Nitrogen
Sound	
Maximum tolerable sound level to human ears	85 dB
Tolerable sound level for Factory workers	90 decibels
Pain in the ear occurs at	140 dB
Repeated exposure to_____ can cause permanent deafness	100 dB
Acceptable noise level in Industries	40–60 dB
Light	
Day light factor in living room should be	>8%
Visible spectrum of light	300–700 nm
Radiation	
State with highest Solar radiation received in India	Rajasthan
Thickness of lead apron of prevent radiation	0.5 mm
Endogenous radiation includes	C-14, K-40, Rb-87, Sr-90
Waste disposal	
Most satisfactory method of Refuse disposal	Sanitary landfill/Controlled tipping
Depth of water seal in sanitary latrine is	2 cm
Sullage consists of	Waste water from kitchen
Biochemical oxygen demand is calculated to know	Organic waste
Sullage in rural area is disposed by	Gobar gas plant
Entomology	
Best approach for arthropod control	Environmental control
Tiger Mosquito	Aedes mosquito
Paris green is a	Stomach poison
Pyrethrum is a	Space spray
Anopheles larvae rest	Parallel to under surface water
Aedes larvae breed in	Artificial collection of water
Mite transmits Rickettsial diseases	Scrub typhus, R pox

Contd...

Contd...

Drug of choice for scabies	5% Permethrin
Number of holes per sq. inch in mosquito net	>150
Mosquito transmitting Dengue hemorrhagic fever	Aedes aegypti
Breteau index is used for	Aedes aegypti
Cyclopropagative transmission is shown by	Plasmodium (malaria)
DDT mechanism of action	Contact poison
Number of scabies mites per person body	10–15
Scabies is transmitted by	Itch mite
Disease transmitted globally by Anopheles, Culex and Aedes	Filariasis
Percentage of para-para isomer in DDT is	70–80%
Black fly transmits	Onchocerciasis
Most prevalent mosquito-borne viral disease in India	Dengue fever
Paris Green is used to eliminate the larva of	Anopheline
Vector of Bancroftian filariasis	Culex quinquefasciatus (C fatigans)
Dengue and Chikungunya fever is transmitted by	Aedes aegypti
Nuisance mosquito is	Culex
KFD is transmitted by	Hemaphysalis spinigera (hard tick)
Scrub typhus is transmitted by	Trombiculid mite
Aedes aegypti (Breteau) index for control of yellow fever	<1%
Mineral oils are used in mosquito control measure as a	Larvicide
Anopheles species MC found in coastal regions	An. stephensi and An. sundaicus
Flight range of Sandfly	50 yards
Number of holes/square inch of a standard mosquito net	>150
Mosquito-net hole diameter is	0.0475 inch
Cigar-shaped eggs are seen in _____ mosquito	Aedes
Trans-stadial transmission is seen in	Ticks
Household insecticide used for malaria	Malathion
Fish is used for larva control of malaria	Gambusia, Lebister, Poecilia

Multiple Choice Questions

WATER

1. The correct method used for collection of tap water sample for the purpose of bacteriological examination for quality of drinking water is: **[NEET PG Pattern 2023]**
   (a) Collect water sample from a leaking tap
   (b) Attach bottle before turning on the tap to avoid splashing
   (c) Allow water to flow for 1 minute, then collect water
   (d) Collect sample from a gentle stream of water to avoid splashing

2. Active disinfectant property of Bleaching powder is mainly due to formation of:
   [NEET PG Pattern January 2020]
   (a) Hydrogen chloride (b) Hypochloric acid
   (c) Hypochlorous acid (d) Chloramines

3. Recommended minimum amount of Residual chlorine in drinking water is: **[JIPMER May 2019]**
   (a) 2 ppm   (b) 0.5 ppm
   (c) 1.5 ppm (d) 4 ppm

4. What is Saturation index? **[JIPMER May 2019]**
   (a) Used to assess the Air quality by measuring concentration of pollutants
   (b) Used to assess the Water quality by estimating hardness, total dissolved solids, alkalinity and pH
   (c) Used to assess the Soil quality that whether it is good for growing crops
   (d) Used to assess the Milk quality by estimating the bacterial count in it

5. Purest water in nature is: **[AIPGME 2000]**
   (a) River water
   (b) Rain water
   (c) Deep well
   (d) Impounding reservoirs

6. All the following statements are true about break point chlorination, *except*: **AIIMS May 2004]**
   (a) Free chlorine is released in water after break point chlorination
   (b) Chlorine demand is the amount needed to kill bacteria, oxidize organic matter and neutralize ammonia
   (c) 1 ppm free chlorine should be present in water after break point has reached
   (d) Contact period of 1 hour is necessary

7. Nitrates in excess of — may cause infantile methaemoglobinaemia: **[AIPGME 1997]**
   (a) 15 mg/l (b) 25 mg/l
   (c) 35 mg/l (d) 45 mg/l

8. All the following provide evidence of faecal pollution *except*: **[AIIMS Sep 1996]**
   (a) Faecal streptococci (b) Coliform
   (c) Cl. Tetani   (d) Enterpathogenic virus

9. Per capita allowance of water per day is recommended at: **[AIIMS Nov 2005]**
   (a) 70–80 lit   (b) 80–120 lit
   (c) 120–150 lit (d) 150–200 lit

10. Horrock's apparatus estimates: **[AIIMS May 2006]**
    (a) Free chlorine   **[NEET Pattern 2017, 2018]**
    (b) Combined chlorine
    (c) (a) + (b)
    (d) Chlorine demand

11. Which one of the following methods is used for the estimation of chlorine demand of water?
    [AIIMS Nov 2006, AIIMS May 2007, 2010, RJ 2001]
    (a) Chlorometer
    (b) Horrock's apparatus
    (c) Berkefeld filter
    (d) Double pot method

12. Ortho-toluidine test is used to determine:
    [AIIMS Nov 1995, AIIMS Nov 2004, WB 2002]
    (a) Nitrates in water   **[AIPGME 2011]**
    (b) Nitrites in water   **[NEET Pattern 2012, 2018]**
    (c) Free and combined chlorine in water
    (d) Ammonia content in water

13. Most desired temperature range for drinking water is:
    (a) 0–5°C   **[AIIMS May 1995]**
    (b) 5–10°C
    (c) 10–15°C
    (d) 15–20°C

14. Most undesirable metal in drinking water is:
    (a) Iron   **[AIIMS June 1991]**
    (b) Copper
    (c) Zinc
    (d) Lead

15. 'Most reliable' evidence of fecal contamination of water is provided by: **[AIPGME 1999]**
    (a) Coliform bacteria (b) Cl. Perfringens
    (c) St. fecalis   (d) Cl. welchii

16. Scabies, an infection of the skin caused by Sarcoptes scabiei, is an example of: **[AIPGME 2002]**
    (a) Water borne disease (b) Water washed disease
    (c) Water based disease (d) Water related disease

17. A daily water supply considered adequate to meet the need for all urban domestic purposes is: [AIIMS Nov 2000]
    [NEET Pattern 2018]
    (a) 10 litres per capita
    (b) 20 litres per capita
    (c) 40–60 litres per capita
    (d) 150–200 litres per capita

18. All are true for Rapid Sand Filters, *except*: [AIPGME 1997]
    (a) No preliminary storage of raw water is required
    (b) Operation requires highly skilled persons
    (c) Frequent washing is not required
    (d) Can be gravity type or pressure type

19. Disinfecting action of chlorine on water is mainly due to:
    [AIPGME 2005]
    (a) Hydrogen chloride [NEET Pattern 2013, 2017, 2018]
    (b) Hypochlorous acid [DNB 2001, 2011, RJ 2001]
    (c) Hypochlorite ions
    (d) Hydrogen ions

20. Which of the following agents have 'residual germicidal effect' when used for disinfection of water:
    [AIIMS Dec 1995]
    (a) Chlorine only
    (b) Chlorine and Ozone gas
    (c) Chlorine and UV radiation
    (d) Chlorine, Ozone gas and UV radiation

21. Proposed guideline values for Radioactivity in Drinking water is: [AIPGME 2001]
    (a) Gross a activity 0.1 Bq/L and Gross b activity 1.0 Bq/L
    (b) Gross a activity 1.0 Bq/L and Gross b activity 0.1 Bq/L
    (c) Gross a activity 1.0 Bq/L and Gross b activity 10.0 Bq/L
    (d) Gross a activity 10 Bq/L and Gross b activity 1.0 Bq/L

22. MPN Multiple Tube Method is done to: [AIIMS Dec 1995]
    (a) Detect the presence of Coliform organisms in a sample of water
    (b) Detect the presence of Faecal streptococci in a sample of water
    (c) Detect the presence of Cl. perfringens in a sample of water
    (d) Do the colony count of bacteria

23. Level of hardness in soft water is ___ mEq/liter:
    [AIIMS Nov 1999]
    (a) Less than 1   (b) 1–3
    (c) 3–6   (d) Over 6

24. The minimum recommended dose of "free" residual chlorine in water for routine chlorination (in mg/lts) is:
    [AIPGME 2002, MP 2003, PGMCET 2015, AIIMS May 1991] [NEET Pattern 2017]
    (a) 0.5 mg/l for a contact period of 1hr [Bihar 2004]
    (b) 0.5 mg/l for a contact period of 1/2 hr [DNB 2008]
    (c) 1.0 mg/l for a contact period of 1hr
    (d) 1.0 mg/l for a contact period of 1/2 hr
    [Karnataka 2009, WB 2004, RJ 2000, 2005]

25. True statement regarding chlorination is: [DPG 2005]
    (a) Orthotolidine test measures combined chlorine separately
    (b) Chlorine acts best when pH is around 7
    (c) It kills bacteria, viruses and spores
    (d) Hypochlorite ions are mainly responsible for disinfecting activity

26. Temporary hardness of water is due to presence of:
    [Karnataka 2004]
    (a) Bicarbonates of calcium and magnesium
    (b) Chlorides of calcium and magnesium
    (c) Nitrates of calcium and magnesium
    (d) Oxides of calcium and magnesium

27. Slow sand filter is differentiated from rapid sand filter by:
    [PGI June 08]
    (a) Bacteria are removed more effectively
    (b) Skilled person is needed
    (c) Cost construction is cheaper
    (d) Sand particle are of smaller size
    (e) Longer duration is needed

28. Indication of Fecal contamination of water is due to presence of: [PGI Dec 03]
    (a) E. coli   (b) Coliform
    (c) Enterococci   (d) Clostridium difficile
    (e) Streptococcus pyogenes

29. NOT seen in fecal pollution: [AIIMS May 2010]
    (a) Staphylococcus
    (b) Streptococcus
    (c) E.coli
    (d) Clostridium perfringens

30. All of the following statements about purification of water are true *except*: [AIIMS May 2010]
    (a) Presence of Clostridial spores indicates recent contamination of water
    (b) Coliforms must not be detectable in any 100 mL sample of drinking water
    (c) Sodium thiosulphate is used to neutralize certain contaminants
    (d) Coliforms may be detected by multiple tube method and indole production

31. All the following statements about purification of water are true *except*: [AIIMS May 2011]
    (a) Presence of clostridial spores indicate recent contamination
    (b) Coliforms must not be detectable in any 100 mL sample of drinking water
    (c) Sodium thiosulphate is used to neutralize chlorine
    (d) Coliforms may be detected by multiple tube method and indole production at 44 degrees

32. True about slow sand filter is: [NEET Pattern 2013]
    (a) Occupies less space
    (b) More expensive
    (c) Requires longer duration
    (d) Sand size 0.4–0.7 mm

33. The vital layer in a slow sand filter is: [DNB June 2011]
    (a) Sand bed
    (b) Under drainage
    (c) Zoogleal layer
    (d) Supernatant

34. Horrock's apparatus determines Chloride which has to have a holding level of: [NEET Pattern 2012]
    (a) 1.0 mg/L
    (b) 1.5 mg/L
    (c) 2.0 mg/L
    (d) 0.5 mg/L

35. Hardness of drinking water should be: [NEET Pattern 2013] [DNB December 2011]
    (a) >3
    (b) <1
    (c) 1–3
    (d) >3

36. Nalgonda technique for defluoridation is in what sequence: [NEET Pattern 2012]
    (a) Lime + Alum
    (b) Soda + Alum
    (c) Alum + Soda
    (d) Alum + Lime

37. Minimum chlorine content of water after chlorination should be: [DNB December 2011] [NEET Pattern 2018]
    (a) 0.5 mg/L
    (b) 5 mg/L
    (c) 0.05 mg/L
    (d) 50 mg/L

38. Safe water criteria include: [PGI November 2013] [AIPGME 1992]
    (a) Free from pathogens
    (b) Free from harmful chemicals
    (c) Free from chlorine
    (d) Free from colour and odour
    (e) Usable for agricultural purposes

39. Method of choice for purification of highly polluted water on a large scale is: [AP 2014]
    (a) Boiling
    (b) Chlorination
    (c) Super chlorination followed by dechlorination
    (d) Ultraviolet light treatment

40. Test for recent contamination of water is [CGPG 2015]
    (a) Nitrates
    (b) Nitrites
    (c) Ammonia
    (d) Chlorides

41. In community well water, Horrock's apparatus first shows 3rd cup blue. What will be the requirement of bleaching powder for disinfecting 9100 liter of water? [NEET Pattern 2015]
    (a) 120 grams
    (b) 160 grams
    (c) 200 grams
    (d) 360 grams

42. Hardness of water is due to all *except*: [NEET Pattern 2018]
    (a) Sulphates
    (b) Chlorides
    (c) Nitrates
    (d) Phosphates

43. Minimum depth for the lining of a Sanitary well is? [NEET Pattern 2018]
    (a) 10 feet
    (b) 20 feet
    (c) 35 feet
    (d) 50 feet

44. All of the following are true about Safe and wholesome water, except: [NEET Pattern 2018]
    (a) It is free from color and odor
    (b) Free from pathogenic agents
    (c) It is unusable for domestic purpose
    (d) Free from harmful chemical pathogens

Review Questions

45. Not a feature of hard water is: [Bihar 2005]
    (a) Increased fuel consumption
    (b) Erosion of lead pipe
    (c) Scaling of boiler
    (d) Decreased soap consumption

46. All are example of water borne disease *except*: [UP 2000]
    (a) Leptospirosis
    (b) Fish tapeworm
    (c) Schistosomiasis
    (d) Brucellosis

47. All the following assess the water-quality-criteria for water pollution are all *except*: [UP 2006]
    (a) Solid particles
    (b) Dissolved oxygen
    (c) Dissolved chloride
    (d) Dissolved nitrogen

48. Maximum permissible chloride level is: [UP 2008]
    (a) 200 mg/litre
    (b) 300 mg/litre
    (c) 500 mg/litre
    (d) 600 mg/litre

49. Vital layer in slow sand filter is seen: [AP 2004]
    (a) Top of water
    (b) On the sand bed
    (c) Near filter valves
    (d) None

50. Most effective water treatment method in rural area: [MP 2002]
    (a) Rapid sand filter
    (b) Slow and filter
    (c) Chlorination of water
    (d) Ozonization

51. Criteria for safe drinking water: [MP 2004]
    (a) pH 6.5–8.5
    (b) Chloride 0.8 g/L
    (c) Nitrate 0.2 g/L
    (d) Solids-12000 mg/L

52. Schmutzdecke refers to the following: [MP 2007]
    (a) Suspended matter in drinking water
    (b) Algae in drinking water
    (c) Alum flocculate on surface of sand bed filter
    (d) Algae, plankton, diatoms and bacteria on surface of sand bed filter

53. Water sample from a well was tested using Horrock's apparatus. It was observed that 3rd white cup showed blue colour after addition of starchiodide indicator: How much bleaching powder is required to disinfect 2275 liters of the well water? [MP 2008]
    (a) 5 gm
    (b) 15 gm
    (c) 25 gm
    (d) 30 gm

54. Criteria for "Problem village" include all *except*: [JIPMER 1998, MH 2006]
    (a) Where no water source in a distance of 1.6 km from community [NEET Pattern 2018]
    (b) Water is more than depth of 15 meter
    (c) There is excess of Na+, K+, F+ salts
    (d) Risk of Guinea worm infection

AIR

55. New Delhi reported the following Air Quality Index during November month last year (as given below):
    20 Nov AQI – 370
    21 Nov AQI – 320
    22 Nov AQI – 360
    23 Nov AQI – 380
    24 Nov AQI – 470
    Which type of air quality was reported on 24 November? [NEET PG Pattern September 2021]
    (a) Moderate
    (b) Poor
    (c) Very poor
    (d) Severe

56. Instrument to measure Low wind velocity measurement and cooling power: [NEET PG Pattern September 2021]
    (a) Kata thermometer
    (b) Wet globe thermometer
    (c) Silvered thermometer
    (d) Globe thermometer

57. Indicators of air pollution are: [NEET PG Pattern January 2020]
    (a) Sulphur dioxide, Lead, Particulate matter
    (b) Carbon dioxide, Hydrogen sulphide, Lead
    (c) Sulphur dioxide, Hydrogen sulphide, Carbon monoxide
    (d) Sulphur dioxide, Smoke, Particulate matter

58. Psychrometer is used to measure: [AIPGME 2008]
    (a) Humidity
    (b) Air velocity
    (c) Room temperature
    (d) Radiant heat

59. All of the following are types of mechanical ventilation *except*: [AIIMS May 1995]
    (a) Perflation and Aspiration
    (b) Exhaust ventilation
    (c) Plenum ventilation
    (d) Air conditioning

60. All are indicators of air pollution, *except*: [AIIMS May 1995]
    (a) Soiling index
    (b) McArdle's index
    (c) Suspended particle count
    (d) SO_2 Concentration

61. McArdle's maximum allowable sweat rate is: [AIIMS June 1997]
    (a) 4 lit/4 hours
    (b) 4 lit/1 hours
    (c) 4.5 lit/4 hours
    (d) 4.5 lit/8 hours

62. Kata thermometer measures: [AIIMS Dec 1998]
    (a) Air temperature only [NEET Pattern 2012, 2017]
    (b) Air temperature and humidity [Karnataka 2004]
    (c) Air temperature, humidity and air movement
    (d) Air velocity only

63. The mechanical system in which fresh air is blown into the room by centrifugal fans so as to create positive pressure and displace the vitiated air is termed as: [Karnataka 2009]
    (a) Balanced ventilation
    (b) Air conditioning
    (c) Exhaust ventilation
    (d) Plenum ventilation

64. The mean radiant temperature is measured by: [Karnataka 2004]
    (a) Dry bulb thermometer
    (b) Wet bulb thermometer
    (c) Six's maximum and minimum thermometer
    (d) Globe thermometer

65. Global warming true is: [AIIMS May 2010]
    (a) CO_2 is a major greenhouse gas
    (b) Stratosphere ozone layer is harmful
    (c) CFC increases stratosphere ozone layer
    (d) Kyoto protocol called for 20% reduction in greenhouse emissions

66. Which of the following is not a source of Indoor Air Pollution? [AIPGME 2011]
    (a) Carbon monoxide
    (b) Nitrogen dioxide
    (c) Radon
    (d) Mercury vapour

67. Indoor air pollution does not cause: [AIIMS PGMEE November 2013]
    (a) Chronic lung disease
    (b) Pregnancy problems
    (c) Childhood pneumonia
    (d) Neuro-developmental problems

68. Which of the following is non-natural gas causing green house effect? [NEET Pattern 2012]
    (a) Carbon dioxide
    (b) Methane
    (c) Ozone
    (d) CFCs

69. The best parameter to measure air pollution is:
    (a) SO_2 *[DNB 2002, 2005, 2006, 2007, UP 2002]*
    (b) CO_2 *[Bihar 2004, RJ 2006]*
    (c) CO   *[NEET Pattern 2018]*
    (d) N_2O

70. Which agency monitors air quality in India? *[NEET Pattern 2012]*
    (a) Central Research Institute
    (b) Ministry if health and Family Welfare
    (c) National Environmental Engineering Research Institute
    (d) Central Pollution Control Board

71. In winter, water vapours and pollutants comes to lie in the lowermost layer of atmosphere by: *[NEET Pattern 2013]*
    (a) Acid rain
    (b) Green house effect
    (c) Temperature inversion
    (d) Ocean effect

72. At which level of heat stress index it is not possible to work comfortably causing threat to health: *[NEET Pattern 2012]*
    (a) 20–40   (b) 40–60
    (c) 60–80   (d) 80–100

73. Which of the following is not a feature of heat stress? *[UPSC CMS 2015]*
    (a) Hyperpyrexia   (b) Syncope
    (c) Cramps   (d) Numbness

74. Green-house gases do not include: *[NEET Pattern 2016, 2017]*
    (a) Carbon dioxide
    (b) Carbon monoxide
    (c) Water vapour
    (d) Methane

75. Not a primary air pollutant *[NEET Pattern 2017]*
    (a) SO_2 (b) CO_2
    (c) Ozone   (d) VOCs

76. Which is an Indoor air pollutant? *[NEET Pattern 2017]*
    (a) Benzene   (b) Ozone
    (c) Asbestos   (d) All of the above

Review Questions

77. Number of air changes in one hour in a work room should be at least: *[DNB 2001]*
    (a) 2–3   (b) 3–4
    (c) 4–6   (d) 5–7

78. In Indoor air pollution, carbon monoxide is produced by: *[UP 2007]*
    (a) Combustion equipment
    (b) Stove
    (c) Gas heaters
    (d) All of the above

79. Kata thermometer is used nowadays to determine: *[AFMC 2000, Karnataka 2004, UPSC 2000, TN 2000]*
    (a) Low Air velocity *[Kolkata 2006]*
    (b) Humidly of air
    (c) Direction of air flow
    (d) Cooling power of air

80. Relative humidity is determined by:
    (a) Kata thermometer *[Karnataka 2005]*
    (b) Anemometer *[MH 2000]*
    (c) Sling psychrometer *[NEET Pattern 2017]*
    (d) Gardbad apparatus

SOUND

81. Whispering produces a sound of: *[AIIMS May 1993]*
    (a) 20–30 dB *[NEET Pattern 2017]*
    (b) 30–40 dB
    (c) 40–50 dB
    (d) 50–60 dB

82. Exposure to following minimum level of sound can cause rupture of tympanic membrane, leading to permanent hearing loss: *[AIPGME 2000]*
    (a) 90 dB
    (b) 110 dB
    (c) 160 dB
    (d) 1600 dB

83. Exposure to noise above ……….. cause permanent loss of hearing: *[DNB 2007]*
    (a) 85 dB   (b) 90 dB *[MH 2002]*
    (c) 100 dB   (d) 160 dB

Review Question

84. The 'acceptable' noise level is: *[UP 2006]*
    (a) 85 dB *[NEET Pattern 2013]*
    (b) 90 dB *[RJ 2004]*
    (c) 95 dB *[MH 2005]*
    (d) 100 dB *[Karnataka 2004]*

LIGHT

85. Brightness of point source of light is measured through SI unit of: *[NEET PG Pattern September 2021]*
    (a) Candela   (b) Lux
    (c) Lumen   (d) Lambert

86. Recommended illumination range for regular work is _____ foot-candles: *[AIPGME 2001]*
    (a) 6–12   (b) 25–50
    (c) 50–75   (d) 75–100

87. SI unit of Luminal intensity is: [NEET Pattern 2016]
    (a) Candela
    (b) Lumen
    (c) Lux
    (d) Coulomb

HOUSING

88. The optimum floor space recommended per adult person in a dwelling place is: [AIIMS Nov 1999]
    (a) 50–100 sq.ft.
    (b) 101–450 sq.ft.
    (c) 151–200 sq.ft.
    (d) 201–250 sq.ft.

WASTE DISPOSAL

89. All of the following are methods of sewage disposal except: [AIPGME 2006]
    (a) River outfall
    (b) Land treatment
    (c) Oxidation ponds
    (d) Bangalore method (Composting)

90. Waste water from kitchen is called: [AIIMS Dec 1997]
    (a) Refuse [AIPGME 2002]
    (b) Garbage [NEET Pattern 2013]
    (c) Sullage
    (d) Sewage

91. The amount of sewage flowing in a system in 24 hours is called: [AIIMS Nov 2000]
    (a) Sewage rate
    (b) Dry weather flow
    (c) RCA index
    (d) Sludge

92. All are features of septic tank except: [AIPGME 92]
    (a) Ideal retention period–48 hrs
    (b) Minimum capacity–500 gallons
    (c) Aerobic oxidation takes place outside
    (d) Sludge is solids setting down

93. Most satisfactory method of Refuse disposal is:
    (a) Dumping [AIIMS May 1993-2003]
    (b) Controlled tipping [AIPGME 1994]
    (c) Incineration [Bihar 2003]
    (d) Manure pits [Kolkata 2008]

94. Strength of sewage is expressed in terms of all except:
    (a) E. Coli Count [AIPGME 2006]
    (b) Suspended particles [JIPMER 1985]
    (c) Chemical oxygen demand [TN 1993]
    (d) Biological oxygen demand [MH 2006]

95. The biological oxygen demand (BOD) indicates:
    (a) Organic matter [AIPGME 2002, AIIMS June 2000]
    (b) Bacterial content
    (c) Anaerobic bacteria
    (d) Chemicals

96. Following latrines are suitable for camps and temporary use, except: [Karnataka 2004]
    (a) Shallow trench latrine
    (b) Pit latrine
    (c) Borehole latrine
    (d) Septic tank

97. Following are the waste types not to be incinerated, except: [Karnataka 2009]
    (a) Pressurized gas containers
    (b) Reactive chemical waste
    (c) Halogenated plastics
    (d) Content of combustible matter above 60%

98. It waste water contain toxic substances, organic load is measured by: [NEET Pattern 2013]
    (a) Biological oxygen demand
    (b) Chemical oxygen demand
    (c) Suspended solid
    (d) None

99. Septic tank true is/are: [PGI November 2014]
    (a) Treatment of household sewage
    (b) Suitable in presence of public sewerage system
    (c) Aerobic oxidation outside septic tank
    (d) Anaerobic digestion inside septic tank
    (e) Retention period 6 hours

100. True about Sewage is/are: [PGI November 2014]
    (a) Does not contain human excreta
    (b) Strength measured by Biological oxygen demand
    (c) BOD >100 mg/L is strong sewage
    (d) Composed of 90% water
    (e) Dry weather flow is measured for 24 hours period

101. Which of the following is/are true about Sewage disposal? [PGI November 2017]
    (a) Biochemical oxygen demand is indicator of the organic content of sewage
    (b) BOD is amount of oxygen absorbed by a sample of sewage
    (c) Undergo both aerobic and anaerobic reaction in sewage purification
    (d) Untreated sewage is thrown into rivers
    (e) None of the above

102. Most important factor in Sewage treatment: [JIPMER May 2018]
    (a) Bacterial count
    (b) Solids
    (c) Nitrite and phosphorus
    (d) Water content

103. For the population of 10000, Trench method sanitary landfill pit of depth 2 m is to be constructed. How much area is required per year? [NEET Pattern 2019]
    (a) 1 acre
    (b) 2 acres
    (c) 3 acres
    (d) 4 acres

Review Questions

104. The sewage ground water is disposed by: [DNB 2002]
    (a) Oxidation pond [NEET Pattern 2018]
    (b) Soakage pit
    (c) Activated sludge process
    (d) Any of the above

105. Not a feature of septic tank: [Bihar 2005]
    (a) Used for personal and small public use
    (b) Water tight compartment
    (c) Used where water supply is adequate
    (d) Used where public sewerage system is adequate

106. Most important prerequisite in sanitary latrine is:
    (a) Water seal [MP 2002]
    (b) Adequate drainage
    (c) Squatting plate/slab
    (d) Smooth slope of the pan

107. Septic tank true is: [MP 2004]
    (a) Always double chamber
    (b) Minimum 200 galon capacity
    (c) Depth is from 5–7 feet
    (d) Retention period is of 24 hrs

108. The function of grit chamber in modern sewage plants is: [MP 2008]
    (a) Formation of sludge
    (b) Removal of floating large objects
    (c) Settlement of heavy objects
    (d) Formation of Zoogleal layer

MISCELLANEOUS (ENVIRONMENT)

109. Which of the following is not a recommended sanitation measure for swimming pool sanitation? [AIIMS May 2005]
    (a) Recommended area per swimmer = 2.2 sq. metre
    (b) Water to be refiltered in less than 6 hours (rapid sand filters)
    (c) Residual level of free chlorine to be >0.5 ppm
    (d) 15% water to be replaced by fresh water every day

110. The permissible dose of man made radiation should not exceed: [Karnataka 2004]
    (a) 3 rads per year
    (b) 5 rads per year
    (c) 8 rads per year
    (d) 10 rads per year

111. 10-days rule is related to: [NEET Pattern 2012]
    (a) Sewage disposal
    (b) Air quality
    (c) Water quality
    (d) Radiation protection in pregnancy

112. Unit of absorbed radiation is: [NEET Pattern 2012]
    (a) Roentgen [NEET Pattern 2013]
    (b) Rad
    (c) Rem
    (d) Sievert

113. Kayakalp award is given for: [JIPMER May 2018]
    (a) Hospital administration
    (b) Hospital hygiene
    (c) Leadership
    (d) Environmental sanitation

Review Questions

114. Venturimeter is used to measure: [Kolkata 2002]
    (a) Air velocity
    (b) Size of suspended particles in the air
    (c) SO_2 content in the atmosphere
    (d) Bed resistance in a slow sand filter

115. Soiling index is a measure of: [MP 2003]
    [NEET Pattern 2013, 2014, 2015]
    (a) Soil pollution (b) Water pollution
    (c) Noise pollution (d) Air pollution

ENTOMOLOGY AND VECTOR CONTROL

116. ASSERTION-REASONING TYPE QUESTION - Assertion (A): Malathion is used as ULV during epidemics; Reasoning (R): ULV fogging has residual effect: [AIIMS November 2019]
    (a) A and R are True statements AND R is the correct explanation of A
    (b) A and R are True statements BUT R is not the correct explanation of A
    (c) A is True BUT R is False
    (d) Both A and R are False

117. Mites are the vectors of the following diseases except: [AIIMS Nov 2003]
    (a) Scabies (b) Scrub typhus
    (c) Rickettsial pox (d) Kyasanur forest disease

118. Pyrethrum is a: [AIIMS Dec 1991]
    (a) Contact poison [NEET Pattern 2013, 2017]
    (b) Stomach poison
    (c) Both of above: a + b
    (d) Space poison

119. Match the following: Method of mosquito control Example:
    I. Biological control   A. Mosquito larvicidal oil [Larvivorous fish) (MLO]
    II. Biological control   B. Bacillus thuringiensis (Bacteria) H14
    III. Chemical control   C. Source reduction
    IV. Environmental control D. Barbados millions

(a) A-I, B-II, C-IV, D-III [AIIMS Nov 06]
(b) A-III, B-IV, C-II, D-I
(c) A-I, B-IV, C-II, D-III
(d) A-III, B-II, C-IV, D-I

120. Mosquitoes that breed in dirty water collection are: [AIIMS Dec 1995]
(a) Anopheles
(b) Culex
(c) Aedes
(d) Mansonia

121. Example of cyclopropagative transmission is:
(a) Plague bacilli in rat flea [AIPGME 2000]
(b) Malarial parasite in mosquito
(c) Microfilaria in mosquito [AIIMS May 1991]
(d) Guineaworm embryo in Cyclops

122. Which of the following is incorrectly matched?
(a) Agent changes in form and number: Cyclopropagative transmission [AIPGME 1992]
(b) Agent merely multiples in vector, but no change in form: Propagative transmission
(c) Agent undergoes only development but no multiplication: Cyclodevelopmental transmission
(d) Agent transmitted from nymph to adult vector: Transovarial transmission

123. All of the following statements about mosquito are true, except: [AIIMS Nov 2004]
(a) It is a definitive host in malaria
(b) It is a definitive host in filaria
(c) Its life cycle is completed in 3 weeks
(d) The female can travel up to 3 kilometers

124. A child has multiple itchy papular lesions on the genitalia and fingers. Similar lesions are also seen in the younger brother. Which of the following is most possible diagnosis? [AIIMS Dec 1997]
(a) Papular urticaria
(b) Scabies
(c) Atopic dermatitis
(d) Allergic contact dermatitis

125. Reduviid bug is a vector for the transmission of:
(a) Relapsing fever [AIPGME 1996, PGMCET 2015]
(b) Lyme's disease [NEET Pattern 2015, 2017]
(c) Scrub typhus
(d) Chagas' disease

126. Babesiosis is transmitted by: [AIPGME 1995]
(a) Tick
(b) Mites
(c) Flea
(d) Mosquito

127. Dengue fever is transmitted by: [AIPGME 1993]
(a) Tiger mosquito
(b) Jackal mosquito
(c) Wolf mosquito
(d) Lion mosquito

128. All of the following diseases are caused by Soft Tick, except: [AIPGME 2008]
(a) Tularemia [MH 2007]
(b) Q fever
(c) Relapsing fever
(d) KFD

129. Spot the wrongly matched pair of arthropod and disease transmitted: [AIIMS Dec 1995]
(a) Housefly–Poliomyelitis
(b) Louse–Epidemic typhus
(c) Itch mite–Scabies
(d) Black fly–Chagas Disease

130. Best approach to control of arthropods is:
(a) Environmental control [AIIMS Sep 1996]
(b) Chemical control
(c) Biological control
(d) Genetic control

131. Flight range for Aedes Mosquito is:
(a) 10 meters [AIPGME 2000]
(b) 100 meters [NEET Pattern 2017]
(c) 400 meters
(d) 11 km

132. Normal life span of mosquitoes is: [AIPGME 2006]
(a) 2–3 days
(b) 5–7 days
(c) 8–34 days
(d) 3–4 months

133. True about Paris green for mosquito control is:
(a) It is used as an anti-adult measure [AIPGME 1999]
(b) It is more effective against Anopheles
(c) In usual doses also it harms fish, man and domestic animals
(d) It is a nerve poison

134. Rat flea transmit following diseases except:
(a) Murine typhus [AIPGME 1995]
(b) Pneumonic plague [NEET Pattern 2017]
(c) Chiggerosis
(d) Hymenolepis dimunita

135. Drug of choice for Scabies is: [AIIMS May 2003]
(a) 25% Benzyl benzoate
(b) 5% Permethrin
(c) 1% HCH
(d) 5% Sulphur ointment

136. Diseases associated with rodents include all except:
(a) Leptospirosis [AIIMS May 2006]
(b) Rat Bite fever
(c) Tularemia
(d) Oriental sore

137. All of the following methods are anti-larval measures except: [AIPGME 2005]
    (a) Intermittent irrigation [AIIMS Nov 2008]
    (b) Paris green
    (c) Gambusia affinis
    (d) Pyrethrum
138. Aedes mosquito transmit the following diseases, except: [Karnataka 2008]
    (a) Yellow fever
    (b) Dengue fever
    (c) Chikungunya fever
    (d) Japanese encephalitis
139. Aedes aegypti transmits following diseases: [PGI 1997]
    (a) Yellow fever
    (b) Dengue
    (c) Japanese encephalitis
    (d) Filariasis
    (e) Malaria
140. Disease transmitted by louse include: [PGI June 02]
    (a) Epidemic typhus [PGI Dec 2008]
    (b) Endemic typhus   (c) Trench fever
    (d) RMSF   (e) Scrub typhus
141. Aedes aegypti transmits: [PGI June 04]
    (a) JE   (b) KFD
    (c) Yellow fever   (d) Filaria
    (e) Dengue
142. Vector borne diseases are: [PGI June 04]
    (a) Syphilis   (b) Typhus
    (c) Dengue   (d) J.E.
    (e) HIV
143. Not spread by louse: [AIIMS May 2010]
    (a) Epidemic typhus   (b) Q fever
    (c) Relapsing fever   (d) Trench fever
144. Aedes- True are A/E: [AIIMS May 2010]
    (a) Recurrent biters
    (b) Eggs can't survive >1 wk without water
    (c) Transmits Dengue
    (d) It takes 7–8 days to develop the parasite and transmit the disease
145. Hard tick is the vector of all the following diseases except: [AIIMS Nov 2010]
    (a) Relapsing fever   (b) KFD
    (c) Indian tick typhus   (d) Tularaemia
146. Which of the following is not DDT-resistant?
    (a) Musca domestica [AIPGME 2011]
    (b) Phlebotomus
    (c) Culex mosquito
    (d) Anopheles stephensi
147. All of the following are deliberate measures of mosquito control except: [AIPGME 2011]
    (a) Use of alkaline soap water in factory
    (b) Use of larvicidal agents
    (c) Community participation
    (d) Use of bed-nets for mosquito
148. Least toxic organophosphorus compound is: [DPG 2011]
    (a) DDT   (b) Paris green
    (c) Malathion   (d) Parathion
149. Which of the following statements regarding DDT is false? [AIIMS May 2011]
    (a) Pyrethrum has synergistic action
    (b) It is a contact poison
    (c) Immediately kills the prey
    (d) Residual effect lasts 18 months
150. Following are larval control measures except?
    (a) DDT [AIIMS May 2011]
    (b) Paris green [AIIMS November 2011]
    (c) Gambusia fish
    (d) Intermittent irrigation
151. Following are used for treatment of Scabies in India, except: [PGI November 2011]
    (a) Crotamiton lotion
    (b) Sulphur ointment
    (c) Tetmosol
    (d) Ivermectin
    (e) Rifampicin
152. Which of the following diseases is transmitted by Mansonoides mosquitoes? [PGMCET 2015]
    (a) Japanese encephalitis   (b) West Nile fever
    (c) Rift Valley fever   (d) Chikungunya fever
153. NOT a feature of Vector of Malaria: [NEET Pattern 2015]
    (a) Spotted wings
    (b) Siphon tube
    (c) Boat shaped eggs
    (d) Rest at an angle, inclined to surface of skin
154. Consider the following diseases:
    1. Yellow fever
    2. Q fever
    3. Chikungunya fever
    4. Relapsing fever
    5. Japanese encephalitis
    6. Sleeping sickness
    Which of the above are transmitted by mosquitoes? [UPSC CMS 2015]
    (a) 1, 2, 3, and 6
    (b) 2, 3 and 5
    (c) 4, 5 and 6
    (d) 1, 3 and 5

155. Disease transmitted by the following vector is:
 [AIIMS November 2015]

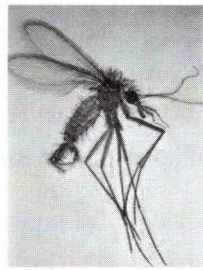

 (a) Japanese encephalitis
 (b) Malaria
 (c) Visceral leishmaniasis
 (d) Dengue

156. Which of the following is NOT true about Hard tick?
 (a) Scutum is present [NEET Pattern 2015]
 (b) Cannot withstand starvation
 (c) They lay hundreds of eggs
 (d) Nymphal stage has seven instars

157. Which is true of pathogenic mosquitoes?
 [NEET Pattern 2016]
 (a) Anopheles has spotted abdomen
 (b) Mansonia lays eggs singly
 (c) Culex cause Yellow fever
 (d) Aedes has striped yellow scales

158. Which is not an Aryl organophosphate?
 [NEET Pattern 2015]
 (a) Malathion   (b) Parathion
 (c) Chlorthion (d) Diazinon

159. True about Culex larvae: [NEET Pattern 2016]
 (a) Rest parallel to surface water
 (b) Long palmate hair
 (c) Siphon tube present
 (d) All are true

160. Synthetic pyrethroid insecticide [NEET Pattern 2016]
 (a) Propoxur   (b) Permethrin
 (c) Cypermethrin (d) Etofenprox

161. True about Mosquito preventive nets are all, except:
 [NEET Pattern 2017]
 (a) Hole size <0.0475
 (b) 150 holes per square inch
 (c) Best pattern in circular
 (d) There should be no rent

162. Western equine encephalitis virus is transmitted by:
 [NEET Pattern 2017]
 (a) Anopheles mosquito
 (b) Culex mosquito
 (c) Sandfly
 (d) Aedes mosquito

Review Questions

163. Mineral oils are used in mosquito control measure as a?
 (a) Personal protection methods [DNB 2008]
 (b) Larvicide
 (c) Adulticide
 (d) Space spray

164. The Anopheles species most commonly found in coastal regions is? [DNB 2008]
 (a) Anopheles philippinensis
 (b) Anopheles stephensi
 (c) Anopheles fluviatilis
 (d) Anopheles minimums

165. Which of the following insecticide is least toxic to man and most toxic to insects? [Bihar 2004]
 (a) Malathion (b) Parathion
 (c) Physostigmine (d) Nicotine

166. True about vector is: [UP 2003]
 (a) Plague is caused by mite
 (b) Sleeping sickness is caused by tsetse flies
 (c) Kala-azar is caused by W. bancrafti
 (d) Epidemic typhus is caused by Flea

167. DDT is: [UP 2003]
 (a) Stomach poison (b) Repellants
 (c) Contact poisons (d) Fumigants

168. An example of Space Spray is: [AP 2001]
 (a) Pyrethrum (b) Malathion
 (c) DDT (d) Paris green

169. All are true regarding DDT, except: [AP 2005]
 (a) It is primarily a contact poison
 (b) It acts as neurotoxin
 (c) It does not cause immediate death, but it takes several hours to kill
 (d) It has repellent action on insects

170. Culex mosquito is associated with transmission of:
 (a) Malaria [AP 1978, MP 2004]
 (b) Typhus [TN 2000]
 (c) Dengue fever [NEET Pattern 2018]
 (d) Japanese encephalitis

171. All belongs to class Insecta, except: [Kolkata 2003]
 (a) Housefly (b) Rat fleas
 (c) Ticks (d) Bedbugs

172. True about sand flea: [MP 2000]
 (a) Not found in India
 (b) Causes ulcers in foot
 (c) Causes bubo in groin
 (d) Vector for Kala-azar

173. Which insecticide is used for space-spray: [MP 2001]
 (a) Pyrethrum (b) DDT
 (c) Malathion (d) BHC

174. Which of the followings is transmitted by ticks: [MP 2001]
(a) H. nana
(b) Babesiosis
(c) Loa-Loa
(d) CJ-disease

175. Mosquito borne diseases are all *except*: [MP 2003]
(a) KFD
(b) Malaria
(c) Filaria
(d) Dengue fever

176. Natural insecticide among following is: [MP 2004]
(a) Malathion
(b) Pyrethrum
(c) Aldrin
(d) BHC

177. Culex is the vector for: [MP 2004]
(a) Filaria
(b) JE
(c) Dengue
(d) Yellow fever

178. Mosquitoes whose larvae lie horizontal on water and thus rest parallel to surface of water: [MH 2006]
(a) Aedes
(b) Anopheles
(c) Culex
(d) Mansonides

179. The nerve gas 'sarin' is: [MH 2007]
(a) Organophosphorous compound
(b) Organchlorine compound
(c) Carbamate
(d) Acridine

180. Which of the following mosquito transmit Japanese encephalitis? [MH 2008]
(a) Culex
(b) Aedes
(c) Mansonides
(d) All of the above

181. Which of the following type of mosquitoes can be controlled by removing and destroying the aquatic plants by herbicides? [MH 2008]
(a) Aedes
(b) Culex
(c) Mansonia
(d) Anopheles

182. All are true about Pyrethrum, *except*: [RJ 2009]
(a) Residual action is similar to DDT
(b) Vegetable origin
(c) Contact poison
(d) Synergistic with DDT

183. Most hazardous pesticide colour coding is: [AIIMS PGMEE November 2013]
(a) Red
(b) Green
(c) Yellow
(d) Black

184. Louse transmitted disease(s) is/are: [PGI November 2012]
(a) Trench fever
(b) Q fever
(c) KFD
(d) Epidemic typhus
(e) Pediculosis

185. Cyclo-propogative cycle is: [DNB June 2011] [DNB December 2011]
(a) Malaria
(b) Plague
(c) Cholera
(d) Filarial

186. Plague undergoes: [DNB December 2011]
(a) Trans-ovarian cycle
(b) Propogative cycle
(c) Cyclo-developmental
(d) Cyclo-propogative

187. Phlebotomus argentipes is killed by:
(a) Pyrethrum [DNB December 2011]
(b) DDT [NEET Pattern 2012]
(c) Malathion [NEET Pattern 2013]
(d) None of the above

188. Mode of transmission of Q fever: [DNB 2008]
(a) Ticks
(b) Mites
(c) Louse
(d) Mosquito

189. Urban malaria is transmitted by? [NEET Pattern 2013]
(a) Anopheles culicifacies
(b) Anopheles stephensi
(c) Anopheles fluviatilis
(d) Anopheles minimus

190. Disease transmitted by Hard tick include all, *except*: [DNB December 2011]
(a) Viral encephalitis
(b) Oriental sore
(c) Tick paralysis
(d) Tularaemia

191. The distance from airport or seaport which has to be kept free from aedes mosquitoes is: [NEET Pattern 2013, 2017]
(a) 400 m
(b) 500 m
(c) 1 km
(d) 100 m

192. Transovarian transmission is seen in: [NEET Pattern 2013]
(a) Rickettsial disease
(b) Malaria
(c) Filariasis
(d) None

193. Cyclodevelopmental stage is seen in: [NEET Pattern 2012, 2013]
(a) Malaria
(b) Filaria
(c) Plague
(d) Cholera

194. Fenthion is: [NEET Pattern 2013]
(a) Space spray
(b) Residual spray
(c) Stomach poison
(d) Fumigant

195. Best way to control houseflies: [NEET Pattern 2013]
(a) Eliminate breeding places
(b) Insecticide spray
(c) BedNet use
(d) Paris green

196. Regarding anopheles mosquito true is all, *except*: [DNB June 2010]
(a) Eggs are laid singly on water
(b) Larva don't have siphon tube
(c) Wings are spotted
(d) Pupa don't have siphon tube

197. Which of the following viral infections is transmitted by tick? [DNB 2007]
    (a) Japanese encephalitis
    (b) Dengue fever
    (c) Kyasanur forest disease
    (d) Yellow fever

198. Ixodes ticks transmit: [NEET Pattern 2012]
    (a) Babesiosis
    (b) Tularaemia
    (c) Lyme's disease
    (d) KFD

199. Disease(s) transmitted by Aedes aegypti include: [PGI November 2013]
    (a) Yellow fever
    (b) Dengue
    (c) Chikungunya fever
    (d) West Nile fever
    (e) Rift valley fever

200. Disease(s) transmitted by Louse include: [PGI November 2013]
    (a) Epidemic typhus
    (b) Scrub typhus
    (c) Relapsing fever
    (d) Trench fever
    (e) Q fever

201. Features of Anopheles mosquito include: [PGI May 2014]
    (a) Stripes on wings
    (b) Larva rests at an angle to water surface
    (c) Adult rests at angle to surface of skin
    (d) Eggs laid in clusters
    (e) No siphon tube in larvae

202. Mansonia mosquito is a vector of all of the following diseases *except*: [JIPMER 2014]
    (a) Malaria
    (b) Brugian filariasis
    (c) Chikungunya fever
    (d) St. Louis Encephalitis

Explanations

WATER

1. **Ans. (d) Collect sample from a gentle stream of water to avoid splashing** [Ref. Park 27/e p834]

   Steps for Water Sample Collection for Bacteriological Examination
   - Use clean sterilized bottles of neutral glass 200–250 mL with a ground glass stopper (Add 0.1 mL Sodium thiosulphate if water is likely to contain chlorine)
   - Take sample from a tap that is in regular use (if tap was not in regular use, heat the tap with blow lamp)
   - Let water to run waste for 2 minutes
   - Hold bottle near base with one hand (and remove stopper and paper)
   - Fill from a gentle stream of water, avoiding splashing (Don't use leaky taps; if you have to use them then first sterilize them properly)

2. **Ans. (c) Hypochlorous acid** [Ref. Park 25/e p775]
   - Disinfecting action of chlorine in water is due to Hypochlorous acid (HOCl–Main role in disinfection) and Hypochlorite ions (OCl–Minor role in disinfection)

3. **Ans. (b) 0.5 ppm** [Ref. Park 25/e p774–775]
   - Recommended minimum amount of Residual chlorine in drinking water is minimum 0.5 ppm (0.5 mg/L), 1.0 ppm for swimming polls, 2.0 ppm for killing Cyclops

4. **Ans. (b) Used to assess the Water quality by estimating hardness, total dissolved solids, alkalinity and pH** [Ref. The Water Dictionary by McTigue 2/e p333]

   Langlier's Saturation Index (LSI)
   - LSI provides an indicator of the degree of saturation of water with respect to calcium carbonate
   - LSI is based on estimating Hardness (calcium concentration), Total dissolved solids (TDS), Alkalinity, pH, Temperature
   - LSI Positive indicates Scaling, LSI negative indicates corrosion

5. **Ans. (b) Rain water** [Ref. Park 27/e p834]
   - Rain:
     - Is the prime source of all water
     - Is the 'purest form of water in nature'
     - Chemically, it is very soft water: contains traces (0.0005%) of solids
     - Gibraltar depends on rain water as a source of supply

> **ALSO REMEMBER**
> - *Safe and wholesome water:* has been defined as water that is
>   - Free from pathogenic agents
>   - Free from harmful chemical substances
>   - Pleasant to taste (free from colour and odour)
>   - Usable for domestic purposes
> - Water is said to be 'polluted' or 'contaminated' if it does not fulfill above criteria
> - *Safe yield of water:* Yield that is adequate for 95% of the year.

6. **Ans. (c) 1 ppm free chlorine should be present in water after break point has reached** [Ref. Park 27/e p841]

   CHLORINATION OF WATER
   - *Disinfecting action of chlorine in water is due to:*
     - Hypochlorous acid (HOCl)–Main role in disinfection
     - Hypochlorite ions (OCl)–Minor role in disinfection
   - *Chlorine has residual germicidal effect (and not Ozone or UV rays):* Provides a margin of safety against subsequent microbial contamination, as may occur during storage and distribution
   - *Phases of Chlorination:*
     - Phase I: Formation of chloramines
     - Phase II: Destruction of chloramines
     - Phase III: Appearance of break-point
     - Phase IV: Accumulation of free residual chlorine
   - *Recommended contact period of free residual chlorine in water:* 1 hour
   - *Level of free residual chlorine (FRC) recommended:*

Water type	Recommended	
	Residual chlorine level*	Contact period
Drinking water	≥ 0.5 mg per litre (ppm)	1 hour
Water bodies, post disaster	≥ 0.7 mg per litre (ppm)	1 hour
Swimming pool sanitation	≥ 1.0 mg per litre (ppm)	1 hour

   *(1 mg per litre = 1 ppm)

   - *Correct dose of chlorine to be applied:* Chlorine demand + FRC 0.5 mg per litre.

ALSO REMEMBER

- *Bleaching powder ($CaOCl_2$) contains:* 33% available chlorine
- *Chlorine acts best as a disinfectant for water at:* pH around 7.0
- *Instruments used in chlorination of water:*

Instrument	Utility
Horrock's Apparatus	Chlorine demand estimation
Chlorinator/Chloronome	Mixing/regulating dose of chlorine
Chloroscope	Measuring residual level of chlorine

- *Tests for chlorination of water:*
  - *Ortho-toluidine (OT) Test:* Measure the levels of,
    1. Free chlorine
    2. Free & Combined chlorine
  - *Ortho-toluidine Arsenite (OTA) Test:* Measure the levels of,
    1. Free chlorine
    2. Combined chlorine
- *OTA test is better than OT test as:*
  - Detects both free and combined chlorine separately
  - Not affected by interfering substances (nitrites, iron, manganese).

7. Ans. (d) 45 mg/l [Ref. Park 27/e p850]

- *Guideline value of nitrate in drinking water:* <50 mg/litre
  - Nitrates in drinking water indicate: Remote contamination
  - Is solely used for prevention of methemoglobinemia
- *Guideline value of nitrite in drinking water:* <3 mg/litre
  - Nitrites in drinking water indicate: Recent contamination
  - May lead to 'Blue baby syndrome'
- Concentration of nitrate/Guideline value of nitrate + Concentration of nitrite/Guideline value of nitrite should be ≤1

8. Ans. (c) Cl. Tetani [Ref. Park 27/e p847–848]

- *Bacteriological indicators of water quality:*
  - Coliforms (E.coli is most important microbiological indicator)
  - Fecal streptococci (Indicator of recent contamination) (Sodium Azide medium)
  - Clostridium perfringens (Indicator of remote contamination)
- *Acceptable level of coliforms in drinking water:* None
  - EXCEPTION: In large urban supplies, up to 5% samples are acceptable to be contaminated, if taken continuously for a period of 12 month

9. Ans. (d) 150–200 lit [Ref. Park 27/e p851]

- *Water supply considered adequate to meet the need for domestic purposes:*
  - *Urban:* 150–200 litres per capita per day
  - *Rural:* 40–60 litres per capita per day
- *Daily drinking water requirement:* 2–3 litres per capita per day.

ALSO REMEMBER

- *Criteria for identification of 'Problem Habitations':*
  - *Not Covered (NC)/No Safe Source (NSS) Habitations:*
    1. Drinking water source point is not within 1.6 kms in plains or 100 m elevation in hilly areas
    2. Water source affected with quality problems like excess salinity, iron, fluoride, arsenic, or other toxic materials or biologically contaminated
    3. Quantum of availability of safe water is not enough to meet drinking and cooking needs
  - *Partially Covered (PC) Habitations:*
    1. Drinking water source point is within 1.6 km in plains or 100 m elevation in hilly areas
    2. Capacity of system is 10–40 lpcd
  - *Fully Covered (FC) Habitations:* include all the remaining habitations.

10. Ans. (d) Chlorine demand [Ref. Park 27/e p855–856]

Horrock's Apparatus

- *Use:* To find out the dose of bleaching powder required for disinfection of water, i.e. 'Chlorine demand estimation of water'
- *Dose of bleaching powder required (Chlorine demand):*
  - n × 2 gm to disinfect 455 litres of water (where n = no. of first cup which shows distinct blue colour).

11. Ans. (b) Horrock's apparatus [Ref. Park 27/e p855–856]

- *Chlorine demand of water:* Is the amount of chlorine that is needed to destroy bacteria, and to oxidize all the organic matter amd ammoniacal substances present in water
  - Is the amount of chlorine added to water minus amount of residual chlorine remaining at the end of a specific period of contact (1 hr)
  - Estimation of chlorine demand of water (or dose of bleaching powder required for disinfection of water) is done by 'Horrock's apparatus'.

12. Ans. (c) Free and combined chlorine in water [Ref. Park 27/e p842]

13. Ans. (b) 5–10°C [Ref. Foundations of Community Medicine, GM Dhaar & I Robbani, 1/e p31]

- Most desired temperature range for drinking water is 40–50° F (5–10°C).

14. Ans. (d) Lead [Ref. Foundations of Community Medicine, GM Dhaar & I Robbani, 1/e p72]

- *Undesirable metals in drinking water:* Iron, manganese, zinc, copper, aluminium, lead
- *MOST undesirable metal in drinking water:* Lead
  - Lead was earlier seen in drinking water when water was being supplied through lead pipes
- *Undesirable salts in drinking water:* Chlorides, Fluorides, Nitrites, Nitrates, Calcium, Magnesium
- *Undesirable gases in drinking water:* Ammonia, Hydrogen sulphide, Methane.

15. **Ans. (a) Coliform bacteria** *[Ref. Park 27/e p847-848]*
    - *Coliform organisms:*
        - Primary & most reliable bacterial indicator for water quality
        - E. coli is most important coliform indicator
        - Reasons for choosing coliforms as indicators of fecal pollution rather than water-Borne pathogens:
            1. Constant presence in great abundance in human intestine; foreign to potable waters
            2. Easily detectable by culture methods
            3. Longer survival period
            4. Greater resistance to forces of natural purification.

16. **Ans. (b) Water washed disease** *[Ref. A Dictionary of Public Health by Dr. J. Kishore; p575-76]*
    - *Water washed diseases:* Include infections of the outer body surface which occur due to inadequate use of water or improper hygiene. Examples: Scabies, Trachoma, Typhus, Bacillary dysentery, Amoebic dysentery

> **ALSO REMEMBER**
> - *Scabies:* Is a transmissible ectoparasite skin infection characterized by superficial burrows, intense pruritus (itching) and secondary infection
>   - Scabies is caused by the mite Sarcoptes scabiei, variety hominis (known as 'Itch mite')
>   - Scabies is usually transmitted by close contact with an infested person; Scabies is transmitted readily, often throughout an entire household, by skin-to-skin contact with an infected person and thus is sometimes classified as a sexually transmitted disease (STD)
>   - Drug of Choice for scabies: 5% Permethrin (Oral systemic DOC: Ivermectin)
>   - Scabies was the first disease of man with known cause.

17. **Ans. (d) 150–200 litres per capita** *[Ref. Park 23/e p724]*

> **ALSO REMEMBER**
> - *Norms of water supply for urban areas:*
>
> | Type of urban area | Norm for water supply |
> | --- | --- |
> | Towns with piped water supply, but no sewerage system | 70 lpcd |
> | Cities with piped water supply & existing/planned sewerage | 135 lpcd |
> | Metropolitan & Megacities with piped water supply & sewerage | 150 lpcd |
> | Public stand post | 40 lpcd |
>
> (lpcd: Litres per capita per day)

18. **Ans. (c) Frequent washing is not required** *[Ref. Park 27/e p841]*
    - *Comparison of Rapid and Slow sand filters:*

	Rapid Sand Filter	Slow Sand Filter
Space	Occupies very little space	Occupies large area
Rate of filtration	200 m.g.a.d.	2–3 m.g.a.d.
Effective size of sand	0.4–0.7 mm	0.2–0.3 mm
Preliminary treatment	Chemical coagulation & sedimentation	Plain sedimentation
Washing	By back-washing	By scraping sand bed
Frequent washing	Required	Not required
Mechanism of action	Essentially physical	Both physical & mechanical
Operation	Highly skilled	Less skilled
Loss of head allowed	6–8 feet	4 feet
Removal of turbidity	Good	Good
Removal of colour	Good	Fair
Removal of bacteria	98–99 percent	99.9–99.99 percent
Suitability	For big cities	For small towns

> **ALSO REMEMBER**
> - *Vital layer (Schmutzdecke, Zoogleal layer or Biological layer):* Slimy, gelatinous layer consisting of algae, planktons, diatoms and bacteria is formed in the slow sand filter
>   - Vital layer is the *'Heart of Slow Sand Filter'*
>   - Formation of vital layer is known as *'Ripening of the filter'*
>   - It removes organic matter, holds back bacteria oxidizes nitrogen to nitrates and helps in yielding bacteria-free water.

19. **Ans. (b) Hypochlorous acid** *[Ref. Park 27/e p841]*
20. **Ans. (a) Chlorine only** *[Ref. Park 27/e p842]*
    - Ozone gas and UV radiation has got no residual action.
    - Free Residual Chlorine (FRC) is allowed to accumulate in water till it reaches a level of 0.5 ppm (mg/litre) when it becomes fit for community supply.
    - FRC has a bactericidal action that takes care of post-chlorination contamination of drinking water.

> **ALSO REMEMBER**
> Chlorine has no effect on bacterial spores, protozoal cysts and helminthic ova (except in higher doses). Viral agents of Infectious hepatitis (Hepatitis A) and Poliomyelitis are also resistant in normal doses, as are cyclops.

21. **Ans. (a) Gross a activity 0.1 Bq/L & Gross b activity 1.0 Bq/L (Now 0.5 Bq/L and 1.0 Bq/L respectively)** *[Ref. Park 27/e p852]*
    - *Key guideline aspects of WHO recommended drinking water quality:*
        - Colour <15 true colour units (TCU)
        - Turbidity <1 nephlometric turbidity units (NTU)
        - pH: 6.5–8.5
        - Total dissolved solids (TDS) <500 mg/litre
        - Zero pathogenic microorganisms
        - Zero infectious viruses

- Absence of pathogenic protozoa and infective stages of helminthes
- Fluoride <1.0 ppm (0.5–0.8 ppm: Optimum level)
- Nitrates <45 mg/litre
- Nitrites <3 mg/litre
- Gross alpha radiological activity <0.5 Bq/litre (New Guideline – WHO)
- Gross beta radiological activity <1.0 Bq/litre (New Guideline – WHO).

22. Ans. (a) Detect the presence of Coliform organisms in a sample of water [Ref. Park 27/e p853]

> **ALSO REMEMBER**
> - Periodicity of water sample collection for bacteriological examination:

Population served	Minimum interval between successive samples
<20,000	1 month
20,001–50,000	2 weeks
50,001–100,000	4 days
>100,000	1 day

23. Ans. (a) Less than 1 [Ref. Park 27/e p854]
- Methods of removal of hardness of water:

Type of hardness	Methods of removal
Temporary hardness	Boiling Addition of lime Addition of sodium carbonate Permutit process
Permanent hardness	Addition of sodium carbonate Base exchange process

- WHO says that 'there does not appear to be any convincing evidence that water hardness causes adverse health effects in humans' (rather it is cardioprotective).

24. Ans. (a) 0.5 mg/l for a contact period of 1 hr [Ref. Park 27/e p842]
25. Ans. (b) Chlorine acts best when pH is around 7 [Ref. Park 27/e p841]
26. Ans. (a) Bicarbonates of calcium and magnesium [Ref. Park 27/e p853–854]
27. Ans. (a) Bacteria are removed more effectively; (c) Cost construction is cheaper; (d); (e) [Ref. Park 27/e p841]
28. Ans. (a) E. coli; (b) Coliform; (c) Enterococci [Ref. Park 27/e p847–848]
29. Ans. (a) Staphylococcus [Ref. Park 27/e p847–848]
30. Ans. (a) Presence of Clostridial spores indicates recent contamination of water [Ref. Park 27/e p847–848]
31. Ans. (a) Presence of clostridial spores indicate recent contamination [Ref. Park 27/e p847–848]
32. Ans. (c) Requires longer duration [Ref. Park 27/e p841]
33. Ans. (c) Zoogleal layer [Ref. Park 27/e p839]
34. Ans. (d) 0.5 mg/L [Ref. Park 27/e p855–856]
35. Ans. (c) 1–3 [Ref. Park 27/e p853–854]
36. Ans. (a) Lime + Alum [Ref. Park 27/e p759]
37. Ans. (a) 0.5 mg/L [Ref. Park 27/e p842]
38. Ans. (a) Free from pathogens; (b) Free from harmful chemicals; (d) Free from colour and odour [Ref. Park 27/e p833]
39. Ans. (c) Super chlorination followed by dechlorination [Ref. Park 27/e p842]
40. Ans. (b) Nitrites [Ref. Park 27/e p850]
41. Ans. (a) 120 grams [Ref. Park 27/e p855–856]
- Dose of bleaching powder required (Chlorine demand): $n \times 2$ gm to disinfect 455 litres of water (where n = no. of first cup which shows distinct blue color in Horrock's apparatus)

In the given question,
- 3rd cup shows blue color so 3×2 grams (6 grams) will disinfect 455 litres of water.
- Hence, 9100 litres will require $6/455 \times 9100 = 120$ grams bleaching powder.

42. Ans. (d) Phosphates [Ref. Park 27/e p853]

Hardness of Water
- Temporary hardness (Carbonate hardness) is due to Calcium & Magnesium salts of Bicarbonates
- Permanent hardness (Non-Carbonate hardness) is due to Calcium & Magnesium salts of Sulfates, Chlorides, Nitrates
- Four main compounds causing Hardness: Calcium bicarbonates, Magnesium bicarbonates, Calcium sulfates, Magnesium sulfates.

43. Ans. (b) 20 feet [Ref. Park 27/e p836]

Sanitary Well Guidelines
- *Location:* <100 m radial distance; >15 m (50 feet) from source of contamination
- *Lining:* >6 m (20 feet) depth; >60–90 cm (2–3 feet) above ground level
- *Parapet wall:* >70–75 cms above ground
- *Platform:* >1 m (3 feet) in all directions
- *Other guidelines:* Pucca drain to a soakage pit/public drain beyond cone of filtration; cement concrete cover; robust hand pump to withdraw water

44. Ans. (c) It is unusable for domestic purpose [Ref. Park 27/e p833]

Safe and Wholesome Water
- Free from pathogenic agents
- Free from harmful chemical substances
- Pleasant to taste (free from colour and odour)
- Usable for domestic purposes

Review Questions

45. Ans. (d) Decreased soap consumption
    [Ref. Park 27/e p853–854]
46. Ans. (d) Brucellosis *[Ref. Park 23/e p710]*
47. Ans. (d) Dissolved nitrogen *[Ref. Park 27/e p848]*
48. Ans. (d) 600 mg/litre *[Ref. Park 27/e p846]*
49. Ans. (b) On the sand bed *[Ref. Park 27/e p839]*
50. Ans. (c) Chlorination of water *[Ref. Park 27/e p841]*
51. Ans. (a) pH 6.5–8.5 *[Ref. Park 27/e p843]*
52. Ans. (d) Algae, plankton, diatoms and bacteria on surface of sand bed filter *[Ref. Park 27/e p839]*
53. Ans. (d) 30 gm *[Ref. Park 27/e p856]*
54. Ans (d) Risk of Guinea worm infection
    [Ref. Park 22/e p347]

AIR

55. Ans. (d) Severe *[Ref. CPCB Website]*

    Air Quality Index (CPCB)
    - AQ sub-index and health breakpoints are evolved for eight pollutants - PM10, PM2.5, NO_2, SO_2, CO, O_3, NH_3, Pb

AQI	Remark	Color Code	Possible Health Impacts
0–50	Good	Green	Minimal impact
51–100	Satisfactory	Light green	Minor breathing discomfort to sensitive people
101–200	Moderate	Yellow	Breathing discomfort to people with lungs, asthma, heart diseases
201–300	Poor	Orange	Breathing discomfort to most people on prolonged exposure
301–400	Very Poor	Red	Respiratory illness on prolonged exposure
401–500	Severe	Dark red	Affects healthy people & seriously impacts those with existing diseases

56. Ans. (a) Kata thermometer *[Ref. Park 26/e p841]*
    - Dry bulb thermometer: Air temperature
    - Wet bulb thermometer: Air temperature
    - Maximum thermometer: Air temperature
    - Minimum thermometer: Air temperature
    - Six's maximum & minimum thermometer: Air temperature
    - Silvered thermometer: Air temperature
    - Globe thermometer: Mean radiant temperature of surroundings
    - Wet globe thermometer: Environment heat
    - Kata thermometer: Low air velocity (earlier colling power)

57. Ans. (d) Sulphur dioxide, Smoke, Particulate matter
    [Ref. Park 27/e p876]
    - The best indicators of Air pollution are Sulphur dioxide, Smoke and Suspended particles

58. Ans. (a) Humidity *[Ref. Foundations of Community Medicine, GM Dhaar & I Robbani, 1/e p54–56, Park 27/e p876]*

    AIR HUMIDITY
    - Air humidity is moisture content of air
    - Air humidity can be measured by:
      - Dry and wet bulb thermometers
      - Hygrometer
      - Sling/Whirling Psychrometer
      - Assman Psychrometer

    Also Refer to Annexure 3

59. Ans. (a) Perflation and Aspiration *[Ref. Park 27/e p866]*
    - Types of ventilation:
      - Natural ventilation:
        1. *Wind:* It blows through a room (Perflation) and may exert a suction at its tail end (Aspiration)
        2. *Diffusion:* When passes through smallest openings
        3. *Inequality of temperature*
      - Mechanical (artificial) ventilation:
        1. *Exhaust ventilation:* Air is extracted to outside by exhaust fans driven by electricity
        2. *Plenum ventilation:* Fresh air is blown into rooms by centrifugal rooms
        3. *Balanced ventilation:* Combination of exhaust and plenum ventilation
        4. *Air conditioning:* Simultaneous control of all factors especially temperature, humidity and air movement

60. Ans. (b) McArdle's index *[Ref. Park 27/e p860–862]*
    - Air pollutants can be of several types:
      - *Primary pollutants:* are emitted directly (SO_2, NO_2, CO, Hydrocarbons, Particulate matter, CFCs, Ammonia, Radioactive materials, Metals like lead, cadmium, copper, volatile organic compounds)
      - *Secondary pollutants:* are formed by interaction between primary pollutants (Ground level ozone, Peroxyacetyl nitrate, Particulate matter formed from primary pollutants)
    - Chemical indicators of air pollution:
      - *Sulphur dioxide:* Best indicator of air pollution
      - *Smoke or Soiling index:* Air strain on a filter paper measured through photoelectric meter
      - Grit & dust measurement
      - Coefficient of haze
      - Air pollution index
    - *BEST Biological indicator of air pollution:* Lichens.

> **ALSO REMEMBER**
> - *Corrected Effective Temperature (CET) is an index of thermal comfort:* Combines effect of temperature, humidity, velocity of air & mean radiant heat
>   - *Mc Ardle's maximum allowable sweat rate:* 4.5 litres/4h
>
> | Zone of comfort | P4SR (Predictable 4 hour sweat rate) |
> |---|---|
> | Comfort zone | 1–3 litres |
> | Just tolerable | 3–4.5 litres |
> | Intolerable | >4.5 litres |
>
> - *The Kyoto protocol:* is a protocol intended to achieve 'stabilization of greenhouse gas concentrations in the atmosphere at a level that would prevent dangerous anthropogenic interference with the climate system'
>   - The protocol was initially adopted for use on 11 December 1997 in Kyoto, Japan and which entered into force on 16 February 2005
>   - The Kyoto Protocol establishes legally binding commitments for the reduction of 6 greenhouse gases (carbon dioxide, methane, nitrous oxide, sulfur hexafluoride, hydrofluorocarbons, and perfluorocarbons) by industrialized nations, as well as general commitments for all member countries
>   - Under Kyoto, industrialized countries agreed to reduce their collective GHG emissions by 5.2%, averaged over the period of 2008–2012, compared to the year 1990.

61. **Ans. (c) 4.5 lit/4 hours** [Ref. Park 27/e p859]
62. **Ans. (c) Air temperature, humidity and air movement** [Ref. Park 27/e p874]
    - Kata thermometer measures 'cooling power of air': Cooling power of air comprises of
        - Air temperature
        - Humidity
        - Air movement
    - Kata thermometer readings as indices of thermal comfort:
        - Dry kata reading >6 (Thermal comfort)
        - Wet kata reading >20 (Thermal comfort)
    - Nowadays it is used to record low air velocity.
63. **Ans. (d) Plenum ventilation** [Ref. Park 27/e p866]
64. **Ans. (d) Globe thermometer** [Ref. Park 27/e p873–874]
    - Instruments used in Air temperature:

Instrument	Measures
Dry bulb thermometer	Air temperature
Wet bulb thermometer	Air temperature
Maximum thermometer	Air temperature
Minimum thermometer	Air temperature
Six's maximum and minimum thermometer	Air temperature
Silvered thermometer	Air temperature
Globe thermometer	Mean radiant temperature
Wet Globe thermometer	Environmental heat
Kata thermometer	Cooling power of Air; Low air velocities

65. **Ans. (a) CO_2 is a major greenhouse gas** [Ref. Wikipedia]
    GREENHOUSE GASES
    - Water vapour (Highest contribution)
    - Carbon dioxide (Second highest contribution)
    - Methane
    - Ozone
        - Ozone layer: Is beneficial as it cuts down UV transmission
    - CFCs depletes ozone layer

66. **Ans. (d) Mercury vapour** [Ref. Park 27/e p863]
    Sources of Indoor Air Pollution: **(Mnemonic: C MORON SCARF)**

Indoor air pollutant	Sources
Respirable particles	Tobacco smoke, Stove, Aerosols
Carbon monoxide	Combustion equipment, Stove, Gas heaters
Nitrogen dioxide	Gas cookers, Cigarettes
Sulphur dioxide	Coal combustion
Carbon dioxide	Combustion, Respiration
Formaldehyde	Particle board, Carpet adhesives, Insulation
Organic vapours (benzene, toulidine)	Solvents, Adhesives, Resins, Aerosols
Ozone	Electric arcing, UV light
Radon & daughters	Building materials
Asbestos	Insulation, Fire-proofing
Mineral fibres	Appliances

Review Questions

67. **Ans. (d) Neuro-developmental problems** [Ref. Park 27/e p863–865]
    Effects of indoor air pollution
    - Acute respiratory tract infections (Pneumonias)
    - Chronic lung disease
    - Lung cancers in adults
    - Adverse pregnancy outcomes (Especially stillbirths)
68. **Ans. (d) CFCs** [Ref. Global Change of Planet Earth OECD, p48]
69. **Ans. (a) SO_2** [Ref. Park 27/e p861, 863]
70. **Ans. (d) Central Pollution Control Board** [Ref. Park 27/e p864]
71. **Ans. (c) Temperature inversion** [Ref. Encyclopedia of Climate and Weather by Schneider, Root & Mastrandrea, 2/e (Volume 3) p392]
72. **Ans. (b) 40–60** [Ref. Park 27/e p874]

Heat Stress Index (HSI)	
HSI %	Consequence of 8 hour exposure
0	No thermal strain
10–30	Mild-Moderate heat stress, Minimal impairment in work

Contd...

Contd...

Heat Stress Index (HSI)	
40–60	Severe heat stress, Threat to health if not fit
70–90	Very severe heat stress, only few can sustain it
100	Maximum heat stress, only young fit acclimatized can sustain it
>100	Varying degrees of stress due to hyperthermia

73. **Ans. (d) Numbness** [Ref. Park 27/e p874]

    EFFECTS OF HEAT STRESS
    - *Heat stroke:* Body temperature >110°F, Delirium, Convulsions, Absence of sweating
    - Heat hyperpyrexia
    - Heat exhaustion
    - Heat cramps
    - Heat syncope

74. **Ans. (b) Carbon monoxide** [Ref. Internet]
    - By their % contribution to Greenhouse effect on earth, 4 major gases:
      – Water vapor, 36–70%
      – Carbon dioxide, 9–26%
      – Methane, 4–9%
      – Ozone, 3–7%

75. **Ans. (c) Ozone** [Ref. Park 27/e p860]
    - Primary pollutants: Emitted directly (SO_2, NO_2, CO, Hydrocarbons, Particulate matter, CFCs, Ammonia, Radioactive materials, Metals - lead, cadmium, copper, Volatile organic compounds)
    - Secondary pollutants: Formed by interaction between primary pollutants (Ground level ozone, Peroxyacetyl nitrate, Particulate matter formed from primary pollutants)

76. **Ans. (d) All of the above** [Ref. Park 27/e p863]
    - Indoor air pollutants include Respirable particles (Tobacco smoke, Aerosols), Carbon monoxide, Nitrogen dioxide, Sulphur dioxide, Carbon dioxide, Formaldehyde, Organic vapours (Benzene, Toulidine), Ozone, Radon & daughters, Asbestos, Mineral fibres

Review Questions

77. **Ans (c) 4–6** [Ref. Park 27/e p866]
78. **Ans. (d) All of the above** [Ref. Park 27/e p863]
79. **Ans. (a) Low Air velocity** [Ref. Park 27/e p874]
80. **Ans. (c) Sling psychrometer** [Ref. Park 27/e p876]

SOUND

81. **Ans. (a) 20–30 dB** [Ref. Park 27/e p869]
    - *Human ear is sensitive to sound frequency:* 20–20,000 Hz
    - Daily maximum tolerable sound level to human ear (without substantial damage to their hearing): 85–90 dB
      – *Auditory fatigue appears in:* 90 dB region (greatest at 4000 Hz)
    - Sound level above which tympanic membrane rupture (permanent mechanical damage): 150–160 dB
    - Sound levels of some noises:
      – Whisper: 20–30 dB
      – Normal conversation: 60–70 dB
      – Mechanical damage: 150–160 dB (e.g., Jet taking off)
    - *Acceptable noise levels:* expressed in dB (A), sound pressure levels conforming to weighting curve (A)

Environment	Place	Acceptable noise level dB (A)
Residential	Bed room	25
	Living room	40
Commercial	Office	35–45
	Conference	40–45
	Restaurants	40–60
Industrial	Workshop	40–60
	Laboratory	40–50
Educational	Class room	30–40
	Library	35–40
Hospitals	Wards	20–35

ALSO REMEMBER
- 20th century has been described as 'Century of noise'
- Basic instruments used in studies of noise:

Instrument	Use
Sound Level Meter	Measures intensity of sound in dB or dB(A)
Octave Band Frequency Analyser	Shows 'sound spectrum', characteristic (pitch)
Audiometer	Measures hearing ability

– *Most Temporary Hearing loss occurs in the frequency range:* 4000–6000 Hz.

82. **Ans. (c) 160 dB** [Ref. Park 27/e p869]
83. **Ans. (c) 100 dB** [Ref. Park 27/e p869]

Review Question

84. **Ans. (a) 85 dB** [Ref. Park 27/e p869]

LIGHT

85. **Ans. (a) Candela** [Ref. Park 27/e p867]

    LIGHT MEASUREMENT UNITS

Unit	Quantity measured	Description
Candela	Luminous intensity	Brightness of source
Lumen	Luminous flux	Flow of light
Lux	Illumination Illuminance	Amount of light reaching surface
Lambert	Brightness Luminance	Amount of light re-emitted by surface

86. **Ans. (a) 6–12** [Ref. Park 27/e p866]
- *Basic minimum illumination for satisfactory vision:* 15–20 foot candles

87. **Ans. (a) Candela** [Ref. Park 27/e p867]

LIGHT MEASUREMENT UNITS

Unit	Quantity measured	Description
Candela	Luminous intensity	Brightness of source
Lumen	Luminous flux	Flow of light
Lux	Illumination Illuminance	Amount of light reaching surface
Lambert	Brightness Luminance	Amount of light re-emitted by surface

HOUSING

88. **Ans. (a) 50–100 sq.ft.** [Ref. Park 27/e p879]
- *Recommend per capita space in urban houses:* 50–100 sq-ft.

> **ALSO REMEMBER**
> - Accepted standards of overcrowding:
>   - Persons per room:
>
> | No. of rooms | Maximum no. of persons |
> | --- | --- |
> | 1 room | 2 persons |
> | 2 rooms | 3 persons |
> | 3 rooms | 5 persons |
> | 4 rooms | 7 persons |
> | 5 rooms (additional 2 for each further room) | 10 persons |
>
>   - *Floor space per person:* Child between 1–10 years is counted as ½ unit; infant is not counted
>
> | Floor space | Maximum no. of persons |
> | --- | --- |
> | >110 sq. ft. | 2 persons |
> | 90–110 sq. ft. | 1½ persons |
> | 70–90 sq. ft. | 1 person |
> | 50–70 sq. ft. | ½ person |
> | <50 sq. ft. | Nil |
>
>   - *Sex separation:* Overcrowding is said to exist if two persons over 9 years of age, not husband and wife, of opposite sexes are obliged to sleep in the same room
> - *Recommended spaces:*
>   - Floor space per person in a house: minimum 70–90 sq. ft.
>   - Floor area per student in a class: >10 sq. ft.
>   - Space per worker in a factory (The Factory Act, 1948): >500 cu. ft.

WASTE DISPOSAL

89. **Ans. (d) Bangalore method (Composting)** [Ref. Park 27/e p882]

> **ALSO REMEMBER**
> - *Composting:* Integrated 'sanitary' method of disposal of refuse & night soil
>   - Bangalore method (Anaerobic hot fermentation process): Alternate layers of refuse & night soil in proportion 3:1, with refuse layer both as lowermost as well as topmost.
>   - Indore Method (Aerobic process).

90. **Ans. (c) Sullage** [Ref. Park 27/e p889]

> **ALSO REMEMBER**
> - *Sullage (Grey water):* Is non-industrial wastewater generated from domestic processes such as kitchen, laundry and bathing
>   - Greywater comprises 50–80% of residential waste water; it consists wastewater generated from all of the house's sanitation equipment except for the toilets
> - 'Black water' is water from toilets
> - 'White water' is groundwater or potable water.

91. **Ans. (b) Dry weather flow** [Ref. Park 27/e p889]
- *Sewage:* Is waste water from a community, containing solid and liquid excreta, derived from houses, street and yard washings, factories and industries
- *Composition of sewage:* 99.9% water + 0.1% solids (organic & inorganic)
- *Dry weather flow:* Is the average amount of sewage that flows in sewerage system in 24 hours
- *Strength of sewage is expressed in terms of:*
  - Biological Oxygen Demand (BOD): Is defined as 'amount of oxygen absorbed by a sample of sewage' during a specified period (Generally 5 days), at a specified temperature (generally 20° C) for aerobic destruction or use of organic matter by living organisms
    1. BOD is most important test done on sewage (done through Dilution method and Manometric method)
    2. Strong Sewage has BOD >300 g/litre and Weak Sewage has BOD <100 g/litre
  - Chemical Oxygen Demand (COD): Measures oxygen equivalent of that portion of organic matter in a sample, which is susceptible to oxidation by a strong chemical oxidizer
    1. Potassium dichromate is best for COD estimation
  - Suspended solids: Amount in domestic sewage varies from 100–500 mg/litre
    1. Strong Sewage has suspended solids amount >500 mg/litre and Weak Sewage has suspended solids amount <100 mg/litre.

92. **Ans. (a) Ideal retention period–48 hrs** [Ref. Park 27/e p887]

SEPTIC TANK:
- Is a water-tight masonary tank into which household sewage is admitted for treatment

- Is a satisfactory method of disposing liquid and excreta wastes from individual dwellings, small groups of houses or institutions which have 'adequate water supply but do not have access to a public sewerage system'
- *Design features of a septic tank:*
  - *Ideal retention period:* 24 hours
- *Steps of purification in a septic tank:*
  - *Anaerobic digestion:* Takes place in septic tank proper
  - *Aerobic oxidation:* Takes place in sub-soil (outside septic tank).

93. **Ans. (b) Controlled tipping** *[Ref. Park 27/e p881]*
    - *Sanitary Landfill (Controlled Tipping):* Laying of dry & condensed refuse in layers with intervening earth partitions & coverings, followed by mechanical compression (Most Satisfactory Method)
      - Trench Method
      - Ramp Method
      - Area Method

94. **Ans. (a) E. Coli Count** *[Ref. Park 27/e p889]*

95. **Ans. (a) Organic matter** *[Ref. Park 27/e p889]*
    - *Biological Oxygen Demand (BOD):* Is defined as 'amount of oxygen absorbed by a sample of sewage' during a specified period (Generally 5 days), at a specified temperature (generally 20° C) for aerobic destruction or use of organic matter by living organisms
      - BOD is most important test done for estimation of strength of sewage (done through Dilution method and Manometric method)
      - Strong Sewage has BOD >300 g/litre and Weak Sewage has BOD <100 g/litre.

96. **Ans. (d) Septic tank** *[Ref. Park 27/e p886]*

97. **Ans. (d) Content of combustible matter above 60%** *[Ref. Park 23/e p754–755]*

98. **Ans. (b) Chemical oxygen demand** *[Ref. Park 27/e p889]*

99. **Ans. (a) Treatment of household sewage; (c) Aerobic oxidation outside septic tank; (d) Anaerobic digestion inside septic tank** *[Ref. Park 27/e p886]*

100. **Ans. (b) Strength measured by Biological oxygen demand; (e) Dry weather flow is measured for 24 hours period** *[Ref. Park 27/e p889]*

101. **Ans. (a) Biochemical oxygen demand is indicator of the organic content of sewage; (b) BOD is amount of oxygen absorbed by a sample of sewage; (c) Undergo both aerobic and anaerobic reaction in sewage purification; (d) Untreated sewage is thrown into rivers** *[Ref. Park 27/e p889–893]*

Sewage Disposal
- Biochemical oxygen demand (BOD)
  - BOD is indicator of the organic content of sewage
  - BOD is amount of oxygen absorbed by a sample of sewage for 5 days at 20 degrees C
- Undergo both aerobic (most efficient method) and anaerobic reaction in sewage purification
- In few countries, untreated sewage is thrown into rivers (though it's not recommended)

> **ALSO REMEMBER**
> **Quantification of Organic Matter in Sewage**
> - *Direct methods:* Total Organic Carbon (TOC)
> - *Indirect methods:* BOD, Ultimate BOD, Chemical oxygen demand (COD)

102. **Ans. (b) Solids** *[Ref. Park 27/e p889]*

Sewage Treatment
- *Primary treatment:* Physical treatment to remove solids (from the liquid)
- *Secondary treatment:* Biological treatment brought about by aerobic and anaerobic bacteria
- *Tertiary treatment:* Improving further the quality of effluent (advanced waste treatment process), sludge (stabilization and dewatering), assist sedimentation and sludge treatment (chemical treatment by the addition of coagulants)

103. **Ans. (a) 1 acre** *[Ref. Park 27/e p881]*

Methods of Sanitary landfill (Controlled tipping)
- Trench method (When ground level is available): Trench sized 2–3 m depth × 4–12 m width (Wherever compacted refuse is available to fell 2 m depth, 1 acre land is required per year for 10000 population)
- Ramp method (Where terrain is moderately sloping)
- Area method (Used for filling land depressions/disused quarries/clay pits): Refuse deposited in uniform layers 2–2.5 m depth, with a mud cover 30 cm thick

> **ALSO REMEMBER**
> - Sanitary landfill is the *'most sanitary method of refuse disposal'*
> - *Mechanism:* Temperature of refuse rises above 60 degrees C in 7 days (kills all pathogens), 2–3 weeks cooling time and 4–6 months for complete decomposition of organic matter
> - *Modified sanitary landfill:* Compaction and covering are accomplished 1–2 times a week

Review Questions

104. **Ans. (c) Activated sludge process** *[Ref. Park 27/e p890]*
105. **Ans. (d) Used where public sewerage system is adequate** *[Ref. Park 27/e p886]*
106. **Ans. (a) Water seal** *[Ref. Park 27/e p884]*
107. **Ans. (d) Retention period is of 24 hrs** *[Ref. Park 27/e p886]*
108. **Ans. (c) Settlement of heavy objects** *[Ref. Park 27/e p889]*

MISCELLANEOUS (ENVIRONMENT)

109. **Ans. (c) Residual level of free chlorine to be >0.5 ppm** *[Ref. Park 27/e p855]*

SANITATION MEASURES FOR SWIMMING POOL SANITATION:
- *Recommended area:* Recommended area is = 2.2 sq. metre (24 sq. ft.) per swimmer

- *Surveillance:* Rules and regulations to be posted in appropriate place
- *Filtration of water:* Water to be refiltered in less than 6 hours (rapid sand filters); 15% water to be replaced by fresh water everyday
- *Chlorination of water:* Residual level of free chlorine to be >1.0 ppm to protect against bacterial and viral agents
- *pH of water:* 7.4–7.8
- *Bacteriological quality of water:* To be as close to standards prescribed for drinking water

> **ALSO REMEMBER**
> - Level of residual chlorine to be maintained in drinking water is >0.5 mg/l (>0.5 ppm) for a contact period of 1 hour
> - Level of residual chlorine to be maintained in all water bodies in post-disaster phase is >0.7 mg/l (>0.7 ppm)
>   - Level of residual chlorine to be maintained for swimming pool sanitation is >1.0 mg/l (>1.0 ppm)

110. Ans. (b) 5 rads per year [Ref. Park 27/e p871]
   - Protection: Maximum permissible radiation exposure is '5 rad per person per year'.

111. Ans. (d) Radiation protection in pregnancy [Ref. An Introduction to Radiobiology by AHW Nias 2/e p86]

112. Ans. (b) Rad [Ref. Park 27/e p871]

113. Ans. (d) Environmental sanitation [Ref. Award to Public Health Facilities KAYAKALP, MOHFW GOI p1]

    KAYAKALP (Launched 15th May 2015)
    - National Initiative to give Awards to Public Health Facilities that demonstrate high levels of cleanliness, hygiene and infection control focuses on promoting cleanliness in public spaces
    - *Parameters used:* Hospital/Facility Upkeep, Sanitation and hygiene, Waste Management, Infection control, Support Services, Hygiene Promotion
    - Objectives
      - To promote Cleanliness, Hygiene & Infection Control Practices in Public Health Care Facilities
      - To incentivize and recognize such public healthcare facilities that show exemplary performance
      - To inculcate a culture of ongoing assessment and peer review of performance
      - To create and share sustainable practices related to improved cleanliness
    - Scope
      - Best District Hospital (DH): [1 in Category A, 2 in Category B, 3 in Category C States]
      - Best Two Community Health Centers (CHC)/Sub District Hospitals (SDH)
      - One Primary Health Centre (PHC) in every district
    - Quantum of Award (INR)
      - Award Winners: 50 Lacs (DH), 15 Lacs (CHC), 10 Lacs (SDH), 2 Lacs (PHC)
      - Certificate of Commendation (at least 70% score): 3 Lacs (DH), 1 Lac (CHC/SDH), 0.5 Lacs (PHC)

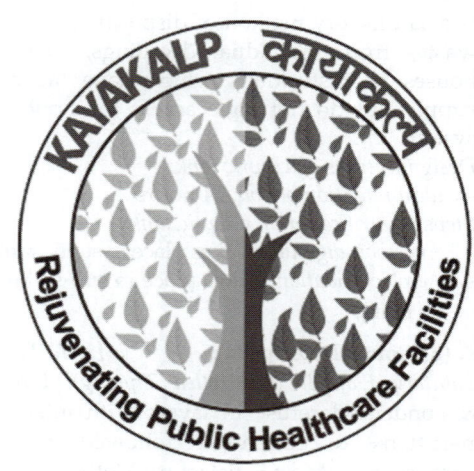

Review Questions

114. Ans. (d) Bed resistance in a slow sand filter [Ref. Park 27/e p839–840]

115. Ans. (d) Air pollution [Ref. Park 27/e p863]

ENTOMOLOGY AND VECTOR CONTROL

116. Ans. (c) A is True BUT R is False [Ref. Park 25/e p843]
   - Malathion is used as ULV during epidemics using aircraft (esp for Aircraft) in dosage 98% pure malathion 1–2 ounces/acre
   - ULV has no diluent (hence its more effective than Thermal fogging)
   - ULV has No residual effect (So multiple applications are required)

117. Ans. (d) Kyasanur forest disease [Ref. Park 27/e p894]

    VECTORS AND DISEASES TRANSMITTED

Vector	Disease (s) transmitted
Housefly (Musca domestica)	Diarrhoeal & dysentrical diseases, Poliomyelitis, Yaws, Anthrax, Trachoma
Sandfly (Phlebotomus argentipes)	Kala azar (Visceral Leishmaniasis), Oriental sore (Cutaneous Leishmaniasis), Sandfly fever, Oroya fever
Tse-Tse fly (Glossina palpalis)	Sleeping sickness of Africa (African Trypanosomiasis)
Reduviid bug (Triatominae)	Chagas Disease (Sleeping sickness of America- American Trypanosomiasis)
Black fly (Simulium)	Onchocerciasis (River Blindness)
Soft tick	Relapsing fever, Q fever, KFD (outside India)
Hard tick	Tularemia, Babesiosis, KFD (India), Tick paralysis, Tick encephalitis, Tick hemorrhagic fever, Indian Tick Typhus, RMSF
Louse	Epidemic typhus, Trench fever, Relapsing fever, Pediculoses
Mite	Scrub typhus, Rickettsial pox
Flea	Plague, Murine typhus

Contd...

Contd...

Vector	Disease (s) transmitted
Anopheles mosquito	Malaria, Filaria (outside India)
Culex mosquito	Bancroftian Filariasis, Japanese Encephalitis, West Nile fever, Viral arthritis
Aedes mosquito	Yellow fever, Dengue, DHF, Chikungunya, Rift Valley fever, Filariasis (Outside India)
Mansonoides mosquito	Malayan (Brugian) filariasis, Chikungunya

ALSO REMEMBER

- *Mites (Chiggers)*: resembles ticks in their general appearance
    - Trombiculid mite (Leptotrombium): transmits Scrub typhus
    - Itch mite (Sarcoptes/Acarus): transmits Scabies
- *Transmission of KFD*:
    - KFD in India is transmitted by: 'Hemophysalis spinigera' (Hard Ticks)
    - KFD outside India is transmitted by: Soft ticks
- *KFD is also known as 'Monkey disease'*
- *Man in KFD*: Incidental, dead-end host (No man-to-man transmission)
- *IP of KFD*: 3–8 days
- *Case fatality rate of KFD*: 5–10%.

118. Ans. (a) Contact poison [Ref. Park 27/e p910]

ALSO REMEMBER

- *Pyrethrum*:
    - Space spray for killing 'adult mosquitoes': Active principal 'pyrethrin'; no residual action–short-lived effect
    - Contact 'nerve' poison
    - Knock-down effect with paralysis
    - *Insecticide of plant origin*: Flowers of Chrysanthemum
    - 5 active principles (all 'nerve poisons'):
        1. Pyrethrin I
        2. Pyrethrin II
        3. Cinerin I
        4. Cinerin II
        5. Jasmoline II
    - *No residual effect*: Short lived effect
    - *Synthetic pyrethroids*: permethrin, allethrin, furethrin, cyclethrin
    - Because of the natural insecticidal properties used as 'companion plants', to repel pest insects from nearby crops.

119. Ans. (d) A-III, B-II, C-IV, D-I [Ref. Park 27/e p909–910]

ALSO REMEMBER

- Experts now recommend an 'integrated approach' for arthropods control
- Best level of prevention of arthropod borne diseases: Primordial prevention (e.g., source reduction)
- Barbados Millions (Lebister reticulates) is a larvivorous fish used for biological control of mosquitoes
- Toxorhynchitis splendens: also known as Predator mosquito are particularly useful biological method for Aedes aegypti
- Mosquito nets are used as personal protection measures:
    - Maximum recommended size of holes in mosquito nets: 0.0475 inch
    - Maximum recommended no. of holes in mosquito nets: 150/sq.inch
- Bacillus thuringiensis H14: Spores and crystalline insecticidal proteins produced by B. thuringiensis are used as specific insecticides. Because of their specificity, these pesticides are regarded as environmentally friendly, with little or no effect on humans, wildlife, pollinators, and most other beneficial insects.

120. Ans. (b) Culex [Ref. Park 27/e p897]

ALSO REMEMBER

- Important culex species in India:

Vector	Disease transmitted
Culex quinquefasciatus (fatigans)	Bancroftian Filariasis
Culex tritaeniorhynchus	Japanese Encephalitis
Culex vishnuii	Japanese Encephalitis
Culex gelidus	Japanese Encephalitis

121. Ans. (b) Malarial parasite in mosquito [Ref. Park 25/e p805]

- *Biological transmission of arthropod-borne diseases*:

Transmission	Definition	Examples
Propagative	Disease agent only multiplies in the body of vector	Plague bacilli in rat fleas Yellow fever virus in Aedes mosquitoes
Cyclo-propagative	Disease agent undergoes cyclical change as well as multiplies in the body of vector	Malarial parasite in anopheline mosquitoes
Cyclo-developmental	Disease agent undergoes only cyclical change in vector	Filarial parasite in culex mosquitoes Guineaworm embryo in cyclops

122. Ans. (d) Agent transmitted from nymph to adult vector: Transovarial transmission [Ref. Park 25/e p817]

- *Trans-stadial transmission*: Agent transmitted from nymph to adult vector
    - Borrelia burgdorferi in ticks

- *Trans-ovarial transmission (vertical transmission):* Female vector passes the infectious agent through her eggs to the next generation
  - Rickettsia rickettsii in ticks.

123. Ans. (b) It is a definitive host in filaria
[Ref. Park 27/e p895–899]
- *In lymphatic and Brugian Filariasis:* Man is the definitive host and mosquito the intermediate host
- *HOST:* A person or other animal, including birds & arthropods, that affords subsistence or lodgement to an infectious agent under natural (as opposed to experimental) conditions
  - Primary (definitive) host: host in which parasite attains maturity or passes its sexual stage
  - Secondary (intermediate) host: host in which parasite is in larval or asexual stage

Disease	Parasite	Host Primary	Host Secondary
Malaria	Plasmodium	Anopheles	Man
Tapeworm	Taenia solium	Man	Pigs
Tapeworm	Taenia saginata	Man	Cattle
Guinea worm	Dracunculus medinensis	Man	Cyclops
Filariasis	Wuchereria bancrofti	Man	Culex
Hydatid Disease	Echinococcus	Dog	Sheep, Cattle, Man
Sleeping sickness	Trypanosomes	Man	Tse tse fly

- *Obligate host:* Only Host for a Parasite. For example, Man in Measles, Man in Typhoid Fever
- *Transport host:* A carrier in which the organism remains alive but does not undergo development
- *Paratenic host:* Is similar to an intermediate host, only that it is not needed for the parasite's development cycle to progress.
  1. The difference between a paratenic and reservoir host is that the latter is a primary host, whereas paratenic hosts serve as "dumps" for non-mature stages of a parasite which they can accumulate in high numbers.
- *Dead-end host:* Is an intermediate host that does generally not allow transmission to the definite host, thereby preventing the parasite from completing its development. For example, humans are dead-end hosts for Echinococcus canine tapeworms.

124. Ans. (b) Scabies [Ref. Park 27/e p907, 908]
- *Diagnosis of scabies:*
  - Itching which worsens at night
  - Follicular lesions at affected site
  - Secondary infection leads to crusted papules and pustules
  - MC sites: Hands & wrists (63%)
  - Other members of the family are affected
  - Confirmation of diagnosis: Search for parasite in skin debris under microscope.

125. Ans. (d) Chagas' disease [Ref. Park 27/e p906]
- *Reduviid bugs (Triatominae):*
  - Also known as 'Cone-nose bugs' or 'Kissing bugs' or 'Assassin bugs'
  - Vectors of Chagas' Disease (American Trypanosomiasis–'Sleeping sickness of America'), caused by Trypanosoma cruzi.

> **ALSO REMEMBER**
> - *Vector for Relapsing fever:* Soft tick
> - *Vector for Lyme's disease:* Hard tick
> - *Vector for Scrub typhus:* Trombiculid mite.

126. Ans. (a) Tick [Ref. Park 27/e p906–907]
- *Hard ticks versus Soft ticks:*

	Hard ticks	Soft ticks
Diseases transmitted	Tick typhus (RMSF) Viral encephalitis Tick fevers Hemorrhagic fevers Tularaemia Tick paralysis Human babesiosis	Q fever (few animal cases) Relapsing fever KFD (outside India) (KFD in India)

- *Mites (Chiggers):* Resembles ticks in their general appearance
  - *Trombiculid mite (Leptotrombium):* transmits Scrub typhus
  - *Itch mite (Sarcoptes/Acarus):* transmits Scabies.

127. Ans. (a) Tiger mosquito [Ref. Park 27/e p897]
- Aedes mosquitoes (Stegomyia) have white stripes on a black body; because of their striped/banded character of legs, they are known as 'Tiger mosquitoes'.

128. Ans. (a) Tularemia [Ref. Foundations of Community Medicine, GM Dhaar & I Robbani, 1/e p235, Park 23/e p780–781, 25/e p818]

> **ALSO REMEMBER**
> - *Q fever is only rickettsial Disease without any vector:* only in few animal cases, soft tick is vector
> - KFD in India is transmitted by 'Hemophysalis spinigera' (Hard Ticks)
> - *Vector of Bancroftian filariasis:* Culex quinquefasciatus (C.fatigans)
> - *Vector of Japanese encephalitis:* Culex tritaeniorhynchus (MC), Culex vishnuii, Culex gelidu

129. Ans. (d) Black fly–Chagas Disease [Ref. Foundations of Community Medicine, GM Dhaar & I Robbani, 1/e p224, Park 27/e p903]

BLACK FLY (SIMULIUM):
- Simulium is vector for Onchocerciasis (River blindness)
- Simulium is also known as 'White socks'

> **ALSO REMEMBER**
> - There are more than 35 species of Black fly in India but none associated with human disease
> - Chagas disease (Sleeping sickness of America) is transmitted by Reduviid bug (Kissing bug).

130. Ans. (a) Environmental control [Ref. Park 27/e p899]

> **ALSO REMEMBER**
> - *Residual sprays for mosquito control:*
>
> | Toxicant | Dosage (gm/m²) | Av. duration of effectiveness (months) |
> |---|---|---|
> | DDT | 1–2 | 6–12 |
> | Lindane | 0.5 | 3 |
> | Malathion | 2 | 3 |

131. Ans. (b) 100 meters [Ref. Park 27/e p895–897]
- Flight range of important mosquito vectors in India:

Mosquito vector	Flight range
Anopheles	3–5 km
Culex	11 km
Aedes	100 m (110 yards)
Mansonia	-

- International measures to restrict spread of Yellow Fever (vector: Aedes aegypti) are specified under International Health Regulations (IHRs):
    – Travellers:
       1. Must possess a valid International certificate of vaccination (validity 10 days–Lifelong) against YF before they enter 'YF receptive areas'
       2. If no such certificate available: Quarantine for 6 days (Max I.P of YF) from date of leaving an infected area
       3. If traveller arrives before certificate becomes valid (10 days after vaccination): Isolate till it becomes valid
    – Mosquitoes:
       1. Aircrafts/ships arriving from endemic areas: Aerosol spray to kill insect vectors
       2. Airports/seaports kept free from vector breeding: at least 400 meters around boundary
       3. Aedes aegypti index: kept below 1
- Simulium (Black fly), vector of Onchocerciasis (River blindness) has a flight range of 100 miles.

132. Ans. (c) 8–34 days [Ref. Park 27/e p895]
- Life span of a mosquito varies from: 8 to 34 days
    – Males, as a rule, are short lived
    – Life of a mosquito is influenced by temperature & humidity
- Egg stage lasts for 1–2 days
- *Gonotrophic cycle:* Period that elapses from the moment a blood meal is taken until the eggs are laid; it is about 48 hrs in hot & humid tropical areas
    – *Larva:* Passes through 4 stages of growth called 'instars', with moulting between each stage
- Larval stage occupies 5–7 days
- Culicine larvae (Culex, Aedes, Mansonia) have a siphon tube
    – *Pupa:* Represents 'resting stage' in life cycle of mosquito
- Pupal stage lasts for 1–2 days
- Have 2 respiratory tubes (trumpets) in thorax
- Does not feed, prefers to stay quiet at the water surface
    – *Adult:* Life cycle from egg to adult is complete in 7–10 days
- Adult mosquito lives for about 2 weeks.

133. Ans. (b) It is more effective against Anopheles
[Ref. Foundations of Community Medicine, GM Dhaar & I Robbani, 1/e p247, Park 27/e p898]

PARIS GREEN (COPPER ACETOARSENITE):
- Emerald green, microcrystalline powder
- Anti-larval measure, kills mainly Anopheles larvae as they are surface feeders
    – Bottom feeding larvae can also be killed, when applied as a special granular formulation
- Paris green is a 'stomach poison'
- Is most widely used larvicide for mosquito control
- *Recommended dose:* 1 kg paris green per hectare water surface
    – In dosage applied, paris green does not harm fish, man or domestic animals

> **ALSO REMEMBER**
> - *Pyrethrum:* Space spray
>   – Anti-adult, nerve poison, kills mainly by 'knock down' effect
>   – *Dosage:* 1oz (0.1% Pyrethrin) per 1000 cu.ft. of space
>   – *Disadvantage:* No residual action; reinfestation occurs within a short time.

134. Ans. (b) Pneumonic plague [Ref. Park 27/e p904–905]

RAT FLEA (XENOPSYLLA):
- *Rat flea acts as a vector for:*
    – Bubonic plague
    – Murine (endemic/flea-borne) typhus
    – Chiggerosis
- *Rat flea acts as a host for:*
    – Hymenolepis diminuta (Rat tapeworm)
    – Hymenolepis nana (Dwarf tapeworm)

> **ALSO REMEMBER**
> - Pneumonic plague is the most virulent and least common form of plague, caused by the Yersinia pestis
>   – Typically, pneumonic form is due to a secondary spread from advanced infection of an initial bubonic form

Contd...

Contd...

- Pneumonic plague is not vector-borne like bubonic plague: results from inhalation of aerosolized droplets and can be transmitted from human to human 'without involvement of fleas or animals'
- Most apparent symptom: coughing, often with hemoptysis
- Human flea (Pulex irritans): can lead to restlessness, and both irritation and scratching of the skin
    - Pulex irritans is also a vector of Yersinia pestis (plague).

135. Ans. (b) 5% Permethrin
[Ref. CMDT 2014, p144, Park 27/e p907–908]

- **Scabies:** Is a transmissible ectoparasite skin infection characterized by superficial burrows, intense pruritus (itching) and secondary infection
    - Scabies is caused by the mite Sarcoptes scabiei, variety hominis (known as 'Itch mite')
    - Scabies is usually transmitted by close contact with an infested person. Scabies is transmitted readily, often throughout an entire household, by skin-to-skin contact with an infected person and thus is sometimes classified as a sexually transmitted disease (STD)
    - Drug of Choice for scabies: 5% Permethrin
    - Other useful treatments:
    - Scabies was the first disease of man with known cause
    - Other treatment modalities for Scabies:
        1. 25% Benzyl benzoate (2 applications)
        2. 1% HCH (Gammaxene; lindane) (2 applications)
        3. 5% Tetmosol solution (3 daily applications)
        4. 10% Sulphur ointment (4 daily applications)
        5. Crotamiton lotion (3 applications)
        6. Malathion (1 application)
        7. Ivermectin (Single dose)—Oral/Systemic Drug of Choice
        8. Neem oil (for persistent cases).

> **ALSO REMEMBER**
> - In scabies, the impregnated female 'tunnels into the stratum corneum of the skin' and deposits eggs in the 'burrows'
> - Scabies is sometimes classified as a sexually transmitted disease (STD): transmitted readily by skin-to-skin contact with an infected person
>   - Scabies transmission cannot be prevented by using condoms.

136. Ans. (d) Oriental sore [Ref. Park 27/e p912–913]
- *Diseases associated with rodents:*

Bacterial	Viral	Rickettsial	Parasitic	Others
Plague Tularaemia Salmonellosis	Lassa fever Hemorrhagic fever Encephalitis	Scrub typhus Murine (Flea-borne) typhus Rickettsial pox	Hymenolepis dimunita Leishmaniasis Amoebiasis Trichinosis Chagas disease	Rat bite fever Leptospirosis Histoplasmosis

> **ALSO REMEMBER**
> - *Rodenticides:* pest control chemicals intended to kill rodents
>   - *Anticoagulants:* 4-hydroxy coumarin
>   - *Phosphides:* Zinc phosphide, aluminium phosphide
>   - *Calciferols:* Vitamin D
>   - *Others:* ANTU (a-naphthylurea), arsenic, barium, thallium, strychnine
> - *Rodenticides dangerous to use:* Arsenic trioxide, Phosphorus, Thallium sulphate, ANTU, Gophacide.

137. Ans. (d) Pyrethrum [Ref. Park 27/e p910]
138. Ans. (d) Japanese encephalitis [Ref. Park 27/e p897]
139. Ans. (a) Yellow fever; (b) Dengue; (d) Filariasis
[Ref. Park 27/e p897]
140. Ans. (a) Epidemic typhus; (c) Trench fever
[Ref. Park 27/e p903]
141. Ans. (c) Yellow fever; (d) Filaria; (e) Dengue
[Ref. Park 27/e p898]
142. Ans. (b) Typhus; (c) Dengue; (d) J.E. [Ref. Park 27/e p898]
143. Ans. (b) Q fever [Ref. Park 27/e p894]
144. Ans. (b) Eggs can't survive >1 wk without water
[Ref. Park 27/e p895–897]
- Egg stage of mosquito life cycle lasts for 1–2 days only, so there is no question of survival more than 1 week
- Aedes mosquitoes are recurrent, fearless biters, chiefly bite during day
- *Aedes mosquitoes transmits*:
    - Dengue
    - Yellow fever
    - Chikungunya fever
- It takes 7–8 days to develop the parasite & transmit the disease (extrinsic incubation period)

145. Ans. (a) Relapsing fever [Ref. Park 27/e p906–907]
146. Ans. (b) Phlebotomus [Ref. Park 27/e p909–910]
DDT (Dichloro-diphenyl-trichloro ethane) Organochlorine
- Synthesised by Zeidler (1874); Insecticidal properties discovered by Noble prize winner Paul Miller (1939)
- *Technical DDT:* 70–80% para-para isomer (most active form)
- *Mechanism of action:* Contact (Nerve) poison (hours to kill) (Acetylcholinesterase inhibitor)
- DDT has 'No repellent action' but 'residual action for 18 months'
- *Dosage:* 100–200 mg per sq.ft.
- Sandflies (Phlebotomus) have not demonstrated resistance to DDT

147. **Ans. (a) Use of alkaline soap water in factory**
[Ref. Internet, Wikipedia]
Alkaline soap water is not used in factories for mosquito control.

148. **Ans. (c) Malathion** *[Ref. Park 27/e p910]*
MALATHION
Is 'least toxic among Organophosphate compounds'
- Because of its low toxicity, it is recommended as 'an alternative to DDT'
- *Dosage:* 100–200 mg per sq. ft. every 3 months
- *ULV spray:* Used to kill adult mosquitoes
- *Mechanism of action:* Interfere with transmission of nerve impulses
- Act by 'inhibiting Acetyl-cholinesterase'

149. **Ans. (c) Immediately kills the prey** *[Ref. Park 27/e p909–910]*

150. **Ans. (a) DDT** *[Ref. Park 27/e p909]*

151. **Ans. (e) Rifampicin** *[Ref. Park 27/e p907–908]*

152. **Ans. (d) Chikungunya Fever** *[Ref. Park 27/e p897]*
- Mansonia can transmit Malayan (Brugian) filariasis, Chikungunya fever

153. **Ans. (b) Siphon tube** *[Ref. Park 27/e p897]*

154. **Ans. (d) 1, 3 and 5** *[Ref. Park 27/e p896]*

155. **(c) Visceral leishmaniasis** *[Ref. Park 27/e p901–902]*
SANDFLY (PHLEBOTOMUS):
- Legs twice as long as body
- Lanceolate (Flame shaped) wings
- Fine hairs on margins of wings

156. **Ans. (d) Nymphal stage has seven instars**
[Ref. Park 27/e p906–907]
HARD TICK Vs SOFT TICK

	Hard tick	Soft tick
	Ixodidae	Argasidae
Scutum	Present	Absent
Head	Situated anteriorly	Lies ventrally
Spiracles	Behind IV coxa	Between III and IV coxa
Eggs	Hundreds-Thousands (1 sitting)	Batches of 100–200 (Long period)
Nymphal stages	One	Five
Habits	Cannot stand starvation	Can stand starvation for 1 year
Diseases transmitted	Tick typhus, Viral encephalitis, Hemorrhagic fever, Tularaemia, Tick paralysis, Babesiosis, KFD in India	Relapsing fever, KFD outside India, Q fever (Animals)

157. **Ans. (d) Aedes has striped yellow scales**
[Ref. Tropical Biology and Conservation Management by Claro 1/e p290]
- Species of Aedes have scales of different colors forming peculiar stripes and spots on their bodies

158. **Ans. (a) Malathion** *[Ref. FMT by Karmakar 5/e p520]*
ORGANOPHOSPHATES
- Alkylphosphates: Malathion, HETP, TEPP, OMPA, Dimefox, Trichlorfon
- Arylphosphates: Parathion, Chlorthion, Diazinon, Paraoxon.

159. **Ans. (c) Siphon tube present** *[Ref. Park 27/e p897]*
- Culex, Aedes larvae: Rest at an angle to water surface, Palmate hair absent, Siphon tube present.

160. **Ans. (a) Propoxur** *[Ref. Park 27/e p910]*
- Synthetic pyrethroids: Permethrin, Cypermethrin, Etofenprox, Allethrin, Cyfluthrin, Resmethrin, Bioresmethrin, Pothrin
- Propoxur is a Carbamate.

161. **Ans. (c) Best pattern in circular** *[Ref. Park 27/e p899]*
MOSQUITO NETS
- Material: White
- Best pattern: Rectangular net
- Hole/rent: Not even a single one should be present
- Size of each hole: <0.0475 inch diameter
- Number of holes/sq. inch: 150

162. **Ans. (b) Culex mosquito**
[Ref. Arbovirus Infections, 2012/e p36]
- Western equine encephalomyelitis virus (WEE virus) is an arbovirus transmitted by mosquitoes of the genera Culex and Culiseta.

Review Questions

163. **Ans. (b) Larvicide** *[Ref: Park 27/e p898]*
164. **Ans. (b) Anopheles stephensi** *[Ref: Park 27/e p896]*
165. **Ans. (a) Malathion** *[Ref. Park 27/e p910]*
166. **Ans. (b) Sleeping sickness is caused by tsetse flies**
[Ref. Park 27/e p902]
167. **Ans. (c) Contact poisons** *[Ref. Park 27/e p909]*
168. **Ans. (a) Pyrethrum** *[Ref. Park 27/e p910]*
169. **Ans. (d) It has repellent action on insects**
[Ref. Park 27/e p909–910]
170. **Ans. (d) Japanese encephalitis** *[Ref. Park 27/e p894]*
171. **Ans. (c) Ticks** *[Ref. Park 27/e p906–907]*
172. **Ans. (b) Causes ulcers in foot** *[Ref. Park 27/e p901–902]*
173. **Ans (a) Pyrethrum** *[Ref. Park 27/e p910]*
174. **Ans. (b) Babesiosis** *[Ref. Harrison's 17/e p1294, Park 27/e p894]*
175. **Ans. (a) KFD** *[Ref. Park 27/e p894]*
176. **Ans. (b) Pyrethrum** *[Ref. Park 27/e p910]*
177. **Ans. (b) JE** *[Ref. Park 27/e p909]*

178. Ans. (b) Anopheles [Ref. Park 27/e p894–896]
179. Ans. (a) Organophosphorous compound [Ref. KDT 5/e p90]
180. Ans. (a) Culex [Ref. Park 27/e p897]
181. Ans. (c) Mansonia [Ref. Park 27/e p897]
182. Ans. (a) Residual action is similar to DDT [Ref. Park 27/e p910]
183. Ans. (a) Red [Ref. Insecticides Rules 1971, Central Insecticides Board, India]
    Toxicity Colour Labels of Pesticides in India
    - *Red label*: Extremely toxic
        - Zinc phosphide
    - *Yellow label*: Highly toxic
        - Endosulphan
    - *Blue label*: Moderately toxic
        - Malathion
    - *Green label*: Slightly toxic
        - Mosquito repellants
184. Ans. (a) Trench fever; (d) Epidemic typhus; (e) Pediculosis [Ref. Park 27/e p903, 904]
185. Ans. (a) Malaria [Ref. Park 27/e p896]
186. Ans. (b) Propogative cycle [Ref. Park 27/e p895]
187. Ans. (b) DDT [Ref. Park 27/e p909–910]
188. Ans. (a) Ticks [MOST COMMON: Inhalation] [Ref. Park 27/e p906–907]
189. Ans. (b) Anopheles stephensi [Ref. Park 27/e p896]
190. Ans. (b) Oriental sore [Ref. Park 27/e p906–907]
191. Ans. (a) 400 m [Ref. Park 27/e p897]
192. Ans. (a) Rickettsial disease [Ref. Rickettsiology and Rickettsial Diseases, 5th International Conference, p146]
193. Ans. (b) Filaria [Ref. Park 27/e p894]
194. Ans. (b) Residual spray [Ref. Park 27/e p899]
195. Ans. (a) Eliminate breeding places [Ref. Park 27/e p900]
196. Ans. (d) Pupa don't have siphon tube [Ref. Park 27/e p897]
197. Ans. (c) Kyasanur forest disease [Ref. Park 27/e p906–907]
198. Ans. (c) Lyme's disease [Ref. Park 27/e p906–907]
199. Ans. (a) Yellow fever; (b) Dengue; (c) Chikungunya fever; (e) Rift valley fever [Ref. Park 27/e p898]
200. Ans. (a) Epidemic typhus; (c) Relapsing fever; (d) Trench fever [Ref. Park 27/e p894]
201. Ans. (c); (e) No siphon tube in larvae [Ref. Park 27/e p897]
202. Ans. (a) Malaria [Ref. Park 27/e p896]

CHAPTER 12: Biomedical Waste Management, Disaster Management, Occupational Health, Genetics and Health, Mental Health

BMW MANAGEMENT

Hospital Waste Composition^Q

- Paper: 15%
- Plastic: 10%
- Rags: 15%
- Metals (Sharps, etc): 1.0%
- Infectious waste: 1.5%
- Glass: 4.0%
- General waste (food waste, sweeping of premises)^Q: 53.5%

Biomedical Waste (BMW) Management in India

- Biomedical Wastes (BMW) in India are handled and managed under *'Biomedical Waste Management (Management and Handling) Rules, 1998'*^Q
    - Exercising powers: *Sections 6, 8, 25 of 'Environmental (Protection) Act, 1986'* (under the Ministry of Environment and Forests)
- *Schedules under Biomedical Waste Management (Management and Handling) Rules, 1998*:
    - Schedule I^Q: *Categories of BMW, treatment and disposal*
    - Schedule II^Q: *Color coding and type of container for BMW disposal*
    - Schedule III^Q: *Labels for BMW containers/bags*
    - Schedule IV: *Label for transport of BMW containers/bags*
    - Schedule V: *Standards for treatment and disposal of BMW*

> **Key points**
> Exercising powers: Sections 6, 8, 25 of 'Environmental (Protection) Act, 1986'.

Types of Biomedical Wastes

Type of Waste	Inclusion(s)
Human Anatomical Waste	Human tissues, organs, body parts and fetus below the viability period (as per The MTP Act 1971)^Q
Animal Anatomical Waste	Experimental animal carcasses, body parts, organs, tissues, including the waste generated from animals used in experiments or testing in veterinary hospitals or colleges or animal houses
Soiled Waste	Items contaminated with blood, body fluids like dressings, plaster casts, cotton swabs and bags containing residual or discarded blood and blood components^Q
Expired or Discarded Medicines	Pharmaceutical waste like antibiotics, cytotoxic drugs including all items contaminated with cytotoxic drugs^Q along with glass or plastic ampoules, vials etc.
Chemical Waste	Chemicals used in production of biological and used or discarded disinfectants

Contd...

Contd...

Type of Waste	Inclusion(s)
Chemical Liquid Waste	Liquid waste generated due to use of chemicals in production of biological and used or discarded disinfectants, Silver X-ray film developing liquid[Q], discarded Formalin, infected secretions, aspirated body fluids, liquid from laboratories and floor washings, cleaning, house-keeping and disinfecting activities[Q]
Discarded linen, mattresses, beddings	Discarded linen, mattresses, beddings contaminated with blood/body fluid[Q]
Microbiology, Biotechnology and other clinical laboratory waste	Blood bags[Q], Laboratory cultures, stocks or specimens of microorganisms, live or attenuated vaccines[Q], human and animal cell cultures used in research, industrial laboratories, production of biological, residual toxins, dishes and devices used for cultures
Waste sharps including Metals	Needles[Q], syringes with fixed needles, needles from needle tip cutter or burner, scalpels, blades, or any other contaminated sharp object that may cause puncture and cuts; this includes both used, discarded and contaminated metal sharps
Glassware	Broken or discarded and contaminated glass including medicine vials and ampoules (Except those contaminated with cytotoxic wastes)
Metallic Body Implants	

NEW Biomedical Waste Management Guidelines 2016[Q]

- *Ministry:* Ministry of Environment and Forests
- *Legislation:* Sections 6, 8 and 25 of Environment (Protection) Act, 1986
- These rules shall not apply to Radioactive wastes, Hazardous chemicals, Municipal solid wastes, Lead acid batteries, Hazardous wastes, e-Waste, Hazardous microorganisms, Genetically engineered microorganisms.

Category	Type of Waste [Older Cat no.]	Bag/Container	Treatment and Disposal options
YELLOW	(a) Human Anatomical Waste [1] (b) Animal Anatomical Waste [2]	Yellow non-chlorinated plastic bags	Incineration/Plasma pyrolysis/Deep burial
	(c) Soiled Waste [6]		Incineration/Plasma pyrolysis/Deep burial OR Autoclaving/Microwaving/Hydroclaving THEN Shredding/Mutilation
	(d) Expired/Discarded Medicines [5] (e) Chemical Waste [10]	Yellow non-chlorinated plastic bags or containers	Incineration/Encapsulation/Plasma pyrolysis
	(f) Chemical Liquid Waste [8]	Separate collection system leading to effluent treatment system	Pretreatment THEN Drain
	(g) Discarded linen, mattresses, beddings contaminated with blood or body fluid	Non-chlorinated yellow plastic bags or suitable packing material	Non-chlorinated chemical disinfection THEN Incineration/Plasma pyrolysis/Energy recovery OR Shredding/Mutilation
	(h) Microbiology, Biotechnology, Clinical laboratory waste [3]	Autoclave safe plastic bags or containers	Pre-treat with Non-chlorinated chemicals THEN Incineration
Red	Contaminated Waste (Recyclable) [7]	Red non-chlorinated plastic bags or containers	Autoclaving/Microwaving/Hydroclaving THEN Shredding/Mutilation THEN Energy recovery/Plastics to diesel or fuel oil/Road making

Contd...

Contd...

Category	Type of Waste [Older Cat no.]	Bag/Container	Treatment and Disposal options
White (Translucent)	Waste sharps including Metals [4]	Puncture proof, Leak proof, Tamper proof containers	Autoclaving/Dry heat THEN Shredding/Mutilation/Encapsulation THEN Iron foundries/Sanitary landfill/Waste sharp pit
Blue	(a) Glassware [4] (b) Metallic Body Implants	Cardboard boxes with blue colored marking	Sodium hypochlorite/Autoclaving/Microwaving/Hydroclaving THEN Recycling

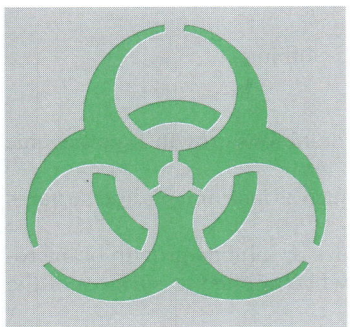

Biohazard symbol

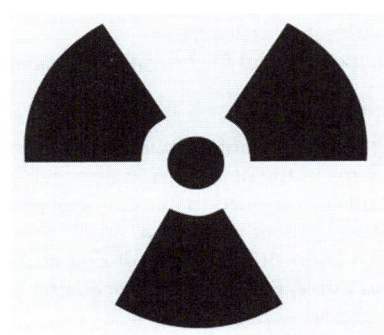

Radiation hazard symbol

Recycling symbol

(Dear Students, although Older Category Numbers 1–10 are NOT USED in Newer classification, I have given them in [ ] so as to help you memorize better).

Inertization

- *Process:* Mixing biomedical waste with cement and other substance before disposal, so as to minimize risk of toxic substances contained in waste to contaminate ground/surface water^Q.
  - Inertization is especially suitable for pharmaceuticals and for incineration ashes with high metal content
- *A typical composition of mixture is*:
  - 65% pharmaceutical waste
  - 15% lime^Q
  - 15% cement^Q
  - 5% water

BMW Management Treatment Modalities

1. Mechanical Processes

- *Compacting:* Reducing size and volume of waste (Useful for general non-hazardous wastes)
- *Shredding:* Breaking the material into smaller pieces by grinding/cutting/granulation (Useful for plastics, rubber and soft metals)
- *Landfill:* Oldest method of waste disposal^Q
  - *Two types:* Open dump or Sanitary landfill
- *Encapsulation*: Filling containers with waste, adding an immobilizing material (plastic foam/bituminous sand/cement mortar/clay material) and sealing containers.
- *Inertization*: Mixing biomedical waste with cement and other substance before disposal.
  - Useful for pharmaceuticals and for incineration ashes with high metal content.

2. Thermal Processes

- *Heat disinfection*: Boiling for 20 minutes^Q
  - Useful for pre-treatment of sharps and plastics waste

> **Key points**
>
> **Hot air oven**: Causes sterilization and mutilation at 160°C^Q

> **Key points**
>
> **Autoclave:** Waste is subjected to 121°C (15 psi) or 135°C (30 psi).

- *Hot air oven*: Causes sterilization and mutilation at 160°C^Q
  - Used for glassware, powders and oils impermeable to steam
- *Autoclave*: Steam-sterilization under pressure is a low-heat thermal process^Q
  - Waste is subjected to 121°C (15 psi) 45 min (vaccum flow AC) – 60 minutes (gravity flow AC)
- *Hydroclave*: Steam-sterilization under pressure causes fragmentation of wastes^Q
  - Waste is subjected to 121°C or 132°C^Q
- *Microwave*: Volumetric heating for microbial hazardous wastes using frequency of 2450 MHz and wavelength 12.24 nm^Q
  - Waste destruction occurs by 'heat conduction'^{Q}
- *Incineration*: High temperature dry oxidation process which reduces waste volume and weight
  - Waste is subjected to 800°C and 1050 ± 50°C^Q
- *Plasma arc*: Ionized gas (electrical discharges) at high temperature causes gasification and molecular dissociation of organic wastes
  - Waste is subjected to 2000°C^Q
- *Gamma irradiation*: Useful for re-usable medical equipments and clothing.

3. Chemical Processes

- *Disinfectants*: A disinfectant is a chemical agent, which destroys or inhibits growth of pathogenic micro-organisms in the non-sporing or vegetative state
  - Disinfectants are applied to inanimate objects and materials such as instruments and surfaces to control and prevent infection.
- *Antiseptics*: An antiseptic is a type of disinfectant, which destroys or inhibits growth of micro-organisms on living tissues without causing injurious effects when applied to surfaces of the body or to exposed tissues^Q.

4. Biological Processes

- *Composting*: Land and cow dung (*gobar*) are used^Q
- *Vermi-composting*: Earth worms (*Eisenia foetida*^{Q}), land, matured cow dung (*khad*) and coconut husk are used
  - Not useful for non-biodegradable wastes
- *Bio-digestion*: Biodegradable kitchen waste or left over food of a hospital is used, which leads to production of manure and methane
  - Useful for rural healthcare institutions.

Incineration

> **Key points**
>
> **Incineration:** Is a 'high temperature dry oxidation' process

- *Incineration*: Is a 'high temperature dry oxidation' process^Q; It leads to significant reduction in waste-volume and weight (up to 70–80%)
  - Incineration does not require pre-treatment^Q
  - Biggest disadvantage of incineration: Generation of smoke^Q
- *Types of Incinerators*:
  - Double-chamber pyrolytic
  - Single-chamber pyrolytic
  - Rotary kilns
- *Temperature in an incinerator*: **(Now >1200°C recommended)**
  - *Primary chamber*: 800° ± 50°C^Q
  - *Secondary chamber*: 1050° ± 50°C^Q
- *Characteristics of wastes suitable for incineration*^{Q}:
  - Low heating volume
  - Combustible matter >60%
  - Non-combustible solids <5%
  - Non-combustible fines <20%
  - Moisture content <30%
- *Wastes types not-to-be incinerated*^{Q}:
  - Pressurized gas containers
  - Reactive chemical wastes (large)
  - Silver/Radiographic/photographic wastes
  - Halogenated plastics (PVC)
  - Wastes with high mercury/cadmium content
  - Sealed ampoules ampoules with heavy metals.
  - Sharps

> **Key points**
>
> **Wastes types not-to-be incinerated**^{Q}:
> - Pressurized gas containers
> - Reactive chemical wastes
> - Silver/Radiographic/photographic wastes
> - Halogenated plastics (PVC)
> - Wastes with high mercury/cadmium content
> - Sealed ampoules ampoules with heavy metals.

Mercury Disposal
- Dispose mercury as a hazardous waste
- 'Never combine it with organic or inorganic waste
- Never dispose it in sink/drain
- Dispose off in 'Recycling units'[Q]

NEW Standards for BMW Treatment in India[Q]
- **Standards for Incineration**
  - Combustion efficiency (CE) ≥ 99.00%.
  - Temperature: >800°C (Primary chamber); ≥1050 ± 50°C (Secondary chamber)
  - Secondary chamber gas residence time: ≥2 seconds
  - Minimum stack height: ≥30 meters above the ground
- **Standards for Plasma Pyrolysis**
  - Combustion efficiency (CE) ≥99.00%.
  - Temperature: >1050 + 50°C (Combustion chamber)
  - Secondary chamber gas residence time: ≥2 seconds (Stack gas ≥3% Oxygen)
  - Minimum stack height: ≥30 meters above the ground
- **Standards for Autoclaving of Bio-Medical Waste**

Gravity Flow Autoclave	Vacuum Autoclave
≥121°C, 15 psi pressure, >60 minutes	≥121°C, 15 psi pressure, >45 minutes
≥135°C, 31 psi pressure, >45 minutes	≥135°C, 31 psi pressure, >30 minutes
≥149°C, 52 psi pressure, >30 minutes	

  - Biological indicator: Geobacillus stearothermophilus (GBS) spores using vials or spore Strips; with at least 1×10^6 spores
- **Standards for Microwaving**
  - Not be used for: Cytotoxic/Hazardous/Radioactive wastes/Contaminated animal carcasses/Body parts/Large metal items
  - Biological indicators: Bacillus atrophaeus spores using vials/Spore strips ($\geq 1 \times 10^4$ spores per detachable strip)
- **Standards for Deep Burial**
  - Pit/Trench >2 meters deep, half filled with waste, then covered with lime within 50 cm of the surface, before filling the rest of the pit with soil
  - When wastes are added to the pit, a layer of 10 cm of soil shall be added to cover the wastes
- **Standards for Efficacy of Chemical Disinfection**
  - ≥ 4 Log10 reduction or greater for Bacillus Subtilis
- **Standards for Dry Heat Sterilization**
  - Waste sharps ≥185°C, ≥150 minutes (each cycle), 90 minutes sterilization period
  - Validation test for Shaprs sterilization unit: Geobacillus Stearothermophillus or Bacillus Atropheaus spores (>$log10^6$ spores per mL)

COVID-19 BMW Management Guidelines: 5th Revision (CPCB 2022–23)
- **Isolation Wards**
  - Double layered bags for collection, storage & handling
  - Bags should be labelled as "COVID-19" waste
  - Wet & dry wastes should be collected in leak proof bags and must be sprayed with sodium hypochlorite spray
  - Yellow bags should not be used for collection of general waste, compostable bags should be used for wet waste
  - Inner as well as outer surface of Bins/Bags/Containers/Trolleys must be sprayed with 1% Hypochlorite spray

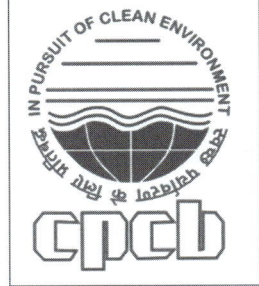

Red Bag	Yellow Bag
Goggles	Masks (N95, Triple layered)
Face shield	Head cover (Cap)
S-P Apron	Shoe cover
Plastic cover all	Disposable linen gown
Hazmat suite	Non plastic cover all
PPE suit	Semi-plastic Cover all
Nitrile Gloves	Used masks/tissue/toiletries of patients

(Table © Dr Vivek Jain 2022–23)

DISASTER MANAGEMENT

Disaster

> **Key points**
>
> **Most commonly reported disease in post-disaster phase** is Gastroenteritis

- *Disaster (WHO):* Is any occurrence that causes damage, ecological disruption, loss of human life or deterioration of health and health services on a scale sufficient to warrant an extraordinary response from outside the affected community or area^Q.
- *Disaster (Colin Grant):* Is catastrophe causing 'injury or illness simultaneously to at least 30 people', who will require hospital emergency treatment^Q.
    - *Most commonly reported disease* in post-disaster phase is Gastroenteritis^Q
    - *Most practical and effective strategy of disease prevention and control* in post-disaster phase is 'supplying safe drinking water and proper disposal of excreta'^{Q}
    - *Foremost step for disease prevention and control* in post-disaster phase is chlorination of all water bodies^Q
    - *Level of residual chlorine to be maintained in all water bodies* in post-disaster phase is >0.7 mg/l (>0.7 ppm) ^{Q}
    - *A common micronutrient deficiency in disasters is Vitamin A deficiency*^{Q}: It occurs due to deficient relief diets, measles and diarrhea (gastroenteritis)
    - Other common deficiencies include scurvy (Vitamin C), anemia (iron) and pellagra (Vitamin B3 –niacin).

> **Key points**
>
> **Foremost step** for disease prevention and control in post-disaster phase is chlorination.

Stages of a Disaster Cycle^Q

- *Disaster impact and response:*
    - Search, rescue and first aid
    - Field care
    - Triage
    - Tagging
    - Identification of dead
- *Stage of health and medical relief:* Disaster containment
    - *Primary phase (0–6 hours):* First aid, medical care
    - *Secondary follow-up (6–24 hours):* Transportation, sanitation and immunization
    - *Tertiary clean up (1–60 days):* Food, clothing, shelter assistance, social service, employment, rehabilitation
- *Rehabilitation:*
    - Water supply
    - Sanitation and personal hygiene
    - Food safety
    - Vector control
- *Mitigation*^{Q}: Measures designed to either prevent hazards from causing emergency or to lessen the effects of emergency
- *Disaster preparedness.*

Triage

> **Key points**
>
> **Triage**^{Q}: Consists of rapidly classifying the injured 'on the basis of LIKELIHOOD OF THEIR SURVIVAL'.

- *Triage*^{Q}: Consists of rapidly classifying the injured NOT *'on the basis of severity of their injuries but on their likelihood of their survival'* with prompt medical intervention^Q
    - First come first serve is NOT followed in emergencies^Q
    - Triage yields best results when carried out at the site of disaster^Q
- *Triage sieve:* Quick survey to separate the dead and the walking from the injured
- *Triage sort:* Remaining casualties are assessed and allocated to categories
- *Triage system:* Most commonly uses FOUR color code system:^{Q}
    - Red (Highest Priority): Immediate resuscitation or limb/life saving surgery in next 6 hours
    - Yellow (High Priority): Possible resuscitation or limb/life saving surgery in next 24 hours (sometimes blue color is used)
    - Green (Low Priority): Minor illness/AMBULATORY patients
    - Black (Least Priority): Dead and moribund patients
- *Tagging:* Is the procedure where identification, age, place of origin, triage category, diagnosis and initial treatment are tagged on to every victim of disaster through a Colour Coding^Q.

Types of Triage

- *Triage is of two types:*
  - *Simple triage*: Simple triage is used in a scene of mass casualty, in order to sort patients into those who need critical attention and immediate transport to the hospital and those with less serious injuries
    - This step is required before transportation becomes available
    - The categorization of patients based on the severity of their injuries can be aided with the use of printed triage tags or colored flagging
  - *Rapid triage*: S.T.A.R.T. (*Simple Triage and Rapid Treatment*[Q]) is a simple triage system that can be performed by lightly-trained lay and emergency personnel in emergencies
    - It is not intended to supersede or instruct medical personnel or techniques
    - It may serve as an instructive example
    - It has been field-proven in mass casualty incidents such as train wrecks and bus accidents
- *Reverse Triage*: In addition to the standard practices of triage as mentioned above, there are conditions where sometimes the less wounded are treated in preference to the more severely wounded. This may arise in,
  - A situation such as war where the military setting may require soldiers be returned to combat as quickly as possible
  - Disaster situations where medical resources are limited in order to conserve resources for those likely to survive but requiring advanced medical care.

> **Key points**
> Black (Least Priority): Dead and moribund patients in Triage

National Institute for Disaster Management (NIDM)

- *Established:* 1995 (under Indian institute of Public Administration)
- *Ministry In-charge:* Ministry of Home Affairs[Q]
- *Head:* Union Home Minister
- *Purpose:*
  - To work as a think tank for Government by providing assistance in policy formulation
  - To facilitate in reducing the impact of disasters

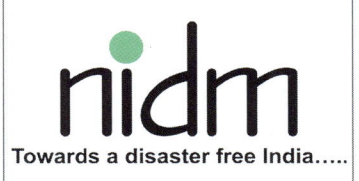

National Disaster Response Force and Civil Defence (NDRF)

- *Established:* 2006
- *Composition:* 10 battalions from CRPF, BSF, ITBP, CISF
- *Purpose:*
  - *Civil defence:* To safeguard the life and property of the civilian population and also to maintain the continuity of productive and economic activity of the nation during war time crisis
  - *Home guards:* To assist the police in controlling civil disturbance and communal riots (maintenance of internal security)
  - *Fire cell:* To organize Fire prevention and Fire fighting services, and to render technical advice on Fire Protection, Fire Prevention and Fire Legislation

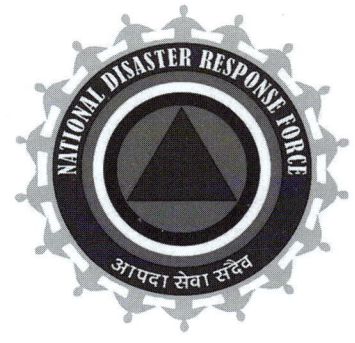

112 - Emergency Response Support System (ERSS), 2019

- Description: Pan-India single number (112) based emergency response system for citizens in emergencies (Voice call, Email, Panic buttons activated calls, 112 India mobile App)
- Utility to the citizens: Emergency assistance from Police, Fire, Health, Disaster management departments or from any other services
- Scope of coverage: Currently rolled out in 18 States/UTs - Andhra Pradesh, Uttarakhand, Punjab, Kerala, Madhya Pradesh, Rajasthan, UP, Telangana, Tamil Nadu, Gujarat, Puducherry, Lakshadweep, Andaman, Dadra & Nagar Haveli, Daman & Diu, J&K, Himachal Pradesh and Nagaland.

OCCUPATIONAL HEALTH

Physical Hazards and Diseases[Q]

- High Temperature
  - Heat cramps
  - Heat hyperpyrexia (body temperature <102°F)

- Heat exhaustion (body temperature >106°F)
- Heat stroke (body temperature up to 110°F)
- Low Temperature
  - Chilblains
  - Trench Foot
  - Frost bite
- Low Pressure
  - Caisson Disease
- Vibration
  - Vibration sickness
  - Neurogenic damage
- Non-ionizing Radiation
- Microwave Injuries
- Laser injuries

Pneumoconioses

> **Key points**
>
> 0.5 to 3.0 microns are the **most dangerous particle size for Pneumoconioses**

- *Pneumoconiosis occur due to:* occupational exposure to dust[Q]
- *Particles size:* 0.5 to 3.0 microns are the most dangerous (as a health hazard causing pneumoconiosis), as they reach the interior of lungs with ease[Q]
- *Particle size and behavior:*

Particle size	Behavior
>10 microns	Settle down by gravity
<10 microns	Remain suspended in air
5–10 microns	Arrested in upper respiratory tract
3–5 microns	Deposited in mid respiratory tract
1–3 microns	Enter alveoli and settle there[Q]
<1 microns	Brownian movement

- *List of Pneumoconioses:*

Disease	Exposure source[Q]
Silicosis	Silica dust
Anthracosis[Q]	Coal dust
Asbestosis	Asbestos dust
Byssinosis[Q]	Cotton fibre
Bagassosis[Q]	Molasses (sugarcane)
Berylliosis	Beryllium
Farmer's Lung[Q]	Mouldy hay
Siderosis	Iron dust
Stannosis	Tin dust
Bird fancier's lung[Q]	Avian/bird droppings
Compost lung	Compost

- *Antigens involved in Pneumoconioses:*

Disease	Antigen[Q]
Bagassosis	Thermoactinomyces sacchari
Farmer's Lung	Micropolyspora faeni
Compost lung	Aspergillus
Chemical workers lung	Isocyanates

Asbestosis

- *Asbestosis is a pneumoconiosis which occurs due to:* Exposure to asbestos
- Asbestosis does not usually appear until after 5–10 years of exposure[Q]
- Sputum shows *'asbestos bodies'*, which are asbestos fibres coated with fibrin
- Asbestos may lead to pulmonary fibrosis, carcinoma of bronchus, mesothelioma of peritoneum/pleura and cancer of GIT[Q]
- Asbestos type most dangerous is *'amphibole'*[Q]

Bagassosis

- *Bagassosis occurs due to:* Occupational exposure to fibrous residue of sugarcane *(bagasse)*; Bagassosis has been shown to be due to *Thermoactinomyces sacchari*^{Q}
  - Bagassosis is a form of extrinsic allergic alveolitis
- *Pathogenesis:*
  - Bagasse contains a percentage of silica, innumerable fungal spores and micro-organisms
  - Bagasse dust blocks bronchioles thus leading to bronchitis and bronchopneumonia
- *Prevention and Bagasse control measures*^{Q}:
  - Keeping moisture content >20%
  - Spraying bagasse with 2% propionic acid (fungicide)
- *Organisms involved in causation of bagassosis:*^{Q}
  - Thermoactinomyces sacchari
  - Thermoactinomyces vulgaris
  - Micropolyspora faeni

Lead Poisoning

- Lead Poisoning is known as *'Plumbism'*, Saturnism or Painter's Colic^Q
- *Greatest source of lead* in Lead Poisoning (*Plumbism*, Saturnism or Painter's Colic) is Gasoline/petrol/vehicular exhaust/automobile exhaust^Q
- *Mode of absorption*: Lead can be absorbed by inhalation (most common mode^Q), ingestion or through skin^Q
- *Clinical picture of lead poisoning*^{Q}:
  - Facial pallor: *Earliest and most consistent sign*^{Q}
  - Anemia: Microcytic hypochromic^Q
  - Punctate basophilia or basophilic stippling of RBCs
  - *Burtonian Line*^{Q}: Lead sulphide line on gums (upper jaw)
  - *Lead colic*: Constipation (but sometimes diarrhea)
  - *Lead Palsy (Peripheral neuropathy)*: Wrist drop or Foot drop^Q
  - *Lead encephalopathy*
  - CNS effects: mostly due to organic lead compounds^Q
- *Diagnosis of lead poisoning*^{Q}:

Laboratory parameter	Remark^Q
Coproporphyrin in Urine (CPU) >150 mcg/l	Exposure to lead
Amino levulinic acid in urine (ALAU) >5 mg/l	Indicates lead absorption
Lead in blood >70 mcg/100 mL	Clinical symptoms appear
Lead in urine >0.8 mg/l	Lead exposure and absorption
Basophilic stippling of RBCs	Punctate basophilia

  - A useful screening test is Coproporphyrin in Urine (CPU).
- *Treatment*: EDTA.

Occupational Dermatitis

- *Causes of occupational dermatitis:*^{Q}

Causes	Agents
Physical	Heat, cold, moisture, pressure, friction, X-rays, other rays
Chemical	Acids, alkalis, dyes, slovents, grease, tar, pitch, chlorinated phenols
Biological	Viruses, bacteria, fungi, parasites
Plant products	Leaves, vegetables, fruits, flowers, vegetable dust
Primary iritants	Acids, alkalis, dyes, solvents
Sensitizers	Sensitization of skin

- *Prevention of occupational dermatitis*: **[Mnemonic: P4]**
  - **Pre-selection**: Similar to pre-placement examination
  - **Protection**: Protective clothing, barrier creams
  - **Personal hygiene**: Washing facilities, water, soap, towel
  - **Periodic inspection**: Post-placement examination

Key points

Greatest source of lead: Gasoline/petrol.

Key points

Burtonian Line^Q: Lead sulphide line on gums (upper jaw).

Occupational Carcinomas

- *Most common*: Nearly 75% of occupational cancers are skin cancers^Q
  - *Type*: Predominantly '*squamous cell carcinomas*'^{Q}
  - *Characteristic feature*: Occurrence on exposed parts of the body (head, neck, hands, arms) that have remained in direct contact with a carcinogenic source
  - *Carcinogens implicated*: UV light, ionizing radiation, coal products, petroleum products, lubricating oils, fuel oils, etc.
- *Occupational cancers affect*: Skin, lungs, bladder and blood forming organs
- *Occupational exposures and cancers*:

> **Key points**
> Nearly 75% of occupational cancers are skin cancers

Agent	Cancer(s) caused^Q
Asbestos^Q	Mesothelioma
Arsenic^Q	Skin. Lung, Liver
Benzene^Q	Leukemia
Benzidine^Q	Urinary bladder
Beryllium	Lung
Cadmium	Lung
Chromium^Q	Nasal sinus, Lung
Ethylene oxide	Leukemia
Ionizing radiation	Skin, Thyroid, Lung
Nickel^Q	Nasal sinus, Lung
Polycyclic aromatic hydrocarbons	Skin, Scrotum, Lung
Radon^Q	Lung
Silica^Q	Lung
Vinyl chloride^Q	Liver
Wood dust^Q	Nasal sinus

Carcinoma Bladder in Occupational Exposures

- Cancer bladder was first noted in man in Aniline industry in 1895
- Now following has been mentioned as possible bladder carcinogens^Q:
  - β-naphthylamines
  - Benzidine
  - Paraamino-diphenyl
  - Auramine
  - Magenta
  - Certain drugs: Cyclophosphamide, Phenacetin
- *Industries associated with cancer bladder*
  - Dye-stuffs and dyeing industry
  - Rubber, gas and electric cable industry
- *Most common symptom*: Blood in the urine (*haematuria*) ^{Q}
- *Most common type*: Transitional Cell (urothelial cell) carcinoma (TCC) [90%]^Q
- Immunotherapy in the form of 'Intravesical (pharmacotherapeutic) BCG instillation' is also used to treat and prevent the recurrence of superficial tumors^Q.

Decompression Sickness (Caisson's Disease)

- *Caisson Disease (Decompression Sickness, DCS^Q)*: Occurs due to low pressure, when a diver ascends rapidly to surface or air passengers ascend too rapidly to high altitudes
- *Manifestations of air expansion^Q*:
  - *Barodontalgia*: Air trapped beneath teeth expands
  - *Barosinusitis*: Compressed air trapped in sinuses expands
  - *Barotitis*: Air under pressure trapped in middle ear expands
  - *Emphysema*: Most 'serious complication^Q (may lead to cerebral embolism)
  - *Abdominal distension*: Air trapped in intestinal canal expands
- *Effects of Nitrogen effervescence^Q*:
  - *Bends*: Steady aching pain in joints^Q

> **Key points**
> Effects of Nitrogen effervescence:
> - Bends
> - Chokes
> - Prickles

- *Chokes*: Rapid, shallow, dyspneic breathing^Q
- *Prickles*: Irritation of nerve terminals in skin
- *Paralysis*: Most Serious Complication^Q
- *Aseptic bone necrosis*: Hip, knee and shoulder joints
- *Gases implicated in DCS*^Q:
  - Nitrogen^Q
  - Trimix (nitrogen + oxygen + helium)
  - Heliox (oxygen + helium)
- Caisson Disease is a type of diving hazard and *dysbarism*.
- *Recompression is the only effective treatment for severe DCS*, although rest and oxygen applied to lighter cases can be effective^Q.

Key points

Gases implicated in DCS^Q:
- Nitrogen^Q
- Trimix
- Heliox Bends

Sickness Absenteeism

- Sickness absenteeism is a *'useful index in industry to assess the state of health of workers'*, and their physical, mental and social well-being^Q
- *Causes of sickness absenteeism may not be entirely due to sickness*:
  - Economic causes
  - Social causes
  - Medical causes
- *Methods of reducing sickness absenteeism*:
  - Good factory management and practices
  - Adequate pre-placement examination
  - Good human relations
  - Application of ergonomics
- *Rate of absenteeism reported in India*^Q: 8–10 days per worker per year.

Occupational Health Examination

- *Pre-placement Examination:* Is the foundation of an efficient occupational health service
  - *Timing*: At the time of employment and includes worker's history (medical, family, occupational and social), physical examination and biological and radiological examinations
  - *Main purpose of Pre-placement Examination* is to place *'the right man in right job'*^Q; so that worker can perform his duties efficiently without detriment to his health *(Ergonomics^Q)*
  - Pre-placement Examination also serves as a useful benchmark for future comparison (examination and epidemiology).
- *Periodic Post-placement Medical Examination*: (for industrial workers) is held at appropriate intervals to test their physical and mental efficiency and to detect any departure from health at the earliest; objective being early diagnosis and prompt treatment *(Secondary level of prevention)*. Frequency of periodic examinations:
  - *Frequency and content depend upon the type of occupational exposure*:^Q
    - *Annual*: for most of occupational exposures
    - *Every 2 months*: Radiation Industry^Q
    - *Monthly*: for lead, dye-stuffs exposure
    - *Daily*: for dichromates exposure.

Ergonomics

- *Ergonomics (human factors):* Is the application of scientific information concerning objects, systems and environment for human use^Q.
- *Physical Ergonomics:* deals with the human body's responses to physical and physiological stress.
- *Cognitive Ergonomics (engineering psychology):* concerns mental processes as they affect interactions among humans and other elements of a system; includes workload, training, interaction, decision-making, errors, etc.
- *Organizational Ergonomics (macroergonomics):* is concerned with the optimization of systems, including their organizational structures, policies, and processes; includes job-satisfaction, motivation, supervision, team work, ethics, etc.

Key points

Employment prohibited for age less than 14 years^Q.

The Factories Act, 1948

- *Scope*: The Act defines factory as an establishment employing 10 or more persons where power is used and 20 or more persons where power is not used^Q
- *Work related norms*:
  - Employment of young persons:
  - Employment prohibited for age less than 14 years^Q
  - 15–18 years old adolescents to be declared fit by 'certifying surgeons'; will work only between 6AM to 7PM
  - Employment prohibited in certain dangerous occupations
  - Hours of work^Q:
    - A maximum of 4½ hours of work per day for adolescents
    - 48 hours per week (9 hrs per day)
    - Maximum 60 hours per week (including overtime)
  - Leave with wages:
    - 1 day per 15 days of work for adolescents
    - Leaves can be accumulated up to 40 days
- *Health, Safety and Welfare recommendations*:
  - A minimum of 500 cubic feet space per worker^Q
  - 1 Safety Officer per 1000 workers^Q
  - 1 Welfare Officer per 500 workers
  - 1 Canteen for greater than 250 workers
  - 1 Crèche for greater than 30 women workers
- Under Factories Act 1948, there are 29 diseases which are notifiable (Schedule 3):^{Q}
  - Silicosis
  - Anthracosis
  - Byssinosis
  - Asbestosis

> **Key points**
> A minimum of 500 cubic feet space per worker^Q.
> 1 Safety Officer per 1000 workers^Q.

> **Key points**
> Diseases which are notifiable
> - Silicosis
> - Anthracosis
> - Byssinosis
> - Asbestosis

The Employees State Insurance (ESI) Act, 1948

- ESI Act is an important measure of social security and health insurance in India
- *Scope of ESI Act*: The act covers all the factories in India *'excluding mines, defence, railways,*^{Q}
  - Coverage: Non-seasonal factories employing 10 or more persons^Q
  - Shops, hotels, restaurants, cinemas including preview theatres, road-motor transport undertakings and newspaper establishments employing 20 or more persons
  - Private Medical and Educational institutions employing 20 or more persons in certain States/UTs
  - *It covers all states except*: Manipur, Sikkim, Arunachal Pradesh and Mizoram; and UTs of Delhi and Chandigarh
  - It covers all employees getting income up to ₹ 21,000/- per month.^{Q}
- *Administration*: The Union Minister of Labour is the Chairman of ESI Corporation
- *Finance*:
  - Employer contributes 4.75% of total wage bill^Q
  - Employee contributes 1.75% of wages (those earning <₹ 100/- per day exempted)
  - State and Central Government share medical expenditure in ration of 1:7^Q
- *Benefits to employees under ESI*:
  - *Medical benefit*: Full medical care^Q
  - *Sickness benefit*: 70% of the average daily wages and is payable for 91 days^Q (in any continuous period of 365 days)
  - *Extended sickness benefit*: Payable for 2 years for a set of 34 diseases^Q (80% wages)
  - *Enhanced sickness benefit*: Full average daily wage for duration upto 7 days in the case of Vasectomy and up to 14 days in the case of the Tubectomy^Q
  - *Maternity benefit*: Full average daily wage for duration upto 26 weeks^Q (NEW GUIDELINE) (confinement) (₹ 5000/- per confinement)
  - *Temporary disablement benefit*: 90% of the average daily wages till recovery^Q
  - *Permanent disablement benefit*: 90% of wages for loss of earning as worked out by a medical board
  - *Dependents' benefit*: Pension at rate of 90% of wages^Q
  - *Funeral expenses*: Cash not exceeding ₹ 10,000/-
  - *Rehabilitation benefit*

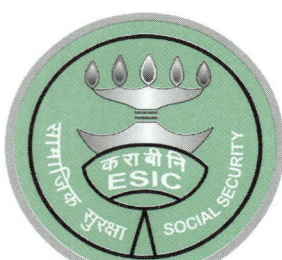

ESIC symbol

> **Key points**
> Employer contributes **4.75%** of total wage bill.

Employees' State Insurance (Central) Amendment Rules, 2017

- Insured woman:
  - A commissioning mother who as biological mother wishes to have a child and prefers to get embryo implanted in any other woman (Surrogacy)
  - A woman who legally adopts a child of up to 3 months of age
- Maternity benefit for Insured woman now enhanced to 26 weeks (6 months) for full confinement^Q
- Insured woman having two or more than two surviving children shall be entitled to receive maternity benefits during a period of 12 weeks of which not more than six weeks shall precede the expected date of confinement

> **Key points**
> **Sickness benefit:** 70% of the average daily wages and is payable for **91 days**.

ESIC 2.0: Health Reforms Agenda of ESIC^Q

- Online availability of electronically-stored health records of the ESI beneficiaries
- Special OPD for Senior citizens and Differently-abled persons
- **Abhiyan Indradhanush:** Change of bed-sheets on daily basis (**VIBGYOR** pattern^Q)

Day	Colour of bedsheet
Sunday	Violet
Monday	Indigo
Tuesday	Blue
Wednesday	Green
Thursday	Yellow
Friday	Orange
Saturday	Red

GENETICS

Definitions

- *Genome:* The sum total of genetic information of an individual which is encoded in structure of DNA
- *Genomics:* Is the study of human genome^Q
- *Gene Therapy:* Introduction of a gene sequence into a cell to modify its behavior
- *DNA Technology:* Development of new diagnostic techniques such as restriction enzymes.

Eugenics and Euthenics

- *Eugenics (Sir Francis Galton^Q):* Is a social philosophy which advocates the improvement of human hereditary traits through various forms of intervention (GENETIC MANIPULATION) ^{Q}
  - *Negative Eugenics^Q:* Is aimed at lowering fertility among the genetically disadvantaged
    - Abortions
    - Sterilizations
    - Other methods of family planning
  - *Positive Eugenics^Q:* Is aimed to encourage reproduction among the genetically advantaged
    - Financial and political stimuli
    - Targeted demographic analyses
    - In vitro fertilization,
    - Egg transplants
    - Gene cloning
- *Euthenics:* Deals with human improvement through altering external factors such as education and the controllable environment, including the prevention and removal of contagious disease and parasites, environmentalism, education regarding home economics, sanitation, and housing (Environmental Manipulation^Q).

Mendelian Diseases Inheritance^Q

Autosomal dominant traits^Q	Autosomal recessive traits^Q
Achondroplasia^Q Huntington's chorea^Q Neurofibromatosis^Q Familial polyposis coli Marfan's Syndrome^Q Retinoblastoma ABO blood group system^Q Hyperlipoproteinemia I, II, III, IV Polycystic kidney Hereditary spherocytosis^Q	Albinism^Q Phenylketonuria^Q Tay sachs disease Alcaptonuria^Q Cystic fibrosis^Q Galactosemia^Q Hemoglobinopathies^Q Maple syrup urine disease^Q Megacolon (Hirschsprung Dis)
Sex-linked dominant traits^Q	**Sex-linked recessive traits^Q**
Vitamin-D resistant rickets Blood group Xg Familial hypophosphatemia	Hemophilia type A & B^Q Duchenne muscular dystrophy Color blindness^Q G6PD deficiency^Q Hydrocephalus Retinitis pigmentosa

Hardy Weinberg Law

> **Key points**
> Hardy Weinberg fails if:
> - Small populations
> - Dynamic populations
> - Non-random mating
> - Assortative mating
> - Mutations
> - Natural selection
> - Gene flow
> - Genetic drift
> - Migration

- *Hardy Weinberg Law^Q:* States that the genotype frequencies in a population remain constant or are in equilibrium from generation to generation unless specific disturbing influences are introduced
  - Genetic equilibrium (HW law) is a basic principle of population genetics; the entire principle is based on Mendelian genetics
  - HW law assumes that human population is static
- *Hardy Weinberg is only applicable for:*^Q
  - Infinitely large populations
  - Random mating populations
  - Static populations
- *Hardy Weinberg fails if:*^Q
  - Small populations
  - Dynamic populations
  - Non-random mating
  - Assortative mating
  - Mutations
  - Natural selection (mortality selection, fecundity selection)
  - Gene flow
  - Genetic drift
  - Migration.

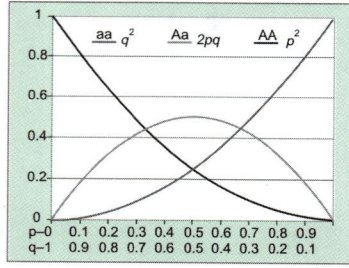

Hardy Weinberg Law

Human Genome Project (HGP)

- *Human Genome Project:* HGP is an international scientific research project
  - Primary goals are *to determine the sequence of chemical base pairs which make up DNA and to identify the approximately 25,000 genes of the human genome*^Q *(Later found 20,500 genes)*
  - *Secondary goals:* To understand human genome and complete a map of all findings
  - Goals of the original HGP were not only to determine more than *3 billion base pairs in the human genome,* but also to identify all the genes in this vast amount of data.
- *Project began in 1990 initially headed by James D. Watson:*
  - Ongoing sequencing led to the announcement of the essentially *complete genome in April 2003*^Q
  - Part of the project is still ongoing, although a preliminary count indicates about **19,000–20,000 genes** in the human genome^Q *(New Update 2017)*
- *The Human Genome Diversity Project (HGDP):* A spinoff research aimed at mapping the DNA that varies between human ethnic groups, to date has yielded new conclusions. In the future, HGDP could possibly expose new data in disease surveillance, human development and anthropology. HGDP could unlock secrets behind and create new strategies for managing the vulnerability of ethnic groups to certain diseases. It could also show how human populations have adapted to these vulnerabilities.

Amniocentesis

- *Amniocentesis*: Examination of a sample of amniotic fluid makes possible the prenatal diagnosis of chromosomal anomalies and certain metabolic defects; The procedure can be used as early as 14th week of pregnancy when abortion of affected fetus is still feasible
  - *Culture and karyotyping of fetal cells* from amniotic fluid is used for diagnosis of fetal anomalies
  - *Biochemical analysis* of amniotic fluid is used for diagnosis of metabolic effects
- Amniocentesis is indicated in following circumstances^Q:
  - A mother aged >35 years (high risk of Down's Syndrome)
  - Patients who have had a child with Down's Syndrome or other chromosomal anomalies
  - Parents known to have chromosomal translocation
  - Patients who have had a child with metabolic defect
  - When sex-determination is warranted.

MENTAL HEALTH

Causes of Mental Health Disorders

- *Organic conditions:* Cerebral arteriosclerosis, neoplasma, metabolic diseases, endocrine diseases and chronic diseases (TB, leprosy, epilepsy)
- *Heredity*: Schizophrenia
- *Socio-pathological:* Worries, anxiety, emotional stress, tension, frustration, unhappy married life, broken homes, poverty, industrialization, urbanization, cruelty, rejection, neglect, etc.

Situational Analysis

- WHO analysis shows *a global point prevalence of neuro-psychiatric conditions is about 10%* for adult
- MCC of DALYs lost: Unipolar depressive disorders^Q
- MCC of deaths: Alzheimer's and other dementias^Q
- Mental morbidity in India: 18–20 per 1000^Q.

> **Key points**
> - MCC of DALYs lost: Unipolar depressive disorders^Q.
> - MCC of deaths: Alzheimer's and other dementias^Q.

DALYs Lost due to Mental Health Disorders

Type of disorder	DALYs lost
Unipolar depressive disorders	64963
Alcohol disorders	18469
Schizophrenia	15686
Bipolar affective disorders	13645
Alzeihmer's dementia	12464
Migraine	7539
Epilepsy	7067

Diagnostic Criteria^Q

- *DSM-IV Criteria:* Diagnostic and Statistical Manual of Mental Disorders, 4th Edition, Text Revision, DSM-IV-TR, is a manual published by the American Psychiatric Association (APA) that includes all currently recognized mental health disorders
- International Classification of Diseases, ICD-10 criteria.

Mental Health Action Plan 2013–2020 (WHO)

- **Goal:** To promote mental well-being, prevent mental disorders, provide care, enhance recovery, promote human rights and reduce the mortality, morbidity and disability for persons with mental disorders.
- **Global Targets by 2020**
  - 80% of countries develop/update policy/plan for mental health
  - 50% of countries develop/updater law for mental health
  - 20% increase in service coverage for severe mental disorders
  - 80% of countries will have ≥2 promotion/prevention programs
  - 10% reduction in rate of suicide in countries
  - 80% of countries collect/report indicators every two years

PYQs: Quick Review for NEET

Biomedical waste management

Yellow bag is used for disposal of BMW categories	1, 2, 3, 5, 6, 8, 10 (New 2016 guidelines)
Category 9 biomedical waste is	Incineration ash (not used now)
Wasted sharps biomedical waste category	Four (now White category)
Sharp waste is disposed in _____ bag	White (translucent) container
Discarded expired medicines are thrown into	Yellow bag (2016 guidelines)
Discarded cytotoxic medicines should be disposed in	Yellow bag (2016 guidelines)
Amount of infectious waste among hospital waste is	1.5%
Disposal of placenta at PHC is	Treat with bleaching powder and burial
BMW bag should not be incinerated as it contains cadmium	Red bag
Animal waste is disposed off by	Incineration
Disposal mechanism for black color BMW bag	None (Incineration: Older classification)
Category 7 BMW contains	Solid waste
Disinfection and mutilation-shredding is TOC for	Sharps waste
Color BMW bag to dispose off human anatomical waste	Yellow bag
BMW rules (1998), temperature of primary chamber of incinerator	800 + 50°C
Puncture-proof bag/container in biomedical waste management in India	White
Disposal mechanism for expired medications	Incineration
Human anatomical waste should be disposed in	Yellow bag
White sharps are classified as _____ category	White (BMW 4) (now White category)

Disaster management

Ambulatory patients in triage	Cat III (GREEN)
Most important step after disaster	Chlorination of water
Colour coding for dead persons in triage	Black color
Color-coded person given first preference in disaster triage	Red
Number of colours in Triage	4
Nodal centre for disaster management	District
Calamity with most amount of damage	Floods
Highest priority is given to _____ color code in Triage	Red color
Least priority color code in triage	Black color

Occupational health

Plumbism is	Lead poisoning
MC occupational cancer	Skin cancer (Squamous cell type)
Preplacement examination is a part of	Ergonomics
Indian Factories Act, 1948 recommends per capita space minimum	500 cu.ft.
Sickness benefit under ESI Act, 1948	91 days
Burtonian line (blue line on gums) is seen in	Lead poisoning (Plumbism)
The Factory Act and ESI Act were passed in	1948
Exposure period required for Anthracosis	12 years
ESI Act came in year	1948
Legal cutoff age for employment in India	14 years
Burtonian line is seen in	Lead poisoning
Pneumoconioses causing mesothelioma	Asbestosis

Contd...

Contd...

Pneumoconioses more prone to develop Tuberculosis	None (Older concept: Silicosis)
Pneumoconioses caused by Thermoactinomyces Sacchari	Bagassosis
"Factory Act, 1948" maximum permissible working hours/week	48 hours (60 hours with overtime)
MC mode of lead poisoning	Inhalation
Extended sickness benefit under ESI is given for	2 years
Bagassosis occurs with exposure to	Bagasse (Sugarcane fibres)
Exposure to cotton dust causes	Byssinosis
Monday fever/Monday sickness is associated with	Byssinosis
Respirable dust for pneumoconiosis	0.5–3 micron
Factory Act, Age for child to work minimum be	14 years
MC heavy metal poisoning in the world	Lead poisoning
Main cause of Farmer's lung is due to microorganism	Micropolyspora faeni
Anthracosis is caused by exposure to	Coal dust
Replacement & periodic examination in radiation industry frequency	Every 2 months
Genetics and health	
Vitamin-D resistant Rickets inheritance	Sex-linked dominant
Hardy Weinberg law failure is seen in	Mutations, Linkage disequilibrium
Human DNA consist of	3 billion base pairs
Hardy Weinberg law is associated with	Population genetics
Human genome has _____ genes	19000–20000 genes
Duffy negative antigen gives protection against	Plasmodium vivax
Darwinism fails to explain	Presence of vestigial organs
MC blood group in Indian population	Blood group 'O'
"Founder effect" describes distribution of diseases on basis of	Genetics
Mental Health	
Prevalence of suicides in India	10.6 per 1 Lac population
'Anonymous group' is a support group for	Alcoholics

Multiple Choice Questions

BMW MANAGEMENT

1. Vacutainers are disposed in: **[INICET May 2023]**
   - (a) Yellow bag
   - (b) Red bag
   - (c) White containers
   - (d) Blue box

2. You were in your lab doing experiment when some of the Mercury got spilled from sphygmomanometer. What should be the proper step in handling? **[INICET May 2022]**
   - (a) Collect using your hand and discard in drain
   - (b) Collect using paper/cardboard and put in water tube/bucket
   - (c) Collect and throw outside in the environment
   - (d) Broom it and discard in dustbin

3. Broken glass vaccine vials at the Vaccination center are supposed to be disposed in which container? **[NEET PG Pattern 2022]**
   - (a) Yellow bag
   - (b) Red bag
   - (c) Sharps container
   - (d) Blue puncture proof container

4. There is H/O pharyngitis in a 4 years old child. Swab was taken and sent for culture. Swab material should be discarded in: **[NEET PG Pattern September 2021]**
   - (a) Yellow bag
   - (b) Red bag
   - (c) White container
   - (d) Blue box

5. As a trauma patient is brought to an emergency, there is blood spill on the floor. Which disinfectant would you use? **[NEET PG Pattern September 2021]**
   - (a) Ethyl alcohol
   - (b) Sodium hypochlorite
   - (c) Sodium hydroxide
   - (d) Chlorhexidine

6. Culture plate is disposed in which BMW bag? **[NEET PG Pattern September 2021]**
   - (a) White container
   - (b) Red bag
   - (c) Yellow bag
   - (d) Blue box

7. Which of the following is discarded in Black bin? **[INI-CET July 2021]**
   - (a) Contaminated gloves
   - (b) Contaminated linen
   - (c) Mattresses
   - (d) Paper/wrapper of gloves

8. As per Bio medical waste management guidelines, Latex gloves after use are discarded into: **[AIIMS June 2020]**
   - (a) Yellow bag
   - (b) Red bag
   - (c) White container
   - (d) Blue bag

9. Cardiac pacemaker is discarded into: **[AIIMS June 2020]**
   - (a) Yellow bag
   - (b) Red bag
   - (c) Blue card board box
   - (d) Puncture proof

10. Liquid chemical waste is discarded in: **[NEET PG Pattern January 2020]**
    - (a) Yellow bag
    - (b) Red Bag
    - (c) White bag
    - (d) Blue bag

11. Blood bag is discarded in: **[NEET PG Pattern January 2020]**
    - (a) Red bag
    - (b) White bag
    - (c) Blue bag
    - (d) Yellow bag

12. Surgical gloves are disposed in which BMW category? **[NEET PG Pattern January 2020]**
    - (a) Yellow
    - (b) Red
    - (c) White
    - (d) Blue

13. MATCH THE FOLLOWING TYPE QUESTION: Match the Biomedical waste with their Colored dustbins (BMW Guidelines)

A. Catheter	1. Blue
B. Torn registration forms	2. Yellow
C. Expired drug	3. Green
D. Antibiotic bottle	4. Red

    Use the following key to mark correct answer **[AIIMS May 2019]**
    - (a) A-2, B-4, C-3, D-1
    - (b) A-1, B-4, C-2, D-3
    - (c) A-4, B-3, C-2, D-1
    - (d) A-4, B-2, C-3, D-1

14. MATCHING TYPE QUESTION: Match the following Biomedical waste and their BMW management disposal bags **[AIIMS May 2019]**

Column 1	Column 2
A. Yellow bag	1. Gloves
B. Red bag	2. Glassware
C. Blue	3. Syringe wrapper
D. White transparent container	4. Scalpel
	5. Chemical waste

    - (a) A5, B1, C2, D4
    - (b) A5, B1, C3, D4
    - (c) A1, B5, C2, D4
    - (d) A3, B5, C1, D4

15. What is the color-coding of bag in hospitals to dispose off human anatomical wastes such as body parts? **[AIPGME 2005, PGMCET 2015]**
    - (a) Yellow
    - (b) Black
    - (c) Red
    - (d) Blue

16. "Inertization" deals with: [AIIMS June 1998]
    (a) Mixing biomedical waste with cement and other substance before disposal
    (b) Incineration of biomedical waste with cement and other substance before disposal
    (c) Dumping of Biomedical waste in sanitary landfills
    (d) Screw feed technology to disinfect sharps

17. HIV (+) patient is being infused amphotericin B for fungal systemic infection patient's iv-cannula and tubing should be managed as which of the following:
    [AIIMS May 2006]
    (a) Disinfect in 1% hypo chlorite, put in blue bag for destruction/shredding
    (b) Put in Red bag for destruction/shredding
    (c) Disinfect in 5% hypochlorite solution and put in yellow bag
    (d) Put in black bag for destruction/shredding

18. What is the color-coding of bag in hospitals to dispose off human anatomical wastes such as appendix:
    [AIIMS May 2004]
    (a) Yellow   (b) Black
    (c) Red   (d) Blue

19. What is the color-coding of bag in hospitals to dispose off waste sharps? [AIIMS Nov 2000]
    (a) Yellow   (b) Black
    (c) Red   (d) Blue

20. Which of the following Categories of Biomedical wastes in India do not require containers/bags for disposal?
    [AIIMS Nov 2005]
    (a) Category 1 (Human anatomical waste)
    (b) Category 4 (Waste sharps)
    (c) Category 5 (Discarded drugs and Cytotoxic medications)
    (d) Category 8 (Liquid waste)

21. Incineration is: [AIPGME 2006]
    (a) High temperature reduction process
    (b) Low temperature reduction process
    (c) High temperature oxidation process
    (d) Low temperature oxidation process

22. Which of the following Biomedical wastes cannot be disposed off in Yellow Bags? [AIIMS Nov 2007]
    (a) Reactive chemical wastes
    (b) Human anatomical wastes
    (c) Microbiology and Biotechnology wastes
    (d) Dressings soiled with blood

23. A known HIV positive patient is admitted in an isolation ward after an abdominal surgery following an accident. The resident doctor who changed his dressing the next day found it to be soaked in blood. Which of the following would be right method of choice of discarding the dressing? [AIIMS Nov 05, DPG 2011]
    (a) Pour 1% hypochlorite on the dressing material and send it for incineration in an appropriate bag
    (b) Pour 5% hypochlorite on the dressing material and send it for incineration in an appropriate bag
    (c) Put the dressing material directly in an appropriate bag and send for incineration
    (d) Pour 2% Lysol on the dressing material and send it for incineration in an appropriate bag

24. Yellow plastic bags containing biomedical wastes are treated by: [Karnataka 2008, UPSC CMS 2015]
    (a) Autoclaving
    (b) Incineration
    (c) Microwaving
    (d) Shredding

25. Hospital waste product accounts: [PGI June 04]
    (a) Paper 40%
    (b) Plastic 10%
    (c) Infectious waste 30%
    (d) Rage 30%
    (e) Glass 4%

26. True about composition of Indian hospital waste products:
    [PGI June 06]
    (a) Metal 1%
    (b) Paper 15%
    (c) Glass 55
    (d) Infectious waste 3%
    (e) Plastics 3%

27. Safe disposal of mercury is: [AIIMS May 2009, 2010]
    (a) Collect carefully and recycle
    (b) Controlled combustion
    (c) Treatment with chemicals
    (d) Deep burial

28. Outdated cytotoxic drugs are best disposed by:
    (a) Disposal in municipal waste [AIIMS Nov 09]
    (b) Destruction and dumping in secured landfill
    (c) Store for months and burial
    (d) Autoclave

29. All of the following statements regarding Biomedical Waste management are true *except*: [AIPGME 2011]
    (a) Human Anatomical waste is thrown in Yellow bag
    (b) Blue bag waste is disposed by Landfill
    (c) Incineration ash is discarded in Black bag
    (d) Material in Red bag could be a source of contamination

30. Not true about Screw feed technique is:
    (a) 80% volume reduction [AIIMS November 2013]
    (b) Pathological waste are removed
    (c) Weight is decreased by 20–30%
    (d) Based on non-burn thermal treatment

31. Biomedical waste(s) to be discarded in Yellow Bag:
    (a) Human anatomical waste [PGI November 2012]
    (b) Animal waste
    (c) Microbiological waste
    (d) Wasted sharps
    (e) Soiled waste

32. Incineration is done for: [NEET Pattern 2013]
    (a) Waste sharps
    (b) Human anatomical waste
    (c) Radiographic waste
    (d) Used batteries

33. Not safe disposal but good for soil building:
    [NEET Patterns 2012, 2013]
    (a) Incineration (b) Controlled tipping
    (c) Composting (d) Dumping

34. Plastic cover of syringes are disposed in:
    [NEET Pattern 2013] [DNB December 2009]
    (a) Red bag [DNB December 2011]
    (b) Yellow bag
    (c) Black bag
    (d) Blue bag

35. Waste sharps should be disposed in: [DNB December 2010]
    (a) Black bag [JIPMER 2014]
    (b) Yellow bag
    (c) White bag
    (d) Yellow bag

36. True about Incinerator is/are: [PGI November 2012]
    (a) Red bag can be incinerated
    (b) No pre-treatment required
    (c) Yellow bag must be incinerated
    (d) Sharps must not be incinerated
    (e) Combustible matter must be above 30%

37. True about Inertization all *except*: [AIIMS November 2014]
    (a) Mixing biomedical waste with cement
    (b) Used for pharmaceutical waste
    (c) Contaminates water sources
    (d) Not useful for infectious waste

38. Incineration is done for BMW categories:
    (a) 1 only [NEET Pattern 2015]
    (b) 3, 6, 7
    (c) 1, 2, 3
    (d) 1, 2, 3, 6

39. Waste disposal of placenta after delivery is done by
    (a) Disposing it in blue bags [UPSC CMS 2015]
    (b) Autoclaving
    (c) Incineration
    (d) Microwaving

40. All are incinerated except: [NEET Pattern 2016]
    (a) Human anatomical waste
    (b) Animal waste
    (c) Infected solid waste
    (d) Broken thermometers

41. Biomedical waste mixing with cement is known as:
    (a) Incineration [NEET Pattern 2017]
    (b) Inertization
    (c) Shredding
    (d) Autoclaving

42. Advantage of Single chamber incinerator:
    [NEET Pattern 2017]
    (a) Low pollutant emissions
    (b) Effective for thermally resistant articles
    (c) Good efficiency
    (d) All of the above

43. Blood spills in Indian Hospitals are disinfected by _____ compounds [AIIMS November 2017]
    (a) Quaternary ammonium
    (b) Chlorine based
    (c) Phenol based
    (d) Alcohol based

44. Cytotoxic Drugs disposal mechanism in India is:
    [NEET Pattern 2018]
    (a) Incineration
    (b) Microwaving
    (c) Autoclaving
    (d) Dry heat

45. According to Biomedical waste rule 2016, Incineration/ Deep burial/Plasma pyrolysis is done for bag having Color code: [PGI November 2017]
    (a) Blue (b) Red
    (c) Yellow (d) White
    (e) None

46. Body fluids and fetuses are classified under this category of waste: [FMGE NEET Pattern 2017]
    (a) Infectious waste
    (b) Pathological waste
    (c) Genotoxic waste
    (d) Humanized waste

47. Cytotoxic drug is disposed in: [NEET Pattern 2018]
    (a) Yellow bag
    (b) Red bag
    (c) Blue bag
    (d) Black bag

48. Following blood transfusion, blood bags are disposed which colour coded bin [PGI November 2018]
    (a) Red (b) Yellow
    (c) Blue (d) White

Review Questions

49. Biodegradable waste products, disposing in which of the colour code of the bags: [UP 2008]
    (a) Blue (b) Black
    (c) Green (d) Yellow

50. According to the BioMedical Waste (Management and Handling) Rules, 1998 of India, schedule II, the waste included in Category 4 are: [MH 2006]
    (a) Human Anatomical Waste
    (b) Waste Sharps
    (c) Animal Waste
    (d) Microbiology and Biotechnology Waste

51. According to biomedical waste, which of the following bag can be incinerated? *[MH 2008]* *[NEET Pattern 2016]*
    (a) Red
    (b) Blue
    (c) Green
    (d) Yellow

52. Soiled waste is seen in the category: *[RJ 2009]*
    (a) 6
    (b) 3
    (c) 5
    (d) 9

DISASTER MANAGEMENT

53. Following an earthquake, the building codes were changed to earthquake-resistant buildings. Which of the following steps of disaster management does this fall under? *[INI-CET November 2022]*
    (a) Disaster response
    (b) Disaster reconstruction
    (c) Disaster rehabilitation
    (d) Disaster mitigation

54. Green color in Triage signifies: *[NEET PG Pattern 2022]*
    (a) Dead patients
    (b) High priority patients
    (c) Ambulatory patients
    (d) Moderate priority patients

55. Things you will not do as a Medical officer of PHC when posted in Seismic areas: *[NEET PG Pattern 2022]*
    (a) Ensure funds and resources are available and can be mobilized at the time of disaster for quick evacuation
    (b) Preparedness to handle emergency
    (c) Disaster simulation practices and then check the response
    (d) Follow the announcements given on loudspeakers

56. Post-flood in Pathanamthitta district of Kerala fever syndrome is being reported. Health authorities distribute Doxycycline along with a Chemical poison spray. Identify the chemical. *[NEET PG Pattern September 2021]*
    (a) Lindane
    (b) Paris green
    (c) Zinc phosphide
    (d) Malathion

57. Definition of Triage is Categorization of Victims of Disaster: *[INI-CET July 2021]*
    (a) Based on 'First come, first treated' principle
    (b) Based on Age of the victims
    (c) Based on Severity of Injury and likelihood of survival
    (d) Based on the Vulnerable groups of victims

58. Vaccine protocol followed after Disaster? *[NEET PG Pattern January 2020]*
    (a) Everyone is given Diphtheria
    (b) Everyone is given Tetanus toxoid
    (c) Everyone is given Cholera vaccine
    (d) Only the health worker given Cholera, Typhoid, Tetanus toxoid

59. ASSERTION-REASONING TYPE QUESTION - Assertion (A): WHO recommends Typhoid vaccine for prophylaxis in Disaster management; Reasoning (R): Vaccines are Cost effective measures of reducing disease outbreak.

    Use the following key to mark correct answer *[AIIMS May 2019]*
    (a) A and R are True statements AND R is the correct explanation of A
    (b) A and R are True statements BUT R is not the correct explanation of A
    (c) A is True BUT R is False
    (d) Both A and R are False

60. Which vaccine is effective for Mass vaccination post-disaster? *[AIIMS May 2019]*
    (a) Cholera
    (b) Typhoid
    (c) Measles
    (d) Scrub typhus

61. Post disaster (earthquake) in Pakistan, which of the following vaccines is recommended by WHO? *[AIPGME 2005]*
    (a) Typhoid
    (b) Cholera
    (c) Tetanus
    (d) None of the above

62. Chernobyl nuclear explosion accident occurred on 26th April, 1986. It resulted in emission of: *[AIIMS Dec 1994]*
    (a) Methyl isocyanate (MI(C)
    (b) Union carbide
    (c) Ur235, Po210
    (d) I131, Cs134, Cs137, Sr90

63. Arrange the following phases of Disaster Cycle in a logical sequence: *[AIIMS Dec 1994][NEET Pattern 2017]*
    (a) Disaster impact–Mitigation–Rehabilitation–Response
    (b) Disaster impact–Response–Rehabilitation– Mitigation
    (c) Rehabilitation–Response–Disaster impact–Mitigation
    (d) Response–Disaster impact–Rehabilitation– Mitigation

64. During a disaster, rapidly classifying the injured on the basis of likelihood of their survival with prompt medical intervention, is a part of: *[AIPGME 2000]*
    (a) Search, rescue and first aid *[NEET Pattern 2017]*
    (b) Triage
    (c) Tagging
    (d) Disaster mitigation

65. Most commonly reported disease in the post disaster period is: *[AIIMS May 2001]*
    (a) Acute Respiratory Infections *[NEET Pattern 2017]*
    (b) Gastroenteritis
    (c) Tetanus
    (d) Malaria

66. As per the most common classification of Triage system that is internationally accepted, the colour code that indicates high priority treatment or transfer is:
    (a) Black *[Karnataka 2007]*
    (b) Yellow *[NEET Pattern 2013]*
    (c) Red
    (d) Blue

67. **Black color in triage is:**
    [NEET Pattern 2012] [NEET Pattern 2013]
    (a) Death   (b) Transfer
    (c) High priority   (d) Low priority

68. **All vaccines are NOT given in disaster, *except*:**
    [NEET Pattern 2013]
    (a) Cholera   (b) Tetanus
    (c) Measles   (d) Tetanus

69. **True about triage is:** [NEET Pattern 2012]
    (a) Yellow-least priority   (b) Red-morbidity
    (c) Green-ambulatory   (d) Blue-ambulatory

70. **Triage is:** [NEET Pattern 2014] [NUPGET 2013]
    (a) A concept in trauma
    (b) A method of breast lump diagnosis
    (c) An investigation for duodenum and pancreas
    (d) Management of old age health problems

71. **Epidemics after disaster are caused by all *except*:**
    (a) Leptospirosis   [AIIMS November 2013]
    (b) Rickettsiosis
    (c) Leishmaniasis
    (d) Acute respiratory infection

72. **The gas responsible for Bhopal gas tragedy was:**
    (a) Methyl isocyanate   [DNB June 2010]
    (b) Potassium isothiocyanate
    (c) Sodium isothiocyanate
    (d) Ethyl isothiocyanate

73. **Which epidemic does not occur after a disaster?**
    [AIIMS May 2014]
    (a) Leptospirosis   (b) Leishmania
    (c) ARTI   (d) Rickettsia

74. **Nodal centre in case of disaster management:**
    (a) PHC   [NEET Pattern 2013, 2014]
    (b) Sub centre
    (c) CHC
    (d) District

75. **During massive disaster what should be done first?**
    (a) Search and rescue, first aid   [NEET Pattern 2014]
    (b) Triage
    (c) Stabilization of victims
    (d) Hospital treatment and redistribution of patients to hospital if necessary

76. **In a disaster management triage, patients who need surgery within 24 hours, are categorized under which color category:** [NEET Pattern 2014]
    (a) Red   (b) Green
    (c) Blue   (d) Black

77. **In disaster management following are practiced *except*:**
    [NEET Pattern 2015]
    (a) Triage   (b) Rehabilitation
    (c) Mass vaccination   (d) Disaster response

78. **Triage category correctly matched is:**
    [AIIMS November 2017]
    (a) Red – Deceased/dead
    (b) Black – Minor injuries
    (c) Green – Immediate intervention needed
    (d) Yellow – Stable patient, Needs observation

79. **Triage means:** [JIPMER May 2018]
    (a) First come first serve basis
    (b) Treating person with better prognosis
    (c) Labeling the death patients
    (d) Identifying seriously ill who needs treatment first

80. **In a Triage black color is for:** [NEET Pattern 2017]
    (a) Immediate resuscitation required
    (b) Ambulatory patients
    (c) Unsalvageable
    (d) Highest priority patients

Review Question

81. **During disaster management the following condition would be classified under international code green signal:** [MP 2007]
    (a) High priority treatment   [NEET Pattern 2017]
    (b) Medium priority treatment
    (c) Ambulatory patient
    (d) Dead patients

OCCUPATIONAL HEALTH

82. **Match the following Pneumoconiosis and Clinical disorder associated with them** [INI-CET May 2023]

Pneumoconioses	Clinical association
A. Asbestosis	1. Caplan's syndrome
B. Silicosis	2. Mesothelioma pleural effusion lower lobe
C. Coal workers' Pneumoconioses	3. Acute diffuse bronchiolitis
D. Bagassosis	4. Crazy pavement pattern on HRCT

    (a) A-2, B-4, C-3, D-1
    (b) A-4, B-2, C-1, D-3
    (c) A-2, B-1, C-4, D-3
    (d) A-2, B-4, C-1, D-3

83. **A 39-year-old cement factory worker presented with X-ray changes suggestive of mesothelioma. Most likely underlying Pneumoconiosis is:** [NEET PG Pattern 2023]
    (a) Silicosis   (b) Anthracosis
    (c) Asbestosis   (d) Byssinosis

84. **A 55-year-old man had been working in a Benzene factory for long time. He got retired 5 years ago. What could be a possible complication?**
    [NEET PG Pattern September 2021]
    (a) Skin cancer   (b) Lung cancer
    (c) Bladder cancer   (d) Blood cancer

85. Most common mode of absorption of Inorganic Lead in industries leading to Lead poisoning is: [INICET July 2021]
    (a) Inhalation
    (b) Skin absorption
    (c) Absorption through hands
    (d) Food and water contamination

86. Maximum working hours' duration including overtime for a person working in a factory, as per The Factory Act' 1948 is: [NEET PG Pattern January 2020]
    (a) 100
    (b) 60
    (c) 48
    (d) 72

87. Under Extended Sickness benefit of ESI Act, Tuberculosis benefit is given for duration of: [NEET PG Pattern January 2020]
    (a) 6 months
    (b) 1 year
    (c) 2 years
    (d) 4 years

88. Following occupational diseases are notifiable under the Indian Factory Act, 1976 except: [AIIMS June 1998]
    (a) Silicosis
    (b) Asbestosis
    (c) Byssinosis
    (d) Bagassosis

89. Ideal periodical examination of worker in an industry is done every: [AIIMS Dec 1995]
    (a) Day
    (b) Month
    (c) Year
    (d) Depends on type of exposure

90. 'Safety officers' have to be appointed in factories where no. of workers is more than: [AIPGME 2001] [NEET Pattern 2017]
    (a) 500
    (b) 1000
    (c) 2000
    (d) 5000

91. Useful screening test for lead is measurement of: [AIIMS Nov 1999]
    (a) Coproporphyrin in urine
    (b) Amino-laevulinic acid in urine
    (c) Lead in blood
    (d) Lead in urine

92. Lead poisoning in industries commonly occurs by: [AIIMS June 1999]
    (a) Inhalation
    (b) Ingestion
    (c) Skin absorption
    (d) Conjunctival route

93. Inhalation of sugarcane dust could cause:
    (a) Bagassosis [AP 1993, 2002, AIIMS Nov 2003]
    (b) Byssinosis [MP 2002, NEET Patterns 2013, 2017]
    (c) Tobacosis [DPG 2004, RJ 2003, DNB 2007, 2011]
    (d) Farmer's lung

94. All are features of Silico-tuberculosis except:
    (a) High sputum AFB +ve [AIPGME 2004]
    (b) Children of such cases do not get disease
    (c) Impairment of total lung
    (d) Nodular fibrosis

95. All are disease manifestations associated with Low Temperature except: [AIPGME 2002]
    (a) Chilblains
    (b) Prickles
    (c) Frostbite
    (d) Trench foot

96. With reference to lead poisoning, various parameters are given below with the levels: [AIIMS Nov 2004]
    A. Coproporphyrin in urine
    B. Aminolevulinic Acid in urine
    C. Lead in urine
    D. Lead in blood
    I. >70 mg/100 mL
    II. >5 mg/L
    III. >150 mg/L
    IV. >0.8 mg/L
    Correct match is:
    (a) A-I B-II C-IV D-III
    (b) A-III B-IV C-II D-I
    (c) A-I B-IV C-II D-III
    (d) A-III B-II C-IV D-I

97. The minimum air space per worker prescribed by Indian Factory (Amendment) Act, 1987 is: [AIPGME 1994, DNB 2011]
    (a) 200 cu ft
    (b) 300 cu ft
    (c) 500 cu ft
    (d) 700 cu ft

98. Maximum permissible level of whole body occupational exposure to ionizing radiation is: [AIIMS Dec 1997]
    (a) 1 rem per year
    (b) 3 rem per year
    (c) 5 rem per year
    (d) 15 rem per year

99. "White Fingers" may result from which of the following occupational hazards: [AIIMS June 1998]
    (a) Heat
    (b) Cold
    (c) UV Radiation
    (d) Vibration

100. Respirable dust, responsible for pneumoconiosis, has a size limit of: [AIPGME 1993]
    (a) <1 micron
    (b) <5 micron
    (c) <10 micron
    (d) <100 micron

101. Which of the following Pneumoconioses is caused by Micropolyspora Faeni? [AIPGME 1996]
    (a) Silicosis
    (b) Byssinosis
    (c) Farmer's lung
    (d) Bagassosis

102. All are true about Lead Poisoning except: [AIPGME 1995]
    (a) Greatest source is drinking water from lead pipes
    (b) Can cause Blue Line on gums
    (c) Measurement of CPU is a useful screening test
    (d) Basophilic stippling of RBCs is a sensitive parameter of hematological response

103. Which of the following are associated with Bladder cancer: [AIIMS May 2008]
    (a) Nickel
    (b) Naphthylamines
    (c) Arsenic
    (d) Lead

104. Pre-placement examination has an important role to play in: [AIIMS May 2008]
    (a) Energy Conservation
    (b) Occupational Health
    (c) Genetic Counselling
    (d) Mental Health

105. Under ESI Act, sickness benefit is given for a period of:
    (a) 17 days [AIPGME 1999, RJ 2006]
    (b) 39 days [NEET Pattern 2017]
    (c) 91 days
    (d) 117 days

106. Sickness absenteeism is a useful index to assess: [AIIMS Nov 1999]
    (a) Working environment
    (b) Sincerity of the workers
    (c) Worker management relationship
    (d) State of health of the workers

107. All of the following are true for occupational lead poisoning except: [AIIMS Nov 02]
    (a) Inhalation is the most common mode of absorption
    (b) Lead in blood and urine provide quantitative indicators of exposure
    (c) Lead poisoning is not a notifiable disease
    (d) Basophilic stippling is a sensitive parameter of hematological response

108. All of the following features are suggestive of asbestosis except: [AIIMS May 2003]
    (a) Occurs within five years of exposure
    (b) The disease progresses even after removal of contact
    (c) Can lead to pleural mesothelioma
    (d) Sputum contains asbestos bodies

109. Bagassosis can be prevented by spraying: [DPG 2005]
    (a) 10% acetic acid
    (b) 5% acetic acid
    (c) 1% propionic acid
    (d) 2% propionic acid

110. Following are the chemical agents, which causes occupational dermatitis by local irritation except: [Karnataka 2009]
    (a) Rubber
    (b) X-rays
    (c) Lime
    (d) Ether

111. Which occupational exposure may cause sterility in females: [NEET Pattern 2012]
    (a) Lead
    (b) Carbon monoxide
    (c) Mercury
    (d) Agricultural insecticides

112. Chairman for ESI in India is: [NEET Patterns 2014, 2017]
    (a) Prime Minister
    (b) Union Minister of Health & Family Welfare
    (c) Union Minister of Labour
    (d) Union Minster of Human Resource Development

113. True about ESI act 1948: [NEET Pattern 2014]
    (a) Applicable on educational institutions also
    (b) Employer employee contribution is 1.75%
    (c) Maternity benefit for 3 months
    (d) Beneficiaries are those having income with >15000/month

114. False about ESI in India: [AIIMS November 2014]
    (a) Centre contribute 7/8 and State contribute 1/8 part on expenditure
    (b) A worker with income less than 70/- per day has to pay only 300/- per month
    (c) Funeral expenses is 50,000/-
    (d) Medical benefit include full medical care

115. Under ESI Act, number of units for which a Family Dispensary must be opened is [NEET Pattern 2015]
    (a) 500
    (b) 1000
    (c) 1500
    (d) 2000

116. Occupational exposure to Benzol may lead to [UPSC CMS 2015]
    (a) Lung cancer
    (b) Leukaemia
    (c) COPD
    (d) Neurofibromas

117. Match List I with List II and select the correct answer: [UPSC CMS 2015]

    List-I (Disease) | List-II (Antigen leading to hypersensitivity pneumonitis)
    A. Bagassosis | 1. Oak, Cedar, Pine dust
    B. Byssinosis | 2. Mouldy hay
    C. Farmer's lung | 3. Cotton
    D. Wood worker's lung | 4. Sugarcane dust

    (a) A4 B3 C2 D1
    (b) A4 B2 C3 D1
    (c) A1 B3 C2 D4
    (d) A1 B2 C3 D4

118. Ministry covering ESI Corporation of India is: [NEET Pattern 2017]
    (a) Ministry of Home Affairs
    (b) Ministry of Health and Family Welfare
    (c) Ministry of Labour
    (d) Ministry of Women and Child Development

119. True about Ergonomics are all except: [NEET Pattern 2017]
    (a) Adjusting the worker to his job
    (b) Designing of machines
    (c) Improvement of efficiency of both man & machines
    (d) Related to criteria for PHC

120. Cash benefits in ESI scheme include? [PGI May 2018]
    (a) Sickness (b) Medical
    (c) Maternal (d) Liability
    (e) Funeral

121. Which of the following is true under Factories Act of 1976? [NEET Pattern 2018]
    (a) Children aged less than 14 years are prohibited from any employment
    (b) Adolescents aged from 15–18 years can work between 7:00pm to 6:00 am
    (c) Women and children can be employed in all type of works
    (d) Adolescents of 16 years need not be duly certified as fit for work by certifying surgeon

Review Questions

122. Byssinosis is seen in: [DNB 2003] [NEET Pattern 2013]
    (a) Cement factories
    (b) Textile industries
    (c) Iron factories
    (d) Grain fields

123. A person working in hot environment who consumes more H_2O without salt is likely to develop: [DNB 200]
    (a) Heat stroke (b) Heat cramps
    (c) Heat exhaustion (d) Heat hyperpyrexia

124. In ESI programme, state government employee contribute to the fund. Employer's contribution is: [DNB 2008]
    (a) 5.75% (b) 4.75%
    (c) 3.75% (d) 2.75%

125. Wrist drop may be caused as industrial hazard in: [UP 2001]
    (a) Battery industry (b) Gas industry
    (c) Asbestos, industry (d) Aniline industry

126. "Snow-storm" appearance are seen in: [UP 2006]
    (a) Anthracosis (b) Silicosis
    (c) Byssinosis (d) Bagassosis

127. ESI Act includes all the following *except*: [AP 2006]
    (a) Small power using factories employing 10–19 persons
    (b) Non power using factories employing 20 or more person
    (c) Newspaper establishment
    (d) Defence establishment

128. All are covered under ESI *except*: [AP 2008]
    (a) News paper workers
    (b) Non power using factories with 18 members
    (c) Small power using factories with 18 members
    (d) Non power using factories with 20 members

129. Which of these is true regarding factories act: [MP 2004]
    (a) It is applicable in establishment employing 20 or more workers where power is used or <20 workers where power is not used
    (b) 500 cubic feet minimum space required per person
    (c) Act has prescribed a maximum of 48 working hrs per week, not exceeding 10 hrs per day
    (d) Act applies to the whole of India including Jammu and Kashmir

130. A 40-year-old man working in a coal mine since 15 years developed couth, dyspnoea on exertion and chest pain. His X-ray showed "snow – storm" appearance in lung fields. The most likely diagnosis is: [MP 2008]
    (a) Anthracosis (b) Silicosis
    (c) Asbestosis (d) Siderosis

131. Which of the following is occupational lung disease but not pneumoconiosis? [MH 2003]
    (a) Brucellosis (b) Silicosis
    (c) Anthracosis (d) Byssinosis

132. Which of the following is not a advantage for employers under ESI act? [MH 2005]
    (a) Exemption from Maternity Benefit ACT 1961
    (b) Rebate under Income Tax Act on contribution deposited in ESI scheme
    (c) Exemption from payment of medical allowance to employees and their dependants or arranging for their medical care
    (d) Exemption from sales tax

133. What are the maximum permissible working hours (in work/person/week) according to the factory act? [MH 2006] [NEET Pattern 2018]
    (a) <42 hours (b) <48 hours
    (c) <56 hours (d) <60 hours

134. Particle size (in micron) at which the dust particles gets lodged in the respiratory tract? [MH 2008]
    (a) 5–10 (b) 0.5–3
    (c) 0.5–0.1 (d) 3–5

135. Under ESIS act, the state government's share of expenditure on medical care is? [MH 2008]
    (a) 1/8 (b) 3/8
    (c) 5/8 (d) 7/8

136. Which is not included in pneumoconiosis? [RJ 2001]
    (a) Byssinosis (b) Bagassosis
    (c) Anthracosis (d) Psittacosis

137. Occupational exposure that may cause sterility in females: [NEET Pattern 2012]
    (a) Aniline (b) Lead
    (c) Radon (d) Nickel

138. The clinical symptoms of lead toxicity are associated with blood levels of: [DNB 2008]
    (a) 30 mcg/100 mL blood (b) 40 mcg/100 mL blood
    (c) 50 mcg/100 mL blood (d) 70 mcg/100 mL blood

139. In ESI programme, state govt, employees contribute to the fund. Employer's contribution is: [DNB 2008]
    (a) 5.75% (b) 4.75%
    (c) 3.75% (d) 2.75%

140. Ergonomics is: [NEET Pattern 2013]
    (a) Adjusting the Worker to his job
    (b) Study of human behaviour
    (c) Study of social mobility
    (d) Study of health of female workers

141. Sickness benefit under ESI act extended into: [DNB December 2011]
    (a) 91 days   (b) 61 days
    (c) 1 year   (d) 2 years

142. All are occupational cancers except: [NEET Pattern 2012]
    (a) Liver ca
    (b) Bladder ca
    (c) Lungs ca
    (d) Breast ca

143. According to The Workmen's Compensation Act, 1992, which of the following is considered an occupational disease? [AIIMS May 2012]
    (a) Typhoid   (b) Anthrax
    (c) Tetanus   (d) Dengue

144. Under ESI, a benefit which is NOT given in cash: [NUPGET 2013]
    (a) Sickness benefit
    (b) Medical benefit
    (c) Maternity benefit
    (d) Dependents' benefit

145. Which is/are not true of ESI Act, 1948? [PGI November 2012]
    (a) Involves those working in restaurants
    (b) 100% wages in temporary disability
    (c) Extended sickness benefit 91 days
    (d) Workers pay 1.75% of income
    (e) Run by Central government

GENETICS

146. Which of the following is false regarding Human genome project? [INICET May 2022]
    (a) HGP is a collaboration of many countries
    (b) More than 20,500 genes were identified
    (c) It uses modern next generation sequencing techniques
    (d) It took more than 2 decades to complete

147. Hardy Weinberg law is related to: [AIIMS May 2005] [NEET Pattern 2012]
    (a) Gene therapy
    (b) Human genome project
    (c) Population genetics
    (d) Eugenics

148. The primary goal of Human Genome Project has been: [AIIMS Nov 2004]
    (a) Introduction of a gene sequence into a cell to modify its behavior
    (b) Development of new diagnostic techniques such as restriction enzymes
    (c) Identify genes and sequence of base pairs in DNA of human genome
    (d) Confirmation of Hardy Weinberg Law

149. Amniocentesis to detect chromosomal abnormalities can be done as early as: [AIIMS Nov 2000]
    (a) 14th week of gestation
    (b) 18th week of gestation
    (c) 22nd week of gestation
    (d) 26th week of gestation

150. Environmental Manipulation which enable genes to express themselves readily is known as: [AIPGME 1998]
    (a) Positive Eugenics
    (b) Negative Eugenics
    (c) Euthenics
    (d) Genetic Counselling

151. In post disaster phase, for ensuring safe water supply, it is advisable to have a Residual Chlorine Level of: [AIPGME June 1997]
    (a) 0.3 mg/litre   (b) 0.5 mg/litre
    (c) 0.7 mg/litre   (d) 3.0 mg/litre

152. Polygenic inheritance seen in: [AIIMS May 99]
    (a) Hypertension
    (b) HOCM
    (c) Manic depressive psychosis
    (d) Familial hyper lipidemia

153. Which of the following does not affect Hardy Weinberg Equation? [AIIMS November 2011]
    (a) Small population
    (b) Natural selection
    (c) Mutation
    (d) Assortative mating

154. All of the following disorders are Autosomal dominant except: [AIPGME 2012]
    (a) Neurofibromatosis
    (b) Retinoblastoma
    (c) Marfan's syndrome
    (d) Ataxia telengiectasia

155. Marriage between two heterozygous individuals for the same disorder is prevented by [UPSC CMS 2015]
    (a) Retrospective genetic counselling
    (b) Prospective genetic counselling
    (c) Legislation
    (d) Mass health education

156. True of consanguineous marriages and genetic abnormalities are all except: [NEET Pattern 2018]
    (a) Phenylketonuria is an example
    (b) Increased risk of premature death
    (c) Increased risk of traits controlled by dominant genes
    (d) Lowering of consanguineous marriages will improve community health

Review Questions

157. "Eugenics" is: [TN 2005]
    (a) The study of hereditary improvement of the human race by controlled selective breeding
    (b) The humane destruction of an animal accomplished by a method that produces rapid unconsciousness and subsequent death without evidence of pain or distress, or a method that utilizes anaesthesia produced by an agent that causes painless loss of consciousness and subsequent death
    (c) A feeling of well-being or elation, may be drug related
    (d) A state of being carried away by overwhelming emotion

158. Population genetics is related with: [MH 2005]
    (a) Mendelian law
    (b) Watson and Crick model
    (c) Hardy Weinberg law
    (d) Weigert Meyer rule

159. All of the following affect the equilibrium in Hardy-Weinberg's law, *except*: [AIIMS May 2012]
    (a) Small population
    (b) Random mating
    (c) Mutations
    (d) Gene outflow

160. Which is/are NOT X-linked disorders? [PGI May 2012]
    (a) Wilson's disease
    (b) Haemophilia
    (c) Thalassemia
    (d) G6PD deficiency
    (e) ABO blood groups system

161. Effect of environment on genes is called: [NEET Pattern 2012]
    (a) Positive Eugenics
    (b) Negative Eugenics
    (c) Euthenics
    (d) Ergonomics

MENTAL HEALTH

162. Most commonly abused agent in India: [AIIMS May 07]
    (a) Cannabis indica [NEET Patterns 2015, 2017]
    (b) Tobacco
    (c) Heroine
    (d) Amphetamine

163. Which one of the following is not a socio-pathological factor associated with mental illness? [AIIMS Nov 1999]
    (a) Emotional stress
    (b) Frustration
    (c) Endocrine diseases
    (d) Anxiety

164. Maximum loss of DALY occurs in which psychiatric disorder? [DPG 2007]
    (a) Schizophrenia
    (b) Depression
    (c) Alcohol dependence
    (d) Bipolar disorder

165. Following are components of District Mental Health Program except: [NEET Pattern 2016]
    (a) Training
    (b) Public awareness
    (c) Record keeping
    (d) Screening

MISCELLANEOUS

166. Punnet's square is used for: [AIPGME 2011]
    (a) Random sampling
    (b) Statistical analysis
    (c) Finding genotype of offspring
    (d) Test of significance

167. Best way to dispose e-waste is: [DNB December 2010]
    (a) Burning
    (b) Incineration
    (c) In a landfill
    (d) Recycling

Explanations

BMW MANAGEMENT

1. **Ans. (b) Red bag** *[Ref. CPCB BMW Guidelines 2018, MOEF Document]*
   - Red category contains Contaminated Waste (Recyclable) including wastes generated from disposable items such as tubing, bottles, intravenous tubes and sets, catheters, urine bags, syringes (without needles and fixed needle syringes) and vacutainers with their needles cut) and gloves

2. **Ans. (b) Collect using paper/cardboard and put in water tube/bucket**
   [Ref. Environmentally Sound Management of Mercury Waste Generated from the Health Care Facilities Mercury Collection Guidelines (CPCB) 2012]
   - Identity visible larger mercury beads and push together using Cardboards and collect using Syringe without needle
   - Store collected Hg beads in an air tight plastic container half filled with water and labelled properly

3. **Ans. (d) Blue puncture proof container** *[Ref. Park 26/e p887]*
   - Under BMW guidelines, Glassware and Metallic Body Implants are disposed in Cardboard boxes with blue colored marking

4. **Ans. (a) Yellow bag** *[Ref. Park 26/e p887]*
   - Items contaminated with blood, body fluids like dressings, plaster casts, cotton swabs and bags containing residual or discarded blood and blood components are types of Soiled waste
   - Soiled waste is disposed off in YELLOW BMW category

5. **Ans. (b) Sodium hypochlorite** *[Ref. Park 26/e p885, 888]*
   - Small volumes (few drops) of Spills: Wipe the spill with a newspaper moistened with hypochlorite solution (1% dilution containing minimum 500 ppm chlorine). Discard the paper as infected waste. Repeat until all visible soiling is removed.
   - Large volumes (>10 mL) of Spills: Flood the spill with 10% hypochlorite solution. Remove and discard the paper as infected waste.

6. **Ans. (c) Yellow bag** *[Ref. Park 26/e p887]*
   - Blood bags, Laboratory cultures, stocks or specimens of microorganisms, live or attenuated vaccines, human and animal cell cultures used in research, industrial laboratories, production of biological, residual toxins, dishes and devices used for cultures are included in Microbiology, Biotechnology and other clinical laboratory waste
   - Microbiology, Biotechnology and other clinical laboratory waste is disposed off in YELLOW BMW category

7. **Ans. (d) Paper/wrapper of gloves**
   [Ref. Improving Municipal Solid Waste Management in India by Asnani. World Bank]
   - Differently colored bins, each per household to promote and ensure segregation:
   - Covered Green Bin: Wet waste
   - Covered White/Blue Bin: Dry waste
   - Covered Black Bin: Domestic Hazardous Waste
   - Paper/wrapper of gloves are disposed in Black bin (municipal waste)

8. **Ans. (b) Red bag** *[Ref. Park 27/e p919]*
   - Under NEW Biomedical Waste Management Guidelines 2016–17, Red bag is used for disposal of Contaminated Waste (Recyclable)
   - It includes wastes generated from disposable items such as tubing, bottles, intravenous tubes and sets, catheters, urine bags, syringes (without needles and fixed needle syringes) and vaccutainers (with their needles cut) and gloves

9. **Ans. (c) Blue card board box** *[Ref. Park 26/e p887]*
   - Blue colour BMW category is used for BMW – Glassware and Metallic Body Implants. Herte, Cardboard boxes with blue colored marking are used for disposal.
   - Disposal mechanism include Sodium Hypochlorite/ Autoclaving/Microwaving/Hydroclaving followed by Recycling

10. **Ans. (a) Yellow bag** *[Ref. Park 25/e p853]*
    - Under BMW Management guidelines in India - Human anatomical waste, Animal anatomical waste, Soiled waste, Expired/Discarded medicines, Chemical waste, Chemical liquid waste, Microbiological/Biotechnological/Clinical-laboratory waste, Discarded line/mattresses/beddings are put into Yellow BMW category

11. **Ans. (d) Yellow bag** *[Ref. Park 25/e p853]*
    - Under BMW Management guidelines in India – Soiled waste (Items contaminated with blood/body-fluids like dressings/plaster-casts/cotton-swabs/bags containing residual or discarded blood) is put into Yellow BMW category

12. **Ans. (b) Red** *[Ref. Park 25/e p853]*
    - Under BMW Management guidelines 2016, Red Contaminated Waste (Recyclable) Category include Wastes generated from disposable items such as tubing, bottles, intravenous tubes and sets, catheters, urine bags, syringes (without needles and fixed needle syringes) and vaccutainers with their needles cut) and gloves

13. **Ans. (c) A-4, B-3, C-2, D-1** *[Ref. Park 25/e p853]*
    - Contaminated recyclable waste (Catheters, tubings, bottles, urine bags, syringes, gloves) are disposed in RED category, Glassware & metallic body implants are disposed in BLUE category

14. **Ans. (a) A5, B1, C2, D4** *[Ref. Park 25/e p853]*
    - Chemical waste is YELLOW category, Glassware is BLUE category, Scalpel is sharp waste in WHITE category, Gloves is contaminated recyclable waste in RED category
    - Syringe wrapper is Black bag Municipal waste

15. Ans. (a) Yellow   *[Ref. BMW Management in India by Dr. J. Kishore and Dr. G. K. Ingle, 1/e p26–28, Park 27/e p919]*

BIOMEDICAL WASTE MANAGEMENT:
- Biomedical Wastes (BMW) in India are handled and managed under 'Biomedical Waste Management (Management and Handling) Rules, 1998'
- The exercising powers are conferred under Sections 6, 8, 25 of 'Environmental (Protection) Act, 1986' (under the Ministry of Environment and Forests)
- *Categories of Bio medical wastes (BMW) (Schedule I):*

Cat	BMW	Wastes included
1.	Human Anatomical Waste	Human tissues, organs, body parts
2.	Animal Waste	Animal tissues, body parts, organs, carcasses, fluids, blood
3.	Microbiology and Biotechnology Waste	Waste from lab cultures, stocks, specimens of microorganisms, live or Attenuated vaccines, cell cultures (human/animal), wastes from production of biologicals, toxins
4.	Waste Sharps	Needles, syringes, blades, scalpels, glass
5.	Discarded Medicines and Cytotoxic Drugs	Outdated contaminated and discarded medicines
6.	Soiled Waste	Items contaminated with blood, and fluids, including cotton, dressings, soiled plaster casts, linen, beddings
7.	Solid Waste	Disposable items (except sharps) including tubings, catheters, intravenous sets
8.	Liquid Waste	Waste generated from lab and washing, cleaning, housekeeping and disinfecting activities
9.	Incineration Ash	Ash from incineration of any BMW
10.	Chemical Waste	Chemical used in disinfection (insecticides) or in production of biologicals

- *Colour coding and Type of container for BMW disposal (Schedule II): Older Guidelines*

Color coding	Type of container	BMW category	Treatment option
Yellow	Plastic bag	1, 2, 3, 6	Incineration/deep burial
Red	Disinfected container/Plastic bag	3, 6, 7	Autoclave/Microwave/Chemical treatment
Blue/White translucent	Plastic bag	4, 7	Autoclave/Microwave/Chemical treatment and Destruction/Shredding
Black	Plastic bag	5, 9, 10 (solid)	Secured landfill

16. Ans. (a) Mixing biomedical waste with cement and other substance before disposal   *[Ref. Park 27/e p918]*
- The process of 'Inertization' involves mixing biomedical waste with cement and other substance before disposal, so as to minimize risk of toxic substances contained in waste to contaminate ground/surface water. Inertization is especially suitable for pharmaceuticals and for incineration ashes with high metal content
- *A typical composition of mixture is:*
  - 65% pharmaceutical waste
  - 15% lime
  - 15% cement
  - 5% water

> **ALSO REMEMBER**
> - *Advantage of Inertization:* Relatively inexpensive
> - *Disadvantage of Inertization:* Not applicable to infectious waste.

17. Ans. NONE [Older Answer-Disinfect in 1% hypo chlorite, put in blue bag for destruction/shredding]   *[Ref. Park 27/e p919]*
- Intravenous cannula and tubing are included in older BMW category 7 (Solid Waste). Earlier it disposed off in blue/white translucent bag (preferable is metal containers which are puncture-proof)

18. Ans. (a) Yellow   *[Ref. Park 27/e p919]*
- Human anatomical wastes (BMW Cat. 1) such as body parts, tissues and organs are disposed off in Yellow bag
- Amputations, cholecystectomised gall bladder, appendix (post appendicectomy) are included in human anatomical wastes

19. Ans. NONE [Older Answer Blue]   *[Ref. Park 27/e p919]*
- Wasted sharps (scalpels, needles, syringes, blades, glass) were included in BMW Category 4 (Schedule I). Category 4 wastes are now disposed off in White translucent container.

> **ALSO REMEMBER**
> - *Schedules under Biomedical Waste Management (Management and Handling) Rules, 1998:*
>   - *Schedule I:* Categories of BMW, treatment and disposal
>   - *Schedule II:* Color coding and type of container for BMW disposal
>   - *Schedule III:* Labels for BMW containers/bags
>   - *Schedule IV:* Label for transport of BMW containers/bags
>   - *Schedule V:* Standards for treatment and disposal of BMW

20. Ans. (d) Category 8 (Liquid waste)   *[Ref. Park 25/e p830]*
- According to Schedule II of Biomedical Waste (Management and Handling) Rules, 1998, following categories do not require containers/bags for disposal:
  - Categories 8 and 10 (liquid)
  - Category 3 (if disinfected locally).

> **ALSO REMEMBER**
> - Chemical treatment before Drainage for category 8 and 10.

21. **Ans. (c) High temperature oxidation process**
 [Ref. Park 27/e p916]

 INCINERATION
 - *Incineration:* Is a 'high temperature dry oxidation' process; It leads to significant reduction in waste-volume and weight (up to 70–80%)
 - Incineration does not require pre-treatment
 - *Biggest disadvantage of incineration:* Generation of smoke
 - *Types of Incinerators:*
   – Double-chamber pyrolytic
   – Single-chamber pyrolytic
   – Rotary kilns
 - *Temperature in an incinerator:*
   – Primary chamber: 800° ± 50°C
   – Secondary chamber: 1050° ± 50°C

 > **ALSO REMEMBER**
 > - *Characteristics of wastes suitable for incineration:*
 >   – Low heating volume
 >   – Combustible matter >60%
 >   – Non-combustible solids <5%
 >   – Non-combustible fines <20%
 >   – Moisture content <30%

 - Red bags should not be incinerated as they contain cadmium (heavy metal).

22. **Ans. (a) Reactive chemical wastes** [Ref. Park 27/e p919]
 - *Yellow color bags are used for disposal of:*
   – BMW Cat. 1: Human anatomical wastes
   – BMW Cat. 2: Animal waste
   – BMW Cat. 3: Microbiological and biotechnology waste
   – BMW Cat. 6: Soiled waste
 - *Container/bags are NOT required for disposal of:*
   – BMW Cat. 8: Liquid waste
   – BMW Cat. 10: Chemical waste
   – BMW Cat. 3 (if disinfected locally): Microbiological and biotechnology waste

23. **Ans. (a) Pour 1% hypochlorite on the dressing material and send it for incineration in an appropriate bag**
 [Ref. Internet, Park 27/e p919]
 - All HIV infected material, i.e. gauge pieces, bandages, cotton swabs, blood units, blood have to be incinerated

24. **Ans. (b) Incineration** [Ref. Park 27/e p916]

25. **Ans. (b) Plastic 10%; (e) Glass 4%** [Ref. Park 27/e p915]
 - Average composition of Hospital waste products in India:
   – Paper: 15%
   – Plastic: 10%
   – Rags: 15%
   – Metals (Sharps, etc): 1.0%
   – Infectious waste: 1.5%
   – Glass: 4.0%
   – General waste (food waste, sweeping of premises): 53.5%

26. **Ans. (a) Metal 1%; (b) Paper 15%** [Ref. Park 27/e p915]

27. **Ans. (a) Collect carefully and recycle**
 [Ref. Guidelines for environmentally sound mercury management in fluorescent lamp sector, CPCB, India]
 MERCURY DISPOSAL:
 - Dispose mercury as a hazardous waste
 - 'Never combine it with organic or inorganic waste
 - Never dispose it in sink/drain
 - Dispose off in 'Recycling units'

28. **Ans. (b) Destruction and dumping in secured landfill**
 [Ref. Park 27/e p919]

29. **Ans. (b) Blue bag waste is disposed by Landfill; (c)**
 [Ref. Park 27/e p919]

30. **Ans. (b) Pathological waste are removed**
 [Ref. Park 27/e p917]

 SCREW-FEED TECHONOLOGY
 - *Principle*: Non-burn dry thermal process
 - *Process*:
   – Shredding of waste
   – Heating in a rotating auger
 - *Reduction in waste*:
   – Reduction in weight: 20–35%
   – Reduction in volume: 80%
 - *Useful for wastes*:
   – Infectious waste
   – Sharps
 - *Not useful for wastes*:
   – Pathological waste
   – Cytotoxic waste
   – Radioactive waste

31. **Ans. (a) Human anatomical waste; (b) Animal waste; (c) Microbiological waste; (e) Soiled waste**
 [Ref. Park 27/e p919]

32. **Ans. (b) Human anatomical waste** [Ref. Park 27/e p919]

33. **Ans. (c) Composting** [Ref. Park 27/e p883]

34. **Ans. (c) Black bag** [Ref. BMW Management Guidelines 2011, Government of India]

35. **Ans. (c) White bag [White translucent puncture-proof container]** [Ref. Park 27/e p919]

36. **Ans. (c) Yellow bag must be incinerated; (d) Sharps must not be incinerated** [Ref. Park 27/e p919]

37. **Ans. (c) Contaminates water sources** [Ref. Park 27/e p916]

38. **Ans. (d) 1, 2, 3, 6 [Now its done for cat 1, 2, 3, 5, 6, 10 and Linen/beddings]** [Ref. Park 27/e p919]

39. **Ans. (c) Incineration** [Ref. Park 27/e p919]

40. **Ans. (d) Broken thermometers** [Ref. Darby's Comprehensive Review of Dental Hygiene 8/e p400]
 - Mercury disposal is through recycling.

41. **Ans. (b) Inertization** [Ref. Park 27/e p917]
 - Inertization process includes mixing biomedical waste with cement and other substance before disposal, so as to minimize risk of toxic substances contained in waste to contaminate ground/surface water
 - Inertization is especially suitable for pharmaceuticals and for incineration ashes with high metal content
 - A typical composition of mixture is: 65% pharmaceutical waste, 15% lime, 15% cement, 5% water.

> **ALSO REMEMBER**
> **CEMENT IN BMW MANAGEMENT**
> - Encapsulation: Filling containers with waste, adding an immobilizing material (plastic foam/bituminous sand/cement mortar/clay material) and sealing containers
> - Inertization: Mixing biomedical waste with cement and other substance (lime) before disposal

42. **Ans. (c) Good efficiency** *[Ref. Park 27/e p918]*
    - Advantages of Single Chamber Incinerators:
      – Good disinfection efficiency
      – Massive reduction of waste's volume and weight
      – Not highly skilled manpower required
      – Low investment, Low operating costs
    - Disadvantages of Single Chamber Incinerators:
      – Atmospheric pollutants emission
      – Require periodic removal of slag and soot
      – Not useful for cytotoxic drugs and thermo-resistant chemicals

43. **Ans. (b) Chlorine based**
    [Ref. Ocular Infections by Sharma 1/e p9]
    Hypochlorites in Hospital waste Management
    - Disinfection of countertops and floors
    - Decontamination of blood spills
    - Irrigating agent in endodontic treatment
    - Disinfectant for manikins, laundry, dental appliances, hydrotherapy tanks
    - Treatment of liquid medical waste before disposal
    - Decontaminating water distribution systems in dialysis

44. **Ans. (a) Incineration** *[Ref. Park 27/e p919]*

45. **Ans. (c) Yellow** *[Ref. Park 27/e p919]*

46. **Ans. (b) Pathological waste**
    [Ref. WHO Guidelines on Medical Waste Chapter 2]
    - **Infectious waste**: Contain pathogens (bacteria, viruses, parasites, or fungi) in sufficient concentration or quantity to cause disease in susceptible hosts. Includes Cultures, Waste from surgery and autopsies on patients with infectious diseases, Waste from infected patients in isolation wards (e.g. excreta, dressings), Waste that has been in contact with infected patients undergoing haemodialysis, Infected animals from laboratories, Any other instruments or materials that have been in contact with infected persons or animals
    - **Pathological waste:** Consists of tissues, organs, body parts, human fetuses and animal carcasses, blood, and body fluids. Within this category, recognizable human or animal body parts are also called Anatomical waste
    - **Pharmaceutical waste:** Includes expired, unused, spilt, and contaminated pharmaceutical products, drugs, vaccines, and sera that are no longer required and need to be disposed of appropriately. The category also includes discarded items used in the handling of pharmaceuticals, such as bottles or boxes with residues, gloves, masks, connecting tubing, and drug vials
    - **Genotoxic waste:** Highly hazardous and may have mutagenic, teratogenic, or carcinogenic properties. Genotoxic waste may include certain cytotoxic drugs, vomit, urine, or faeces from patients treated with cytostatic drugs, chemicals, and radioactive material

47. **Ans. (a) Yellow bag** *[Ref. Park 27/e p919]*

48. **Ans. (b) Yellow** *[Ref. Park 27/e p919]*
    - Soiled waste includes Items contaminated with blood, body fluids like dressings, plaster casts, cotton swabs and bags containing residual or discarded blood and blood components
    - Soiled waste is discarded in Yellow Category (NEW BMW Management Guidelines 2016–17)
    - Soiled waste (Yellow category disposal): Incineration/Plasma Pyrolysis/Deep burial (In absence of above facilities, Autoclaving/Micro-waving/Hydroclaving followed by Shredding/Mutilation Or combination of Sterilization and Shredding; Treated waste should be sent for energy recovery)

Review Questions

49. **Ans. (d) Yellow** *[Ref. Park 27/e p919]*
50. **Ans. (b) Waste Sharps** *[Ref. Park 27/e p919]*
51. **Ans. (d) Yellow** *[Ref. Park 27/e p919]*
52. **Ans. (a) 6 [Now Yellow Category]** *[Ref. Park 27/e p919]*

DISASTER MANAGEMENT

53. **Ans. (d) Disaster mitigation** *[Ref. Park 27/e p925]*
    - Disaster mitigation: Includes measures that are taken to prevent disasters from causing emergencies or to lessen the likely effects of emergencies
    - Disaster mitigation measures aim to reduce the vulnerability of the system; It complements disaster preparedness and response activities and includes measures taken to lessen the likely effects of emergencies. Some of these measures are,
      – Flood mitigation
      – Land-use planning
      – Improved building codes
      – Reduction and protection of vulnerable populations or structures.

54. **Ans. (c) Ambulatory patients** *[Ref. Park 26/e p891]*
    - Triage system include Red (Highest Priority - Immediate resuscitation or limb/life-saving surgery in next 6 hours), Yellow (High Priority - Possible resuscitation or limb/life-saving surgery in next 24 hours), Green (Low Priority - Minor illness/AMBULATORY patients) and Black (Least Priority - Dead and moribund patients)

55. **Ans. (d) Follow the announcements given on loudspeakers** *[Ref. Assam State Disaster Management Plan 2022]*
    Roles and responsibilities of Medical officer of PHC when posted in Seismic areas
    - Ensure funds and resources are available and can be mobilized at the time of disaster for quick evacuation
    - Preparedness to handle emergency
    - Disaster simulation practices and then check the response

56. **Ans. (c) Zinc phosphide** *[Ref. Park 26/e p881]*

LEPTOSPIROSIS CONTROL
- The most effective preventive measure is avoidance of high-risk exposure (i.e. wading in floods and contaminated water, contact with animal's body fluid). It includes wearing boots, goggles, overalls, and rubber gloves. [GRADE-A]
- Pre-exposure antibiotic prophylaxis is NOT ROUTINELY RECOMMENDED. It may be considered for short-term exposures. [GRADE-B]. Doxycycline (hydrochloride and hyclate) 200 mg once weekly, to begin 1 to 2 days before exposure and continued throughout the period of exposure
- Zinc phosphide is used for chemical control of rodents due to its good safety record, low cost and high effectiveness

57. Ans. (c) Based on Severity of Injury and likelihood of survival [Ref. Park 26/e p891]
- Triage is Categorization of Victims of Disaster based on likelihood of survival

58. Ans. (d) Only the health worker given Cholera, Typhoid, Tetanus toxoid [Ref. Park 25/e p858]
- WHO does not recommend Typhoid, Cholera and Tetanus Toxoid vaccinations in routine use in endemic areas post-disaster, However, these vaccinations are recommended for health workers

59. Ans. (d) Both A and R are False [Ref. Park 25/e p858]
- WHO does not recommend Vaccination in Post-disaster phase especially Typhoid, Cholera, Tetanus vaccine
- Vaccination has not been proven effective, as a large scale Public health measure

60. Ans. (c) Measles [Ref. Park 25/e p858]
- Vaccination is generally C/I Post-disaster especially Typhoid, Cholera, Tetanus
- Only Measles vaccine is permitted Post-disaster

61. Ans. (d) None of the above [Ref. Park 27/e p924–925]
- WHO does not recommend Typhoid, Cholera and Tetanus Toxoid vaccinations in routine use in endemic areas post-disaster
  - However, these vaccinations are recommended for health workers
- Because measles can deplete Vitamin A stores in children, 'measles is the highest priority among vaccinations for children' living in congregate care after a disaster

ALSO REMEMBER
- *Clean water supply in post-disaster phase:* UNHCR recommends 15 liters/person/day clean water be provided
- *A common micronutrient deficiency in disasters is Vitamin A deficiency:* It occurs due to deficient relief diets, measles and diarrhea (gastroenteritis)
- Other common deficiencies include scurvy (Vitamin C), anemia (iron) and pellagra (Vitamin B4 –niacin)

62. Ans. (d) I131, Cs134, Cs137, Sr90 [Ref. Park 27/e p928]
- Chernobyl nuclear explosion accident occurred on 26th April, 1986 in Russia (now Ukraine)
  - It resulted in emission of I131, Cs134, Cs137, Sr90
- Chernobyl nuclear explosion accident is the 'largest accidental release of radioactive material in the history of nuclear power'
- It is the only instance so far of level 7 on the International Nuclear Event Scale for nuclear accidents

ALSO REMEMBER
- *World's worst man-made disaster is Bhopal gas Tragedy, 3rd December 1984:*
  - Methylisocyanate (MIC) gas leaked from Union Carbide pesticide plant in Bhopal, India
  - It resulted in resulting in the death of about 3,000 people according to the Indian Supreme Court
  - *Fukushima Daichii Tragedy, 11 March 2011:* I_{131}, Cs_{134}, Cs_{137}.

63. Ans. (b) Disaster impact – Response – Rehabilitation – Mitigation [Ref. Park 27/e p923]

ALSO REMEMBER
- Disaster (Colin Grant): Is catastrophe causing 'injury or illness simultaneously to at least 30 people', who will require hospital emergency treatment
- For every 1 disaster registered (in official database), there are 20 other unacknowledged smaller emergencies with destructive impact
- During the phase of search, rescue and first aid, most immediate help cover is derived from uninjured survivors
- 'Most crucial phase of disaster management' is the stage of health and medical relief
- World Disaster Reduction Day: 2nd Wednesday of October **(now 13th October)**
- Greatest need for emergency care in immediate post disaster occurs in first few hours.

64. Ans. (b) Triage [Ref. Park 27/e p923]
- *Triage:* Consists of rapidly classifying the injured 'on the basis of severity of their injuries and likelihood of their survival' with prompt medical intervention
- First come first serve is NOT followed in emergencies
- *Triage sieve:* Quick survey to separate the dead and the walking from the injured
- *Triage sort:* Remaining casualties are assessed and allocated to categories
- *Triage system:* Most commonly uses FOUR color code system:
  - Red (Highest Priority): Immediate resuscitation or limb/life saving surgery in next 6 hours
  - Yellow (High Priority): Possible resuscitation or limb/life saving surgery in next 24 hours
  - Green (Low Priority): Minor illness/ambulatory patients
  - Black (Least Priority): Dead and moribund patients
- *Tagging:* Is the procedure where identification, age, place of origin, triage category, diagnosis and initial treatment are tagged on to every victim of disaster through a colour coding
- *Mitigation:* Measures designed to either prevent hazards from causing emergency or to lessen the effects of emergency.

ALSO REMEMBER
- **TRIAGE:**
- Triage yields best results when carried out at the site of disaster
- *Triage is of two types:*
  - Simple triage: Simple triage is used in a scene of mass casualty, in order to sort patients into those who need critical attention and immediate transport to the hospital and those with less serious injuries.
    1. This step is required before transportation becomes available
    2. The categorization of patients based on the severity of their injuries can be aided with the use of printed triage tags or colored flagging
  - *Rapid triage:* S.T.A.R.T. (Simple Triage and Rapid Treatment) is a simple triage system that can be performed by lightly-trained lay and emergency personnel in emergencies.
    1. It is not intended to supersede or instruct medical personnel or techniques
    2. It may serve as an instructive example
    3. It has been field-proven in mass casualty incidents such as train wrecks and bus accidents
  - *Reverse Triage:* In addition to the standard practices of triage as mentioned above, there are conditions where sometimes the less wounded are treated in preference to the more severely wounded. This may arise in,
    - A situation such as war where the military setting may require soldiers be returned to combat as quickly as possible
    - Disaster situations where medical resources are limited in order to conserve resources for those likely to survive but requiring advanced medical care.

65. Ans. (b) Gastroenteritis [Ref. Park 27/e p925]
- Most commonly reported disease in post-disaster phase is Gastroenteritis
- Most practical and effective strategy of disease prevention and control in post-disaster phase is 'supplying safe drinking water and proper disposal of excreta'
- Foremost step for disease prevention and control in post-disaster phase is chlorination of all water bodies
- Level of residual chlorine to be maintained in all water bodies in post-disaster phase is >0.7 mg/l (>0.7 ppm)

ALSO REMEMBER
- *A common micronutrient deficiency in disasters is Vitamin A deficiency:* It occurs due to deficient relief diets, measles and diarrhea (gastroenteritis)
  - Other common deficiencies include scurvy (Vitamin C), anemia (iron) and pellagra (Vitamin B4 –niacin).

66. Ans. (c) Red [Ref. Park 27/e p923]
- Categories in Triage:

Category	Tagging color	Priority
I	Red	High
II	Yellow	Medium
III	Green	Low
IV	Black	Least

67. Ans. (a) Death [Ref. Park 27/e p923]
68. Ans. (c) Measles [Ref. Park 27/e p924–925]
69. Ans. (c) Green-ambulatory [Ref. Park 27/e p923]
70. Ans. (a) A concept in trauma [Ref. Park 27/e p923]
71. Ans. (c) Leishmaniasis [Ref. Park 27/e p924]
    Diseases common in Post-disaster Phase
    - Gastroenteritis (MC)
    - Acute respiratory tract infections (Pneumonias)
    - Leptospirosis
    - Rickettsiosis
    - Rabies
    - Equine encephalitis
72. Ans. (a) Methyl isocyanate [Ref. Park 27/e p928–929]
73. Ans. (b) Leishmania [Ref. Park 27/e p924]
    Diseases common in Post-disaster Phase: Gastroenteritis (MC), Acute respiratory tract infections (Pneumonias), Leptospirosis, Rickettsiosis, Rabies, Equine encephalitis
74. Ans. (d) District [Ref. National Health Programmes in India by Dr Jugal Kishore, 9/e p457]
75. Ans. (a) Search and rescue, first aid [Ref. Park 27/e p923]
76. Ans. (c) Blue [Ref. Park 27/e p923]
77. Ans. (c) Mass vaccination [Ref. Park 27/e p924–925]
    - WHO does not recommend routine vaccines viz. Typhoid, Cholera and Tetanus Toxoid vaccinations in routine use in endemic areas post-disaster.
78. Ans. (d) Yellow – Stable patient, Needs observation [Ref. Park 27/e p923]
79. Ans. (d) Identifying seriously ill who needs treatment first [Ref. Park 27/e p923]
80. Ans. (c) Unsalvageable [Ref. Park 27/e p923]

Review Question
81. Ans. (c) Ambulatory patient [Ref. Park 27/e p923]

OCCUPATIONAL HEALTH
82. Ans. (d) A-2, B-4, C-1, D-3 [Ref. Park 27/e p933–934]
    - Malignant pleural mesothelioma is an aggressive malignancy of the pleural surface, predominantly caused by prior asbestos exposure
    - Multiple bilateral centrilobular densities, multifocal patchy ground-glass densities, and consolidation with 'crazy paving pattern' (superimposition of reticular and ground-glass opacities,) constitute the HRCT findings seen in Acute silicosis
    - Caplan syndrome (Rheumatoid pneumoconiosis) is the combination of seropositive rheumatoid arthritis and a characteristic pattern of fibrosis. It was first described in coal miners (coal workers' pneumoconiosis)
    - Bagassosis may lead to breathlessness, cough, haemoptysis, slight fever and acute diffuse bronchiolitis
83. Ans. (c) Asbestosis [Ref. Park 27/e p934]
    - Asbestos may lead to pulmonary fibrosis, carcinoma of bronchus, mesothelioma of peritoneum/pleura and cancer of GIT

84. **Ans. (d) Blood cancer** *[Ref. Park 26/e p903–904]*
    - IARC classifies benzene as "carcinogenic to humans," based on sufficient evidence that benzene causes acute myeloid leukemia (AML)
    - IARC also notes that benzene exposure has been linked with acute lymphocytic leukemia (ALL), chronic lymphocytic leukemia (CLL), multiple myeloma, and non-Hodgkin lymphoma

85. **Ans. (a) Inhalation** *[Ref. Park 26/e p902]*

    Modes of Lead Absorption
    - *Inhalation:* MC mode in Industries
    - *Ingestion:* Less common
    - *Skin:* Only for organic compounds of Lead

86. **Ans. (b) 60** *[Ref. Park 25/e p876]*
    - Under The Factories Act 1948, work hours duration includes maximum 48 hours per week (9 hours per day) which could be increased up to 60 hours per week (including paid overtime)

87. **Ans. (c) 2 years** *[Ref. Park 25/e p878]*
    - Extended Sickness Benefit (ESB): For 34 long term diseases, ESI have a provision for paying Sickness Benefit for an extended period (Extended Sickness Benefit) of up to 2 years in a ESB period of 3 years

88. **Ans. (d) Bagassosis** *[Ref. National Health programs of India by Dr. J Kishore, 5/e p430]*

> **ALSO REMEMBER**
> - Under Factories Act 1948, there are 29 diseases which are notifiable (Schedule 3) including Silicosis, Anthracosis, Byssinosis, Asbestosis.

89. **Ans. (d) Depends on type of exposure** *[Ref. Park 27/e p930]*
    - The frequency and content of periodic medical examinations depend upon the type of occupational exposure
    - *Periodic Medical Examination:* (for industrial workers) is held at appropriate intervals to test their physical and mental efficiency and to detect any departure from health at the earliest; objective being early diagnosis and prompt treatment (Secondary level of prevention). Frequency of periodic examinations:
        - Annual: for most of occupational exposures
        - Monthly: for lead, radium and dye-stuffs exposure
        - Daily: for dichromates exposure

90. **Ans. (b) 1000** *[Ref. Park 27/e p942]*
    - *The Factories Act, 1948:*
        - Health, Safety and Welfare recommendations:
            1. A minimum of 500 cubic feet space per worker
            2. 1 Safety Officer per 1000 workers
            3. 1 Welfare Officer per 500 workers
            4. 1 Canteen for greater than 250 workers
            5. 1 Crèche for greater than 30 women workers

91. **Ans. (a) Coproporphyrin in urine** *[Ref. Park 27/e p934–935]*
    - Diagnosis of lead poisoning:

Laboratory parameter	Remark
Coproporphyrin in Urine (CPU) >150 mcg/l	Exposure to lead
Amino levulinic acid in urine (ALAU) >5 mg/l	Indicates lead absorption
Lead in blood >70 mcg/100 mL	Clinical symptoms appear
Lead in urine >0.8 mg/l	Lead exposure and absorption
Basophilic stippling of RBCs	Punctate basophilia

> **ALSO REMEMBER**
> - A useful screening test is Coproporphyrin in Urine (CPU)
> - Lead Poisoning is known as 'Plumbism', Saturnism or Painter's Colic
> - *Clinical picture of lead poisoning:*
>   - Facial pallor: Earliest and most consistent sign
>   - Anemia: Microcytic hypochromic
>   - Punctate basophilia or basophilic stippling of RBCs
>   - Burtonian Line: Lead sulphide line on gums (upper jaw)
>   - Lead colic: Constipation (but sometimes diarrhea)
>   - Lead Palsy (Peripheral neuropathy): Wrist drop or Foot drop
>   - Lead encephalopathy
>   - CNS effects: mostly due to organic lead compounds
> - Clinical symptoms of plumbism occur when lead level in blood >70 mcg/100 mL
> - A sensitive parameter of hematological response is Basophilic stippling of RBCs.

92. **Ans. (a) Inhalation** *[Ref. Park 27/e p934]*
    - Greatest source of lead in Lead Poisoning (Plumbism, Saturnism or Painter's Colic) is Gasoline/petrol/vehicular exhaust/automobile exhaust
    - Mode of absorption: Lead can be absorbed by inhalation (most common mode), ingestion or through skin

93. **Ans. (a) Bagassosis** *[Ref. Park 27/e p934]*
    - Bagassosis occurs due to occupational exposure to fibrous residue of sugarcane (bagasse); Bagassosis has been shown to be due to Thermoactinomyces sacchari
    - Bagasse contains a percentage of silica, innumerable fungal spores and micro-organisms; Bagasse dust blocks bronchioles thus leading to bronchitis and bronchopneumonia
    - *Prevention and Bagasse control measures:*
        - Keeping moisture content >20%
        - Spraying bagasse with 2% propionic acid (fungicide).

> **ALSO REMEMBER**
> - Bagassosis is a form of extrinsic allergic alveolitis
> - *Organisms involved in causation of bagassosis:*
>   - Thermoactinomyces sacchari
>   - Thermoactinomyces vulgaris
>   - Micropolyspora faeni.

94. **Ans. (a) High sputum AFB +ve** *[Ref. Park 27/e p933]*
    - Patients with silicosis are particularly susceptible to tuberculosis (TB) infection, known as 'Silicotuberculosis' (ST)
        - The reason for the increased risk, 10–30 fold increased incidence, is not well understood
        - It is thought that silica damages pulmonary macrophages, inhibiting their ability to kill mycobacteria

- In recent years doubts have risen in the association between silicois and tuberculosis as:
  - Sputum is rarely AFB+
  - Children and women of STs do not develop tuberculosis
  - Post mortem of STs fail to prove existence of tuberculosis
  - Radiological evidence of both conditions is similar.

> **ALSO REMEMBER**
> - Among the occupational diseases, silicosis is the major cause of permanent disability and mortality
> - Particles of the size 0.5–3 microns are most dangerous for causation of silicosis
> - IP: Few months to 6 years
> - X-ray shows 'snow storm appearance'
> - No effective treatment is available
> - Silicosis is a notifiable disease under Factories Act, 1948 and Mines Act 1952.

95. Ans. (b) Prickles

[Foundations of Community Medicine, 1/e p318]

- Disease manifestations associated with physical hazards:
  - High Temperature
    1. Heat cramps
    2. Heat hyperpyrexia (body temperature <102°F)
    3. Heat exhaustion (body temperature >106°F)
    4. Heat stroke (body temperature up to 110°F)
  - Low Temperature
    1. Chilblains
    2. Trench Foot
    3. Frost bite
  - Low Pressure
    1. Caisson Disease
  - Vibration
    1. Vibration sickness
    2. Neurogenic damage
  - Non-ionizing Radiation
  - Microwave Injuries
  - Laser injuries
- Prickles: Irritation of nerve terminals in skin due to nitrogen bubbles as seen in Caisson Disease (low pressure).

> **ALSO REMEMBER**
> - *Caisson Disease (Decompression Sickness, DCS):* Occurs due to low pressure, when a diver ascends rapidly to surface or air passengers ascend too rapidly to high altitudes
>   - Manifestations of air expansion:
>   1. *Barodontalgia:* Air trapped beneath teeth expands
>   2. *Barosinusitis:* Compressed air trapped in sinuses expands
>   3. *Barotitis:* Air under pressure trapped in middle ear expands
>   4. *Emphysema:* Most serious complication (may lead to cerebral embolism)
>   5. *Abdominal distension:* Air trapped in intestinal canal expands
>
> *Contd...*

Contd...
> - Effects of Nitrogen effervescence:
>   1. Bends: Steady aching pain in joints
>   2. Chokes: Rapid, shallow, dyspneic breathing
>   3. Prickles: Irritation of nerve terminals in skin
>   4. Paralysis: Most serious complication
>   5. Aseptic bone necrosis: Hip, knee and shoulder joints
> - Caisson Disease is a type of diving hazard and dysbarism.
> - Recompression is the only effective treatment for severe DCS, although rest and oxygen applied to lighter cases can be effective.
> - Gases implicated in DCS:
>   - Nitrogen
>   - Trimix (nitrogen + oxygen + helium)
>   - Heliox (oxygen + helium).

96. Ans. (d) A-III B-II C-IV D-I [Ref. Park 27/e p944]

97. Ans. (c) 500 cu ft [Ref. Park 27/e p942]

- *The Factories Act, 1948:*
  - Scope: The Act defines factory as an establishment employing 10 or more persons where power is used and 20 or more persons where power is not used.

98. Ans. (c) 5 rem per year [Ref. Park 27/e p870–872]

RADIATION EXPOSURE:

- International Commission of Radiological Protection (ICRP) has set the maximum permissible level of whole body occupational exposure to ionizing radiation at '5 rem per year for workers' AND at '0.5 rem per year for general public'
- *ICRPs set of recommendations for radiation exposure:*
  - Any tissue or organ dose less than 50 rem per year
  - Lens of the eye dose less than 15 rem per year
  - Whole body dose less than 5 rem per year
  - Lifetime average dose less than 1 rem per year.

> **ALSO REMEMBER**
> - Radiation poisoning, also called 'radiation sickness' or a 'creeping dose', is a form of damage to organ tissue due to excessive exposure to ionising radiation
> - 1 Sv = 100 rem
>   1 Gray = 100 rad
> - For b–particles, X-rays and g-rays, rad and rem are equivalent
>   For α–particles, 1 rad is equivalent to 20 rem
> - Cow's milk contain a soluble radioactive substance: ^{90}Sr
> - *Radiation exposure and effects:*
>
> | Dose (rem) | Effects | Signs and symptoms |
> |---|---|---|
> | 5–20 | No symptoms | — |
> | 20–50 | No symptoms generally | Temporary ↓ in RBC count |
> | 50–100 | Mild radiation sickness | Headache, ↑ infection risk, temporary male sterility |
> | 100–200 | Light radiation poisoning | Vomiting, fatigue, ↓ immunity, spontaneous abortion, stillbirth |
>
> *Contd...*

Contd...

Dose (rem)	Effects	Signs and symptoms
200–300	Moderate radiation poisoning	Loss of hair, massive leucopenia, permanent female sterility
300–400	Severe radiation poisoning	-do-
		Uncontrollable bleeding in mouth, under skin, kidneys
400–600	Acute radiation poisoning (severity)	-do-
600–1,000	Acute radiation poisoning	Complete bone marrow failure
1000–5000	Acute radiation poisoning	Massive diarrhea, bleeding, dyselectrolytemia, delirium, death
>5000	Acute radiation poisoning	Death

99. Ans. (d) Vibration *[Ref. Park 27/e p931]*
- After some months or years of exposure to vibrations (10–500 Hz), the fine blood vessels of fingers may become extremely sensitive to spasm, known as 'White fingers'.
- White fingers are a form of Raynaud's Disease. Vibration white finger is the vascular component of 'hand-arm vibration syndrome (HAVS)'.

100. Ans. (b) <5 micron *[Ref. Park 27/e p933]*
- Pneumoconiosis occur due to occupational exposure to dust. Particles size 0.5 to 3.0 microns are the most dangerous (as a health hazard causing pneumoconiosis), as they reach the interior of lungs with ease.
- *Particle size and behavior:*

Particle size	Behavior
>10 microns	Settle down by gravity
<10 microns	Remain suspended in air
5–10 microns	Arrested in upper respiratory tract
3–5 microns	Deposited in mid respiratory tract
1–3 microns	Enter alveoli and settle there (cause pneumoconioses)
<1 microns	Brownian movement

101. Ans. (c) Farmer's lung *[Ref. Park 27/e p934]*
- Farmer's Lung is due to inhalation of mouldy hay or grain dust. Micropolyspora faeni (Saccharopolyspora rectivirgula) is the main cause of farmer's lung.

102. Ans. (a) Greatest source is drinking water from lead pipes *[Ref. Park 27/e p934]*
- *Source of lead:* Greatest source of environmental (non-occupational) lead is Gasoline/petrol/vehicular exhaust/automobile exhaust
- *Mode of absorption:* Lead can be absorbed by inhalation (most common), ingestion or through skin.

ALSO REMEMBER
- A useful screening test is Coproporphyrin in Urine (CPU)
- A sensitive parameter of hematological response is Basophilic stippling of RBCs
- Plumbism (lead poisoning) can cause Burtonian's line (Blue Line on gums).

103. Ans. (b) Naphthylamines *[Ref. Park 27/e p935]*
- Cancer bladder was first noted in man in Aniline industry in 1895
- *Now following has been mentioned as possible bladder carcinogens:*
  - β-naphthylamines
  - Benzidine
  - Paraamino-diphenyl
  - Auramine
  - Magenta
- Industries associated with cancer bladder are dye-stuffs and dyeing industry, rubber, gas and electric cable industry

ALSO REMEMBER
- The most common symptom of cancer of the bladder is blood in the urine (haematuria)
  - Most common type of Ca-bladder (90%) is Transitional Cell (urothelial cell) carcinoma (TCC)
- Tobacco use (specifically cigarette smoking) is thought to cause 50% of bladder cancers discovered in male patients and 30% of those found in female patients
- Certain drugs such as cyclophosphamide and phenacetin are known to predispose to bladder TCC
- Immunotherapy in the form of 'Intravesical (pharmacotherapeutic) BCG instillation' is also used to treat and prevent the recurrence of superficial tumors.

104. Ans. (b) Occupational Health *[Ref. Park 27/e p939]*
- Pre-placement Examination: Is the foundation of an efficient occupational health service. It is done at the time of employment and includes worker's history (medical, family, occupational and social), physical examination and biological and radiological examinations.
- Main purpose of Pre-placement Examination is to place 'the right man in right job'; so that worker can perform his duties efficiently without detriment to his health (Ergonomics).
- Pre-placement Examination also serves as a useful benchmark for future comparison (examination and epidemiology).

ALSO REMEMBER
- *Ergonomics (human factors):* Is the application of scientific information concerning objects, systems and environment for human use.

105. Ans. (c) 91 days *[Ref. Park 27/e p943]*

THE EMPLOYEES STATE INSURANCE (ESI) ACT, 1948: (NEW GUIDELINES)
- *Scope of ESI Act:* The act covers all the factories in India 'excluding mines, defence, railways'. The Act in the first

instance applies to all non-seasonal factories, employing 10 or more persons, for wages on any day in implemented areas. (Now included education)
- It covers all employees getting up to ₹ 21,000/- per month
- *Finance:* The employer contributes 4.75% of total wage bill; the employee contributes 1.75% of wages. State and Central Government share medical expenditure in ration of 1:7
- *Sickness Benefits to employees under ESI:*
  - *Sickness benefit:* 90% of the average daily wages and is payable for 91 days (in any continuous period of 365 days).
  - *Extended sickness benefit:* Payable for 2 years for a set of 34 diseases
  - *Enhanced sickness benefit:* Full average daily wage for duration upto 7 days in the case of Vasectomy and up to 14 days in the case of the Tubectomy.

ALSO REMEMBER
- The per capita cost of medical benefit under ESI scheme was ₹ 905/- in 2001–02
- To become eligible to Sickness Benefit, one should have paid contribution for not less than 78 days during the corresponding contribution period
- Employees in receipt of a daily average wage up to ₹ 100/- are exempted from payment of contribution; Employers will however contribute their own share in respect of these employees
- Rajiv Gandhi Shramik Kalyan Yojana (under ESI): Unemployment allowance (at 50% wages for maximum 2 years) for employees who are rendered unemployed involuntarily due to closure of factory.

106. Ans. (d) State of health of the workers *[Ref. Park 27/e p937]*

SICKNESS ABSENTEEISM:
- Sickness absenteeism is a 'useful index in industry to assess the state of health of workers', and their physical, mental and social well-being
- Rate of absenteeism reported in India: 8–10 days per worker per year.

107. Ans. (c) Lead poisoning is not a notifiable disease
[Ref. Park 27/e p934–935]

108. Ans. (a) Occurs within five years of exposure
[Ref. Park 27/e p934]
- Asbestosis is a pneumoconiosis which occurs due to exposure to asbestos
- Asbestosis does not usually appear until after 5–10 years of exposure. Once established, the disease is progressive even after removal of worker from contact
- Sputum shows 'asbestos bodies', which are asbestos fibres coated with fibrin
- Asbestos may lead to pulmonary fibrosis, carcinoma of bronchus, mesothelioma of peritoneum/pleura and cancer of GIT
- Asbestos type most dangerous is 'amphibole'.

ALSO REMEMBER
- *List of Pneumoconioses:*

Disease	Exposure source
Silicosis	Silica dust
Anthracosis	Coal dust
Asbestosis	Asbestos dust
Byssinosis	Cotton fibre
Bagassosis	Molasses (sugarcane)
Berylliosis	Beryllium
Farmer's Lung	Mouldy hay
Siderosis	Iron dust
Stannosis	Tin dust
Bird fancier's lung	Avian/bird droppings
Compost lung	Compost

- *Antigens involved in Pneumoconioses:*

Disease	Antigen
Bagassosis	Thermoactinomyces sacchari
Farmer's Lung	Micropolyspora faeni
Compost lung	Aspergillus
Chemical workers lung	Isocyanates

- Pneumoconioses occur due to occupational exposure to dust, especially of the size 0.5–3.0 microns diameter Most Dangerous particle size)
- Coal workers lung is known as 'black lung'
- Silicosis is known as 'grinder's disease'.

109. Ans. (d) 2% propionic acid *[Ref. Park 27/e p934]*

110. Ans. (d) Ether *[Ref. Davidson's, 20/e p1285, Park 27/e p936]*

111. Ans. (a) Lead; (d) Agricultural insecticides
[Ref. Sittig's Handbook of Pesticides and Agricultural Chemicals by Stanley A. Greene, 1/e p319]

112. Ans. (c) Union Minister of Labour *[Ref. Park 27/e p943]*

113. Ans. (a) Applicable on educational institutions also
[Ref. Park 27/e p942–943]

114. Ans. (b) A worker with income less than 70/- per day has to pay only 300/- per month; (c) Funeral expenses is 50,000/- *[Ref. Park 27/e p942–945]*
- Under ESI, a worker with income below 100/- per day is exempted from payment of contribution
- Under ESI, Funeral expenses are Rs 10000/-

115. Ans. (b) 1000 *[Ref. Park 27/e p943]*

ESI NORMS:
- Setting up of one Doctor Dispensary: ≥1000 Family units
- Setting up of Two Doctor Dispensary: ≥2000 Family units
- Setting up of Diagnostic centers: ≥5000 Family units
- Setting up of 100 Bedded Hospital: ≥15000 Family units

116. Ans. (b) Leukaemia *[Ref. Park 25/e p845–846]*
- *Occupational exposures leading to Leukemia:*
  - Benzol
  - X-rays
  - Radioactive substances

117. **Ans. (a) A4 B3 C2 D1** *[Ref. Master Differential Diagnosis: Internal Medicine by Argento 1/e p101]*
- Wood worker's lung is associated with Oak, Cedar, Pine, Mahogany dust.

118. **Ans. (c) Ministry of Labour** *[Ref. Park 25/e p853]*
- Chairperson of ESI Corporation: Union Minister of Labour
- Vice-chairperson of ESI Corporation: Secretary to Govt. of India, Minister of Labour

> **ALSO REMEMBER**
> - Chief executive officer of ESI Corporation: Director General, assisted by 4 principal officers:
>   - Insurance commissioner
>   - Medical commissioner
>   - Financial commissioner
>   - Actuary

119. **Ans. (d) Related to criteria for PHC** *[Ref. Park 27/e p930]*

120. **Ans. (a) Sickness; (c) Maternal; (e) Funeral** *[Ref. Park 25/e p853]*
- ESI benefits include Sickness benefit (and Extended sickness benefit, Enhanced sickness benefit), Maternity benefit, Disablement benefit (Temporary disablement benefit, Permanent disablement benefit), Dependent's benefit, Funeral expenses, Rehabilitation expenses, Confinement expenses.

121. **Ans. (a) Children aged less than 14 years are prohibited from any employment** *[Ref. Park 27/e p942]*
   The Factory Act, 1948
- No child <14 years age shall be required or allowed to work in any factory
- A child >14 years age or an adolescent (15–18 years age) shall allowed to work in any factory if they get a certificate of fitness from a Surgeon
- No child shall be employed to work in any factory for >4 ½ hours in any day and during night
- No female child shall be allowed to work in any factory except between 8AM to 7PM
- No female/male adolescent shall be allowed to work except between 6AM to 7PM
- Women and children cannot be employed in dangerous works

Review Questions

122. **Ans. (b) Textile industries** *[Ref. Park 27/e p933]*
123. **Ans. (b) Heat cramps** *[Ref. Internet]*
124. **Ans. (b) 4.75%** *[Ref. Park 27/e p943]*
125. **Ans. (a) Battery industry** *[Ref. Park 27/e p934–935]*
126. **Ans. (b) Silicosis** *[Ref. Park 27/e p933]*
127. **Ans. (d) Defence establishment** *[Ref. Park 27/e p942–943]*
128. **Ans. (b) Non power using factories with 18 members** *[Ref. Park 27/e p942–943]*
129. **Ans. (b) 500 cu. feet minimum space required per person** *[Ref. Park 27/e p942]*
130. **Ans. (b) Silicosis** *[Ref. Park 27/e p933]*
131. **Ans. (a) Brucellosis** *[Ref. Park 27/e p933]*
132. **Ans. (d) Exemption from sales tax** *[Ref. Park 27/e p943–945]*
133. **Ans. (b) <48 hours** *[Ref. Park 27/e p942]*
134. **Ans. (b) 0.5–3** *[Ref. Park 27/e p933]*
135. **Ans. (a) 1/8** *[Ref. Park 27/e p943]*
136. **Ans. (d) Psittacosis** *[Ref. Park 27/e p933–934]*
137. **Ans. (b) Lead** *[Ref. Reproductive Endocrinology and Infertility by Carrell & Peterson, /e p800]*
138. **Ans. (d) 70 mcg/100 mL blood** *[Ref. Park 27/e p935]*
139. **Ans. (b) 4.75%** *[Ref. Park 27/e p943]*
140. **Ans. (a) Adjusting the Worker to his job** *[Ref. Park 27/e p930]*
141. **Ans. (d) 2 years** *[Ref. Park 27/e p944]*
142. **Ans. (d) Breast ca** *[Ref. Park 27/e p935–936]*
143. **Ans. (b) Anthrax** *[Ref. Workman's Compensation Act, 1923 document]*
144. **Ans. (b) Medical benefit** *[Ref. Park 27/e p943–945]*
145. **Ans. (b) 100% wages in temporary disability; (c) Extended sickness benefit 91 days** *[Ref. Park 27/e p942–945]*

GENETICS

146. **Ans. (c) It uses modern next generation sequencing techniques; (d) It took more than 2 decades to complete** *[Ref. Park 26/e p921]*

   Human Genome Project (HGP) 1 Oct 1990–14 Apr 2003
- Project began in 1990 initially headed by James D. Watson
- Primary goals: To determine the sequence of chemical base pairs which make up DNA and to identify the approximately 25,000 genes of the human genome (Later found 19,500 genes)
- Ongoing sequencing led to the announcement of the essentially complete genome in April 2003
- International Human Genome Sequencing Consortium: The sequencing of the human genome involved researchers from 20 separate universities and research centers across 6 countries - United States, United Kingdom, France, Germany, Japan and China
- Two techniques used in HGP: Maxam gilbert technique (breaking the DNA strands at specific bases) and Sanger technique (chain-termination technique)

147. **Ans. (c) Population genetics** *[Ref. Park 27/e p954]*
- *Hardy Weinberg Law*: States that the genotype frequencies in a population remain constant or are in equilibrium from generation to generation unless specific disturbing influences are introduced.
- Genetic equilibrium (HW law) is a basic principle of population genetics; the entire principle is based on Mendelian genetics.
- *Deviations in HW law*: HW law fails to apply in:
  - Non-random mating (assortative mating)

- New mutations
- Genetic drift
- Gene flow
- Natural selection (mortality selection, fecundity selection)
- Small populations
- Migrations
- Dynamic populations
- HW law assumes that human population is static, large and has random mating.

148. **Ans. (c) Identify genes and sequence of base pairs in DNA of human genome** [Ref. Park 27/e p953]

    HUMAN GENOME PROJECT (HGP)
    - *Human Genome Project:* HGP is an international scientific research project
    - Primary goals were to determine the sequence of chemical base pairs which make up DNA and to identify the approximately 25,000 genes of the human genome
      - They also want to understand it and complete a map of all their findings
    - The project began in 1990 initially headed by James D. Watson
    - Ongoing sequencing led to the announcement of the essentially complete genome in April 2003
    - The goals of the original HGP were not only to determine more than 3 billion base pairs in the human genome, but also to identify all the genes in this vast amount of data
      - This part of the project is still ongoing, although a preliminary count indicates about 22,000–23,000 genes in the human genome.

    ALSO REMEMBER
    - *Genome:* The sum total of genetic information of an individual which is encoded in structure of DNA
    - *Genomics:* Is the study of genome
    - *Gene Therapy:* Introduction of a gene sequence into a cell to modify its behavior
    - Development of new diagnostic techniques such as restriction enzymes is a component of DNA Technology

149. **Ans. (a) 14th week of gestation** [Ref. Park 27/e p956]
    - *Amniocentesis:* Examination of a sample of amniotic fluid makes possible the prenatal diagnosis of chromosomal anomalies and certain metabolic defects; The procedure can be used as early as 14th week of pregnancy when abortion of affected fetus is still feasible
      - Culture and karyotyping of fetal cells from amniotic fluid is used for diagnosis of fetal anomalies
      - Biochemical analysis of amniotic fluid is used for diagnosis of metabolic effects
    - *Amniocentesis is indicated in following circumstances:*
      - A mother aged >35 years (high risk of Down's Syndrome)
      - Patients who have had a child with Down's Syndrome or other chromosomal anomalies
      - Parents known to have chromosomal translocation
      - Patients who have had a child with metabolic defect
      - When sex-determination is warranted

ALSO REMEMBER
- Various genetic testing may be performed, but the three most common abnormalities tested for are
  - Down's syndrome
  - Trisomy 18
  - Spina bifida

150. **Ans. (c) Euthenics** [Ref. Park 27/e p955]
    - *Eugenics (Sir Francis Galton):* Is a social philosophy which advocates the improvement of human hereditary traits through various forms of intervention (Genetic Manipulation).
    - *Euthenics:* Deals with human improvement through altering external factors such as education and the controllable environment, including the prevention and removal of contagious disease and parasites, environmentalism, education regarding home economics, sanitation, and housing (Environmental Manipulation).

    ALSO REMEMBER
    - Earlier proposed means of achieving eugenic goals focused on selective breeding, while modern ones focus on prenatal testing and screening, genetic counseling, birth control, in vitro fertilization, and genetic engineering
    - Euthenics is a pre-requisite for Eugenics
    - *Dysgenics:* Is a term describing the progressive evolutionary 'weakening' or genetic deterioration of a population of organisms relative to their environment.

151. **Ans. (c) 0.7 mg/litre** [Ref. Internet]
    - Level of residual chlorine to be maintained in all water bodies in post-disaster phase is >0.7 mg/l (>0.7 ppm).

    ALSO REMEMBER
    - Level of residual chlorine to be maintained in drinking water is >0.5 mg/l (>0.5 ppm) for a contact period of 1 hour
    - Level of residual chlorine to be maintained for swimming pool sanitation is >1.0 mg/l (>1.0 ppm).

152. **Ans. (a) Hypertension; (c) Manic depressive psychosis** [Ref. Park 21/e p762, Park 22/e p766]
153. **Ans. None** [Ref. Park 27/e p954]
154. **Ans. (d) Ataxia telengiectasia** [Ref. Park 27/e p950]
155. **Ans. (b) Prospective genetic counselling** [Ref. Park 27/e p955]

    GENETIC COUNSELLING:
    - *Prospective genetic counselling*: Identify heterozygous individuals for any particular defect (though screening) and explaining to them risk if having affected children, if they marry another heterozygote for same gene
      - *Useful in*: Thalassemia, Sickle cell anemia
    - *Retrospective genetic counselling*: Seeking genetic advice after hereditary disorder has already occurred in the family
      - *Useful in*: Congenital anomalies, Mental retardation, Psychiatric illness, Inborn errors of metabolism

156. **Ans. (c) Increased risk of traits controlled by dominant genes** [Ref. Park 27/e p979]

    Consanguineous Marriages
    - When blood relatives marry each other
    - Increased risk in offspring of traits controlled by recessive genes, determined by polygenes
    - Increased risk of premature death
    - Lowering of consanguineous marriages will improve community health
    - Examples: Albinism, Alkaptonuria

Review Questions

157. **Ans. (a) The study** [Ref. Park 27/e p954–955]
158. **Ans. (c) Hardy Weinberg law** [Ref. Park 27/e p954]
159. **Ans. (b) Random mating** [Ref. Park 27/e p954]
160. **Ans. (a) Wilson's disease; (c) Thalassemia; (e) ABO blood groups system** [Ref. Park 27/e p950]
161. **Ans. (c) Euthenics** [Ref. Park 27/e p955]

MENTAL HEALTH

162. **Ans. (b) Tobacco** [Ref. Park 27/e p962]
    - In India, about 47% of males and about 17% of females smoke.

    > **ALSO REMEMBER**
    > - *Cannabis:*
    >   - Is the *'most widely used drug today'* (Most commonly abused Narcotic substance)
    >   - *Most common reaction:* Dreamy state of altered consciousness
    >   - *Forms of Cannabis:*
    >   1. *Bhang:* Dried leaves and flowering shoots
    >   2. *Hashish/Charas:* Resinous exudates from flowering tops of the female plant
    >   3. *Ganja:* Resinous mass from small leaves and brackets of inflorescence
    >   4. *Marijuana:* Refer to any part of plant that induces somatic and psychic changes in man
    > - *Heroin:*
    >   - *'Heroin addiction is worst type of addiction'*
    >   - Heroin is Di-acetyl-morphine
    > - *Amphetamine:*
    >   - Synthetic drug structurally similar to adrenaline
    >   - Known as *'Superman drugs'*: Tremendous boost to energy and self-confidence.

163. **Ans. (c) Endocrine diseases** [Ref. Park 25/e p869]
    - Causes of mental health disorders:
      - *Organic conditions:* Cerebral arteriosclerosis, neoplasma, metabolic diseases, endocrine diseases and chronic diseases (TB, leprosy, epilepsy)
      - *Heredity:* Schizophrenia
      - *Socio-pathological:* Worries, anxiety, emotional stress, tension, frustration, unhappy married life, broken homes, poverty, industrialization, urbanization, cruelty, rejection, neglect, etc.

    > **ALSO REMEMBER**
    > - WHO analysis shows a global point prevalence of neuropsychiatric conditions is about 10% for adult
    >   - *MCC of DALYs lost:* Unipolar depressive disorders
    >   - *MCC of deaths:* Alzheimer's and other dementias
    >
    > *Contd...*
    >
    > - WHO analysis shows a global point prevalence of neuropsychiatric conditions is about 10% for adult
    >   - *MCC of DALYs lost:* Unipolar depressive disorders
    >   - *MCC of deaths:* Alzheimer's and other dementias
    > - *Mental morbidity in India:* 18–20 per 1000
    > - *DSM-IV Criteria:* Diagnostic and Statistical Manual of Mental Disorders, 4th Edition, Text Revision, DSM-IV-TR, is a manual published by the American Psychiatric Association (APA) that includes all currently recognized mental health disorders. The coding system utilized by the DSM-IV is designed to correspond with codes from the International Classification of Diseases, ICD.

164. **Ans. (b) Depression** [Ref. Park 27/e p959]
    - *DALYs lost due to mental disorders:*

Type of disorder	DALYs lost
Unipolar depressive disorders	64963
Alcohol disorders	18469
Schizophrenia	15686
Bipolar affective disorders	13645
Alzeihmer's dementia	12464
Migraine	7539
Epilepsy	7067

165. **Ans. (d) Screening** [Ref. Park 25/e p497]

    DISTRICT MENTAL HEALTH PROGRAM (DMHP)
    - Launched under NMHP in 1996 (IX Five Year Plan)
    - DMHP was based on 'Bellary Model' with the following components:
      - Early detection and treatment
      - Training: Imparting short-term training to general physicians for diagnosis and treatment of common mental illnesses with limited number of drugs under guidance of specialist; Health workers are being trained in identifying mentally ill persons
      - IEC: Public awareness generation
      - Monitoring: The purpose is for simple Record Keeping.

MISCELLANEOUS

166. **Ans. (c) Finding genotype of offspring** [Ref. Internet, Wikipedia]

    PUNNETT SQUARE
    - Is a diagram that is used to predict the result of a cross/breeding experiment
    - Is representing summary of every possible combination of each maternal allele with paternal allele for each gene studied in square
    - Is used by biologists 'to determine the probability of an offspring having a particular genotype'
    - Can be used for both monohybrid and dihybrid cross
    - Are standard tools for genetic counsellors
    - *Typical example of a Punnett square:*

	Y	y
Y	YY	Yy
y	Yy	yy

167. **Ans. (d) Recycling** [Ref. Electronic Waste Management by RE Hester, Volume 27, p111]

CHAPTER 13

Health Education and Communication

HEALTH COMMUNICATION

Communication Process
- *Communication process:* Process of exchanging ideas, feelings and information
- *Components of communication process^Q:*
  - Sender (source)
  - Message (content)
  - Feedback (effect)
  - Receiver (audience)
  - Channel(s) (medium)

TYPES OF COMMUNICATION

1. *One-way Communication Vs Two-way Communication:*
   - *One-way communication (Didactic Method^Q):* Flow of communication is one way–from communicator to audience
     - *Disadvantages of one-way communication^Q:*
       a. Knowledge is imposed and learning authoritative
       b. Little audience participation and no feedback
       c. Does not influence human behaviour
       d. Makes no attempt at removing misconceptions and misunderstandings
       e. Communicates message even if unintelligible or unacceptable
       f. Autocratic process
     - *Examples of one-way communication^Q:*
       a. Lecture method (Chalk and talk method)
       b. Television
       c. Radio
       d. Newsprint

   > **Key points**
   > One-way communication
   > **(Didactic Method)**

   - *Two-way communication (Socratic Method^Q):* Two way communication in which both the communicator and the audience take part
     - *Advantages of two-way communication^Q:*
       a. Active participatory and democratic process
       b. More likely to influence human behaviour
       c. Better audience participation and feedback
     - *Examples of two-way communication^Q:*
       a. Focus Group Discussion (FGD)
       b. Symposium
       c. Panel discussion

   > **Key points**
   > Two-way communication
   > **(Socratic Method)**

2. *Verbal Communication Vs Non-verbal Communication:*
   - *Verbal Communication:* Face-to-Face communication
     - *Advantages of verbal communication:*
       a. May be loaded with hidden meanings
       b. Persuasive
   - *Non-verbal Communication:* Indirect interaction
     - *Advantages of non-verbal communication:*
       a. Silence speaks louder than words
3. *Other Types of Communication:*
   - *Formal Communication:* Follows line of authority

- *Non-formal Communication:* Grape-vine communications
- *Advantages:* May be more active than formal channels
- *Visual Communication:* Comprises charts, graphs, pictograms, tables, maps, posters.

COMMUNICATION METHODS

Audio-visual Aids

- *Audiovisual aids:* No health education can be effective without audiovisual aids
- *Auditory aids:* Radio, cassette tape-recorder, microphone, amplifier, earphone, public address system, disks
- *Visual aids:*
  - *Not requiring projection:* Chalk-board, leaflets, posters, charts, flannelgraph, exhibits, models, specimens, diagrams, photographs
  - *Requiring projection:* Slides, filmstrips, overhead projector, epidiascope
- *Combined A-V aids[Q]:* Television, sound films (cinema, synchronized slide-tape combination, multimedia, videotape system, drama, skits)

Delphi Method

- *Delphi method[Q]:* Is a 'systematic interactive forecasting method' for obtaining consensus forecasts from a panel of independent geographically dispersed experts
- *Method:*
  - Carefully selected experts answer questionnaires in two or more rounds
  - After each round, a facilitator provides an anonymous summary of the experts' forecasts from the previous round as well as the reasons they provided for their judgments
  - Thus, participants are encouraged to revise their earlier answers in light of the replies of other members of the group
  - Range of the answers decrease and the group will converge towards the 'correct' consensual answer
  - Finally, the process is stopped after a pre-defined stop criterion (e.g. number of rounds, achievement of consensus, stability of results) and the mean or median scores of the final rounds determine the results
- *The objective of most Delphi applications:* Reliable and creative exploration of ideas or the production of suitable information for decision making

Counselling

- *Definition:* Counselling is face-to-face communication through which a person is helped to make a decision or solve a problem[Q]
- Counselling helps clients make informed choices
- COUNSELLING IS DIFFERENT FROM ADVICE: In Counselling, 'Choice is given to clients'[Q]
- *Elements of Counselling:* (**GATHER** Approach[Q])
  - *G:* Greet the clients (make them comfortable, give attention)
  - *A:* Ask/ascertain needs/problems or reasons for coming
  - *T:* Telling different methods/options/choices to solve the problem
  - *H:* Help client to make voluntary decisions
  - *E:* Explain fully the chosen decision/action/method
  - *R:* Return for follow-up visit
- GATHER Approach can be used for counselling about contraceptives

Group Approach to Health Education

1. *Chalk and Talk (Lecture):*
   - For effective communication through lecture method[Q]:
     - Group size should be <30

> **Key points**
> Counselling helps clients make informed choices

> **Key points**
> Elements of Counselling:
> **G:** Greet
> **A:** Ask
> **T:** Tell
> **H:** Help
> **E:** Explain
> **R:** Return visit

- Talk duration <15–20 minutes
- Combine with flip charts, flannelgraphs, exhibits, films and charts
- *Advantages of lecture method*^Q:
  - Most economical method
  - Information transfer in a short time to a large group
  - Less preparation and minimal resources
- *Disadvantages of lecture method:*
  - Learning is passive; does not motivate
  - Suitable only for small groups
  - Students are involved to minimal extent
  - Do not stimulate thinking or problem solving capacity
  - Comprehension and retention varies with student
  - Health behaviour of listeners not necessarily affected

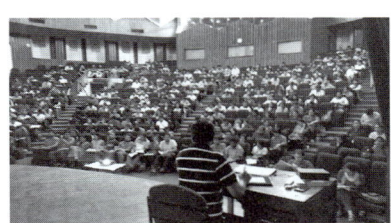
Lecture

2. *Demonstrations:*
   - *Definition:* Is a carefully planned presentation to show how to perform a skill or procedure
   - *Method:* Demonstrator carries out step-by-step in font of an audience and involves them
   - *Advantages:*
     - Dramatises by arousing interest
     - Persuades onlookers to adopt
     - Upholds principles of 'seeing is believing' and 'learning by doing'^Q
     - Can bring desirable changes in behaviour
     - High motivational value
   - *Utility:*
     - Environmental sanitation (hand pump installation, use of sanitary latrine)
     - MCH (ORS technique^Q)
     - Control of disease (Scabies)

Key points
Demonstrations: Upholds principles of 'seeing is believing' and 'learning by doing'

3. *Group Discussion:*
   - *Description:* A group is an aggregation of people interacting in a face-to-face situation^Q
   - *Advantages of group discussion:*
     - A very effective method of health communication
     - Well conducted group discussion is 'effective to change health behaviour and attitudes'^Q
     - Permits learning by free exchange of ideas, knowledge and opinions
     - Provides a wider interaction among members
     - Valuable to ensure long term compliance
   - *Ensuring an effective discussion:*
     - Group size of '6–12 members', including^Q
     - *1 group leader:* Initiates discussion, helps discussion in a proper manner, prevents side conversations, encourages everyone to participate and sums up the discussion
     - *1 recorder:* Record, report on issues discussed and agreements reached
     - *Rules to be followed*^Q:
     - Listen to what others are saying
     - Express ideas clearly and concisely
     - Do not interrupt when others are saying
     - Make only relevant remarks
     - Accept criticism gracefully
     - Help to reach conclusions
   - *Limitations of group discussion:*
     - *Unequal participation:* Those shy may not take part in discussion while some may dominate the discussion
     - Some may deviate from the subject and make the GD irrelevant or unprofitable

Key points
Well conducted group discussion is 'effective to change health behaviour and attitudes'

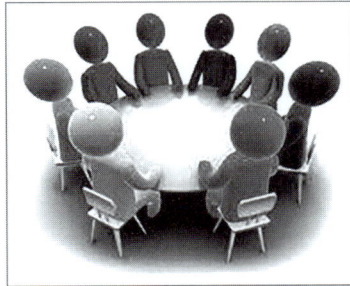
Focus group discussion

4. *Panel Discussion:*
   - *Features of a panel discussion:*
     - '4–8 persons' who are qualified to talk about the topic sit and discuss a given problem/topic in front of a target group or audience^Q
     - Panel comprises,
     - A chairman or moderator
     - 4–8 expert speakers
   - *Method of Panel discussion:*
     - The chairman introduces topic briefly and invites panel members to speak

Key points
Panel discussion: 'no specific agenda, no order of speaking and no set speeches'

- There is 'no specific agenda, no order of speaking and no set speeches'[Q]
- The success of panel depends on chairman; he makes it going and provides train of thought
- After speakers explore the topic, audience is invited to take part
- Panelists may have to have a preliminary meeting and prepare the material on the subject
- *Advantages of a panel discussion*[Q]:
  - Flexible, spontaneous; better understanding of various aspects, keeps audience alert
  - If properly planned and guided, panel discussion can be 'an extremely effective method of education'
- *Disadvantages of a panel discussion*[Q]:
  - Needs a thorough planning and preparation in advance
  - Panelists need to be of sufficient experience
  - Audience is usually passive

5. **Symposium:**
   - *Features of a symposium:*
     - A series of speeches/lectures on a selected subject[Q]
     - Each person or expert presents an aspect briefly
     - There is no discussion among symposium members[Q]
     - Audience may raise questions in the end
     - Chairman makes a comprehensive summary at the end of symposium
     - In an ideal symposium, there is no discussion in between presentations of speakers
   - *Advantages of a symposium*[Q]:
     - Transfers concise information to audience at one time
     - Audience remains alert (frequent change of speakers)
     - Analysis of different aspects of a topic at one time
     - Good tool for integrated teaching
   - *Disadvantage of a symposium:*
     - No discussion during symposium (Q and A at end)

6. **Workshop:**
   - *Features of workshop:*
     - A series of meetings usually >4[Q]
     - Emphasis is on individual work within the group to impart training[Q]
     - Help sought from consultants and resource personnel
     - Total workshop may be divided in to smaller groups; each group will choose a chairman and a recorder
     - Individuals solve a problem through personal effort with help of consultants, contribute to group work and group discussion and leave workshop with concrete suggestions and a 'plan of action' on problem[Q]
   - *Advantages of workshop:*
     - Learning takes place in a friendly, happy and democratic atmosphere, under expert guidance
     - Provides each participant an opportunity to improve his effectiveness a s a professional worker
   - *Disadvantages of workshop:*
     - Needs a lot of baseline ground work[Q]
     - Benefits a small no. of people

7. **Role-Playing (Socio-Drama):**
   - *Features of role-playing:*
     - Situation is dramatized by a group
     - Group enact as if they have observed/experienced it
     - Audience not passive; actively concerned with drama; can suggest alternative solutions at request of leader
     - Followed by discussion of the problem
     - *Ideal size of the group:* 25[Q]
   - *Advantages of role-playing:*
     - Useful to discuss problems of human relationships[Q]
     - Useful educational device for school children[Q]

8. **Conferences and Seminars:**
   - *Features of conferences and seminars:*
     - Contains a large component of commercialized continuing education
     - Usually held on a regional, state or national level[Q]
     - ½ day to 1 week in length
     - May cover a single topic in depth or be broadly comprehensive
     - Use variety of teaching formats: self instruction to mass media

> **Key points**
> **Symposium:** Series of speeches/lectures on a selected subject

> **Key points**
> **Workshop:** A series of meetings usually >4 to impart training

HEALTH EDUCATION

Health Education

- *Health Education:* The process by which individuals and groups of people learn to behave in a manner conducive to the promotion, maintenance or restoration of health (John M. Last)[Q]
- Changing concepts of Health Education (Alma – Ata Declaration, 1978):

Older emphasis	New emphasis[Q]
Prevention of disease	Promotion of healthy lifestyles
Modification of individual behaviour	Modification of social environment
Community participation	Community involvement
	Promotion of individual & community self reliance

Approaches to Health Education[Q]

- *Regulatory approach (Managed prevention):*
  - Defined as any Governmental intervention
  - Coercive approach or Legislative approach
  - Useful in times of emergency
- *Service approach:*
  - Providing health services at peoples' door step
  - Not based o felt needs
- *Health education approach:*
  - Slow but enduring results
- *Primary healthcare approach:*
  - Radically new approach[Q]
  - Community involvement and intersectoral coordination
  - Help individuals becomes self reliant in health

> **Key points**
> Primary healthcare approach: Radically new approach

Principles of Health Education[Q]

- Credibility
- Interest
- Participation
- Motivation
- Comprehension
- Reinforcement
- Learning by doing
- Known to unknown
- Setting an example
- Good human relations
- Feedback
- Leaders

Health Education versus Propaganda/Publicity

	Health education	Health propaganda
Knowledge and skills[Q]	Actively acquired	Instilled in minds
Promotion of thought process[Q]	Present	Absent
Primitive desires	Disciplines	Arouses
Behaviour developed[Q]	Reflective behaviour	Reflexive behaviour
Appeals to[Q]	Reason	Emotion
Develops	Individuality, personality	Set attitudes, behaviour
Knowledge acquired by	Self-reliant activity	Passive spoon-feeding
Process[Q]	Behaviour centred	Information centred

MISCELLANEOUS

Mass Media

- *Mass media:* TV, radio, printed media
  - Mass media are mainly a one-way communication (Didactic Methods)

> **Key points**
>
> Advantages of mass media: Reaches a relatively larger population in a shorter time

- *Advantages of mass media*[Q]:
  - Reaches a relatively larger population in a shorter time than with other means
  - Useful for message transmission even in remote areas
  - More influential with average and below average education level
  - Get public attention
- *Disadvantages of mass media*[Q]:
  - Being impersonal, not usually effective in changing established modes of behaviour if used alone
  - *One way communication:* Carry messages from centre to periphery; feedback mechanisms are poorly organized

Methods of Mass Media

> **Key points**
>
> *Television:* Most popular of all media

- *Television:*
  - Most popular of all media[Q]
  - Creates awareness, influence public opinions and introduce new ways of life
  - Raise levels of understanding
  - Has much potential for health communication
  - Not much opportunity for feedback and discussion
- *Radio:*
  - Purely didactic medium
  - Valuable aid in putting across health information
- *Internet*:
  - Fast growing communication media[Q]
  - Holds very large potential to become a major health education tool
- *Newspapers:*
  - Most widely disseminated of all forms of literature[Q]
  - Reach only to limited population (literates)
- *Printed material:*
  - Can convey detailed information
  - Produced in bulk at low cost, can be shared
- *Direct mailing:*
  - New innovation in health communication
- *Posters, billboards, signs:*
  - Can be displayed at public places
  - Less effective in changing behaviour
- Health museums and exhibitions
- Folk media

PYQs: Quick Review for NEET

Focus group discussion should have	6–12 members
Group addressed and lectures on specific topic by experts is	Symposium
A group of health experts discuss a health topic and audience	Panel discussion
Gather approach is used in	Contraceptive counseling
Series of speeches by experts but no discussion among speakers	Symposium
Education charts serially flashed to group as talk is being given	Flip charts

Multiple Choice Questions

HEALTH COMMUNICATION

1. Which of the following is the correct sequence of various components of the 'communication process'? [AIIMS Nov 1993]
   (a) Receiver, Message, Channel, Feedback, Sender
   (b) Sender, Feedback, Message, Channel, Receiver
   (c) Sender, Message, Channel, Receiver, Feedback
   (d) Message, Sender, Channel, Feedback, Receiver

TYPES OF COMMUNICATION

2. Lecture Method of teaching is a type of: [AIIMS June 92]
   (a) Socratic Method
   (b) Didactic Method
   (c) Non-verbal communication
   (d) Visual Communication

3. All of the following involve a two-way communication except: [AIIMS Dec 1991]
   (a) Symposium [Karnataka 2008]
   (b) Lecture [DNB 2010]
   (c) Panel discussion [NEET Pattern 2017]
   (d) Workshop

4. Which of the following is/are didactic methods of health communication? [PGI November 2013]
   (a) Group discussion   (b) Workshop
   (c) Demonstration   (d) Lecture
   (e) Panel discussion

5. Which of the following is the socratic method of teaching? [DNB 2008]
   (a) Lecture   (b) Films
   (c) Exhibition   (d) Panel discussion

6. In one of the method of health communication, 4 to 8 persons who are qualified to talk about the topic sit and discuss a given problem/topic in front of a large group or audience, this method is called as [PGMCET 2015] [DNB December 2011]
   (a) Symposium
   (b) Panel discussion
   (c) Workshop
   (d) Seminar

7. Total communication means: [NEET Pattern 2016]
   (a) Use of all methods of communication for advertisement
   (b) Use of all methods of communication for school teaching
   (c) Use of all methods of communication for community participation
   (d) Using every communication option to teach deaf child

Review Questions

8. An example of a two-way discussion is: [DNB 2003]
   (a) A seminar [NEET Pattern 2017]
   (b) Role playing
   (c) Symposium
   (d) Group discussion

9. Which of the following is the Socratic method of teaching? [DNB 2008]
   (a) Lecture   (b) Films
   (c) Exhibition   (d) Panel discussion

10. True about mass media education except: [RJ 2001]
    (a) Rapid
    (b) High rich content
    (c) Distorted information
    (d) Local community needs

11. Which is incorrect about socratic method? [RJ 2008]
    (a) Two way communication
    (b) Audience can raise question
    (c) Active and democratic
    (d) Audience can take part

COMMUNICATION METHODS

12. A tool for increasing consensus among a large no. of people is: [AIPGME 2006]
    (a) Chalk and talk (lecture)
    (b) Delphi method
    (c) Television
    (d) Interpersonal communication (IPC)

13. The most effective method for motivating a couple for adopting family planning practices is: [AIIMS Nov 01]
    (a) Printed material
    (b) Films and television
    (c) Group discussion
    (d) Interpersonal communication

14. All are a type of audio-visual aids except: [AIIMS June 1992]
    (a) Television
    (b) Cinema
    (c) Flannelgraph
    (d) Slide-tape combination

15. All are true for a group discussion except: [AIPGME 1991]
    (a) Not a very effective method of health communication
    (b) Ideally a group should comprise of 6–12 members
    (c) Can lead to change in health attitudes and behaviour
    (d) Allows free exchange of ideas and opinions

16. **Best method of teaching an urban slum about ORS is:**
    (a) Lecture [DPG 2005]
    (b) Role play [NEET Pattern 2013]
    (c) Demonstration
    (d) Flash cards

17. **All of the following facts are true with group discussion** *except*: [Karnataka 2006]
    (a) Group discussion is very effective method of health education
    (b) Group members should not have known each other before
    (c) The group should sit in a circle
    (d) There should be a group leader to initiate

18. **Panel discussion can be defined as:** [Karnataka 2007]
    (a) Series of speeches
    (b) Discussion by 4–8 qualified persons
    (c) Groups describing individual experiences
    (d) Stage wise formatted teaching

19. **All are true about Panel discussion** *except*: [NEET Pattern 2012]
    (a) Panel of 4–8 experts discuss a health topic
    (b) Audience is present
    (c) Specific order, Set speeches
    (d) Audience can take part

20. **Workshop is:** [NEET Pattern 2016]
    (a) Discussion of 4–8 experts in front of audience
    (b) Discussion between 6–12 members
    (c) Series of four or more meetings
    (d) Series of speeches on given subject

21. **'Cafeteria approach' is related with** [NEET Pattern 2018]
    (a) Diet program
    (b) Child and maternal health
    (c) National vector borne disease control program
    (d) Contraception

22. **SPIKES protocol is used for** [AIIMS November 2018]
    (a) Triage
    (b) Communication with patients/attendants regarding bad news
    (c) Writing death certificate
    (d) RCT

Review Questions

23. **Which method is used for HIV pretest counselling:** [DNB 2002]
    (a) Individual approach (b) Group approach
    (c) Mass media (d) All of the above

24. **Which method is used for HIV postest counselling:** [DNB 2005]
    (a) Individual approach (b) Group approach
    (c) Mass media (d) All of the above

HEALTH EDUCATION

25. **All of the following are approaches to health education** *except*: [AIIMS May 09]
    (a) Service approach
    (b) Regulatory approach
    (c) Health education approach
    (d) Mass media

26. **All of the following can be done with Individual as a unit** *except*: [AIPGME 2012]
    (a) Drug administration
    (b) Vaccination
    (c) Health education
    (d) Case report

27. **Which of the following statements refers to propaganda?** [Karnataka 2011]
    (a) Appeals to emotion
    (b) Develops individuality
    (c) The process is behaviour centered
    (d) Makes people think for themselves

28. **In which model of health education does 'internalization' occurs:** [AP 2014]
    (a) Medical model
    (b) Socio-environmental model
    (c) Service model
    (d) Motivation model

29. **Propaganda is defined as:** [NEET Pattern 2017]
    (a) Knowledge by active learning
    (b) Knowledge forced into the mind
    (c) Facilitates learning
    (d) Develops reflective behaviour

MISCELLANEOUS

30. **All are advantages of using mass media** *except*:
    (a) More influential with average and below average education level [AIPGME 1996]
    (b) Gives greater support for concentrated programmes
    (c) Get public attention
    (d) Reaches the widest population

31. **Most popular media for mass education of general public is:** [AIPGME 1998]
    (a) Television
    (b) Radio
    (c) Newspaper
    (d) Internet

32. **Loss of Interpersonal communication is managed by** [JIPMER November 2017]
    (a) Group counseling
    (b) Individual counseling
    (c) Check telecommunications
    (d) Improving language

Explanations

HEALTH COMMUNICATION

1. **Ans. (c) Sender, Message, Channel, Receiver, Feedback** *[Ref. Park 27/e p982]*
   - *Communication process*: Process of exchanging ideas, feelings and information
   - *Components of communication process*:
     – Sender (source)
     – Receiver (audience)
     – Message (content)
     – Channel(s) (medium)
     – Feedback (effect)

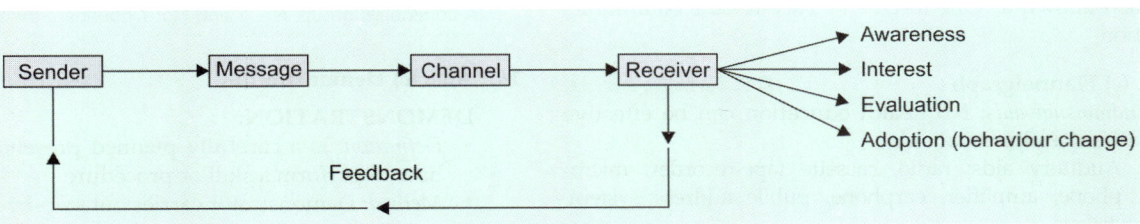

Communication process

TYPES OF COMMUNICATION

2. **Ans. (b) Didactic Method** *[Ref. Park 27/e p983]*

   TYPES OF COMMUNICATION:
   - *One-way communication (Didactic Method):* Flow of communication is one way – from communicator to audience
     – Disadvantages of one way communication:
       - Knowledge is imposed and learning authoritative
       - Little audience participation and no feedback
       - Does not influence human behaviour
       - Makes no attempt at removing misconceptions and misunderstandings
       - Communicates message even if unintelligible or unacceptable
       - Autocratic process
     – Examples of one way communication:
       - Lecture method (Chalk and talk method)
       - Television
       - Radio
       - Newsprint
   - *Two-way communication (Socratic Method):* Two way communication in which both the communicator and the audience take part
     – Advantages of two way communication:
       - Active participatory and democratic process
       - More likely to influence human behaviour
       - Better audience participation and feedback
     – Examples of two way communication:
       - Focus Group Discussion (FGD)
       - Symposium
       - Panel discussion
   - *Verbal Communication*: Face-to-Face communication
     – Advantages of verbal communication:
       - May be loaded with hidden meanings
       - Persuasive
   - *Non-verbal Communication:* Indirect interaction
     – Advantages of non-verbal communication:
       - Silence speaks louder than words
   - *Formal Communication*: Follows line of authority
   - *Non-formal Communication*: Grape-vine communications
   - Advantages: May be more active than formal channels
   - *Visual Communication*: Comprises charts, graphs, pictograms, tables, maps, posters

3. **Ans. (b) Lecture** *[Ref. Park 27/e p983, 992]*

4. **Ans. (c) Demonstration; (d) Lecture** *[Ref. Park 27/e p983, 992]*

5. **Ans. (d) Panel discussion** *[Ref. Park 27/e p983, 993]*

6. **Ans. (b) Panel discussion** *[Ref. Park 27/e p993]*
   - *Features of a panel discussion*: '4–8 persons' who are qualified to talk about the topic sit and discuss a given problem/topic in front of a target group or audience
   - Panel comprises, A chairman or moderator, 4–8 expert speakers

7. **Ans. (d) Using every communication option to teach deaf child** *[Ref. Hearing in Children by Northern 1/e p366]*
   - Total communication, as it is stressed by its advocates, is a philosophy and not simply another method for teaching deaf children.

Review Questions

8. **Ans. All choices** *[Ref. Park 27/e p983, 992]*
9. **Ans. (d) Panel discussion** *[Ref. Park 27/e p993]*
10. **Ans. (b) High rich content** *[Ref. Park 27/e p993]*
11. **Ans. None** *[Ref. Park 27/e p983]*

COMMUNICATION METHODS

12. **Ans. (b) Delphi method** [*Ref. Simple Biostatistics by Indrayan and Indrayan, 1/e p31, 222*]

    Refer to Theory

    > **ALSO REMEMBER**
    > - *Mini-Delphi* or *Estimate-Talk-Estimate* (*ETE*): The delphi technique when adapted for use in face-to-face meetings

13. **Ans. (d) Interpersonal communication** [*Ref. Park 27/e p983, 992*]
    - Also known as One-to-One or Face-to-face communication

14. **Ans. (c) Flannelgraph** [*Ref. Park 27/e p992*]
    - *Audiovisual aids*: No health education can be effective without audiovisual aids
        - Auditory aids: radio, cassette tape-recorder, microphone, amplifier, earphone, public address system, disks
        - Visual aids:
            - *Not requiring projection*: Chalk-board, leaflets, posters, charts, flannelgraph, exhibits, models, specimens, diagrams, photographs
            - *Requiring projection*: Slides, filmstrips, overhead projector, epidiascope
        - Combined A-V aids: Television, sound films (cinema), synchronized slide-tape combination, multimedia, videotape system, drama, skits

15. **Ans. (a) Not a very effective method of health communication** [*Ref. Park 27/e p992–993*]

    > **ALSO REMEMBER**
    > - *Sociogram*: Graphical representation of interaction among participants in a FGD
    >   - Sociogram helps in understanding whether there was equal participation from all participants in a FGD

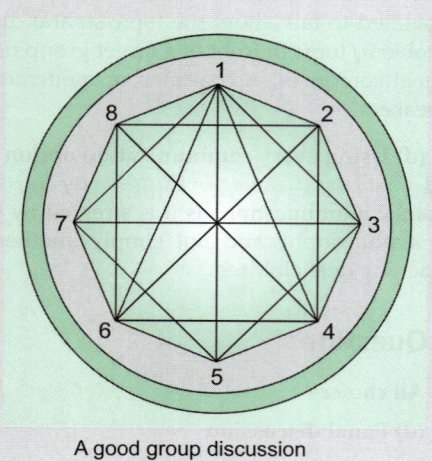

A good group discussion

Contd...

Contd...

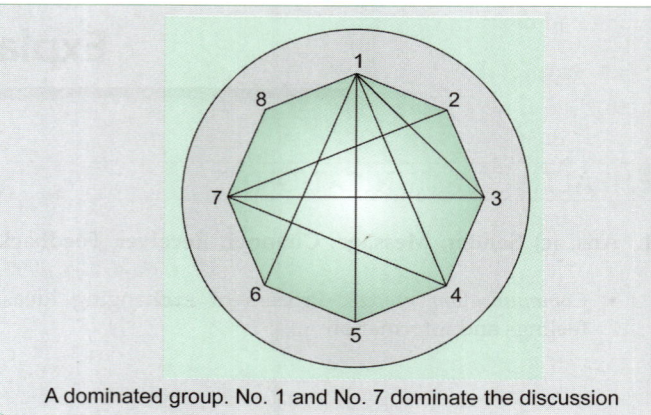

A dominated group. No. 1 and No. 7 dominate the discussion

16. **Ans. (c) Demonstration** [*Ref. Park 27/e p992*]

    DEMONSTRATION:
    - *Definition*: Is a carefully planned presentation to show how to perform a skill or procedure
    - *Method*: Demonstrator carries out step-by-step in font of an audience and involves them
    - *Advantages*:
        - Dramatises by arousing interest
        - Persuades onlookers to adopt
        - Upholds principles of 'seeing is believing' and 'learning by doing'
        - Can bring desirable changes in behaviour
    - *Utility*:
        - Environmental sanitation (hand pump installation, use of sanitary latrine)
        - MCH (ORS technique)
        - Control of disease (Scabies)

17. **Ans. (b) Group members should not have known each other before** [*Ref. Park 27/e p992*]

18. **Ans. (b) Discussion by 4–8 qualified persons** [*Ref. Park 27/e p993*]

19. **Ans. (c) Specific order, Set speeches** [*Ref. Park 27/e p993*]

20. **Ans. (c) Series of four or more meetings** [*Ref. Park 27/e p993*]

    WORKSHOP
    - Series of meetings usually >4 with mphasis is on individual work within the group to impart training
    - Advantages of workshop: Learning takes place in a friendly, happy and democratic atmosphere, under expert guidance
    - Disadvantages of workshop: Needs a lot of baseline ground work, Benefits a small no. of people.

21. **Ans. (d) Contraception** [*Ref. Community Medicine by Sunder Lal 2/e p48*]

    Cafeteria Approach
    - India's public sector program claims to provide a "Cafeteria approach" with a "basket of choices" for Contraceptives available under RCH Program
    - It includes 5 official methods: Female sterilization, Male sterilization, IUD, OCPS, Condoms
    - Currently the term has been replaced by GATHER Approach

22. **Ans. (b) Communication with patients/attendants regarding bad news** [Ref. Oncology in Primary Care by Rose 1/e p197]

SPIKES Technique'
- Used for communication of Cancer prognosis (or other adverse outcomes)
- It has been found quite useful for communication of Breast cancer prognosis
- SPIKES Technique is,
  - **S** Setting up an interview
  - **P** Assessing Perceptions
  - **I** Invitation to explain
  - **K** Imparting Knowledge
  - **E** Addressing Emotions
  - **S** Summary and Strategy

Review Questions

23. **Ans. (a) Individual approach** [Ref. Park 27/e p991]
24. **Ans. (a) Individual approach** [Ref. Park 27/e p991]

HEALTH EDUCATION

25. **Ans. (d) Mass media** [Ref. Park 27/e p991]
26. **Ans. (c) Health education** [Ref. Park 27/e p991]
    - Health education can be done individually BUT limitation is that the numbers we reach is really small, and health education is given to only those who come in contact with health system

27. **Ans. (a) Appeals to emotion** [Ref. Park 27/e p987]
    - Health education versus propaganda/publicity:

	Health education	Health propaganda
Knowledge and skills	Actively acquired	Instilled in minds
Promotion of thought process	Present	Absent
Primitive desires	Disciplines	Arouses
Behaviour developed	Reflective behaviour	Reflexive behaviour
Appeals to	Reason	Emotion
Develops	Individuality, personality	Set attitudes, behaviour
Knowledge acquired by	Self-reliant activity	Passive spoon-feeding
Process	Behaviour centred	Information centred

28. **Ans. (d) Motivation model** [Ref. Park 27/e p987]
    Motivation Model of Health education (Adoption Model)
    - Three stages in process of behavioural change:
      - Awareness: Interest
      - Motivation: Evaluation, Decision-making
      - Action: Adoption, Acceptance
    - Internalization: New idea/acquired behavior becomes part of own existing values

29. **Ans. (b) Knowledge forced into the mind** [Ref. Park 27/e p987]

    Health propaganda
    - Spread of systemized doctrine
    - Knowledge instilled in minds of people
    - Knowledge spoon-fed (Passive reception)

MISCELLANEOUS

30. **Ans. (b) Gives greater support for concentrated programmes** [Ref. Park 27/e p933]
    - *Mass media*: TV, radio, printed media
      - Advantages of mass media:
        - Reaches a relatively larger population in a shorter time than with other means
        - Useful for message transmission even in remote areas
        - More influential with average and below average education level
        - Get public attention
      - Disadvantages of mass media:
        - Being impersonal, not usually effective in changing established modes of behaviour if used alone
        - One way communication: Carry messages from centre to periphery; feedback mechanisms are poorly organized

31. **Ans. (a) Television** [Ref. Park 27/e p933]
    - *Mass media* are mainly a one-way communication (Didactic Methods):
      - *Television:*
        - Most popular of all media
        - Creates awareness, influence public opinions and introduce new ways of life
        - Raise levels of understanding
        - Has much potential for health communication
        - Not much opportunity for feedback and discussion
      - *Radio:*
        - Purely didactic medium
        - Valuable aid in putting across health information
      - *Internet:*
        - Fast growing communication media
        - Holds very large potential to become a major health education tool
      - *Newspapers:*
        - Most widely disseminated of all forms of literature
        - Reach only to limited population (literates)
      - *Printed material:*
        - Can convey detailed information
        - Produced in bulk at low cost, can be shared
      - *Direct mailing:*
        - New innovation in health communication
      - *Posters, billboards, signs:*
        - Can be displayed at public places
        - Less effective in changing behaviour
      - Health museums and exhibitions
      - Folk media

32. **Ans. (c) Check telecommunications** [Ref. Park 25/e p893]
    Telecommunications
    - Telecommunications is the process of communication over distance using designated electromagnetic instruments
      - Mass communication media: TV, Internet, Radio
      - Point-to-point system: Telephone, Mobile (Point to point systems are more closer to Interpersonal communication)

CHAPTER 14

Health Care in India, Health Planning and Management

HEALTH CARE IN INDIA

Health Planning Committees In India

1. *Bhore Committee (1946^Q):*
    - Also known as 'Health Survey and Development Committee'^Q
    - *Short term measure*^Q: 1 PHC per 40,000 population^Q, 30 beds, 3 subcentres and 2 medical officers
    - *Long term measure (3 Million Plan^Q):* Primary health units with 75-bedded hospitals per 10,000–20,000 population; Secondary health units with 650-bedded hospitals; Regional health units with 2,500 beds
    - Prepare 'Social Physicians'^Q (3 months training in preventive and social medicine in medical education)
    - School Health^Q
    - Comprehensive Health Care Concept^Q
2. *Mudaliar Committee (1962):*
    - Also known as 'Health Survey and Planning Committee'^Q
    - 1 PHC per 40,000 population maximum^Q
    - Constitution of 'All India Health Service'^Q
    - Strengthen district hospitals with specialist services
    - Regional organizations in each state
3. *Chadah Committee (1963):*
    - Constituted to study arrangements necessary for the 'Maintenance Phase of National Malaria Eradication Programme (NMEP)'^Q
    - Vigilance operations of NMEP should be the responsibility of general health services (PHCs at block level)
    - 1 Basic Health Worker per 10,000 population (for malaria vigilance, collection of vital statistics and family planning) ^Q
    - Family Planning Health Assistants to supervise 3–4 basic health workers
4. *Mukherji Committee (1965):*
    - 'Delink malaria activities from family planning'^Q
    - Separate staff for family planning programme
5. *Mukherji Committee (1966):*
    - BASIC HEALTH SERVICE should be provided at block level^Q
6. *Jungalwalla Committee (1967):*
    - Also known as 'Committee on Integration of Health Services'^Q
    - Unified cadre, common seniority, recognition of extra qualifications, 'equal pay for equal work', special pay for specialized work, 'no private practice' and good service conditions^Q
7. *Kartar Singh Committee (1973):*
    - Also known as 'Committee on Multipurpose Workers under Health and Family Planning'^Q
    - ANMs to be replaced by 'Female Health Workers'; Basic health workers, Malaria surveillance workers, Vaccinators, Health education assistants and family planning health assistants be replaced by 'Male Health Workers'^Q
    - 1 PHC for 50,000 population, 15–16 subcentres each for 3,000–3,500 population
    - Each subcentre be staffed by team of one male and one female health worker
    - 1 Male Health Supervisor per 3–4 male health workers and 1 Female Health Supervisor per 4 female health workers^Q
    - Lady Health Visitors be designated as Female Health Supervisors
    - Doctor in charge of PHC should have overall charge of supervisors and health workers in his area

> **Key points**
> **Bhore Committee (1946^Q):** Short term measure: 1 PHC per 40,000 population

> **Key points**
> **Kartar Singh Committee (1973):** 'Committee on Multipurpose Workers.

8. *Shrivastava Committee (1975):*
   - Also known as 'Group on Medical Education and Support Manpower'^Q
   - Create 'Bands of Para-professionals and Semi-professional health workers' from within the community^Q
   - Establish 2 cadre of health workers—Village health guides and Health Assistants.
   - Development of 'Referral Services Complex' (between PHCs and higher level referral and services centers) ^Q
   - Establishment of 'Medical and Health Education Commission'^Q
   - 'Reorientation of Medical Education' (ROME) Scheme^Q
   - 'Village Health Guide (Community Health Worker) Scheme'^Q
9. *Krishnan Committee (1983):*
   - 'Urban Revamping Scheme'^Q
10. *Bajaj Committee (1986):*
    - Formulation of 'National Medical and Health Education Policy'^Q
    - Formulation of 'National Health Manpower Policy'
    - 'Education Commission'
    - Health Manpower Cells

Key points

Shrivastava Committee (1975):
'Group on Medical Education and Support Manpower'
ROME Scheme
'Village Health Guide'

Health Care and System

Health Care Characteristics	Health System Components
• Appropriateness • Comprehensiveness • Adequacy • Availability • Accessibility • Affordability • Feasibility	• Concepts (Health, Disease) • Ideas (Equity, Coverage, Effectiveness, Impact) • Objects (Health centres, Health programs) • Persons (Providers, Consumers)

Primary Health Care

- *Definition:* Essential health care, based on practical, scientifically sound, and socially acceptable methods and technology, made universally accessible to individuals and families in the community, through their full participation and at a cost that the community and country can afford^Q
- *Hallmarks of Primary Health Care^Q:* 4 A's
  - Affordability
  - Acceptability
  - Accessibility
  - Availability
- *4 Principles/Pillars of Primary Health Care^Q:*
  - Equitable distribution
  - Community Participation
  - Intersectoral Coordination
  - Appropriate Technology

Key points

Hallmarks of Primary Health Care:
- Affordability
- Acceptability
- Accessibility
- Availability

Elements/Components of Primary Health Care (Alma-Ata Declaration, 1978)^Q

- **E:** Education concerning health problems and their control
- **L:** Locally endemic diseases prevention and control
- **E:** Essential drugs
- **M:** Maternal and child health care including family planning
- **E:** EPI (Immunization) against Vaccine Preventable Diseases
- **N:** Nutrition and promoting proper food supply
- **T:** Treatment of common diseases and injuries
- **S:** Safe water supply and sanitation

Key points

Elements/Components of Primary Health Care
ELEMENTS

Functions of Primary Health Centre[Q]

- Medical care
- MCH including family planning
- Safe water supply and sanitation
- Locally endemic diseases prevention and control
- Collection and reporting of vital statistics
- Education concerning health
- National Health Programs
- Referral services
- Training of health personnel
- Basic laboratory services

> **Key points**
> Primary Level of Health Care:
> 1. Sub-centre
> 2. Primary Health Centre

Levels of Primary Health Care System in India[Q]

- *Primary Level of Health Care:*
  - Is 'first level of contact between population and health care system' in India[Q]
  - Health services are delivered through[Q]:
    - Sub-centre
    - Primary Health Centre
- *Secondary Level of Health Care:*
  - Is 'First referral level of health care' in India[Q]
  - Health services are delivered through: Community Health Centre[Q]
- *Tertiary Level of Health Care:*
  - Is 'Second referral level of health care' in India[Q]
  - Health services are delivered through: Medical Colleges and Hospitals

> **Key points**
> - Staff of PHC: 13–14
> - PHC has provision of '4–6 beds'

Sub-centre

- Type A subcentre: Will provide all recommended services except that the facilities for conducting delivery
- Type B (MCH) Sub-centre[Q]: Will provide all recommended services PLUS facilities for conducting delivery (Centrally/better located with good connectivity to catchment areas, having good physical infrastructure and a good case load of deliveries from catchment areas with no nearby higher level delivery facilities)
- Staff at Sub-centre[Q]:

Staff	Sub-centre A	Sub-centre B
ANM/Health Worker (Female)	1	2
Health Worker (Male)	1	1
Safai-Karamchari	1 (part time)	1 (full time)
Total	3	4

- Is 'most peripheral and first contact point' between primary health care system and community[Q]
- Ministry of Health and Family Welfare is providing '100% Central assistance'[Q]
- No. of Sub-centres in India: 158, 417 [2018]

Sub-centres (NEW IPHS Guidelines 2022)

- HWC – SHC Rural
  - 1/5000 plains
  - 1/3000 hilly, tribal areas
- UHWC – URBAN – 1/15,000–20,000

Primary Health Centre (PHC)

- *Type A PHC[Q]:* PHC with delivery load of <20 deliveries in a month
- *Type B PHC[Q]:* PHC with delivery load of >20 deliveries in a month

- *Staff at PHC:*

STAFF	TYPE A PHC		TYPE B PHC	
	Essential	Desirable	Essential	Desirable
Medical Officer – MBBS	1		1	+1*
Medical Officer – AYUSH		1		1
Accountant cum Data Entry Operator	1		1	
Pharmacist	1		1	
Pharmacist AYUSH		1		1
Nurse-midwife (Staff-Nurse)	3	+1	4	+1
Health worker (Female)	1		1	
Health Assistant (Male)	1		1	
Health Assistant (Female)/Lady Health Visitor	1		1	
Health Educator		1		1
Laboratory Technician	1		1	
Cold Chain and Vaccine Logistic Assistant		1		1
Multi-skilled Group D worker	2		2	
Sanitary worker cum watchman	1		1	+1
Total	13	18	14	21

(*If delivery case-load >30 per month)

- PHC is 'First contact point' between village community and the Medical Officer^Q
- Each PHC acts as a 'Referral centre for 6 Sub-centers'^{Q}
- Medical officer is the 'Leader of team at PHC'
- PHCs are established and maintained by State Governments under Minimum Needs Program (MNP)/Basic Minimum Services Program (BMS)^Q
- PHC has provision of '4–6 beds'^{Q}
- No. of PHCs in India^Q: 25,743 [2018]

Key points

Staff of CHC: 46–52

HWC - PHC (NEW IPHS Guidelines 2022)

- Rural PHC:
  - 1/30,000 (Plains)
  - 1/20,000 (Hilly/Tribal)
- Urban PHC 1/50,000
- Polyclinic 1/2,50,000–3,00,000

Community Health Centre (CHC)

- Staff of CHC: 46–52 (Essential-Desirable)
  - Block Medical Officer/Medical Superintendent 1
  - Public Health Specialist 1
  - Physician 1
  - Surgeon 1
  - Obstetrician and Gynecologist 1
  - Pediatrician 1
  - Anesthetist 1
  - Dental Surgeon 1
  - General Duty Medical Officer 2
  - Medical Officer AYUSH 1
  - Ophthalmologist 0–1 (1 Ophthalmologist is recommended for 5 CHCs)
  - Public Health Nurse 1
  - Staff Nurse 10
  - Other Staff
- Each CHC acts as a 'Referral centre for 4 PHCs'^{Q}
- CHCs are established and maintained by State Government under MNP/BMS program
- Bed strength of CHC^Q: 30
- No. of CHCs in India: 5624 [2018]

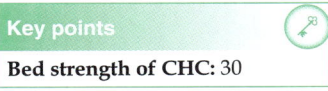

Key points

Bed strength of CHC: 30

Key Facts about Primary Health Care System

	Sub-centre	PHC	CHC
Level of care^Q	Primary	Primary	Secondary
Population norm^Q Plains	5000	30,000	1,20,000
Hilly/tribal areas	3000	20,000	80,000
Staff	3	13–21	46–52
Maintenance	Central govt.	State govt.	State govt.
Rural area covered	21 sq. km.	140 sq. km.	770 sq. km.
Radial distance covered	2.6	6.6	15.6
Average no. of villages covered^Q	4	29	158

> **Key points**
> - Health Assistant 1 per 30,000 population in plain area
> - Multi-purpose worker 1 per 5,000 population in plain area

Population Norms for Health Workers in India^Q [See Annexure 18 for Current Norms]

- *Suggested norm for Health Assistant (male and female)^Q:*
  - 1 per 30,000 population in plain area
  - 1 per 20,000 population in tribal and hilly areas
- *Suggested norm for Health Worker/Multi-purpose worker (male and female)^Q:*
  - 1 per 5,000 population in plain area
  - 1 per 3,000 population in tribal and hilly areas
- *Suggested norm for Anganwadi worker^Q:*
  - 1 per 400–800 population in plain area
  - 1 per 300–800 population in tribal and hilly areas

> **Key points**
> - Doctor 1 per 1000
> - Nurse^Q 3 per Doctor
> - ASHA 2 per 1000

Suggested Population Norms for Health Personnel

Health personnel	Norm suggested^Q
Doctor^Q	1 per 1000
Nurse^Q	3 per 1 Doctor
Health worker (male and female)- MPW^Q	1 per 5000 (plains) or 3000 (hilly)
Health assistant (male and female)^Q	1 per 30000 (plains) or 20000 (hilly)
Pharmacist^Q	1 per 10,000
Lab technician	1 per 10,000
ASHA^Q	2 per 1000 (village)
Trained dai/TBA^Q	1 per 1000 (village)
Village health guide (VHG)^Q	1 per 1000 (village)
Anganwadi worker (AWW)	1 per 400–800 (plains) or 300–800 (hilly)

Rural Health Statistics 2018

- Number of Sub-centres: 158, 417
- Number of PHCs^Q: 25, 743
- Number of CHCs: 5, 624
- Number of District Hospitals: 764
- Number of Districts^Q: 701
- Number of Villages: 640, 867
- Rural Population^Q: 68.9% [Census 2011]
- CBR: 20.4 [SRS 2017]
- CDR: 6.4 [SRS 2017]
- IMR^Q: 34 [Highest MP 47; Lowest Goa 8] [SRS 2017]

Job Responsibilities of Health Worker – Female^Q

- *Maternal and child health:* Register pregnant, Urine and Hb test, Refer, Conduct deliveries, 3–4 post-natal visits
- *Family planning:* Maintain eligible couple registers, distribute conventional and oral contraceptives, establish female depot holders

- *Medical termination of pregnancy:* Identification and referral
- *Nutrition:* Identify and referral, IFA, Vitamin A
- *Immunization:* TT in pregnancy, VPDs in children
- *Dai training:* List dais, Help health assistant in training
- *Communicable diseases:* Notify the medical officer as per guidelines
- Vital events record maintenance
- Record keeping
- Treatment of minor ailments
- Team activities

Job Responsibilities of Health Worker – Male[Q]

- Maintenance of records
- Making Malaria slides[Q]
- Identifying suspected cases of Malaria, Filariasis, Japanese encephalitis, Kala azar
- Identify diarrhoea/dysentery cases; give ORS
- Identify suspect Leprosy, TB cases; sputum collection; supervise MDT, DOTS
- Chlorinate water bodies; educate public
- Administer vaccines
- Distribute conventional contraceptives

> **Key points**
> Job Responsibilities of Health Worker – Male
> Making Malaria slides

Panchayati Raj Institutions (PRIs)

- *Panchayati Raj System:* Is a 3-tier system of rural local self-government in India, linking village to the district[Q]
- *Panchayati Raj Institutions were strengthened in India by Constitution[Q]:*
  - 73rd amendment
  - 74th amendment
- *The 3 level PRIs:*[Q]
  - *Panchayat:* Village level
  - *Panchayat Samiti/Janapada Panchayat:* Block level
  - *Zila Parishad/Zila Panchayat:* District level
- *Panchayati Raj at Village Level comprises of:*[Q]
  - Gram Sabha
  - Gram Panchayat
  - Nyaya Panchayat

> **Key points**
> **Panchayati Raj Institutions** were strengthened in India by Constitution[Q]:
> 73rd amendment
> 74th amendment

District

- The principal unit of administration in India is the 'District under the Collector'[Q]
- Within each district there are 6 types of administrative areas:
  - Sub-divisions (each under a Sub-Collector or Assistant Collector)
  - Tehsils/Talukas (each under a Tehsildar; a tehsil comprises 200–600 villages)
  - Community Development Blocks (each under a Block Development Officer; a block comprises 100 villages and 80,000–1,20,000 population)
  - Municipalities and Corporations
  - Villages
  - Panchayats (Institutions of rural local self governments)

HEALTH PLANNING

Objectives and Goals of a Health Program

- *Objective:* Is planned end-point of all activities[Q]
  - Is precise[Q]
  - Is concerned with the problem itself
- *Target:* A discrete activity which helps measure the extent of attainment of objectives[Q]
  - Is a concept of achievement[Q]
  - Is concerned with the factors involved in a problem
- *Goal:* Ultimate desired state towards which objectives and resources are directed[Q]
  - Is not constrained by time or existing resources
  - Is not necessarily attainable[Q]

> **Key points**
> **Objective:** Is planned end-point of all activities

- *Mission:* Is a description of fundamental principle of existence of a programme
  - Is usually time bound^Q
  - Is a statement of purpose
- *Impact:* Is an expression of the positive effect of a programme, service or institution on the overall health development and on related social and economic development

National Population Policy (NPP) 2000
National Health Policy 2017

Refer to Annexure 9 and 10

Steps of Planning Cycle^Q

- *Pre-planning:*
  - Government interest
  - Legislation
  - Organization for planning
  - Administrative capacity
- *Step 1:* 'Analysis of health situation'
- *Step 2:* Establishment of goals and objectives
- *Step 3:* Assessment of resources
- *Step 4:* Fixing priorities
- *Step 5:* Write-up of formulated plan
- *Step 6:* Programming and implementation
- *Step 7:* Monitoring
- *Step 8:* Evaluation

NITI (National Institute for Transforming India) Aayog

- *Description:* National Planning Commission (1951) of India has been renamed as NITI Aayog, 1st January 2015 onwards
- *Chairperson:* Prime Minister of India
- *Functions:*
  - Promote a rapid rise in the standard of living of the people by efficient exploitation of the resources of the country, increasing production and offering opportunities to all for employment in the service of the community
  - Assessment of all resources of the country, augmenting deficient resources, formulating plans for the most effective and balanced utilization of resources and determining priorities

> **Key points**
> Cost Effectiveness Analysis (CEA)^Q: Benefits are measured in natural units

HEALTH MANAGEMENT

Modern Management Techniques

- *Cost Minimization Analysis (CMA):* Comparison of costs of different interventions that are assumed to provide equivalent benefits
- *Cost Effectiveness Analysis (CEA)^Q:* Benefits are measured in natural units (e.g. Life years gained, heart attacks avoided)
  - CEA is an expression of the desired effect of a programme, service, institution or support activity in reducing a health problem
  - CEA measures the degree of attainment of pre-determined objectives and targets
  - *Most comprehensive indicator of CEA:* Quality adjusted life years (QALYs) gained^Q
- *Cost Utility Analysis (CUA):* Comparison of costs and benefits of health technologies that impact both quality and quantity of life
  - CUA measures health benefits as healthy years; QALYs, DALYs (Disability adjusted life years), healthy year equivalent are used
  - CUA is multi-dimensional
  - *Most widely used measure of benefit in CUA:* Quality adjusted life years (QALYs)
- *Cost Benefit Analysis (CBA):* Benefits are measured in monetary terms^Q
  - Human capital approach
  - Willingness to pay approach
- *Cost Accounting:* A quantitative management technique which provides basic data on cost structure of any programme^Q

- *Input-Output Analysis:* An economic technique which enables calculations to be made of the effects of changing the inputs
- *Network Analysis:* Is the graphic plan of all events and activities to be completed in order to reach an end objective[Q]
    - *Programme Evaluation and Review Technique (PERT):* An arrow diagram representing the logical sequence in which events must take place. It aids in planning, scheduling and monitoring the project; allows better communication between various levels and helps furnish timely, updated progress reports[Q]
    - *Critical Path Method (CPM):* The 'longest path' of the network is called as critical path. If any activity along the critical path is delayed, entire project will be delayed[Q]
- *Systems Analysis:* Is a management technique of finding out the cost-effectiveness of the available alternatives[Q]
- *Planning Programming Budgeting System (PPBS):* It helps decision makers to allocate resources so as to help achieve objectives in the most efficient way
    - It allows grouping of activities related to each objective
    - *Zero Budget Approach:* All budgets start at zero and no one gets any budget that he cannot specifically justify on a year-to-year basis[Q]
- *Work Sampling:* Systematic observation and recording of activities of one or more individuals, carried out at pre-determined or random intervals[Q]
    - It provides quantitative measurement of various activities

> **Key points**
> Critical Path Method **(CPM)**: The 'longest path' of the network

MISCELLANEOUS

Evaluation of Health Services[Q]

- *Relevance:* Appropriateness (need) of a health service
- *Adequacy:* Sufficient attention to pre-determined course of action
- *Accessibility:* Proportion of population expected to use the service
- *Acceptability:* Socially and culturally acceptable
- *Effectiveness:* Extent of prevention/alleviation of underlying problem
- *Efficiency:* How well resources are utilized
- *Impact:* Overall effect of programme/service on health and development

PYQs: Quick Review for NEET

Health Care in India	
1 PHC is for a population of	30,000 in plains
International Conference at Alma-Ata (1978) gave concept of	Primary Health Care
SDGs have to be achieved by	2030
MPW is located at	Subcentre level
No. of PHCs in India	>25000
One urban-PHC is for population	50,000
1 PHC in tribal area for a population of	20,000
Kit B is kept at	Subcentres
Hospice is for	Old and terminally ill patients
Minimum number of beds at CHC	30 beds
A Sub-centre in backward area is for	3000 population
Population covered by PHC in tribal areas	20,000
First referral level is	Secondary level of care
ASHA is located/posted at	Village level
ASHA population norm	2 per 1000 population
Female MPW is per _____ population	5000 population
Total population covered by CHC is	80,000–120,000
One health assistant male/female posted for _____ population	30,000 population
A sub-centre is manned by	Multipurpose worker
Suggested norm for nurses in Indian population	3 nurses per doctor
How many beds are there in PHC for indoor patients	4–6
Community health centre covers a population of	80,000–120,000
Minimum number of beds in Community Health Centre	30 beds
One village health guide is for population of	1000
Vaccine can be stored at sub-centre for	1 day
Village health guide scheme in introduced in	1980
In India under norms Doctor-population ratio is	1 Doctor per 1000 population
In Hilly area PHC caters population of	20,000
A trained Dai caters for a population of	1000
First Referral level in Health care system in India is	Secondary level
Population norms for CHC in difficult areas is	80,000
One village health guide is for population of	1000
Population covered by Primary health center is	30000
Multipurpose worker covers a population of (Plains)	5000
Community health centers provide _____ care	Secondary health care
Training period for Anganwadi worker	4 months

Contd...

Contd...

Health Planning in India	
Bhore Committee (1946) recommended	'3 Million Plan' and 'Social Physicians'
'Multi-purpose Workers' introduced by	Kartar Singh Committee
Bhore Committee was established in	1943
3 divisions of Planning Commission	General secretariat, Technical divisions, Program advisors
ROME scheme recommended by	Srivastava Committee
Rural Health Scheme was recommended by	Srivastava Committee
Ultimate aim in health program is	To attain the goal of Health
Concept of multipurpose workers was given by	Kartar Singh committee
Health Survey and Development Committee is given by	Sir Joseph Bhore
3 month training of doctors in PSM suggested by	Bhore committee
PHC was introduced as result of report by	Bhore committee
Democratic-decentralization was recommended by	Balwant Rai Mehta Committee (1957)
3-tier Panchayati Raj system was proposed by	Balwant Rai Mehta Committee (1957)
Ultimate desired state of a Health Program	Goal
Health Management in India	
'Inventory' (of materials) means	Stock on hand at anytime
Longest path in network analysis (PERT)	Critical path
PERT technique is used in	Network analysis
Economic benefits of program is evaluated in terms of money by	Cost benefit analysis
PERT is a component of	Network analysis

Multiple Choice Questions

HEALTH CARE IN INDIA

1. A 23 years old pregnant woman, 30 weeks POG, presented to a subcenter with a suspicion of abortion of the child. The woman gave a history of avoiding eating papaya, mango and other foods as she had a belief that they could act aa abortifacients. She is referred to primary health centre for examination and confirmation if her pregnancy is safe. Which of the following worker will counsel and educate her to dispel these myths?
   [NEET PG Pattern 2023]
   (a) ANM
   (b) Anganwadi worker
   (c) ASHA worker
   (d) Traditional birth attendant

2. Criteria for establishing Urban CHC to ensure facilities *[NEET PG Pattern 2022]*
   (a) Where subdistrict or district hospital are not present
   (b) Referral centre for 2–3 Urban primary health centers
   (c) For city with 1–1.5 Lac population
   (d) 100 bedded in Metro cities

3. School health is the responsibility of *[NEET PG Pattern September 2021]*
   (a) Sub-centre
   (b) PHC
   (c) Sub-district hospital
   (d) District hospital

4. One PHC is located for a population of: *[AIPGME 1999]*
   (a) 5000
   (b) 30,000
   (c) 100,000
   (d) 500

5. A subcentre in a hilly area caters to a population of:
   (a) 1000 *[AIPGME 2001]*
   (b) 2000 *[NEET pattern 2013]*
   (c) 3000
   (d) 5000

6. Eligible Couple Register is maintained at:
   (a) Subcentre *[AIIMS Dec 1997]*
   (b) PHC
   (c) CHC
   (d) District headquarters

7. Three-Tier system of Health care delivery in rural areas in India is based on the recommendations of:
   [AIIMS May 1993]
   (a) Bhore Committee
   (b) Chadah Committee
   (c) Srivastava Committee
   (d) Mudalair Committee

8. Elements of primary health care include all of the following *except*: *[NEET pattern 2014] [AIIMS Dec 1994]*
   (a) Adequate supply of safe water and basic sanitation
   (b) Prevention & control of local endemic diseases
   (c) Providing employment to every youth
   (d) Immunization against major infectious diseases

9. Panchayati Raj System is a 3-tier system of rural local self-government in India. Match the institutions with levels: *[AIPGME 1996]*
   A – Panchayat,   I – Village level
   B – Panchayat Samiti,   II – District level
   C – Zila Parishad,   III – Block level
   (a) A-III, B-II, C-I   (b) A-II, B-III, C-I
   (c) A-I, B-III, C-II   (d) A-I, B-II, C-III

10. Match list A with List B: *[AIPGME 2000]*
    List A | List B
    A. Shrivastava Committee | 1. Malaria workers to look after FP work too
    B. Chadah Committee | 2. Integration of health services
    C. Kartar Singh | 3. Led to creation of Committee Health guides
    D. Jungalwallah | 4. Led to creation of Committee MPW
    (a) A3; B4; C1; D2   (b) A3; B1; C4; D2
    (c) A2; B1; C4; D3   (d) A2; B4; C1; D3

11. Elements of primary health care include all of the following *except*: *[AIIMS May 1994; AIPGME 03]*
    (a) Adequate supply of safe water and basic sanitation
    (b) Providing essential drugs *[AIIMS May 2014]*
    (c) Sound referral system
    (d) Health education

12. All of the following are Pillars of primary health care *except*: *[NEET pattern 2014] [AIPGME 1999]*
    (a) Equitable distribution *[UPSC CMS 2015]*
    (b) Community participation
    (c) Health education
    (d) Intersectoral coordination

13. Alma Ata conference was held in: *[DPG 2005]*
    (a) 1948   (b) 1956
    (c) 1977   (d) 1978

14. Health man power indicated by which of the following?
    [PGI June 2005]
    (a) Doctor 1 per 3500 population
    (b) ANM 1 per >1000 population
    (c) Lab technician 1 per 10000 population
    (d) Pharmacist 1 per 100000 population
    (e) MPW

15. Population of 1000 is covered by: [PGI Dec 2K]
    (a) Anganwadi worker (b) Health assistant
    (c) Trained Dai (d) Village health guide
16. Function of PHC are: [PGI June 03]
    (a) Referral services
    (b) Family planning & referral services
    (c) Basic laboratory services
    (d) Specialist service
    (e) Collection and reporting of viral statistics
17. All of the following are state responsibility for health except: [DPG 2006]
    (a) Vital statistics
    (b) Promotion of research through research centers & their bodies
    (c) Prevention of adulteration
    (d) Prevention of communicable disease
18. Which of the following is a new concept in primary Health Care? [AIPGME 2010]
    (a) Equitable distribution
    (b) Community participation
    (c) Qualitative enquiry
    (d) Primary health care
19. Principles of Primary Health Care includes all except:
    (a) Intersectoral coordination [NEET pattern 2013]
    (b) Appropriate technology [DNB 2009]
    (c) Mainly coordinated by doctors
    (d) Community participation
20. Following is/are the job(s) of Health worker male:
    (a) Sputum collection [PGI May 2011]
    (b) ORS distribution
    (c) DOTS supervision
    (d) Growth monitoring
    (e) Environmental sanitation
21. Staff at PHC include: [PGI November 2012]
    (a) Pharmacist (b) Clerk
    (c) Radiologist (d) Laboratory technician
    (e) Paediatrician
22. Which of the following is not a work of female multipurpose health worker? [NEET pattern 2012]
    (a) Malaria surveillance (b) Distribution of condoms
    (c) Immunization (d) Dots activities
23. With of the following is at sub-centre level? [DNB December 2011]
    (a) Zila parishad (b) Panchayat samiti
    (c) Gram panchayat (d) Gram sabha
24. Which of the following is true about female health worker? [DNB June 2011]
    (a) Acts at PHC level
    (b) Covers a population of 5000 population
    (c) Chlorinates well at regular intervals
    (d) Makes at least 3 post natal visits for each delivery
25. Emphasis shifted from urban to rural services:
    (a) Equitable distribution [NEET pattern 2013]
    (b) Community participation
    (c) Intersectoral coordination
    (d) Appropriate technology
26. Which of the following is not a work of anganwadi worker? [DNB 2012]
    (a) Immunization of children
    (b) Non formal preschool education
    (c) Sanitation
    (d) Health education
27. Most common operation done by an Ophthalmologist in district hospital: [AIIMS May 2013]
    (a) Phacoemulsification
    (b) Trabeculectomy
    (c) Bilateral lamellar tarsal rotation
    (d) Dacryocystorhinostomy
28. Staff at PHC include: [PGI November 2013]
    (a) Radiographer (b) Pharmacist
    (c) Anesthetist (d) Pediatrician
    (e) Laboratory technician
29. Functions of female health worker includes:
    (a) Visit 4 sub-centers/month [NEET pattern 2014]
    (b) Collection of blood sample
    (c) Conduct 50% delivery
    (d) Chlorination of water
30. Following are Objectives of Indian Public Health Standards for Primary Health Centres except: [UPSC CMS 2015]
    (a) Provision of comprehensive primary health care
    (b) Achievement of an acceptable quality of health care
    (c) Provision of accident and emergency care
    (d) Making services more responsive to the needs of the community
31. Following is a principle of primary health care: [NEET pattern 2015]
    (a) Safe water supply and sanitation
    (b) Free medical care
    (c) Equitable distribution
    (d) Local endemic disease prevention and control
32. One eye surgeon is recommended for: [NEET pattern 2015]
    (a) 1 CHC (b) 2 CHC
    (c) 3 CHC (d) 5 CHC
33. Number of ASHA visits after home delivery is: [NEET pattern 2015, 2016]
    (a) 4 (b) 5
    (c) 6 (d) 7
34. Community health guide is selected by: [NEET pattern 2015]
    (a) Block Development Officer
    (b) ASHA
    (c) Zila Parishad
    (d) Medical officer-in-charge

35. True about broad principles of PHC are all *except*: [NEET pattern 2015]
    (a) Self-reliance
    (b) Social equity
    (c) Nationwide coverage
    (d) Health education

36. Which of the following are the criteria used for selecting village health guides? [NEET pattern 2016]
    i. Permanent residents of the local community
    ii. Women are preferred to men
    iii. Minimum formal education up to VI standard
    iv. Should be able to spare 8 hours daily for community health work
    v. Should be acceptable to all sections of the community
    (a) i, iii ,v only
    (b) ii, iv, v only
    (c) i, ii ,iii ,v only
    (d) i, iii, iv, v only

37. Urban social health activist (USHA) workers are proposed to work for population of: [NEET pattern 2016]
    (a) 1000–2500
    (b) 2500–3500
    (c) 4000–5000
    (d) 5000–10000

38. Female health worker in Plains is for a population of: [NEET pattern 2017]
    (a) 1000
    (b) 3000
    (c) 5000
    (d) 30000

39. Standpipe in rural areas is an example of which Principle of Primary health care? [NEET pattern 2017]
    (a) Equitable distribution
    (b) Community participation
    (c) Intersectoral coordination
    (d) Appropriate technology

40. Not criteria of First referral unit: [NEET pattern 2017]
    (a) Covers a population of 1 lac
    (b) Provide secondary care
    (c) Has 30 beds
    (d) Community health officer is medical graduate or post-graduate

41. Not true about First referral unit in urban areas: [NEET pattern 2017]
    (a) 30–50 beds
    (b) Covers 2.5 lakh population
    (c) Salary is given by state government
    (d) Setting up cost is given by state government

42. Use of Shakir's tape for measuring arm circumference is: [NEET pattern 2017]
    (a) Equitable distribution
    (b) Community participation
    (c) Intersectoral coordination
    (d) Appropriate technology

43. True about population coverage of Primary health center: [PGI 2017]
    (a) 20000 in plains area
    (b) 30000 in plains area
    (c) 10000 in tribal area
    (d) 20000 in tribal area
    (e) 30000 in tribal area

44. If someone goes to a Sub-center as part of an audit, how many infants should be registered with a health worker working there? [AIIMS May 2018]
    (a) 50
    (b) 100
    (c) 150
    (d) 200

45. Which of the following is included in Concurrent list by Government of India? [NEET Pattern 2019]
    (a) Landmine injuries
    (b) Medical emergencies
    (c) Adulteration of food prevention
    (d) Road traffic accidents

Review Questions

46. At the village level, the Panchayati Raj consists of all of the following *except*? [DNB 2003]
    (a) Zila Parishad
    (b) Nyaya Panchayat
    (c) Gram Panchayat
    (d) Gram Sabha

47. Primary health care involves all *except*: [UP 2000]
    (a) Sanitation & water supply
    (b) Sound referral center
    (c) Supply of essential drugs
    (d) Health education

48. "Mobile medical care" is provided services to all *except*: [UP 2005]
    (a) Primary health care
    (b) Secondary health care
    (c) Tertiary health care
    (d) Near home based

49. Community health centres covering a population of:
    (a) 40–60,000 [UP 2007]
    (b) 60–80,000 [DNB 2000, 2012]
    (c) 80–120,000
    (d) None

50. Which of the following is not a function of primary health center in India? [MP 2008]
    (a) Medical Care
    (b) Safe water supply
    (c) Collection of vital statistics
    (d) Supplementary functioning of under six children

51. Recommended numbers of population for primary Health Centres for a tribal area is: [MH 2002] [MP 2003, RJ 2006]
    (a) 50,000
    (b) 30,000
    (c) 20,000
    (d) 10,000

52. Recommended number of populations for primary health centers & subcenters for tribal area is: [MH 2003]
    (a) 30,000 & 5000 respectively
    (b) 20,000 & 3000 respectively
    (c) 30,000 & 3000 respectively
    (d) 20,000 & 5000 respectively

53. Panchayati Raj includes the following *except*: [MH 2007]
    (a) Gram Panchayat
    (b) Gram Sabha
    (c) Nyaya Panchayat
    (d) Nyaya sabha

54. Anganwadi worker demonstrating preparation of home made ORS to the mothers of under five children, is an example of: [MH 2008]
    (a) Intersectoral coordination
    (b) Community participation
    (c) Appropriate technology
    (d) All of the above

55. All are grass root level worker *except*: [RJ 2001]
    (a) Anganwadi worker
    (b) Village health assistant
    (c) Dai
    (d) Health assistant

HEALTH PLANNING

56. Which of the following is a set point framed for long term plans but is yet something that cannot be quantified or measured? [AIPGME 2009]
    (a) Target   (b) Goal
    (c) Objective   (d) Mission

57. The National Population Policy of India has set the following goals *except*: [AIPGME 04]
    (a) To bring down total fertility rate (TFR) to replacement levels by 2015
    (b) To reduce the infant mortality rate to 30 per 1000 live births
    (c) To reduce the maternal mortality rate to 100 per 100,000 live births
    (d) 100 percent registration of births, deaths, marriages and pregnancies

58. "3-Million Plan" was proposed by: [AIPGME 1991]
    (a) Kartar Singh Committee
    (b) Mudaliar Committee
    (c) Srivastava Committee
    (d) Bhore Committee

59. Under the National Population Policy 2000, it is aimed to reduce the maternal mortality ratio to below: [MP 2007]
    (a) 100 per 100,000 live births
    (b) 200 per 100,000 live births
    (c) 50 per 100,000 live births
    (d) 150 per 100,000 live births

60. All of the following goals under NHP 2002 have to be achieved by 2010 *except*: [AIIMS May 2004]
    (a) Reduce prevalence of blindness to 0.5%
    (b) Reduce IMR to 30/100 and MMR to 100/Lakh
    (c) Increase utilization of Public health facilities from <20% to >75%
    (d) Eliminate Lymphatic Filariasis

61. Recommendations of Bhore Committee include:
    (a) Constitution of All India Health Service on the pattern of IAS [AIIMS May 1995]
    (b) Separate staff for Family Planning Programme
    (c) Creation of "Bands of para-professionals & semi-professional health workers"
    (d) Major changes in Medical education to prepare "Social Physicians"

62. Multi-purpose worker scheme in India was introduced following the recommendation of: [AIPGME 2004]
    (a) Srivastava Committee [NEET pattern 2012]
    (b) Bhore Committee [NEET pattern 2014]
    (c) Kartar Singh Committee
    (d) Mudaliar Committee

63. Match the following names of health committees in India: [AIPGME 1991]
    A Bhore Committee
    B Mudaliar Committee
    C Jungalwallah Committee
    D Kartar Singh Committee
    I Health Survey & Development Committee
    II Committee on MPWs under Health & Family Planning
    III Committee on Integration of Health Services
    IV Health Survey & Planning Committee
    (a) A-I, B-III, C-II, D-IV   (b) A-I, B-IV, C-III, D-II
    (c) A-IV, B-I, C-III, D-II   (d) A-I, B-IV, C-II, D-III

64. A group on Medical Education & Support Manpower was popularly known as: [AIIMS Sep 1996]
    (a) Kartar Singh Committee
    (b) Mudaliar Committee
    (c) Srivastava Committee
    (d) Bhore Committee

65. Planning Cycle has got several steps: [AIPGME 1993]
    Monitoring & evaluation – a
    Programming & implementation – b
    Assessment of resources – c
    Analysis of existing health situation – d
    Logical sequence in planning cycle would be
    (a) a b c d   (b) d c b a
    (c) d b c a   (d) c d b a

66. A 3 year graduate MBBS programme was suggested by which committee? [AIIMS May 2013]
    (a) Sundar Committee
    (b) Srivastava Committee
    (c) Expert Level Committee on Universal Health Coverage
    (d) Krishnan Committee

67. Planning cycle includes: [NEET pattern 2013]
    (a) Analysis of situation (b) Evaluation
    (c) Resource assessment (d) All

68. Set of statement for monitoring Progress towards goal is referred as: [DNB December 2011] [DNB December 2010]
    (a) Target (b) Objective
    (c) Programme (d) Procedure

69. Bajaj committee, true is: [NEET pattern 2013]
    (a) Constituted in 1946
    (b) Recommends formation of PHC
    (c) Recommends health manpower policy
    (d) None

70. Bajaj committee in 1986 proposed: [DNB December 2010]
    (a) Multipurpose health worker
    (b) Manpower and planning
    (c) Rural health service
    (d) Integrated health services

71. Rural health scheme introduced by: [DNB June 2011]
    (a) Bhore committee
    (b) Mukherjee committee
    (c) Shrivastava committee
    (d) Mudaliar committee

72. Universal Health Coverage of India was recently approved by which health committee? [AIIMS May 2014]
    (a) Medical education health group
    (b) MPW in health and family planning
    (c) High level expert group
    (d) Health survey and development committee

73. Which article of Indian Constitution confers 'Right to life' to citizens of India? [NEET pattern 2014]
    (a) Article 11 (b) Article 21
    (c) Article 23 (d) Article 25

Review Questions

74. Concept of multipurpose workers was given by:
    (a) Mudaliar committee [DNB 2008] [RJ 2006]
    (b) Srivastava committee
    (c) Kartar Singh committee
    (d) Mukherjee committee

75. All are included in health sector policy in India except: [UP 2000]
    (a) Nutritional supplements
    (b) Medical education
    (c) Family welfare programme
    (d) Control of communicable disease

76. 3 month's training in preventive and social medicine during internship is recommended by: [UP 2005]
    (a) Bhore committee (b) Chadha committee
    (c) Mudaliar committee (d) Mukherji committee

77. Each subcenter should be staffed by one male and one female health worker. It was recommended by:
    (a) Bhore committee [MP 2001]
    (b) Mudaliar committee
    (c) Chadha committee
    (d) Kartar Singh committee

78. Recommendation of the Krishnan committee was for:
    (a) Local dai [MP 2003]
    (b) Village health guides
    (c) Integration of PHCs
    (d) Abolition of private practise

79. Which of the following health committee recommended a medical and health education commission for reform in health and medical education on the times of University Grants Commission? [MP 2008]
    (a) Shrivastav Committee
    (b) Mukherji Committee
    (c) Chadha Committee
    (d) Kartar Singh Committee

80. Who among the following is Chairman of Central Council for Health? [MH 2003]
    (a) Prime minister
    (b) Secretary of health
    (c) Union health minister
    (d) Director General of Health Sciences

81. Correct sequence of cycle is: [RJ 2007]
    (a) Planning, Evaluation, Object, Goal
    (b) Planning, Object, Goal, Evaluation
    (c) Planning, Object, Evaluation, Goal
    (d) Planning, Goal, Evaluation, Object

82. Chadha committees recommended all except: [RJ 2007]
    (a) PHC at the block level
    (b) Concept of multipurpose worker
    (c) One basic health worker per 10,000 populations
    (d) The family planning Health assistants were to supervise 3 to 4 of this basic health worker

HEALTH MANAGEMENT

83. Monetary benefit is measured in?
    [NEET PG Pattern January 2020]
    (a) Planning Program budgeting system
    (b) Cost benefit analysis
    (c) Network analysis
    (d) Cost effective analysis

84. Which of the following is a technique based on Behavior sciences methods? [NEET PG Pattern January 2020]
    (a) Network analysis
    (b) Management by objective
    (c) Systems analysis
    (d) Decision making

85. Most comprehensive indicator of Cost Effectiveness Analysis is: [AIIMS Dec 1997]
    (a) No. of life years gained
    (b) No. of heart attacks avoided
    (c) QALYs gained
    (d) Cost per life year gained

86. Which one of the following is not a source of manager's power? [AIPGME 2005]
    (a) Reward (b) Coercive
    (c) Legal   (d) Efferent

87. The management technique which is more promising tool for application in health field is: [AIPGME 2008]
    (a) Cost effective analysis (b) Cost benefit analysis
    (c) Cost accounting   (d) Input output analysis

88. Economic/monetary benefits of any programme are compared with the costs incurred in:
    [AIIMS Nov 2007][Karnataka 2007]
    (a) Cost benefit analysis   (b) Cost effective analysis
    (c) Cost accounting   (d) Network analysis

89. All are true regarding Critical Path Method (CPM) except: [AIIMS May 1994]
    (a) Is a part of Input-Output analysis
    (b) Visualised in graphical representation of all events/activities carried out
    (c) Is the longest part of the network
    (d) Any delay in CP delays whole project

90. In Management "Goal" refers to: [Karnataka 2007]
    (a) Planned end point of all activity
    (b) Discrete activity
    (c) Ultimate desired state towards which objectives and resources are directed
    (d) Analysis of health Situation

91. In health management, Cost benefit analysis is an example of: [NUPGET 2013]
    (a) Critical path method
    (b) Program evaluation and review technique
    (c) Management by objectives
    (d) Total Quality management

92. Systemic observation and recording of activities of one/more individuals carried out at predetermined/random intervals: [NEET pattern 2012]
    (a) Decision making   (b) Systems analysis
    (c) Network analysis   (d) Work sampling

93. Analysis done for expenditure of large proportion for small number and vice versa: [NEET pattern 2012]
    (a) ABC   (b) SDE
    (c) VED   (d) FSN

94. "Critical Path" in Network Analysis is: [AP 2014]
    (a) Most expensive path in a network
    (b) Congested path in a network
    (c) Shortest path in a network
    (d) Longest path in a network

95. Which one of the following is a quantitative method of health management? [UPSC CMS 2015]
    (a) Cost effectiveness analysis
    (b) Human Resource Management
    (c) Communication management
    (d) Supportive supervision and leadership

96. In the management of stores VED, D stands for: [NEET Pattern 2016]
    (a) Discrete   (b) Desirable
    (c) Decide   (d) Definite

97. In primary health care, ABC and VED are related to: [AIIMS May 2016]
    (a) National program evaluation at PHC level
    (b) Drug inventory management at PHC
    (c) Staff management at PHC
    (d) Vaccination coverage assessment in PHC area

98. Which of the following is true about Six-sigma: [PGI November 2017]
    (a) Developed by Motorola
    (b) Only practiced in Motorola Company
    (c) Represents an ideology that focuses on statistical improvements to a business process
    (d) It is a quality-control program
    (e) It can used in Health care sector

Review Questions

99. All of the following are included in methods based an behavioural sciences except: [DNB 2002, 2005]
    (a) Personal management
    (b) System analysis
    (c) Management by objectives
    (d) Communication

100. PERT is a technique for: [DNB 2003]
    (a) Network analysis   [Karnataka 2006]
    (b) Cost-effective analysis [DNB 2011]
    (c) Input-output analysis [NEET pattern 2011]
    (d) System analysis

101. Qualities of a leader are all except: [Kolkata 2008]
    (a) Leading from the front
    (b) Burning/breaking of bridges
    (c) Courageous
    (d) Fights instantly

102. PERT is associated with: [Kolkata 2009]
    (a) Qualitative analysis
    (b) Quantitative analysis
    (c) Behavioral analysis
    (d) None

103. PERT & critical path methods are employed in:
    (a) Community education   [MP 2003]
    (b) Healthy planning
    (c) Management
    (d) Health survey

104. True about rural health services in India: [MP 2004]
    (a) Pharmacists are more than lab technician
    (b) Male health worker are more than female health worker
    (c) Doctors are more than nurses
    (d) Pediatricians are more than Gynecologist

105. A study was conducted among nursing staff to find out time taken in different aspects of patient care viz., bed preparation, monitoring of vital diagnosis, attending doctor's rounds, blood sampling, drug administration. Which management technique would be applied for the analysis? [MP 2008]
    (a) Critical path method
    (b) Input-output analysis
    (c) Systems analysis
    (d) Work sampling

MISCELLANEOUS

106. For analysis of functioning of a health centre with respect to evaluation, which of the following is the most important for assessing clinical management?
    (a) Input   [NEET PG Pattern September 2021]
    (b) Output
    (c) Process
    (d) Structure

107. You are a Medical Officer at a PHC. 50 patients requiring anti-hypertensive are being transferred to your PHC from periphery. 40 people need Amlodipine (5 mg PO). 10 people have contraindication to use of Amlodipine so those people have to be started with Lisinopril (10 mg PO). Drugs will come at PHC once a month. So how many drugs will you order combined, and what will be the reorder factor? [INICET July 2021]
    (a) 800, 3
    (b) 1000, 2
    (c) 1600, 3
    (d) 3000, 2

108. Drugs A & B are both used for treating a particular skin infection. After one standard application, drug A eradicates the infection in 95% of both adults and children. Drug B eradicates the infection in 47% of adults & 90% of children. There are otherwise no significant pharmacological differences between the two drugs, and there are no significant side effects. However, the cost of drug A is twice that of drug B. Dr Sunil, a general practitioner, always uses drug B for the first treatment, and resorts to drug A if the infection persists. Dr Sudhir, another general practitioner, always uses drug A for adults and drug B for children. Ignoring indirect costs, which of the following statement is incorrect? [AIPGME 02]
    (a) Drug A is more effective than B for treating children
    (b) Drug A is more cost-effective than drug B for treating children
    (c) Drug A is more cost-effective than drug B for treating adults
    (d) Dr Sudhir's regime achieves a higher level of cost-effectiveness than Dr. Sunil's

109. According to the World Health report 2000, India's health expenditure is: [AIPGME 2006]
    (a) 4.8% of G.D.P
    (b) 5.2% of G.D.P
    (c) 6.8% of G.D.P
    (d) 7% of G.D.P

110. Indian (economic) real GDP growth for the year 2003 is:
    (a) 6.0
    (b) 6.5   [AIPGME 2006]
    (c) 7.8
    (d) 10.5

111. All the following are health policy indicators except:
    (a) Political commitment to health for all
    (b) Resource allocation   [AIIMS June 1997]
    (c) Disability prevalence
    (d) Community involvement

112. All are Elements of Evaluation except:
    (a) Repeatability   [AIIMS May 2005]
    (b) Relevance
    (c) Acceptability
    (d) Effectiveness

113. Which of the following are referred to as "Ivory Towers of Disease"? [AIIMS Nov 1993]
    (a) Small health centres
    (b) Large hospitals
    (c) Private practitioners
    (d) Health Insurance Companies

Review Question

114. All of the following are peripheral level health workers except: [TN 2003]
    (a) Village Health Guide
    (b) Gram Sevak
    (c) Anganwadi worker
    (d) Local Dai

Explanations

HEALTH CARE IN INDIA

1. **Ans. (b) Anganwadi worker** [Ref. Park 27/e p701]
   The trainings of Anganwadi workers is localized to incorporate specific local challenges that
   - Prevent healthy behaviors, cultural practices, breaking myths, local food availability, dietary practices

2. **Ans. (d) 100 bedded in Metro cities**
   [Ref. National URBAN Health Mission – Framework for Implementation, MoHFW 2013 p54]

   Urban Community Health Centre (U-CHC)
   - U-CHC may be set up as a satellite hospital for every 4–5 U-PHCs
   - One U-CHC to be established for every 2.5 lakh population with an inpatient facility that is 30–50 bedded
   - In metro cities, One U-CHC to be established for every 5 lakh population with an inpatient facility that is 100 bedded

3. **Ans. (b) PHC** [Ref. Park 26/e p667]
   School Health Committee (Renuka Roy Committee) 1960
   - School health services should be an integral part of General health services
   - General health care services are delivered through PHCs in India (rural areas) so School health services is an important function of PHCs

4. **Ans. (b) 30,000** [Ref. Park 27/e p700]
   Primary Health Care System In India:
   - **Primary Level of Health Care**:
     - Is 'first level of contact between population and health care system' in India
     - Health services are delivered through:
       - Sub-centre
       - Primary Health Centre
   - **Secondary Level of Health Care**:
     - Is 'First referral level of health care' in India
     - Health services are delivered through: Community Health Centre
   - **Tertiary Level of Health Care**:
     - Is 'Second referral level of health care' in India
     - Health services are delivered through: Medical Colleges and Hospitals
   - **Key Facts About Primary Health Care System:**

	Sub-centre	PHC	CHC
Level of care	Primary	Primary	Secondary
Population norm			
Plains	5000	30,000	1,20,000
Hilly/tribal areas	3000	20,000	80,000

	Sub-centre	PHC	CHC
Staff	3–4	13–18	46–52
Maintenance	Central govt.	State govt.	State govt.
Rural area covered	21 sq. km.	140 sq. km.	770 sq. km.
Radial distance covered	2.6	6.6	15.6
Average no. of villages covered	4	29	158

5. **Ans. (c) 3000** [Ref. Park 25/e p960]
   - *Population norms for Health centres in India*:

	Primary health care system			ICDS system
Centre	Sub-centre	PHC	CHC	Anganwadi
Level of care	Primary	Primary	Secondary	–
Population norm				
Plain	5000	30,000	1,20,000	400–800
Hilly/tribal areas	3000	20,000	80,000	300–800

   ALSO REMEMBER
   - Suggested norm for Health Assistant (male and female):
     - 1 per 30,000 population in plain area
     - 1 per 20,000 population in tribal and hilly areas
   - Suggested norm for Health Worker/Multi-purpose worker (male and female):
     - 1 per 5,000 population in plain area
     - 1 per 3,000 population in tribal and hilly areas
   - Suggested norm for Anganwadi worker:
     - 1 per 400–800 population in plain area
     - 1 per 300–800 population in tribal and hilly areas

6. **Ans. (a) Subcentre** [Ref. Park 27/e p706]

   ALSO REMEMBER
   - Eligible Couple Register is maintained at subcentre, primarily by female multipurpose health worker
   - 'Eligible Couple Register' is a basic document for organizing family planning work. It is regularly updated by each functionary of the family planning programmer, for the area falling within his jurisdiction
   - 'Each subcentre is manned by one male and one female multipurpose worker'

7. **Ans. (c) Srivastava Committee** [Ref. Park 25/e p938]
   - Three-Tier system of Health care delivery in rural areas in India is based on the recommendations of Srivastava Committee

> **ALSO REMEMBER**
>
> - **Shrivastava Committee (1975):** *'Group on Medical Education and Support Manpower'*
>   - Create *'Bands of Para-professionals and Semi-professional health workers'* from within the community
>   - Establish 2 cadre of health workers – Multipurpose Workers and Health Assistants between community level workers and doctors at PHCs
>   - Development of *'Referral Services Complex'* (between PHCs and higher level referral and services centers)
>   - Establishment of *'Medical and Health Education Commission'*
>   - *'Reorientation of Medical Education'* (ROME) Scheme
>   - *'Village Health Guide (Community Health Worker) Scheme'*
>   - '3-tier system of Health care delivery – Subcentre, PHC, CHC

8. **Ans. (c) Providing employment to every youth**
   [Ref. Park 27/e p693]
   - 8 essential **ELEMENTS**/components of Primary Health Care (as outlined by the *'Alma-Ata Declaration, 1978'*):
     - E: Education concerning health problems and their control
     - L: Locally endemic diseases prevention and control
     - E: Essential drugs
     - M: Maternal and child health care including family planning
     - E: EPI (Immunization) against Vaccine Preventable Diseases
     - N: Nutrition and promoting proper food supply
     - T: Treatment of common diseases and injuries
     - S: Safe water supply and sanitation

9. **Ans. (c) A-I, B-III, C-II** *[Ref. Park 27/e p1006–1007]*
   - **The Panchayati Raj System:** Is a 3-tier system of rural local self-government in India, linking village to the district. The 3 institutions are:
     - *Panchayat:* Village level
     - *Panchayat Samiti/Janapada Panchayat:* Block level
     - *Zila Parishad/Zila Panchayat:* District level

> **ALSO REMEMBER**
>
> - *Panchayati Raj at Village Level comprises of:*
>   - Gram Sabha
>   - Gram Panchayat
>   - Nyaya Panchayat
> - *Panchayati Raj Institutions were strengthened in India by Constitution:*
>   - 73rd amendment
>   - 74th amendment

10. **Ans. (b) A3; B1; C4; D2**
    [Ref. Park 23/e p873–875, 25/e p937–939]

11. **Ans. (c) Sound referral system**
    [Ref. Park 27/e p693]
    Primary health care:
    - *Definition:* Essential health care, based on practical, scientifically sound, and socially acceptable methods and technology, made universally accessible to individuals and families in the community, through their full participation and at a cost that the community and country can afford

> **ALSO REMEMBER**
>
> - *Hallmarks of Primary health care:* **4 A's**
>   - Affordability
>   - Acceptability
>   - Accessibility
>   - Availability
> - 4 Principles/Pillars of Primary Health Care:
>   - Equitable distribution
>   - Community Participation
>   - Intersectoral Coordination
>   - Appropriate Technology

12. **Ans. (c) Health education** *[Ref. Park 27/e p963–964]*

13. **Ans. (d) 1978** *[Ref. Park 27/e p963]*
    Alma-Ata Conference:
    - Took place in USSR in 1978
    - It gave the concept of 'Primary Health Care' (and its 8 elements)
    - Called for WHO goal of 'Health for All by 2000'
    - India is a signatory

14. **Ans. (c) Lab technician 1 per 10000 population**
    [Ref. Park 27/e p699]
    - *Suggested norm for health personnel:*

Health personnel	Norm suggested
Doctor	1 per 1000
Nurse	3 per 1 Doctor
Health worker (male and female)- MPW	1 per 5000 (plains) or 3000 (hilly)
Trained dai/TBA	1 per 1000 (village)
Health assistant (male and female)	1 per 30000 (plains) or 20000 (hilly)
Pharmacist	1 per 10,000
Lab technician	1 per 10,000
ASHA	2 per 1000 (village)
Village health guide (VHG)	1 per 1000 (village)
Anganwadi worker (AWW)	1 per 400–800 (plains) or 300–800 (hilly)

15. **Ans. (c) Trained Dai; (d) Village health guide**
    [Ref. Park 27/e p699]
    - *Population covered by health workers:*

Health worker	Population covered
Anganwadi worker	400–800
Trained Dai	1000
Village Health Guide	1000
ASHA (NRHM)	1000 (2 ASHAS per 1000 population)
USHA (NUHM)	1000–2500
Health Assistant	30000 (20000 in Hilly areas)
Multi-purpose worker	5000 (3000 in Hilly areas)

16. Ans. (a) Referral services; (b) Family planning & referral services; (c) Basic laboratory services; (e) Collection and reporting of vital statistics   *[Ref. Park 27/e p706]*

17. Ans. (b) Promotion of research through research centres & other bodies   *[Ref. Park 27/e p1005-1006]*
    - *Concurrent list under Union Ministry of Health and Family Welfare includes*: [responsibility of both Union and State governments] **[Mnemonic: V CLAPPED]**
      - **V**ital statistics
      - **C**ommunicable diseases spread prevention
      - **L**abour welfare
      - **A**dulteration of food prevention
      - **P**orts other than major
      - **P**opulation control and family planning
      - **E**conomic and social planning
      - **D**rugs and poisons control

18. Ans. (c) Qualitative enquiry   *[Ref. Internet]*
    - 'Qualitative enquiry' in primary health care avoids advance decisions about what exactly is to be discovered and asks open questions to explore new interpretations.

19. Ans. (c) Mainly coordinated by doctors   *[Ref. Park 27/e p700-701]*

20. (a) Sputum collection; (b) ORS distribution; (c) DOTS supervision; (e) Environmental sanitation   *[Ref. Park 27/e p715]*

21. Ans. (a) Pharmacist; (d) Laboratory technician   *[Ref. Park 27/e p706]*

22. Ans. (a) Malaria surveillance   *[Ref. Park 27/e p714]*

23. Ans. (c) Gram Panchayat   *[Ref. Park 27/e p1007]*

24. Ans. (b) Covers a population of 5000 population; (d) Makes at least 3 post natal visits for each delivery   *[Ref. Park 27/e p713]*

25. Ans. (a) Equitable distribution   *[Ref. Park 27/e p693]*

26. Ans. (c) Sanitation   *[Ref. Park 25/e p960]*

27. Ans. (a) Phacoemulsification   *[Ref. IPHS Standards: Guidelines for District Hospitals 2012, Government of India, 2012, p 10]*

Ophthalmologic services at District hospital

OPD Procedures	IPD Procedures
Refraction (by using Snellen's chart)	Examination under GA
Refraction (by auto refractometer)	Canthotomy
Syringing and Probing	Paracentesis
Foreign Body Removal (conjunctival)	Air Injection & Resuturing
Foreign Body Removal (Corneal)	Enucleation with Implant
Epilation	Enucleation without Implant
Suture Removal	Perforating Coneo Scleral Injury Repair
Sub-conjunctival Injection	
Retrobulbar Injection (Alcohol etc.)	Cataract Extraction with IOL
Tonometry	Glaucoma (Trabeculectomy)
Biometry/Keratometry	

OPD Procedures	IPD Procedures
Automated Perimetry	Cutting of Iris Prolapse
Pterygium Excision	Small Lid Turnour Excision
Syringing & Probing	Conjunctival Cyst
I & C of chalazion	Capsulotomy
Wart Excision	Ant. Chamber Wash
Stye	Evisceration
Cauterization (Thermal)	
Conjunctival Resuturing	
Corneal Scarping	
I & D Lid Abscess	
Uncomplicated Lid Tear	
Indirect Ophthalmoscopy	
Retinoscopy	

- Cataract surgery with IOL implantation is the most common surgery at District hospital
- ECCE +IOL is Most common followed by Phacoemulsification

[PLEASE NOTE: After consultations with few Ophthalmologists at District level, in my opinion, Phacoemulsification at district level is much more common than other choices (though no written reference could be located on web or in library books/journals)]

28. Ans. (b) Pharmacist; (e) Laboratory technician   *[Ref. Park 27/e p706]*

29. Ans. (b) Collection of blood sample; (c) Conduct 50% delivery   *[Ref. Park 27/e p713]*

30. Ans. (c) Provision of accident and emergency care   *[Ref. Park 27/e p705]*

    Objectives of IPHs for PHCs:
    - Provision of comprehensive primary health care through PHCs
    - Achievement and maintenance of an acceptable standard of quality of health care
    - Making services more responsive and sensitive to the needs of community

31. Ans. (c) Equitable distribution   *[Ref. Park 27/e p693]*

32. Ans. (d) 5 CHC   *[Ref. Indian Public Health Standards (IPHS) Guidelines for Community Health Centres Revised 2012, MOHFW, GOI p5]*
    - According to IPHS, One ophthalmologist is being envisaged for every 5 lakh population, i.e. one ophthalmologist will cater to 5 CHCs in India.

> **ALSO REMEMBER**
> - According to WHO, One ophthalmologist is being envisaged for every 50000 population in every Asian country by 2020

33. Ans. (d) 7   *[Ref. Park 25/e p496]*
    - ASHA 6 visits in Institutional deliveries: Day 3, 7, 14, 21, 28, 42
    - ASHA 7 visits in Home based deliveries: Day 1, 3, 7, 14, 21, 28, 42

34. **Ans. (d) Medical officer-in-charge**
    [Ref. Community Health Care by Goel 1/e p239]
    - Village community is requested to recommended 2–3 persons suitable to be Health guides
    - Final selection is made by Medical officers of PHC jointly after consulting with Block Development Officer and Field staff of several government organisations

35. **Ans. (d) Health education**
    [Ref. Declaration of Alma Ata, International Conference on Primary Health Care, Alma-Ata, USSR, 6–12. 1978]

    Primary health care concept
    - Background: One year after the World Health Assembly stated its "Health for All" goal, WHO came up with the concept of primary health care at Alma-Ata Conference, USSR, in 1978
    - Broad principles: Social equity, National coverage, Self-reliance and Inter-sectoral coordination
    - Aim: To put the people's health in the people's hand
    - Definition: Essential health care based on practical, scientifically sound and socially acceptable methods and technology made universally accessible to individuals and families in the community through their full participation and at a cost that the community and the country can afford to maintain at every stage of their development in the spirit of self-reliance and self-determination

36. **Ans. (c) i, ii, iii, v only** *[Ref. Park 23/e p902]*

    Village health guide (VHG)
    - VHG scheme launched 2 October 1977
    - Work: Treatment of simple ailments, First aid, MCH including family planning, Health education Sanitation
    - National target norm: I VHG per 1000 population
    - Selection criteria:
      - *Preferably women, permanent residents of local community*
      - *Minimum VI standard education, able to read and write*
      - *Acceptable to all sections of community*
      - *Able to spare 2–3 hours of work every day*
    - Training at nearby PHC, 200 hours (3 months) duration
    - Stipend: 3000/- per month

37. **Ans. (a) 1000–2500** *[Ref. NUHM Document, MOHFW. GOI p4]*

    Urban Social Health Activist (USHA)
    - Frontline community worker expected to deliver services at the doorstep in community
    - Link between Urban Primary Health Centre (UPHC) and urban slum population
    - 1 UHSA worker per 1000–2500 population (250–500 households)
    - Woman who resides in the slum, preferably 25–45 years age
    - Chosen through a community driven process involving urban local body of counselors, self-help groups, Anganwadis.

38. **Ans. (c) 5000** *[Ref. Park 27/e p699]*
    - Sub-centre in Plains is for 5000 population (and for 3000 population in hilly/tribal areas)
    - Health worker (male), Health worker (Female) are located at Sub-centre

39. **Ans. (d) Appropriate technology** *[Ref. Park 27/e p694]*

    Appropriate Technology
    - Definition: Technology that is scientifically sound, adaptable to local needs and acceptable to those who apply it and those for whom it is used and that can be maintained by the people themselves in keeping with the principle of self-reliance with the resources the community and country can afford
    - Examples:
      - ORS instead of expensive IV fluids in mild and moderate dehydration
      - Growth charts: Can be maintained by health workers or even mothers
      - Vaccine Vial Monitor (VVM) instead of lab testing of potency of vaccine
      - Biogas system in a small community rather than Piped natural gas or LPG cylinders
      - Standpipe: Socially acceptable, financially more feasible than house-to-house connections.

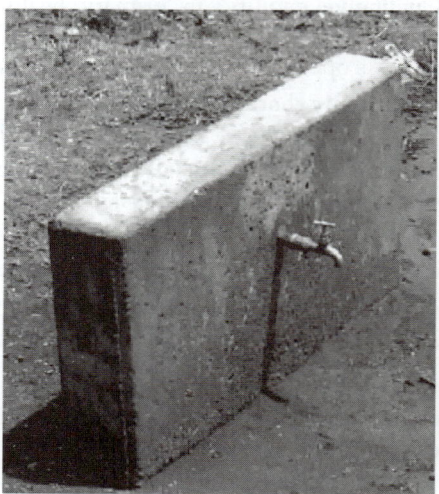

Standpipe in a village

40. **Ans. (d) Community health officer is medical graduate or post-graduate** *[Ref. Park 27/e p709]*

    Community Health Officer (CHO) at CHC (First referral unit)
    - Non-medical post created at CHC
    - Selected from supervisory category of staff at PHC and District level
    - Minimum 7 years' experience in Rural health programs
    - States who have not opted for CHO-scheme, appoint Second Medical officer at CHC

41. **Ans. (d) Setting up cost is given by state government**
    [Ref. NHM Guidelines, MoHFW, GOI. 2013. P54]

    Urban Community Health Centre (U-CHC)
    - First referral unit in Urban areas under NUHM
    - To provide medical care, minor surgical facilities and facilities for institutional delivery
    - May be set up as a satellite hospital for every 4–5 U-PHCs
      - In non-metro cities: 1 U-CHC per 250,000 population with in-patient services with 30–50 bedded facility
      - In metro cities: 1 U-CHCs per 5 lakh population with 100 bedded facility

- For setting up the U-CHCs the Central Govt. would provide only a one time capital cost
  - Recurrent costs including the salary of the staff would be borne by the respective state governments.

42. Ans. (d) Appropriate technology [Ref. Park 27/e p694]
43. Ans. (b) 30000 in plains area; (d) 20000 in tribal area [Ref. Park 27/e p705]
44. Ans. (b) 100 [Ref. Indian Public Health Standards for Sub-Centres 2006 Guidelines p3]
    - Total population catered by a Subcentre = 5000
    - Crude birth rate (CBR) India = 20.4 per 1000 Mid-year population (SRS 2016)
    - So, estimated number of births in a year = 20.4/1000 × 5000 = 102 births per year
    - Also, current Infant mortality rate (IMR) India = 34 per 1000 Live births
    - So, Expected number of infant deaths in a year in that population = 34/1000 × 100 = 3.4 deaths
    - So, total number of expected alive infants = 102–3.4 = 99 Infants approximately
45. Ans. (c) Adulteration of food prevention [Ref. Park 25/e p964]

    Inclusions in Concurrent list (MoHFW) [Mnemonic: V CLAPPED]
    - Vital statistics
    - Communicable diseases spread prevention
    - Labour welfare
    - Adulteration of food prevention
    - Ports other than major
    - Population control and family planning
    - Economic and social planning
    - Drugs and poisons control

Review Questions

46. Ans. (a) Zila Parishad [Ref. Park 27/e p1006–1007]
47. Ans. (b) Sound referral center [Ref. Park 27/e p706–709]
48. Ans. (c) Tertiary health care [Ref. Internet]
49. Ans. (c) 80–1.20,000 [Ref. Park 27/e p709]
50. Ans. (d) Supplementary functioning of under six children [Ref. Park 27/e p706]
51. Ans. (c) 20,000 [Ref. Park 27/e p705]
52. Ans. (b) 20,000 & 3000 respectively [Ref. Park 27/e p705]
53. Ans. (d) Nyaya sabha [Ref. Park 27/e p1006]
54. Ans. (c) Appropriate technology [Ref. Park 27/e p694]
55. Ans. (d) Health assistant [Ref. Park 27/e p693]

HEALTH PLANNING

56. Ans. (b) Goal [Ref. Park 27/e p996]
    - *Goal*: Ultimate desired state towards which objectives and resources are directed
    - Is not constrained by time or existing resources
    - Is not necessarily attainable

> **ALSO REMEMBER**
> - *National Rural Health Mission (NRHM) was launched in*: 2005
> - *Target years for important health related goals*:
>   - National socio-demographic goals of *'National Population Policy 2000'* have to be achieved by 2010
>   - Goals of *'National Health Policy 2002'* have to be achieved by 2015 (Few goal(s) each for 2005, 2007, 2010 and 2015)
>   - 8 Millennium Development Goals (MDGs) have to achieved by 2015
>   - 3 out of 8 goals, 8 out of 18 targets required to achieve them and 18 out of 48 indicators of progress are *'directly health related'*
>   - Goal 4, 5 and 6 are *'directly health related'*
>   - Goal 2 and 3 *'do not pertain to health'*
> - *3 next diseases targeted for eradication globally*:
>   - Poliomyelitis
>   - Guinea worm/Dracunculiasis
>   - Measles
> - *Disease next targeted for elimination from India*: Poliomyelitis

57. Ans. (a) To bring down total fertility rate (TFR) to replacement levels by 2015 [Ref. Park 27/e p568]
58. Ans. (d) Bhore Committee [Ref. Park 25/e p937]
    - Bhore Committee (1946) gave along term plan known as "3-million Plan". It envisaged setting up 'Primary health units' with 75-bedded hospitals for each 10,000–20,000 population and 'Secondary health units' with 650-bedded hospitals, again regionalized around district hospitals with 2,500 beds

> **ALSO REMEMBER**
> - Bhore Committee (1946), also known as *'Health Survey & Development Committee'* was appointed by Government of India, with Sir Joseph Bhore as chairman *'in 1943'*

59. Ans. (a) 100 per 100,000 live births [Ref. Park 27/e p568]
    - Under the National Population Policy (NPP) 2000, it is aimed to reduce the maternal mortality ratio (MMR) to below 100 per 100,000 live births
60. Ans. (d) Eliminate Lymphatic Filariasis [Ref. Park 27/e p1001]
    - Under National Health Policy (NHP)–2002, *'Lymphatic Filariasis has to be eliminated by 2015'*

> **ALSO REMEMBER**
> - National socio-demographic goals of 'National Population Policy 2000' have to be achieved by 2010
> - 'Millennium Development Goals' (MDGs) have to be achieved by 2015
> - Previous National Health Policy, India was formulated in 1983

61. **Ans. (d) Major changes in Medical education to prepare "Social Physicians"** [Ref. Park 25/e p937]
    - Bhore Committee (1946) recommended preparing 'Social physicians' (3 months internship training in medical education of Preventive and Social Medicine)
    - Constitution of All India Health Service on the pattern of IAS: Recommendation of *Mudaliar Committee* (1962)
    - Separate staff for Family Planning Programme: Recommendation of *Mukherji Committee* (1965)
    - Creation of "Bands of para-professionals & semi-professional health workers":
    - Recommendation of *Srivastav Committee* (1975)

62. **Ans. (c) Kartar Singh Committee** [Ref. Park 25/e p938]
    - Kartar Singh Committee was known as 'The Committee on Multi purpose Workers under Health and Family Planning'

63. **Ans. (b) A-I, B-IV, C-III, D-II** [Ref. Park 25/e p937-939]
    - Bhore Committee: *Health Survey & Development Committee*
    - Mudaliar Committee: *Health Survey & Planning Committee*
    - Jungalwallah Committee: *Committee on Integration of Health Services*
    - Kartar Singh Committee: *Committee on MPWs under Health & Family Planning*

64. **Ans. (c) Srivastave Committee:** [Ref. Park 25/e p938]
    - Srivastava Committee (1975) was set up as the 'Group on Medical Education & Support Manpower'

65. **Ans. (b) d c b a** [Ref. Park 27/e p997]
    - *Planning Cycle consists of following steps*:
      – Pre-planning: Government interest, Legislation, Organization for planning and Administrative capacity
      – *Step 1:* 'Analysis of health situation'
      – *Step 2:* Establishment of goals and objectives
      – *Step 3:* Assessment of resources
      – *Step 4:* Fixing priorities
      – *Step 5:* Write-up of formulated plan
      – *Step 6:* Programming and implementation
      – *Step 7:* Monitoring
      – *Step 8:* Evaluation

66. **Ans. (c) Expert Level Committee on Universal Health Coverage** [Ref. Universal Health Coverage in India, Planning Commission, Government of India, 2010]
    HLEG Recommendations
    - High Level Expert Group (HLEG, Planning Commission, GOI) on Universal health Coverage has suggested 3½ year MBBS course for serving rural population
    - HLEG was developed for XII Five Year Plan
    - Rural doctors will be called as 'Community Health Officers'
    - 3½ Degree given: B.Sc. Community Health

67. **Ans. (d) All** [Ref. K. Park 27/e p997]

68. **Ans. (d) Procedure** [Ref. Park 27/e p997]

69. **Ans. (c) Recommends health manpower policy** [Ref. India Health Report 2010, p132]

70. **Ans. (b) Manpower and planning** [Ref. India Health Report 2010, p132]

71. **Ans. (c) Shrivastava committee** [Ref. K. Park 25/e p939]

72. **Ans. (c) High level expert group** [Ref. Universal Health Coverage in India, Planning Commission, Government of India, 2010]

73. **Ans. (b) Article 21** [Ref. Ideas of Being Indians and Making of Indians by Varugghhese, 1/e]

Review Questions

74. **Ans. (c) Kartar Singh committee** [Ref. Park 23/e p873-875, 25/e p938]

75. **Ans. (a) Nutritional supplements** [Ref. Park 27/e p1002]

76. **Ans. (a) Bhore committee** [Ref. Park 25/e p937]

77. **Ans. (d) Kartar Singh committee** [Ref. Park 23/e p874-875, 25/e p938-939]

78. **Ans. (c) Integration of PHCs** [Ref. Internet]

79. **Ans. (a) Shrivastav Committee** [Ref. Park 25/e p938]

80. **Ans. (c) Union health minister** [Ref. Park 27/e p1005]

81. **Ans. (b) Planning, Object, Goal, Evaluation** [Ref. Park 27/e p997]

82. **Ans. (b) Concept of multipurpose worker** [Ref. Park 25/e p937]

HEALTH MANAGEMENT

83. **Ans. (b) Cost benefit analysis** [Ref. Park 25/e p934]
    Evaluation of Efficiency
    - *Cost-benefit analysis:* Both input as well as output is in monetary terms
    - *Cost-effectiveness analysis:* Input is in monetary terms whereas output is in terms of 'results achieved'

84. **Ans. (b) Management by objective** [Ref. Park 25/e p934]
    - Behavioural sciences methods include Organizational design, Personal management, Communication, Information system. Management by Objectives (MBO)
    - Quantitative methods include Cost benefit analysis, Cost effective analysis, Cost accounting, Input-output analysis, Model, Systems analysis, Network analysis (PERT/CPM), Planning programming budget system, Work sampling, Decision making

85. **Ans. (c) QALYs gained** [Ref. Textbook of Community Medicine by Sunder Lal, 2/e p56-57; Park 27/e p999]
    - *Cost Effectiveness Analysis (CEA):* Benefits are measured in natural units (e.g. Life years gained, heart attacks avoided)
      – CEA is an expression of the desired effect of a programme, service, institution or support activity in reducing a health problem

- CEA measures the degree of attainment of pre-determined objectives and targets
- Most comprehensive indicator of CEA: Quality adjusted life years (QALYs) gained
• Cost Benefit Analysis (CBA): Benefits are measured in monetary terms
  – Approaches for CBAL:
    a. Human capital approach
    b. Willingness to pay approach

86. **Ans. (d) Efferent** [Ref. Internet; www.cliffnotes.com]

Power of a Manager:
• A manager has two sources of 'Power' (ability to influence or use the authority entrusted):
  – Positional sources of power:
    - *Reward*: A manager can reward (monetary, promotion) his subordinates
    - *Coercive* (Punishment): A manager can punish his subordinates
    - *Legal*: A manager has legal authority and power over subordinates
    - *Contractual*: A manager has power over subordinates by virtue of signed contract by his employees
  – Personal sources of power:
    - *Expertise*: A manager can assert greater power if he has expertise in his field of work
    - *Referent*: A manager has greater power if he has good inter-personal relationships with his subordinates

87. **Ans. (a) Cost effective analysis** [Ref. Park 27/e p999]
• *Cost Effective Analysis*: A management technique where benefits are expressed in terms of results achieved, e.g., number of lives saved or number of days free from disease
  – It is a more promising tool than cost benefit analysis in the health field
• *Cost Benefit Analysis*: A management technique where economic benefits of any programme are compared with cost of that programme
  – The 'benefits are expressed in monetary terms'
  – Main drawback: All benefits in field of heath cannot be expressed in monetary terms
• *Cost Accounting*: A quantitative management technique which provides basic data on cost structure of any programme
• *Input-Output Analysis*: An economic technique which enables calculations to be made of the effects of changing the inputs

88. **Ans. (a) Cost benefit analysis** [Ref. Park 27/e p999]

89. **Ans. (a) Is a part of Input-Output analysis** [Ref. Park 27/e p999]

90. **Ans. (c) Ultimate desired state towards which objectives and resources are directed** [Ref. Park 27/e p996]

91. **Ans. (d) Total Quality management** [Ref. Park 27/e p999]

92. **Ans. (d) Work sampling** [Ref. Park 27/e p1000]

93. **Ans. (a) ABC** [Ref. Inventory management by DC Bose, 1/e p32]

94. **Ans. (d) Longest path in a network** [Ref. Park 27/e p1000]

95. **Ans. (a) Cost effectiveness analysis** [Ref. Park 27/e p999]

Health Management Techniques/Methods:

Behavioural sciences methods	Quantitative methods
Organizational design	Cost benefit analysis
Personal management	Cost effective analysis
Communication	Cost accounting
Information system	Input-output analysis
Management by Objectives (MBO)	Model
	Systems analysis
	Network analysis (PERT/CPM)
	Planning programming budget system
	Work sampling
	Decision making

96. **Ans. (b) Desirable** [Ref. Inventory Management by Bose 1/e p36]

VED analysis
• Vital drugs: Items whose absence cannot be tolerated (10% of total items)
• Essential drugs: Items whose absence can be tolerated for some time (40% of total items)
• Desirable drugs: Items whose absence can be tolerated for long time (50% of total items)

ALSO REMEMBER
• ABC analysis: Always Better Control

Category	Label	Quantity (%)	Cost (%)
A	Outstandingly important	15	70
B	Average importance	30	25
C	Relatively unimportant	55	5

• SDE analysis: Scarce- Difficult- Easy- availability
• FSN analysis: Fast- Slow- Non- moving
• HML analysis: High Cost Items-Medium Cost Items- Low Cost Items
• SOS analysis: Seasonal items-Off seasonal items
• GOLF analysis: Government-Open market-Local-Foreign source of supply

97. **Ans. (b) Drug inventory management at PHC** [Ref. Inventory Management by Bose 1/e p36]

Inventory management
• Science primarily about specifying the shape and placement of stocked goods
• It is required at different locations within a facility or within many locations of a supply network to precede the regular and planned course of production and stock of materials

- Right stock at right quantity, in right place, at right time, and at right cost
- Minimize costs and minimize wastage.

98. **Ans. (a) Developed by Motorola; (c) Represents an ideology that focuses on statistical improvements to a business process; (d) It is a quality-control program; (e) It can used in Health care sector**
    [Ref. Improving Healthcare Quality and Cost with Six Sigma by Trusko 1/e p35]

Six Sigma (6σ)

Introduced by Bill Smith (Motorola, 1980)

- A set of techniques and tools that seek to improve the quality of the output of a process by identifying and removing the causes of defects in manufacturing and business processes (99.99966% of all opportunities statistically expected to be free of defects)
- Specific value targets: Reduce process cycle time, reduce pollution, reduce costs, increase customer satisfaction, and increase profits
- Utility in fields of Manufacturing, Engineering and construction, Finance, Supply chain, Healthcare (Inventory control)
- Two Methodologies (Deming's Plan-Do-Study-Act Cycle)

1. **DMAIC:** Used for projects aimed at improving an existing business process

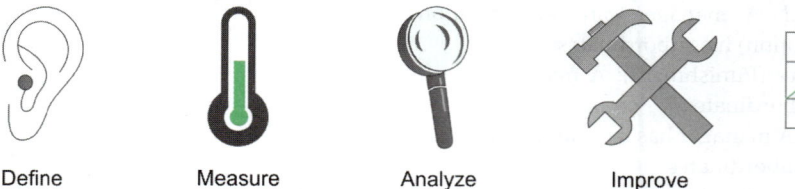

Define — Measure — Analyze — Improve — Control

2. **DMADV:** Used for projects aimed at creating new product or process design

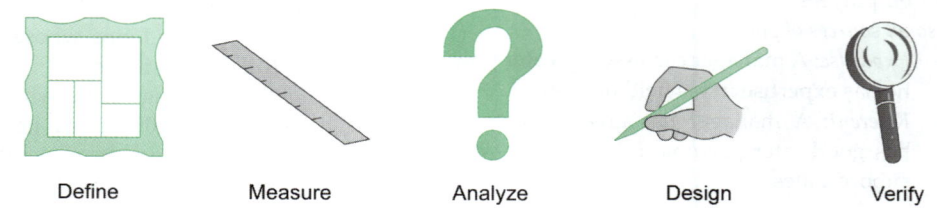

Define — Measure — Analyze — Design — Verify

Review Questions

99. Ans. (b) Systems analysis *[Ref. Park 27/e p1000]*
100. Ans. (a) Network analysis *[Ref. Park 27/e p1000]*
101. Ans. (b) Burning/breaking of bridges *[Ref. Logical reasoning]*
102. Ans. (b) Quantitative analysis *[Ref. Park 27/e p999]*
103. Ans. (c) Management *[Ref. Park 27/e p1000]*
104. Ans. (a) Pharmacists are more than lab technician *[Ref. Park 27/e p999]*
105. Ans. (d) Work sampling *[Ref. Park 27/e p1000]*

MISCELLANEOUS

106. **Ans. (a) Input** *[Ref. Park 26/e p976]*

    Three types of Evaluation for Health Services
    - *Structure:* If facilities, equipment, manpower and organization meet good standards
    - *Process:* Recognition, diagnostic procedures, treatment & clinical management, care and prevention is compared with a pre-determined standard (Medical/Nursing audit: An objective and systematic way of evaluation of Physician/Nurse's performance)
    - *Outcome:* If persons using health services experience measure benefits like improved survival, reduced disability (5Ds of Ill-Health: Disease, Discomfort, Dissatisfaction, Disability, Death)

107. **Ans. (d) 3000, 2** *[Ref. Financing and Cost Recovery 1/e p48]*

    - *Reorder factor:* Help us calculate the actual order to be placed (Stock as well as buffer taken into account). Though RF values vary in literature, most common ones used are given below:

Frequency of drug supply	Reorder factor
Monthly	2
Every 3 months	6
Every 6 months	12

    In the given question,
    - Total Tab Amlodipine requirement: 40 people × 1 tablet per day × 30 days = 1200 tablets
    - Total Tab Lisinopril requirement: 10 people × 1 tablet per day × 30 days = 300 tablets
    - Total tablets combined requirement: 1200 + 300 = 1500 tablets

- Drugs will come at PHC once a month, so Reorder factor will be 2

    So, Total drugs to be ordered: 1500 tablets × 2 = 3000 tablets

108. **Ans. (b) Drug A is more cost-effective than drug B for treating children** *[Logical Reasoning]*
    - In the given question

Drug	Cost	Effectiveness	
		Children	Adults
Drug A	2X	95%	95%
Drug B	X	90%	47%

    Also,
    - Dr. Sunil, a general practitioner, always uses drug B for the first treatment, and resorts to drug A if the infection persists WHEREAS,
    - Dr. Sudhir, another general practitioner, always uses drug A for adults and drug B for children

    Therefore,
    - Drug A is more effective than B for treating children (A - 95% *versus* B - 90%)
    - Drug A is more cost-effective than drug B for treating adults (A – 2X cost with 95% effectiveness *versus* B – X cost with 47% effectiveness)
    - Dr. Sudhir's regime achieves a higher level of cost-effectiveness than Dr. Sunil's (Dr. Sudhir – A for adults and B for children *versus* Dr. Sunil – B for initial treatment and A if infection persists)
    - However, Drug B is more cost effective for treating children (B – Cost X with 90% effectiveness *versus* A – Cost 2x with 95% effectiveness i.e., marginal increase)

109. **Ans. (b) 5.2% of GDP** *[Ref. World Health Report, 2000]*
    - *According to the World Health report 2000, India's total health expenditure on health as % of GDP: 5.2%*

110. **Ans. (c) 7.8** *[Ref. Internet]*

111. **Ans. (c) Disability prevalence** *[Ref. Park 23/e p27]*
    - *Crucial factors for realization of goals of a National Health Policy*:
        – A political commitment
        – Financial implications
        – Administrative reforms
        – Community participation
        – Basic legislation

112. **Ans. (a) Repeatability** *[Ref. Park 27/e p1008–1009]*
    - Components/elements of evaluation process in health services are:
        – *Relevance:* Appropriateness (need) of a health service
        – *Adequacy:* Sufficient attention to pre-determined course of action
        – *Accessibility:* Proportion of population expected to use the service
        – *Acceptability:* Socially and culturally acceptable
        – *Effectiveness:* Extent of prevention/alleviation of underlying problem
        – *Efficiency:* How well resources are utilized
        – *Impact:* Overall effect of programme/service on health and development

113. **Ans. (b) Large hospitals** *[Ref. Park 23/e p48, 25/e p55]*
    - Hospitals are known as *'Ivory Towers of Disease'*, as they exist in splendid isolation in the community, absorb vast proportion (50–80%) of the health budget, are not people-oriented, are inflexible in procedures and styles and treatment is expensive

Review Question

114. **Ans. (b) Gram Sevak** *[Ref. Park 21/e p839–40]*

CHAPTER 15

International Health

INTERNATIONAL HEALTH AGENCIES

World Health Organization (WHO)

> **Key points**
>
> Headquarters of WHO: Geneva, Switzerland

WHO

- *Description:* WHO is a specialized, non-political health agency of United Nations
- *Constitution of WHO:*
  - Drafted by 'Technical Preparatory Committee' in 1946
  - Came into force on 7th April, 1948^Q
- *Objective of WHO:* Is attainment by all people of the highest level of health^Q
- *First Constitutional function of WHO:* To act as the directing and co-coordinating authority on all International health work^Q
- *Headquarters of WHO:* Geneva, Switzerland^Q
- *Broad areas of work of WHO:*
  - Prevention and control of specific diseases
  - Development of comprehensive health services
  - Family health
  - Environmental health
  - Health statistics
  - Bio-medical research
  - Health literature and information
  - Cooperation with other organisations
- *Structure of WHO^Q:*
  - *The World Health Assembly (WHA):* Is the 'Health Parliament' and supreme governing body of the organization^Q; Functions of WHA:
    - To determine International health policies and programmes
    - To review work of past year
    - To approve budget for the following year
    - To elect member states to designate persons for Executive Board
    - *The Executive Board*
    - *The Secretariat:* Is the 'Chief technical and administrative unit of WHO'^{Q}
- WHO has established 6 regional organizations:

Region	Headquarters
Southeast Asia^Q	New Delhi, India
Africa	Brazzaville, Congo
The Americas	Washington DC, USA
Europe	Copenhagen, Denmark
Eastern Mediterranean	Alexandria, Egypt
Western Pacific	Manila, Philippines

World Health Day (WHD) Themes

Year	World Health Day (WHD) Theme
2010	Urbanization and health (1000 cities – 1000 lives)
2011	Antimicrobial resistance

Contd...

Contd...

Year	World Health Day (WHD) Theme
2012^Q	Ageing and health
2013^Q	High blood pressure
2014^Q	Vector borne diseases
2015^Q	Food Safety
2016	Diabetes
2017	Depression (Let's Talk)
2018, 2019*	Universal Health Coverage
2020	Support nurses and midwives
2021	Building a fairer, healthier world for everyone
2022	Our planet, our health
2023	Health for All – 75 years of public Health

> **Key points**
> **Theme 2018, 2019 WHD:** UHC

World Health Day 2023 (WHD 2023)

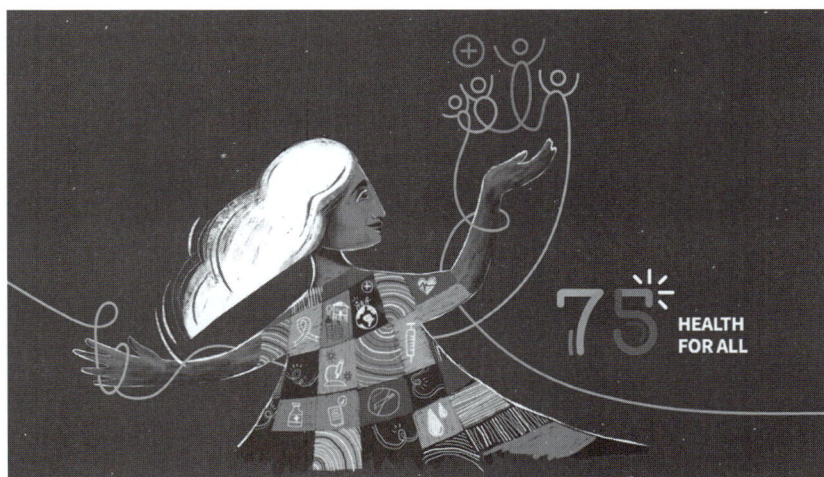

Health Agencies Headquarters

Health agencies	Headquarters
WHO (World Health Organization)^Q	Geneva, Switzerland
UNICEF (United Nations Children Fund)^Q	New York, USA
UNDP (United Nations Development Programme)	New York, USA
FAO (Food and Agricultural Organization)	Rome, Italy
ILO (International Labour Organization)	Geneva, Switzerland

> **Key points**
> UNICEF (United Nations Children Fund) New York, USA

UNICEF's GOBI-FFF Campaign^Q

- UNICEF is promoting 'GOBI Campaign' to encourage 4 strategies for a 'Child Health Revolution':
  - **G:** Growth Charts (to better monitor child development)
  - **O:** Oral Rehydration (to treat mild and moderate dehydration)
  - **B:** Breast Feeding
  - **I:** Immunization (against TB, Polio, Diphtheria, Pertussis, Tetanus and Measles)
- 'Three F's' have now been incorporated in 'UNICEF's GOBI-FFF Campaign':
  - **F:** Female Education
  - **F:** Family Spacing
  - **F:** Food Supplements

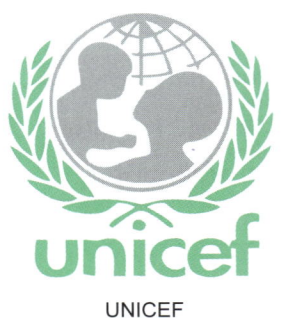

UNICEF

MISCELLANEOUS

Updated International Health Regulations (WHO IHR)

Immediately notifiable diseases	List of quarantinable diseases
• Small pox • Human Influenza • Wild Poliomyelitis • SARS *Note:* Immediately notifiable diseases must be notified "within 24 hours"	• Diphtheria • Infectious TB • Plague • Small pox • Yellow fever • SARS • Viral Haemorrhagic Fevers • Flu • Cholera

Potentially notifiable diseases
1. Public Health Importance
  • Cholera
  • Plague
  • Yellow fever
  • Viral Haemorrhagic fevers*
  • Dengue
  • West Nile Fever
  • Rift Valley Fever
  • Meningococcal disease
2. Biological/Chemical/Radiological Events
3. Serious Illness of Unknown Origin
	Diseases under training & research
	• Malaria
	• Filariasis
	• Leprosy
	• Leishmaniasis
	• Trypanosomiasis
	• Schistosomiasis
	• Onchocerciasis
	• TB
	• Vector borne diseases$
	• Ebola
	• Helminthiasis

(Table © Dr Vivek Jain 2022–23) (* Ebola, Marburg, Lassa) ($ Dengue, Zika, Chikungunya fever) (Based on WHO, CDC Guidelines)

Bio-Terrorism Agents

> **Key points**
> Most dangerous BT Agent: Smallpox

Category A^Q	Category B	Category C^Q
Can be easily disseminated	Moderately easy to disseminate	Emerging pathogens
High mortality rates	Moderate morbidity + low mortality	Available
Public panic & disruption	Require enhanced diagnostic capacity	Ease of production
	Require enhanced surveillance	High morbidity and mortality
Botulism **T**ularaemia **A**nthrax **S**mall pox **P**lague **V**iral hemorrhagic fevers [**Mnemonic: Bio T**errorism **A**gents include **S**mall **P**ox **V**irus]	Brucellosis Clostridium perfringens Food safety threats Water safety threats Glanders Meliodoses Psittacosis Q fever Ricin toxin Staphylococcal enterotoxin B Epidemic typhus Viral encephalitis	Nipah virus Hantavirus

List of Few Nobel Laureates in Physiology or Medicine

> **Key points**
> *Sir Ronald Ross:* Life cycle of Plasmodium
> *F.G. Banting & J.J.R. McLeod:* Insulin
> *Paul H. Muller*: DDT
> *Har Gobind Khorana*: Interpretation of genetic code

- *Sir Ronald Ross:* Life cycle of Plasmodium^Q
- *I.P. Pavlov:* Physiology of digestion
- *Robert Koch:* Discoveries in Tuberculosis^Q
- *Paul Ehrlich:* Immunity
- *F.G. Banting & J.J.R. McLeod:* Insulin^Q
- *Willem Einthoven:* ECG^Q
- *Karl Landsteiner:* Human blood groups^Q
- *Sir Alexander Fleming:* Penicillin^Q
- *Paul H. Muller:* DDT^Q

- *S.A. Waksman:* Streptomycin (First antibiotic, against TB)^Q
- *Har Gobind Khorana:* Interpretation of genetic code^Q
- *Sir Godfrey N. Hounsfield:* CT scan^Q
- *J.E. Murray & E.D. Thomas:* Organ and cell transplantation
- *Sir Peter Mansfield:* MRI^Q
- *B.J. Marshall & J.R. Warren:* H. pylori; its role in peptic ulcer disease
- *H.Z. Hausen:* HPV causing cervical cancer
- *F.B. Sinoussi & L. Montagnier:* HIV
- *Robert G. Edwards:* In-vitro fertilization

PYQs: Quick Review for NEET

World Health Day	7 April
'O' in GOBI Campaign (UNICEF) stands for	Oral Rehydration therapy
Diseases under International Health Regulations	Cholera, Plague and Yellow fever (and Smallpox, Wild Polio, Human Influenza and SARS)
Area around airports kept free of Aedes	400 m
District border cluster strategy is supported by	UNICEF
Headquarters of UNICEF is at	New York
Emporiatrics deals with the health of	International travelers
World Anti-tobacco day is celebrated on	31st May
According to IHR, pregnant woman can take air travel up to POG	36 weeks (32 weeks if Twins)
World Health Day of WHO is on	7th April
World AIDS day is on	1 December
Monitoring area in and around airports helps in control of disease	Yellow fever
Theme of World Health Day celebrated on 7th April 2015	From farm to plate, make food safe!
Headquarter of UNICEF are located at	New York, USA
International Red Cross was founded by	Henry Dunant
National Epilepsy day is	17th November
World Heart day is celebrated on	29 September
World Anaesthesia day is celebrated on	16 October
Declaration of Lisbon is related to	Right of patient
The last case of Small pox was reported in the world in	1977 (Somalia)
World breastfeeding week is celebrated in	1st week of August

Multiple Choice Questions

INTERNATIONAL HEALTH AGENCIES

1. Following is correct about the Colombo Plan: [NEET PG Pattern 2023]
   (a) Chemotherapy units
   (b) Health manpower strengthening
   (c) PET scans for cancer diagnosis
   (d) Cobalt therapy units

2. For applied nutrition program, seeds and manure supply under school health services has been done by: [NEET PG Pattern 2022]
   (a) WHO
   (b) UNICEF
   (c) CARE
   (d) UNDP

3. Which of the following statements is incorrect about WHO? [AIPGME 1999]
   (a) Objective of WHO is attainment by all people of the highest level of health
   (b) Headquarters of WHO are located in Geneva
   (c) WHO is a non-specialized, political agency of United Nations
   (d) World Health Assembly is the 'Health Parliament' and supreme governing body of the organization

4. Match the following health agencies and the location of their headquarters:
   Health agency Headquarters
   A. WHO I – Rome, Italy
   B. UNICEF–II – New York, USA
   C. FAO III – Geneva, Switzerland
   (a) A – I, B – II, C – III [AIIMS Nov 1999]
   (b) A – III, B – II, C – I [RJ 2000]
   (c) A – III, B – I, C – II
   (d) A – I, B – III, C – II

5. WHO was established in: [AIIMS Dec 95]
   (a) 1945
   (b) 1948
   (c) 1950
   (d) 1956

6. International Red Cross is based in: [AIIMS Dec 97]
   (a) Geneva
   (b) New York
   (c) New Delhi
   (d) Rome

7. In UNICEF's GOBI Campaign, 'O' stands for:
   (a) Oral Contraceptives [DPG 2006]
   (b) Oral Rehydration Therapy
   (c) Obesity
   (d) Occupational hazards

8. Members of southeast Asia of WHO are: [PGI June 01]
   (a) Japan
   (b) Afghanistan
   (c) India
   (d) Pakistan
   (e) Sri Lanka

9. Highest funding for reproductive health is by:
   (a) UNFPA [NEET Pattern 2013]
   (b) UNICEF
   (c) ILO
   (d) WHO

10. Which of the following international health agencies promoted a GOBI campaign? [PGMCET 2015]
    (a) USAID
    (b) UNICEF
    (c) UNDP
    (d) UNFPA

11. Surveillance Reporting System used by WHO is: [NEET Pattern 2015]
    (a) Technical Report Series
    (b) Weekly Epidemiological Report
    (c) Morbidity and Mortality Weekly Report
    (d) WHO Bulletin

12. 'Clean care is safer care' guideline given by WHO is for: [NEET Pattern 2015]
    (a) Hand hygiene
    (b) Obstetric care
    (c) Cord care
    (d) Injection practices

Review Questions

13. UNICEF provides all except: [UP 2000]
    (a) Child nutrition
    (b) Child health education
    (c) Immunization
    (d) Family planning

14. World bank gives loans for: [UP 2005]
    (a) For economic growth
    (b) Cobalt therapy of radiotherapy department
    (c) Purchase of microscope for tuberculosis investigation
    (d) To change of the social justice

15. All of the following activities of Junior Red Cross except: [UP 2007]
    (a) Military hospital worker
    (b) Village uplift
    (c) Prevent epidemic work
    (d) Any of the above

16. All of the following organizations have their head quarter at Geneva except: [MH 2006] [(MH 2008]
    (a) UNICEF
    (b) WHO
    (c) ILO
    (d) International red cross

17. All disease are included in internationally notifiable disease except: [RJ 2004]
    (a) Plague
    (b) Cholera
    (c) Yellow fever
    (d) TB

MISCELLANEOUS

18. All are true about categories of bioterrorism agents except: *[INICET May 2023]*
    (a) Category A is most dangerous
    (b) Category B is less dangerous
    (c) Category C is new emerging pathogens
    (d) Category D is highly lethal agents

19. Type-A bioterrorism agent include: *[NEET PG Pattern January 2020]*
    (a) Coxiella burnetii
    (b) Bacillus anthracis
    (c) Clostridium perfringens
    (d) NIPAH virus

20. According to Sustainable Development Goal 3 – "Ensure healthy life and promote well being for all at all ages", Target 3.1 is to reduce Maternal mortality ratio by 2030 is less than: *[NEET PG Pattern January 2020]*
    (a) 100   (b) 50
    (c) 90   (d) 70

21. Diseases under International Surveillance includes all except: *[AIPGME 1991, 992]*
    (a) Louse borne typhus fever *[AIIMS May 1991]*
    (b) Relapsing fever *[NEET Pattern 2013, 2017]*
    (c) Paralytic polio
    (d) Yellow fever

22. Tropical diseases targeted for research and training by WHO include all except: *[JIPMER 2008]*
    (a) Trypanosomiasis   (b) Filariasis
    (c) Schistosomiasis   (d) Onchocerciasis

23. Finger Print Bureau was first established in: *[AIPGME 06]*
    (a) England   (b) China
    (c) India   (d) Singapore

24. Emporiatrics refers to study of: *[AIIMS May 95]*
    (a) Occupational disease (b) Air pollution
    (c) Environmental factor (d) Health of travelers

25. Disease excluded and re-included from International Health Regulations till date is: *[AIPGME 2006]*
    (a) Small pox   (b) Guinea worm
    (c) Typhoid   (d) HIV/AIDS

26. World Health Day is observed every year on:
    (a) January 11 *[AIIMS Dec 92]*
    (b) April 7 *[NEET Pattern 2013]*
    (c) June 5 *[RJ 2000]*
    (d) December 1

27. Only certificate of vaccination required for international travel is: *[Karnataka 2009]*
    (a) Hepatitis B *[MP 2003]*
    (b) BCG
    (c) Tetanus
    (d) Yellow fever

28. Contribution of Germany to pubic health: *[PGI June 05]*
    (a) Germ theory   (b) Pasteurization
    (c) Quarantine ship   (d) Social medicine
    (e) Compulsory sickness benefit

29. All of the following are most important and potential agents which can be used for Bio-terrorism except: *[AIIMS Dec 97]*
    (a) Smallpox   (b) Plague
    (c) Botulism   (d) Tuberculosis

30. Which of the following is not true about World Health Report 2008? *[AIPGME 2011]*
    (a) Service delivery reforms (b) Leadership reforms
    (c) Public Policy reforms   (d) Economic reforms

31. For studying the complete amino acid sequence of two polypeptide chains of Insulin, Nobel Prize was awarded to: *[AIIMS November 2011]*
    (a) Frederick Sanger   (b) Banting and Macleod
    (c) Paul Muller   (d) Alexander Fleming

32. Bioterrorism group-A agent is? *[NEET Pattern 2012, 2013]*
    (a) Q fever   (b) Typhus fever
    (c) Anthrax   (d) Brucellosis

33. Maximum damage to Napoleon's army during his march to Moscow was done by: *[DNB June 2010]*
    (a) Typhus   (b) Plague
    (c) Diarrhea   (d) Typhoid

34. According to International Health regulation (IHR) Act, a pregnant woman, with the following duration of pregnancy (in weeks), can't travel by air to other country: *[DNB 2007]*
    (a) 20   (b) 28
    (c) 32   (d) 36

35. Patient of which disease need not be quarantined? *[NEET Pattern 2015]*
    (a) Avian flu   (b) Ebola virus disease
    (c) Infectious TB   (d) Tetanus

36. Millennium development Goals are based upon: *[NEET Pattern 2016]*
    (a) WHO health records
    (b) UNICEF health criteria
    (c) United Nation Millennium Declaration
    (d) SEARO Millennium Declaration

37. Organism included in Category 'A' Bio-terrorism is/are: *[PGI May 2018]*
    (a) Vibrio cholera   (b) Clostridium botulinum
    (c) Yersinia pestis   (d) Bacillus anthracis
    (e) Burkholderia mallei

Review Question

38. International Notification is must in the following except: *[TN 2003]*
    (a) Cholera   (b) Plague
    (c) Yellow fever   (d) Paralytic polio

Explanations

INTERNATIONAL HEALTH AGENCIES

1. **Ans. (d) Cobalt therapy units** [Ref. Park 27/e p1031]
   Colombo Plan 1950
   - Drawn up for cooperative economic development of South and South East Asia (20 countries) with main aim to improve living standards of people
   - Industrial and agricultural development
   - Support for Health Promotion (mostly via fellowships)
   - AIIMS, New Delhi was established with financial assistant from New Zealand
   - Canada supplied Cobalt therapy units to medical institutions in India

2. **Ans. (b) UNICEF** [Ref. Evaluation Study of the Applied Nutrition Programme 1976 p1]
   Applied Nutrition Program
   - UNICEF promoted the scheme by supplying basic equipment for production and training while FAO and WHO were involved in providing technical advice
   - UNICEF provided seeds, manure and water supply equipment for developing school gardens, to be utilized in school feeding programs

3. **Ans. (c) WHO is a non-specialized, political agency of United Nations** [Ref. Park 27/e p1026]
   WORLD HEALTH ORGANIZATION (WHO):
   - WHO is a specialized, non-political health agency of United Nations
   - *Constitution of WHO*:
     – Drafted by 'Technical Preparatory Committee' in 1946
     – Came into force on 7th April, 1948
   - *Objective of WHO*: Is attainment by all people of the highest level of health
   - *First Constitutional function of WHO*: To act as the directing and co-coordinating authority on all International health work
   - *Headquarters of WHO*: Geneva, Switzerland
   - *Structure of WHO*:
     – The World Health Assembly (WHA): Is the 'Health Parliament' and supreme governing body of the organization; Functions of WHA:
       - To determine International health policies and programmes
       - To review work of past year
       - To approve budget for the following year
       - To elect member states to designate persons for Executive Board
     – The Executive Board
     – The Secretariat: Is the 'Chief technical and administrative unit of WHO'
   - WHO has established 6 regional organizations:

Region	Headquarters
Southeast Asia	New Delhi, India
Africa	Brazzaville, Congo
The Americas	Washington DC, USA
Europe	Copenhagen, Denmark
Eastern Mediterranean	Alexandria, Egypt
Western Pacific	Manila, Philippines

   ALSO REMEMBER
   - *WHO is unique among UN specialized agencies*: It has its own constitution, own governing bodies, own membership and own budget
   - *7th April every year is celebrated every year as World Health Day (WHD)*:
   - WHD 2017: Depression (Let's Talk).

4. **Ans. (b) A – III, B – II, C – I** [Ref. Park 27/e p1026–1029]
   - Health agencies and the location of their headquarters:

Health agencies	Headquarters
IRC (International Red Cross)	Geneva, Switzerland
WHO (World Health Organization)	Geneva, Switzerland
UNICEF (United Nations Children Fund)	New York, USA
UNDP (United Nations Development Programme)	New York, USA
FAO (Food and Agricultural Organization)	Rome, Italy
ILO (International Labour Organization)	Geneva, Switzerland

5. **Ans. (b) 1948** [Ref. Park 27/e p1026]
   - WHO has its origin in April 1945, whereas formal existence began on 7th April 1948

6. **Ans. (a) Geneva** [Ref. Park 27/e p1032]
   - International Red Cross was founded by 'Henry Dunant'
   - Head quarters: Geneva, Switzerland

7. **Ans. (b) Oral Rehydration Therapy** [Ref. Park 27/e p1029]
   - UNICEF is promoting 'GOBI Campaign' to encourage 4 strategies for a 'Child Health Revolution':
     – **G:** *Growth Charts (to better monitor child development)*
     – **O:** *Oral Rehydration (to treat mild and moderate dehydration)*
     – **B:** *Breast Feeding*
     – **I:** *Immunization (against TB, Polio, Diphtheria, Pertussis, Tetanus and Measles)*

ALSO REMEMBER

- In addition, recent research in the developing world has highlighted three kinds of support for women. These changes 'the three F's' have now been incorporated in 'UNICEF's GOBI-FFF Campaign':
  - F: Female Education
  - F: Family Spacing
  - F: Food Supplements

8. Ans. (c) India; (e) Sri Lanka [Ref. Park 27/e p1027]
   - Members of WHO South East Asian Region (WHO SEARO):
     - Bangladesh
     - Bhutan
     - India
     - Indonesia
     - Korea
     - Maldives Islands
     - Myanmar
     - Nepal
     - Sri Lanka
     - Thailand

ALSO REMEMBER

- Members of SAARC Region:
  - Afghanistan
  - Bangladesh
  - Bhutan
  - India
  - Maldives Islands
  - Nepal
  - Pakistan
  - Sri Lanka

9. Ans. (a) UNFPA [Ref. Park 27/e p1030]
10. Ans. (b) UNICEF [Ref. Park 27/e p1029]
11. Ans. (b) Weekly Epidemiological Report [Ref. Park 27/e p1027]
    - WHO routinely collects and disseminated Communicable disease International surveillance information through:
      - ATRS (Automated Telex Reply Service)
      - WER (Weekly Epidemiological Record)

ALSO REMEMBER

- *WHO Technical Report Series (TRS)*: Publishes views and recommendations of WHO Expert Committee on Biological Standardization and Provide updated information on the establishment, discontinuation and replacement of the WHO International Biological Reference Preparations as well on the adoption of Guidelines and Recommendation
- *WHO Bulletin*: A monthly public health journal published by WHO which aims to give public health policy and practice guidance based on the best evidence available, while encouraging closer links between scientific investigation and the art of helping populations to lead healthier lives

Contd...

- *Morbidity and Mortality Weekly Report (MMWR) series is prepared by the Centers for Disease Control and Prevention (CDC)*: Agency's primary vehicle for scientific publication of timely, reliable, authoritative, accurate, objective, and useful public health information and recommendations

12. Ans. (a) Hand hygiene [Ref. WHO Guidelines on Hand Hygiene in Health Care 2009 p4]

CLEAN CARE IS SAFER CARE

- Launched in 2005, targeted the important aspect of reducing health care-associated infections (HCAIs)
- HCAI is the most frequent harmful event in health-care delivery and occurs worldwide in both developed and developing countries
- Initial focus was to promote best hand hygiene practices globally, at all levels of health care, as a first step in ensuring high standards of infection control and patient safety
- WHO campaign, SAVE LIVES: Clean Your Hands, launched in 2009, aims to maintain the global profile

Review Questions

13. Ans. (d) Family planning [Ref. Park 27/e p1029–1030]
14. Ans. (a) For economic growth [Ref. Park 27/e p1030]
15. Ans. (a) Military hospital worker [Ref. Park 27/e p1032]
16. Ans. (a) UNICEF [Ref. Park 27/e p1029]
17. Ans. (d) TB [Ref. Park 23/e p841, 25/e p904]

MISCELLANEOUS

18. Ans. [Ref. Mandell, Douglas, and Bennett's Principles and Practice of Infectious Diseases E-Book 1/e p186]
    - Category A bioterrorism agents can be easily disseminated, have high mortality rates and lead to public panic & disruption
    - Category B bioterrorism agents are moderately easy to disseminate, cause moderate morbidity with low mortality, require enhanced diagnostic capacity with enhanced surveillance
    - Category C bioterrorism agents are new emerging pathogens that are available, have ease of production and exhibit high morbidity and mortality

19. Ans. (b) Bacillus anthracis [Ref. Community Health Nursing by Lundy 3/e p558]
    - Category A Bioterrorism agents include Botulism, Tularaemia, Anthrax, Small pox, Plague, Viral hemorrhagic fevers

20. Ans. (d) 70 [Ref. Park 25/e p524]
    - Sustainable Development Goal 3 – "Ensure healthy life and promote well being for all at all ages", Target 3.1 is to reduce Maternal mortality ratio by 2030 is less than 70 per 100,000 live births

21. **Ans. (d) Yellow fever** *[Ref. Park 23/e p841, 25/e p904]*
    - *Diseases under International Surveillance (WHO):*
        - *Louse borne typhus fever*
        - *Relapsing fever*
        - *Poliomyelitis*
        - *Malaria*
        - *Human Influenza*
        - *Rabies*
        - *Salmonellosis*

    ALSO REMEMBER
    - Most of the *'national health programmes in India rely on Passive Surveillance'* for morbidity and mortality data collection
    - Active Surveillance in National Health Programmes of India is done in:
        - NVBDCP (Health worker goes house to house every fortnight to detect fever cases, collect blood slides and provide presumptive treatment under malaria component)
        - National Leprosy Elimination Programme (Modified Leprosy Elimination Campaigns)
    - Sentinel Surveillance in National Health Programmes of India is done in National AIDS Control Programme (STD Clinics, ANC Clinics have been identified as sentinel sites to monitor trends of HIV/AIDS)
    - *Monitoring versus Surveillance*:

MONITORING	SURVEILLANCE
Performance and analysis of routine measurements to detecting changes in environment or health status of a population	Continuous scrutiny of the factors that determine the occurrence and distribution of disease and other conditions of ill-health
One Time linear activity No feedback present No inbuilt action component present Stops once disease is eliminated/eradicated Smaller concept	*Continuous Cycle* Feedback present *'Inbuilt action component'* present Continues even after disease is eliminated/eradicated Broader concept

22. **Ans. (d) Onchocerciasis**
    [Ref. Park 20/e p818, Park 21/e p983]

• Tropical diseases targeted for research and training by WHO:	• Diseases under International Health Regulations (IHRs):
– Trypanosomiasis	– Cholera
– Filariasis	– Plague
– Schistosomiasis	– Yellow Fever
– Leishmaniasis	– Wild Poliomyelitis
– Malaria	– Human Influenza
– Leprosy	– SARS
	– Smallpox

    Contd...

    Contd...

• Tropical diseases targeted for research and training by WHO: • Diseases under International Surveillance (WHO):	• Diseases under International Health • Current *'List of Quarantinable Diseases'* (CDC):
– Louse borne typhus fever	– Diphtheria
– Relapsing fever	– Plague
– Poliomyelitis	– Yellow Fever
– Malaria	– Smallpox
– Human Influenza	– Infectious TB
– Rabies	– Viral Hemorrhagic Fevers
– Salmonellosis	– Severe Acute Respiratory Syndrome (SARS)

23. **Ans. (c) India** *[Ref. Internet]*
    - *Fingerprint*: Is an impression of the friction ridges of all part of the finger
    - *World's first Fingerprint Bureau*: opened in Calcutta (Kolkata), India in 1897 after the Council of the Governor General approved a committee report that fingerprints should be used for classification of criminal records
        - *Sir Williams James Herschel initiated fingerprinting in India*
    - *Dermatoglyphics*: Is the scientific study of human fingerprints
    - *Some firsts in Public Health*:
        - *First country to introduce Socialized medicine: Russia*
        - *First country to introduce Compulsory Sickness Insurance: Germany*
        - *First country to introduce Family Planning programme: India*
        - *First country to introduce Blindness Control programme: India*
        - *First country to introduce Fingerprint Bureau: India*

24. **Ans. (d) Health of travelers**
    [Ref: A Dictionary of Public Health by Dr Jugal Kishore, 2002; p165, Park 23/e p126, 25/e p138]
    - Travel medicine or *'Emporiatrics'* is the branch of medicine that deals with the prevention and management of health problems of international travelers

    ALSO REMEMBER
    - *Nosology*: Branch of medicine dealing with classification of diseases

25. **Ans. (a) Small pox** *[Ref. World Health Organization]*
    - The *'International Health Regulations'* (IHR, 2005) are an international law which helps countries working together to save lives and livelihoods caused by the international spread of diseases and other health risks
    - The IHR (1969) were primarily intended to monitor and control six serious infectious diseases: cholera, plague, yellow fever, smallpox, relapsing fever and typhus

- Under the IHR (1969), *'only cholera, plague and yellow fever remain notifiable'*, meaning that States are required to notify WHO if and when these diseases occur on their territory

> **ALSO REMEMBER**
> - The IHR (2005) broaden the scope of the 1969 Regulations to cover existing, new and re-emerging diseases, including emergencies caused by non-infectious disease agents
> - Under the IHR (2005), all cases of the following four diseases must also be automatically notified to WHO:
>   - Smallpox
>   - Poliomyelitis due to wild-type poliovirus
>   - SARS
>   - Human influenza

26. Ans. (b) April 7   [Ref. Park 27/e p1026]
27. Ans. (d) Yellow fever   [Ref. Park 23/e p282–309]
28. Ans. (e) Compulsory sickness benefit
    [Ref. Internet, Park 21/e p10]
    - *Germ theory:* France (Louis Pasteur)
    - *Pasteurisation:* France (Louis Pasteur)
    - *Quarantine:* Croatia
    - *Socialised medicine:* Russia
    - *Compulsory sickness insurance:* Germany

29. Ans. (d) Tuberculosis
    [Ref. CDC Atlanta Website; http://emergency.cdc.gov/agent/agentlist-category.asp]
    - Categories of bio-terrorism agents:

Category A	Category B	Category C
Can be easily disseminated	Moderately easy to disseminate	Emerging pathogens
High mortality rates	Moderate morbidity + low mortality	Available
Public panic and disruption	Require enhanced diagnostic capacity	Ease of production
	Require enhanced surveillance	High morbidity and mortality
Botulism	Brucellosis	Nipah virus
Tularaemia	Clostridium perfringens	Hantavirus
Anthrax	Food safety threats	
Smallpox	Water safety threats	
Plague	Glanders	
Viral hemorrhagic fevers	Meliodoses	
[**Mnemonic:**	Psittacosis	
Bio **T**errorism **A**gents	Q fever	
include **S**mall **P**ox **V**irus]	Ricin toxin	
	Staphylococcal enterotoxin B	
	Epidemic typhus	
	Viral encephalitis	

30. Ans. (d) Economic reforms
    [Ref. World Health Report 2008, WHO, Pg XVI]
    - World Health Report 2008 ("Primary Health Care – Now More Than Ever") structures Primary health care reforms into 4 sets: [**Mnemonic: PLUS**]
      - **P**ublic policy reforms (promote and protect community health)
      - **L**eadership reforms (reliable health authorities)
      - **U**niversal coverage reforms (health equity)
      - **S**ervice delivery reforms (people-centred, health systems)
    - World Health Report 2010 ("Health Systems Financing – The Path To Universal Coverage") recommends 4 strategies: [**Mnemonic: BIRD**]
      - **B**udgets (Governmental) reprioritization
      - **I**nnovative financing
      - **R**evenue collection efficiency increase
      - **D**evelopment assistance

31. Ans. (a) Frederick Sanger   [Ref. Wikipedia]
    LIST OF FEW NOBEL LAUREATES IN PHYSIOLOGY OR MEDICINE
    - *Sir Ronald Ross*: Life cycle of Plasmodium
    - *I.P. Pavlov*: Physiology of digestion
    - *Robert Koch*: Discoveries in Tuberculosis
    - *Paul Ehrlich*: Immunity
    - *F.G. Banting & J.J.R. McLeod*: Insulin
    - *Willem Einthoven*: ECG
    - *Karl Landsteiner*: Human blood groups
    - *Sir Alexander Fleming*: Penicillin
    - *Paul H. Muller*: DDT
    - *S.A. Waksman*: Streptomycin (First antibiotic, against TB)
    - *Har Gobind Khorana*: Interpretation of genetic code
    - *Sir Godfrey N. Hounsfield*: CT scan
    - *J.E. Murray & E.D. Thomas*: Organ and cell transplantation
    - *Sir Peter Mansfield*: MRI
    - *B.J. Marshall & J.R. Warren*: H. pylori; its role in peptic ulcer disease
    - *H.Z. Hausen*: HPV causing cervical cancer
    - *F.B. Sinoussi & L. Montagnier*: HIV
    - *Robert G. Edwards*: In-vitro fertilization

32. Ans. (c) Anthrax
    [Ref. Bioterrorism Preparedness by N Khardori, 1/e p12]

33. Ans. (a) Typhus   [Ref. Contagion and Chaos by AT PriceSmith, 1/e p166]

34. Ans. (d) 36   [Ref. International Health Regulations, WHO 2011]

35. Ans. (d) Tetanus   [Ref. CDC, Atlanta website]
    - *Quarantinable diseases*: Cholera, Diphtheria, Infectious Tuberculosis, Plague, Smallpox, Yellow Fever, Viral Haemorrhagic Fevers (Lassa, Marburg, Ebola, Crimean-Congo, South American, and others not yet isolated or named), Severe Acute Respiratory Syndrome (SARS 2003), Novel/Re-emergent influenza viruses (2005 Latest addition)

36. **Ans. (c) United Nation Millennium Declaration**
    [Ref. Park 23/e p893, 25/e p]
    - The Millennium Development Goals (MDGs) were the eight international development goals for the year 2015 that had been established following the Millennium Summit of the United Nations in 2000, following the adoption of the United Nations Millennium Declaration
    - All 189 United Nations member states at that time, and at least 22 international organizations, committed to help achieve MDGs by 2015

37. **Ans. (b) Clostridium botulinum; (c) Yersinia pestis; (d) Bacillus anthracis**
    [Ref. Preparedness by Khardori, 1/e p12]
    - Category A Bioterrorism agents (WHO) include Botulism, Tularaemia, Anthrax, Smallpox, Plague, Viral hemorrhagic fevers (Filoviruses – Ebola & Marburg; Arenaviruses – Lassa, Machupo)

Review Question

38. **Ans. NONE** *[Ref: Park 23/e p841, 25/e p904]*

CHAPTER 16

Biostatistics

DATA, VARIABLES AND SCALES

Data Presentation

Quantitative data[Q]	Qualitative data[Q]
Histogram[Q]	Bar diagram[Q]
Frequency polygon	Pie/Sector diagram
Frequency curve	Pictogram/Picture diagram
Line chart/graph	Map diagram/Spot map
Cumulative frequency diagram (Ogive)	
Scatter/Dot diagram[Q]	

STATISTICAL DATA GRAPHS

- **Histogram**
  - Is graphical presentation for 'continuous quantitative data'[Q]
  - Continuous groups are marked on x-axis (abscissa) while frequencies are marked on y-axis (ordinate).

> **Key points**
> **Histogram**
> Is graphical presentation for 'continuous quantitative data'

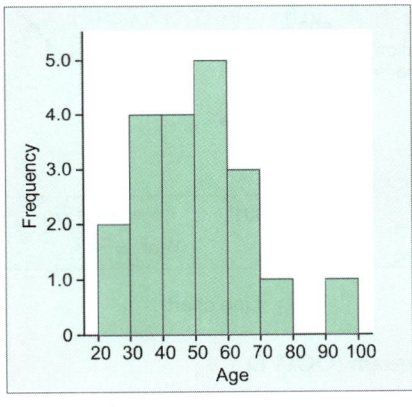

Histogram

- **Frequency Polygon**
  - Is an area diagram of frequency distribution developed over a histogram: Made by joining mid-points of class intervals at the heights of frequencies[Q]

> **Key points**
> **Frequency Polygon**
> Made by joining mid-points of class intervals at the heights of frequencies[Q]

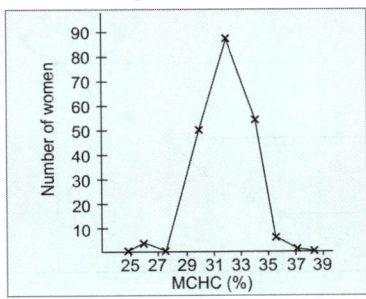

Frequency polygon

- **Frequency Curve**
  - When no. of observations is large and group-interval is reduced: Frequency polygon loses its angulations to become a curve^Q.

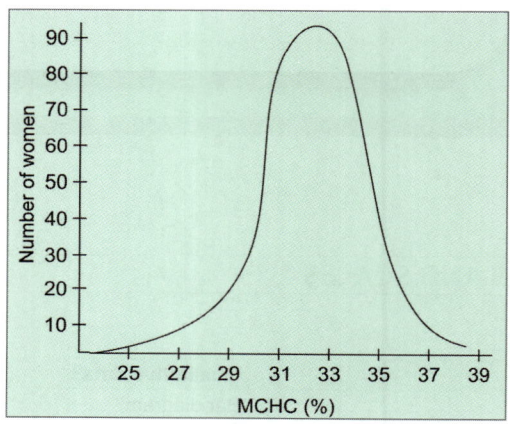

Frequency curve

> **Key points**
>
> **Line Chart/Graph:** It shows the trend of an event over a period of time^Q.

- **Line Chart/Graph**
  - Is a frequency polygon presenting variations by line
  - It shows the trend of an event over a period of time^Q.

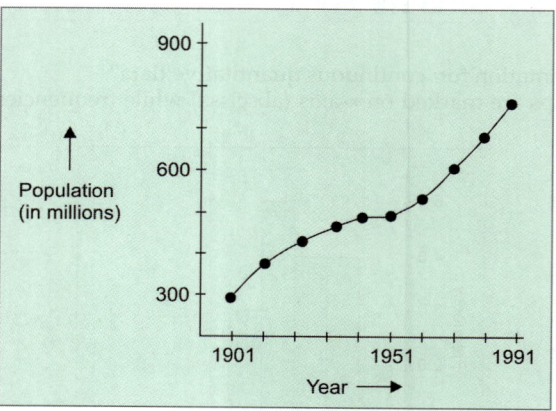

Line chart

> **Key points**
>
> **OGIVE:** Cumulative relative frequency distribution^Q.

- **Cumulative Frequency Diagram (OGIVE)**
  - Is graph of cumulative relative frequency distribution^Q.

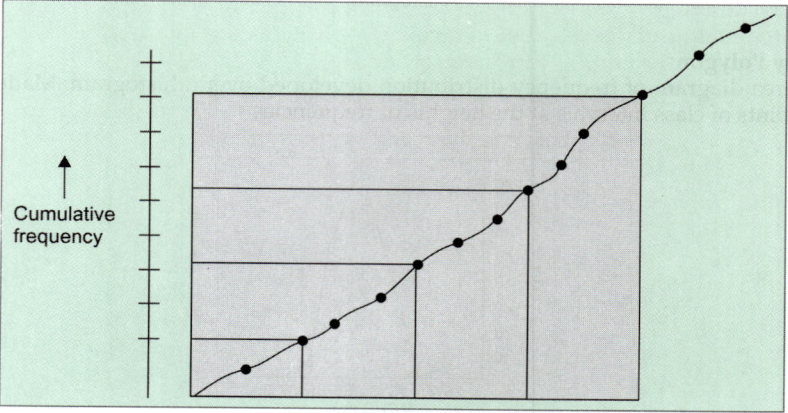

OGIVE (Cumulative frequency diagram)

- **Scatter/Dot Diagram**
  - Also known as 'Correlation diagram'[Q]
  - Is used to depict 'correlation (relationship) between 2 quantitative variables'[Q]
  - Vertical axis in scatter diagram: should be the dependent or the outcome variable
  - In a scatter diagram, 2 imaginary lines are drawn along the distribution of dots/scatter.

> **Key points**
> Scatter/Dot Diagram: Is used to depict correlation

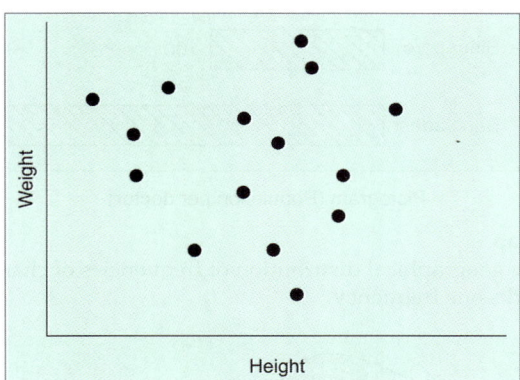

Scatter/dot diagram

- **Bar Diagram**
  - Is for visual comparison of magnitude of different frequencies in discrete data
  - Is 'the most versatile of all statistical diagrams'[Q]
  - Bar diagram is of 3 types:
    - Simple bar diagram
    - Multiple bar diagram
    - Proportional bar diagram.

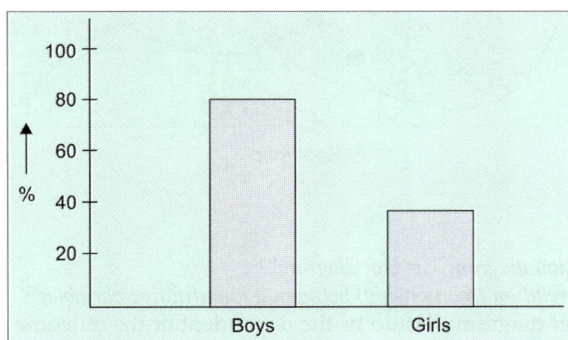

Bar diagram

- **Pie/Sector Diagram**
  - Is for 'presentation of discrete data of qualitative characteristics'[Q]
  - All pie categories are mutually exclusive, with a total of 100% (360°)[Q].

> **Key points**
> Pie/Sector Diagram: All pie categories are mutually exclusive, with a total of 100%

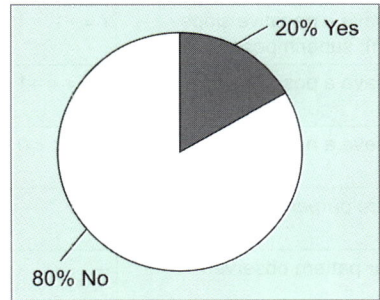

Pie (Sector) diagram

- **Pictogram/Picture Diagram**
  - Is a method to impress the frequency of occurrence of events to common man[Q]

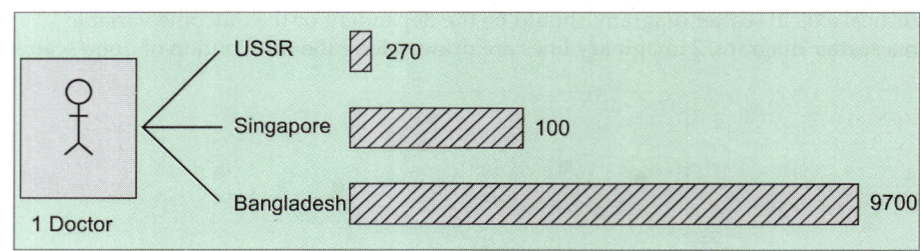

Pictogram (Population per doctor)

- **Map diagram/Spot Map**
  - Is prepared to show geographical distribution of frequencies of characteristic[Q]
  - Each spot (dot) marks one frequency.

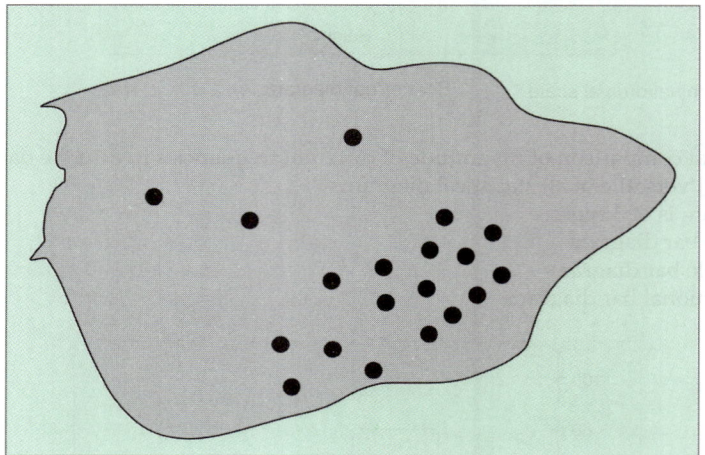

Spot map

Scatter Diagram

Also known as 'Correlation diagram' or 'Dot diagram'[Q]
- Is used to depict 'correlation (relationship) between 2 quantitative variables'[Q]
- Vertical axis in scatter diagram: should be the dependent or the outcome variable
- In a scatter diagram, 2 imaginary lines are drawn along the distribution of dots/scatter
- *Types of correlation:*

Types of correlation	Scatter diagram[Q]	Correlation coefficient[Q]	Interpretation[Q]
Perfectly positive correlation	Both lines have a positive slope (at 45° each); superimposed	r = +1	Rise in one variable leads to proportionate rise in other
Perfectly negative correlation	Both lines have a negative slope (at 45° each); superimposed	r = −1	Rise in one variable leads to proportionate fall in other
Moderately positive correlation	Both lines have a positive slope	0 < r < +1	Rise in one variable leads to rise in other
Moderately negative correlation	Both lines have a negative slope	−1 < r < 0	Rise in one variable leads to fall in other
No (absent) correlation	Both lines are perpendicular	r = 0	Rise/fall in one variable leads to no change in other
Spurious (false) correlation	No particular pattern observed	–	No particular pattern observed

Variables

- *Definition:* Is a characteristic or attribute that vary from person to person, from time to time and from person to person.

Quantitative variable^Q	Qualitative variable^Q
Is a variable that can be measured directly	Is a variable that cannot be measured directly
Measured on ordinal/metric scale	Measured on a nominal scale
Examples: Weight Height Mid-arm circumference Blood sugar level ºC/ºF temperature scale Body mass index (BMI) Hemoglobin level Serum cholesterol level	Examples: ABO blood group Gender Sites of lymphadenopathy Presence of Diabetes Weather Obesity Type of anemia

Discrete variable^Q	Continuous variable^Q
Is a variable that has few possible values & no in-between values	Is a variable that has large no. of possible values & several in-between values
Measured on nominal/ordinal scale	Measured on a metric scale
Examples: ABO blood group Gender Sites of lymphadenopathy Presence of Diabetes Parity Obesity No. of living children in a family	Examples: Weight Height Mid-arm circumference Blood sugar level ºC/ºF temperature scale Body mass index (BMI) Hemoglobin level Serum cholesterol level

> **Key points**
> **Continuous variable:** Is a variable that has large no. of possible values & several in-between values

Dichotomous (Binary) variable^Q	Polytomous variable^Q
Is a variable that has only 2 possible values	Is a variable that has >2 possible values
Examples: Rh blood group Weight >80 kg Gender Presence of Diabetes Obesity Temperature <12ºC Blood group B	Examples: ABO blood group Weight Height Mid-arm circumference Blood sugar level ºC/ºF temperature scale Body mass index (BMI) Hemoglobin level Serum cholesterol level

> **Key points**
> **Dichotomous (Binary) variable:** Is a variable that has only 2 possible values

Scales of Measurement

	Categorical scales		Dimensional scales
	Nominal scale^Q	Ordinal scale^Q	Metric scale^Q
Definition	Based on NOM (names); no specific order	Based on ORD (order); grading into categories	Based on ME (measurement); in terms of quantities
Variables	Qualitative	Qualitative	Quantitative
Examples	Race Religion Country of birth Clinical features Sites of lymphadenopathy Sex of child Type of anemia ABO blood group Site of malignancy	TNM staging (cancers) Severity of a disease Social classes	Blood glucose Hemoglobin level Serum cholesterol Weight Height Mid-arm circumference Blood pressure Pulse rate Temperature (ºC, ºF, K) scale

> **Key points**
> **Nominal scale:** Based on NOM (names)

Contd...

Contd...

	Categorical scales		Dimensional scales
	Nominal scale[Q]	**Ordinal scale**[Q]	**Metric scale**[Q]
	Counting	> or < operations	Interval scale: +/– Ratio scale: X/÷
	Mode, Chi–square	Median, Percentile	Interval scale: Mean, SD, Correlation, Regression, ANOVA Ratio scale: Geometric mean, Harmonic mean, Coefficient of variation

- *Metric scale is of 2 types*[Q]:
  - *Interval scale (Absence of absolute zero; no ratios are possibl(e):* **Examples:** Centigrade/Fahrenheit temperature scale[Q].
  - *Ratio scale (Presence of absolute zero; thus ratios are possibl(e):* **Examples:** Weight, Height, Blood glucose, Hemoglobin level, Serum cholesterol, Mid-arm circumference, Blood pressure, Pulse rate, Kelvin temperature scale[Q].

Likert Scale

> **Key points**
>
> **Likert Scale:** 'Responses are graded on a continuum'

- Is also known as 'Summative scale'[Q]
- Is a 'type of Ordinal scale'[Q]
- Is generally used to quantify attitudes and behaviour
- 'Responses are graded on a continuum' (For example: Strongly agree – Agree – Neutral – Disagree – Strongly disagree)[Q]
- No. of responses are usually 3, 5 or 7
- Likert scale is 'usually a bipolar scaling' method: It measures positive or negative response to a statement
- *Likert response can be:*
  - Collated into bar charts
  - Central tendency summarized as median or mode (NOT mean)
  - Dispersion summarized by range (NOT standard deviation)
  - Analyzed by non-parametric tests.

MEASURES OF CENTRAL TENDENCY

Measures of Central Tendency[Q]

> **Key points**
>
> **Median:** Middlemost value in a distribution arranged in an ascending or descending order

- *Mean (Average):* Is obtained as sum of all values divided by the no. of values[Q].

$$\text{Mean} = \Sigma x / n$$

- *Median:* Middlemost value in a distribution arranged in an ascending or descending order of values[Q].
  - *In a distribution with odd no. of total values:* Middlemost value in a distribution arranged in an ascending or descending order of values[Q].

$$\text{Median} = ((n + 1)/2)\text{th value in ascending order}$$

  - *In a distribution with even no. of total values:* Such a distribution has 2 middlemost values; median is the average of two middlemost values when arranged in an ascending or descending order of values[Q].

$$\text{Median} = \text{Mean (average) of } (n/2)\text{th and } (n/2 + 1)\text{th value in ascending order}$$

> **Key points**
>
> **Mode:** Most frequent or most commonly occurring value in a distribution

- *Mode:* Most frequent or most commonly occurring value in a distribution
  - *In a distribution with one most frequent value:* Mode is the most frequent or most commonly occurring value in the distribution[Q].
  - *In a distribution with two most frequent values:* 2 Modes (2 most frequent values in the distribution) known as Bimodal distribution; thus Mode = Average of 2 modes.

Central Tendency in Various Distributions

Distribution	Central tendency^Q
Normal (Gaussian) distribution	Mean = Median = Mode (coincide)
Right (Positive) skew distribution	Mean > Median > Mode
Left (Negative) skew distribution	Mean < Median < Mode

- *In a bimodal series*, Mode = 3 Median – 2 mean
- *In distribution with extreme values (Outliers)*:
  - Most affected measure of central tendency: Mean^Q
  - Least affected measure of central tendency: Mode^Q
  - Most preferable measure of central tendency: Median^Q.

> **Key points**
> **Right (Positive) skew** distribution
> Mean > Median > Mode

OTHER MEASURES OF LOCATION

Various Measures of Location

	Divides distribution into	No. of intercepts
Tertile	3 equal parts	2
Quartile^Q	4 equal parts	3
Pentile (Quintile^Q)	5 equal parts	4
Hextile	6 equal parts	5
Heptile	7 equal parts	6
Octile	8 equal parts	7
Decile	10 equal parts	9
Centile (Percentile^Q)	100 equal parts	99

> **Key points**
> - Quartile: 4 equal parts
> - Quintile: 5 equal parts

Tertile

- *Tertile:* Divides a distribution into 3 equal parts, so the number of intercepts required will be 2, i.e. T1, T2
  - T1 (1st tertile) divides a distribution in a ratio of 33 : 66 OR 1 : 2
  - T2 (2nd tertile) divides a distribution in a ratio of 66 : 33 OR 2 : 1.

Quartile

- *Quartile:* Divides a distribution into 4 equal parts, so the number of intercepts required will be 3, i.e. Q1, Q2, Q3
  - Q1 (1st Quartile^Q) divides a distribution in a ratio of 1 : 3
  - Q2 (2nd Quartile^Q) divides a distribution in a ratio of 1 : 1
  - Q3 (3rd Quartile^Q) divides a distribution in a ratio of 3 : 1.

> **Key points**
> Q2 (2nd Quartile^Q) divides a distribution in a ratio of 1 : 1

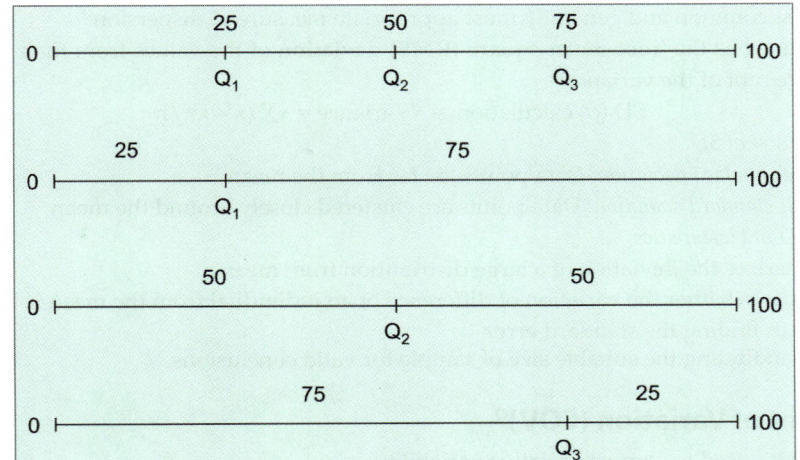

Quartiles

Pentile

- **Pentile (QUINTILE):** Divides a distribution into 5 equal parts, so the number of intercepts required will be 4, i.e. P1, P2, P3, P4
  - P1 (1st pentile) divides a distribution in a ratio of 20 : 80 OR 1 : 4
  - P2 (2nd pentile) divides a distribution in a ratio of 40 : 60 OR 2 : 3
  - P3 (3rd pentile) divides a distribution in a ratio of 60 : 40 OR 3 : 2
  - P4 (4th pentile) divides a distribution in a ratio of 80 : 20 OR 4 : 1.

Centile (Percentile)

> **Key points**
> **Centile (Percentile):** Divides a distribution into 100 equal parts.

- Divides a distribution into 100 equal parts, AFTER arranging in an ascending order, SUCH THAT each part/segment has equal number (n/100) of subjects^Q.
- Requires 99 intercepts (cut-off points) for division into 100 parts
- *Total percentiles:* 99^Q.
- *The nth percentile implies:* When all values are arranged in ascending order, n% are below this value
- *Methods for location of percentiles:*
  - *Graphical method:* Cumulative frequency diagram (Ogive)
  - *Arithmetic method:* Cumulative frequency table
- *Applications and uses of percentiles^Q:*
  - Location of a percentile
  - Preparation of a standard percentile (Q2, Median) for particular age, sex, etc.
  - Comparison of a percentile value of a variable (between samples or populations)
  - To study growth in children (using growth charts)
  - As a measure of dispersion (interquartile/semi-interquartile range).

VARIABILITY

Measures of Variability

Measures of Variability^Q	
Individual observations	**Samples**
Range	Standard error of mean
Inter-quartile range	Standard error of difference between 2 means
Mean deviation	Standard error of proportion
Standard deviation	Standard error of difference between 2 proportions
Coefficient of variation	Standard error of correlation coefficient
	Standard deviation of regression coefficient

Standard Deviation (SD)

> **Key points**
> - SD is most common and generally most appropriate measure of dispersion^Q
> - SD is defined as the 'root-mean-square (RMS) deviation

- SD is most common and generally most appropriate measure of dispersion^Q
- SD is defined as the **'root-mean-square (RMS) deviation** of the values from their mean', or as the square root of the variance^Q

$$SD\ (\sigma)\ \text{calculation:} = \sqrt{\text{Variance}} = \sqrt{\sum (x - \bar{x})^2 / n}$$

- *Interpretation of SD:*
  - *A large standard deviation:* Data points are far from the mean
  - *A small standard deviation:* Data points are clustered closely around the mean
- *Uses of SD in biostatistics:*
  - Summarizes the deviation of a large distribution from mean
  - Indicates whether the variation of difference of an individual from the mean is by chance
  - Helps in finding the standard error
  - Helps in finding the suitable size of sample for valid conclusions.

Coefficient of Variation (COV)^Q

> **Key points**
> COV = SD/Mean × 100 = σ/μ × 100

- Is a measure used to compare relative variability
- Is a unit-free measure to compare dispersion of one variable with another

- Is SD expressed as percentage of mean
$$COV = SD/Mean \times 100 = \sigma/\mu \times 100$$

Standard Error of Mean (SE Mean)

SE mean is the measure of difference between sample and population values: Whatever be the sampling procedure or the care taken while selecting sample, the sample estimates (statistics) will differ from population values (parameters)
- SE is a measure of variability of sample summaries: SEmean is the SD of sample means[Q]
- SE is a 'measure of chance variation', and IT DOESNOT mean an error or mistake[Q]
$$SE\ mean = Standard\ deviation\ (SD)/\sqrt{Sample\ size} = \sigma/\sqrt{n}$$
- *Importance of SE mean:*
  - Greater the standard deviation (σ), greater will be the standard error (SE), especially in small samples
  - SE can be minimized by reducing SD: By taking a large sample
  - SE is a measure of variability of sample summaries: SEmean is the SD of sample means
- *Uses of standard error of mean (SEmean) in large samples:*
  - To work out limits of desired confidence within which population mean would lie
  - To determine if sample is drawn from a known population or not
  - To find SE of difference between 2 means (to know if difference is real and statistically significant)
  - To calculate sample size (within desired confidence limits)

Key points

SE mean = Standard deviation (SD)/√Sample size = $\sigma/\sqrt{n}$

Standard error of difference between 2 means[Q]:
$$SE\ difference\ between\ means = \sqrt{\sigma_1^2/n_1 + \sigma_2^2/n_2}$$

Standard error of proportion[Q]:
$$SE\ proportion = \sqrt{pq/n}\ ;\ where\ q = (1-p)$$

Standard error of difference between 2 proportions[Q]:
$$SE\ difference\ between\ proportions = \sqrt{(p_1q_1/n_1) + (p_2q_2/n_2)}$$

Z Score (Standard Score)

- Is also known as 'normal deviate'[Q]
- Is difference of a value from group mean, in terms of how many times of SD (σ)
$$Z\ score = (Individual\ level - Mean)/Standard\ deviation = (x - \mu)/\sigma$$
- Standard score indicates how many standard deviations an observation is above or below the mean
- Z scores are frequently used in assessing how far a child is in his relative growth to a standard
- Z score = 2: Any measurement of atleast 2 SD away is considered too far away to be normal.

Key points

Z score = (Individual level − Mean)/Standard deviation = $(x - \mu)/\sigma$

DISTRIBUTIONS—NORMAL AND SKEWED

Poisson Distribution

- Is a 'discrete probability distribution' that expresses the 'probability of a number of events occurring in a fixed period of time'[Q] (if these events occur with a known average rate and independently of the time since the last event).
- It can also be used for the number of events in other specified intervals such as distance, area or volume.
- Is generally used to model the number of events occurring within a given time interval.
- Is a discrete distribution which takes on the values X = 0, 1, 2, 3,….

Normal Distribution

- Is also known as 'Gaussian distribution' or 'Standard distribution'[Q]
- Type of distribution: Is the distribution of values of a quantitative variable such that they are symmetric with respect to a middle value with same mean, median and mode, and then the frequencies taper off rapidly and symmetrically on both sides – 'bell shaped distribution'.

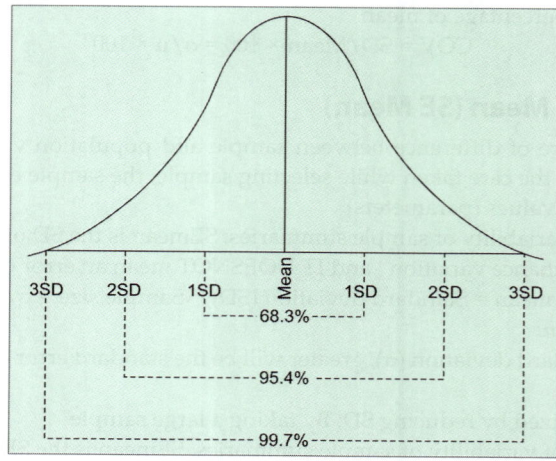

Normal curve showing distribution of values

- Is 'bilaterally symmetrical, bell-shaped'^{Q}
- Is based on mean (μ) and standard deviation (σ)
- Mean, Median and Mode coincide (Mean = Median = Mode)^Q
- Has Mean (μ) = 0 and SD (μ) = 1^Q
- SD = √Variance OR Variance = σ²
  - In Normal distribution, SD (σ) = 1, thus Variance = 1^Q
- Mean ± 1SD (μ ± 1σ) covers 68% values^Q
- Mean ± 2SD (μ ± 2σ) covers 95% values^Q
- Mean ± 3SD (μ ± 3σ) covers 99% values^Q
- Actual parameters in a Normal (Gaussian) distribution:
  - Mean ± 1SD (μ ± 1σ) limits include 68.27% values
  - Mean ± 2SD (μ ± 2σ) limits include 95.45% values
  - Mean ± 1.96SD (μ ± 1.96σ) limits include 95% values
  - Mean ± 3SD (μ ± 3σ) limits include 99.73% values
  - Mean ± 2.58SD (μ ± 2.58σ) limits include 99% values.

> **Key points**
>
> Normal Distribution
> - (μ ± 1σ) covers 68% values^Q
> - (μ ± 2σ) covers 95% values^Q
> - (μ ± 3σ) covers 99% values^Q

Skewness of Central Tendency

- *Description:* Is measure of asymmetry of a probability distribution of a random variable
- *Measures of skewness:*
  - Pearson's mode or First Skewness coefficient^Q = (Mean − Mode)/SD
  - Pearson's median or Second Skewness coefficient = 3(Mean − Median)/SD
  - Quartile skewness = (Q3−2Q2 + Q1)/Q3 − Q1
- *Asymmetrical distributions:*
  - *Right (positive) skew:* Mean > Median > Mode^Q
  - *Left (negative) skew:* Mean < Median < Mode^Q

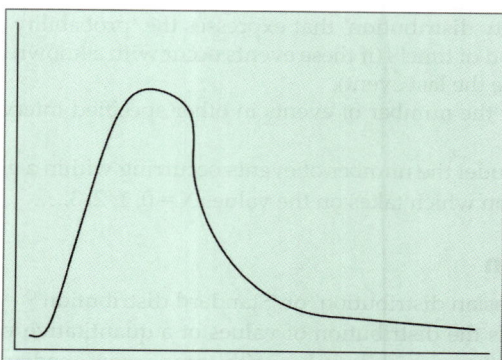

Right skewed curve

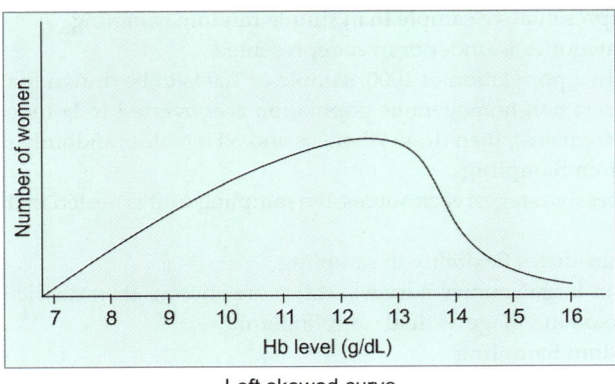

Left skewed curve

SAMPLING

Sample Size Estimation

- *Sample size depends upon^Q:*
  - the effect size (usually the difference between 2 groups)
  - the population standard deviation (for continuous data)
  - the desired power of the experiment to detect the postulated effect (Power = $1-\beta$)
  - the significance level (α).

Types of Sampling

	Random Sampling^Q	**Non-random sampling^Q**
Synonyms	Probability sampling^Q Non-purposive sampling	Non-probability sampling Purposive sampling^Q
Types	Simple random sampling Systematic random sampling Stratified random sampling Multistage random sampling Multiphase random sampling Cluster random sampling	Convenience sampling Quota sampling Snow-ball sampling Clinical trial sampling

Types of Random Sampling

- **Simple Random Sampling**
  - Every unit of population has equal and known chance of being selected^Q
  - Is also known as 'unrestricted random sampling'
  - Applicable for small, homogenous and readily available populations
  - Used in clinical trials
  - Methods of Simple random sampling^Q:
    - Lottery method
    - Random no. tables
    - Computer software.
- **Systematic Random Sampling**
  - Based on sampling fraction: Every Kth unit is chosen in the population list, where K is chosen by sampling interval
  - Sampling Interval (K) Q = Total no. of units in population/Total no. of units in sample
  - Applicable for large, non-homogenous populations where complete list of individuals is available
  - For example, if there is a population of 1000 from which sample of 20 is to be chosen, then K = 1000/20 = 50; thus every 50th unit will be included in the sample (i.e. 1st, 51st, 101st, so on…) First unit among first 50 is chosen by simple random sampling.
- **Stratified Random Sampling**
  - Non-homogenous population is converted to homogenous groups/classes (strata); sample is drawn from each strata at random, in proportion to its size^Q
  - Applicable for large non-homogenous population

- Gives more representative sample than simple random sampling
- None of the categories is under or over-represented
- For example, In a population of 1000, sample of 100 is to be drawn for Hemoglobin estimation; first convert non-homogenous population is converted to homogenous strata (i.e. 700 males and 300 females), then draw 70 males and 30 females randomly respectively.

- **Multistage Random Sampling**
  - Is done in successive stages; each successive sampling unit is nested in the previous sampling unit^Q
  - Advantage: Introduces flexibility in sampling
  - For example, in large country surveys, states are chosen, then districts, then villages, then every 10th person in village as final sampling unit
- **Multiphase Random Sampling**
  - Is done in successive phases; part of information is obtained from whole sample and part from the sub-sample^Q
  - For example, in a TB survey, Mantoux test done in first phase, then X-ray done in all Mantoux positives, then sputum examined in all those with positive X-ray findings.
- **Cluster Random Sampling**
  - Applicable when units of population are natural groups or clusters
  - *Use in India:* Evaluation of immunization coverage^Q
  - *WHO technique used:* 30 × 7 technique (total = 210 children)^Q
  - *WHO technique used in CRS:* 30 × 7 technique (total = 210 children)
    - 30 clusters, each containing
    - 7 children who are 12–23 months age and are completely immunized for primary immunization (till Measles vaccine)^Q
    - Clusters are heterogeneous within themselves but homogenous with respect to each other
    - Sampling interval is also calculated in CRS
  - *Accuracy^Q:* Low error rate of only ± 5%
  - *Limitation:* Clusters cannot be compared with each other^Q.

> **Key points**
> **CRS**
> - *Use in India:* Evaluation of immunization coverage
> - 30 × 7 technique

Types of Non-Random Sampling^Q

- *Convenience Sampling*
  - Patients are selected, in part or in whole, at the convenience of the researcher; no/limited attempt to ensure that sample is an accurate representation of population^Q
  - For example, standing at a shopping mall and selecting shoppers as they walk by to fill out a survey.
- *Quota Sampling^Q*
  - Population is first segmented into mutually exclusive sub-groups (quotas), just as in stratified sampling; then judgment is used to select the units from each group non-randomly
  - Is a type of convenience sampling.
- *Snow-ball Sampling^Q*
  - A technique for developing a research sample where existing study subjects recruit future subjects from among their acquaintances; thus the sample group appears to grow like a rolling snowball
  - Is often used in hidden populations which are difficult for researchers to access, e.g. drug users or commercial sex workers^Q.
- *Clinical Trial Sampling.*

> **Key points**
> **Snow-ball Sampling:** Is often used in hidden populations

PROBABILITY AND ODDS

Bayes' Theorem

Refer to Chapter 4, Theory.

Probability

- Probability: Is the chance that some event will occur
- Probability range: 0 to +1 (0% to 100%)
  - Probability can never be zero^Q
  - Probability cannot exceed one^Q.

Addition Rule of Probability

- *Rule of addition*^{Q}: Probabilities are added for mutually exclusive events i.e. P(Total) = P(A) + P(B)
- For example, If probability of having birth weight <2500 grams (P (A)) is 0.50 (50%), birth weight 2500–2999 grams (P(B)) is 0.30 (30%) and birth weight >3 kg (P (C)) is 0.20 (20%),
  - Probability of having birth weight <3 kg (P (T1)) will be; P (T1) = P (A) + P (B) = 0.50 + 0.30 = 0.80 (80%) as both events are mutually exclusive
  - Similarly, probability of having birth weight >2500 (P (T2)) will be; P (T2) = P (B) + P (C) = 0.30 + 0.20 = 0.50 (50%) as both events are mutually exclusive

Multiplication Rule of Probability

- *Rule of multiplication*^{Q}: Probabilities are multiplied for obtaining joint occurrence of two or more independent events i.e. P(Total) = P(A) × P(B)
- For example, If probability of having birth weight <3 kg (P (C)) is 0.70 (70%), probability of having birth weight >3 kg (P (D)) is 0.30 (30%) AND Probability of being of male sex (P (E)) is 0.50 (50%), and probability of being of female sex (P (F)) is 0.50 (50%)
  - Probability of having a child with birth weight <3 kg and of male sex will be P (T3) = P (C) × P (E) = 0.70 × 0.50 = 0.35 (35%) as both are independent events
  - Similarly, Probability of having a child with birth weight <3 kg and of female sex will be P (T4) = P (C) × P (F) = 0.70 × 0.50 = 0.35 (35%) as both are independent events
  - Probability of having a child with birth weight >3 kg and of male sex will be P (T5) = P (D) × P (E) = 0.30 × 0.50 = 0.15 (15%) as both are independent events
  - Probability of having a child with birth weight >3 kg and of female sex will be P (T6) = P (D) × P (F) = 0.30 × 0.50 = 0.15 (15%) as both are independent events
  - Total probability of a child being borne with any characteristic (P (T)) will be P (T) = P (T3) + P (T4) + P (T5) + P (T6) = 0.35 + 0.35 + 0.15 + 0.15 = 1 (100%).

Odds

- *Odds:* Odds are the chance of frequency of occurrence of a characteristic relative to its non-occurrence (expressed as a ratio of occurrence to non-occurrence)^Q

$$\text{Odds} = \text{Probability}/(1 - \text{Probability})$$
$$\text{Probability} = \text{Odds}/(1 + \text{Odds})$$

> **Key points**
> **Probability** = Odds/(1 + Odds)

TESTS OF STATISTICAL SIGNIFICANCE

Parametric Tests and Non-parametric Tests

	Parametric tests^Q	**Non-parametric tests**^{Q}
Based on^Q	Gaussian/Normal distributions	Non-normal distributions
Type of data^Q	Quantitative	Qualitative
Compares^Q	Means (+ SD)	Percentage, proportions & fractions
Examples^Q	Students (paired) t - test Students (unpaired) t - test ANOVA F - test	Sign test Chi-square test (χ^2 - test) Wilcoxan test (signed rank) Wilcoxan test (rank sum)

Parametric Tests^Q

- *Paired Student's t-test*^{Q}: Comparing means (+ SD) in paired data (in same group of individuals before and after an intervention)
  - Example: Mean serum albumin level of dengue patients before treatment was 3.6 g/dL and after treatment was 3.2 g/dL; Comparison of mean levels can be done by Paired Student's t-test
- *Unpaired Student's t-test*^{Q}: Comparing means (+ SD) in two different group of individuals
  - Example: Mean Hb level of anemia patients was 9.6 g/dL and those of hookworm patients was 7.2 g/dL; Comparison of mean levels can be done by Unpaired Student's t-test
  - Z - test: Is a variant of student's t-test which is used when sample size is >30
- *ANOVA test (F-test/F-ratio)*^{Q}: Comparing means (+ SD) in more than two different group of individuals
  - Example: Mean weight of students in class A is 50 kg, those of class B is 44.6 kg and those of class C is 52.7 kg; Comparison of mean weights can be done by ANOVA test.

> **Key points**
> **Paired Student's t-test**^{Q}: Comparing means (+ SD) in paired data

> **Key points**
>
> **Chi-square test (χ^2 – test^Q)**: Comparing percentage, proportions & fractions in two or more different group of individuals

Non-parametric Tests^Q

- *Sign test^Q*: Comparing percentage, proportions & fractions in paired data (in same group of individuals before and after an intervention)
    - Example: 30% of students in a class are anaemic, after 6 months of IFA therapy, now 20% of students are anaemic; Test of significance to be applied is Sign test
- *Chi-square test (χ^2 – test)^Q*: Comparing percentage, proportions & fractions in two or more different group of individuals
    - Example: Three-fourth of students in a class are underweight whereas another class has two-thirds anaemic; test of significance to be used is Chi-square test
    - Fischer's test: Is a variant of Chi-square test when sample size is <30
- *Wilcoxan tests^Q*:
    - *Wilcoxon (signed rank) test:* Comparing percentage, proportions & fractions in matched paired data
    - *Wilcoxon (rank sum) test:* Comparing percentage, proportions & fractions in two unpaired samples
    - *Mann-Whitney (Wilcoxon) test:*
        - MWW is same as Wilcoxon (rank sum) test
        - Is used for assessing whether two set of observations come from same distribution (if 2 independent 'nonpaired' samples come from the same population)
        - 'MWW is analogous to parametric two-sample t-test' on the data after ranking over the combined samples
        - MWW requires calculation of 'U statistic'.

Chi-Square Test (χ^2 Test)

> **Key points**
>
> **CHI-SQUARE TEST**
> Is used to 'test significance of association between 2 or more qualitative characteristics'^{Q}

- Is a 'non-parametric test' of significance^Q
- Is used to 'test significance of association between 2 or more qualitative characteristics'^{Q}
- Is used to compare proportions in 2 or more groups^Q
- Is used for non-Normal (non-Gaussian) distributions
- *Applications of Chi-square test:^{Q}*
    - Test of proportions
    - Test of association
    - Test of goodness of fit
- *Essential requirements for calculation of Chi-square test:^{Q}*
    - Random sample
    - Qualitative data
    - Lowest expected frequency not <5.

Degrees of Freedom

> **Key points**
>
> dof = (c – 1) (r – 1)

- *Degree of freedom:* Is the no. of observations in a dataset that can freely vary once the parameters have been estimated.
- *Used in Chi-square test and t-test:*
    - In a Chi-square test, contingency table, dof = (c – 1) (r – 1) (where c = no. of columns and r = no. of rows)^Q
    - In a Student's t-test (one-sample data/paired test), dof v = n – 1 (where n = no. of units in the sample)
    - In a Student's t-test (two-sample data/unpaired test), dof v = ($n_1 + n_2$) – 1 (where n1 and n_2 = no. of units in the two samples).

CORRELATION AND REGRESSION

Correlation

> **Key points**
>
> **Correlation coefficient (r)** lies between: –1 to +1 (–1 < r < +1)^Q

- *Description:* Is relationship between 2 quantitative or continuous variables^Q
- *Correlation is represented by:* 'Scatter diagram'^{Q}
- *Correlation coefficient (r):* Measures the degree or strength of relationship in a correlation
    - Correlation coefficient (r) lies between: –1 to +1 (–1 < r < +1)^Q
- *Strength of correlation:*
    - Weak positive correlation: 0 < r < 0.3
    - Moderate positive correlation: 0.4 < r < 0.6
    - Strong positive correlation: r >0.7

- *Correlation is represented by:* 'Scatter diagram'
- *Correlation coefficients:*
  - *Pearson's Correlation coefficient^Q:*
    - Is used in ungrouped series
    - Is used when associated variables are normally distributed
    - Symbol is 'r'
  - *Spearman's Rank Correlation coefficient^Q:*
    - Is used in grouped series
    - Is used when associated variables are not normally distributed
    - Symbol is 'rho (ρ)'
  - *Multiple correlation coefficient:* Is used for calculation of correlation between one variable (dependent) and the combination of two or more variables (independents)
- *Coefficient of determination:^{Q}*
  - Is the percentage of variation in a variable that is explained by one or more of the others^Q
  - Is generally obtained in a regression setup
  - Coefficient of determination^Q = (Correlation coefficient)^2 = r^2. ($0 < r^2 < +1$)

Regression

- *Description:* Is change in measurements of a variable
  - Provides structure of relationship between 2 quantitative variables^Q
- *Regression Coefficient (b):* Measure of change of one dependent variable (y) with change in independent variable (x) or variables (x_1, x_2, x_3......)
- *Equations of regression,*
  $y = a + b(x)$
  $y = a + b(x_1) + c(x_2) + d(x_3)$,
  where y is a dependent variable and x, x_1, x_2, x_3 are independent variables; a is a constant and b, c, d are regression coefficients
- *Types of regressions^Q:*
  - *Simple linear regression:* Only one dependent variable and one independent variable
  - *Multiple linear regression:* Only one dependent variable and more than one independent variable
  - *Simple curvilinear regression:* Only one dependent variable and one independent variable, with some power of independent variable
  - *Multiple curvilinear regression:* Only one dependent variable and more than one independent variables, with some power of independent variables).
- *Types of regression equations:*

Types of regression	Equation^Q
Simple linear regression	$y = a + b(x)$
Multiple linear regression	$y = a + b(x_1) + c(x_2) + d(x_3)$
Simple curvilinear regression	$y = a + b(x)^6$
Multiple curvilinear regression	$y = a + b(x_1)^2 + c(x_2)^4 + d(x_3)^3$

> **Key points**
> Simple linear regression
> $y = a + b(x)$

Other types of regressions:

Types of regressions	Features	
	Dependent variables	Independent variables
Logistic regression^Q	Qualitative, dichotomous	Qualitative/Quantitative/Mixed
ANOVA	Quantitative	Qualitative
ANCOVA	Quantitative	Qualitative + Quantitative
Multivariate multiple regression	Set of Quantitative	Set of Quantitative
MANOVA	Set of Quantitative	Set of Qualitative
Multivariate logistic regression	Set of Qualitative	Qualitative/Quantitative

ERRORS AND P-VALUE

Null Hypothesis

- *Hypothesis (H):* Is an assumption about the status of a phenomenon
- *Null Hypothesis (H_0):* In Biostatistics, when we have to prove a particular hypothesis about difference between 2 regimens, we make Null Hypothesis (For examples, If we have to prove that new treatment is better than older treatment, H_0 = new treatment is not better than older treatment)^Q.

Statistical Errors & P-value

- *Statistical errors*^{Q}: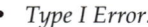

	H_0 rejected	H_0 not rejected
Null Hypothesis (H_0) true	Type I error	No error
Null Hypothesis (H_0) false	No error	Type II error

- *Type I Error:*
    - Null hypothesis is true but rejected^Q
    - Probability of Type I error is given by 'P – value' (probability of declaring a significant difference when actually it is not present)^Q
    - Significance (α) level: is the maximum tolerable probability of Type I error^Q
    - Alpha is fixed in advance: P – value calculated can be less than, equal to or greater than alpha (α)
    - Keep Type I error to be minimum (P < α): Then results are declared statistically significant^Q.
- *Type II Error:*
    - Null hypothesis is false but not rejected (or accepted)^Q
    - Probability of Type II error is given by beta (β) (probability of declaring no significant difference when actually it is present)^Q
    - Type I error is more serious than Type II error^Q.

Power of a Test

- *Description:* Is probability of rejecting a Null hypothesis when a predetermined clinically significant difference is indeed present
    - Measures the ability to demonstrate an association, when one really exists
- *Power of a statistical test:* 1–β (1–Probability of Type II error)^Q
- *Power of a statistical test is a numeric representation of:* Sensitivity
- *Power of a statistical test can be increased by*^{Q}:
    - Increasing the no. of subjects in a trial (sample size)
    - Reducing β (probability of Type II error)
    - Increasing sensitivity
- Power of a statistical test is also used for calculation of sample size for a study^Q.

MISCELLANEOUS

Validity

- *Validity:* Refers to what extent the test measures which it purports to measure (adequacy of measurement)^Q
- *Validity has 2 components*^{Q}:
    - Sensitivity
    - Specificity
- *Types of Validity:*
    - *Conclusion validity:* Defines if there is a relationship between 2 variables
    - *Internal validity:* Assuming relationship between 2 variables, defines if it is causal
        - Is free of bias
        - Valid conclusions can be drawn for individuals in a sample

---

Key points

Type I Error:
- Null hypothesis is true but rejected^Q
- Probability of Type I error is given by 'P – value'

Key points

Type II Error: Null hypothesis is false but not rejected

Key points

Power of a statistical test: 1–β

- *Construct validity:* Assuming causal relationship between 2 variables, defines if our theory is best to our constructs
- *External validity:* Assuming causal relationship between 2 variables, defines if our theory can be generalized to the broader population
- *Concurrent validity:* refers to the degree of correlation with other measures of the same construct measured at the same time
- *Face (Logical) validity:* Relevance of a measurement appear obvious
- *Content validity:* Measurement of all variable components
- *Consensual validity:* If no. of experts agree to a parameter
- *Criterion validity:* If compared with a reference or gold standard
  - Is best measure of validity[Q]
  - Usually expressed as sensitivity & specificity[Q]
- *Discriminant validity:* If not showing strong correlation between 2 variables.

> **Key points**
> **Criterion validity:** If compared with a reference or gold standard
> - Is best measure of validity[Q]
> - Usually expressed as sensitivity & specificity[Q]

Delphi Method

- *Delphi method:* Is a 'systematic interactive forecasting method' for obtaining consensus forecasts from a panel of independent experts[Q]
- *Method:* The carefully selected experts answer questionnaires in two or more rounds; After each round, a facilitator provides an anonymous summary of the experts' forecasts from the previous round as well as the reasons they provided for their judgments; Thus, participants are encouraged to revise their earlier answers in light of the replies of other members of the group.
  - The range of the answers decrease and the group will converge towards the 'correct' consensual answer; Finally, the process is stopped after a pre-defined stop criterion (e.g. number of rounds, achievement of consensus, stability of results) and the mean or median scores of the final rounds determine the results.
  - Objective of most Delphi applications: The reliable and creative exploration of ideas or the production of suitable information for decision-making
  - Delphi Method is based on: A structured process for collecting and distilling knowledge from a group of experts by means of a series of questionnaires interspersed with controlled opinion feedback
  - Delphi method is an exercise in group communication among a panel of geographically dispersed experts
  - In general, the Delphi method is useful in answering one, specific, single-dimension question
- *Mini-Delphi or Estimate-Talk-Estimate (ETE):* The delphi technique when adapted for use in face-to-face meetings.

Confidence Intervals, Levels, Limits

- *Confidence interval (CI):* Is the interval within which a parameter value is expected to lie with certain confidence levels, as could be revealed by repeated samples
  - Is the 'range that is likely to contain the population mean when so obtained for repeated samples'[Q].
  - A narrow CI is always preferable: as it tells more precisely what might be the population mean BUT also it will have higher chances of not containing the population mean[Q].
  - Larger the sample size, narrower is CI[Q].
  - Smaller the SD (σ), narrower is CI

> **Key points**
> - Larger the sample size, narrower is CI[Q].
> - Smaller the SD (s), narrower is CI

- *Confidence level:*
  - Is the level of hope or expectation fixed at a sufficiently high level while dealing with samples, to ensure high reliability
  - Is the 'degree of assurance for an interval to contain the value of the parameter'[Q]
  - There is NO WAY to achieve 100% confidence[Q]
  - Internationally acceptable confidence level: 95%[Q]
  - Maximum tolerance of probability of Type I error (α) is the probability that CI would not contain the population mean[Q]
  - Confidence level[Q] = $1 - \alpha$
- *Confidence limits:* Are the upper and lower boundaries of a confidence interval[Q].

PYQs: Quick Review for NEET

Variables and Scales

Likert scale is a type of	Ordinal scale
Most frequently occurring value in a group of data	Mode
Number of observations 25, number of class intervals must be	5
Anemia is classified into mild, moderate and severe on _____ scale	Ordinal scale

Statistical diagrams

Scatter/Dot Diagram represents	Correlation
Histogram represent data	Continuous quantitative data
Graph showing relation between 2 variables is	Scatter diagram
Trends can be best represented by	Line diagram
Scatter diagram represents	Correlation
Histogram is used for _____ data	Continuous, quantitative data

Central tendency and Dispersion

Standard deviation is a measure of	Dispersion
1, 3, 6, 7, 8, 9, 11 Median is	7
Most frequently occurring value in a data distribution	Mode
MC deviation used in social medicine is	Standard deviation
Median of data 10, 9, 8, 8, 7 is	8
Confidence limit in 2 S.D.	95%
S.D. is 1.96, the confidence limit is	95%
Square root of deviation is called	Standard deviation
Standard error of mean is called as	Standard deviation
'Z score' is for which type of distribution	Normal distribution
For Deviation, modify denominator if population size is below	30
Most commonly used measure of Central tendency is	Mean

Normal distribution

Normal Distribution Curve shape is	Bell Shaped Symmetric
Mean ± 1 SD in Normal distribution covers	68% of total values
Mean ± 2 SD in Normal distribution covers	95% of total values
In a Normal distribution, central tendency relation	Mean = Median = Mode
3 SD from mean covers _____ area under normal distribution curve	99%

To test significance of Difference between two proportions	Chi-Square test
Statistical test to compare means between 2 groups	Unpaired students t-test
Chi-square Test is test of Significance of association b/w	2 qualitative characteristics
Degrees of freedom for 3X6 table (Chi-square) is	10
Degrees of freedom in Chi-square test	(c-1) (r-1)

Sampling methods

Word 'Random' means	Equal and known chance
Use of Cluster Random Sampling	Evaluation of Immunization Coverage
Random in Random sampling means	Equal and known chance
Cluster sampling for immunization coverage, age group is	12–23 months
Maternal and child welfare program, sampling is	Cluster-30
Probability that confounding factor fall to the right of 95%	1 in 40

Multiple Choice Questions

DATA, VARIABLES AND SCALES

1. Methods to describe collection of data can be included under? [INICET May 2022]
   (a) Applied statistics   (b) Theoretic statistics
   (c) Descriptive statistics (d) Inferential statistics

2. Glasgow coma scale is type of: [AIIMS June 2020]
   (a) Nominal   (b) Ordinal
   (c) Metric   (d) Alpha-numeric

3. Histogram is used to describe: [AIIMS Dec 1995]
   (a) Quantitative data of a group of patients
   (b) Qualitative data of a group of patients
   (c) Data collected on nominal scale
   (d) Data collected on ordinal scale

4. Which of the following variables is measured on the ordinal scale? [AIPGME 1996]
   (a) Type of anemia   (b) Severity of anemia
   (c) Hemoglobin level   (d) Serum ferritin level

5. Measurement of blood pressure is which type of data: [AIPGME 1996]
   (a) Nominal   (b) Ordinal
   (c) Interval   (d) Continuous

6. Histogram is used to present which kind of the data:
   (a) Nominal   [AIIMS May 2010] [AIIMS May 2006]
   (b) Continuous   [AP 2006] [MP 2002]
   (c) Discrete
   (d) Any of above

7. All of the following are quantitative variables except:
   (a) Serum cholesterol   [AIPGME 1996]
   (b) Weight
   (c) Gender
   (d) Celsius temperature scale

8. All of the following methods can show relationship between two variables except: [AIPGME 1995]
   (a) Histogram   (b) Line diagram
   (c) Bar chart   (d) Scatter plot

9. A physician, after examining a group of patients of a certain disease, classifies the condition of each one as 'Normal', 'Mild', 'Moderate' or 'Severe'. Which one of the following is the scale of measurement that is being adopted for classification of the disease condition?
   [AIIMS Nov 92 Dec 98, May 94, AIPGME 04, 07]
   (a) Normal   (b) Interval
   (c) Ratio   (d) Ordinal

10. In statistical literature data are broadly classified as interval scale data, ordinal scale data & categorical data. Blood groups will be an example for: [AIIMS Dec 1994]
    (a) Interval scale data   (b) Ordinal scale data
    (c) Categorical data   (d) None of the above

11. An investigator into the life expectancy of IV drug abusers divides a sample of patients into HIV- positive and HIV-negative groups. What type of data does this division constitute? [AIIMS June 2000]
    (a) Nominal   (b) Ordinal
    (c) Interval   (d) Ratio

12. A Scatter diagram is drawn to study: [AIIMS June 1997]
    (a) Trend of a variable over a period of time
    (b) Frequency of occurrence of events
    (c) Mean & median values of the given data
    (d) Relationship between two given variables

13. In a study following interpretation are obtained: Satisfied, Very satisfied, Dissatisfied. Which type of scale is this? [AIIMS May 2010, AIPGME 2003]
    (a) Nominal   (b) Ordinal
    (c) Interval   (d) Ratio

14. All of the following are example of nominal scale except: [NEET Pattern 2012]
    (a) Race   (b) Sex
    (c) Body weight   (d) Socio-economic status

15. Best way to plot the change of incidence of disease over time is: [NEET Pattern 2012]
    (a) Histogram   (b) Line chart
    (c) Scatter diagram (d) Ogive

16. Best method to show trend of events with passage of time is: [DNB December 2010]
    (a) Line diagram   [NEET Patterns 2013, 2017]
    (b) Bar diagram
    (c) Histogram
    (d) Pie chart

17. Graph to correlate two quantitative data is: [DNB June 2009]
    (a) Histogram   (b) Scatter diagram
    (c) Line diagram   (d) Frequency curve

18. A Doctor is taking history from a Diabetes patient and decides to make a chart to assess joint involvement. Which chart should he make? [AIIMS November 2015]
    (a) Pie chart   (b) Venn diagram
    (c) Histogram   (d) Tree diagram

19. Identify the Statistical diagram shown in Photograph: [AIIMS November 2015]

```
52 │ 0
53 │ 2 4
54 │ 0 2 8
55 │ 0 0 4 4 5 5 5 6 6 7 9
56 │ 0 0 0 0 0 2 4 5 6 8 9 9
57 │ 0 0 0 7 8 9
58 │ 0 0 0 0 4 7
59 │ 0 0 0 0
60 │ 0 0 0 0 3 3 7 8
61 │ 0 5
```

(a) Funnel plot
(b) Forest plot
(c) Stem and Leaf plot
(d) Box and Whisker plot

20. Identify the Statistical diagram shown in Photograph
 [AIIMS November 2015] [NEET Pattern 2015]

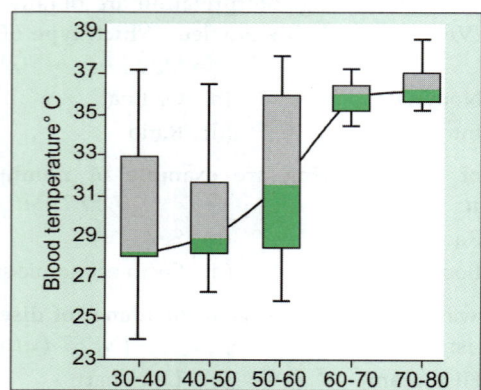

(a) Funnel plot
(b) Forest plot
(c) Stem and Leaf plot
(d) Box and Whisker plot

21. Value of one parameter can be estimated from another related parameter by: [NEET Pattern 2015]
(a) Bar chart
(b) Correlation
(c) Scatter diagram
(d) Regression

22. All of the following are Continuous variable *except*: [AIIMS May 2016]
(a) Weight in kgs
(b) Blood group (A, B, AB, O)
(c) Age in years and months
(d) Height in cm

23. All of the following show relationship between two variables, *except*: [NEET Pattern 2017]
(a) Correlation coefficient
(b) Regression
(c) Scatter diagram
(d) Line diagram

24. True about Bar chart is: [NEET Pattern 2017]
(a) Width of bar is proportional to representative values
(b) Used for Quantitative data
(c) Same as histogram
(d) Rectangular bars are used to represent data

25. Child Pugh Score for Chronic liver disease classified patients into three categories, namely, Category A (5–6), Category B (7–9) and Category C (10–15). This is a type of ____ variable/data now. [AIIMS November 2017]
(a) Nominal
(b) Ordinal
(c) Metric
(d) Quantitative

26. Pictorial diagram of Frequency distribution is: [NEET Pattern 2017]
(a) Histogram
(b) Scatter diagram
(c) Pie chart
(d) Bar Chart

27. Best statistical data diagram to depict Incidence change over a period of time is: [NEET Pattern 2019]
(a) Pie chart
(b) Histogram
(c) Scatter diagram
(d) Line diagram

Review Question

28. Which type of variable "Social Class" is, if it has four categories-I to V and Class I is the highest social class and Class V is the lowest? [MP 2006]
(a) Dichotomous
(b) Nominal
(c) Ordinal
(d) Interval

STATISTICAL DATA GRAPHS

29. Flow cytometry Immunohistochemistry in PNH is plotted through (CD markers) [INICET July 2021]
(a) Pie chart and Dot plot
(b) Bar chart and Dot plot
(c) Line chart and Dot plot
(d) Histogram and Dot plot

MEASURES OF CENTRAL TENDECY

30. True about Central tendency is [INICET May 2023]
(a) Median is qualitative
(b) Median affected by extremes of data
(c) Mode is qualitative
(d) Arithmetic mean is not affected by extreme values

31. Out of 11 births in a hospital, 5 babies weighed over 2.5 kg and 5 weighed less than 2.5 kg. What value do 2.5 represent?
    [AIPGME 2001]
    (a) Geometric average
    (b) Arithmetic average
    (c) Median
    (d) Mode

32. The number of malaria cases reported during the last 10 years in a town is given below, 250, 320, 190, 300, 5000, 100, 260, 350, 320, and 160 The epidemiologist wants to find out the average number of malaria cases reported in that town during the last 10 years. The most appropriate measure of average for this data will be:
    [AIIMS Nov 2004], [AIIMS May 2001]
    (a) Arithmetic mean
    (b) Mode
    (c) Median
    (d) Geometric mean

33. The incidence of malaria in an area is 20, 20, 50, 56, 60, 5000, 678, 898, 345, 456. Which of these methods is the best to calculate the average incidence?
    [AIIMS Nov 01, June 2000]
    (a) Arithmetic mean
    (b) Geometric mean
    (c) Median
    (d) Mode

34. In a bimodal series, if mean is 2 and median is 3, what is the mode? [AIIMS June 1999]
    (a) 5
    (b) 2.5
    (c) 4
    (d) 3

35. Mean value of weight of a group of 10 boys was found to be 18.2 kg. Later it was found that weight of one of the boys was wrongly recorded as 2.0 kg that should have been 20 kg. The true mean weight of the group is:
    (a) 18.2 kg [AIPGME 1998]
    (b) 20.2 kg
    (c) 16.4 kg
    (d) 20 kg

36. Central tendency is given by: [PGI Dec 01]
    (a) Mean [NEET Pattern 2017]
    (b) Median
    (c) Mode
    (d) Range
    (e) Variance

37. Median is important for all *except*: [AIPGME 2012]
    (a) Blood pressure
    (b) Survival time
    (c) Incubation period
    (d) Health expenses

38. Which of the following statements is/are correct about the distribution of weights of a group of students: 70, 70, 70, 75, 79, 83, 84, 85? [PGI May 2014]
    (a) Mean 77
    (b) Median 77
    (c) Mode 70
    (d) Range 12
    (e) Normal distribution

39. A smoker states that he has been smoking for 6 years. In the first year he was taking up to 5 sticks per day only. In the next 3 years he increased it to half pack per day. In the 5th year, his habits worsened to 1 pack per day. In the last year he stated that his daily sticks consumption is 2 packs per day. Select the correct statement Mean, median and mode of number of sticks are: [NEET Pattern 2014]
    (a) 16,10, 15
    (b) 16, 10, 10
    (c) 10, 10, 15
    (d) 16, 10, 15

40. In a survey of Sleep apnea scores among 10 persons, the highest value obtained of 58 was wrongly recorded as 85. This will affect the final results as: [AIIMS PG May 2015]
    (a) No change in Mean, Increased Median
    (b) Increased Mean, No change in median
    (c) Increased Mean, Increased Median
    (d) Increased Mean, Decreased Median

41. Which can have more than one value?
    [NEET Pattern 2016, 2018]
    (a) Mean
    (b) Median
    (c) Mode
    (d) Any of the above

42. In set of date with highly variable values (very high & low), the best measure of central tendency is:
    (a) Mean [NEET Pattern 2017]
    (b) Median
    (c) Mode
    (d) SD

43. Bimodal distribution is represented by:
    (a) Mode = 3 median – 2 mean [NEET Pattern 2017]
    (b) Mode = 3 median + 2 mean
    (c) Mode = 2 median + 2 mean
    (d) Mode = 3 mode – 3 median

44. 18, 20, 22, 24, 26, 28 and 30, Best central tendency is determined by: [NEET Pattern 2018]
    (a) Mean
    (b) Median
    (c) Mode
    (d) Range

Review Questions

45. What is true among given data 20, 31, 31, 31, 25, 28, 35, 38, 31: [MP 2004]
    (a) Mean is 31
    (b) Range is 20–38
    (c) Median is 15
    (d) Mode is 15

46. Commonly used measures of central tendency are all of the following *except*: [MP 2005]
    (a) Mean
    (b) Median
    (c) Mode
    (d) Chi-square test

OTHER MEASURES OF LOCATION

47. 'Centile' divides data into: [AIPGME 01]
    (a) 100 equal parts [NEET Pattern 2017]
    (b) 4 equal parts
    (c) 10 equal parts
    (d) 20 equal parts

48. 50th percentile is equivalent to: [AIIMS Sep 1996]
    (a) Mean
    (b) Median
    (c) Mode
    (d) Range

49. A bacterium can divide every 20 minutes. Beginning with a single individual, how many bacteria will be there in the population if there is exponential growth for 3 hours? [AIIMS May 05]
    (a) 18
    (b) 440
    (c) 512
    (d) 1024

50. For a group of n = 250 subjects, 40th percentile would be the following value (after arranging in ascending order): [AIPGME 2000]
    (a) 7th
    (b) 40th
    (c) 100th
    (d) 140th

51. Central value of a set of 180 values can be obtained by:
    (b) 90th percentile [AIIMS Nov 2000]
    (a) 2nd tertile
    (c) 9th decile
    (d) 2nd quartile

52. Blood pressure data of 200 persons were collected. The first quartile BP of data was 94 mm Hg and third quartile was 110 mm Hg. How many patients lie between the 3rd and 4th quartile? [AIIMS PG May 2015]
    (a) 25
    (b) 50
    (c) 100
    (d) 200

53. A physician recorded Diastolic BP in 125 women aged 18–60 years and found the Mean to be 70 mm Hg with SD of 10 mm Hg. What will be the 5th Percentile value? [AIIMS November 2015]
    (a) 40
    (b) 53.6
    (c) 67.5
    (d) 89.4

VARIABILITY

54. Given formula is used for: [INICET November 2022, May 2023]

    $$s = \sqrt{\frac{\Sigma(X-\bar{x})^2}{n-1}}$$

    (a) Mean
    (b) Mean deviation
    (c) Standard deviation
    (d) Precision

55. Difference between lowest and highest value in a data distribution is known as: [INICET November 2020]
    (a) Quartile range
    (b) Range
    (c) Coefficient of variation
    (d) Variance

56. Variation in a given data set can be compared with another data set with different mean and SD by [NEET PG Pattern January 2020]
    (a) Coefficient of correlation
    (b) Coefficient of regression
    (c) Coefficient of variation
    (d) Standard deviation

57. MULTIPLE COMPLETION TYPE QUESTION: Village-1 (1000 population total) has Mean age of population 20 years and SD 2 years; Village 2 (2000 population total) has Mean age of population 40 years and SD 1 year.
    A. Variation in Village-1 age is 10
    B. Variation in Village-2 is 2.5
    C. Village-1 has higher variation
    D. Village-2 has higher variation

    Use the following key to mark correct answer [AIIMS May 2019]
    (a) If A, B, C are correct
    (b) If A and C are correct
    (c) If B and D are correct
    (d) If all four (A, B, C, & D) are correct

58. Standard deviation is the measure of: [AIPGME 08]
    (a) Chance
    (b) Central tendency
    (c) Deviation from mean value
    (d) None

59. Median weight of 100 children was 12 kg. The standard deviation was 3. Calculate the percent coefficient of variance: [AIIMS May 1994]
    (a) 25%
    (b) 35%
    (c) 45%
    (d) 55%

60. While calculating the incubation period for measles in a group of 25 kids, standard deviation is 2 and the mean incubation period is 8 days, calculate standard error: [AIPGME 1993]
    (a) 0.4
    (b) 1.0
    (c) 2.0
    (d) 0.5

61. Standard deviation of means measures: [AIIMS May 01]
    (a) Non-sampling errors
    (b) Sampling errors
    (c) Random errors
    (d) Conceptual errors

62. If the birth weight of each of the 10 babies born in a hospital in a day is found to be 2.8 kg, then the standard deviation of this sample will be:
    (a) 2.8   *[AIIMS May 2006, Dec 97, AIPGME 01]*
    (b) 0   *[NEET Pattern 2013]*
    (c) 1
    (d) 0.28

63. Among a 100 women with average Hb of 10 gm%, the standard deviation was 1, what is the standard error?
    (a) 0.01   *[AIIMS May 01, 04, 07]*
    (b) 0.1
    (c) 1
    (d) 10

64. The Hb level in healthy women has mean 13.5 g/dl and standard deviation 1.5 g/dl, what is the Z score for a woman with Hb level 15.0 g/dl: *[AIPGME 2005]*
    (a) 9.0
    (b) 10.0
    (c) 2.0
    (d) 1.0

65. In a sample of 100 pregnant females, Mean haemoglobin level estimated was 10 gm% with a Standard deviation of 1 gm%. What is the Standard error?   *[AIPGME 2012]*
    (a) 1 gm%
    (b) 10 gm%
    (c) 0.1 gm%
    (d) 100 gm%

66. Following denotes measures of variability?
    (a) Range   *[PGI November 2011]*
    (b) Mean deviation
    (c) Standard deviation
    (d) Median
    (e) Mode

67. In a population of 100 prevalence of candida glabrata was found to be 80%. If the investigator has to repeat the study with 95% confidence what will the prevalence estimate likely be?   *[AIIMS PGMEE May 2013]*
    (a) 78–82%
    (b) 76–84%
    (c) 72–88%
    (d) 74–86%

68. How much population falls between median and median plus one standard deviation in a normal distribution?
         [AIIMS PGMEE November 2013]
    (a) 0.34   (b) 0.68
    (c) 0.17   (d) 0.47

69. There is a population of 20000 people with mean hemoglobin being 13.5 gm% having a normal distribution. What proportion of population constitutes proportion more than 13.5 gm%?   *[AIIMS PGMEE November 2013]*
    (a) 0.25   (b) 0.50
    (c) 1   (d) 0.34

70. True about Standard deviation is/are:
    (a) 1 SD covers 95% values   *[PGI November 2014]*
    (b) Indicated distribution of variables
    (c) Most common method used for dispersion
    (d) Better indicator of variance than range
    (e) Should be used only in normal distributions

71. If sample size is < 30, then formula for Standard deviation is: *[NEET Pattern 2015]*
    (a) $\sqrt{\Sigma (x-\bar{x})/\eta}$ (b) $\sqrt{\Sigma (x-\bar{x})/\eta-1}$
    (c) $\sqrt{\Sigma (x-\bar{x})^2/\eta}$ (d) $\sqrt{\Sigma (x-\bar{x})^2/\eta-1}$

72. Variation of Sample mean from Population mean is:
         [JIPMER November 2017]
    (a) Standard error of the mean
    (b) Standard error of proportion
    (c) Standard error of difference between two means
    (d) Standard error of difference between two proportions

Review Questions

73. Mean is 230 & SD = 10, then 95% confidence limits is:
         [Bihar 2003]
    (a) 210–250   (b) 250–290
    (c) 290–330   (d) 330–370

74. Measures of dispersion all *except*:   *[UP 2006]*
    (a) Range   *[UPSC CMS 2015]*
    (b) Mean or average deviation
    (c) Standard deviation
    (d) Correlation and regression

75. Confidence limit is calculated by using: *[AP 2006]*
    (a) Mean and standard error
    (b) Mean and standard deviation
    (c) Median and standard deviation
    (d) Median

76. Correct relation between S = standard deviation & V = variance is: *[MH 2003]*
    (a) V = square root of S
    (b) S = square root of V
    (c) V = 2S
    (d) S = 2V

77. Standard deviation does not depend on: *[RJ 2001]*
    (a) Mean   (b) Median
    (c) Range   (d) Sample size

DISTRIBUTIONS – NORMAL AND SKEWED

78. Tests for Normalcy of data include: *[INICET May 2023]*
    1. Histogram
    2. Box and whisker plot
    3. Shapiro wilk test
    4. Q-Q plot
    (a) 1,2   (b) 1,3
    (c) 1,2,3   (d) 1,2,3,4

79. Discrete probability distribution that describes probability of given number of events occurring in a fixed interval of time is known as: [INICET November 2020]
    (a) Normal probability distribution
    (b) Gaussian distribution
    (c) Poisson's distribution
    (d) Binomial distribution

80. A study generated a Normal distribution with the median value as 200 and standard deviation 20. 68% will fall between [NEET PG Pattern January 2020]
    (a) 160–240
    (b) 180–220
    (c) 190–210
    (d) 170–230

81. Which is the best distribution to study the daily admission of head injury patients in a trauma care centre? [AIIMS May 2008]
    (a) Normal distribution
    (b) Binomial distribution
    (c) Uniform distribution
    (d) Poisson distribution

82. The standard normal distribution:
    (a) Is skewed to the left [NEET Pattern 2012, 2017]
    (b) Has mean = 1.0 [AIPGME 05, AIIMS Nov 99]
    (c) Has standard deviation = 0.0 [Bihar 2005]
    (d) Has variance = 1.0

83. The fasting blood levels of glucose for a group of diabetics is found to be normally distributed with a mean of 105 mg per 100 mL of blood and a standard deviation of 10 mg per 100 mL of blood. From this data is can be inferred that approximately 95% of diabetics will have their fasting blood glucose levels within the limits of: [AIIMS Nov 2003]
    (a) 75 and 135 mg
    (b) 85 and 125 mg
    (c) 95 and 115 mg
    (d) 65 and 145 mg

84. In a group of 100 children, the mean weight of children is 15 kg. The standard deviation is 1.5 kg. Which one of the following is true? [AIIMS May 2007]
    (a) 95% of all children weight between 12 and 18 kg
    (b) 95% of all children weight between 13.5- and 16.5kg
    (c) 99% of all children weight between 12 and 18 kg
    (d) 99% of all children weight between 13.5 and 16.5kg

85. Which of the following statements is incorrect about standard normal distribution? [AIIMS Dec 1997]
    (a) Shows a 'bath tub distribution'
    (b) Has mean = 0.0
    (c) Is bilaterally symmetrical bell shaped
    (d) Has variance = 1.0

86. For a negatively skewed data mean will be:
    (a) Less than median [AIIMS May 02, 05]
    (b) More than median [NEET Pattern 2013]
    (c) Equal to median
    (d) One

87. The distribution of random blood glucose measurements from 50 first year medical students was found to have a mean of 3.0 mmol/litre with a standard deviation of 3.0 mmol/litre. Which of the following is a correct statement about the shape of the distribution of random blood glucose in these first year medical students? [AIIMS Nov 2005]
    (a) Since both mean and standard deviation are equal, it should be a symmetric distribution
    (b) The distribution is likely to be positively skewed
    (c) The distribution is likely to be negatively skewed
    (d) Nothing can be said conclusively

88. A chest physician observed that the distribution of forced expiratory volume (FEV) in 300 smokers had a median value of 2.5 litres with the first and third quartiles being 1.5 and 4.5 litres respectively. Based on this data how many persons in the sample are expected to have a FEV between 1.5 and 4.5 litres? [AIIMS Nov 05]
    (a) 7.5
    (b) 150
    (c) 225
    (d) 300

89. If the distribution of intra-ocular pressure (IOP) seen in 100 glaucoma patients has an average 30 mm with a SD of 1.0, what is the lower limit of the average IOP that can be expected 95% of times? [AIIMS Nov 05, AIPGME 99]
    (a) 28
    (b) 26
    (c) 32
    (d) 259

90. How much of the sample is included in 1.95 SD?
    (a) 99% [AIIMS May 1995, AIPGME 1997]
    (b) 95% [JIPMER 2015]
    (c) 68% [Kolkata 2004]
    (d) 65% [NEET Pattern 2019]

91. For a given set of values, Mean = 20, Median = 24 & Mode = 26. The given distribution is: [AIPGME 1998]
    (a) Symmetric
    (b) Right-skewed
    (c) Left-skewed
    (d) Can be either symmetric or skewed

92. A population study showed a mean glucose of 86 mg/dL. In a sample of 100 showing normal curve distribution, what percentage of people have glucose above 86 mg/dL? [AIIMS Dec 94, AIPGME 02]
    (a) 34
    (b) 50
    (c) NIL
    (d) 68

93. Systolic blood pressure of a group of normal people between the age of 25–27 years was taken and a mean of 120 mm Hg was found. What will be the expected number of individuals among a group of 100 people taken for study whose systolic blood pressure will be below 120 mm Hg: [AIIMS May 2001]
    (a) 25
    (b) 50
    (c) 75
    (d) 100

94. The PEFR of a group of 11 year old girls follow a normal distribution with mean 300 l/min and standard deviation 20 l/min: [AIPGME 05]
    (a) About 95% of the girls have PEFR between 260 and 340 l/min
    (b) The girls have healthy lungs
    (c) About 5% of girls have PEFR below 260 l/min
    (d) All the PEFR must be less than 340 l/min

95. Normal distribution curve: [PGI June 08]
    (a) Mean, median, mode are same
    (b) B/L symmetrical
    (c) bell shape
    (d) SD is zero
    (e) Mean is one

96. Regarding the normal curve, which of the following statements is true: [PGI Dec 01]
    (a) Both limbs of the curve touch the baseline
    (b) The curve is bilaterally symmetrical
    (c) There is a skew to the right
    (d) There is a skew to the left
    (e) Mean, median and mode coincide

97. Pearson's Skewness Coefficient is given by:
    (a) Mean-Mode/SD [AIPGME 2011]
    (b) Mode-Mean/SD
    (c) SD/Mean-Median
    (d) SD/Median-Mean

98. Mean value of marks in a distribution of 100 students in a class is 105 and Standard deviation is 10. How many students will have their marks in the range 85–125?
    (a) 50%   (b) 68% [AIPGME 2012]
    (c) 95%   (d) 99.7%

99. In a left skewed curve, true statement is:
    (a) Mean = Median [DNB June 2011]
    (b) Mean < Mode
    (c) Mean > Mode
    (d) Mean = Mode

100. Mean hemoglobin of a group of pregnant females is found to be 10.6 gm/dL with Standard deviation of 2 gm/dL. 5% pregnant females in this group will have their hemoglobin level below: [AIIMS May 2014]
    (a) 8.6 gm/dL
    (b) 7.31 gm/dL
    (c) 6.6 gm/dL
    (d) 5.0 gm/dL

101. A researcher has selected all possible samples from a population and plotted the Mean of each sample on a linear graph. It is a type of [AIIMS November 2015]
    (a) Population distribution
    (b) Parametric distribution
    (c) Sample distribution
    (d) Sampling distribution

102. An obstetrician used APGAR score to assess health of 30 newborn infants. The result showed most of them with score >7. Then correct statement is [AIIMS May 2016]
    (a) Data is symmetrical
    (b) Data is negatively skewed
    (c) Data is positively skewed
    (d) Data is symmetrically skewed

103. Area under Standard normal distribution curve: [NEET Pattern 2017]
    (a) 0.5   (b) 1
    (c) 1.5   (d) 2.0

104. In positive skewed deviation, what is true? [NEET Pattern 2017]
    (a) Mode < Median < Mean
    (b) Mode > Median > Mean
    (c) Median > Mean > Mode
    (d) Mode > Mean > Median

105. Mean < Median < Mode is seen in _____ curve: [NEET Pattern 2017]
    (a) Negative skewed
    (b) Positively skewed
    (c) Normal distribution
    (d) No correlation

SAMPLING

106. What happens to minimum sample size when range of allowable error is doubled? [JIPMER May 2019]
    (a) Reduced to 1/2
    (b) Reduced to 1/4
    (c) Sample size does not depend on acceptable error
    (d) Cannot to be calculated

107. For calculation of sample size for a prevalence study all of the following are necessary *except*: [AIPGME 03]
    (a) Prevalence of disease in population
    (b) Power of the study
    (c) Significance level
    (d) Desired precision

108. In the WHO recommended EPI Cluster sampling for assessing primary immunization coverage, the age group of children to be surveyed is: [AIIMS Nov 2005]
    (a) 0–12 months
    (b) 6–12 months
    (c) 9–12 months
    (d) 12–23 months

109. Sampling method used in assessing immunization status of children under immunization program is:
    (a) Systematic sampling [AIIMS May 2004,
    (b) Stratified sampling   AIPGME 07]
    (c) Group sampling
    (d) Cluster sampling

110. Following are the sampling techniques used to conduct community health surveys, *except*: [AIIMS May 1994]
    (a) Simple random
    (b) Systematic random
    (c) Stratified random
    (d) Cluster testing

111. The number of patients required in a clinical trial to treat a specify disease increases as: [AIPGME 05, AIIMS Nov 02]
    (a) The incidence of the disease decreases
    (b) The significance level increases
    (c) The size of the expected treatment effect increased
    (d) The drop-out rate increases

112. In a study, people are separated into certain sub-groups and then some are selected randomly from each of these sub-groups. What type of sampling is being done? [AIPGME 2011]
    (a) Simple random sampling
    (b) Cluster random sampling
    (c) Systematic random sampling
    (d) Stratified random sampling

113. True about cluster sampling all *except*: [AIIMS May 2011]
    (a) Sample size same as simple random
    (b) It is two stage sampling
    (c) Cheaper than other methods
    (d) It is a method for rapid assessment

114. For which of the following sampling, a Design effect is used? [AIPGME 2012]
    (a) Simple random sampling
    (b) Systematic random sampling
    (c) Stratified random sampling
    (d) Cluster random sampling

115. 50% population having disease with estimated prevalence to be 45–55% with 95% of probability of identifying them minimum sample size required is:
    (a) 100 [AIIMS PGMEE May 2013]
    (b) 200
    (c) 300
    (d) 400

116. Stratified sampling is ideal for: [NEET Pattern 2012]
    (a) Heterogenous data
    (b) Homogenous data
    (c) Both
    (d) None

117. Children surveyed in cluster sampling for coverage of national immunization programme in: [DNB June 2011]
    (a) 30 cluster of 5 children
    (b) 20 cluster of 5 children
    (c) 30 cluster of 10 children
    (d) 30 cluster of 7 children

118. In a study first schools are sampled, then sections, and finally students. This type of sampling is known as: [AIIMS PGMEE November 2012]
    (a) Stratified sampling
    (b) Simple random sampling
    (c) Cluster sampling
    (d) Multistage sampling

119. All of following comes under random sampling method *except*: [DNB December 2011]
    (a) Quota sampling
    (b) Simple random sampling
    (c) Stratified sampling
    (d) Cluster sampling

120. For an epidemiological study, every 10th person is selected from a population. This type of sampling is known as: [NEET Pattern 2017] [AIIMS November 2014]
    (a) Simple random sampling
    (b) Stratified random sampling
    (c) Systematic random sampling
    (d) Cluster random sampling

121. If subjects are assigned according to the potential factor that will influence the outcome of the study, then the sampling is:
    (a) Systemic random sampling
    (b) Stratified random sampling
    (c) Simple random sampling
    (d) Clustered random sampling

122. In a study with prevalence of 10%. Calculate the sample size for a cross-sectional study if relative precision of 20%, alpha error -5% and power of the study 80%.
    (a) 3600 [AIIMS May 2016]
    (b) 400
    (c) 900
    (d) 600

123. Stratified sampling is ideal for: [NEET Pattern 2017]
    (a) Small homogenous population
    (b) Natural population group
    (c) Hidden population
    (d) When subpopulation vary considerably

124. In a psychiatric hospital, all patients are arranged chronologically according to height [from lower to higher]. Than every 4th patient is taken into study. Type of sampling: [NEET Pattern 2017]
    (a) Simple random sampling
    (b) Stratified random sampling
    (c) Systematic random sampling
    (d) All of the above

125. All of the following are true regarding Increasing sample size *except*: [JIPMER November 2017]
    (a) Decreases power of test
    (b) Standard error of mean decreases
    (c) Confidence interval narrows
    (d) Decreases alpha error

PROBABILITY AND ODDS

126. You have diagnosed a patient clinically as having SLE and ordered 6 tests. Out of which 4 tests have come positive and 2 are negative. To determine the probability of SLE at this point, you need to know: [AIPGME 05, AIIMS May 2006] [AIPGME 2007]
    (a) Prior probability of SLE; sensitivity and specificity of each test
    (b) Incidence of SLE and predictive value of each test
    (c) Incidence and prevalence of SLE
    (d) Relative risk of SLE in this patient

127. If prevalence of diabetes is 10%, the probability that three people selected at random from the population will have diabetes is: [AIPGME 04]
    (a) 0.01
    (b) 0.03
    (c) 0.001
    (d) 0.003

128. Chance of passing a Genetic disease "y" trait by the affected parents to children is 0.16. They plan to have two children. Probability of both the children having "y" trait is: [AIIMS Dec 1994]
    (a) Zero
    (b) 0.16
    (c) 0.32
    (d) 0.0256

129. For Mrs Rekha, probability of having a baby of BW <2500 gms is 0.50 and of having a BW 2500–2999 gms is 0.20. So the probability for Mrs Rekha to have a baby of BW <3 kg is: [AIPGME 05]
    (a) 0.30
    (b) 0.70
    (c) 0.10
    (d) 1.0

130. Probability of Mr Ram developing Acute MI in his lifetime is 0.75. What are his Odds of developing Acute MI in his lifetime? [AIPGME 04]
    (a) 3:4
    (b) 3:1
    (c) 4:3
    (d) 1:3

131. The events A and B are mutually exclusive, so: [AIPGME 05]
    (a) Prob (A or B) = Prob (A) + Prob (B)
    (b) Prob (A and B) = Prob (A) X Prob (B)
    (c) Prob A) = Prob (B)
    (d) Prob A) + Prob (B) = 1

Review Question

132. There were 50 patients in a ward 20 girls and 30 boys of them 10 girls and 20 boys required surgery. What is the probability of each patient being selected correctly for surgery: [DNB 2008]
    (a) 2/6
    (b) 3/5
    (c) 6/25
    (d) 1/6

STATISTICAL TESTS

133. Which is a non-parametric test? [AIIMS June 2020]
    (a) Student's t test
    (b) Pearson's test
    (c) ANOVA test
    (d) Friedman test

134. A study was undertaken to assess the malnutrition among young children. A sample of 100 children were selected each from rural and urban area. Out of these, 40 children among rural and 30 children among urban were found to be malnourished. Which of the following statistical test is used to compare the data sets? [NEET PG Pattern January 2020]
    (a) Paired t test
    (b) Chi-square test
    (c) ANOVA
    (d) Standard error of mean

135. Study is done on a group of children to check Seasonal variation of Sudden infant death syndrome (SIDS) in summer season from June to July, and from August to September in another group with similar characteristics from same area. Which test is used to compare the data? [AIIMS May 2019]
    (a) Chi-square test
    (b) Paired T test
    (c) Wilcoxon Rank test
    (d) ANOVA

136. Square root of $p_1q_1/n_1 + p_2q_2/n_2$ is a measure of:
    (a) Mean [AIIMS Dec 1995]
    (b) Standard error of difference between two means
    (c) Standard error of difference between two proportions
    (d) Normal deviate

137. A cardiologist wants to study the effect of an atrovastatin drug. He notes down the initial cholesterol levels of 50 patients and then administers the drug on them. After a month's treatment, he measures the cholesterol level again. Which of the following is the most appropriate to test the statistical significance of the change in blood cholesterol? [AIPGME 02]
    (a) Paired t-test
    (b) Unpaired or independent t-test
    (c) Analysis of variance
    (d) Chi-square test

138. A chi-square test would be most appropriate for testing which one of the following hypotheses? [AIPGME 2000]
    (a) That the mean AIPGE score of Delhi students is greater than that of mumbai students
    (b) That a smaller proportion of people who were immunized against chickenpox subsequently develop zoster than those who were not immunized
    (c) That the mean blood pressure of black and white male-hypertensive patients taking ACE inhibitors is the same as that of black and white female-hypertensive patients taking ACE inhibitors and that of black and white males and females taking diuretics and placebos
    (d) That the mean cost of treating a patient with coronary artery disease with angioplasty is greater than the mean cost of providing medical treatment

139. In a particular trial, the association of lung cancer with smoking is found to be 40% in one sample and 60% in another. What is the best test to compare the results?
    [AIIMS May 2001]
    (a) Chi-square test
    (b) Fischer test
    (c) Paired t test
    (d) ANOVA test

140. Height of group of 20 Boys aged 10 years was 140 + 13 cm & 20 girl of same age was 135 cm ± 7cm to test the statistical significance of difference in height, test applicable is:
    [AIIMS Nov 05]
    (a) X^2
    (b) Z
    (c) t
    (d) F

141. The mean B.P. of a group of persons was determined and after an interventional trial, the mean BP was estimated again. The best test to be applied to determine the significance of intervention is: [AIIMS Dec 1997]
    (a) Chi-square
    (b) Paired 't' test
    (c) Correlation coefficient
    (d) t-test

142. An investigator wants to study the association between maternal intake of iron supplements (Yes or No) and incidence of low birth weight (<2500 or >2500) gm). He collects relevant data from 100 pregnant women as to the status of usage of iron supplements and the status of low birth weight in their newborns. The appropriate statistical test of hypothesis advised in this situation is:
    (a) Paired-t-test [AIIMS Nov 03]
    (b) Unpaired or independent t-test
    (c) Analysis of variance
    (d) Chi-Square test

143. In a 3 × 4 contingency tables, the number of degrees of freedom equals to: [AIIMS Nov 2004]
    (a) 1
    (b) 5
    (c) 6
    (d) 12

144. A cardiologist wants to study the effect of an anti-hypertensive drug. He notes down the initial systolic blood pressure (mm Hg) of 50 patients and then administers the drug on them. After a week's treatment, he measures the following is the most appropriate statistical test of significance to test the statistical significance of the change in blood pressure:
    [AIIMS June 1997, AIIMS May 1995, AIIMS Nov 2004]
    (a) Paired t-test
    (b) Unpaired or independent t-test
    (c) Analysis of variance
    (d) Chi-square test

145. A study was undertaken to assess the effect of a drug in lowering serum cholesterol levels. 15 obese women and 10 non-obese women formed the 2 limbs of the study. Which test would be useful to correlate the results obtained? [AIIMS Nov 01]
    (a) ANOVA test
    (b) Student's t-test
    (c) Chi-square test
    (d) Fischer test

146. Not required for Chi-square test is: [AIIMS Dec 1997]
    (a) Mean & SD of the groups
    (b) Each expected cell frequency >5
    (c) Large sample
    (d) Contingency table

147. Appropriate statistical method to compare two means is:
    [AIPGME 2000]
    (a) Chi-square test [NEET Pattern 2013]
    (b) Student's t-test [NEET Pattern 2019]
    (c) Odds ratio
    (d) Correlation coefficient

148. Appropriate statistical method to compare two proportions is: [AIPGME 1995]
    (a) Chi-square test [NEET Pattern 2019]
    (b) Student's t-test
    (c) Odds ratio
    (d) Correlation coefficient

149. In a given data, degree of freedom will be:
    [AIIMS May 06]

Duration of developing AIDS	Blood group			
	A	B	AB	O
0–5 years	20	30	48	7
5–10 years	110	12	37	12
10–15 years	12	9	8	3

    (a) 12
    (b) 6
    (c) 9
    (d) 20

150. Not true about Chi-square test is:
    [AIPGME 03, AIIMS June 99]
    (a) Tests the significance of difference between two proportions
    (b) Tells about presence or absence of an association between two variables
    (c) Directly measures the strength of association
    (d) Can be used when more than two groups are to be compared

151. Mean bone density amongst 2 group of 50 people each is compared, which would be the best test?
    [AIIMS May 2008]
    (a) Chi-square
    (b) Student t test
    (c) McNemar chi-square test
    (d) Fischer test

152. An antihypertensive drug is studied before and after using it for treatment of a patient, what is this study: [PGI Dec 2K]
    (a) Chi-square test
    (b) Paired 't' test
    (c) Student 't' test
    (d) Regression
    (e) Co-relation

153. What will be the degree of freedom in no. of row 3 and col. 4: [PGI Dec 2002]
    (a) 3
    (b) 6
    (c) 4
    (d) 9
    (e) 10

154. An investigator finds out that 5 independent factors influence the occurrence of a disease. Comparison of multiple factors that are responsible for the disease can be assessed by: [AIIMS May 2011]
    (a) ANOVA
    (b) Multiple linear regression
    (c) Chi-square test
    (d) Multiple logistic regression

155. Mean blood alcohol levels are measured in patients before and after using an interventional drug. The statistical test of significance to be applied is: [AIPGME 2012]
    (a) Chi-square test
    (b) ANOVA
    (c) Paired students t-test
    (d) Unpaired students t-test

156. In a study, Two groups of newborns are checked for their weights based on whether mothers received food supplements or not. Appropriate statistical test that can be used is [AIIMS PG May 2015]
    (a) Paired t test
    (b) Unpaired t test
    (c) Fischer's exact test
    (d) Chi-square test

157. Not a Parametric test of significance: [NEET Pattern 2017]
    (a) Z-test
    (b) ANOVA
    (c) Student 't-test'
    (d) Chi-square test

158. Non-parametric tests in Biostatistics are better than parametric tests because: [NEET Pattern 2018]
    (a) Useful for non-normal (skewed) data
    (b) Calculations are more accurate
    (c) More powerful in nature
    (d) Require less data

159. Quantitative test for same group of individuals before and after study is: [NEET Pattern 2018]
    (a) Paired t - test
    (b) Unpaired t - test
    (c) Z - test
    (d) Chi- square test

160. All of the following are nonparametric test, *except:* [NEET Pattern 2018]
    (a) Chi-square test
    (b) Z-test
    (c) Wilcoxon rank sum test
    (d) Kruskal – Wallis 'H' test

161. Appropriate statistical test to find out Obesity as a significant risk factor for Breast cancer is: [NEET Pattern 2018]
    (a) Student's paired 't' test
    (b) Student's unpaired 't' test
    (c) Chi-square test
    (d) Wilcoxon's signed rank test

162. All of the following can be analyzed with Chi-square test except? [AIIMS May 2018]
    (a) Sex and stage of cancer
    (b) Heart rate/min and age
    (c) Benign or malignant, and type of surgery
    (d) Age group and cancer stage

163. In a clinical trial, blood pressure was measured between 2 independent groups following treatment, which of the following test will be suitable as at test of significance? [AIIMS November 2018]
    (a) Paired t-test
    (b) Unpaired t-test
    (c) ANOVA
    (d) Chi-square

164. In a clinical trial, blood pressure was measured between in a group of patients before and after treatment, which of the following test will be suitable as at test of significance? [AIIMS November 2018]
    (a) Paired t-test
    (b) Mann Whitney U test
    (c) Student test
    (d) ANOVA

165. Test of significance for comparing Means of 2 groups is: [NEET Pattern 2019]
    (a) Paired t-test
    (b) Unpaired t-test
    (c) Chi-square test
    (d) ANOVA

Review Questions

166. In a table of 2 × 2, the degree of freedom is: [UP 2001]
    (a) 4
    (b) 1
    (c) 8
    (d) 7

167. 1 degree of freedom in chi-square test, the value of x^2 for a probability of 0.05 is: [UP 2007]
    (a) 0.45
    (b) 2.41
    (c) 3.84
    (d) 4.34

168. Test of association between two qualitative variables is done by: [AP 2004]
    (a) Chi-square test
    (b) Correlation
    (c) Regression
    (d) None

169. About chi-square test, true is: [MP 2000]
    (a) <0.001 is statistically significant
    (b) Less no. of samples are associated with less error
    (c) Categories of data used in test need not be mutually exclusive and discrete
    (d) Tests correlation and regression

170. A study who planned to find out the effect of iron supplementation during pregnancy on the birth weight of new born children. Two groups, one with iron supplementation and the other without iron supplementation during pregnancy were compared. Birth weight of new borns were recorded as means + SD. Which significant test (statistical) is appropriate for comparison of birth weights between the two groups? [MP 2008]
    (a) Unpaired 't' test
    (b) Paired 't' test
    (c) McNemar's chi-square test
    (d) Chi-square test

171. A study measures a patient's serum cholesterol before and after a new lipid-lowering therapy has been gives. What type of significance test should be used to analyze the data? [MH 2007]
    (a) Paired t-test
    (b) Student's t-test
    (c) Chi-squared test
    (d) Pearson's test

172. Chi-square test 5 rows/4 columns, degree of freedom is:
    (a) 9 [NEET Pattern 2012, 2013]
    (b) 12 [DNB 2009, 2011] [RJ 2009]
    (c) 16
    (d) 20

173. Not required for chi-square test: [NEET Pattern 2012]
    (a) Null hypothesis
    (b) Degrees of freedom
    (c) Means in different groups
    (d) Proportions in different groups

174. Chi-square test is for: [DNB December 2010]
    (a) Standard error of mean
    (b) Standard error of proportion
    (c) Standard error of difference between 2 means
    (d) Standard error of difference between proportions

175. Test is used to compare Kaplan-Meier survival curve: [NEET Pattern 2012]
    (a) ANOVA
    (b) Bland-Altman analysis
    (c) Chi-square test
    (d) Cox proportional hazards test

176. Test(s) used to compare two proportions is/are: [PGI November 2013]
    (a) Paired t-test
    (b) Unpaired t-test
    (c) ANOVA
    (d) Fischer's exact test
    (e) Chi-square test

CORRELATION AND REGRESSION

177. The correlation between variables A and B in a study was found to be 1.1. This indicates: [AIPGME 02]
    (a) Very strong correlation
    (b) Moderately strong correlation
    (c) Weak correlation
    (d) Computational mistake in calculating correlation

178. A lecturer states that the correlation coefficient between prefrontal blood flow under cognitive load and the severity of psychotic symptoms in schizophrenic patients is – 1.24. You can therefore conclude that: [AIIMS June 2000]
    (a) Pre-frontal blood flow under cognitive load is a good predictor of the severity of psychotic symptoms in schizophrenic patients
    (b) Prefrontal blood flow under cognitive load accounts for a large proportion of the variance in psychotic symptoms in schizophrenic patients
    (c) Psychosis or schizophrenia is in some way a cause or partial cause of low prefrontal blood flow under cognitive load
    (d) The lecturer has reported the correlation coefficient incorrectly

179. A cardiologist found a highly significant correlation coefficient (r = 0.90, p = 0.01) between the systolic blood pressure values and serum cholesterol values of the patients attending his clinic. Which of the following statements is a wrong interpretation of the correlation coefficient observed? [AIPGME 05]
    (a) Since there is a high correlation, the magnitudes of both the measurements are likely to be close to each other
    (b) A patient with a high level of systolic BP is also likely to have a high level of serum cholesterol
    (c) A patient with a low level of systolic BP is also likely to have a low level of serum cholesterol
    (d) About 80% of the variation in systolic blood pressure among his patients can be explained by their serum cholesterol values and vice a versa

180. Best way to study relationship between two variables is: [AIPGME 02]
    (a) Bar chart
    (b) Scatter diagram
    (c) Histogram
    (d) Pie chart

181. If we know the value of one variable in an individual & wish to know the value of another variable, we calculate:
    [AIIMS June 1997]
    (a) Coefficient of correlation
    (b) Coefficient of regression
    (c) SE of mean
    (d) Geometric mean

182. If the correlation of height with age is given by the equation y = a + biopsy, what would be the nature of the graph? [AIPGME 05]
    (a) Straight line   (b) Parabola
    (c) Hyperbola   (d) Sigmoid curve

183. What can be true regarding the coefficient of correlation between IMR and economic status? [AIIMS May 2001]
    (a) r = + 1
    (b) r = – 1
    (c) r = + 0.22
    (d) r = – 0.8

184. The Correlation Coefficient between Smoking & Lung Cancer was found to be 1.4. This indicates:
    (a) Weak correlation   [AIIMS Feb 1997]
    (b) Moderate correlation
    (c) Strong correlation
    (d) Mistake in calculation

185. Study finds a correlation coefficient of + 0.7 between self reported work satisfaction & expectancy of life in a random sample of 5000 corporate workers. (p = 0.01). This means that: [AIIMS Dec 1997]
    (a) Work satisfaction improves life expectancy
    (b) Strong statistically significant (+) association between work satisfaction and life expectancy
    (c) 70% people who enjoy work shall live longer
    (d) 70% association between work satisfaction & life expectancy

186. Total Cholesterol level = a + b (calorie intake) + c (physical activity) + d (body mass index); is an example of:
    [AIPGME 05]
    (a) Simple linear regression
    (b) Simple curvilinear regression
    (c) Multiple linear regression
    (d) Multiple logistic regression

187. Mosquitoes decrease as height increases in:
    (a) Positive correlation   [NEET Pattern 2013]
    (b) Negative correlation
    (c) Bidirectional
    (d) Zero correlation

188. Strong correlation is signified by a correlation coefficient of: [DNB June 2011]
    (a) Zero
    (b) 1
    (c) Less than 1
    (d) More than 1

189. Four populations had Correlation coefficients of + 0.6 each for Weight and Height when plotted together. What would be Net coefficient of correlation?
    [AIIMS November 2015]

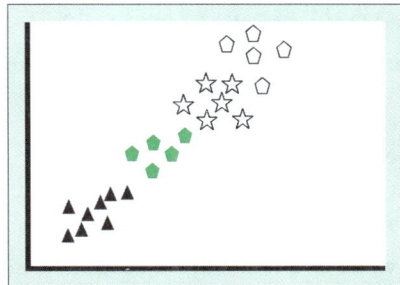

    (a) Same
    (b) Smaller
    (c) Greater
    (d) Cannot be predicted

190. Correlation between Height and Weight is best depicted by: [NEET Pattern 2017]
    (a) Histogram
    (b) Line chart
    (c) Scatter diagram
    (d) Ogive

Review Questions

191. If R = 2.86, it means: [Kolkata 2009]
    (a) Positive correlation
    (b) Negative correlation
    (c) No correlation
    (d) It is a wrong statement

192. Correlation coefficient varies between: [MP 2000]
    (a) 0 to + 1
    (b) -1 to 0
    (c) -1 to + 1
    (d) + 1 to +2

ERRORS AND P-VALUE

193. MULTIPLE RESPONSE TYPE QUESTION: Two studies were undertaken to assess the effect of an Intervention for a certain disease. Study A 'p' value is 0.02 and Study B 'p' value is 0.001, using test X and Y with a control group respectively. Confidence limit in both studies is within 95%. The analysis of the above data is as follows:
    A. Study B is more precise than Study A and test Y is more significant as compared to X.
    B. Study A is more precise than Study B and test X is more significant as compared to Y.
    C. Both X and Y show same variation but Study B is more significant than Study A
    D. Both Study A and B show a significant variation and both test have similar statistical significance

Which of the following options is correct?
[AIIMS May 2019]
(a) A, B, C are correct
(b) A and C are correct
(c) All are correct
(d) A and D are correct

194. Rejection of True Null Hypothesis is known as:
[JIPMER May 2019]
(a) Type II error
(b) Type I error
(c) Both
(d) None

195. The "P" value of a randomized controlled trial comparing operation A (new procedure) & Operation B (Gold standard) is 0.04. From this, we conclude that:
[AIPGME 2003]
(a) Type II error is small & we can accept the findings of the study
(b) The probability of false negative conclusion that operation A is better than operation B, when in truth it is not, is 4%
(c) The power of study to detect a difference between operation A & B is 96%
(d) The probability of a false positive conclusion that operation 'Operation A is better that Operation B', when in truth it is not, is 4%

196. Power of study can be increased by: [AIPGME 2002]
(a) Increasing alpha error [AIIMS May 2014]
(b) Decreasing beta error
(c) Decreasing alpha error
(d) Increasing beta error

197. In assessing the association between maternal nutritional status and the birth weight of the newborns, two investigators A and B studied separately and found significant results with p values 0.02 and 0.04 respectively. From this information, what can you infer about the magnitudes of association found by the two investigations?
[AIIMS Nov 2004]
(a) The magnitude of association found by investigator A is more than that found by B
(b) The magnitude of association found by investigator B is more than that found by A
(c) The estimates of association obtained by A and B will be equal, since both are significant
(d) Nothing can be concluded as the information given is inadequate

198. A randomized trial comparing efficacy of two regimens showed that difference is statistically significant with p < 0.001 but in reality the two drugs do not differ in their efficacy. This is an example of:
[AIIMS May 2006]
(a) Type-I error (alpha error)
(b) Type – II error (beta error)
(c) 1-alpha
(d) 1-beta

199. After applying a statistical test, an investigator gets the 'P value' as 0.01. it means that:
[AIIMS Nov 2003, AIIMS May 05, 08]
(a) The probability of finding a significant difference is 1%
(b) The probability of declaring a significant difference is 1%
(c) The difference is not significant 1% times and significant 99% times
(d) The power of the test used is 99%

200. All are true about P-value except: [AIPGME 03]
(a) Is the probability of committing Type-I error
(b) Is equal to 1-beta
(c) Is the chance that the presence of difference is concluded when actually there is none
(d) When P-value is less than a, the result is statistically significant

201. All are true except: [AIIMS May 04]
(a) Alpha is the maximum tolerable probability of type-I error
(b) Beta is the probability of type-II error
(c) When Null Hypothesis is true but is rejected, it is Type-II error
(d) P-value can be more or less than alpha

202. P-value is the probability of: [AIIMS June 2000]
(a) Not rejecting a null hypothesis when true
(b) Rejecting a null hypothesis when true
(c) Not rejecting a null hypothesis when false
(d) Rejecting a null hypothesis when false

203. An investigator wants to study the association between maternal intake of iron supplements (Yes/No) and birth weights (in gms) of newborn babies. He collects relevant data from 100 pregnant women and their newborns. What statistical test of hypothesis would you advise for the investigator in this situation? [AIIMS May 03]
(a) Chi-square test
(b) Unpaired or independent t-test
(c) Analysis of Variance
(d) Paired t-test

204. A randomized trial comparing the efficacy of two drugs showed a difference between the two with a p-value of <0.005. In reality, however the two drugs do not differ. This therefore is an example of: [AIIMS Nov 02]
(a) Type I error (alpha error)
(b) Type II error (beta error)
(c) 1 – α (alpha)
(d) 1 – β

205. The risk factor association of smoking with pancreatic cancer was studied in a case control study. The values are:

Group	Odds ratio	95% Confidence limits
A	2.5	1.0–3.1
B	1.4	1.1–1.7
C	1.6	0.9–1.7

Which of the following is correct [AIIMS Nov 09]
   (a) Risk is more associated with Group A
   (b) Risk is more associated with Group B
   (c) Risk is more associated with Group C
   (d) Risk is equally associated with all three groups

206. All of the following are true about Standard error except? [AIIMS Nov, 09]
   (a) As the sample size increases, Standard error will also increase
   (b) Based on Normal distribution
   (c) It depends on Standard deviation of mean
   (d) Is used to estimate confidence limit

207. P-value is defined as: [AIPGME 2012]
   (a) Probability of declaring a significant difference when actually it is not present
   (b) Probability of declaring a significant difference when actually it is present
   (c) Probability of not declaring a significant difference when actually it is not present
   (d) Probability of not declaring a significant difference when actually it is present

208. Rejecting a null hypothesis when it is true is called as:
   (a) Type 1 error [DNB December 2010]
   (b) Type 2 error
   (c) Type 3 error
   (d) Type 4 error

209. Type I Statistical error occurs if: [JIPMER 2015]
   (a) Null hypothesis is true but rejected
   (b) Null hypothesis is true and accepted
   (c) Null hypothesis is false but accepted
   (d) Null hypothesis is false and rejected

210. If we say that there is no significant association between two variable and if truly an association exists. Then it is called: [AIIMS May 2016]
   (a) Type I error
   (b) Type II error
   (c) Systematic error
   (d) Random error

Review Questions

211. P-value significant indicates: [UP 2003]
   (a) Probability of Type I Error is <0.05
   (b) Probability null hypothesis is correct
   (c) Probability null hypothesis is false
   (d) To find out meaning of regression

212. In a test of significance, P value is 0.023 the observed difference in study can be considered as: [MH 2005]
   (a) Null hypothesis accepted and the study is rejected
   (b) Null hypothesis rejected and the study is accepted
   (c) Null hypothesis accepted and the study is accepted
   (d) Null hypothesis rejected and the study is also rejected

MISCELLANEOUS

213. Confidence interval is not increased by: [INICET May 2022]
   (a) Increasing sample size
   (b) Decreasing sample size
   (c) Increasing confidence level
   (d) Increasing variance

214. Which is the best method to compare the results obtained by a new test and a gold standard test? [AIIMS May 07]
   (a) Correlation study
   (b) Regression study
   (c) Bland and Altman analysis
   (d) Kolmogorov-Smirnov test

215. Which of the following statements about Delphi method is true? [AIPGME 2008]
   (a) Method involves formation of a team to undertake and monitor a Delphi on a given subject
   (b) Selection of one or more panels to participate in the exercise. Customarily, the panelists are experts in the area to be investigated
   (c) The first round in Delphi method involves development of a questionnaire
   (d) All are true

216. A researcher draws unbiased sample of 100 adult delhites and finds that their mean weight is 72 kg with a standard deviation of 1.5. 95% of wt of delhites shall between: [AIPGME 1996]
   (a) 66 and 78 kg   (b) 69 and 75 kg
   (c) 70.5 and 73.5 kg   (d) None of the above

217. In a drug trial A 50-year-old patient with CAD is being interviewed about his dietary & smoking habits. The possible bias that might be introduced might be: [AIIMS Feb 1997]
   (a) Selection bias   (b) Berkesonian bias
   (c) Recall bias   (d) No possibility of bias

218. If a 95% Confidence Interval for prevalence of Cancer in Smokers aged >65 years is 56% to 76%, the chance that the prevalence could be less than 56% is: [AIIMS May 07]
   (a) Practically NIL   (b) 44%
   (c) 2.5%   (d) 5%

219. Receiver Operator Characteristic (ROC) curve is usually drawn between: [AIPGME 06]
   (a) Sensitivity & Specificity
   (b) (1 – Sensitivity) & Specificity
   (c) Sensitivity & (1 – Specificity)
   (d) (1 – Sensitivity) & (1 – Specificity)

220. Mean, Medium and Mode are: [Karnataka 2004]
   (a) Measure of dispersion
   (b) Measure association between two variables
   (c) Test of significance
   (d) Measure of central tendency

221. Association can be measured by all *except*:
[AIIMS May 2009]
(a) Correlation coefficient
(b) Cronbach's alpha
(c) P value
(d) Odds ratio

222. Method used for comparison of a new test with an available gold-standard test is: [AIIMS November 2011]
(a) Regression analysis/Likelihood test
(b) Correlation analysis/Bland and Altmann test
(c) Baltin and Altimore method
(d) Kimorov and Samletor technique

223. If confidence limit is increased, then:
[AIIMS PGMEE May 2013]
(a) Previously insignificant data becomes significant
(b) Previously significant data becomes insignificant
(c) No effect on significance
(d) Any change can happen

224. In a group of 100 people, the average GFR is 85 mL/min with a Standard deviation of 25. What is the range for 90% Confidence Intervals? [AIIMS May 2015]
(a) 70–100
(b) 75–95
(c) 81–89
(d) 80–90

225. Intraocular pressure (IOP) was measured in 400 people. Mean was found to be 25 mm Hg and Standard deviation was recorded 10 mm Hg. 95% Confidence Interval would be? [AIIMS November 2016]
(a) 22–28
(b) 23–27
(c) 24–26
(d) 21–29

226. What will be the 95% confidence interval in a study estimated prevalence of 10% and 100 being their sample size? [AIIMS May 2016]
(a) 4–16
(b) 2–18
(c) Inadequate information to calculate 95% CI
(d) 7–13

227. To see if Sample mean is an accurate estimate of Population mean, we use [NEET Pattern 2016]
(a) Geometric mean
(b) Range
(c) Deviation
(d) Standard error

228. Cronbach alpha is a measure of: [JIPMER May 2018]
(a) Criterion validity
(b) Internal consistency
(c) Values are between 1 and 100
(d) Content validity

229. Confidence limit includes: [NEET Pattern 2018]
(a) Range and standard deviation
(b) Median and standard error
(c) Mean and standard error
(d) Mode and standard deviation

Explanations

DATA, VARIABLES AND SCALES

1. **Ans. (c) Descriptive statistics** *[Ref. Descriptive and Inferential Statistics by Lacort, 1/e 2014]*
   - Descriptive Statistics:
     - Data is summarised through the given observations; summarisation is done from a sample of population using parameters such as the mean or standard deviation
     - Descriptive statistics is a way to organise, represent and describe a collection of data using tables, graphs, and summary measures
   - Inferential Statistics:
     - This type of statistics is used to interpret the meaning of Descriptive statistics; so once the data has been collected, analysed and summarised then we use these stats to describe the meaning of the collected data
     - Inferential Statistics allows us to use information collected from a sample to make decisions, predictions or inferences from a population
   - Applied Statistics:
     - Pure statistics focuses primarily on the numbers, math, and problems themselves (theoretical)
     - Applied statistics on the other hand, can be thought of as "statistics-in-action" or using statistics with an eye toward real-world problems and what their solutions might be

2. **Ans. (b) Ordinal** *[Ref. Simple Biostatistics by Indrayan & Indrayan, 1/e p51-52]*
   - Glasgow Coma Scale (GCS) is a clinical scale used to reliably measure a person's level of consciousness after a brain injury
   - GCS measures three functions - EVM, namely, Eye Opening (E), Verbal Response (V) and Motor Response (M). Each function has scoring based on patient response. GCS score for a patient can range from 3 (completely unresponsive) to 15 (responsive)
   - Finally, brain injury is classified as Severe (GCS <8-9), Moderate (GCS 9-12) or Minor, (GCS ≥ 13). Since head injury outcome in GCS is represented as a continuum of outcome for a variable, thus is measured on an ordinal scale

3. **Ans. (a) Quantitative data of a group of patients** *[Ref. Simple Biostatistics by Indrayan & Indrayan, 1/e p104 and Methods in Biostatistics by Mahajan, 9/e p26; Park 27/e p973]*
   - *Data presentation:*

Quantitative data	Qualitative data
Histogram	Bar diagram
Frequency polygon	Pie/Sector diagram
Frequency curve	Pictogram/Picture diagram
Line chart/graph	Map diagram/Spot map
Cumulative frequency diagram (Ogive)	
Scatter/Dot diagram	

   - *Histogram:*
     - Is graphical presentation for 'continuous quantitative data'
     - Continuous groups are marked on x-axis (abscissa) while frequencies are marked on y-axis (ordinate).

   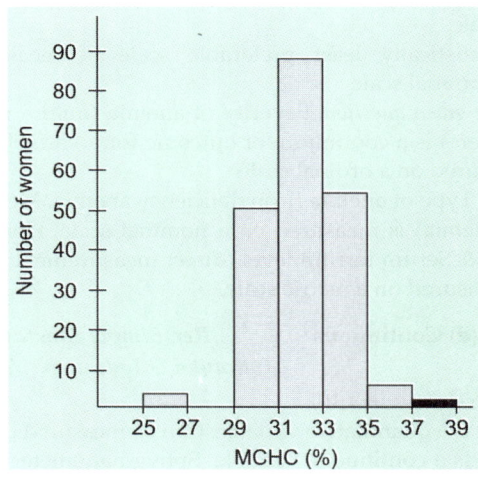

   Histogram

4. **Ans. (b) Severity of anemia** *[Ref. Simple Biostatistics by Indrayan & Indrayan, 1/e p51-52]*
   - *Scales of measurement:*

	Categorical scales		Dimensional scales
	Nominal scale	**Ordinal scale**	**Metric scale**
Definition	Based on NOM (names); no specific order	Based on ORD (order); grading into categories	Based on ME (measurement); in terms of quantities
Variables	Qualitative	Qualitative	Quantitative
Examples	Race	TNM staging (cancers)	Blood glucose
	Religion	Severity of a disease	Hemoglobin level

Contd...

Contd...

	Categorical scales		Dimensional scales
	Nominal scale	**Ordinal scale**	**Metric scale**
	Country of birth	Social classes	Serum cholesterol
	Clinical features		Weight
	Sites of lymphadenopathy		Height
	Sex of child		Mid-arm circumference
	Type of anemia		Blood pressure
	ABO blood group		Pulse rate
	Site of malignancy		Temperature (°C, °F, K) scale
Permissible arithmetic	Counting	> or < operations	Interval scale: +/–
			Ratio scale: ×/÷
Permissible statistics	Mode, Chi–square	Median, Percentile	Interval scale: Mean, SD, Correlation, Regression, ANOVA Ratio scale: Geometric mean, Harmonic mean, Coefficient of variation

- Metric scale is of 2 types:
  - Interval scale (Absence of absolute zero; no ratios are possibl(e): Examples: Centigrade/Fahrenheit temperature scale
  - Ratio scale (Presence of absolute zero; thus ratios are possibl(e): Examples: Weight, Height, Blood glucose, Hemoglobin level, Serum cholesterol, Mid-arm circumference, Blood pressure, Pulse rate, Kelvin temperature scale
- Statistically most preferable scale of measurement: Metric scale
- Statistically least preferable scale of measurement: Nominal scale

In the given question, Severity of anemia (mild – moderate – severe) is a continuum of outcome for a variable, thus is measured on a ordinal scale
Also, Type of anemia (Iron deficiency anemia, Megaloblastic anemia) is measured on a nominal scale, Hemoglobin level & Serum ferritin level (direct measurement possible) is measured on a metric scale.

5. **Ans. (d) Continuous**   *[Ref. Simple Biostatistics by Indrayan & Indrayan, 1/e p53–54]*

- *Blood pressure (BP):*
  - Is a quantitative variable: Can be measured directly
  - Is a continuous variable: Sphygmanometer can only measure with a minimum count of 2 mm Hg; but it has several in-between values
  - Is a polytomous variable: BP can have several values possible.

> **ALSO REMEMBER**
> - *Weight:* Is a quantitative, continuous, polytomous variable
> - *Height:* Is a quantitative, continuous, polytomous variable
> - *Pulse rate (PR):* Is a quantitative, continuous, polytomous variable
> - *Blood pressure (BP):* Is a quantitative, continuous, polytomous variable
> - *Temperature:* Is a quantitative, continuous, polytomous variable

Contd...

> Contd...
> - *ABO blood group:* Is a qualitative, discrete, polytomous variable
> - *Rhesus (Rh) blood group:* Is a qualitative, discrete, dichotomous variable
> - *Gender:* Is a qualitative, discrete, dichotomous variable.

6. **Ans. (b) Continuous**   *[Ref. Simple Biostatistics by Indrayan & Indrayan, 1/e p104 and Methods in Biostatistics by Mahajan, 9/e p26; Park 27/e p973]*

> **ALSO REMEMBER**
> - *Frequency polygon:* Is an area diagram of frequency distribution developed over a histogram (by joining mid-points of class intervals at heights of frequencies)
> - *Frequency curve:* When no. of observations is large and group-interval is reduced, then frequency polygon loses its angulations to become a curve
> - *Line chart/graph:* Is a frequency polygon presenting variations by line; shows the trend of an event over a period of time
> - *Cumulative frequency diagram (Ogiv(e):* Is graph of cumulative relative frequency distribution
> - *Scatter/Dot diagram (Correlation diagram):* Is used to depict 'correlation (relationship) between 2 quantitative variables'
> - *Bar diagram:* Is for visual comparison of magnitude of different frequencies in discrete data
> - *Pie/Sector diagram:* Is for 'presentation of discrete data of qualitative characteristics'; all pie categories are mutually exclusive, with a total of 100% (360°)
> - *Pictogram/Picture diagram:* Is a method to impress the frequency of occurrence of events to common man
> - *Map diagram/Spot map:* Is prepared to show geographical distribution of frequencies of characteristic; Each spot (dot) marks one frequency.

7. **Ans. (c) Gender** [Ref. Simple Biostatistics by Indrayan & Indrayan, 1/e p53]

- Variable: Is a characteristic or attribute that vary from person to person, from time to time and from person to person

Quantitative variable	Qualitative variable
Is a variable that can be measured directly	Is a variable that cannot be measured directly
Measured on ordinal/metric scale	Measured on a nominal scale
Examples:	Examples:
Weight	ABO blood group
Height	Gender
Mid-arm circumference	Sites of lymphadenopathy
Blood sugar level	Presence of Diabetes
ºC/ºF temperature scale	Weather
Body mass index (BMI)	Obesity
Hemoglobin level	Type of anemia
Serum cholesterol level	

> **ALSO REMEMBER**
- *BP is a continuous variable:* Sphygmanometer can only measure with a minimum count of 2 mm Hg; but it has several in-between values.
- *Pulse rate (PR) is a continuous variable:* Human mind can only process 72 or 73 beats per minute (and not 72.3 beats per minute); but if PR is counted as 216 in 3 minutes then PR will be 72.3 beats per minute.

8. **Ans. (c) Bar chart** [Ref. Simple Biostatistics by Indrayan & Indrayan, 1/e p101–02 and Methods in Biostatistics by Mahajan, 9/e p36; Park 27/e p972]

- Bar diagram/chart:
  - Is for visual comparison of magnitude of different frequencies in discrete data
  - Is a diagram appropriate for disjoint categories (nominal or ordinal) to show the no. of subjects or mean or rates by bars of corresponding height
  - Is 'the most versatile of all statistical diagrams'
  - *Bar diagram is of 3 types:*
    1. Simple bar diagram
    2. Multiple bar diagram
    3. Proportional bar diagram

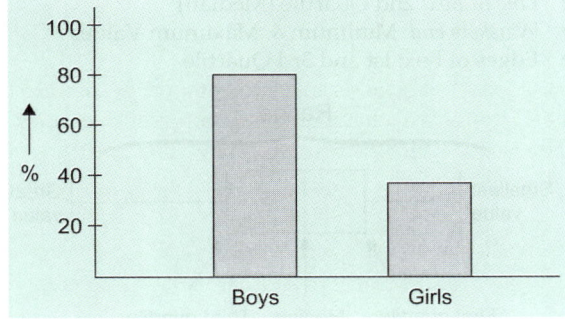

Bar diagram

9. **Ans. (d) Ordinal** [Ref. Simple Biostatistics by Indrayan & Indrayan, 1/e p51–52]

In the given question, a physician, after examining a group of patients of a certain disease, classifies the condition of each one as 'Normal', 'Mild', 'Moderate' or 'Severe'. 'Normal-mild-moderate-severe' is a continuum of outcome for a variable, thus is measured on a ordinal scale.

> **ALSO REMEMBER**
- *Likert Scale:*
  - Is also known as 'Summative scale'
  - Is a 'type of Ordinal scale'
  - Is generally used to quantify attitudes and behaviour
  - 'Responses are graded on a continuum' (For example: Strongly agree – Agree – Neutral – Disagree – Strongly disagree)
  - No. of responses are usually 3, 5 or 7
  - Likert scale is 'usually a bipolar scaling' method: It measures positive or negative response to a statement
  - *Likert response can be:*
    1. Collated into bar charts
    2. Central tendency summarized as median or mode (NOT mean)
    3. Dispersion summarized by range (NOT standard deviation)
    4. Analyzed by non-parametric tests.

10. **Ans. (c) Categorical data** [Ref. Simple Biostatistics by Indrayan & Indrayan, 1/e p51–52]

11. **Ans. (a) Nominal** [Ref. Simple Biostatistics by Indrayan & Indrayan, 1/e p51]

In the given question, an investigator into the life expectancy of IV drug abusers divides a sample of patients into HIV- positive and HIV- negative groups; Since there is no order of characteristic and it cannot be measured directly, it can't be an ordinal data or metric data respectively.

Thus it is nominal data (based only on names, i.e. HIV-positive and HIV- negative groups).

12. **Ans. (d) Relationship between two given variables** [Ref. Park 27/e p974]

Scatter Diagram
- Also known as 'Correlation diagram' or 'Dot diagram'
- Is used to depict 'correlation (relationship) between 2 quantitative variables'
- Vertical axis in scatter diagram: should be the dependent or the outcome variable
- In a scatter diagram, 2 imaginary lines are drawn along the distribution of dots/scatter

- *Types of correlation:*

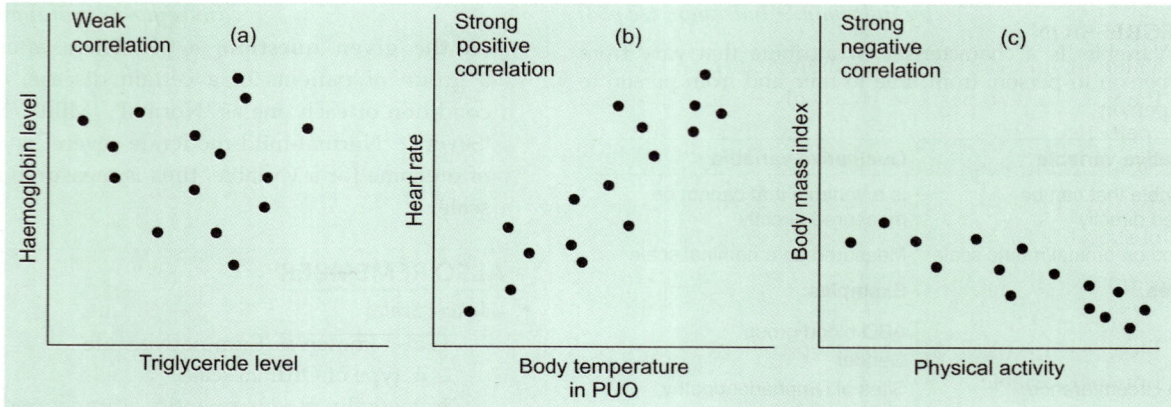

Scatter Diagrams in the cases in weak, strong positive and strong negative correlation

Types of correlation	Scatter diagram	Correlation coefficient	Interpretation
Perfectly positive correlation	Both lines have a positive slope (at 45° each); superimposed	$r = +1$	Rise in one variable leads to proportionate rise in other
Perfectly negative correlation	Both lines have a negative slope (at 45° each); superimposed	$r = -1$	Rise in one variable leads to proportionate fall in other
Moderately positive correlation	Both lines have a positive slope	$0 < r < +1$	Rise in one variable leads to rise in other
Moderately negative correlation	Both lines have a negative slope	$-1 < r < 0$	Rise in one variable leads to fall in other
No (absent) correlation	Both lines are perpendicular	$r = 0$	Rise/fall in one variable leads to no change in other
Spurious (false) correlation	No particular pattern observed	–	No particular pattern observed

13. **Ans. (b) Ordinal**   *[Ref. A Dictionary of Public Health by J Kishore, p475–76]*
14. **Ans. (c) Body weight**   *[Ref. Simple Biostatistics by Indrayan & Indrayan, 1/e p51–52]*
15. **Ans. (b) Line chart**   *[Ref. Park 27/e p974]*
16. **Ans. (a) Line diagram**   *[Ref. Park 27/e p974]*
17. **Ans. (b) Scatter diagram**   *[Ref. Park 27/e p974]*
18. **Ans. (d) Tree diagram**
    - A tree diagram is simply a way of representing a sequence of events along with their probabilities
    - Tree diagrams are particularly useful in probability since they record all possible outcomes in a clear and uncomplicated manner

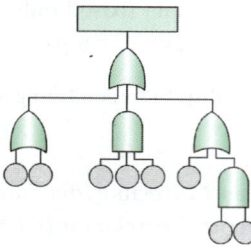

    - **In the given question,** Branches can indicate different joints involvement in the case of Diabetes; Further branches can indicate if test conducted was positive or not
    - It can further help in Decision making for treatment joint wise and overall

19. **Ans. (c) Stem and Leaf plot**   *[Ref. Basic Statistics by Hatcher, 1/e p187]*
    STEM AND LEAF PLOT
    - *Description*: A special table where each data value is split into a "stem" (the first digit or digits) and a "leaf" (usually the last digit)
      - *Stem*: Vertical column of numbers listed downwards
      - *Leaves*: Each horizontal row of numbers
    - *Utility*: Detailed quantitative data presentation, a method for showing the frequency with which certain classes of values occur

20. **Ans. (d) Box and Whisker plot**   *[Ref. Business Statistics by Black, 7/e p85]*
    Box and whisker plot
    - *Description*: A convenient way of graphically depicting groups of numerical data through their quartiles
    - *Line in Box*: 2nd Quartile (Median)
    - *Whiskers end*: Minimum & Maximum Values
    - *Edges of box*: Ist and 3rd Quartile

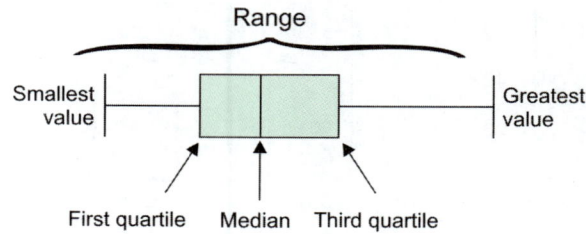

21. **Ans. (d) Regression** [Ref. Park 27/e p981]

    REGRESSION
    - Value of one variable in an individual case knowing the value of another, can be calculated by Regression-coefficient of one measurement to another
    - Simple regression equation y = a + bx

    where, y is Dependent variable, x is Independent variable c is Constant b is Regression coefficient of y upon x

22. **Ans. (b) Blood group (A, B, AB, O)**
    [Ref. Statistics by Healey 1/e p9]
    - Blood groups (A, B, AB, O) is a type of Discrete (Discontinuous) variable
    - There are few fixed possible values with no in-between values

23. **Ans. (d) Line diagram** [Ref. Park 27/e p974]
    - Correlation: Relationship between two quantitative variables
      – Correlation coefficient (r): Indicates the strength and direction of a linear relationship between two random variables
      – Scatter diagram: Is a statistical diagram used to depict correlation between two quantitative variables
    - Regression: Is change in measurements of a variable, provides structure of relationship between 2 quantitative variables
      – Regression coefficient: Measure of change of one dependent variable with change in independent variable or variables.

24. **Ans. (d) Rectangular bars are used to represent data**
    [Ref. Park 27/e p972–973]

    Bar chart
    - Is used for qualitative data representation
    - A visual tool that uses bars to compare data among categories
    - Bar graph may run horizontally or vertically
    - Length of each bar is proportional to the magnitude to be represented

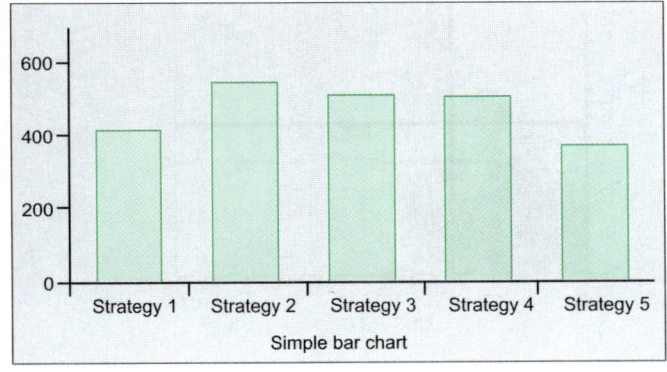

Simple bar chart

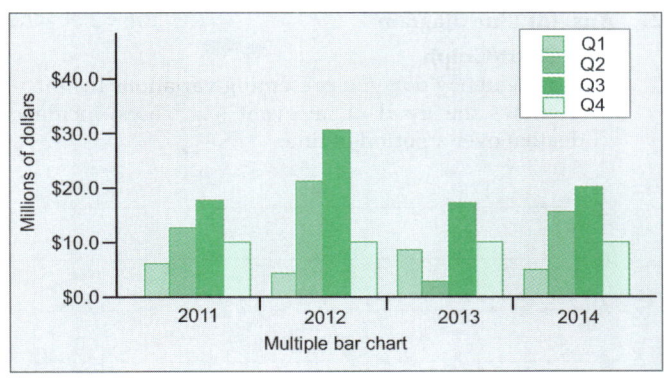

Multiple bar chart

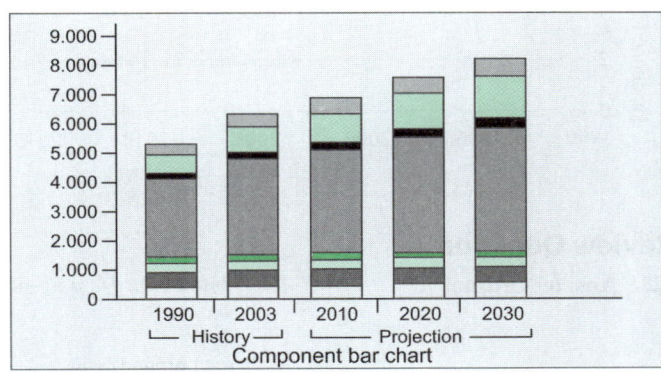

Component bar chart

25. **Ans. (b) Ordinal** [Ref. Biostatistics by Norman 3/e p5]
    - Ordinal data is a categorical, statistical data type where the variables have ordered categories (like Categories A, B, C in the given question)
    - If CP Score is expressed individually as number, then it'd become Metric quantitative data.

26. **Ans. (a) Histogram** [Ref. Park 27/e p973]
    - Histogram is pictorial diagram of Frequency distribution
    - Depicts continuous quantitative data (Continuous data takes the form of class intervals)
    - Class intervals or attributes as the base (x-axis) and frequency as the height (y-axis)

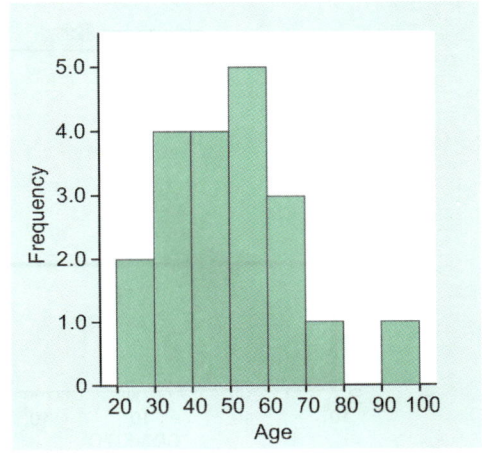

Histogram

27. Ans. (d) Line diagram [Ref. Park 27/e p972]

Line Chart/Graph
- Is a frequency polygon presenting variations by line
- It shows the trend of an event (e.g. cases, incidence, deaths) over a period of time

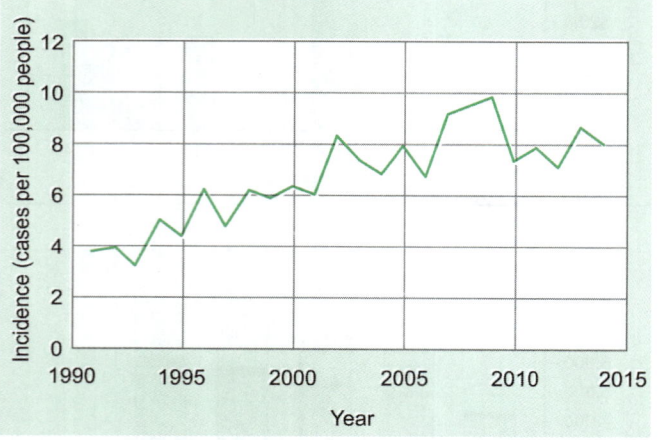

Review Question

28. Ans. (c) Ordinal [Ref. Indrayan, 1/e p 51–52]

STATISTICAL DATA GRAPHS

29. Ans. (d) Histogram and Dot plot
[Ref. Practical Flow Cytometry by Shapiro 4/e p32]

- Flow cytometry is a popular analytical cell-biology technique that utilizes light to count and profile cells in a heterogenous fluid mixture
- Flow cytometry data is typically represented in one of two ways
  - *Histograms:* Measure or compare only a single parameter (A histogram typically plots the intensity detected in a single channel along one axis and the number of events detected at that intensity is in a separate axis. A large number of events detected at one particular intensity will be displayed as a spike on the histogram)
  - *Dot-plots:* Compare 2 or 3 parameters simultaneously on a two- or three-dimensional scatter-plot (each event is represented as a single point on a scatter-plot. Intensity of 2 or 3 different channels are represented along the various axes. Events with similar intensities will cluster together in the same region on the scatter-plot.)

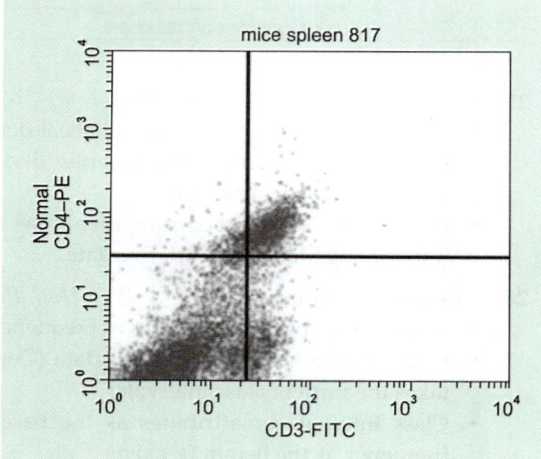
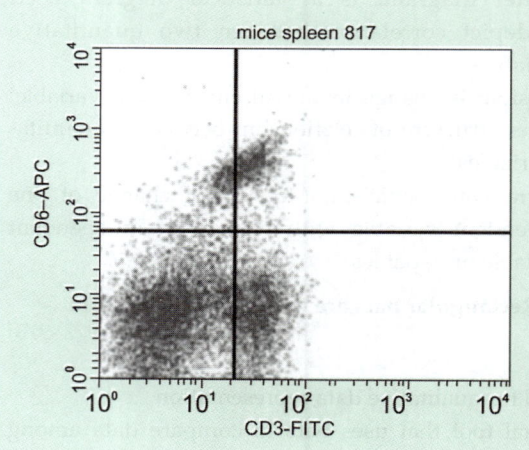
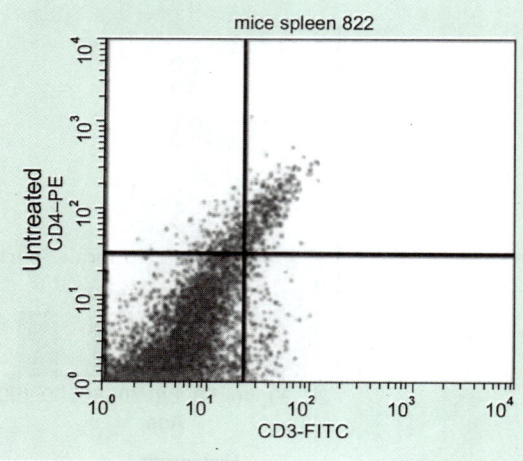
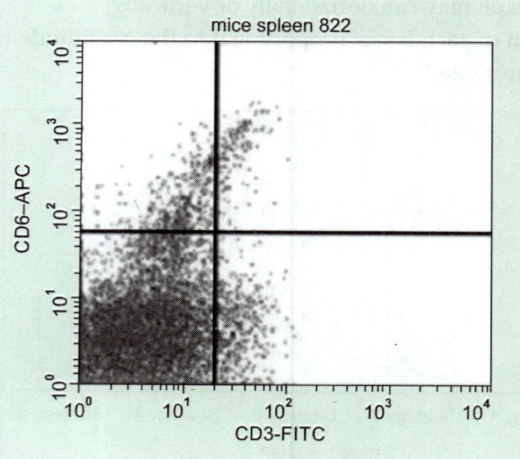

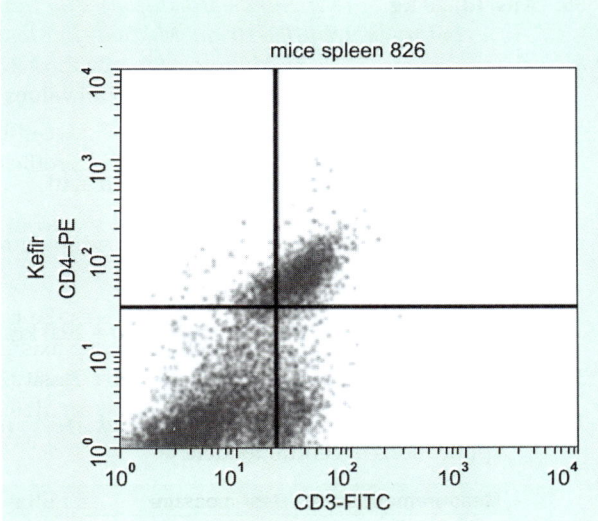
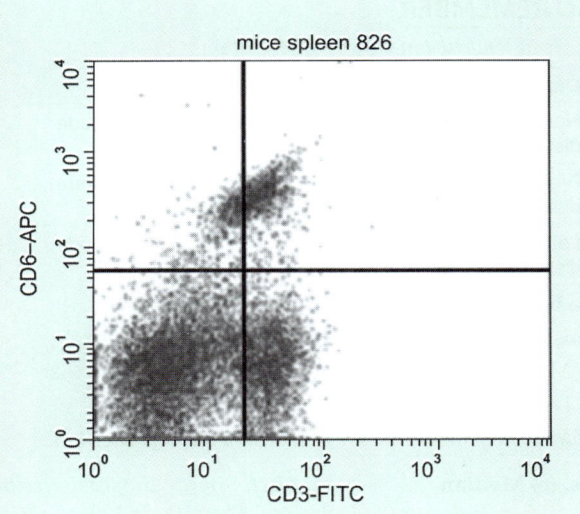
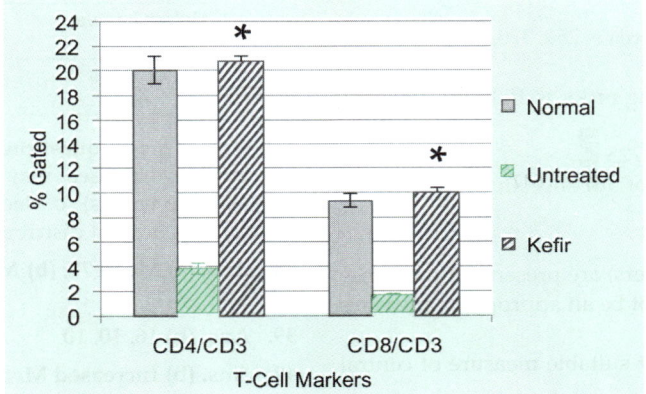

MEASURES OF CENTRAL TENDENCY

30. Ans. (c) Mode is qualitative   *[Ref. Park 27/e p975]*
- Mean and Median are determined only for quantitative data
- Mode can be determined for both quantitative as well as qualitative data
- Mean is affected by outliers (extreme values)
- Median and mode are generally not affected by outliers

31. Ans. (c) Median   *[Ref. Simple Biostatistics by Indrayan & Indrayan, 1/e p108–11 and Methods in Biostatistics by Mahajan, 9/e p42–44; Park 27/e p975]*

Measures of central tendency
- Mean (Average): Is obtained as sum of all values divided by the no. of values.
- Mean = $\Sigma x/n$
- *Median*: Middlemost value in a distribution arranged in an ascending or descending order of values
  - *In a distribution with odd no. of total values:* Middlemost value in a distribution arranged in an ascending or descending order of values

$$\text{Median} = (n+1)/2\text{th value}$$

  - *In a distribution with even no. of total values:* Such a distribution has 2 middlemost values; median is the average of two middlemost values when arranged in an ascending or descending order of values

Median = Mean (average) of $(n/2)$th and $(n/2 + 1)$th value

- *Mode:* Most frequent or most commonly occurring value in a distribution
  - *In a distribution with one most frequent value:* Mode is the most frequent or most commonly occurring value in the distribution
  - *In a distribution with two most frequent values:*
    1. There will be 2 Modes (2 most frequent values in the distribution): Bimodal distribution
    2. Mode = Average of 2 modes

In the given question, out of 11 births in a hospital, 5 babies weighed over 2.5 kg and 5 weighed less than 2.5 kg, Thus, when arranged in ascending or descending order, 2.5 kg will be the central value,
So, value do 2.5 represent Median.

> **ALSO REMEMBER**
> - *Central tendency in various distributions:*
>
> | Distribution | Central tendency |
> |---|---|
> | Normal (Gaussian) distribution | Mean = Median = Mode (coincide) |
> | Right (Positive) skew distribution | Mean > Median > Mode |
> | Left (Negative) skew distribution | Mean < Median < Mode |
>
> - In a bimodal series, Mode = 3 Median – 2 mean
> - *In distribution with extreme values (Outliers):*
>   - *Most affected measure of central tendency:* Mean
>   - *Least affected measure of central tendency:* Mode
>   - *Most preferable measure of central tendency:* Median.

32. **Ans. (c) Median** *[Ref. Simple Biostatistics by Indrayan & Indrayan, 1/e p111 and Methods in Biostatistics by Mahajan, 9/e p42–44; Park 27/e p975]*

    In the given question,
    - Incidence of malaria in an area is 250, 320, 190, 300, 5000, 100, 260, 350, 320, and 160
    - And, incidence in ascending order is 100, 160, 190, 250, 260, 300, 320, 320, 350, 5000
    - Mean = $\Sigma x/n$ = 7250/10 = 725
    - Median = Mean (average) of 5th and 6th value = (260 + 300)/2 = 280
    - Mode = 320
    - Since extreme values (outliers) are present for incidence (20 and 5000), mean will not be an appropriate measure of central tendency,

    Thus median will be the most suitable measure of central tendency.

33. **Ans. (c) Median** *[Ref. Simple Biostatistics by Indrayan & Indrayan, 1/e p111 and Methods in Biostatistics by Mahajan, 9/e p43; Park 27/e p975]*

    In the given question
    - Incidence of malaria in an area is 20, 20, 50, 56, 60, 5000, 678, 898, 345, 456
    - And, incidence in ascending order is 20, 20, 50, 56, 60, 345, 456, 678, 898, 5000
    - Mean = $\Sigma x/n$ = 7583/10 = 758.3
    - Median = Mean (average) of 5th and 6th value = (60 + 345)/2 = 202.5
    - Mode = 20
    - Since extreme values (outliers) are present for incidence (20 and 5000), mean will not be an appropriate measure of central tendency,

    Thus median will be the most suitable measure of central tendency.

34. **Ans. (a) 5** *[Ref. Elementary statistical methods by Gupta, 1/e p191; Park 27/e p975]*
    - In a bimodal series Mode = 3 Median – 2 mean
      In the given question, mean is 2 and median is 3 in a bimodal series
      Thus Mode = 3(3) – 2(2) = 9 – 4 = 5

35. **Ans. (d) 20 kg** *[Ref. Simple Biostatistics by Indrayan & Indrayan, 1/e p109–10 and Methods in Biostatistics by Mahajan, 9/e p42; Park 27/e p975]*
    - *Mean (Average):* Is obtained as sum of all values divided by the no. of values
      Mean = $\Sigma x/n$
      In the given question, = 18.2 kg and n = 10
      Thus Σx = 182
      Also, weight of one of the boys was wrongly recorded as 2.0 kg that should have been 20 kg
      True Σx = 182 + (20 – 2.0) = 200
      So true Mean = Σx (true)/n = 200/10 = 20.0 kg.

36. **Ans. (a) Mean; (b) Median; (c) Mode** *[Ref. Park 27/e p975]*

37. **Ans. (a) Blood pressure** *[Ref. Quick MBA statistics]*
    - Applications of central tendency

Measurement scale	Best measure
Nominal	Mode
Ordinal	Median
Metric: Interval	*Symmetrical data:* Mean *Skewed data:* Median
Metric: Ratio	*Symmetrical data:* Mean *Skewed data:* Median

    In the given question, Survival time, Incubation period, Health expenses may present with skewed data (few extreme values) so Median is suitable; BUT Blood pressure follows normal distribution so Mean is more suitable.

38. **Ans. (a) Mean 77; (b) Median 77; (c) Mode 70** *[Ref. Park 27/e p975]*

39. **Ans. (b) 16, 10, 10** *[Ref. Park 27/e p975]*

40. **Ans. (b) Increased Mean, No change in median** *[Ref. Park 27/e p975]*

    In the given question, Sleep apnea scores of 10 students is recorded. If the highest value (obtained 58) is wrongly recorded as 85 then,
    - *Mean will Increase:* As total sum in numerator will increase while denominator (number of persons 10) remain same
    - *Median will not change:* As only the highest value changes, Middle value in the distribution (Ascending order) remains same
    - *Mode:* Is unlikely to change (unless 58 was the mode, the it may change)

41. **Ans. (c) Mode** *[Ref. Park 27/e p975]*

    Mode
    - Most frequently occurring value in a data distribution
    - May be multiple (Bimodal, trimodal, etc.)
    - *Advantages:* Easy to understand, Unaffected by extreme values
    - *Disadvantages:* Exact location is uncertain, often not clearly defined
    - Not used in biological or medical studies

42. **Ans. (b) Median** *[Ref. Park 27/e p975]*
    - Best measure of Central tendency in a distribution: Mean

- In statistics, an outlier is an observation point that is distant from other observations (i.e. abnormally/ excessively low or high value)
- When a distribution includes Outliers, the Median is often used as a better measure of central tendency.

43. Ans. (a) Mode = 3 median – 2 mean
    [Ref. Statistics by RSN Pillai, 7/e p172]
44. Ans. (a) Mean   [Ref. Park 27/e p975]
    - Given data is Metric (and Non-skewed), so best measure of Central tendency is Mean

Review Questions

45. Ans. (b) Range is 20–38   [Ref. Park 27/e p976]
46. Ans. (d) Chi-square test   [Ref. Park 27/e p975]

OTHER MEASURES OF LOCATION

47. Ans. (a) 100 equal parts   [Ref. Simple Biostatistics by Indrayan & Indrayan, 1/e p111–12 and Methods in Biostatistics by Mahajan, 9/e p56–57; Park 21/e p785–86, Park 22/e p789–90]

    CENTILE (PERCENTILE):
    - Divides a distribution into 100 equal parts, AFTER arranging in an ascending order, SUCH THAT each part/segment has equal number (n/100) of subjects
    - Requires 99 intercepts (cut-off points) for division into 100 parts
    - Total percentiles: 99
    - The nth percentile implies: When all values are arranged in ascending order, n% are below this value
    - Methods for location of percentiles:
      - Graphical method: Cumulative frequency diagram (Ogive)
      - Arithmetic method: Cumulative frequency table
    - Applications and uses of percentiles:
      - Location of a percentile
      - Preparation of a standard percentile (Q2, Median) for particular age, sex, etc.
      - Comparison of a percentile value of a variable (between samples or populations)
      - To study growth in children (using growth charts)
      - As a measure of dispersion (interquartile/semi-interquartile range).

ALSO REMEMBER
- Division of distributions:

	Divides distribution into	No. of intercepts
Tertile	3 equal parts	2
Quartile	4 equal parts	3
Pentile (Quintile)	5 equal parts	4
Hextile	6 equal parts	5
Heptile	7 equal parts	6
Octile	8 equal parts	7
Decile	10 equal parts	9
Centile (Percentile)	100 equal parts	99

Contd...

Contd...
- *Quartile:* Divides a distribution into 4 equal parts, so the number of intercepts required will be 3, i.e. Q_1, Q_2, Q_3.
  - Q_1 (1st Quartile) divides a distribution in a ratio of 1 : 3
  - Q_2 (2nd Quartile) divides a distribution in a ratio of 1 : 1
  - Q_3 (3rd Quartile) divides a distribution in a ratio of 3 : 1

ALSO REMEMBER
- Median (middlemost point in an ascending/descending distribution) divides a distribution in the ratio of 1 : 1
  - Is equivalent to second quartile (Q_2)
  - Is equivalent to 50th percentile (P50)
  - Each segment has n/2 subjects.

48. Ans. (b) Median   [Ref. Simple Biostatistics by Indrayan & Indrayan, 1/e p112 and Methods in Biostatistics by Mahajan, 9/e p56; Park 27/e p975]

49. Ans. (c) 512   [Ref. Mathematics, Class X]
    $P = C (1 + r)^n$
    where, P = Final value
    C = Initial value
    r = fraction increase
    n = no. of times increase
    In the given question, A bacterium can divide every 20 minutes and exponential growth is for 3 hours,
    Thus, C = 1
    And r = 1 (it doubles every time)
    n = 3 hours/20 minutes = 9 times
    Thus $P = C (1 + r)^n = 1 (1 + 1)^9 = 2^9 = 512$

    One Other Simple Way of Doing IT
    - Given information: A bacterium can divide every 20 minutes (3/hour)
    - Thus in 3 hours, it will total divide 3/hour × 3 hours = 9 times
    - Thus 9 times multiplication will successively yield 2, 4, 8, 16, 32, 64, 128, 256, 512 bacteria.
    - So at end of 9 hours, there will be 512 bacteria.

50. Ans. (c) 100th   [Ref. Mahajan 9/e p56]
    Percentiles (Centiles):
    - Are values in a series of observations arranged in an ascending order of magnitude 'which divides a distribution into 100 equal parts'
    - In all there are a 'total of 99 percentiles'
    - Median is 50th centile (50th percentile has 50% observations on either side)
    - Percentile and Percentage:
      - 'x' percentile implies: x% values are below this value
      - For example, 40th percentile implies 40% values are below it
    - In general:
      - kth percentile = (k × n/100)th value
      - In the given question, n = 250 subjects, thus 40th percentile would be,
      - 40th percentile = (40 × 250/100) th value = 100th value

51. **Ans. (d) 2nd quartile** [Ref. Simple Biostatistics by Indrayan & Indrayan, 1/e p112–13 and Methods in Biostatistics by Mahajan, 9/e p56]

- *Quartile:* Divides a distribution into 4 equal parts, so the number of intercepts required will be 3, i.e. Q_1, Q_2, Q_3
  - So, Zero – Q_1 covers 25% values
  - Similarly, $Q_2 – Q_1$, $Q_3 – Q_2$ and $100 – Q_3$ all cover 25% values each
  - Thus, Q_2 – Zero, $100 – Q_2$ and $Q_3 – Q_1$ all cover 50% values each
  - Q_1 divides a distribution in a ratio of 25 : 75 OR 1 : 3
  - Q_2 divides a distribution in a ratio of 50 : 50 OR 1 : 1, Thus second quartile is equivalent to median
  - Q_3 divides a distribution in a ratio of 75 : 25 OR 3 : 1.

In the given question, n = 180

Thus Q_2 which is equivalent to median, divides a distribution in a ratio of 50 : 50 OR 1 : 1.

52. **Ans. (b) 50** [Ref. Simple Biostatistics by Indrayan & Indrayan, 1/e p112–13; Methods in Biostatistics by Mahajan, 9/e p56]
- Among 200 persons, $Q_1, Q_2,$ and Q_3 would be located at 50th, 100th and 150th person respectively
- This would divide data of 200 persons into Four equal parts of 50 each
- Also, Q_3 (3rd Quartile) divides a distribution in a ratio of 3 : 1 i.e., 150:50
- So last quarter would include 50 persons

53. **Ans. (b) 53.6** [Ref. Research by Thomas, 6/e p136]

Percentile calculation
- Standard normal distribution is also be useful for computing percentiles:
  - *Median*: 50th percentile
  - *First quartile*: 25th percentile
  - *Third quartile*: 75th percentile
- Percentile formula,
X = μ + Zσ (where μ is Mean, σ is SD and Z is Value from Normal distribution for Desired percentile)
- Z values for commonly used percentiles:

Percentile	Z value
1st	– 2.326
2.5 th	– 1.960
5th	– 1.645
10th	– 1.282
25th	– 0.675
50th	0
75th	0.675
90th	1.282
95th	1.645
97.5th	1.960
99th	2.326

- In the given question, Mean = 70 mm Hg, SD = 10 mm Hg, Z = – 1.645 and X = 5th percentile value
- So, X_5 = 70 + (– 1.645) 10 = 53.6 mm Hg

VARIABILITY

54. **Ans. (c) Standard deviation** [Ref. Park 27/e p976]
- Standard deviation formula (SD) = $\sqrt{\sum (x_i - \bar{x})^2 / N}$
- Standard deviation formula (SD) for smaller samples (<30) = $\sqrt{\sum (x_i - \bar{x})^2 / N-1}$
- SD is a measure of how dispersed the data is in relation to the mean
- SD is Root mean square deviation

55. **Ans. (b) Range** [Ref. Park 26/e p944]
- Range of a set of data is the difference between the largest and smallest values
- Difference is the result of subtracting the sample maximum and minimum values
- Range is the *'Simplest measure of dispersion'*

56. **Ans. (c) Coefficient of variation** [Ref. Business Statistics by Sharma 2/e p157]]
- Coefficient of Variation (COV) is a measure used to compare relative variability (a unit-free measure to compare dispersion of one variable with another)
- COV is SD expressed as percentage of mean = SD/Mean × 100

57. **Ans. (a) If A, B, C are correct** [Ref. Statistics for Business and Financial Economics (Volume 1) by Lee 2/e p103]
- Coefficient of variation, COV = SD/Mean × 100

In the given question, So in Village-1, COV-1 = 2/20 × 100 = 5%
- And in Village-2, COV-2 = 1/40 × 100 = 2.5%

58. **Ans. (c) Deviation from mean value** [Ref. Simple Biostatistics by Indrayan & Indrayan, 1/e p114–15 and Methods in Biostatistics by Mahajan, 9/e p69–84; Park 27/e p976]
- *Measures of variability:*

Measures of variability	
Individual observations	**Samples**
Range	Standard error of mean
Inter-quartile range	Standard error of difference between 2 means
Mean deviation	Standard error of proportion
Standard deviation	Standard error of difference between 2 proportions
Coefficient of variation	Standard error of correlation coefficient
	Standard deviation of regression coefficient

Standard deviation (SD)
- SD is most common and generally most appropriate measure of dispersion
- SD is defined as the 'root-mean-square (RMS) deviation of the values from their mean', or as the square root of the variance
- SD calculation: = $\sqrt{(Variance)} = \sqrt{\dfrac{\sum (x - \bar{x})^2}{n}}$
- *Interpretation of SD:*
  - A large standard deviation: Data points are far from the mean
  - A small standard deviation: Data points are clustered closely around the mean

- *Uses of SD in biostatistics:*
  - Summarizes the deviation of a large distribution from mean
  - Indicates whether the variation of difference of an individual from the mean is by chance
  - Helps in finding the standard error
  - Helps in finding the suitable size of sample for valid conclusions

> **ALSO REMEMBER**
- *Measures of chance:*
  - Probability
  - Odds (& Odds ratio)
  - Likelihood ratio
- *Measures of Central tendency:*
  - Mean
  - Median
  - Mode

59. Ans. (a) 25% *[Ref. Simple Biostatistics by Indrayan & Indrayan, 1/e p115 and Methods in Biostatistics by Mahajan, 9/e p82; Park 21/e p787, Park 22/e p791]*

- *Coefficient of variation:*
  - Is a measure used to compare relative variability
  - Is a unit-free measure to compare dispersion of one variable with another
  - Is SD expressed as percentage of mean

$$CV = \frac{SD}{Mean} \times 100 = \frac{\sigma}{\mu} \times 100$$

In the given question, Median weight (μ) = 12 kg, n = 100, Standard deviation (σ) = 3, Thus, coefficient of variance = $\sigma/\mu \times 100 = 3/12 \times 100 = 25\%$.

> **ALSO REMEMBER**
- *Multiple correlation coefficient:* Is used for calculation of correlation between one variable (dependent) and the combination of two or more variables (independents)
- *Coefficient of determination:*
  - Is the percentage of variation in a variable that is explained by one or more of the others
  - Is generally obtained in a regression setup
  - Coefficient of determination = (Correlation coefficient)^2 = r^2
- *Correlation coefficient (r):* Measures the degree or strength of relationship in a correlation
  - Correlation coefficient (r) lies between: –1 to + 1 (–1 < r < + 1).

60. Ans. (a) 0.4 *[Ref. Simple Biostatistics by Indrayan & Indrayan, 1/e p140 and Methods in Biostatistics by Mahajan, 9/e p189]*

STANDARD ERROR OF MEAN (SE$_{MEAN}$)
- SEmean is the measure of difference between sample and population values: Whatever be the sampling procedure or the care taken while selecting sample, the sample estimates (statistics) will differ from population values (parameters)
- SE is a 'measure of chance variation', and it does not mean an error or mistake.

$$SE_{mean} = \frac{\text{Standard deviation (SD)}}{\text{Sample size}} = \frac{\sigma}{\sqrt{n}}$$

- **In the given question,** n = 25 kids, Standard deviation (σ) = 2, Mean incubation period (μ) = 8 days,
- Thus, standard error = 0.4.
- Greater the standard deviation (σ), greater will be the standard error (SE), especially in small samples
- *SE can be minimized by reducing SD:* By taking a large sample
- *SE is a measure of variability of sample summaries:* SE$_{mean}$ is the SD of sample means
- *Uses of standard error of mean (SEmean) in large samples:*
  - To work out limits of desired confidence within which population mean would lie
  - To determine if sample is drawn from a known population or not
  - To find SE of difference between 2 means (to know if difference is real and statistically significant)
  - To calculate sample size (within desired confidence limits)
- Standard error of difference between 2 means:

$$SE_{\text{diff bet means}} = \sqrt{(\sigma_1^2/n_1 + \sigma_2^2/n_2)}$$

61. Ans. (b) Sampling errors *[Ref. Simple Biostatistics by Indrayan & Indrayan, 1/e p139–40 and Methods in Biostatistics by Mahajan, 9/e p73–74; Park 27/e p978]*

> **ALSO REMEMBER**
- Sampling errors are not errors in conventional sense
- Standard error of difference between 2 means:

$$SE_{\text{diff bet means}} = \sqrt{(\sigma_1^2/n_1 + \sigma_2^2/n_2)}$$

- Standard error of proportion: $SE_{\text{proportion}} = \sqrt{pq/n}$ where q = (1 – p)
- Standard error of difference between 2 proportions:

$$SE_{\text{diff bet proportions}} = \sqrt{(p_1 q_1/n_1) + (p_2 q_2/n_2)}$$

62. Ans. (b) 0 *[Ref. Simple Biostatistics by Indrayan & Indrayan, 1/e p114–15 and Methods in Biostatistics by Mahajan, 9/e p73–74; Park 27/e p976]*

In the given question, the birth weight of each of the 10 babies born in a hospital in a day is found to be 2.8 kg, thus, SD = ZERO

So the standard deviation of this sample will be, SD (σ) =

$$\sqrt{\text{(Variance)}} = \sqrt{\frac{\Sigma(x-\bar{x})^2}{n}} = \text{Zero}.$$

63. **Ans. (b) 0.1** *[Ref. Simple Biostatistics by Indrayan & Indrayan, 1/e p139–40 and Methods in Biostatistics by Mahajan, 9/e p167–168; Park 27/e p978]*

In the given question, n = 100 women, mean Hemoglobin (μ) = 10 gm%, standard deviation (σ) = 1,

Thus standard error (SE)

$$= \frac{SD}{\sqrt{\text{sample size}}} = \frac{\sigma}{\sqrt{n}} = \frac{1}{\sqrt{100}} = 0.1$$

64. **Ans. (d) 1.0** *[Ref. Simple Biostatistics by Indrayan &Indrayan, 1/e p115–16]*

Z Score (Standard Score):
- Is also known as 'normal deviate'
- Is difference of a value from group mean, in terms of how many times of SD (σ)

$$Z \text{ score} = \frac{\text{Individual level} - \text{Mean}}{SD} = \frac{(x-\mu)}{\sigma}$$

- The standard score indicates how many standard deviations an observation is above or below the mean
- Z scores are frequently used in assessing how far a child is in his relative growth to a standard
   - Z score = 2: Any measurement of at least 2SD away is considered too far away to be normal.

In the given question,
x = 15.0 g/dL, μ = 13.5 g/dl, σ = 1.5 g/dL
Thus, Z score = (x – μ)/σ = (15.0 – 13.5)/1.5 = 1

65. **Ans. (c) 0.1 gm%** *[Ref. Park 27/e p978]*

66. **Ans. (a) Range; (b) Mean deviation; (c) Standard deviation** *[Ref. Methods in Biostatistics by Mahajan, 9/e p65]*

67. **Ans. (c) 72–88%** *[Ref. Simple Biostatistics by Indrayan, 1/e p146]*

Confidence Intervals for Population proportions (For 95% Confidence)
CI = P ± 2 SEP = P ± 2 √pq/n
In the given question, P=0.80 (80%); p=0.80; q= 1-p = 1–0.80 = 0.20; n=100
CI = 0.80 ± 2 √0.8*0.2/100 = 0.80 ± 0.08 = 0.72, 0.88 (72%, 88%)

68. **Ans. (a) 0.34** *[Ref. Park 27/e p977]*

Normal distribution
- Shape is bilaterally symmetrical
- Mean = Median = Mode (coincide)
- 50% of all values lie above Mean (or Median or Mode)
- Mean ± 1SD cover 68% values (Mean + 1SD cover 34% values)
- Mean ± 2SD cover 95% values (Mean + 2SD cover 47.5% values)
- Mean ± 3SD cover 99% values (Mean + 3SD cover 49.5% values)

69. **Ans. (b) 0.50** *[Ref. Park 27/e p977]*
- *In a Normal distribution, 50% of values lie above Mean (or Median or Mode)*

70. **Ans. (b) Indicated distribution of variables; (c) Most common method used for dispersion; (d) Better indicator of variance than range** *[Ref. Park 27/e p976]*

71. **Ans. (d) $\sqrt{\Sigma (x-\bar{x})^2/\eta\text{-}1}$** *[Ref. Statistics Unplugged by Caldwell 3/e p45]*

Standard deviation
- Is 'Root mean square deviation', a measure of dispersion
- SD (Larger samples) = $\sqrt{\Sigma (x-\bar{x})^2/\eta}$
- SD (Smaller sample size <30) + $\sqrt{\Sigma (x-\bar{x})^2/\eta\text{-}1}$

72. **Ans. (a) Standard error of the mean** *[Ref. Park 27/e p976]*
- Standard deviation of the sample is the degree to which individuals within the sample differ from the Sample mean
- Standard error is an estimate of how far the Sample mean is likely to be from the Population mean

Review Questions

73. **Ans. (a) 210–250** *[Ref. 23/e p849]*
74. **Ans. (d) Correlation and regression** *[Ref. Park 27/e p980]*
75. **Ans. (a) Mean and standard error** *[Ref. Park 27/e p978]*
76. **Ans. (b) S = square root of V** *[Ref. An Introduction to Medical Statistics by Bland, 2/e p60]*
77. **Ans. (b) Median** *[Ref. Park 27/e p976]*

DISTRIBUTIONS – NORMAL AND SKEWED

78. **Ans. (d) 1,2,3,4** *[Ref. Encyclopedia of Research Design 2010 (Volume 1) 1/e p933]*
- Methods available to test the normality of the continuous data
   - Shapiro–Wilk test
   - Kolmogorov–Smirnov test
   - Skewness, Kurtosis
   - Histogram,
   - Box plot
   - P–P Plot, Q–Q Plot
   - Mean with SD

79. **Ans. (c) Poisson's distribution** *[Ref. Business Statistics Using Excel by Davis 1/e p155]*

POISSON DISTRIBUTION
- Is a 'discrete probability distribution' that expresses the 'probability of a number of events occurring in a fixed period of time' (if these events occur with a known average rate and independently of the time since the last event)
- It can also be used for the number of events in other specified intervals such as distance, area or volume
- Is generally used to model the number of events occurring within a given time interval
- Is a discrete distribution which takes on the values X = 0, 1, 2, 3,….

80. **Ans. (b) 180–220** *[Ref. Park 25/e p912]*
    - Mean ± 1SD covers 68% values in Normal distribution
    - So, 200 ± 1(20) = 200 ± 20 = 180 – 220 will cover 68% values in Normal distribution

81. **Ans. (d) Poisson distribution** *[Ref. Internet]*

    Poisson distribution:
    - Is a 'discrete probability distribution' that expresses the 'probability of a number of events occurring in a fixed
    - Period of time' (if these events occur with a known average rate and independently of the time since the last event)
    - It can also be used for the number of events in other specified intervals such as distance, area or volume
    - Is generally used to model the number of events occurring within a given time interval
    - Is a discrete distribution which takes on the values X = 0, 1, 2, 3,….

    In the given question, one has to study the daily admission of head injury patients in a trauma care centre,
    Since, it describes the no. of events in time (no. of head injury patients admitted per day,
    Therefore, it is a Poisson distribution.

    > **ALSO REMEMBER**
    > - *Binomial distribution:*
    >   - Is the 'discrete probability distribution' of the number of successes in a sequence of n independent yes/no experiments, each of which yields success with probability p (Success/Failure experiment)
    >   - Is also called a Bernoulli experiment or Bernoulli trial: In fact, when n = 1, the binomial distribution is a 'Bernoulli distribution'
    >   - Is the basis for the popular binomial test of statistical significance
    > - *Normal distribution:*
    >   - Is also known as 'Gaussian distribution' or 'Standard distribution'
    >   - Is the distribution of values of a quantitative variable such that they are symmetric with respect to a middle value with same mean, median and mode, and then the frequencies taper off rapidly and symmetrically on both sides – 'bell shaped distribution'
    > - *Uniform distribution:*
    >   - All values of the distribution are equally probable.
    >   - Is of 2 types: Discrete and Continuous.

82. **Ans. (d) Has variance = 1.0** *[Ref. Simple Biostatistics by Indrayan & Indrayan, 1/e p117; Park 27/e p977]*

    Normal Distribution:
    - Is also known as 'Gaussian distribution' or 'Standard distribution'
    - *Type of distribution:* Is the distribution of values of a quantitative variable such that they are symmetric with respect to a middle value with same mean, median and mode, and then the frequencies taper off rapidly and symmetrically on both sides – 'bell shaped distribution'.

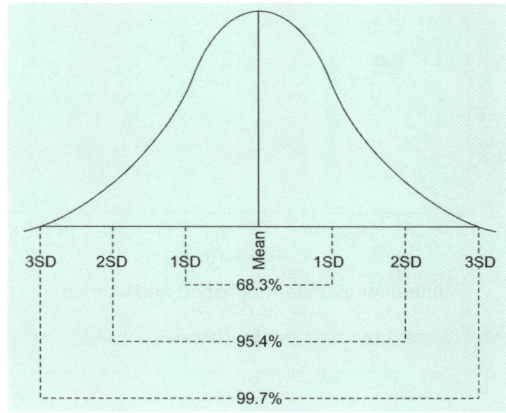

Normal curve showing distribution of values

- *Normal/Gaussian curve:*
    - Is 'bilaterally symmetrical, bell-shaped'
    - Is based on Mean & standard deviation
    - Mean, Median and Mode coincide (Mean = Median = Mode)
    - Has Mean (μ) = 0 and SD (σ) = 1
        1. Mean ± 1SD ($\mu \pm 1\sigma$) covers 68% values
        2. Mean ± 2SD ($\mu \pm 2\sigma$) covers 95% values
        3. Mean ± 3SD ($\mu \pm 3\sigma$) covers 99% values
    - In normal distribution, 50% values lie above mean & 50% below mean.

> **ALSO REMEMBER**
> - SD = i.e. σ = OR Variance = σ^2
>   - In Normal distribution, SD(σ) = 1, thus Variance = 1
> - Normal range: Is the range of Mean ± 2SD ($\mu \pm 2\sigma$)
> - Inflections in a Normal curve: Central part is convex, while at the points of inflection, the curve changes from convexity to concavity
>   - Perpendicular from point of inflection will cut he base at distance of 1SD (1σ) from mean (μ) on either side
> - Asymmetrical distributions:
>   - *Right (positive) skew:* Mean > Median > Mode
>
>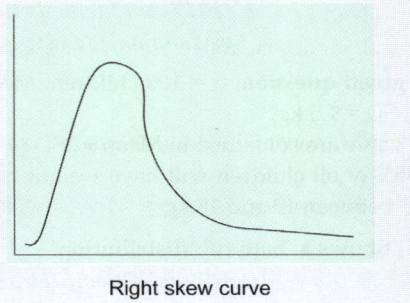
>
> Right skew curve

Contd…

Contd...

- *Left (negative) skew:* Mean < Median < Mode

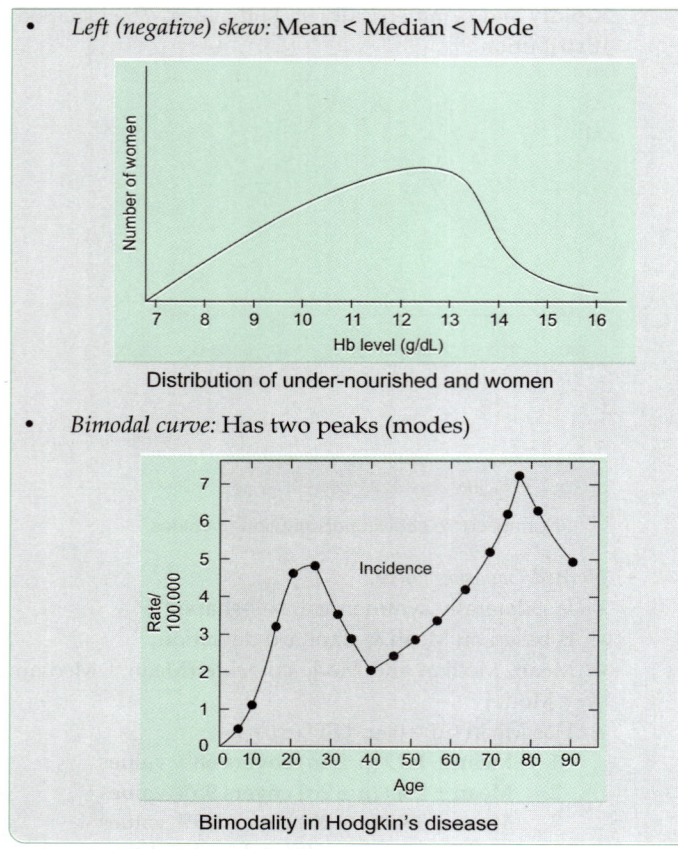

Distribution of under-nourished and women

- *Bimodal curve:* Has two peaks (modes)

Bimodality in Hodgkin's disease

ALSO REMEMBER
- *Bath tub distribution:*
  - Is a distribution where the curve shows trough (depression) in the middle instead of peak.
  - Example: No. of deaths in various age groups in India (Deaths in India are high in infancy and above the age of >50 years).

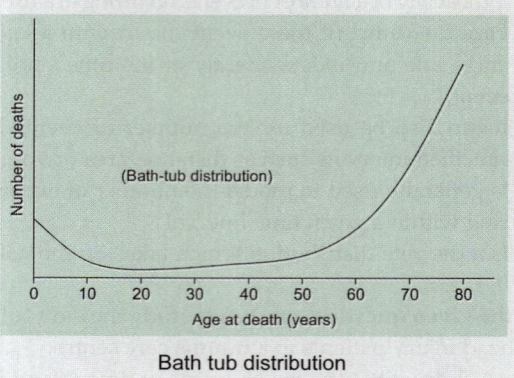

Bath tub distribution

---

83. Ans. (b) 85 and 125 mg [Ref. Simple Biostatistics by Indrayan & Indrayan, 1/e p117 and Methods in Biostatistics by Mahajan, 9/e p99; Park 27/e p976]

In the given question, the fasting blood levels of glucose for a group of diabetics is found to be normally distributed with a mean of 105 mg per 100 mL of blood and a standard deviation of 10 mg per 100 mL of blood,
Thus, Mean (μ) = 105 mg/dl and SD (σ) = 10 mg/dl
95% of diabetics will have their fasting blood glucose levels within the limits of Mean ± 2SD ($\mu \pm 2\sigma$)
i.e. within 105 ± 2(10) or between 85–125 mg per 100 mL.

84. Ans. (a) 95% of all children weight between 12 and 18 kg
[Ref. Simple Biostatistics by Indrayan & Indrayan, 1/e p117 and Methods in Biostatistics by Mahajan, 9/e p99; Park 27/e p976]

In the given question, n = 100 children, Mean weight (μ) =15 kg, SD = 1.5 kg,
95% of value are contained in Mean ± 2SD ($\mu \pm 2\sigma$),
Thus 95% of all children will have weight between 15 ± 2 (1.5) i.e. between 12 and 18 kg.

85. Ans. (a) Shows a 'bath tub distribution'
[Ref. Simple Biostatistics by Indrayan & Indrayan, 1/e p104–05 and Methods in Biostatistics by Mahajan, 7/e p72–79; Park 27/e p976]

86. Ans. (a) Less than median [Ref. Simple Biostatistics by Indrayan & Indrayan, 1/e p111]

- *Central tendency in various distributions:*

Distribution	Central tendency
Normal (Gaussian) distribution	Mean = Median = Mode (coincide)
Right (Positive) skew distribution	Mean > Median > Mode
Left (Negative) skew distribution	Mean < Median < Mode

- *In distribution with extreme values (Outliers):*
  - *Most affected measure of central tendency:* Mean
  - *Least affected measure of central tendency:* Mode
  - *Most preferable measure of central tendency:* Median

87. Ans. (d) Nothing can be said conclusively
[Ref. Simple Biostatistics by Indrayan & Indrayan, 1/e p35–36 and Methods in Biostatistics by Mahajan, 9/e p109; Park 27/e p977]

- In a normal distribution, Mean (μ) = 0 and SD (σ) = 1
- In a right (positive) skew, Mean > Median > Mode
- In a left (negative) skew, Mean < Median < Mode

In the given question, Mean = 3.0 mmol/litre and Standard deviation = 3.0 mmol/litre,
Thus nothing can be said conclusively.

88. Ans. (b) 150 [Ref. Simple Biostatistics by Indrayan & Indrayan, 1/e p112–13 and Methods in Biostatistics by Mahajan, 9/e p56; Park 21/e p787–88, Park 22/e p791–92]

- *Quartile:* Divides a distribution into 4 equal parts, so the number of intercepts required will be 3, i.e. Q_1, Q_2, Q_3
  - So, Zero – Q_1 covers 25% values
  - Similarly, $Q_2 – Q_1$, $Q_3 – Q_2$ and $100 – Q_3$ all cover 25% values each
  - Thus, Q_2 – Zero, $100 – Q_2$ and $Q_3 – Q_1$ all cover 50% values each
  - Q_1 divides a distribution in a ratio of 25 : 75 OR 1 : 3

- Q_2 divides a distribution in a ratio of 50 : 50 OR 1 : 1, Thus second quartile is equivalent to median
- Q_3 divides a distribution in a ratio of 75 : 25 OR 3 : 1

In the given question, n = 300, Q_3 = 4.5 litres and Q_1 = 1.5 litres

Thus $Q_3 - Q_1$ will cover 50% values, i.e. 50% of 300 = 150 values.

89. **Ans. (a) 28** *[Ref. Simple Biostatistics by Indrayan & Indrayan, 1/e p117 and Methods in Biostatistics by Mahajan, 9/e p101; Park 27/e p976]*

In the given question, Mean (μ) = 30 mm and SD (σ) = 1.0 mm

Thus, 95% values are contained in the range of Mean ± 2 SD (μ ± 2σ) or 30 ± 2 (1)

So, 95% values are contained in the range 30 – 2 mm and 30 + 2 mm OR between 28 and 30 mm.

90. **Ans. (b) 95%** *[Ref. Simple Biostatistics by Indrayan & Indrayan, 1/e p117–19 and Methods in Biostatistics by Mahajan, 9/e p101; Park 27/e p976]*

- *In a Normal (Gaussian) distribution:*
  - Mean ± 1SD (μ ± 1σ) limits include 68.27% values
  - Mean ± 2SD (μ ± 2σ) limits include 95.45% values
  - Mean ± 1.96SD (μ ± 1.96σ) limits include 95% values
  - Mean ± 3SD (μ ± 3σ) limits include 99.73% values
  - Mean ± 2.58SD (μ ± 2.58σ) limits include 99% values
- Values that differ from the mean by more than 2SD are rare, being only 4.55%
- Values higher or lower than the Mean ± 3SD (μ ± 3σ) are very rare, being only 0.27%
- 6 SD (3 on either side of mean) cover almost the entire range of a variable character
  - SD divides the range into 6 equal sub-ranges
- Minimum sample size required for establishment of normal range for any health parameter: 300 healthy subjects.

91. **Ans. (c) Left-skewed** *[Ref. Simple Biostatistics by Indrayan & Indrayan, 1/e p111]*

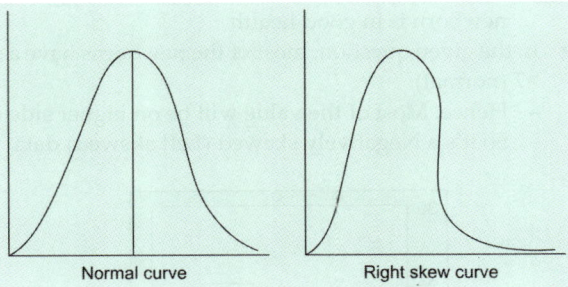

Normal curve   Right skew curve

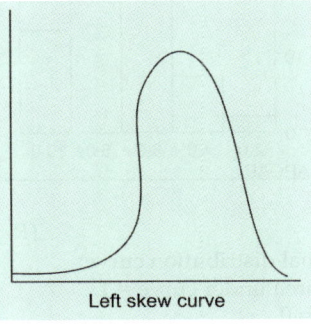

Left skew curve

Central tendency

In the given question, Mean = 20, Median = 24 & Mode = 26

Thus Mean < Median < Mode, making it a Left (Negative) skew distribution.

92. **Ans. (b) 50** *[Ref. Simple Biostatistics by Indrayan and Indrayan, 1/e p105 and Methods in Biostatistics by Mahajan, 9/e p101; Park 27/e p976]*

In the given question
- Mean glucose (μ) = 86 mg/dL,
- Thus, 50% of people will have glucose above 86 mg/dL and 50% of people will have glucose below 86 mg/dL.

> **ALSO REMEMBER**
> - Statistical tests based on Gaussian distribution are known as 'Parametric tests'
>   - Student's t - test
>   - ANOVA - F test

93. **Ans. (b) 50** *[Ref. Simple Biostatistics by Indrayan and Indrayan, 1/e p117 and Methods in Biostatistics by Mahajan 9/e 9101; Park 27/e p976]*

In the given question, Mean Systolic blood pressure (SBP) = 120 mm Hg,

So 50% of values (50% of n) i.e. 50 individuals will have their SBP below 120 mm Hg, and a similar no. will have value of SBP above 120 mm Hg.

94. **Ans. (a) About 95% of the girls have PEFR between 260 and 340 l/min** *[Ref. Simple Biostatistics by Indrayan & Indrayan, 1/e p117; Park 27/e p976]*

- *In Normal distribution,*
  - Mean ± 1SD (μ ± 1σ) covers 68% values
  - Mean ± 2SD (μ ± 2σ) covers 95% values
  - Mean ± 3SD (μ ± 3σ) covers 99% values

In the given question,
- Mean of PEFR (μ) = 300 l/min
- Standard deviation of PEFR (σ) = 20 l/min

Thus,
- 68% of girls will have PEFR in the range Mean ± 1SD (μ ± 1σ) = 300 ± 20 l/min, i.e. between (300 – 20) and (300 + 20) l/min
  - 280 – 320 l/min range covers 68% of girls
- 95% of girls will have PEFR in range Mean ± 2SD (μ ± 2σ) = 300 ± 2(20) l/min, i.e. between (300 – 40) and (300 + 40) l/min
  - 260 – 340 l/min range covers 95% of girls
- 99% of girls will have PEFR in range Mean ± 3SD (μ ± 3σ) = 300 ± 3(20) l/min, i.e. between (300 – 60) and (300 + 60) l/min
  - 240 – 360 l/min range covers 99% of girls
- Now, 260 – 340 l/min range covers 95% of girls, thus rest 5% of girls are outside this range, i.e. they have PEFR either <260 l/min or >340 l/min
  - Even this will be symmetrically distributed (Normal curve is bilaterally symmetrical), thus
    1. 2.5% girls will have PEFR <260 l/min
    2. 2.5% girls will have PEFR >340 l/min
  - Girls having PEFR less than 340 l/min: 97.5%
- Since the normal range of PEFR for girls is not given in the question, it cannot be concluded that all girls have healthy lungs.

> **ALSO REMEMBER**
> - In a Normal distribution, 50% of values lie above the mean and 50% lie below the mean
>   - In the given question,
>   1. 50% of girls will have PEFR >300 l/min
>   2. 50% of girls will have PEFR <300 l/min
> - In a Normal distribution, Mean ± 1SD ($\mu \pm 1\sigma$) covers 68% values, so 32% of girls are outside this range
>   - Even this will be symmetrically distributed (Normal curve is bilaterally symmetrical), thus in the given question,
>   1. 16% girls will have PEFR <280 l/min
>   2. 16% girls will have PEFR >320 l/min
> - In a Normal distribution, Mean ± 3SD ($\mu \pm 3s$) covers 99% values, so 1% of girls are outside this range
>   - Even this will be symmetrically distributed (Normal curve is bilaterally symmetrical), thus in the given question
>   1. 0.5% girls will have PEFR <240 l/min
>   2. 0.5% girls will have PEFR >360 l/min

95. **Ans. (a) Mean, median and mode are same; (b) B/L symmetrical (c) Bell shape** *[Ref. Park 27/e p977]*

96. **Ans. (b) The curve is bilaterally symmetrical; (e) Mean, Median and Mode coincide** *[Ref. Park 27/e p977]*

97. **Ans. (a) Mean-Mode/SD** *[Ref. Quantitative methods by TR Jain and AS Sandhu, Latest ed., 2009–10, p3.4]*

   Skewness:
   - Is measure of asymmetry of a probability distribution of a random variable
   - Measures of skewness:
     - Pearson's mode or First Skewness coefficient = (Mean – Mode)/SD
     - Pearson's median or Second Skewness coefficient = 3(Mean – Median)/SD
     - Quartile skewness = $(Q_3 - 2Q_2 + Q_1)/Q_3 - Q_1$.

98. **Ans. (c) 95%** *[Ref. Park 27/e p976]*
   In the given question, n = 100, Mean = 105 marks, SD = 10 marks
   So, Mean ± 1SD = 105 ± 10 = 95–115 marks covers 68% students
   Mean ± 2SD = 105 ± 20 = 85–125 marks covers 95% students, and
   Mean ± 3SD = 105 ± 30 = 75–135 marks covers 99% students.

99. **Ans. (b) Mean < Mode** *[Ref. Simple Biostatistics by Indrayan & Indrayan, 1/e p111]*

100. **Ans. (b) 7.31 gm/dL** *[Ref. Park 27/e p976]*
    - Mean ± 1SD covers 68% values; So, Hb of 68% pregnant females will lie between 10.6 ± 2 gm/dL or between 8.6–12.6 g/dL
      - So, 16% will lie below 8.6 gm/dL
    - Similarly, Mean ± 2SD covers 95% values; So, Hb of 95% pregnant females will lie between 10.6 ± 2(2) gm/dL or between 6.6–14.6 gm/dL
      - So, 2.5% will lie below 6.6 gm/dL

- So 5% pregnant females will have Hb below 7.31 gm/dL (most appropriate answer)

101. **Ans. (d) Sampling distribution** *[Ref. Research Design and Methods by Bordens, 6/e p392]*
    - *Sample distribution*: A distribution resulting from the collection of actual data, after drawing a sample from the population
      - A major characteristic of a sample is that it contains a finite (countable) number of scores
    - *Population distribution*: A distribution made up of all the classes or values of variables which we would observe if we were to conduct a census of all members of the population
    - *Sampling distribution*: Sampling distribution is a distribution of a sample statistic
      - It is a model of a distribution of scores, like the population distribution, except that the scores are not raw scores, but statistics
      - If we draw a number of samples from the same population, then compute sample statistics for each, we can construct a distribution consisting of the values of the sample statistics we've computed
      - This is a kind of "second-order" distribution
      - Whereas the population distribution and the sample distribution are made up of data values, the sampling distribution is made up of values of statistics computed from a number of sample distributions

102. **Ans. (b) Data is negatively skewed** *[Ref. Simple Biostatistics by Indrayan & Indrayan, 1/e p111]*
    - The Apgar score is based on a total score of 1 to 10
      - The higher the score, the better the baby is doing after birth
      - A score of 7, 8, or 9 is normal and is a sign that the newborn is in good health
    - In the given question, most of the newborns have a score >7 (normal)
      - Hence, Most of the value will be on higher side
      - So it's a Negatively skewed (Left skewed) data

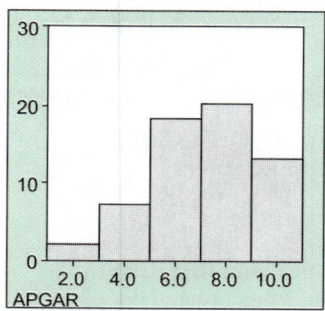

103. **Ans. (b) 1** *[Ref. Park 27/e p976]*
    - In a Normal distribution curve:
      - Total area under curve = 1
      - Mean = 0
      - Standard deviation = 1

Biostatistics

104. Ans. (a) Mode < Median < Mean
[*Ref. Essentials of Statistics by Gravetter, 9/e p75*]

Central tendency in distributions
- Right skew (Positive skew) distribution: Mean > Median > Mode
- Left skew (Negative skew) distribution: Mean < Median < Mode
- Normal (Gaussian) distribution: Mean = Median = Mode

105. Ans. (a) Negative skewed [*Ref. Essentials of Statistics by Gravetter 9/e p75*]

Central tendency in Various Distributions
- Normal (Gaussian) distribution Mean = Median = Mode (coincide)
- Right (Positive) skew distribution Mean > Median > Mode
- Left (Negative) skew distribution Mean < Median < Mode

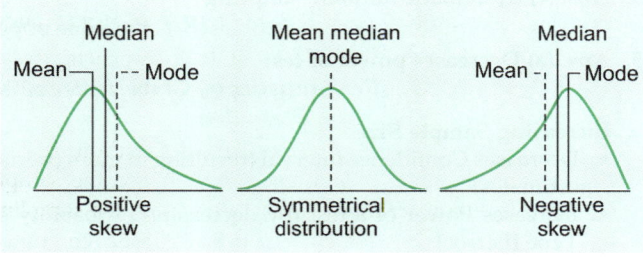

SAMPLING

106. Ans. (b) Reduced to 1/4 [*Ref. Essentials of Marketing Research by Babin 6/e p382*]
- Sample size is Inversely related to the Square of allowable error
- So, if allowable error is doubled, Sample size required will be reduced to $1/4^{th}$

107. Ans. (d) Desired precision [*Ref. Clinical Epidemiology by Fletcher, p177–78*]
- Sample size depends upon:
  - The effect size (usually the difference between 2 groups)
  - The population standard deviation (for continuous data)
  - The desired power of the experiment to detect the postulated effect (Power = 1 – β)
  - The significance level (α).

108. Ans. (d) 12–23 months [*Ref. Simple Biostatistics by Indrayan & Indrayan, 1/e p35–36 and Methods in Biostatistics by Mahajan, 9/e p133–134*]

Cluster random sampling (CRS)
- Applicable when units of population are natural groups or clusters
- Use of CRS in India: Evaluation of immunization coverage
- WHO technique used in CRS: 30 × 7 technique (total = 210 children)
  - 30 clusters, each containing
  - 7 children who are 12–23 months age and are completely immunized for primary immunization (till Measles vaccine)
- Clusters are heterogeneous within themselves but homogenous with respect to each other
- Sampling interval is also calculated in CRS
- Accuracy: Low error rate of only ± 5%
- Limitation: Clusters cannot be compared with each other.

> **ALSO REMEMBER**
> - Main objective of cluster sampling is to reduce costs by increasing sampling efficiency; this contrasts with stratified sampling where the main objective is to increase precision.

109. Ans. (d) Cluster sampling [*Ref. Simple Biostatistics by Indrayan & Indrayan, 1/e p35–36 and Methods in Biostatistics by Mahajan, 9/e p133–134*]

110. Ans. (d) Cluster testing [*Ref. Simple Biostatistics by Indrayan & Indrayan, 1/e p34–37 and Methods in Biostatistics by Mahajan, 9/e p133–134*]

Types of sampling:

	Random Sampling	**Non-random sampling**
Synonyms	Probability sampling Non-purposive sampling	Non-probability S Purposive sampling
Types	Simple random sampling Systematic random sampling Stratified random sampling Multistage random sampling Multiphase random sampling Cluster random sampling	Convenience S Quota sampling Snow-ball sampling Clinical trial S

Refer to Theory.

111. Ans. (d) The drop-out rate increases [*Ref. Internet*]

112. Ans. (d) Stratified random sampling [*Ref. Park 27/e p980–981*]

Refer to Theory.

113. Ans. (a) Sample size same as simple random [*Ref. Methods in Biostatistics by Mahajan, 9/e p133–134*
- *Cluster random sampling:*
  - Sample size (total 210): Is much smaller than that of random sampling
  - Is a 2-satge sampling procedure:
    1. First stage: Choosing 30 clusters in an area
    2. Second stage: Choosing 12–23 months children (7 in each cluster)
  - Cheaper quick method: Lesser time, lesser population coverage, lesser sample size.

114. Ans. (d) Cluster random sampling [*Ref. Designing and Conducting Health Surveys: A Comprehensive Guide, p175*]

Design effect
- *Definition:* Adjustment used in few study/sampling designs to allow for design structure, especially to allow for correlations among cluster of observations

- *Uses:*
  - Cluster randomised trials
  - Cluster random sampling
  - Multistage sampling
  - Health facility cluster survey

115. **Ans. (d) 400**   *[Ref. Applied Statistics in Health Sciences by Rao & Murthy, 1/e p105]*
- Minimum sample size for prevalence calculation in Cross-sectional studies (Field surveys):

Sample size = $4pq/L^2$
Where, p= prevalence; q=1-p; l=error in estimation of prevalence
In the given question, p = 50% (50/100); q = 1-p = 1–0.50 = 0.50 (50/100); L=5% (5/100 as range permissible is 45–50% i.e. +5%)
So, Sample size = $[4*50/100*50/100]/[5/100]^2$ = 400

116. **Ans. (a) Heterogenous data**   *[Ref. Park 27/e p988]*

117. **Ans. (d) 30 cluster of 7 children** *[Ref. Simple Biostatistics by Indrayan & Indrayan, 1/e p35–36]*

118. **Ans. (d) Multistage sampling** *[Ref. The Practice of Social Research by E Babbie, 12/e p218]*

119. **Ans. (a) Quota sampling**   *[Ref. Park 23/e p850]*

120. **Ans. (c) Systematic random sampling** *[Ref. Park 27/e p988]*

121. **Ans. (b) Stratified random sampling** *[Ref. Comparative Effectiveness Research by Rogers 1/e Chap3, 25/e p887]*

Stratified randomization
- Procedure conducted to minimize differences in the study arms based on patient characteristics that are known at the start of trial
- Study groups are balanced for that characteristic(s)
- Best method when studying a large random non-homogenous population
- Gives a more representative sampling population compared to other methods

122. **Ans. (c) 900** *[Ref. Applied Statistics in Health Sciences by Rao & Murthy, 1/e p105]*

$$N = \frac{Z_{\alpha/2}^2 * P * (1-p) * D}{E^2}$$

- Where N is the minimum sample size required in a Cross-sectional study, P is Prevalence, D is Design effect (1 for Simple random sampling, Higher values for other types of Random sampling), E is Precision (Permissible error) of prevalence, $Z\alpha/2$ is normal deviate for two-tailed alternative hypothesis at a level of significance

Alpha	Zα/2
0.20	1.28
0.15	1.44
0.10	1.64
0.05	1.96
0.01	2.58
0.001	3.29

In the given question,
- P = 10% (0.10); 1-p = 0.90
- D = 1
- Zα/2 = 1.96 (for alpha error 5%)
- So N = $(1.96)^2 * 0.10 * 0.90 * 1/(0.20 * 0.10)^2$ = 864

> **ALSO REMEMBER**
> - Shortened version of this formula is N = $4pq/L^2$
> - So, N = $4 * 0.10 * 0.90/(0.20 * 0.20)^2$ = 900

123. **Ans. (d) When subpopulation vary considerably** *[Ref. Park 27/e p988]*

Stratified sampling
- Method of sampling from a heterogeneous population after diving them into homogenous strata/groups
- When subpopulations within an overall population vary, it is advantageous to sample each subpopulation (stratum) independently

124. **Ans. (c) Systematic random sampling** *[Ref. Park 27/e p988]*

125. **Ans. (a) Decreases power of test** *[Ref. Statistics by Gravetter 8/e p270]*

Increasing Sample Size
- Decreases Confidence interval (resulting in more precise estimates)
- Increases Power of a test (by decreasing probability of Type II error)
- Decreases Alpha error (maximum probability threshold of Type I error)
- Decreases Standard error of mean

PROBABILITY AND ODDS

126. **Ans. (a) Prior probability of SLE; sensitivity and specificity of each test** *[Ref. Simple Biostatistics by Indrayan & Indrayan, 1/e p107–08]*
- PPV is also known as 'post-test probability of a disease' or 'precision rate'
- *Baye's Theorm:* Gives relationship between PPV of a screening test and Sensitivity, Specificity & Prevalence of disease in a population

$$PPV = \frac{Sensitivity \times Prevalence}{Sensitivity \times Prevalence + [(1 - Specificity)(1 - Prevalence)]} \times 100$$

- *Actual Baye's Theorm:* Gives relationship between Post-test probability of a disease in a population (PTP = PPV) and Sensitivity, Specificity & Post-test probability of a disease in a population (pTP = Prevalence)
  - Post-test probability of a disease in a population (pTP) IS SAME AS PPV
  - Pre-test probability of a disease in a population (pTP) IS SAME AS Prevalence.

In the given question, a patient is clinically diagnosed as having SLE and ordered 6 tests; out of which 4 tests have come positive and 2 are negative;

Thus, to determine the probability of SLE at this point (Post-test probability of SLE OR PPV), one would need to know Prior probability of SLE (Pre-test probability OR Prevalence of SLE); sensitivity and specificity of each test.

 ALSO REMEMBER
- *Positive predictive value (PPV)*: Ability of a screening test to identify correctly all those who have the disease, out of all those who test positive on a screening test

  $PPV = \dfrac{a}{a+b} \times 100 = \dfrac{TP}{TP+FP} \times 100$
- *PPV of a screening test depends on:*
  - Sensitivity
  - Specificity
  - Prevalence of disease in the population
- PPV of a screening test is directly proportional to prevalence of disease in the population.

127. Ans. (c) 0.001   *[Ref. Simple Biostatistics by Indrayan & Indrayan, 1/e p106–07 and Methods in Biostatistics by Mahajan, 9/e p144–147]*

- *Probability:* Is the chance that some event will occur
- *Probability range:* 0 to +1 (0% to 100%)
  - Probability can never be zero
  - Probability cannot exceed one
- *Probability rules:*
  - Rule of addition: Probabilities are added for mutually exclusive events i.e. P(Total) = P(A) + P(B)
  - Rule of multiplication: Probabilities are multiplied for obtaining joint occurrence of two or more independent events i.e. P(Total) = P(A) × P(B)

In the given question, Prevalence diabetes in a population is 10%,
Thus each individual has a probability of having diabetes P(A) = 10% = 0.10
If three people selected at random from the population, then each will have a probability of having diabetes as P(A) = 0.10
As all 3 events are independent of each other, so probability of all 3 having diabetes will be

$P(T)_1 = P(A) \times P(A) \times P(A) = 0.10 \times 0.10 \times 0.10 = 0.001$ (0.1%)

Also, the probability of either one of them having diabetes will be

$P(T)_2 = P(A) + P(A) + P(A) = 0.30$ (30%).

128. Ans. (d) 0.0256   *[Ref. Simple Biostatistics by Indrayan & Indrayan, 1/e p105–07]*

In the given question, Chance of passing a Genetic disease 'y' trait by the affected parents to children is 0.16 and they plan to have two children,
Probability of 1st child having 'y' trait, P(A) = 0.16 (16%)
Probability of 2nd child having 'y' trait, P(B) = 0.16 (16%)
Thus, Probability of both the children having 'y' trait (both events are independent of each other) is
$P(Total)_1 = P(A) \times P(B)$
$P(Total)_1 = 0.16 \times 0.16 = 0.0256$ (2.56%)

Also,
Probability of 1st child not having 'y' trait, P(C) = 0.84 (84%)
Probability of 2nd child not having 'y' trait, P(D) = 0.84 (84%)
Thus, Probability of both the children not having 'y' trait (both events are independent of each other) is
$P(Total)_2 = P(C) \times P(D)$
$P(Total)_2 = 0.84 \times 0.84 = 0.7056$ (70.56%)
Also, probability of having 1st child with 'y' trait and 2nd child without 'y' trait (both events are independent of each other) will be:
$P(Total)_3 = P(A) \times P(D)$
$P(Total)_3 = 0.16 \times 0.84 = 0.1344$ (13.44%)
Also, probability of having 1st child without 'y' trait and 2nd child with 'y' trait (both events are independent of each other) will be:
$P(Total)_4 = P(B) \times P(C)$
$P(Total)_4 = 0.16 \times 0.84 = 0.1344$ (13.44%)
Total probability = $P(Total)_1 + P(Total)_2 + P(Total)_3 + P(Total)_4$
P (Total) = 0.0256 + 0.7056 + 0.1344 + 0.1344 = 1.0 (100%),
These are the only four possibilities with both child births.

129. Ans. (b) 0.70   *[Ref. Simple Biostatistics by Indrayan & Indrayan, 1/e p105–07]*

In the given question, for Mrs Rekha, probability of having a baby of BW <2500 gms, P(A) is 0.50 and of having a BW 2500–2999 gms, P(B) is 0.20
Thus, the probability for Mrs. Rekha to have a baby of BW <3 kg is

$P(Total) = P(A) + P(B) = 0.50 + 0.20 = 0.70$ (70%)

There is one more possibility, i.e. probability of having a baby of BW >3 kg, whose probability P(C) will be 1 – (P(A) + P(B)) = 0.30 (30%).

130. Ans. (b) 3:1   *[Ref. CMDT, 41/e p1676]*

ALSO REMEMBER
- Odds: Odds are the chance of frequency of occurrence of a characteristic relative to its non-occurrence (expressed as a ratio of occurrence to non-occurrence)
  - Odds = Probability/(1 – Probability)
  - Probability = Odds/(1 + Odds)

131. Ans. (a) Prob (A or B) = Prob (A) + Prob (B)
    [Ref. Simple Biostatistics by Indrayan & Indrayan, 1/e p105–07]

- *Probability:* Is the chance that some event will occur
- *Probability range:* 0 to + 1 (0% to 100%)
  - Probability can never be zero
  - Probability cannot exceed one
- *Probability rules:*
  - Rule of addition: Probabilities are added for mutually exclusive events i.e. P(Total) = P(A) + P(B)

For example, If probability of having birth weight <2500 grams (P (A)) is 0.50 (50%), birth weight 2500–2999 grams (P(B)) is 0.30 (30%) and birth weight ≥ 3 kg (P (C)) is 0.20 (20%),
Then,
- Probability of having birth weight <3 kg (P (T1)) will be

- P (T1) = P (A) + P (B) = 0.50 + 0.30 = 0.80 (80%) as both events are mutually exclusive
- Similarly, probability of having birth weight >2500 (P (T2)) will be
- P (T2) = P (B) + P (C) = 0.30 + 0.20 = 0.50 (50%) as both events are mutually exclusive
  - Rule of multiplication: Probabilities are multiplied for obtaining joint occurrence of two or more independent events i.e. P(Total) = P(A) × P(B).

For example,
- If probability of having birth weight <3 kg (P (C)) is 0.70 (70%),
- Probability of having birth weight ≥ 3 kg (P (D)) is 0.30 (30%) AND
- Probability of being of male sex (P (E)) is 0.50 (50%), and probability of being of female sex (P (F)) is 0.50 (50%).

Then,
- Probability of having a child with birth weight <3 kg and of male sex will be

P (T_3) = P (C) × P (E) = 0.70 × 0.50 = 0.35 (35%) as both are independent events

- Similarly, Probability of having a child with birth weight <3 kg and of female sex will be

P (T_4) = P (C) × P (F) = 0.70 × 0.50 = 0.35 (35%) as both are independent events

- Probability of having a child with birth weight ≥ 3 kg and of male sex will be

P (T_5) = P (D) × P (E) = 0.30 × 0.50 = 0.15 (15%) as both are independent events

- Probability of having a child with birth weight ≥ 3 kg and of female sex will be

P (T_6) = P (D) × P (F) = 0.30 × 0.50 = 0.15 (15%) as both are independent events

- Total probability of a child being borne with any characteristic (P (T) will be

P (T) = P (T_3) + P (T_4) + P (T_5) + P (T_6) = 0.35 + 0.35 + 0.15 + 0.15 = 1 (100%)

Odds: Odds are the chance of frequency of occurrence of a characteristic relative to its non-occurrence (expressed as a ratio of occurrence to non-occurrence).

$$Odds = \frac{Probability}{1 - Probability}$$

$$Probability = \frac{Odds}{1 + Odds}$$

For example, if probability of occurrence of CHD in a man in lifetime is 0.75 (75%) i.e. P (CHD),
Then odds of CHD development in lifetime will be,
P (CHD)/(1 − P (CHD)) = 0.75/(1 − 0.75) = 0.75/0.25 = 3 (3 : 1).

Review Question

132. Ans. (a) 2/6 *[Ref: Park 25/e p912]*

STATISTICAL TESTS

133. Ans. (d) Friedman test *[Ref. Research in Health Care by Sim & Wright, 1/e p296]*

Friedman Test
- Non-parametric alternative to One-way ANOVA (One-Way Repeated Measure Analysis of Variance by Ranks)
- This nonparametric test is used to compare three or more matched groups
- An ideal statistic to use for a repeated measures type of experiment to determine if a particular factor has an effect

134. Ans. (b) Chi-square test *[Ref. Park 25/e p915]*
- Since we are comparing qualitative data (proportion of malnourished children) among two different groups (children in Rural Vs Urban area), Chi-square test is most appropriate

135. Ans. (a) Chi-square test *[Ref. Park 25/e p915]*
- **In the given question,** there are two different in dependent groups in the study one group of children in Summer season and another group in Rainy season with similar characteristics from same area
- We will compare proportion of children with SIDS in Summer season Vs those in Rainy season
- Hence, Chi-square test would be most appropriate

136. Ans. (c) Standard error of difference between two proportions *[Ref. Simple Biostatistics by Indrayan & Indrayan, 1/e p146–47 and Methods in Biostatistics by Mahajan, 9/e p218; Park 25/e p888–889]*

> **ALSO REMEMBER**
> - *Mean (Average):*
>   - Is a measure of central tendency
>   - Is obtained as sum of all values divided by the no. of values
> - Mean = $\Sigma x/n$
> - *Normal deviate:*
>   - Is also known as Z score (Standard score)
>   - Is difference of a value from group mean, in terms of how many times of SD (σ)
> - Z score = $\frac{Individual\ level - Mean}{SD} = \frac{x - \mu}{\sigma}$
> - The standard score indicates how many standard deviations an observation is above or below the mean
> - Z scores are frequently used in assessing how far a child is in his relative growth to a standard
> - Z score = 2: Any measurement of atleast 2SD away is considered too far away to be normal.

137. Ans. (a) Paired t-test *[Ref. Simple Biostatistics by Indrayan & Indrayan, 1/e p164 and Methods in Biostatistics by Mahajan, 9/e p184]*
- **In the given question**, a cardiologist wants to study the effect of an atrovastatin drug; he notes down the initial cholesterol levels of 50 patients and then administers the drug on them and after a month's treatment, he measures the cholesterol level again

- Since mean cholesterol levels are being measured in the same group of individuals before and after an intervention, this is PAIRED DATA
- Thus, the most appropriate to test the statistical significance of the change in blood cholesterol will be Students (paire(d) t-test.

> **ALSO REMEMBER**
> - *Mann-Whitney (Wilcoxon) test:*
>   - MWW is same as Wilcoxon (rank sum) test
>   - Is used for assessing whether two set of observations come from same distribution (if 2 independent 'non-paired' samples come from the same population)
>   - 'MWW is analogous to parametric two-sample t-1test' on the data after ranking over the combined samples
>   - MWW requires calculation of 'U statistic'.

138. Ans. (b) That a smaller proportion of people who were immunized against chickenpox subsequently develop zoster than those who were not immunized
[Ref. Simple Biostatistics by Indrayan & Indrayan, 1/e p170–72 and Methods in Biostatistics by Mahajan, 9/e p230; Park 27/e p80]

In the given question,
- Choice (a): Mean score of 2 groups are compared, thus most appropriate test of significance would be 'Unpaired Students t-test'
- Choice (b): Two proportions are compared, thus most appropriate test of significance would be 'Chi-square test'
- Choice (c): Mean score of 3–4 groups are compared, thus most appropriate test of significance would be 'ANOVA (F ratio) test'
- Choice (d): Mean score of 2 groups are compared, thus most appropriate test of significance would be 'Unpaired Students t-test'

139. Ans. (a) Chi-square test [Ref. Simple Biostatistics by Indrayan & Indrayan, 1/e p170–72 and Methods in Biostatistics by Mahajan, 9/e p215; Park 27/e p980]

Chi-square test (χ^2 – Test):
- Is a 'non-parametric test' of significance
- Is used to 'test significance of association between 2 or more qualitative characteristics'
- Is used to compare proportions in 2 or more groups
- Is used for non – Normal (non –Gaussian) distributions
- Applications of Chi-square test:
  - Test of proportions
  - Test of association
  - Test of goodness of fit
- Essential requirements for calculation of Chi-square test:
  - Random sample
  - Qualitative data
  - Lowest expected frequency not <5

In the given question, in a particular trial, the association of lung cancer with smoking is found to be 40% in one sample and 60% in another, Sincw two proportions are to be compared best test will be Chi-square test.

> **ALSO REMEMBER**
> - *Degree of freedom:* Is the no. of observations in a dataset that can freely vary once the parameters have been estimated
>   - Used in Chi-square test and t-test
>   1. In a contingency table, dof = (c – 1) (r – 1) (where c = no. of columns and r = no. of rows)
>   2. In a Student's t-test (one-sample data/paired test), dof v = n – 1 (where n = no. of units in the sample)
>   3. In a Student's t –test (two-sample data/unpaired test), dof v = (n1 + n2) – 1 (where n1 and n2 = no. of units in the two samples)
> - *Paired Student's t-test:* Comparing means (± SD) in paired data (in same group of individuals before and after an intervention)
> - *Fischer's test:* Is a variant of Chi-square test when sample size is <30
> - *ANOVA test (F-test/F-ratio):* Comparing means (± SD) in more than two different group of individuals.

140. Ans. (c) t [Ref. Simple Biostatistics by Indrayan & Indrayan, 1/e p160–63 and Methods in Biostatistics by Mahajan, 9/e p184]

- *Student's t-test:*
  - Paired Student's t-test: Comparing means (± SD) in paired data (in same group of individuals before and after an intervention)
  - Unpaired Student's t-test: Comparing means (± SD) in two different group of individuals
  - Z-test: Is a variant of student's t-test which is used when sample size is **>30.**

In the given question, mean ± SD of 20 boys (140 ± 13 cm) and 20 girls (135 cm ± 7 cm) of the same age are compared, Thus most appropriate statistical test of significance would be Unpaired Student's t-test.

> **ALSO REMEMBER**
> - *Chi-square test (χ^2 - test):* Comparing percentage, proportions & fractions in two or more different group of individuals
>   - Fischer's test: Is a variant of Chi-square test when sample size is <30
> - *ANOVA test (F - test/F -ratio):* Comparing means (± SD) in more than two different group of individuals.

141. Ans. (b) Paired 't' test [Ref. Simple Biostatistics by Indrayan & Indrayan, 1/e p160–63 and Methods in Biostatistics by Mahajan, 9/e p184]

- *Student's t-test:*
  - Paired Student's t-test: Comparing means (± SD) in paired data (in same group of individuals before and after an intervention)
  - Unpaired Student's t-test: Comparing means (± SD) in two different group of individuals
  - Z-test: Is a variant of student's t-test which is used when sample size is >30.

In the given question, the mean B.P. of a group of persons was determined and after an interventional trial, the mean BP was estimated again. The best test to be applied to determine the significance of intervention would be Paired Student's t-test.

142. **Ans. (d) Chi-Square test** *[Ref. Simple Biostatistics by Indrayan & Indrayan, 1/e p168–85 and Methods in Biostatistics by Mahajan, 9/e p215; Park, 25/e p915]*
    - Chi-square test as a test of association between 2 events in binomial or multinomial samples is its' 'most important application'

    In the given question, an investigator wants to study the association between maternal intake of iron supplements (Yes or No) and incidence of low birth weight (<2500 or >2500) gms),
    Thus, association is to be studied between 2 qualitative variables, i.e. status of usage of iron supplements and status of low birth weight in their newborns,
    So, most appropriate test would be Chi-square test.

143. **Ans. (c) 6** *[Ref. Simple Biostatistics by Indrayan & Indrayan, 1/e p171 and Methods in Biostatistics by Mahajan, 9/e p215, 9/e p215]*
    - In a Student's t-test (one-sample data/paired test):
      - Degree of freedom, $v = n - 1$
      - where n = no. of units in the sample
    - In a Student's t -test (two-sample data/unpaired test):
    Degree of freedom, $v = (n_1 + n_2) - 1$
    where n_1 and n_2 = no. of units in the two samples.

144. **Ans. (a) Paired t-test** *[Ref. Simple Biostatistics by Indrayan & Indrayan, 1/e p164 and Methods in Biostatistics by Mahajan, 9/e p215]*

    In the given question, a cardiologist wants to study the effect of an anti-hypertensive drug. So he will compare mean BP of 50 patients before and after administering the drug. Thus Paired t-test will be most appropriate test of significance.

145. **Ans. (b) Student's t-test** *[Ref. Simple Biostatistics by Indrayan & Indrayan, 1/e p162–63]*
    - Student's t-test:
      - *Paired Student's t - test:* Comparing means (± SD) in paired data (in same group of individuals before and after an intervention)
        Example: Mean serum albumin level of dengue patients before treatment was 3.6 g/dL and after treatment was 3.2 g/dL; Comparison of mean levels can be done by Paired Student's t-test
      - *Unpaired Student's t-test:* Comparing means (± SD) in two different group of individuals
        Example: Mean Hb level of anemia patients was 9.6 g/dL and those of hookworm patients was 7.2 g/dL; Comparison of mean levels can be done by Unpaired Student's t-test
      - *Z-test:* Is a variant of student's t-test which is used when sample size is >30

    In the given question, the study to assess the effect of a drug in lowering serum cholesterol levels was undertaken in 15 obese women and 10 non-obese women (2 limbs of the study)
    Thus mean lowering of serum cholesterol would be obtained in the two samples, thereby making 'two-sampled student's t –test' as the test of choice.

146. **Ans. (a) Mean & SD of the groups** *[Ref. Simple Biostatistics by Indrayan & Indrayan, 1/e p170–72 and Methods in Biostatistics by Mahajan, 9/e p230; Park 27/e p980]*

147. **Ans. (b) Student's t-test** *[Ref. Simple Biostatistics by Indrayan & Indrayan, 1/e p160–64 and Methods in Biostatistics by Mahajan 9/e p215]*

ALSO REMEMBER

- *Odds ratio (OR):* Ratio of odds that cases were exposed to a risk factor to the odds that the controls were exposed
  - Is used to 'measure strength of association in a case control study'
  - Is also known as 'Cross product ratio' or 'Relative odds'
  - Is an 'estimate of Relative risk (RR)', which is used to measure strength of association in a cohort study (RR is more accurate than OR' as a measure of strength of association)
  - OR calculation: Correct table construction in a case control study requires that table will have disease at the top (row) and history of exposure/risk factor on the left (column).

	Disease	
	Present (cases)	Absent (Controls)
Exposure present	a	b
Exposure absent	c	d

  - Odds Ratio (Cross Product Ratio) = ad/bc
  - Interpretation of Odds ratio is just like relative risk: OR can be >1 (associated), = 1 (no association) or <1 (protective effect)
- *Correlation coefficient (r):* Measures the degree or strength of relationship in a correlation
  - Correlation coefficient (r) lies between: –1 to +1 ($-1 < r < +1$)
  - Correlation is represented by: 'Scatter diagram'
  - Correlation coefficients:
    1. Pearson's Correlation coefficient
    2. Spearman's Rank Correlation coefficient
- *Chi-square test (χ^2 – TEST):*
  - Is a 'non-parametric test' of significance
  - Is used to 'test significance of association between 2 or more QUALITATIVE characteristics'
  - Is used for non – Normal (non–Gaussian) distributions
  - Applications of Chi-square test:
    1. Test of proportions
    2. Test of association
    3. Test of goodness of fit.

148. **Ans. (a) Chi-square test** *[Ref. Simple Biostatistics by Indrayan & Indrayan, 1/e p170 and Methods in Biostatistics by Mahajan, 9/e p230; Park 27/e p980]*

149. **Ans. (b) 6** [Ref. Simple Biostatistics by Indrayan & Indrayan, 1/e p171 and Methods in Biostatistics by Mahajan, 9/e p230; Park 27/e p980]

In the given question, there are 3 rows and 4 columns (we only count those rows and columns which are filled with frequencies),
Thus, dof = (c – 1) (r – 1) = (4 – 1) (3 – 1) = 6.

150. **Ans. (c) Directly measures the strength of association** [Ref. Simple Biostatistics by Indrayan & Indrayan, 1/e p170–73 and Methods in Biostatistics by Mahajan, 9/e p230; Park 27/e p980]

CHI-SQUARE TEST (χ^2-TEST):
- Is a 'non-parametric test' of significance
- Is used to 'test significance of association between 2 or more qualitative characteristics'
- Is used for non – Normal (non–Gaussian) distributions
- Applications of Chi-square test:
  – Test of proportions
  – Test of association
  – Test of goodness of fit
- Essential requirements for calculation of Chi-square test:
  – Random sample
  – Qualitative data
  – Lowest expected frequency not <5

In a 2 × 2 contingency table,

a	b
c	d

$\chi^2 = \Sigma (O - E)^2 / E$

where O = Observed frequency and E = Expected frequency in each cell

OR $\chi^2 = \dfrac{[(ab - bc)^2 (a + b + c + d)]}{[(a + b)(c + d)(a + c)(c + d)]}$.

> **ALSO REMEMBER**
> - Advantages of χ^2 – test over 'Standard error of difference between two proportions' test as a test of proportions has:
>   – Can be used to compare values of 2 binomial samples even if they are less than size of 30.
>   1. Apply correction factor – Yates correction
>   2. Expected value must not be <5 in any cell
>   – Can be used to compare frequencies of 2 multinomial samples
> - Chi-square test as a test of association between 2 events in binomial or multinomial samples is its' 'most important application'
>   – χ^2-test tells about the presence or absence of association between 2 events/characteristics but 'do not tell about strength of association'
>   – If strength of association (Relative Risk or Odds Ratio) found in a study is close to value of 1: Chi-square test can be used to find whether or not RR/OR is really statistically significantly different from value of 1.
> - If in any cell frequency is <5: Fischer's exact test is used.

151. **Ans. (b) Student t test** [Ref. Simple Biostatistics by Indrayan & Indrayan, 1/e p164 and Methods in Biostatistics by Mahajan, 9/e p215]
- In the given question, mean bone density amongst 2 groups of 50 people each is compared,
- Thus means are to be compared in 2 different groups,
- So, Unpaired Student's t-test is most appropriate to test significance of association.

> **ALSO REMEMBER**
> - McNemar's Chi-square test: is a non-parametric test used to test significance of association between 2 sampled paired data or for paired nominal data in sample.

152. **Ans. (b) Paired 't' test** [Ref. Indrayan, 1/e p164]

153. **Ans. (b) 6** [Ref. Park 27/e p980]

154. **Ans. (d) Multiple logistic regression** [Ref. Principles of Medical Statistics by Alvan R Feinstein, p612]
- *ANOVA:* Analysis of Variance is a parametric test used for polytomous independent variable
- *Chi-square test:* Is non-parametric test used for testing association between 2 or more qualitative variables
- *Multiple linear regression:* Is used if the target variables are dimensional having multiple possible values (e.g. blood pressure, serum cholesterol, body temperature)
- *Multiple logistic regression:* Is used if the target variables are binary having only two possible values (e.g. hypertension, smoking, geriatric age group)

In the given question, the investigator finds out that 5 independent factors influence the occurrence of a disease. So to compare these 5 factors (each factor being dichotomous) one should use Multiple logistic regression.

155. **Ans. (c) Paired students t-test** [Ref. Biostatistics by Mahajan, 9/e p215]

156. **Ans. (d) Chi-square test** [Ref. Park 27/e p980]
- **In the given question,** Significance has to be tested between Receipt of Maternal food supplements (Yes/No) and Subsequent weights of newborns (Values or Categories), hence Chi-square test would be more appropriate

157. **Ans. (d) Chi-square test** [Ref. Biomedical Research Methodology by Das 1/e p144]

Parametric tests	Non-parametric tests
Gaussian/Normal distributions	Non–normal distributions
Quantitative data	Qualitative data
Compares Means (+ SD)	Compares Proportions & fractions
Students (paired) t - test Students (unpaired) t - test ANOVA F – test Z test	Sign test Chi-square test (c2 - test) Wilcoxan test (signed rank) Wilcoxan test (rank sum) Fischer's exact test

158. **Ans. (a) Useful for non-normal (skewed) data**
    [Ref. Applied Engineering Statistics by Bethea 1/e p248]

    Parametric tests Vs Non-parametric tests

	Parametric tests	Non-parametric tests
Based on data type	Normal/Gaussian distributions	Non-normal distributions
Applicability	Narrow	Wider
Nature	More powerful	Less powerful
Data requirements	Fewer data requirements	More data requirements
Data type	Metric	Nominal/Ordinal
Calculations	Difficult	Easy
Accuracy, Precision	More	Less

159. **Ans. (a) Paired t-test**
    [Ref. Essentials of Biostatistics by Saha 1/e p109]

    Parametric Tests
    - Paired Student's t-test: Comparing means (+ SD) in paired data (in same group of individuals before and after an intervention)
    - Unpaired Student's t-test: Comparing means (+ SD) in two different group of individuals
    - ANOVA test (F-test/F-ratio): Comparing means (+ SD) in more than two different group of individuals

160. **Ans. (b) Z-test**

161. **Ans. (c) Chi-square test** *[Ref. Park 27/e p980]*

162. **Ans. (b) Heart rate/min and age** *[Ref. Park 25/e p889]*
    - Heart rate/min and Age are both quantitative data (2 different groups) so Parametric type test, i.e., Unpaired Students' t-test would be used
    - Sex and stage of cancer, Benign/malignant and type of surgery, Age group and cancer stage are Qualitative data (2 different groups) so Non parametric test, Chi square would be used

163. **Ans. (b) Unpaired t-test**
    [Ref. Statistical and Methodological Aspects of Oral Health Research by Lesaffre, 1/e p170]

    In the given question,
    - Blood pressure is compared between 2 groups; Blood pressure is a Metric type data, so Means would be the most appropriate measure of Central tendency to be compared
    - Comparison of Means in 2 different groups of populations require Unpaired Students' t-test

164. **Ans. (a) Paired t-test**
    [Ref. Statistical and Methodological Aspects of Oral Health Research by Lesaffre, 1/e p170]

    In the given question,
    - Blood pressure is compared within 1 group before and after treatment
    - Blood pressure is a Metric type data, so Means would be the most appropriate measure of Central tendency to be compared
    - Before and after BP measurements with intervention (treatment) in between, within 1 group, makes it a Paired data
    - Comparison of Means in Paired data require Paired Students' t-test

165. **Ans. (b) Unpaired t-test**
    [Ref. Statistical and Methodological Aspects of Oral Health Research by Lesaffre, 1/e p170]

    Statistical Tests of Significance

Tests	Use in Biostatistics (Test of significance for)
Paired students' t-test	Comparison of Means in paired data (1 group)
Unpaired students' t-test	Comparison of Means in unpaired data (2 groups)
ANOVA test	Comparison of Means in unpaired data (≥ 3 groups)
Sign test	Comparison of Proportions/fractions in paired data (1 group)
Chi-square test	Comparison of Proportions/fractions in unpaired data (≥ 2 groups)

Review Questions

166. **Ans. (b) 1** *[Ref. Park 27/e p980]*
167. **Ans. (c) 3.84** *[Ref. Park 27/e p980]*
168. **Ans. (a) Chi-square test** *[Ref. Park 27/e p980]*
169. **Ans. (a) <0.001 is statistically significant**
    [Ref. Park 27/e p980]
170. **Ans. (a) Unpaired t-test** *[Ref. Park 20/e p753–54]*
171. **Ans. (a) Paired t-test** *[Ref. Indrayan, 1/e p164]*
172. **Ans. (b) 12** *[Ref. Park 27/e p980]*
173. **Ans. (c) Means in different groups** *[Ref. Park 27/e p980]*
174. **Ans. (d) Standard error of difference between proportion**
    [Ref. Park 27/e p978]
175. **Ans. (d) Cox proportional hazards test**
    [Ref. Cholesterol: New Insights by A Acton, 1/e p511]
176. **Ans. (d) Fischer's exact test; (e) Chi-square test**
    [Ref. Park 27/e p980]

CORRELATION AND REGRESSION

177. **Ans. (d) Computational mistake in calculating correlation**
    [Ref. Simple Biostatistics by Indrayan & Indrayan, 1/e p127–30 and Methods in Biostatistics by Mahajan, 9/e p248; Park 27/e p980–981]

    Correlation:
    - Is relationship between 2 quantitative or continuous variables
    - *Correlation coefficient (r):* Measures the degree or strength of relationship in a correlation
      – Correlation coefficient (r) lies between: –1 to +1 ($-1 < r < +1$)
    - *Correlation is represented by:* 'Scatter diagram'
      – In a scatter diagram, 2 imaginary lines are drawn along the distribution of dots/scatter.

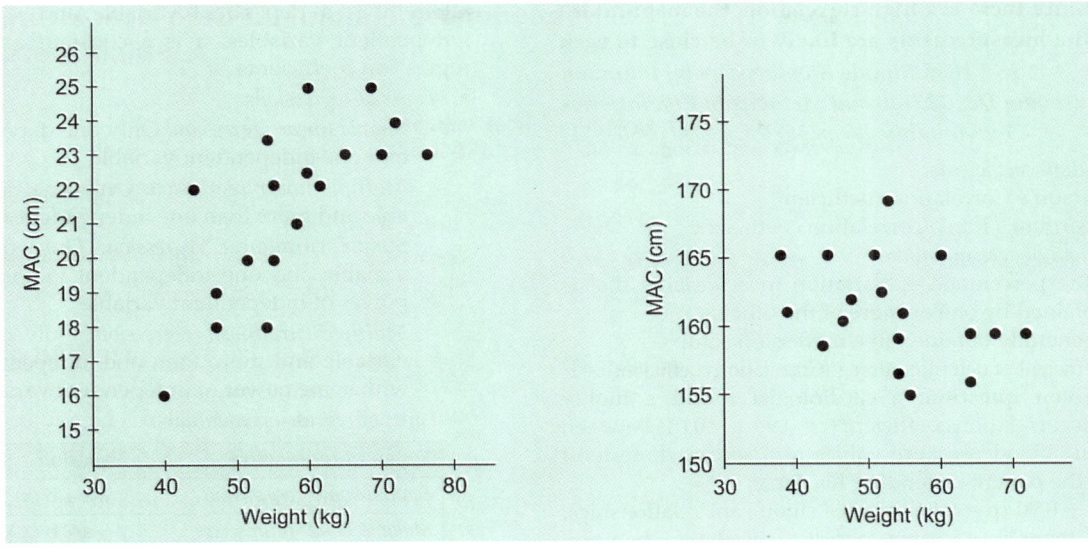

Scatter showing positive correlation between weight and mix-arm circumference of male medical students

Scatter diagram showing negative correlation between weight and height of male medial students

- *Correlation coefficients:*
  - *Pearson's Correlation coefficient:*
    1. Is used in ungrouped series
    2. Is used when associated variables are normally distributed
    3. Symbol is 'r'
  - *Spearman's Rank Correlation coefficient*
    1. Is used in grouped series
    2. Is used when associated variables are not normally distributed
    3. Symbol is 'rho (r)'.

> **ALSO REMEMBER**
- *Multiple correlation coefficient:* Is used for calculation of correlation between one variable (dependent) and the combination of two or more variables (independents)
- *Coefficient of determination:*
  - Is the percentage of variation in a variable that is explained by one or more of the others
  - Is generally obtained in a regression setup
  - Coefficient of determination = (Correlation coefficient)^2 = r^2
- *Coefficient of variation:*
  - Is a measure used to compare relative variability
  - Is a unit-free measure to compare dispersion of one variable with another
    CV = SD/Mean × 100 = σ/μ × 100.

178. **Ans. (d) The lecturer has reported the correlation coefficient incorrectly** *[Ref. Simple Biostatistics by Indrayan & Indrayan, 1/e p127 and Methods in Biostatistics by Mahajan, 9/e p248; Park 27/e p980–981]*

Correlation coefficient (r):
- Measures the degree or strength of relationship in a correlation (relationship between 2 quantitative or continuous variables)
- Correlation coefficient (r) lies between: –1 to +1 (–1 < r < +1)
- Strength of correlation:
  - Weak positive correlation: 0 < r < 0.3
  - Moderate positive correlation: 0.4 < r < 0.6
  - Strong positive correlation: r > 0.7
- Correlation is represented by: 'Scatter diagram'

In the given question, a lecturer states that the correlation coefficient between prefrontal blood flow under cognitive load and the severity of psychotic symptoms in schizophrenic patients is –1.24
Since correlation coefficient (r) lies between –1 to +1 only, a value of r = –1.24 IS NOT POSSIBLE. There is some computational mistake in calculation.

> **ALSO REMEMBER**
- *Few important ranges in public health:*

Parameter	Range (Lies between)
Correlation coefficient (r)	–1 to +1 (–1 < r < +1)
Coefficient of determination (r2)	0 to +1 (0 < r2 < +1)
Physical quality of life index (PQLI)	0 to +100 (0 < PQLI < +100)
Human development index (HDI)	0 to +1 (0 < HDI < +1)
Probability	0 to +1 (0% < Probability < 100%)
Sensitivity (screening test)	0% < Sensitivity < 100%
Specificity (screening test)	0% < Specificity < 100%
PPV (screening test)	0% < PPV < 100%
NPV (screening test)	0% < NPV < 100%

179. **Ans. (a) Since there is a high correlation, the magnitudes of both the measurements are likely to be close to each other**
    [*Ref. Simple Biostatistics by Indrayan & Indrayan, 1/e p127–30 and Methods in Biostatistics by Mahajan, 9/e p248; Park 27/e p980–981*]
    - *Correlation coefficients:*
        - Pearson's Correlation coefficient:
        - Spearman's Rank Correlation coefficient
    - *Coefficient of determination:*
        - Is the percentage of variation in a variable that is explained by one or more of the others
        - Is generally obtained in a regression setup
        - Coefficient of determination = (Correlation coefficient)^2 = r^2

    In the given question, a cardiologist found a highly significant correlation coefficient (r = 0.90, p = 0.01) between the systolic blood pressure values and serum cholesterol values of the patients attending his clinic,

    Since r = + 0.90 (p = 0.01; implies significant relationship), it means there is a strong positive correlation between systolic blood pressure (SBP) and serum cholesterol (SC); therefore as SBP increases, SC will also increase and vice-versa.

    Thus, a patient with a high level of systolic BP is also likely to have a high level of serum cholesterol AND a patient with a low level of systolic BP is also likely to have a low level of serum cholesterol.

    Since r = + 0.9; Coefficient of determination = r^2 = $(0.9)^2$ = 0.81
    Interpretation of r^2: 0.81 or 81% of variation in systolic blood pressure among patients can be explained by their serum cholesterol values and vice-versa.

180. **Ans. (b) Scatter diagram**
    [*Ref. Simple Biostatistics by Indrayan & Indrayan, 1/e p103 and Methods in Biostatistics by Mahajan, 9/e p26; Park 27/e p980–981*]
    - *Scatter/Dot diagram:*
        - Also known as 'Correlation diagram'
        - Is used to depict 'correlation (relationship) between 2 quantitative variables'
        - Vertical axis in scatter diagram: should be the dependent or the outcome variable
        - In a scatter diagram, 2 imaginary lines are drawn along the distribution of dots/scatter
        - Correlation coefficient (r): Lies between –1 to +1

181. **Ans. (b) Coefficient of regression**
    [*Ref. Simple Biostatistics by Indrayan & Indrayan, 1/e p125 and Methods in Biostatistics by Mahajan, 9/e p248; Park 27/e p980–981*]

    Regression:
    - Is change in measurements of a variable
    - Provides structure of relationship between 2 quantitative variables
    - Regression Coefficient (b): Measure of change of one dependent variable (y) with change in independent variable (x) or variables (x_1, x_2, x_3……)
    Equations of regression,
    y = a + b (x)
    y = a + b (x_1) + c (x_2) + d (x_3),

    where y is a dependent variable and x, x_1, x_2, x_3 are independent variables; a is a constant and b, c, d are regression coefficients
    - *Types of regressions:*
        - *Simple linear regression:* Only one dependent variable and one independent variable
        - *Multiple linear regression:* Only one dependent variable and more than one independent variable
        - *Simple curvilinear regression:* Only one dependent variable and one independent variable, with some power of independent variable
        - *Multiple curvilinear regression:* Only one dependent variable and more than one independent variables, with some power of independent variables).
    - *Types of regression equations:*

Types of regression	Equation
Simple linear regression	y = a + b (x)
Multiple linear regression	y = a + b (x_1) + c (x_2) + d (x_3)
Simple curvilinear regression	y = a + b $(x)^6$
Multiple curvilinear regression	y = a + b $(x_1)^2$ + c $(x_2)^4$ + d $(x_3)^3$

    - Other types of regressions:

Types of regressions	Features	
	Dependent variables	Independent variables
Logistic regression	Qualitative, dichotomous	Qualitative/ Quantitative/Mixed
ANOVA	Quantitative	Qualitative
ANCOVA	Quantitative	Qualitative + Quantitative
Multivariate multiple regression	Set of Quantitative	Set of Quantitative
MANOVA	Set of Quantitative	Set of Qualitative
Multivariate logistic regression	Set of Qualitative	Qualitative/ Quantitative

> **ALSO REMEMBER**
> - *Relationships of variables:*
>   - Association: Simultaneous existence of 2 variables
>   - Correlation: Relationship between 2 quantitative or continuous variables
>   1. Correlation coefficient (r): Lies between –1 to +1 (measures relationship between 2 variables)
>   - Regression: Provides structure (quantification) of relationship between 2 quantitative variables
> - *SE of mean:*
>   - 'SE is a measure of chance variation,' and it does not mean error or mistake
>   - SE is SD or variability of sample means
>
> $$SE = \frac{SD}{\sqrt{\text{sample size}}} = \frac{\sigma}{\sqrt{n}}$$

Contd...

Contd...

> **Uses of standard error:**
> 1. To work out limits of desired confidence within which population mean would lie
> 2. To determine if sample is drawn from a known population or not
> 3. To find SE of difference between 2 means (to know if difference is real and statistically significant)
> 4. To calculate sample size (within desired confidence limits).

182. Ans. (a) Straight line *[Ref. Simple Biostatistics by Indrayan & Indrayan, 1/e p125–27 and Methods in Biostatistics by Mahajan, 9/e p260; Park 27/e p980–981]*

In the given question, the correlation of height with age is given by the equation y = a + biopsy, thus it is a Simple linear regression (equation: y = a + bx)
Nature of the graph will be a straight line.

183. Ans. (d) r = –0.8 *[Ref. Simple Biostatistics by Indrayan & Indrayan, 1/e p127–29 and Methods in Biostatistics by Mahajan, 9/e p248; Park 27/e p980–981]*

In the given question, correlation between IMR and economic status has to be inversely proportional (as economic status increases, IMR reduces and vice-versa)
But perfectly negative linear relation (r = –1) will not be seen (as IMR will also depend on other factors like available health services, literacy level, etc.)
Thus, it will show a moderately negative correlation (–1 < r < 0).

184. Ans. (d) Mistake in calculation *[Ref. Simple Biostatistics by Indrayan & Indrayan, 1/e p127 and Methods in Biostatistics by Mahajan, 9/e p248; Park 27/e p980]*

185. Ans. (b) Strong statistically significant (+) association between work satisfaction and life expectancy *[Ref. Simple Biostatistics by Indrayan & Indrayan, 1/e p127–30 and Methods in Biostatistics by Mahajan, 9/e p248; Park 27/e p980–981]*

- *Correlation coefficients:*
  – Pearson's Correlation coefficient:
  – Spearman's Rank Correlation coefficient
- *Coefficient of determination:*
  – Is the percentage of variation in a variable that is explained by one or more of the others
  – Coefficient of determination = (Correlation coefficient)^2 = r^2

In the given question, a study finds a correlation coefficient of + 0.7 between self reported work satisfaction & expectancy of life in a random sample of 5000 corporate workers. (p = 0.01)
Since r = + 0.70 (p = 0.01; implies significant relationship), it means there is a strong positive correlation between self reported work satisfaction (SRWS) & expectancy of life (LE); therefore as SRWS increases, LE will also increase. Thus, a patient with a high level of SRWS will have a high LE.

Since r = + 0.7; Coefficient of determination = r^2 = $(0.7)^2$ = 0.49
Interpretation of r^2: 0.49 or 49% of variation in expectancy of life can be explained by their self reported work satisfaction
Thus INCREASE in work satisfaction will improve life expectancy.

186. Ans. (c) Multiple linear regression *[Ref. Simple Biostatistics by Indrayan & Indrayan, 1/e p125–27 and Methods in Biostatistics by Mahajan, 9/e p248; Park 27/e p980–981]*

In the given question,
Total Cholesterol level = a + b (calorie intake) + c (physical activity) + d (body mass index) is an example of Multiple linear regression equation y = a + b (x_1) + c (x_2) + d (x_3).

> **ALSO REMEMBER**
> - *Relationships of variables:*
>   – *Association:* Simultaneous existence of 2 variables
>   – *Correlation:* Relationship between 2 quantitative or continuous variables
>   – *Regression:* Provides structure (quantification) of relationship between 2 quantitative variables

187. Ans. (b) Negative correlation *[Ref. Park 27/e p981]*

188. Ans. (b) 1 *[Ref. Park 27/e p981]*

189. Ans. (a) Same *[Ref. Statistics by Lewicki, 1/e p24, 27/e p981]*
- Generally different correlation coefficients (r) cannot be averaged directly: As Value of 'r' is not a linear function of magnitude of relation between 2 variables
- Average can be taken directly for Coefficient of determination (r^2)

In the given question (and graph), all correlation coefficients are same (+ 0.6), so their Coefficients of determinations would also be same (+ 0.6^2 = + 0.36 for each distribution)
Hence, they can be averaged to come out to be exactly "+ 0.6"
Combined correlation coefficient = $\sqrt{(0.36 + 0.36 + 0.36 + 0.36)/4}$ = + 0.6

190. Ans. (c) Scatter diagram *[Ref. Park 27/e p974]*
- Correlation is best depicted by Scatter diagram
- Height and weight show a Positive correlation (0 < r <+1)
- As Height increase, weight will increase (Positive slope of line in Scatter diagram)

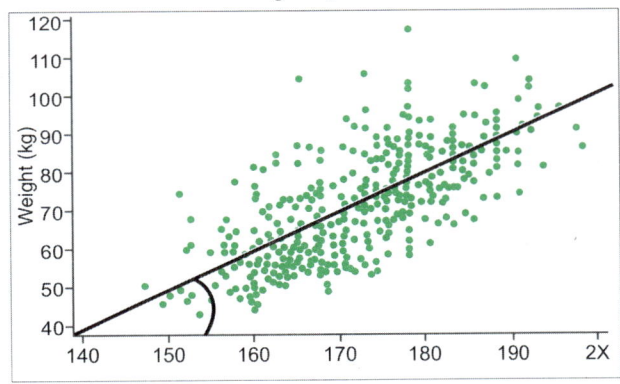

Scatter diagram (Height Vs Weight)

Review Questions

191. Ans. (d) It is a wrong statement [Ref: High yield biostastistics 2/e p50–52; Park 25/e p820]

192. Ans. (c) –1 to +1 [Ref. Park 27/e p980–981]

ERRORS AND P-VALUE

193. Ans. (b) A and C are correct [Ref. A Guide to the Scientific Career by Shoja 1/e p597]
- Narrow p-value function would result from a large study with high precision
- Lesser the p-value, higher the significance of test results

194. Ans. (b) Type I error [Ref. Statistics Explained by McKillup 1/e p104]
- Null hypothesis true (in reality) but rejected (based on our study results) lead to Type I error
- Null hypothesis false (in reality) but accepted (based on our study results) lead to Type II error

195. Ans. (d) The probability of a false positive conclusion that operation 'Operation A is better that Operation B', when in truth it is not, is 4% [Ref. Simple Biostatistics by Indrayan & Indrayan, 1/e p155–56 and Methods in Biostatistics by Mahajan, 9/e p179]

In the given question, the "P" value of a randomized controlled trial comparing operation A (new procedure) & Operation B (Gold standard) is 0.04;

Thus the probability of committing Type I error is 0.04 or 4% (i.e. probability of declaring a false positive conclusion that operation 'Operation A is better that Operation B', when in truth it is not, is 4%).

> **ALSO REMEMBER**
> - *Type I error:*
>   - Significance (α) level: is the maximum tolerable probability of Type I error
>   - Alpha is fixed in advance: P – value calculated can be less than, equal to or greater than alpha (α)
>   - Keep Type I error to be minimum (P < α): Then results are declared statistically significant.
> - Type I error is more serious than Type II error
> - *Power of a test:* 1 – β
>   - Is probability of rejecting a Null hypothesis when a predetermined clinically significant difference is indeed present
>   - Power can be increased by increasing the no. of subjects in a trial
> - A test with a high specificity has a low Type I error rate
>   - False positive rate (α) = 1 – specificity
>   - False negative rate (β) = 1 – sensitivity

196. Ans. (b) Decreasing β error [Ref. Simple Biostatistics by Indrayan & Indrayan, 1/e p156–60]

- *Power of a Test:*
  - Is probability of rejecting a Null hypothesis when a predetermined clinically significant difference is indeed present
  - Measures the ability to demonstrate an association, when one really exists
  - Power of a statistical test: 1 – β (1 – probability of Type II error)
  - Power of a statistical test is complimentary to β (probability of Type II error)
  - Power of a statistical test is a numeric representation of: Sensitivity
  - Power of a statistical test can be increased by:
    1. Increasing the no. of subjects in a trial (sample size)
    2. Reducing b (probability of Type II error)
    3. Increasing sensitivity
  - Power of a statistical test is also used for calculation of sample size for a study

- *Statistical errors:*

	H0 rejected	H0 not rejected
Null Hypothesis (H0) true	Type I error	No error
Null Hypothesis (H0) false	No error	Type II error

- *Types of Statistical errors:*

Type I Error	Type II Error
Null hypothesis is true but rejected	Null hypothesis is false but not rejected
Probability of Type I error is given by 'P – value' (probability of declaring a significant difference when actually it is not present)	Probability of Type II error is given by beta (β) (probability of declaring no significant difference when actually it is present)
Significance (α) level: is the maximum tolerable probability of Type I error	
Keep Type I error to be minimum (P < α): Results are declared statistically significant Type I error is more serious	Power of a test: (1 – β) Is probability of rejecting a Null hypothesis when a predetermined clinically significant difference is indeed present

> **ALSO REMEMBER**
> - A test with a high specificity has a low Type I error rate
>   - False positive rate (α) = 1 – specificity
>   - False negative rate (β) = 1 – sensitivity

197. Ans. (d) Nothing can be concluded as the information given is inadequate [Ref. Simple Biostatistics by Indrayan & Indrayan, 1/e p141 and Methods in Biostatistics by Mahajan, 9/e p179]

In the given question, In assessing the association between maternal nutritional status and the birth weight of the newborns, two investigators A and B studied separately and found significant results with p values 0.02 and 0.04 respectively

Only levels of significance are given, thus we can only conclude that investigator A has 98% chance of being correct whereas investigator B has 96% chance of being correct.

198. **Ans. (a) Type-I error (α error)**
    [Ref. Simple Biostatistics by Indrayan & Indrayan, 1/e p155–56 and Methods in Biostatistics by Mahajan, 9/e p179]

    In the given question, a randomized trial comparing efficacy of two regimens showed that difference is statistically significant with p <0.001 (null hypothesis is rejected) but in reality the two drugs do not differ in their efficacy (null hypothesis is true),
    Thus it is Type-I error (α error).

199. **Ans. (b) The probability of declaring a significant difference is 1%**
    [Ref. Simple Biostatistics by Indrayan & Indrayan, 1/e p155–56]

200. **Ans. (b) Is equal to 1-β**
    [Ref. Simple Biostatistics by Indrayan & Indrayan, 1/e p155]
    - 'Type I error is usually fixed in advance' by the choice of level of significance employed in the test
    - Type I error is more serious than Type II error
    - Power of a test: 1 – β
      - Is probability of rejecting a Null hypothesis when a predetermined clinically significant difference is indeed present
      - Power can be increased by increasing the no. of subjects in a trial
    - There is no mathematical relationship between α and β.

201. **Ans. (c) When Null Hypothesis is true but is rejected, it is Type-II error**
    [Ref. Simple Biostatistics by Indrayan & Indrayan, 1/e p155–57 and Methods in Biostatistics by Mahajan, 9/e p179]

202. **Ans. (b) Rejecting a null hypothesis when true**
    [Ref. Simple Biostatistics by Indrayan & Indrayan, 1/e p156]
    - P-value:
      - Is the 'Probability of Type I error' (Null hypothesis is true but rejected)
      - Significance (α) level: is the maximum tolerable probability of Type I error
      - P- value is calculated (on basis of data while Alpha is fixed in advance: by the choice of level of significance employed in the test
      - P – value calculated can be less than, equal to or greater than alpha (α)
      - Keep Type I error to be minimum (P < α): Then results are declared statistically significant.

203. **Ans. (a) Chi-square test**
    [Ref. Simple Biostatistics by Indrayan & Indrayan, 1/e p170–73 and Methods in Biostatistics by Mahajan, 9/e p179]

    In the given question, association is to be studied between maternal intake of iron (yes/no) and birth weights of newborns (to see the proportion of low birth weight) i.e. between 2 qualitative characteristics, thus Chi-square test is most suitable

204. **Ans. (a) Type I error (alpha error)**
    [Ref. Simple Biostatistics by Indrayan & Indrayan, 1/e p155–57 and Methods in Biostatistics by Mahajan, 9/e p179]
    - A test with a high specificity has a low Type I error rate
      - False positive rate (α) = 1 – specificity
      - False negative rate (β) = 1 – sensitivity

205. **Ans. (b) Risk is more associated with Group B**
    [Ref. Internet]
    In the given question. Both Group A Confidence interval (1.0–3.1) as well as Group C Confidence interval (0.9–1.7) contains 1 in their range. So, there is a possibility of true value of strength of association being 1 (implying no association) Whereas Group B (CI = 1.1–1.7) has no such possibility, so this value of Odds ratio (1.4) may be least in all three groups but shows more association.

206. **Ans. (a) As the sample size increases, Standard error will also increase**
    [Ref. Simple Biostatistics by Indrayan & indrayan, 1/e p139–40 and Methods in Biostatistics by Mahajan, 9/e p179]

207. **Ans. (a) Probability of declaring a significant difference when actually it is not present**
    [Ref. Methods in Biostatistics by Mahajan, 9/e p179]

208. **Ans. (a) Type 1 error**
    [Ref. Simple Biostatistics by Indrayan & Indrayan, 1/e p155–57]

209. **Ans. (a) Null hypothesis is true but rejected**
    [Ref. Simple Biostatistics by Indrayan & Indrayan, 1/e p155–57 and Methods in Biostatistics by Mahajan, 7/e p111–113]

    Statistical errors

	H0 rejected	H0 not rejected
Null Hypothesis (H0) true	Type I error	No error
Null Hypothesis (H0) false	No error	Type II error

210. **Ans. (b) Type II error**
    [Ref. Simple Biostatistics by Indrayan & Indrayan, 1/e p155–56 and Methods in Biostatistics by Mahajan, 9/e p179]
    - Null hypothesis (H0) There is No significant association
      In the given question,
    - In reality an association exists, So Null hypothesis is False
    - We say no significant association exists, So we are accepting Null hypothesis
    - Hence its Type II error

Review Questions

211. **Ans. (a) Probability of Type I Error is <0.05**
    [Ref. K.S. Negi Biostatistics, 7/e p105]

212. **Ans. (b) Null hypothesis rejected and the study is accepted**
    [Ref. Park 25/e p889]

MISCELLANEOUS

213. Ans. (a) Increasing sample size
[Ref. Simple Biostatistics by Indrayan, 1/e p146]
- A smaller sample size or a higher variability will result in a wider confidence interval with a larger margin of error
  - As sample size increases, the margin of error decreases
  - As the variability in the population increases, the margin of error increases
- As you increase the confidence level (e.g., 95% to 99%) while holding the sample size and variability constant, the confidence interval widens
- Smaller the SD, narrower is Confidence interval

214. Ans. (c) Bland and Altman analysis [Ref. Internet]

Bland-Altman analysis:
- Is not a statistical test measured with a p-value
- Is a process used to assess agreement between two methods of measurement
- Is used to 'assess level of agreement between 2 methods' to compare a new technique with an established one.

> **ALSO REMEMBER**
> - *Kolmogorov-Smirnov test:*
>   - Is one of the most useful and general nonparametric methods for comparing two samples
>   - KS-test tries to determine if two datasets differ significantly

215. Ans. (d) All are true [Ref. Simple Biostatistics by Indrayan & Indrayan, 1/e p31, 222]

Delphi method
- Delphi method: Is a 'systematic interactive forecasting method' for obtaining consensus forecasts from a panel of independent experts
  - Method: The carefully selected experts answer questionnaires in two or more rounds; After each round, a facilitator provides an anonymous summary of the experts' forecasts from the previous round as well as the reasons they provided for their judgments; Thus, participants are encouraged to revise their earlier answers in light of the replies of other members of the group
  - The range of the answers decrease and the group will converge towards the 'correct' consensual answer; Finally, the process is stopped after a pre-defined stop criterion (e.g. number of rounds, achievement of consensus, stability of results) and the mean or median scores of the final rounds determine the results
- The objective of most Delphi applications: The reliable and creative exploration of ideas or the production of suitable information for decision-making.
- The Delphi Method is based on: A structured process for collecting and distilling knowledge from a group of experts by means of a series of questionnaires interspersed with controlled opinion feedback
- The Delphi method is an exercise in group communication among a panel of geographically dispersed experts
- In general, the Delphi method is useful in answering one, specific, single-dimension question.

> **ALSO REMEMBER**
> - *Mini-Delphi or Estimate-Talk-Estimate (ETE):* The delphi technique when adapted for use in face-to-face meetings.

216. Ans. (b) 69 and 75 kg [Ref. Simple Biostatistics by Indrayan & Indrayan, 1/e p141 and Methods in Biostatistics by Mahajan, 9/e p99; Park 25/e p912]

95% range = Mean ± 2SD ($\mu \pm 2\sigma$)

In the given question, n = 100 adult Delhites, Mean weight (μ) = 72 kg, Standard deviation (σ) = 1.5
95% range for of wt of Delhites = Mean ± 2SD ($\mu \pm 2\sigma$)
= 72 ± 2 (1.5) = 72 – 3, 72 + 3 = 69, 75 kg.

> **ALSO REMEMBER**
> - *Confidence level:*
>   - Is the level of hope or expectation fixed at a sufficiently high level while dealing with samples, to ensure high reliability
>   - Is the 'degree of assurance for an interval to contain the value of the parameter'
>   - There is NO WAY to achieve 100% confidence
>   - Internationally acceptable confidence level: 95%
>   - Maximum tolerance of probability of Type I error (σ) is the probability that CI would not contain the population mean
>   - Confidence level = 1 – α
> - *Confidence limits:* Are the upper and lower boundaries of a confidence interval.

217. Ans. (c) Recall bias [Ref. Simple Biostatistics by Indrayan & Indrayan, 1/e p236; Park 27/e p81]

Refer to chapter 3, Theory.

In the given question, in a drug trial a 50 yr old patient with CAD is being interviewed about his dietary & smoking habits.
Since history is being recalled regarding exposure, it can introduce recall bias.

218. Ans. (c) 2.5% [Ref. Simple Biostatistics by Indrayan & Indrayan, 1/e p141–42 and Methods in Biostatistics by Mahajan, 9/e p99; Park 27/e p976]
- In Normal distribution,
  - Mean ± 1SD ($\mu \pm 1\sigma$) covers 68% values
  - Mean ± 2SD ($\mu \pm 2\sigma$) covers 95% values
  - Mean ± 3SD ($\mu \pm 3\sigma$) covers 99% values

In the given question, 95% Confidence Interval (CI) for prevalence of Cancer in Smokers aged >65 years is 56% to 76%

Thus, 56% to 76% range covers 95% CI, thus rest 5% probability is of being OUTSIDE THIS RANGE, i.e. prevalence will be either <56% or >76%

Even this will be symmetrically distributed (Normal curve is bilaterally symmetrical), thus, 2.5% probability will be of having prevalence <56%

And 2.5% probability will be of having prevalence >76%.

ALSO REMEMBER

- *Confidence interval (CI):*
  - Is the interval within which a parameter value is expected to lie with certain confidence levels, as could be revealed by repeated samples
  - Is the 'range that is likely to contain the population mean when so obtained for repeated samples'
  - A narrow CI is always preferable: as it tells more precisely what might be the population mean BUT also it will have higher chances of not containing the population mean.
    1. Larger the sample size, narrower is CI
    2. Smaller the SD (s), narrower is CI
       95% CI for population mean = Mean ± 2SD ($\mu \pm 2\sigma$)
- *Confidence level:*
  - Is the level of hope or expectation fixed at a sufficiently high level while dealing with samples, to ensure high reliability
  - Is the 'degree of assurance for an interval to contain the value of the parameter'
  - There is NO WAY to achieve 100% confidence
  - Internationally acceptable confidence level: 95%
  - Maximum tolerance of probability of Type I error (α) is the probability that CI would not contain the population mean Confidence level = $1 - \alpha$
- *Confidence limits:*
  - Are the upper and lower boundaries of a confidence interval
- *Central limit theorem:*
  - Means that 'sample means have a tremendous tendency to follow a Gaussian (Normal) form of distribution, especially for large samples'.
  - Is observed even when distribution of individual values is highly skewed.

219. Ans. (c) Sensitivity & (1 – Specificity) *[Ref. A Dictionary of Public Health by J Kishore, p446–47]*

RECEIVER OPERATOR CHARACTERISTIC (ROC) CURVE:
- Is a graphical representation between sensitivity and specificity of a diagnostic test
- ROC curve is 'drawn between Sensitivity and (1 – Specificity)'
  - ROC curve is drawn between True positives and False positive error rate
- In clinical tests, ROC curve is 'used to determine a cut-off point'
- ROC curve is 'equivalent to Likelihood ratio for a positive result (LR+)'
- Types of ROC curves:
  - Straight line at 45° (Line a): No benefit by this test/cut-off
  - Straight lines above line a (Lines b and c): Fair, Good results by this test/cut-off
  - Uppermost line touching Y-axis and then horizontal line (Line d): Excellent results by this test/cut-off (Perfect ROC: 100% sensitivity & 100% specificity).

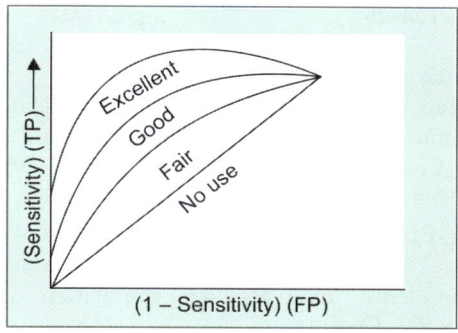

Receiver operating characteristic (ROC) curve

220. Ans. (d) Measure of central tendency *[Ref. Park 25/e p884]*

221. Ans. (b) Cronbach's alpha *[Ref. Wikipedia]*
- *Association:* Is any relationship between two measured quantities that render them statistically dependent
  - Correlation coefficient
  - Odds ratio
  - Good man's and Kruskal's Lambda
  - P value
  - Cronbach's alpha: is a measurement of internal consistency or reliability
  - Is particularly useful for Likert Scales (grading of continuum).

222. Ans. (b) Correlation analysis/Bland and Altmann test *[Ref. Statistical analysis quick reference guide, 1/e p78]*

223. Ans. (b) Previously significant data becomes insignificant *[Ref. Defence Counsel Journal, Vol. 66, p55]*
If Confidence limit is increased:
- Then degree of assurance of intervals containing the population mean is increased, BUT getting the value of population mean become less precise
- Previously significant data will now become less significant

224. Ans. (c) 81–89 *[Ref. Research Methods by Pittenger, 1/e p214]*

Confidence intervals
- A confidence interval gives an estimated range of values which is likely to include an unknown population parameter, the estimated range being calculated from a given set of sample data
- Confidence Intervals (CI) = Mean ± Z (Standard error), where 'Z' is the Critical value for the given CI, and

SE = SD/$\sqrt{n}$ (SD Standard deviation, n = Sample size)
- Critical value for 90% Confidence level (Z_{68}) = 1.0
- Critical value for 90% Confidence level (Z_{90}) = 1.645
- Critical value for 95% Confidence level (Z_{95}) = 1.96
- Critical value for 98% Confidence level (Z_{98}) = 2.33
- Critical value for 99% Confidence level (Z_{99}) = 2.575

In the given question, Mean (μ) = 85 mL/min, Standard deviation (σ) = 25, and Z_{90} = 1.645 (as we are asked 90% CI)
So, Confidence intervals (CI_{90}) = Mean ± Z_{90} (SE)
CI_{90} = 85 ± 1.645 (25/$\sqrt{100}$) = 81 – 89

225. **Ans. (c) 24–26**
[Ref. Research Methods by Pittenger, 1/e p214]
- In the given question,
- Mean (μ) = 25 mm Hg, Standard deviation (σ) = 10 mm Hg, and Z95 = 1.96 (as we are asked 95% CI)
- So, Confidence intervals (CI95) = Mean ± Z95 (SE)
- CI95 = 25 ± 1.96 (10/√400) = 24–26 mm Hg

226. **Ans. (a) 4–16**
[Ref. Simple Biostatistics by Indrayan, 1/e p146]
- Confidence Intervals for Population proportions (For 95% Confidence)
- CI = P ± 2 SEP = P ± 2 √pq/n

In the given question, P = 0.10 (10%)
- So, p=0.10; q= 1-p = 1–0.10 = 0.90; n=100
- CI = 0.10 ± 2 √0.1*0.9/100 = 0.10 ± 0.06 = 0.04, 0.16 (4%, 16%)

227. **Ans. (d) Standard error**
[Ref. Conducting Research in Human Geography by Kitchin 1/e p58]

Standard error (SE)
- Used to determine, for a given confidence level, the distance by which a sample mean is within a stated range of its true value
- It gives accuracy of sample mean vis-a-vis estimate of Population mean

228. **Ans. (b) Internal consistency**
[Ref. Statistics by Leung, 1/e p84]

Cronbach's alpha

Syn. Coefficient alpha, Guttman's lambda 3, Hoyt method, KR-20
- A measure of Internal consistency, that is, how closely related a set of items are as a group
- It is considered to be a measure of scale reliability
- Value lies between 0 to +1: Higher the alpha coefficient, the more the items have shared covariance and probably measure the same underlying concept (Internal consistency)
- Interpretation: + 0.7 or more is considered satisfactory

229. **Ans. (c) Mean and standard error**
[Ref. Research Methods by Pittenger 1/e p214]
- Confidence Intervals (CI) = Mean ± Z (Standard error),
- Where 'Z' is the Critical value for the given CI, and SE = SD/√n (SD Standard deviation, n = Sample size)

Notes

Notes

SECTION 4

PYQs (2012–2018): Image-based Questions

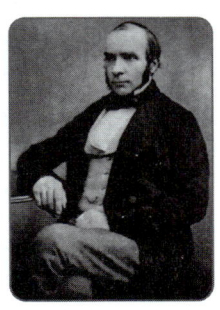
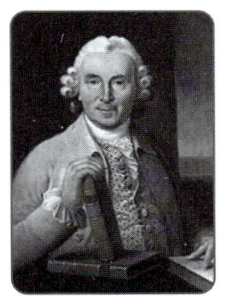
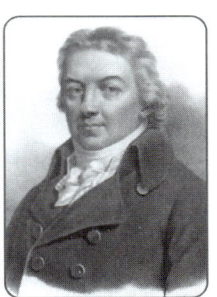

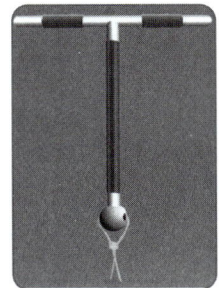
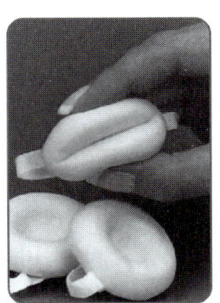

Image-based Questions

CHAPTER–1

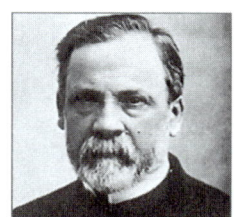

Q1. Identify the scientist as given in photograph:
[NEET Pattern 2013, 2016]
(a) Louis Pasteur
(b) Edward Jenner
(c) James Lind
(d) Hippocrates

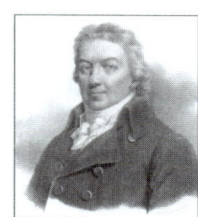

Q2. Identify the scientist as given in photograph:
[NEET Pattern 2014, 2015]
(a) Louis Pasteur
(b) Edward Jenner
(c) James Lind
(d) Hippocrates

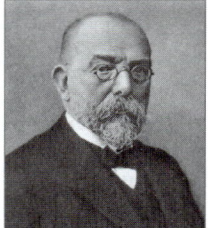

Q3. Identify the scientist as given in photograph:
[NEET Pattern 2012]
(a) John Snow
(b) Edward Jenner
(c) James Watson
(d) Robert Koch

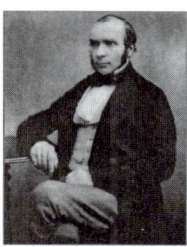

Q4. Identify the scientist as given in photograph:
[NEET Pattern 2012]
(a) John Snow
(b) Alexander Fleming
(c) James Lind
(d) Hippocrates

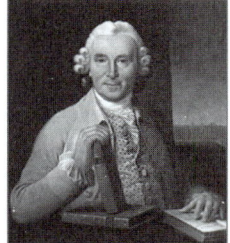

Q5. Identify the scientist as given in photograph:
[NEET Pattern 2012]
(a) John Snow
(b) Alexander Fleming
(c) James Lind
(d) Hippocrates

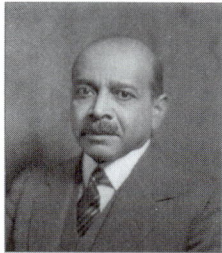

Q6. Identify the public health figure as given in photograph:
[NEET Pattern 2012]
(a) Hargobind Khorana
(b) Alexander Fleming
(c) Joseph Bhore
(d) Hippocrates

CHAPTER-2

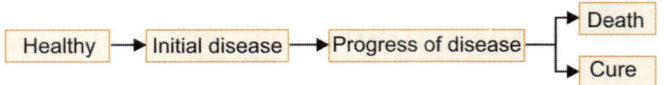

Q1. The image given below depicts: *[NEET Pattern 2019]*
(a) Causation of disease
(b) Pathogenicity of disease
(c) Natural history of disease
(d) Interventions taken

CHAPTER-3

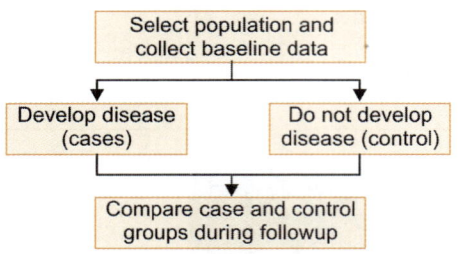

Q1. Identify the study design given in photograph:
[NEET Pattern 2015]
(a) Prospective cohort study
(b) Retrospective cohort study
(c) Case control study
(d) Nested case control study

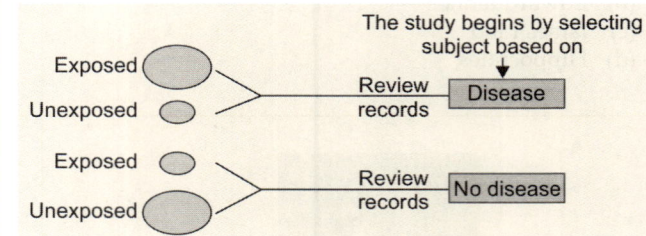

Q2. Identify the study design given in photograph:
[NEET Pattern 2016]
(a) Prospective cohort study
(b) Retrospective cohort study
(c) Case control study
(d) Nested case control study

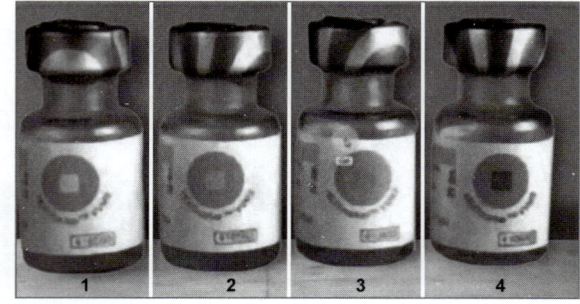

Q3. Which of the following OPV vials are usable?
[NEET Pattern 2017]
(a) Only 1
(b) Only 1, 2
(c) Only 1, 2, 3
(d) Only 3, 4

CHAPTER-4

Q1. In course of a disease, A (disease onset), B (detected by screening), C (usual time of diagnosis) and D (final outcome) is given. B----C is known as:
[NEET Pattern 2015, 2016]
(a) Lag time
(b) Lead time
(c) Screening time
(d) Latent period

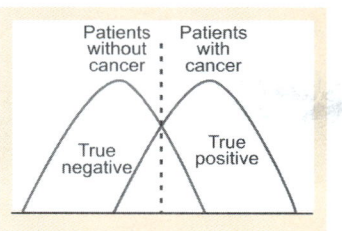

Q2. If a test has cut off value at point A, it will have:
[NEET Pattern 2016]
(a) High PPV
(b) Low sensitivity
(c) Low PPV
(d) High specificity

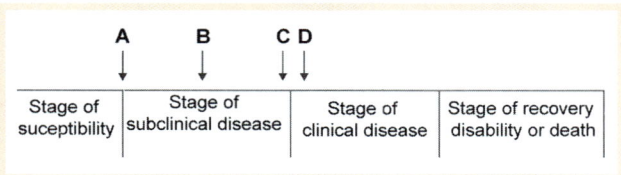

Q3. Which point in the below natural history of disease marks the onset of symptoms? *[AIIMS May 2017]*
(a) A
(b) B
(c) C
(d) D

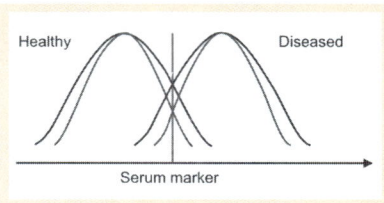

Q4. Observe the following curves. What will happen to Sensitivity and Specificity if curve changes from Blue to Red? *[AIIMS May 2017]*
(a) Both Sensitivity & Specificity increase
(b) Both Sensitivity & Specificity decrease
(c) Sensitivity increase & Specificity decrease
(d) Sensitivity decrease & Specificity increase

CHAPTER-5

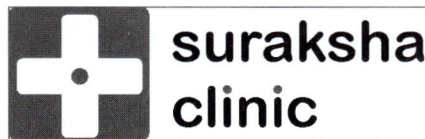

Q1. Identify services provided at clinic shown in symbol in photograph:
(a) ARI
(b) Diarrhoea
(c) RTI/STI
(d) Blood transfusion

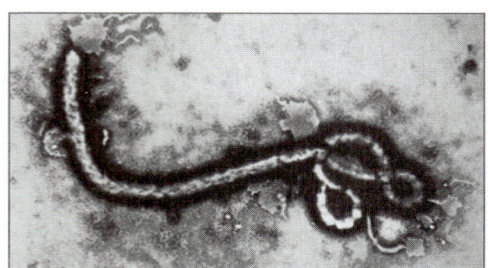

Q2. Identify organism shown in the photograph:
(a) H7N9 virus
(b) Ebola virus
(c) H1N1 virus
(d) H5N1 virus

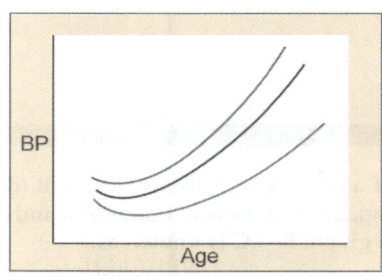

Q3. Identify the photograph shown:
[NEET Pattern 2015]
(a) Growth chart
(b) Tracking phenomena
(c) Rule of Halves
(d) Line chart

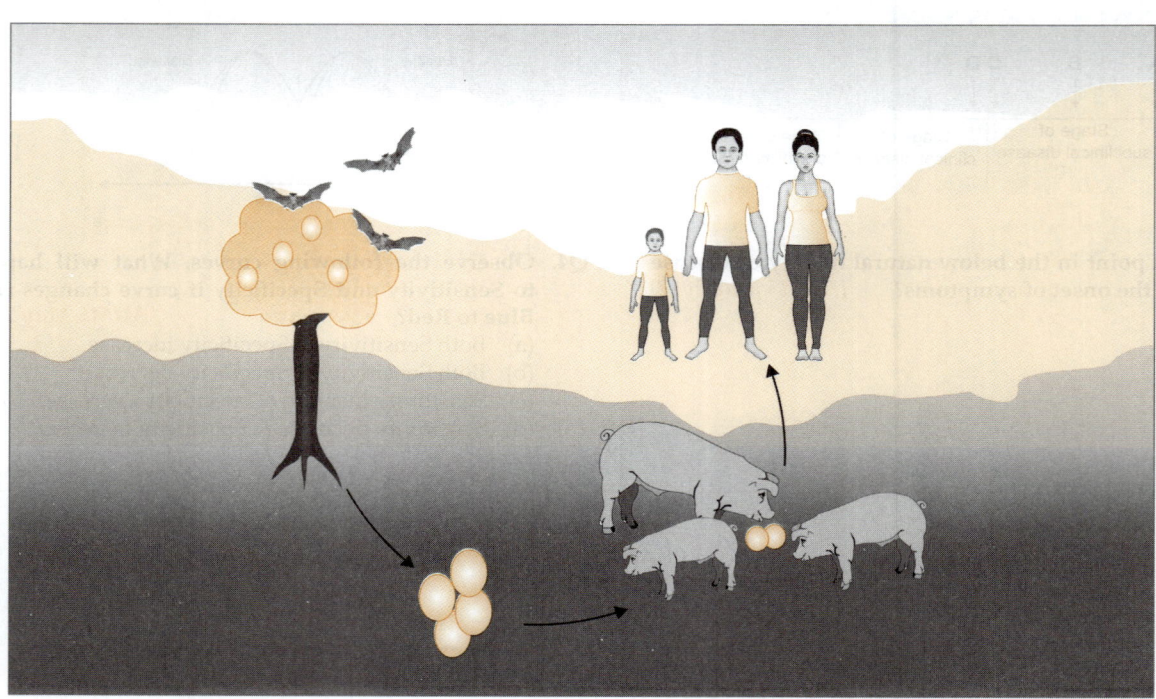

Q4. Life cycle shown in the image above represents: [AIIMS November 2018]
(a) JE virus
(b) Influenza virus
(c) Chandipura virus
(d) NIPAH virus

CHAPTER-6

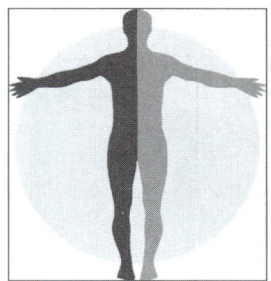

Q1. Identify the symbol as given in photograph:
 [*NEET Pattern 2012, 2015*]
(a) MDT
(b) DOTS
(c) ART
(d) ASHA

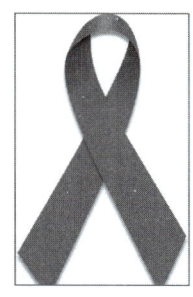

Q2. Identify the symbol as given in photograph:
 [*NEET Pattern 2013*]
(a) Tuberculosis
(b) Malaria
(c) Leprosy
(d) HIV/AIDS

Q3. Identify the National Health Program symbol as given in photograph: [*NEET Pattern 2012, 2014*]
(a) RNTCP
(b) NLEP
(c) NVBDCP
(d) NACP

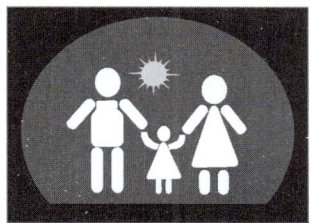

Q4. Identify the National Health Program symbol as given in photograph: [*NEET Pattern 2012, 2014*]
(a) RNTCP
(b) NLEP
(c) NRHM
(d) NACP

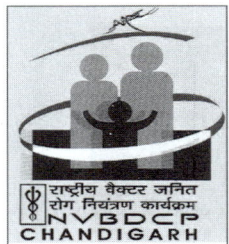

Q5. Identify the National Health Program symbol as given in photograph: [*NEET Pattern 2015*]
(a) NRHM
(b) NVBDCP
(c) RCH
(d) NPCDCS

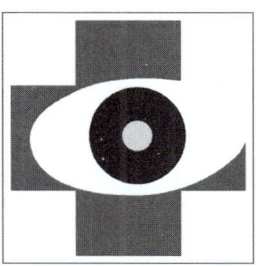

Q6. Identify the National Health Program symbol as given in photograph: [*NEET Pattern 2015*]
(a) NRHM
(b) NPCB
(c) NPCDCS
(d) RCH

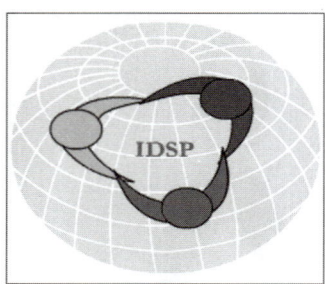

Q7. Identify the National Health Program symbol as given in photograph: [NEET Pattern 2016]
(a) NUHM
(b) PMJDY
(c) NPCDCS
(d) IDSP

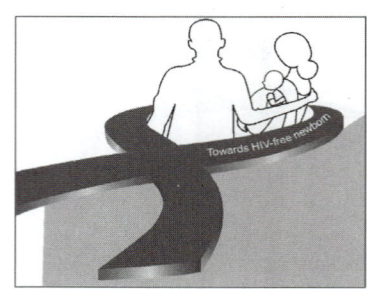

Q8. Identify component of NACP as shown in photograph: [NEET Pattern 2016]
(a) ART
(b) ICTC
(c) PPTCT
(d) Blood transfusion

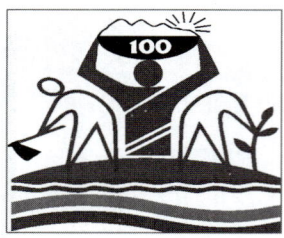

Q9. Identify the symbol as given in photograph: [NEET Pattern 2013]
(a) Organ Transplantation Act 1994
(b) RTI Act 2005
(c) MTP Act 1971
(d) NREGA Act 2005

CHAPTER–7

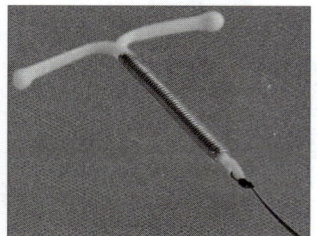

Q1. Identify contraceptive shown in the photograph: [NEET Pattern 2013, 2015]
(a) Diaphragm
(b) Vaginal ring
(c) Vaginal sponge
(d) IUD

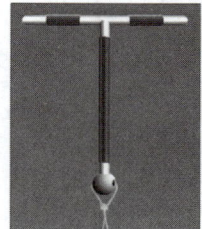

Q2. Identify the IUD shown in the photograph: [NEET Pattern 2015]
(a) Multiload CuT 375
(b) NOVA-T
(c) CuT 380 A
(d) LNG-IUD

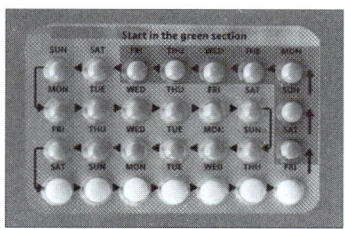

Q3. Identify contraceptive shown in the photograph:
 [*NEET Pattern 2014, 2015*]
 (a) Iron folic acid (IFA) tablets
 (b) DOTS category 1
 (c) MDT PBL blister
 (d) Combined OCPs

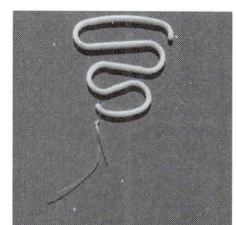

Q4. Identify contraceptive shown in the photograph:
 [*NEET Pattern 2012*]
 (a) CuT 380 A
 (b) Progestasert
 (c) Lippes loop
 (d) Mirena

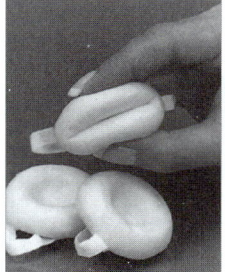

Q5. Identify contraceptive shown in the photograph:
 (a) DMPA
 (b) Vaginal ring
 (c) Diaphragm
 (d) Vaginal sponge

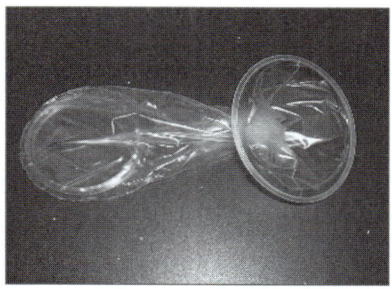

Q6. Identify contraceptive shown in the photograph:
 [*NEET Pattern 2016*]
 (a) Male condom
 (b) Female condom
 (c) Diaphragm
 (d) Vaginal sponge

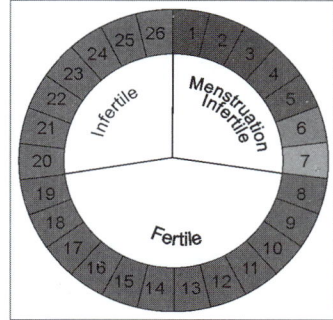

Q7. Identify contraceptive method shown in the photograph:
 (a) Rhythm method
 (b) Cervical mucus method
 (c) BBT method
 (d) Coitus interruptus

CHAPTER-11

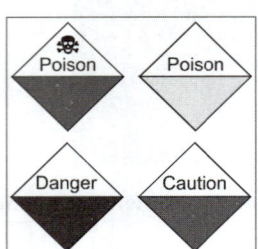

Q1. Symbol shown in photograph is that of:
[AIIMS November 2013]
(a) Vaccine safety labels
(b) Contraceptive efficacy labels
(c) Drugs toxicity labels
(d) Pesticide toxicity labels

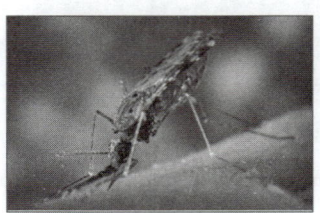

Q2. Identify the vector shown in the photograph:
[NEET Pattern 2012, 2013, 2014, 2015]
(a) Sandfly
(b) Anopheles mosquito
(c) Aedes mosquito
(d) Culex mosquito

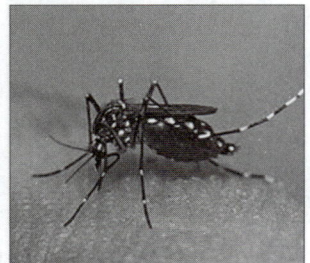

Q3. Identify the vector shown in the photograph:
[NEET Pattern 2013, 2015]
(a) Sandfly
(b) Anopheles mosquito
(c) Aedes mosquito
(d) Culex mosquito

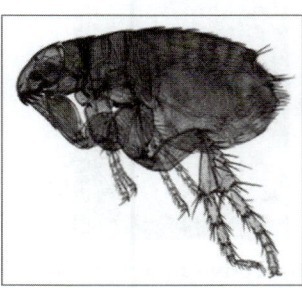

Q4. Identify the vector shown in the photograph:
[NEET Pattern 2015]
(a) Sandfly
(b) Housefly
(c) Hard tick
(d) Rat flea

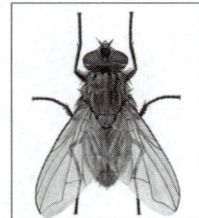

Q5. Identify the vector shown in the photograph:
[NEET Pattern 2013, 2015]
(a) Simulium
(b) Musca domestica
(c) Phlebotomus
(d) Reduviid bug

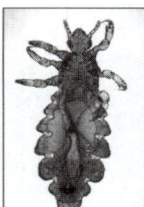

Q6. Identify the vector shown in the photograph:
[NEET Pattern 2013, 2015]
(a) Soft tick
(b) Hard tick
(c) Louse
(d) Rat flea

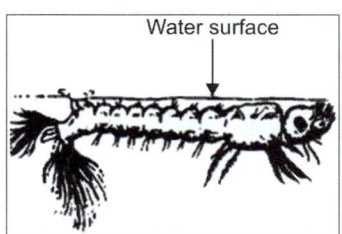

Q7. Identify larva of mosquito shown in the photograph: [NEET Pattern 2014, 2016]
(a) Anopheles
(b) Culex
(c) Aedes
(d) Mansonia

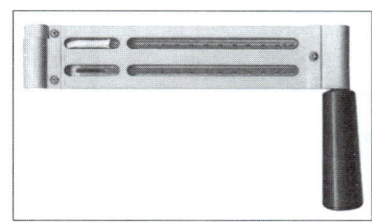

Q8. Instrument shown in photograph is sued to assess: [NEET Pattern 2016]
(a) Environmental heat measurement
(b) Cooling power of air
(c) Mean radiant temperature of surroundings
(d) Relative humidity of air

CHAPTER-12

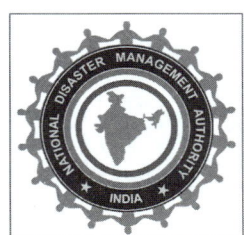

Q1. Chairman of agency shown in photograph is: [NEET Pattern 2013]
(a) Minister of Labour
(b) Defence Minister
(c) Prime Minister
(d) Minister of Health-FW

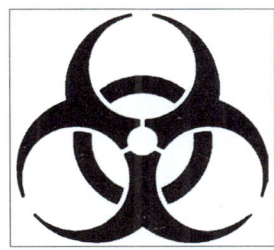

Q2. Identify symbol shown in the photograph: [NEET Pattern 2012, 2015]
(a) Disaster management
(b) Occupational health
(c) Biomedical waste management
(d) Family planning and contraception

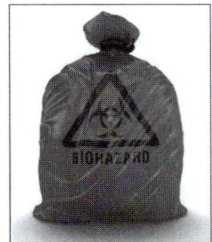

Q3. Which of the following wastes are disposed in the bag shown below? [AIIMS May 2017]
(a) Anatomical waste
(b) Sharp waste
(c) Urine bags
(d) Soiled waste

Q4. Identify symbol shown in the photograph: [NEET Pattern 2012, 2015]
(a) Recycling
(b) Organic matter
(c) Biomedical waste management
(d) Radiation hazard

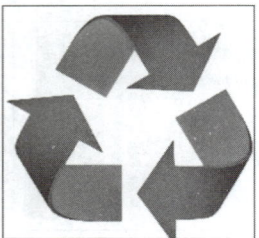

Q5. Identify symbol shown in the photograph:
[NEET Pattern 2013]
(a) Recycling
(b) Green-house effect
(c) Afforestation
(d) Radiation hazard

Q6. The depicted image above represents:
[AIIMS November 2018]
(a) Biomedical waste
(b) Cytotoxic waste
(c) Radiation hazard
(d) Bioterrorism

CHAPTER–15

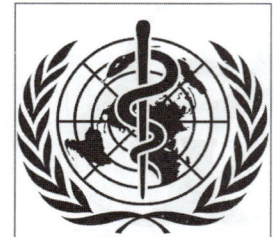

Q1. Identify the organization depicted by symbol as given in photograph: [NEET Pattern 2012, 2013, 2014, 2015]
(a) WHO
(b) UNICEF
(c) UNDP
(d) UNAIDS

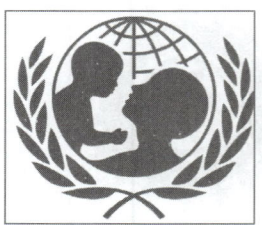

Q2. Identify the organization depicted by symbol as given in photograph: [NEET Pattern 2012, 2015]
(a) WHO
(b) UNICEF
(c) UNDP
(d) UNAIDS

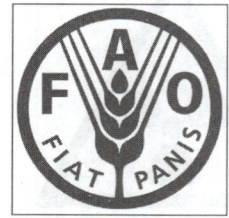

Q3. Headquarters location of International health agency depicted in photograph: [NEET Pattern 2014]
(a) New Delhi
(b) Geneva
(c) New York
(d) Rome

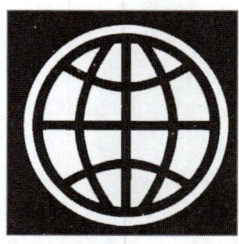

Q4. Identify International organization depicted in photograph: [NEET Pattern 2014]
(a) DFID
(b) World Bank
(c) UNDP
(d) UNAIDS

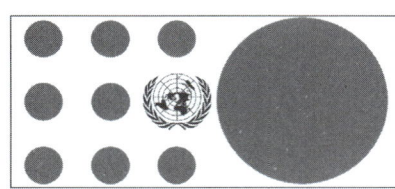

Q5. Identify International organization depicted in photograph: *[NEET Pattern 2014]*
(a) UNAIDS
(b) World Bank
(c) UNDP
(d) UNFPA

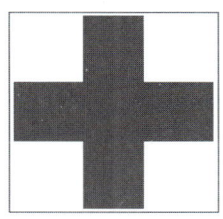

Q6. Identify symbol shown in the photograph: *[NEET Pattern 2014]*
(a) Medical professionals
(b) Nursing staff
(c) International Red Cross
(d) Colombo plan

CHAPTER–16

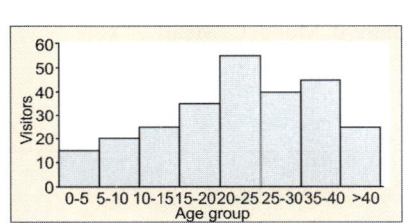

Q1. Identify the statistical diagram shown in photograph: *[NEET Pattern 2012, 2013, 2015]*
(a) Bar chart
(b) Histogram
(c) Frequency polygon
(d) OGIVE

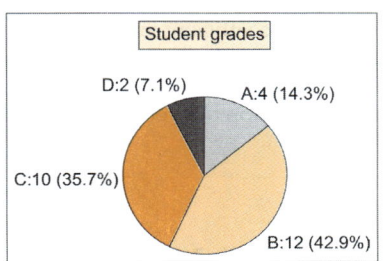

Q2. Identify the statistical diagram shown in photograph: *[NEET Pattern 2014]*
(a) Pie chart
(b) Pictogram
(c) Scatter diagram
(d) OGIVE

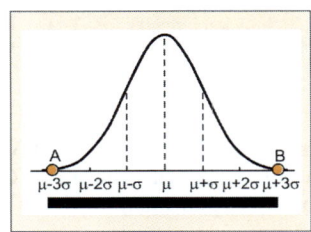

Q3. In the diagram depicted here, how much is the area between points A and B, on either side of the mean? *[NEET Pattern 2016]*
(a) 68.3%
(b) 95.4%
(c) 99.7%
(d) 102.5%

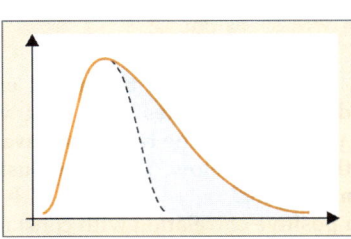

Q4. In the following type of distribution: *[NEET Pattern 2016]*
(a) Mean = Median = Mode
(b) Mean > Median > Mode
(c) Mode > Median > Mean
(d) Median > Mode > Mean

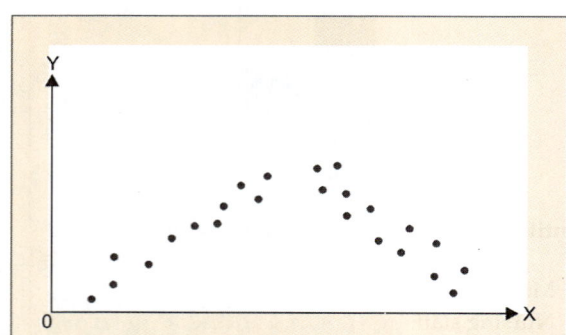

Q5. A scatter diagram was plotted as shown below to study the relationship between two quantitative variables. What is the correct interpretation?
[AIIMS November 2016]
(a) There is correlation between the two variables and the Pearson's coefficient is 1
(b) There is correlation between the two variables and the Pearson's coefficient is – 1
(c) There is no linear correlation between the two variables
(d) There is no association between the two variables

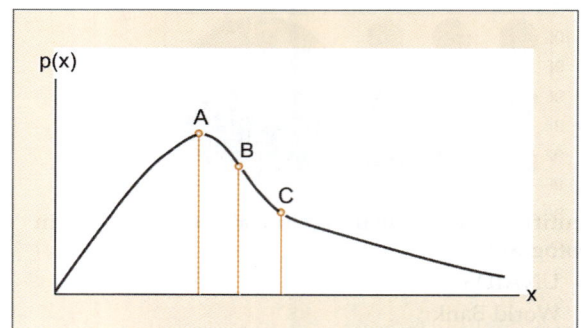

Q6. A study was conducted to find out number of positive lymph nodes in a population of breast cancer patients who underwent axillary dissection. A graph was plotted between the number and frequency of positive nodes as below. Which of the following is the correct statement? *[AIIMS November 2016]*
(a) A: Mode; B: Median; C: Mean
(b) A: Mode; B: Mean; C: Median
(c) A: Median; B: Mode; C: Mean
(d) A: Mean; B: Median; C: Mode

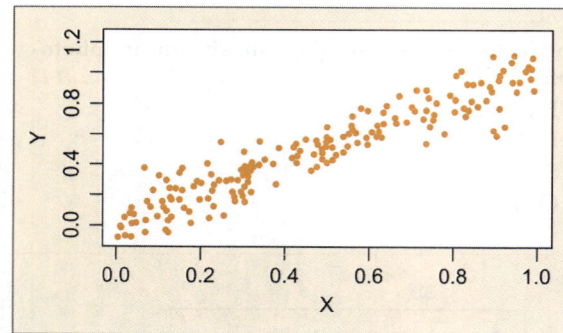

Q7. A study was conducted to see the effect of pulse oximeter readings in neonates with and without micropore. A plot between the two values was made as shown in the figure below. What conclusion can be drawn from the plot? *[AIIMS November 2016]*
(a) There is a positive correlation with constant 3% increase in Y-axis value
(b) There is a constant negative correlation between two variables
(c) There is a constant positive correlation between two variables
(d) There is no correlation

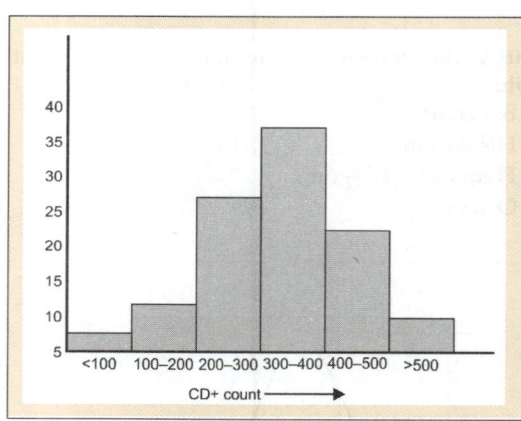

Q8. Below is the graph of CD4 count in HIV patients. From the graph below identify the mean CD4 count (Normal CD4 count is up to 1500). *[AIIMS May 2017]*
(a) 300
(b) Above 300
(c) Below 300
(d) Between 300 and 400

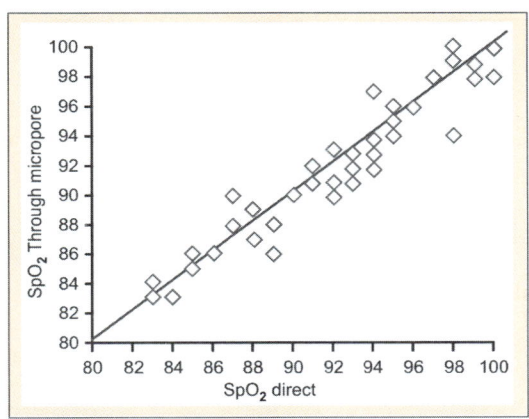

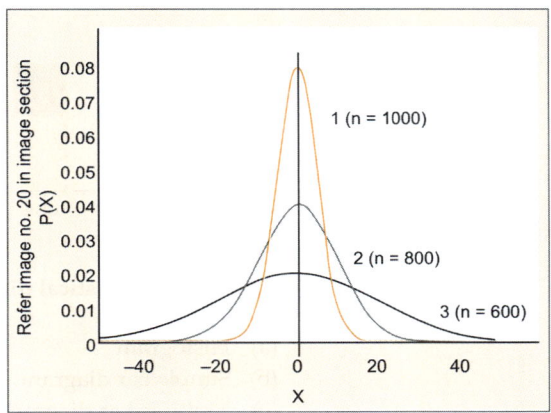

Q9. In an agreement between SpO$_2$ of two groups with and without micropore in a pediatric population the values spotted is as below. Which of the following is true?
[AIIMS November 2016]
(a) There is no agreement between the two groups
(b) The two groups have a constant relation with a variation of 3%
(c) The is no association between the two groups
(d) The curve shows a regression line means co-relation

Q10. Order for the Margin of error in the graph given above is?
[AIIMS May 2018]
(a) 3>2>1
(b) 3>1>2
(c) 1>3>2
(d) 1=2=3

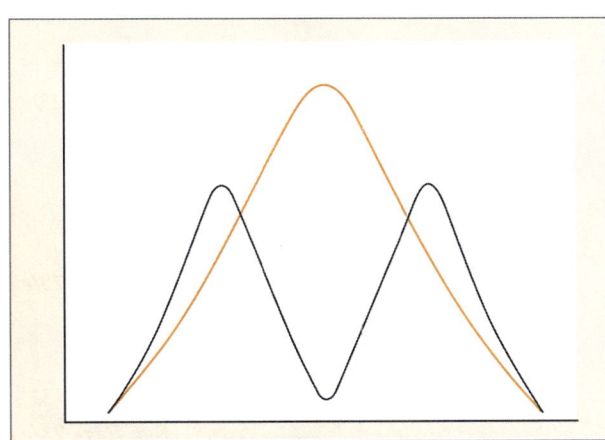

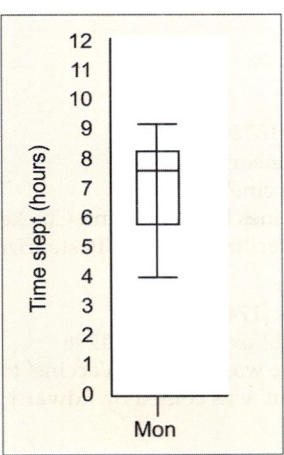

Q11. Which of the following true regarding the following two curves (Thin and Thick) overall?
[AIIMS November 2018]
(a) Mean = Median = Mode
(b) Mean = Median, not equal to Mode
(c) Mean = Mode, not equal to Median
(d) Mean, Median and Mode are not equal

Q12. Not true about the image given above is:
[AIIMS November 2018]
(a) Negatively skewed
(b) Positively skewed
(c) Mean < Median
(d) Mean < Mode

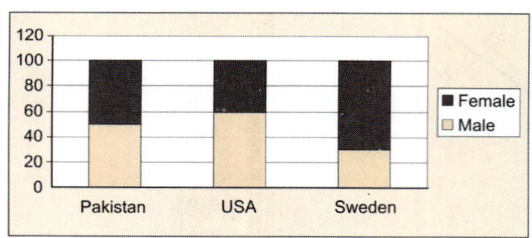

Q13. Identify the statistical diagram given above:
[NEET Pattern 2019]
- (a) Histogram
- (b) Simple bar diagram
- (c) Multiple bar diagram
- (d) Component bar diagram

Explanations

CHAPTER 1

Ans. 1 (a) Louis Pasteur *[Ref. Park 23/e p6]*
LOUIS PASTEUR [1822-1895]
- Gave the 'Germ theory of disease'
- Coined term 'Vaccine'
- Developed 'Vaccines for Rabies and Chicken Cholera'
- Techniques of 'Sterilization' and 'Pasteurization'.

Ans. 2 (b) Edward Jenner *[Ref. Park 23/e p6]*
EDWARD JENNER [1749-1823]
- Discovered Small Pox vaccine in 1796
- Small pox vaccine was the 'First Vaccine' to be discovered
- Term 'Vaccination' was coined by Edward Jenner.

Ans. 3 (d) Robert Koch *[Ref. Park 23/e p6]*
ROBERT KOCH [1843-1910]
- Discovered causative agents of TB, Cholera, Anthrax
- Gave experimental support for concept of infectious disease
- Koch's postulates, a series of four generalized principles linking specific microorganisms to specific diseases that remain today the "gold standard" in medical microbiology
- Nobel Prize in Physiology or Medicine in 1905.

Ans. 4 (a) John Snow *[Ref. Park 23/e p5]*
JOHN SNOW [1813-1858]
- English epidemiologist, studied cholera (1848-54) and established the role of drinking water in its spread (causative agent was identified much later)
- Father of Epidemiology/Modern Epidemiology
- Greatest doctor
- Calculated dosages for use of ether and chloroform as surgical anesthesia.

Ans. 5 (c) James Lind [Ref. Park 23/e p6]
- James Lind gave the concept that Citrus fruits can prevent/cure Scurvy (Later found to be due to deficiency of Vitamin-C/Ascorbic Acid).

Ans. 6 (c) Joseph Bhore [Ref. Park 23/e p873]
BHORE COMMITTEE (1946)
- 'Health Survey and Development Committee'
- Short term measure: 1 PHC per 40,000 population, 30 beds, 3 sub-centres and 2 medical officers
- Long-term measure (3 Million Plan): Primary health units with 75-bedded hospitals per 10,000-20,000 population; Secondary health units with 650-bedded hospitals; Regional health units with 2,500 beds
- Prepare 'Social Physicians' (3 months training in PSM in internship).

CHAPTER 2

1. **Ans. 1 (c) Natural history of disease** [Ref. Park 27/e p41]
   - Natural history of disease is the course a disease takes in individual people from its pathological onset (inception) until its eventual resolution through complete recovery or death, in absence of any intervention

CHAPTER 3

Ans. 1 (d) Nested case control study [Ref. Epidemiology by Gordis, 4/e p172; Basic Epidemiology by Beaglehole, WHO; p40-41]
NESTED CASE CONTROL STUDY
- Only exposure has occurred when the study begins; when the disease develops in a population, then 2 groups of cases (diseased) and controls (non-diseased) are formed and their exposure status is compared
- A population is identified and baseline data is obtained from interviews, blood or urine tests, etc.
- Population is then followed up for a period of time (Cohort study) for development for the disease under study
- A case control study is then carried out:
  - Cases: people who developed the disease
  - Controls: sample from those who did not develop the disease
  - Samples/history collected at baseline are then examined.

Ans. 2 (c) Case control study [Ref. Park 27/e p79]
- Case control study: A study that compares patients who have a disease or outcome of interest (cases) with patients who do not have the disease or outcome (controls), and looks back retrospectively to compare how frequently the exposure to a risk factor is present in each group to determine the relationship between the risk factor and the disease.

Ans. 3 (b) Only 1, 2 [Ref. Park 27/e p122]
Rules for VVM use in India
- Rule 1: If the inner square is lighter than the outer circle, the vaccine may be used (Vials 1, 2)
- Rule 2: If the inner square is the same colour as, or darker than, the outer circle, the vaccine must not be used (Vials 3, 4).

CHAPTER 4

Ans. 1 (b) Lead time [Ref. Park 27/e p151]
- Lead time is the advantage gained by screening (leading the time of diagnosis)
- Early detection of disease due to screening (B rather than C) will ensure earlier institution of treatment, thus better prognosis.

Ans. 2 (c) Low PPV [Ref. Epidemiology for Public Health Practice by Friis 5/e p482; Park 27/e p156]
- If cut-off point is kept at A then,
  - Lower cut-off for disease
  - False positives increase
  - False negatives decrease
  - Sensitivity increased (as those now declared positives have more chances of actually having the disease)
  - Specificity decreased (as more non-diseased are classified as diseased)
  - PPV will be lowered as False positives will increase
  - NPV shall increase.

Ans. 3 (c) C [Ref. Park 27/e p41]
- Point A marks the entry of infectious agent into the host
- Point B marks the subclinical phase where symptoms and signs are not visible, but the disease agent induces tissue and physiological changes

- Point C marks the Clinical horizon when symptoms and signs appear
- Point D is present inside the Clinical phase after the Clinical horizon.

> **ALSO REMEMBER**
> **NATURAL HISTORY OF DISEASE**
> - Prepathogenesis phase
> - Pathogenesis phase:
>   Begins with the entry of disease agent into the host
>   Final outcome of the disease may be Recovery, Disability or Death
>   Pathological changes are essentially below the level of Clinical horizon
>   Clinical stage begins when signs and symptoms appear

Ans. 4 (a) Both Sensitivity & Specificity increase *[Ref. Park 27/e p157]*

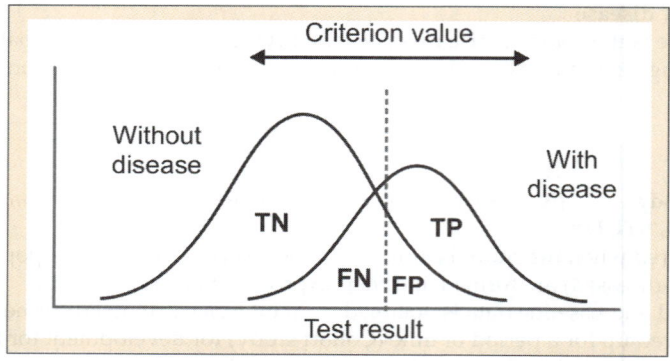

- If Blue colour curve changes to Red colour curve (see **Photograph in Question**), then
  - FN will reduce, Sensitivity will increase (see Photograph given in Answer)
  - FP will reduce, Specificity will increase (see Photograph given in Answer).

CHAPTER 5

Ans. 1 (c) RTI/STI *[Ref. http://naco.gov.in/sti-rti-services]*
SURAKSHA CLINICS
- 1160 designated STI/RTI clinics (situated at government health care facilities at district level and above) under NACP
- Providing free standardized STI/RTI services
- Provide sexual and reproductive health services
- Standardized training to the medical and paramedical personnel based on syndromic case management approach
- Counseling services from trained counselors
- Colour coded syndromic drug kits and RPR test kits.

Ans. 2 (b) Ebola virus *[Ref. Park 27/e p407]*
EBOLA VIRUS DISEASE
- Incubation period: 2-21 days
- Route of transmission: Body fluids (including semen, breast milk)
- Source: Cases
- Reservoir: Bats
- Case fatality rate: 40%
- Treatment: Rehydration, symptomatic.

Ans. 3 (b) Tracking phenomena *[Ref. Park 27/e p427]*
TRACKING OF BLOOD PRESSURE
- If BP of individuals were followed up over a period of years from early childhood into adult life, then those having high BP would continue into same 'track' as adults
- Low BP tends to remain low and high BP tends to become higher as individuals grow older.

Ans. 4 (d) NIPAH virus *[Ref. Park 27/e p330]*
NIPAH Virus Transmission
- Occurrence: West Bengal, Kerala

- Route of transmission:
  - Direct contact with infected bats, infected pigs, infected people
  - Consumption of fruits/raw date palm sap contaminated with bats (Pteropus: 'Flying foxes') secretions

CHAPTER 6

Ans. 1 (b) DOTS *[Ref. RNTCP, PIB, GOI]*

DOTS LOGO
- Tagline: "Pura course, Pakka Ilaj"
  - Mark the emphasis on completion of full course of treatment
  - Signifies a response to the emerging challenges regarding tuberculosis and its manifestations in the form of MDR-TB and co-infection with HIV
- Progression from previous DOTS logo with the slogan (DOTS: "Sure Cure for TB")
- Visual element in the old logo has been retained as the old logo had already successfully established connect with communities.

Ans. 2 (d) HIV/AIDS *[Ref. Strategic Communication in the HIV/AIDS Epidemic by McKee 1/e p270]*

INVERTED RED RIBBON
- Red ribbon is the universal symbol of awareness and support for those living with HIV:
  - It was first developed in 1991 under the Ribbon Project by Visual AIDS Artists Caucus in New York, a New York-based charity group of art professionals that to recognise and honour friends and colleagues either died or are dying of AIDS
  - Color red was chosen for its "connection to blood and the idea of passion—not only anger, but love, like a valentine"
  - The tails of the ribbon pointing down was chosen to symbolise life flowing away
  - It represents Care, Hope and Care and support
- Red ribbon has inspired other charities to utilize the symbol by changing the color (like Pink ribbon for Breast cancer awareness).

Ans. 3 (b) NLEP *[Ref. www.nlep.nic.in]*

THE NLEP EMBLEM
- Symbolizes beauty and purity in lotus
- Leprosy can be cured and a leprosy patient can be a useful member of the society in the form of a partially affected thumb
- A normal fore-finger and the shape of house
- Symbol of hope and optimism in a rising sun
- Captures the spirit of hope positive action in the eradication of Leprosy.

Ans. 4 (c) NRHM *[Ref. www.nrhm.gov.in]*

NRHM/NUHM/NHM LOGO
- National Health Mission (NHM) encompasses its two Sub-Missions:
  - National Rural Health Mission (NRHM)
  - National Urban Health Mission (NUHM)
- Main programmatic components include Health System Strengthening in rural and urban areas- Reproductive-Maternal-Neonatal-Child and Adolescent Health (RMNCH+A), and Communicable and Non-communicable Diseases
- NHM envisages achievement of universal access to equitable, affordable and quality health care services that are accountable and responsive to people's needs.

Ans. 5 (b) NVBDCP *[Ref. www.nvbdcp.gov.in]*

NATIONAL VECTOR BORNE DISEASE CONTROL PROGRAM (NVBDCP)
- Program for prevention and control of vector borne diseases
  - Malaria
  - Dengue
  - Lymphatic Filariasis
  - Kala-azar
  - Japanese Encephalitis
  - Chikungunya.

Ans. 6 (b) NPCB *[Ref. www.npcb.nic.in]*

NATIONAL PROGRAM FOR CONTROL OF BLINDNESS (NPCB)
- Launched in the year 1976
- 100% Centrally Sponsored scheme
- Goal: To reduce the prevalence of blindness from 1.4 to 0.3%.

Ans. 7 (d) IDSP [Ref. www.idsp.nic.in]

INTEGRATED DISEASE SURVEILLANCE PROJECT (IDSP)
- Launched in November 2004 for a period up to March 2010
  - Project was restructured and extended up to March 2012
  - Project continues in the 12th Plan under NHM for all States.
- Objective: To strengthen/maintain decentralized laboratory based IT enabled disease surveillance system for epidemic prone diseases to monitor disease trends and to detect and respond to outbreaks in early rising phase through trained Rapid Response Team (RRTs).

Ans. 8 (c) PPTCT [Ref. http://naco.gov.in/prevention-parent-child-transmissionpptct]

PREVENTION OF PARENT TO CHILD TRANSMISSION OF HIV/AIDS (PPTCT) PROGRAM
- Launched in the country in 2002
- Aims to prevent the perinatal transmission of HIV from an HIV infected pregnant mother to her newborn baby
- Entails counselling and testing of pregnant women in the ICTCs.

Ans. 9 (d) NREGA Act 2005 [Ref. NREGA and Quality of Life of Beneficiaries by Thomas 1/e p34]

NATIONAL RURAL EMPLOYMENT GUARANTEE ACT (NREGA) 2005
- Provide for '100 days of guaranteed wage employment in every year' to every household whose adult members volunteer to do 'unskilled manual work'
- A household is entitled for '100 days of work in a year'
- 'Job card' to be given to every registered household (valid for 5 years)
- Allotment for work 'within 15 days', else he/she shall be provided unemployment allowance
- Work will be provided 'within 5 km' of applicant's residence
- The 'panchayats' have the principal responsibility for planning, implementation and monitoring.

CHAPTER 7

Ans. 1 (d) IUD [Ref. Park 27/e p570]

Ans. 2 (c) CuT 380 A [Ref. Park 27/e p571]

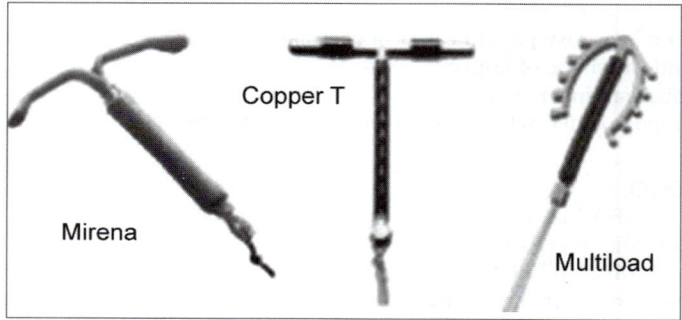

Ans. 3 (d) Combined OCPs [Ref. Park 27/e p574]

Ans. 4 (c) Lippes loop [Ref. Park 27/e p570]

INTRAUTERINE DEVICES (IUDs)

1st Generation IUDs	2nd Generation IUDs	3rd Generation IUDs
Non-medicated IUDs Inert IUDs	Medicated IUDs Bioactive IUDs	
No medication is added to the IUD	Metallic ions (Copper) are added to IUD	Hormones are added to IUD
Lippes Loop Grafenberg's Ring	CuT 7 CuT 220 B CuT 380 A or Ag	Progestasert LNG – IUD

Ans. 5 (d) Vaginal sponge [Ref. Park 27/e p570]

VAGINAL SPONGE: TODAY
- Sponge a barrier method of contraception: It actually combines barrier and spermicidal methods to prevent conception
- Saturated with 1000 mg of spermicide 'Nonoxynol-9'

- Pearl Index: 9-20/HWY
- Disadvantages of sponge:
  - Sponge provide no protection from STIs
  - Can lead to Toxic Shock Syndrome.

Ans. 6 (b) Female condom [Ref. Park 27/e p569]

FEMALE CONDOMS
- A contraceptive device that is used during sexual intercourse by women
- Invented by Danish MD Lasse Hessel
- It is worn internally by the receptive partner and physically blocks ejaculated semen from entering that person's body
- Prevent pregnancy and transmission of STIs
- Pearl Index: 5-21/HWY.

Ans. 7 (a) Rhythm method [Ref. Park 27/e p582]

SAFE PERIOD (RHYTHM METHOD/CALENDAR METHOD)
- Fertile period: Shortest cycle minus 18 days (Last day of fertile period: Longest cycle minus 10 days)
- Drawbacks:
  - Difficult to predict safe period in irregular cycles
  - Only suitable for educated couples with high motivation
  - PROGRAMMED SEX: Abstinence required for ½ month
  - Not useful in postnatal period
  - High failure rate: 9 per HWY
  - Medical complications: Ectopic pregnancies and embryonic abnormalities.

CHAPTER 11

Ans. 1 (d) Pesticide toxicity labels [Ref. Insecticides Rules 1971, Central Insecticides Board, India]

TOXICITY COLOUR LABELS OF PESTICIDES IN INDIA
- Red label: Extremely toxic (e.g. Zinc phosphide)
- Yellow label: Highly toxic (e.g. Endosulfan)
- Blue label: Moderately toxic (e.g. Malathion)
- Green label: Slightly toxic (e.g. Mosquito repellants).

Ans. 2 (b) Anopheles mosquito [Ref. Park 27/e p896]

ADULT MOSQUITOES

Anopheles	Culex	Aedes	Mansonia
Inclined at an angle to surface Long palpi Spotted wings	'Hunch back' rest Short palpi (Female)	Stripes on body & legs Short palpi (Female)	Speckling on body & legs Short palpi (Female)

Ans. 3 (c) Aedes mosquito [Ref. Park 27/e p897]

Ans. 4 (d) Rat flea [Ref. Park 27/e p904]

RAT FLEA (XENOPSYLLA)
- Rat flea acts as a vector for:
  - Bubonic plague
  - Murine (endemic/flea-borne) typhus
  - Chiggerosis.
- Rat flea acts as a host for:
  - Hymenolepis diminuta (Rat tapeworm)
  - Hymenolepis nana (Dwarf tapeworm).

Ans. 5 (b) Musca domestica [Ref. Park 27/e p900]

HOUSEFLY
- Regarded as a sign of insanitation' (and their number as Index of sanitation)
- Important species: Musca domestica, M. vicinia, M. nebula, M. sorbens
- Life span: 15-25 days
- Important breeding places (in order of importance): Fresh horse manure, Human excreta, Manure of other animals, Garbage
- Modes of disease transmission:
  - Mechanical transmission: Houseflies are known as 'Porters of infection'
  - Vomit-drop
  - Defecation.

Ans. 6 (c) Louse [Ref. Park 27/e p903]
- LICE (singular LOUSE)
- Wingless insects, also known as 'Fly babies'
- Lice as the vectors of diseases:
  - Epidemic typhus (Rickettsia prowazekii)
  - Relapsing fever (Borrelia recurrentis)
  - Trench fever (Rickettsia Quintana)
  - Dermatitis (Due to scratching and secondary infection)

Ans. 7 (a) Anopheles [Ref. Park 27/e p896]
MOSQUITO LARVAE

Anopheles	Culex	Aedes	Mansonia
No siphon tube	Siphon tube	Siphon tube	Siphon tube
Rest parallel to undersurface of water	Rest perpendicular to undersurface of water	Rest in dark bottom corners	Rest attached to rootlets of plants

Ans. 8 (d) Relative humidity of air [Ref. Park 27/e p874]
INSTRUMENTS USED IN AIR PARAMETERS

Instrument	Use
Kata Thermometer	Cooling power of air, Low air velocity
Anemometer	Air/wind velocity
Hygrometer, Sling Psychrometer (Photograph) Assman Psychrometer	Air humidity (moisture content)
Mercurial Barometer	Atmospheric pressure
Aneroid Barometer	Atmospheric pressure
Wind Vane	Air/wind direction

CHAPTER 12

Ans. 1 (c) Prime Minister [Ref. http://www.ndma.gov.in/en/about-ndma/ndma-logo.html]
- National Disaster Management Authority (NDMA)
- Headed by the Prime Minister of India
- Apex body for Disaster Management in India
- Mandated by the Disaster Management Act, 2005.
- The NDMA Logo reflects the aspirations of this National Vision, of empowering all stakeholders to improve the effectiveness of Disaster Management in India:
  - Map of India circumscribed by the National Tricolor represents aspiration to contain potential threat of disasters through capacity development
  - Outer circle is a Golden Ring of Partnership of all Stakeholders
  - NDMA in the inner circle in tranquil Blue integrates the entire process by empowering all stakeholders at the local, district, state and national levels.

Ans. 2 (c) Biomedical waste management [Ref. Park 27/e p920]
THE BIOHAZARD SYMBOL
- An image that warns people of possible exposure to biological substances that are harmful to living organisms
- These biohazards can be viruses, toxins or medical waste
- Symbol was created by Charles Baldwin in 1966.

Ans. 3 (c) Urine bags [Ref. Park 27/e p919]
- BMW Bag shown here is of Red colour
- It is used for contaminated plastic/rubber solid wastes: Tubings, bottles, intravenous tubes, catheters, syringes without needles, gloves.

Ans. 4 (d) Radiation hazard [Ref. Phlebotomy Essentials by McCall 4/e p107]
INTERNATIONAL RADIATION SYMBOL (TREFOIL)
- Central circle of radius R, an internal radius of 1.5R and an external radius of 5R for the blades, which are separated from each other by 60°
- Trefoil is black in the international version
- Commonly referred to as a Radioactivity warning sign, but it is actually a warning sign of ionizing radiation
- Includes X-ray apparatus, medical beam cannons and particle accelerators.

Ans. 5 (a) Recycling [Ref. The EU Directive Handbook by Bailey 1/e p60]
RECYCLING SYMBOL
- Required on any product that can be recycled
- By international agreement, the Recycling Symbol is used on most plastic products.

Ans. 6 (c) Radiation hazard [Ref. Phlebotomy Essentials by McCall 4/e p107]
TREFOIL
- Radiation hazard symbol
- For inner circle of radius R, the inside radius of the blades is 1.5R and the outer radius of the blades is 5R
- The blades are separated by 60°

CHAPTER 15

Ans. 1 (a) WHO [Ref. World Health Organization by Burci 1/e p1]
WORLD HEALTH ORGANIZATION (WHO)
- WHO is a specialized, non-political health agency of United Nations
- Constitution of WHO: Came into force on 7th April, 1948Q
- Objective of WHO: Is attainment by all people of the highest level of health
- First Constitutional function of WHO: To act as the directing and co-coordinating
- Authority on all International health work
- Headquarters of WHO: Geneva, Switzerland.

Ans. 2 (b) UNICEF [Ref. Park 27/e p1029]
UNICEF LOGO
- One element that unifies and represents UNICEF
- It has been specially designed to symbolize name, but also what UNICEF stand for children
- Lower case letters of 'unicef' used in the logo are friendly and approachable
- Parent and child symbol: Child as central purpose while the laurel leaves provide a link to UNICEF's history with United Nations
- Headquarters: New York.

Ans. 3 (d) Rome [Ref. Park 27/e p1030]
FOOD AND AGRICULTURAL ORGANISATION (FAO)
- Prime objective: Increase food production in relation to growing world population
- FAO of the UN leads international efforts to defeat hunger
- Serving both developed and developing countries, FAO acts as a neutral forum where all nations meet as equals to negotiate agreements and debate policy
- Headquarters: Rome, Italy.

Ans. 4 (b) World Bank [Ref. World Bank Literature by Kumar 1/e p12]
WORLD BANK (WB)
- An international financial institution that provides loans to developing countries for capital programs
- A component of the World Bank Group, which is part of the United Nations system
- Comprises two institutions:
  - International Bank for Reconstruction and Development (IBRD)
  - International Development Association (IDA).
- Official goal is the reduction of poverty
- Commitment: Promotion of foreign investment and international trade and facilitation of Capital investment.

Ans. 5 (d) UNFPA [Ref. The UN in Moldova by UN Resident Coordinator, 1/e p1]
UNITED NATIONS POPULATION FUND (UNFPA)
- Lead UN agency for delivering a world where every pregnancy is wanted, every childbirth is safe and every young person's potential is fulfilled

- Work involves the improvement of reproductive health; including creation of national strategies and protocols, and providing supplies and services
- Organization has recently been known for its worldwide campaign against obstetric fistula and female genital mutilation

Ans. 6 (c) International Red Cross [Ref. Park 27/e p1032]
INTERNATIONAL RED CROSS
- Founded by 'Henry Dunant'
- Headquarters: Geneva, Switzerland
- The Red Cross logo was designed by Henri Dunant in 1863
- The emblem of a red cross with arms of equal length on a white background is the visible sign of protection under the 1949 Geneva Conventions
- As such, it is the emblem of the armed forces' medical services.

CHAPTER 16

Ans. 1 (b) Histogram [Ref. Park 27/e p973]
- HISTOGRAM
- Graphical presentation for 'continuous quantitative data'
- Continuous groups are marked on X-axis (abscissa) while frequencies are marked on Y-axis (ordinate).

Ans. 2 (a) Pie chart [Ref. Park 27/e p974]
PIE CHART
- Qualitative data diagram
- Each qualitative category is represented as pie of a circle
- Each category drawn as % of 360 degrees
- Categories is mutually-exclusive and total of all categories is 100%.

Ans. 3 (c) 99.7% [Ref. Park 27/e p977]
NORMAL DISTRIBUTION (Photograph)
- Is also known as 'Gaussian distribution' or 'Standard distribution'
- Type of distribution: Is the distribution of values of a quantitative variable such that they are symmetric with respect to a middle value with same mean, median and mode, and then the frequencies taper off rapidly and symmetrically on both sides – 'bell shaped distribution'
  - Is 'bilaterally symmetrical, bell-shaped'
  - Mean, Median and Mode coincide (Mean = Median = Mode)
  - Has mean (μ) = 0 and SD (σ) = 1
  - Mean $\pm$ 1SD ($\mu \pm 1\sigma$) covers 68.3% values
  - Mean $\pm$ 2SD ($\mu \pm 2\sigma$) covers 95.4% values
  - Mean $\pm$ 3SD ($\mu \pm 3\sigma$) covers 99.7% values.

Ans. 4 (b) Mean > Median > Mode [Ref. The Basic Practice of Statistics by Moore 5/e p71]
- In Right skew curve (Photograph): Mean > Median > Mode
- In Left skew curve: Mean < Median < Mode
- In Normal distribution: Mean = Median = Mode.

Ans. 5 (c) There is no linear correlation between the two variables [Ref. Agricultural Statistics by Rangaswamy 1/e p142]
NON-LINEAR CORRELATION
- On rare occasions, a scatter plot will indicate a relationship that is not a simple linear relationship, but rather shows a complex relationship that changes at different points in the scatter plot
- Scatter plot (Photograph in Question) illustrates a nonlinear relationship, in which Y increases as X increases, but only up to a point; after that point, the relationship reverses direction
- Using a simple correlation coefficient for such a situation would be a mistake, because the correlation cannot capture accurately the nature of a nonlinear relationship.

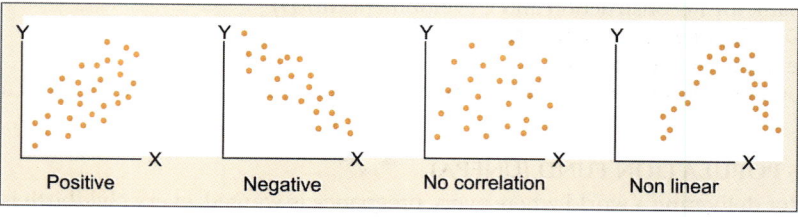

Ans. 6 (a) A: Mode; B: Median; C: Mean [Ref. Business Statistics by Alagar 1/e p253]
- In the photograph given,
- There is clustering of values towards left side, longer tail towards right side
- Hence it's a Right (Positively) skewed curve
- So, Mean > Median > Mode
- Therefore, A is Mode (Maximum repeated value), B is Median (in middle) and C is Mean.

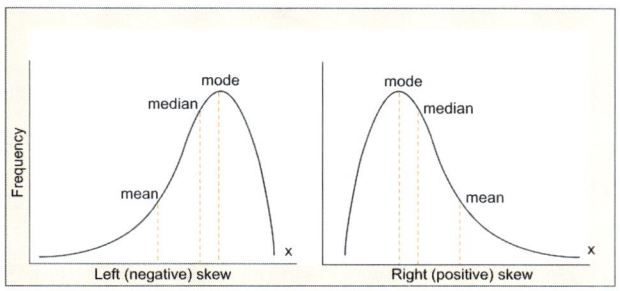

Ans. 7 (c) There is a constant positive correlation between two variables [Ref. Park 27/e p981]
- PEARSON CORRELATION COEFFICIENT (r)
- A value of r = 0 indicates that there is no association between the two variables
- A value 0 < r < +1 indicates a positive association; that is, as the value of one variable increases, so does the value of the other variable
- A value −1 < r < 0 indicates a negative association; that is, as the value of one variable increases, the value of the other variable decreases.

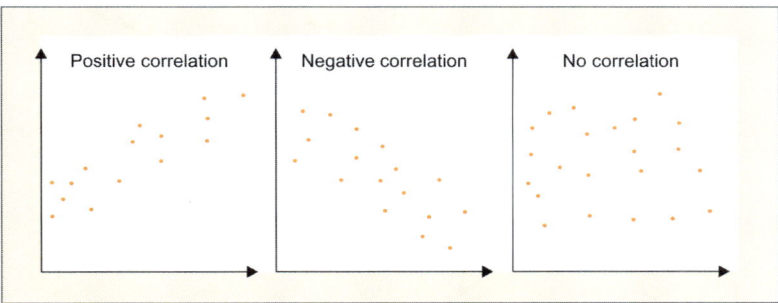

Ans. 8 (d) Between 300 and 400 [Ref. Statistical Methods (Combined) by Das, 1/e p71]
- **In the given question,** Class intervals are given (CD4 count on X-axis)
- Calculation of mean from Class-interval data:
  - Find the midpoint of each interval (x)
  - Get the sum of all the frequencies (f) and the sum of all the fx
  - Divide 'sum of fx' by 'sum of f' to get the mean

CD4 count interval	Mid-point (x)	Frequencies (f)	fx
<100	50	5	250
100-200	150	10	1500
200-300	250	25	6250
300-400	350	35	12250
400-500	450	20	9000
500-1500	1000	5	5000
TOTAL		**100**	**34250**

Therefore Mean = $\sum fx / \sum f$ = 34250/100 = 342.5 CD4 count

Ans. 9 (d) The curve shows a regression line means co-relation [Ref. Statistical Analysis by Elliott, 1/e p107]
BLAND-ALTMAN PLOT
- Difference plot
- A graphical method to compare two measurements techniques

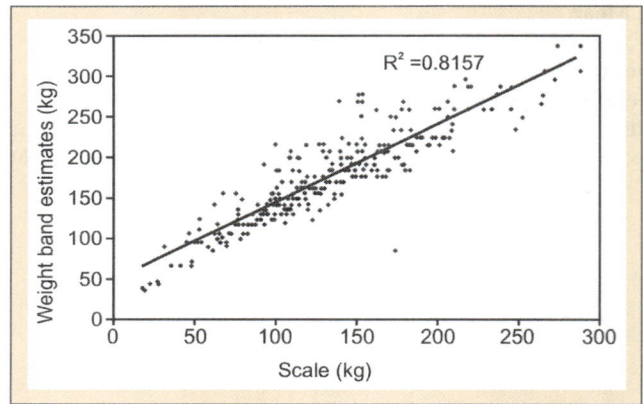

- The differences/ratios between the two techniques are plotted against the averages of the two techniques
- Alternatively the differences can be plotted against one of the two methods, if this method is a reference or "Gold standard" method

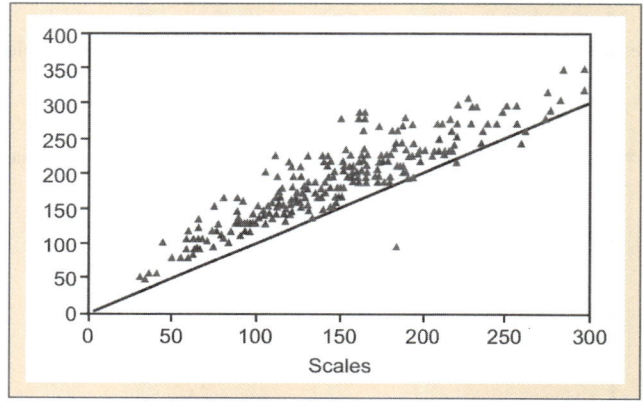

- Horizontal lines are drawn at the mean difference, and at the limits of agreement, which are defined as the mean difference plus and minus 1.96 times the standard deviation of the differences
- Interpretation of Bland-Altman Plot:
  - Perfect correlation if the points lie perfectly along any straight line
  - Regression line indicates Correlation: (See previous page)
  - Perfect agreement only if they lie perfectly along the line of equality
  - Line of equality does not indicate perfect agreement: (See above)

Ans. 10 (a) 3>2>1 [Ref. Statistics by LeBlanc 1/e p161]
- Margin of Error: Amount of random sampling error in a survey's results
- Margin of error is simply the "radius" (or half the width) of a confidence interval
- Margin of error = Critical value × Standard error
- Standard error is inversely related to sample size (SEmean = SD/√Sample size)
- Margin of error is inversely related to the Sample size

Ans. 11 (b) Mean = Median, not equal to Mode [Ref. Park 27/e p975]
In the given question,
- Thick curve is Bilaterally symmetrical, bell shaped curve, hence it's a Normal distribution
  - In Normal distribution, Mean = Median = Mode (Green vertical line)
- Thin curve has two modes (both symmetrical too), hence it's a Bimodal distribution
  - Since Bimodal curve is symmetrical, its Mean and Mode would lie at intersection 'X', so Mean = Median (Black arrow)

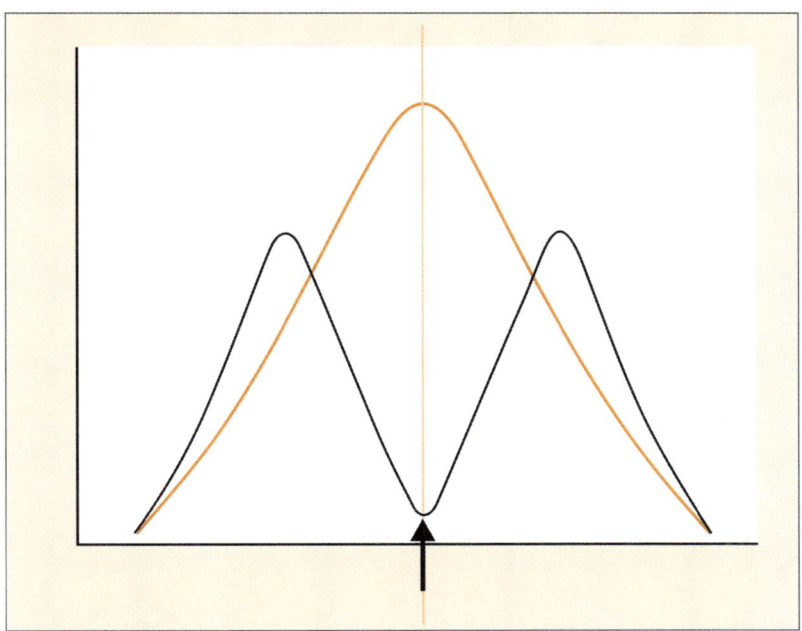

Ans. 12 (b) Positively skewed *[Ref. Essentials of Statistics by Gravetter 9/e p75]*
  In the given question,
- Plot shown is 'Box and Whisker Plot'
  - Sides of boxes represent Quartiles 1st and 3rd; Line inside the Box is 2nd Quartile (Median)
  - Whiskers on the side represent Minimum and Maximum value
- If Median line (Q_2) in exact centre of box, Its bilaterally symmetrical Normal distribution
  - But if Median line is towards a side of the box, Its skewed distribution

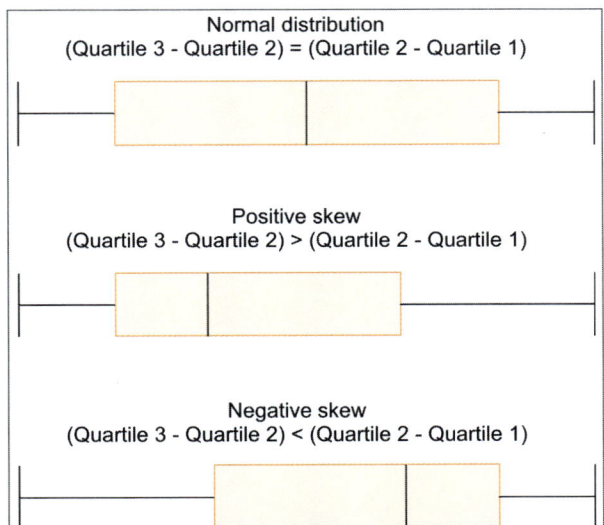

- So the graph shown in the question is negatively skewed distribution (Mean < Median < Mode) as it shows Downward skewness

Ans. 13 (d) Component bar diagram *[Ref. Park 27/e p973]*
  Component Bar Chart
  Syn. Sub-divided bar chart
- Represent data in which the total magnitude is divided into different or components
- First we make simple bars for each class taking the total magnitude in that class and then divide these simple bars into parts in the ratio of various components